Textbook of
Assisted Reproductive
Techniques

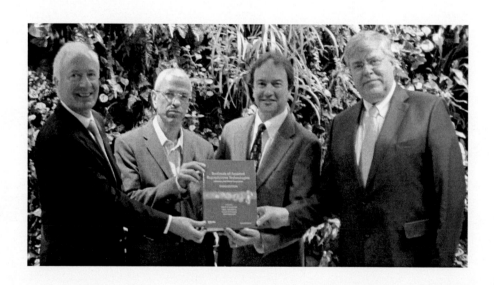

The editors (from left to right: Colin M. Howles, Ariel Weissman, David K. Gardner, and Zeev Shoham) at the annual meeting of ESHRE, Stockholm, July 2011

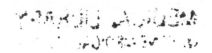

Textbook of Assisted Reproductive Techniques

Fourth Edition

Volume 2: Clinical Perspectives

Edited by

David K. Gardner DPhil
Chair of Zoology, University of Melbourne, Australia

Ariel Weissman MD
Senior Physician, IVF Unit, Department of Obstetrics and Gynecology,
Edith Wolfson Medical Center, Holon and Sackler Faculty of Medicine,
Tel Aviv University, Tel Aviv, Israel

Colin M. Howles PhD, FRSM
Vice President, Regional Medical Affairs Fertility, External Scientific Affairs,
Global Development and Medical, Merck Serono SA, Geneva, Switzerland

Zeev Shoham MD
Director, Reproductive Medicine and Infertility Unit, Department of Obstetrics and
Gynecology, Kaplan Medical Center, Rehovot, Israel

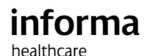

informa
healthcare

This edition published in 2012 by Informa Healthcare, 119 Farringdon Road, London EC1R 3DA, UK. Simultaneously published in the USA by Informa Healthcare, 52 Vanderbilt Avenue, 7th Floor, New York NY 10017, USA. Informa Healthcare is a trading division of Informa UK Ltd.

Registered Office: Informa House, 30–32 Mortimer Street, W1W 7RE. Registered in England and Wales number 1072954.

A CIP record for this book is available from the British Library.
Library of Congress Cataloging-in-Publication Data available on application.

Volume 1: ISBN 978-1-84184-970-6; eISBN 978-1-84184-971-3
Volume 2: ISBN 978-1-84184-972-0; eISBN 978-1-84184-973-7
Two volume set: 978-1-84184-974-4; eISBN 978-1-84184-975-1

Orders may be sent to: Informa Healthcare, Sheepen Place, Colchester, Essex CO3 3LP, UK
Telephone: +44 (0)20 7017 6682; Email: Books@Informa.com; www.informahealthcarebooks.com; www.informa.com

For corporate sales please contact: CorporateBooksIHC@informa.com
For foreign rights please contact: RightsIHC@informa.com
For reprint permissions please contact: PermissionsIHC@informa.com

Typeset by Exeter Premedia Services Pvt Ltd, India
Printed and bound in the United Kingdom

Contents

List of contributors

Michael Alper
Boston IVF, Waltham, Massachusetts, USA

Joseph P. Alukal
Clinical Assistant Professor of Urology,
Department of Urology, NYU School of Medicine
New York, New York, USA

Marli Amin
Department of Obstetrics and Gynecology, David Geffen
School of Medicine, Los Angeles, California, USA

Claus Yding Andersen
Laboratory of Reproductive Biology, Copenhagen
University Hospital, Copenhagen, Denmark

Usama Bajouh
Faculté de médecine, Université Paris Descartes,
Paris Sorbonne-Cité, and Department of Obstetrics,
Gynecology, and Reproductive Medicine, Assistance
Publique Hôpitaux de Paris, CHU Cochin,
Paris, France

Juan Balasch
Department of Obstetrics and Gynecology, Faculty of
Medicine, Hospital Clinic, University of Barcelona,
Barcelona, Spain

Adam H. Balen
Leeds Centre for Reproductive Medicine, Seacroft
Hospital, Leeds, UK

Vera Baukloh
Fertility Center Hamburg, Hamburg, Germany

Ido Ben-Ami
Fertility and IVF Unit, Assaf Harofeh Medical Center,
Tel Aviv University, Tel Aviv, Israel

Zion Ben-Rafael
Sackler Faculty of Medicine, Tel Aviv University,
Tel Aviv, Israel

Juliane Berdah
Faculté de médecine, Université Paris Descartes,
Paris Sorbonne-Cité, and Department of Obstetrics,
Gynecology, and Reproductive Medicine, Assistance
Publique Hôpitaux de Paris, CHU Cochin,
Paris, France

Inna Berin
Fertility Institute of New Jersey and New York
Westwood, New Jersey, USA

Isaac Blickstein
Department of Obstetrics and Gynecology, Kaplan
Medical Center, Rehovot, Israel

Andrea Mechanick Braverman
Director, The Braverman Center for Health Journeys
Bala Cynwyd, Pennsylvania, USA

Christopher Brewer
Leeds Centre for Reproductive Medicine, Seacroft
Hospital, Leeds, UK

Peter R. Brinsden
Bourn Hall Clinic International, Bourn, Cambridge, UK

Frank J. Broekmans
Department of Reproductive Medicine and Gynecology,
Division of Woman and Baby, University Medical
Center Utrecht, Utrecht, The Netherlands

Simone L. Broer
Department of Reproductive Medicine and Gynecology,
Division of Woman and Baby, University Medical
Center Utrecht, Utrecht, The Netherlands

Isabelle Cédrin-Durnerin
University of Paris XIII, Division of Reproductive
Medicine, Hôpital Jean Verdier, Bondy, France

Peter Chan
Division of Reproductive Endocrinology and Infertility,
Department of Obstetrics and Gynecology, McGill
University, Montreal, Quebec, Canada

Charles Chapron
Faculté de médecine, Université Paris Descartes,
Paris Sorbonne-Cité, and Department of Obstetrics,
Gynecology, and Reproductive Medicine, Assistance
Publique Hôpitaux de Paris, CHU Cochin, Paris, France

Tim J. Child
Oxford Fertility Unit, Institute of Reproductive
Sciences, and Nuffield Department of Obstetrics and
Gynaecology, John Radcliffe Hospital, University of
Oxford, Oxford, UK

Matthew A. Cohen
Department of Obstetrics and Gynecology, College of
Physicians & Surgeons, Columbia University, New York,
New York, USA

Sharon N. Covington
Psychological Support Services, Shady Grove
Fertility Reproductive Science Center, Rockville,
Maryland, USA

Mark A. Damario
Department of Obstetrics, Gynecology and Women's
Health, University of Minnesota, Minneapolis,
Minnesota, USA

Alan H. DeCherney
Department of Obstetrics and Gynecology, David Geffen
School of Medicine, Los Angeles, California, USA

Patricio Donoso
Centre for Reproductive Medicine, Clinica Alemana de
Santiago, Santiago, Chile

Robert G. Edwards
Duck End Farm, Dry Drayton, Cambridge, UK

Shmuel Evron
Obstetric Anesthesia Unit, Wolfson Medical Center, and
Sackler Faculty of Medicine, Tel Aviv University,
Tel Aviv, Israel

Tiberiu Ezri
Department of Anesthesiology, Wolfson Medical Center,
and Sackler Faculty of Medicine, Tel Aviv University,
Tel Aviv, Israel

Bart C. J. M. Fauser
Departments of Reproduction and Gynecology, Division
of Woman and Baby, University Medical Center Utrecht,
Utrecht, The Netherlands

Robert Fischer
Fertility Center Hamburg, Hamburg, Germany

Shevach Friedler
Fertility and IVF Unit, Assaf Harofeh Medical Center,
Tel Aviv University, Tel Aviv, Israel

David K. Gardner
Department of Zoology, University of Melbourne,
Victoria, Australia

Vanessa Gayet
Faculté de médecine, Université Paris Descartes,
Paris Sorbonne-Cité, and Department of Obstetrics,
Gynecology, and Reproductive Medicine, Assistance
Publique Hôpitaux de Paris, CHU Cochin,
Paris, France

Yarev Gidoni
Fertility and IVF Unit, Assaf Harofeh Medical Center,
Tel Aviv University, Tel Aviv, Israel

Carole Gilling-Smith
The Agora Gynaecology and Fertility Centre, Hove, UK

Ingrid Granne
Oxford Fertility Unit, Institute of Reproductive
Sciences, and Nuffield Department of Obstetrics and
Gynaecology, John Radcliffe Hospital, University of
Oxford, Oxford, UK

Tine Greve
Laboratory of Reproductive Biology, Copenhagen
University Hospital, Copenhagen, Denmark

Georg Griesinger
Department of Reproductive Medicine and
Gynecological Endocrinology, University Hospital of
Schleswig-Holstein, Luebeck, Germany

Torbjörn Hillensjö
Fertility Centre Scandinavia, Carlander's Hospital,
Göteborg, Sweden

Hananel Holzer
Division of Reproductive Endocrinology and Infertility,
Department of Obstetrics and Gynecology, McGill
University, Montreal, Quebec, Canada

Outi Hovatta
Karolinska Institute, Karolinska University Hospital
Huddinge, Stockholm, Sweden

Colin M. Howles
External Scientific Affairs, Global Development and
Medical, Merck Serono SA, Geneva,
Switzerland

Andy Huang
Department of Obstetrics and Gynecology, David Geffen
School of Medicine, Los Angeles, California, USA

Jean-Noël Hugues
University of Paris XIII, Division of Reproductive
Medicine, Hôpital Jean Verdier, Bondy, France

Judith A. F. Huirne
Department of Obstetrics and Gynecology, Division of
Reproduction and Fertility Investigation, IVF Center,
Vrije Universiteit Medical Center, Amsterdam, The
Netherlands

Kathleen Hwang
Assistant Professor of Surgery (Urology),
Division of Urology, Alpert Medical School
of Brown University Providence, Rhode Island, USA

Osamu Ishihara
Department of Obstetrics and Gynaecology, Saitama
Medical University, and Saitama Medical Centre
Hospital, Kawagoe, Japan

Martin H. Johnson
The Anatomy School, Department of Physiology,
Development and Neuroscience, and The Centre for
Trophoblast Research, University of Cambridge,
Cambridge, UK

Christoph Keck
IVF Group, Endokrinologikum, Hamburg, Germany

Efstratios M. Kolibianakis
Unit for Human Reproduction, First Department of
Obstetrics and Gynaecology, Medical School, Aristotle
University of Thessaloniki, and Papageorgiou General
Hospital, Thessaloniki, Greece

Gab Kovacs
Monash IVF, Richmond, Victoria, Australia

Stine Gry Kristensen
Laboratory of Reproductive Biology, Copenhagen
University Hospital, Copenhagen, Denmark

Dolores J. Lamb
Division of Male Reproductive Medicine and Surgery,
Scott Department of Urology, Baylor College of
Medicine, Houston, Texas, USA

Zalman Levine
Fertility Institute of New Jersey and New York,
Westwood, New Jersey, USA

Joanne L. Libraro
Center for Reproductive Medicine and Infertility, Weill
Medical College, New York, New York, USA

Larry I. Lipshultz
Division of Male Reproductive Medicine and Surgery,
Scott Department of Urology, Baylor College of
Medicine, Houston, Texas, USA

Nick S. Macklon
Department of Obstetrics and Gynaecology,
University of Southampton, and Complete Fertility
Centre Southampton, Princess Anne Hospital,
Southampton, UK

Ragaa Mansour
The Egyptian IVF Center, Cairo, Egypt

Lisa J. Moran
Robinson Institute and School of Paediatrics and
Reproductive Health, University of Adelaide, Adelaide,
South Australia, Australia

Daniel Navot
Fertility Institute of New Jersey and New York,
Westwood, New Jersey, USA

Scott M. Nelson
Department of Obstetrics and Gynaecology,
School of Medicine, University of Glasgow,
Glasgow, UK

Susie Nicholas
Leeds Centre for Reproductive Medicine, Seacroft
Hospital, Leeds, UK

Robert J. Norman
Robinson Institute and School of Paediatrics and
Reproductive Health
University of Adelaide, Adelaide, South Australia,
Australia

Karl G. Nygren
Karolinska Institute, Institute of Medical Epidemiology
& Biostatistics, Stockholm, Sweden

Raoul Orvieto
Infertility and IVF Unit, Department of Obstetrics
and Gynecology, Barzilai Medical Center, Ashkelon,
and Faculty of Health Sciences, Ben Gurion University
of the Negev, Beer Sheva, Israel

Arie Raziel
Fertility and IVF Unit, Assaf Harofeh Medical Center,
Tel Aviv University, Tel Aviv, Israel

Botros Rizk
Reproductive Endocrinology and Infertility,
Department of Obstetrics and Gynecology,
University of South Alabama, Mobile,
Alabama, USA

Sarah A. Robertson
Robinson Institute and School of Paediatrics and
Reproductive Health, University of Adelaide, Adelaide,
South Australia, Australia

Raphael Ron-El
Fertility and IVF Unit, Assaf Harofeh Medical Center,
Tel Aviv University, Tel Aviv, Israel

Zev Rosenwaks
Center for Reproductive Medicine and Infertility,
Weill Medical College of Cornell University, New York,
New York, USA

Isabelle Roux
Division of Reproductive Endocrinology
and Infertility, Department of Obstetrics and
Gynecology, McGill University, Montreal,
Quebec, Canada

Mark V. Sauer
Department of Obstetrics and Gynecology, College of
Physicians & Surgeons, Columbia University, New York,
New York, USA

Roel Schats
Department of Obstetrics and Gynecology, Division of
Reproduction and Fertility Investigation, IVF Center,
Vrije Universiteit University Medical Center,
Amsterdam, The Netherlands

Machelle M. Seibel
Department of Obstetrics and Gynecology, University of
Massachusetts School of Medicine, Worcester,
Massachusetts, USA

Zeev Shoham
Reproductive Medicine and Infertility Unit, Department
of Obstetrics and Gynecology, Kaplan Medical Center,
Rehovot, Israel

Cecilia Sjöblom
Westmead Fertility Centre, University of Sydney,
Western Clinical School, Westmead Hospital,
Westmead, New South Wales, Australia

Laurel Stadtmauer
The Jones Institute for Reproductive Medicine, Eastern
Virginia Medical School, Norfolk, Virginia, USA

Annika Strandell
Department of Obstetrics and Gynecology, Institute of
Clinical Sciences, Sahlgrenska Academy, University of
Göteborg, Göteborg, Sweden

Isabelle Streuli
Faculté de médecine, Université Paris Descartes,
Paris Sorbonne-Cité, and Department of Obstetrics,
Gynecology, and Reproductive Medicine, Assistance
Publique Hôpitaux de Paris, CHU Cochin, and Cochin
Institute, Paris, France

Thomas H. Tang
Leeds Centre for Reproductive Medicine, Seacroft
Hospital, Leeds, UK

Basil C. Tarlatzis
Unit for Human Reproduction, First Department of
Obstetrics and Gynaecology, Medical School, Aristotle
University of Thessaloniki, and Papageorgiou General
Hospital, Thessaloniki, Greece

Herman Tournaye
Center for Reproductive Medicine, University Hospital
of the Brussels Free University, Brussels, Belgium

Togas Tulandi
Division of Reproductive Endocrinology and Infertility,
Department of Obstetrics and Gynecology, McGill
University, Montreal, Quebec, Canada

Ilan Tur-Kaspa
Institute for Human Reproduction (IHR), and
the Department of Obstetrics and Gynecology,
The University of Chicago, Chicago, Illinois, USA

Ariel Weissman
IVF Unit, Department of Obstetrics and Gynecology,
Edith Wolfson Medical Center, Holon, and Sackler
Faculty of Medicine, Tel Aviv University, Tel Aviv,
Israel

Matts Wikland
Fertility Centre Scandinavia, Carlander's Hospital,
Göteborg, Sweden

Fernando Zegers-Hochschild
Unit of Reproductive Medicine, Clínica las Condes,
Santiago, Chile

Dominique de Ziegler
Faculté de médecine, Université Paris Descartes,
Paris Sorbonne-Cité, and Department of Obstetrics,
Gynecology, and Reproductive Medicine,
Assistance Publique Hôpitaux de Paris, CHU Cochin,
Paris, France

The beginnings of human *in vitro* fertilization

Robert G. Edwards

In vitro fertilization (IVF) and its derivatives in preimplantation diagnosis, stem cells, and the ethics of assisted reproduction continue to attract immense attention scientifically and socially. All these topics were introduced by 1970. Hardly a day passes without some public recognition of events related to this study, and clinics spread ever further worldwide. Now we must be approaching 1.5 million IVF births, it is time to celebrate what has been achieved by so many investigators, clinical, scientific, and ethical.

While much of this chapter "Introduction" covers the massive accumulation of events between 1960 and 2000, it also briefly discusses new perspectives emerging in the 21st century. Fresh advances also increase curiosity about how these fields of study began and how their ethical implications were addressed in earlier days. As for me, I am still stirred by recollections of those early days. Foundations were laid in Edinburgh, London, and Glasgow in the 1950s and early 1960s. Discoveries made then led to later days in Cambridge, working there with many PhD students. It also resulted in my working with Patrick Steptoe in Oldham. Our joint opening of Bourn Hall in 1980, which became the largest IVF clinic of its kind at the time, signified the end of the beginning of assisted human conception and the onset of dedicated applied studies.

INTRODUCTION

First of all, I must express in limited space my tributes to my teachers, even if inadequately. These include investigators from far-off days when the fundamental facts of reproductive cycles, surgical techniques, endocrinology, and genetics were elicited by many investigators. These fields began to move in the 20th century, and if one pioneer of these times should be saluted, it must be Gregory Pincus. Famous for the contraceptive pill, he was a distinguished embryologist, and part of his work dealt with the maturation of mammalian oocytes in vitro. He was the first to show how oocytes aspirated from their follicles would begin their maturation in vitro, and how a number matured and expelled a first polar body. I believe his major work was done in rabbits, where he found that the 10 to 11-hour timings of maturation in vitro accorded exactly with those occurring in vivo after an ovulatory stimulus to the female rabbit.

Pincus et al. also studied human oocytes (1). Extracting oocytes from excised ovaries, they identified chromosomes in a large number of oocytes and interpreted this as evidence of the completion of maturation in vitro. Many oocytes possessed chromosomes after 12 hours, the proportion remaining constant over the next 30 hours and longer. Twelve hours was taken as the period of maturation. Unfortunately, chromosomes were not classified for their meiotic stage. Maturing oocytes would be expected to display diakinesis or metaphase-I chromosome pairs. Fully mature oocytes would display metaphase-II chromosomes, signifying they were fully ripe and ready for fertilization. Nevertheless, it is well known that oocytes can undergo atresia in the ovary involving the formation of metaphase-II chromosomes in many of them. These oocytes complicated Pincus' estimates, even in controls, and were the source of his error which led later workers to inseminate human oocytes 12 hours after collection and culture in vitro (2,3). Work on human fertilization in vitro, and indeed comparable studies in animals, remained in abeyance from then and for many years. Progress in animal IVF had also been slow. After many relatively unsuccessful attempts in several species in the 1950s and 1960s, a virtual dogma arose that spermatozoa had to spend several hours in the female reproductive tract before acquiring the potential to bind to the zona pellucida and achieve fertilization. In the late 1960s, Austin and Chang independently identified the need for sperm capacitation, identified by a delay in fertilization after spermatozoa had entered the female reproductive tract (4,5). This discovery was taken by many investigators as the reason for the failure to achieve fertilization in vitro, and why spermatozoa had to be exposed to secretions of the female reproductive tract. At the same time, Chang reported that rabbit eggs that had fully matured in vitro failed to produce normal blastocysts, none of them implanting normally (6).

MODERN BEGINNINGS OF HUMAN IVF, PREIMPLANTATION GENETIC DIAGNOSIS, AND EMBRYO STEM CELLS

My PhD began at the Institute of Animal Genetics, Edinburgh University in 1952, encouraged by Professor Conrad Waddington, the inventor of epigenesis, and supervised by Dr Alan Beatty. At the time, capacitation was gaining in significance. My chosen topic was the genetic control of early mammalian embryology, specifically the growth of preimplantation mouse embryos with altered chromosome complements.

Achieving these aims included a need to expose mouse spermatozoa to x-rays, ultraviolet light, and various chemicals in vitro. This would destroy their chromatin and prevent them from making any genetic contribution to the embryo, hopefully without impairing their capacity to fertilize eggs in vivo. Resulting embryos would become gynogenetic haploids. Later, my work changed to exposing ovulated mouse oocytes to colchicine in vivo, in order to destroy their second meiotic spindle in vivo. This treatment freed all chromosomes from their attachment to the meiotic spindle, and they then became extruded from the egg into tiny artificial polar bodies. The fertilizing spermatozoon thus entered an empty egg, which resulted in the formation of androgenetic haploid embryos with no genetic contribution from the maternal side. For three years, my work was concentrated in the mouse house, working at midnight to identify mouse females in estrus by vaginal smears, collecting epididymal spermatozoa from males, and practicing artificial insemination with samples of treated spermatozoa. This research was successful, as mouse embryos were identified with haploid, triploid, tetraploid, and aneuploid chromosomes. Moreover, the wide range of scientific talent in the Institute made it a perfect place for fresh collaborative studies. For example, Julio Sirlin and I applied the use of radioactive DNA and RNA precursors to the study of spermatogenesis, spermiogenesis, fertilization, and embryogenesis, and gained knowledge unavailable elsewhere.

An even greater fortune beckoned. Allen Gates, who arrived newly from the United States, brought commercial samples of Organon's pregnant mares' serum (PMS) rich in follicle-stimulating hormone (FSH), and human chorionic gonadotropin (hCG) with its strong luteinizing hormone (LH) activity to induce estrus and ovulation in immature female mice. Working with Mervyn Runner (7), he had used low doses of each hormone at an interval of 48 hours to induce oocyte maturation, mating, and ovulation in immature mouse females. He now wished to measure the viability of three-day embryos from immature mice by transferring them to an adult host to grow to term (8). I was more interested in stimulating adult mice with these gonadotropins to induce estrus and ovulation at predictable times of the day. This would help my research, and I was by now weary of taking mouse vaginal smears at midnight. My future wife, Ruth Fowler, and I teamed up to test this new approach to superovulating adult mice. We chose PMS to induce multifolliculation and hCG to trigger ovulation, varying doses and times from those utilized by Allen Gates. PMS became obsolete for human studies some time later, but its impact has stayed with me from that moment, even till today.

Opinion in those days was that exogenous hormones such as PMS and hCG would stimulate follicle growth and ovulation in immature female mammals, but not in adults because they would interact badly with an adult's reproductive cycles. In fact, they worked wonderfully well. Doses of 1–3 IU of PMS induced the growth of numerous follicles, and similar doses of hCG 42 hours later invoked estrus and ovulation a further 6 hours later in almost all of them. Often, 70 or more ovulated oocytes crowded the ampulla, most of them being fertilized and developing to blastocysts (9). Oocyte maturation, ovulation, mating, and fertilization were each closely timed in all adults, another highly unusual aspect of stimulation (10). Diakinesis was identified as the germinal vesicle regressed, with metaphase I a little later and metaphase II, expulsion of the first polar body, and ovulation at 11.5–12 hours after hCG. Multiple fertilization led to multiple implantation and fetal growth to full term, just as similar treatments in anovulatory women resulted in quintuplets and other high-order multiple pregnancies a few years later. Years afterward, germinal vesicle breakdown and diakinesis were to prove equally decisive in identifying meiosis and ovulation in human oocytes in vivo and in vitro. Even as these results were gained, Ruth and I departed in 1957 from Edinburgh to the California Institute of Technology, where I switched over immunology and reproduction, a topic that was to dominate my life for five or six years on my return to the United Kingdom.

The Institute at Edinburgh had given me an excellent basis not only in genetics, but equally in reproduction. I had gained considerable knowledge about the endocrine control of estrus cycles, ovulation, and spermatozoa; the male reproductive tract; artificial insemination; the stages of embryo growth in the oviduct and uterus; superovulation and its consequences; and the use of radiolabeled compounds. Waddington had also been deeply interested in ethics and the relationships between science and religion, and instilled these topics in his students. I had been essentially trained in reproduction, genetics, and scientific ethics, and all of this knowledge was to prove to be of immense value in my later career. A visit to the California Institute of Technology widened my horizons into the molecular biology of DNA and the gene, a field then in its infancy.

After a year in California, London beckoned me, to the National Institute for Medical Research to work with Drs Alan Parkes and Colin (Bunny) Austin. I was fortunate indeed to have two such excellent colleagues. After two intense years in immunology, my curiosity returned to maturing oocytes and fertilization in vitro. Since they matured so regularly and easily in vivo, it should be easy to stimulate maturation in mouse oocytes in vitro by using gonadotropins. In fact, to my immense surprise, when liberated from their follicles into culture medium, oocytes matured immediately in vast numbers in all groups, with exactly the same timing as those maturing in vivo following an injection of hCG. Adding hormones made no difference. Rabbit, hamster, and rat oocytes also matured within 12 hours, each at their own species' specific rates. But to my surprise, oocytes from cows, sheep, and rhesus monkeys, and the occasional baboon, did not mature in vitro within 12 hours. Their germinal vesicles persisted unmoved, arrested in the stage known as diffuse diplotene. Why had they not responded like those of rats, mice, and rabbits? How would human oocytes respond? A unique opportunity emerged to collect pieces of human ovary, and to aspirate human oocytes from their occasional follicles. I grasped it with alacrity.

MOVING TO HUMAN STUDIES

Molly Rose was a local gynecologist in the Edgware and District Hospital who delivered two of our daughters. She agreed to send me slithers or wedges of ovaries such as those removed from patients with polycystic disease, as recommended by Stein and Leventhal, or with myomata or other disorders demanding surgery. Stein–Leventhal wedges were the best source of oocytes, with their numerous small Graafian follicles lined up in a continuous rim just below the ovarian surface. Though samples were rare, they provided enough oocytes to start with. These oocytes responded just like the oocytes from cows, sheep, and pigs, their germinal vesicles persisting and diakinesis being absent after 12 hours in vitro.

This was disappointing, and especially so for me, since Tjio and Levan, and Ford had identified 46 diploid chromosomes in humans, while studies by teams in Edinburgh (Scotland) and France had made it clear that many human beings were heteroploid. This was my subject, because chromosomal variations mostly arose during meiosis and this would be easily assessed in maturing oocytes at diakinesis. Various groups also discovered monosomy or disomy in many men and women. Some women were XO or XXX; some men were XYY and XYYY. Trisomy 21 proved to be the most common cause of Down's syndrome, and other trisomies were detected. All this new information reminded me of my chromosome studies in the Edinburgh mice.

For human studies, I would have to obtain diakinesis and metaphase I in human oocytes, and then continue this analysis to metaphase II when the oocytes would be fully mature, ready for fertilization. Despite being disappointed at current failure with human oocytes, it was time to write my findings for *Nature* in 1962 (11). There was so much to write regarding the animal work, and describing the new ideas then taking shape in my mind. I had heard Institute lectures on infertility, and realized that fertilizing human oocytes *in vitro* and replacing embryos into the mother could help to alleviate this condition. It could also be possible to type embryos for genetic diseases when a familial disposition was identified. Pieces of tissue, or one or two blastomeres, would have to be excised from blastocysts or cleaving embryos, but this did not seem to be too difficult. There were few genetic markers available for this purpose in the early 1960s, but it might be possible to sex embryos by their XX or XY chromosome complement by assessing mitoses in cells excised from morulae or blastocysts. Choosing female embryos for transfer would avert the birth of boys with various sex-linked disorders such as hemophilia. Clearly, I was becoming totally committed to human IVF and embryo transfer.

While looking in the library for any newly published papers relevant to my proposed *Nature* manuscript, I discovered those earlier papers of Pincus and his colleagues described earlier. They had apparently succeeded 30 years earlier in maturing human oocytes cultured for 12 hours, where I had failed. My *Nature* paper (11) became very different from that originally intended, even though it retained enough for publication. Those results of Pincus et al. had to be repeated. After trying hard, I failed completely to repeat them, despite infusing intact ovaries in vitro with gonadotropin solutions, using different culture media to induce maturation, and using joint cultures of maturing mouse oocytes and newly released human oocytes. Adding hormones to culture media also failed. It began to seem that menstrual cycles had affected oocyte physiology in a different manner than in nonmenstruating mammalian species. Finally, another line of inquiry emerged after two years of fruitless research on the precious few human oocytes available. Perhaps the timing of maturation in mice and rabbits differed from that of those oocytes obtained from cows, baboons, and humans. Even as my days in London were ending, Molly Rose sent a slither of human ovary. The few oocytes were placed in culture just as before. Their germinal vesicles remained static for 12 hours as I already knew, and then after 20 hours in vitro. Three oocytes remained, and I waited to examine them until they had been in vitro for 24 hours. The first contained a germinal vesicle, so did the second. There was one left and one only. Its image under the microscope was electrifying. I gazed down at chromosomes in diakinesis and at a regressing germinal vesicle. The chromosomes were superb examples of human diakinesis with their classical chiasmata. At last, I was on the way to human IVF, to completion of the maturation program and the onset of studies on fertilization in vitro.

This was the step I had waited for, a marker that Pincus had missed. He never checked for diakinesis, and apparently confused atretic oocytes, which contained chromosomes, with maturing oocytes. Endless human studies were opening. It was easy now, even on the basis of one oocyte in diakinesis, to calculate the timing of the final stages of maturation because the postdiakinesis stages of maturation were not too different from normal mitotic cycles in somatic cells. This calculation provided me with an estimate of about 36 hours for full maturation, which would be the moment for insemination. All these gaps in knowledge had to be filled. But now, my research program was stretching far into the future.

At this wonderful moment, John Paul, an outstanding cell biologist, invited me to join him and Robin Cole at Glasgow University to study differentiation in early mammalian embryos. This was exciting, to work in biochemistry with a leading cell biologist. He had heard that I was experimenting with very early embryos, trying to grow cell lines from them. He also wanted to grow stem cells from mammalian embryos and study them in vitro. This began one of my most memorable 12 months of research. John's laboratory had facilities unknown outside, with CO_2 incubators, numerous cell lines in constant cultivation, cryopreservation facilities, and the use of media droplets held under liquid paraffin. We decided to start with rabbits. Cell lines did not grow easily from cleaving rabbit embryos. In contrast, stem cells migrated out in massive numbers from cultures of rabbit blastocysts, forming muscle, nerves, phagocytes, blood islands, and other tissues in vitro (12). Stem cells were differentiating in vitro into virtually all the tissues of the body. In contrast, dissecting the inner cell mass from blastocysts and culturing it intact or as disaggregated cells produced lines of cells which divided and divided, without ever differentiating. One line of these embryonic stem cells expressed specific enzymes, diploid chromosomes, and a fibroblastic structure as it grew over 200 and more generations. Another was epithelioid and had different enzymes but was similar in other respects. The ability to make whole-embryo cultures producing differentiating cells was now combined with everlasting lines of undifferentiated stem cells which replicated over many years without changing. Ideas of using stem cells for grafting to overcome organ damage in recipients began to emerge. My thoughts returned constantly to growing stem cells from human embryos to repair defects in tissues of children and adults.

Almost at my last moment in Glasgow, with this new set of ideas in my mind, a piece of excised ovary yielded several oocytes. Being placed in vitro, two of them had reached metaphase II and expelled a polar body at 37 hours. This showed that another target on the road to human IVF had been achieved as the whole pattern of oocyte maturation continued to emerge but with increasing clarity.

Cambridge University, my next and final habitation, is an astonishing place. Looking back on those days, it seems that the Physiological Laboratory was not the ideal place to settle in that august university. Nevertheless, a mixture of immunology and reproduction remained my dominant theme as I rejoined Alan Parkes and Bunny Austin there. I had to do immunology to obtain a grant to support my family, but thoughts of human oocytes and embryos were never far away. One possible model of the human situation was the cow and other agricultural species, and large numbers of cow, pig, and sheep oocytes were available from ovaries given to me by the local slaughterhouse. Each species had its own timing, all of them longer than 12 hours (13). Pig oocytes were closest to humans, requiring 37 hours. In each species, maturation timings in vitro were exactly the same as those arising in vivo in response to an hCG injection. This made me suspect that a woman ovulated 36–37 hours after an injection of hCG. Human oocytes also trickled in, improving my provisional timings of maturation, and one or two of them were inseminated, but without signs of fertilization.

More oocytes were urgently needed to conclude the timings of oocyte meiosis. Surgeons in Johns Hopkins Hospital, Baltimore performed the Stein–Leventhal operation, which would allow me to collect ovarian tissue, aspirate oocytes from their follicles, and retain the remaining ovarian tissues for pathology if necessary.

I had already met Victor McKusick, who worked in Johns Hopkins, at many conferences. I asked for his support for my request to work with the hospital gynecologists for six weeks. He found a source of funds, made laboratory space available, and a wonderful invitation that introduced me to Howard and Georgeanna Jones. This significant moment was equal to my meeting with Molly Rose. The Joneses proved to be superb and unstinting in their support. Sufficient wedges and other ovarian fragments were available to complete my maturation program in human oocytes. Within three weeks, every stage of meiosis was classified and timed (14). We also undertook preliminary studies on inseminating human oocytes that had matured in vitro, trying to achieve sperm capacitation by using different media or adding fragments of ampulla to the cultures, and even attempting fertilization in rhesus monkey oviducts. Two nuclei were found in some inseminated eggs, resembling pronuclei, but sperm tails were not identified so no claims could be made (15). During those six weeks, however, oocyte maturation was fully timed at 37 hours, permitting me now to predict with certainty that women would ovulate at 37 hours after an hCG injection.

A simple means of access to the human ovary was now essential in order to identify human ovarian follicles in vivo and to aspirate them 36 hours after hCG, just before the follicular rupture. Who could provide this? And how about sperm capacitation? Only in hamsters that fertilization in vitro had been achieved, using in vivo matured oocytes and epididymal spermatozoa (16). I met Victor Lewis, my third clinical colleague, and we noticed what seemed to be anaphase II in some inseminated eggs. Again, no sperm tails were seen within the eggs.

An attempt to achieve human capacitation in Chapel Hill, North Carolina, United States, working with Robert McGaughey and his colleagues, also failed (17). A small intrauterine chamber lined with porous membrane was filled with washed human spermatozoa, sealed, and inserted overnight into the uterus of human volunteers at mid-cycle. Molecules entering it could react with the spermatozoa. No matured human eggs were fertilized. Later evidence indicated that the chamber contained inflammatory proteins, perhaps explaining the failure.

DECISIVE STEPS TO CLINICAL HUMAN IVF

Back in the United Kingdom, my intention to conceive human children in vitro had grown even stronger. So many medical advantages could flow from it. A small number of human embryos had been flushed from human oviducts or uteri after sexual intercourse, providing slender information on these earliest stages of human embryology. It was time to attain human fertilization in vitro, in order to move close to working with infertile patients. Ethical issues and moral decisions would emerge, one after the other, in full public view. Matters such as cloning and sexing embryos, the risk of abnormalities in the children, the clinical use of embryo stem cells, the ethics of oocyte donation and surrogate pregnancy, and the right to initiate human embryonic life in vitro would never be very far away. These issues were all acceptable, since I was confident that studies of human conception were essential for future medicine, and correct ethically, medically, and scientifically. The increasing knowledge of genetics and embryology could assist many patients if I could achieve human fertilization and grow embryos for replacement into their mothers.

Few human oocytes were available in the United Kingdom. Despite this scarcity, one or two of those matured and fertilized in vitro possessed two nuclei after insemination. But there were no obvious sperm tails. I devised a cow model for human fertilization, using in vitro matured oocytes and insemination in vitro with selected samples of highly active, washed bull spermatozoa extracted from neat semen. It was a pleasure to see some fertilized bovine eggs, with sperm tails and characteristic pronuclei, especially using spermatozoa from one particular bull. Here was a model for human IVF and a prelude to a series of events, which implied that matters in my research were suddenly changing. A colleague had stressed that formalin fixatives were needed to detect sperm tails in eggs. Barry Bavister joined our team to study for his PhD and designed a medium of high pH, which gave excellent fertilization rates in hamsters. We decided to collaborate by using it for trials on human fertilization in vitro.

Finally, while browsing in the library of the Physiological Laboratory, I read a paper in *The Lancet* which instantly caught my attention. Written by Dr P C Steptoe of the Oldham and District General Hospital (18), it described laparoscopy, with its narrow telescope and instruments and the minute abdominal incisions. He could visualize the ampulla and place small amounts of medium there, in an operation lasting 30 minutes or less and maybe even without using anesthesia. This is exactly what I wanted, because access to the ampulla was equivalent to gaining access to ovarian follicles. Despite advice to the contrary from several medical colleagues, I telephoned him about collaboration and stressed the uncertainty in achieving fertilization in vitro. He responded most positively, just as Molly, Howard and Georgeanna, and Victor had done. We decided to get together.

Last but by no means least, Molly Rose sent a small piece of ovary to Cambridge. Its dozen or more oocytes were matured in vitro for 37 hours, when Barry and I added washed spermatozoa suspended in his medium. We examined them a few hours later. To our delight, spermatozoa were pushing through the zona pellucida, into several of the eggs. Maternal and paternal pronuclei were forming beautifully. We saw polar bodies and sperm tails within the eggs. That evening in 1969, we watched in delight virtually all the stages of human fertilization in vitro (Fig. I.1). One fertilized egg had fragments, as Chang had forecast from his work on oocyte maturation and fertilization in vitro of rabbit eggs. This evidence strengthened the need to abandon oocyte maturation in vitro and replace it by stimulating maturation by means of exogenous hormones. Our 1969 paper in *Nature* surprised a

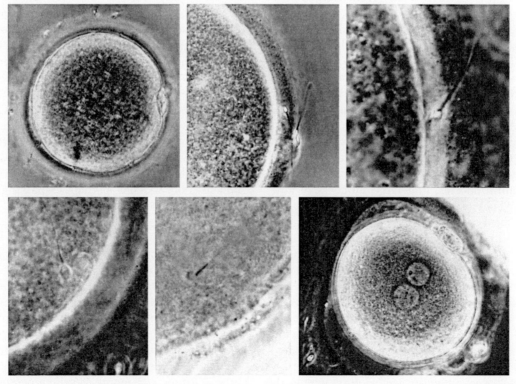

Figure I.1 A composite picture of the stages of fertilization of the human egg. (*Upper left*) An egg with a first polar body and spermatozoa attached to the outer zona pellucida. (*Upper central*) Spermatozoa are migrating through the zona pellucida. (*Upper right*) A spermatozoon with a tail beating outside the zona pellucida is attaching to the oocyte vitelline membrane. (*Lower left*) A spermatozoon in the ooplasm, with enlarging head and distinct mid-piece and tail. (*Lower central*) Further development of the sperm head in the ooplasm. (*Lower right*) A pronucleate egg with two pronuclei and polar bodies. Notice that the pronuclei are apparently aligned with the polar bodies, although more dimensions must be scored to ensure that polarity has been established in all axes.

world unaccustomed to the idea of human fertilization in vitro (19).

Incredibly fruitful days followed in our Cambridge laboratory. Richard Gardner, another PhD candidate, and I excised small pieces of trophectoderm from rabbit blastocysts and sexed them by staining the sex chromatin body. Those classified as female were transferred into adult females and were all correctly sexed at term. This work transferred my theoretical ideas of a few years earlier into the practice of preimplantation diagnosis of inherited disease, in this case for sex-linked diseases (20). Alan Henderson, a cytogeneticist, and I analyzed chiasmata during diakinesis in mouse and human eggs, and explained the high frequencies of Down's syndrome in offspring of older mothers as a consequence of meiotic errors arising in oocytes formed last in the fetal ovary, which were then ovulated last at later maternal ages (21). Dave Sharpe, a lawyer from Washington, joined forces to write an article in *Nature* (22) on the ethics of IVF, the first ever paper in the field. I followed this up with a detailed analysis of ethics and law in IVF covering scientific possibilities, oocyte donation, surrogacy by embryo transfer, and other matters (22). So the first ethical papers were written by scientists and lawyers and not by philosophers, ethicists, or politicians.

THE OLDHAM YEARS

Patrick and I began our collaboration six months later in the Oldham and District General Hospital, almost 200 miles north of Cambridge. He had worked closely with two pioneers, Palmer in Paris (23) and Fragenheim in Germany (24). He improved the pneumoperitoneum to gain working space in the abdominal cavity and used carbon fibers to pass cold light into the abdomen from an external source (25). By now, Patrick was waiting in the wings, ready to begin clinical IVF in distant Oldham. We had a long talk about ethics and found our stances to be very similar.

Work started in the Oldham and District General Hospital and moved later to Kershaw's Hospital, set up by my assistants, especially Jean Purdy. We knew the routine. It was based on my Edinburgh experiences with mice. Piero Donini from Serono Laboratories in Rome had purified urinary human menopausal gonadotropins (hMG) as a source of FSH and the product was used clinically to stimulate follicle growth in anovulatory women by Bruno Lunenfeld (26). It removed the need for PMS, thus avoiding the use of nonhuman hormones. We used low-dosage levels in patients, that is, 2–3 vials (a total of 150–225 IU) given on days 3 and 5, and 5000–7000 IU of hCG on day 10. Initially, the timing of oocyte maturation in vitro was confirmed, by performing laparoscopic collections of oocytes from ovarian follicles at 28 hours after hCG to check that they were in metaphase I (27). We then moved to 36 hours to aspirate mature metaphase II oocytes for fertilization. Those beautiful oocytes were surrounded by masses of viscous cumulus cells and were maturing exactly as predicted. We witnessed follicular rupture at 37 hours through the laparoscope. Follicles could be classified from their appearance as ovulatory or nonovulatory, this diagnosis being confirmed later by assaying several steroids in the aspirated follicular fluids (Fig. I.2).

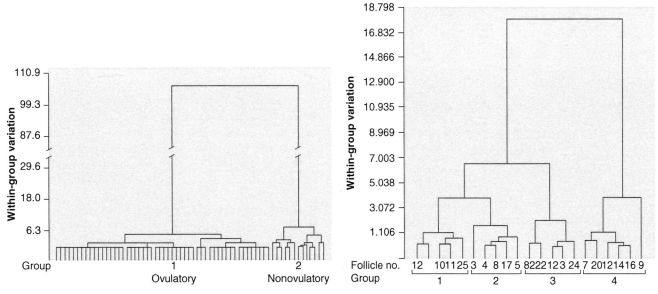

Figure I.2   Eight steroids were assayed in fluids extracted from human follicles aspirated 36–37 hours after the human chorionic gonadotropin (hCG) shot. The follicles had been classified as ovulating or nonovulating by laparoscopic examination in vivo. Data were analyzed by cluster analysis, which groups follicles with similar features. The upper illustration shows data collected during the natural menstrual cycle. Note that two sharply separated groups of follicles were identified, each with very low levels of within-group variance. Attempting to combine the two groups resulted in a massive increase of within-group variation, indicating that two sharply different groups had been identified. These different groups accorded exactly with the two groups identified by means of steroid assays. The lower figure shows the same analysis during stimulated cycles on fluids collected 36–37 hours after injecting hCG. With this form of stimulation, follicle growth displays considerable variation within groups. Attempts to combine all the groups result in a moderately large increase in variation. This evidence suggests that follicles vary considerably in their state of development in simulated cycles using human menopausal gonadotropin (hMG) and hCG.

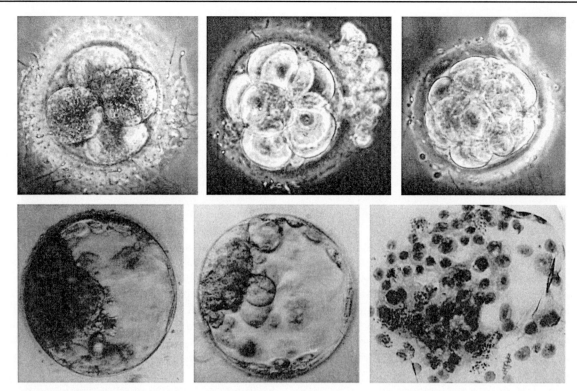

Figure I.3   Successive stages of human preimplantation development in vitro in a composite illustration made in Oldham in 1971. (*Upper left*) 4-cell stage showing the crossed blastomeres typical of most mammals. (*Upper middle*) 8-cell stage showing the even outline of blasto-meres and a small piece of cumulus adherent to the zona pellucida. (*Upper right*) A 16 to 32-cell stage, showing the onset of compaction of the outer blastomeres. Often, blastocelic fluid can be seen accumulating between individual cells to give a "stripey" appearance to the embryo. (*Lower left and middle*) Two living blastocysts showing a distinct inner cell mass, single-celled trophectoderm, blastocelic cavity, and thinning zona pellucida. (*Lower right*) A fixed preparation of a human blastocyst at 5 days, showing more than 100 even-sized nuclei and many mitoses.

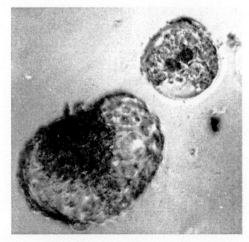

Figure I.4   A hatched human blastocyst after 9 days in culture. Notice the distinct embryonic disc and the possible bilaminar struc-ture of the membrane. The blastocyst has expanded considerably, as shown by comparing its diameter with that of the shed zona pellu-cida. The zona contains dying and necrotic cells and its diameter provides an estimate of the original oocyte end embryo diameters.

It was a pleasure and a new duty to meet the patients searching for help to alleviate their infertility. We did our best, driving from Cambridge to Oldham and arriving at noon to prepare the small laboratory there. Patrick had stimulated the patients with hMG and hCG, and he and his team led by Muriel Harris arrived to prepare for surgery.

Patrick's laparoscopy was superb. Ovarian stimulation, even though mild, produced five or six mature follicles per patient, and ripe oocytes came in a steady stream into my culture medium for insemination and overnight incuba-tion. The next morning, the formation of two pronuclei and sperm tails indicated fertilization had occurred, even in simple media, now with a near-neutral pH. Complex culture media, Ham's F10 and others, each with added serum or serum albumin, sustained early and later cleav-ages (28), and, even more fascinating, was the gradual appearance of morulae and then light, translucent blasto-cysts (Fig. I.3) (29). Here was my reward—growing embryos was now a routine, and examinations of many of them convinced me that the time had come to replace them into the mothers' uterus. I had become highly familiar with the teratologic principles of embryonic development, and knew many teratologists. The only worry I had was the chance of chromosomal monosomy or trisomy, on the basis of our mouse studies, but these conditions could be detected later in gestation by amniocentesis. Our human studies had surpassed work on all animals, a point rubbed in even more when we grew blastocysts to day 9 after they had hatched from their zona pellucida (Fig. I.4) (30). This beautifully expanded blastocyst had a large embryonic disc which was shouting that it was a potential source of embryonic stem cells.

When human blastocysts became available, we tried to sex them using the sex chromatin body as in rabbits.

Unfortunately, they failed to express either sex chromatin or the male Y body so we were unable to sex them as female or male embryos. Human preimplantation genetic diagnosis would have to wait a little longer.

During these years there were very few plaudits for us, as many people spoke against IVF. Criticism was mostly aimed at me, as usual when scientists bring new challenges to society. Criticism came not only from the Pope and archbishops, but also from scientists who should have known better, including James Watson (who testified to a U.S. Senate Committee that many abnormal babies would be born), and Max Perutz, who supported him. These scientist critics knew virtually nothing about my field, so who advised them to make such ridiculous charges? Cloning football teams or intelligentsia was always raised by ethicists, which clearly dominated their thoughts rather than the intense hopes of our infertile patients. Yet one theologian, Gordon Dunstan, who became a close friend, knew all about IVF from us, and wrote an excellent book on its ethics. He was far ahead of almost every scientist in my field of study. Our patients also gave us their staunch support, and so did the Oldham Ethical Committee, Bunny Austin back home in Cambridge, and Elliott Philip, a colleague of Patrick's.

Growing embryos became a routine, so we decided to transfer one each to several patients. Here again we were in untested waters. Transferring embryos via the cervical canal, the obvious route to the uterus, was virtually a new and untested method. We would have to do our best. From now on, we worked with patients who had seriously distorted tubes or none whatsoever. This step was essential, since no one would have believed we had established a test-tube baby in a woman with near-normal tubes. This had to be a condition of our initial work. Curiously, it led many people to make the big mistake of believing that we started IVF to bypass occluded oviducts. Yet we already knew that embryos could be obtained for men with oligozoospermia or antibodies to their gametes, and for women in various stages of endometriosis.

One endocrinological problem did worry me. Stimulation with hMG and hCG shortened the succeeding luteal phase, to a very short time for embryos to implant before the onset of menstruation. Levels of urinary pregnanediol also declined soon after oocyte collection. This condition was not a result of the aspiration of granulosa and cumulus cells, and luteal support would be needed, preferably progesterone. Csapo et al. stressed how this hormone was produced by the ovaries for the first 8–10 weeks before the placenta took over this function (31). Injections of progesterone in oil given over that long period of time seemed unacceptable since it would be extremely uncomfortable for patients. While mulling over this problem, my attention turned to those earlier endocrinologists who believed that exogenous hormones would distort the reproductive cycle, although I doubt they even knew anything about a deficient luteal phase.

This is how we unknowingly made our biggest mistake in early IVF days. Our choice of Primolut (Sigma Chemical co., St Louis, USA) depot, a progestogen, meant it should be given every five days to sustain pregnancies, since it was supposed to save threatened abortions. So, we began embryo transfers to patients in stimulated cycles, giving this luteal phase support. Even though our work was slowed down by having to wait to see whether pregnancies arose in one group of patients before stimulating the next, enough patients had accumulated after two to three years. None of our patients was pregnant, and disaster loomed. Our critics were even more vociferous as the years passed, and the mutual support between Patrick and me had to pull us through.

Twenty or more different factors could have caused our failure, for example cervical embryo transfers, abnormal embryos, toxic culture dishes or catheters, inadequate luteal support, incompatibility between patients' cycles and that imposed by hMG and hCG, inherent weakness in human implantation, and many others. We had to glean every scrap of information from our failures. I knew Ken Bagshawe in London, who was working with improved assay methods for gonadotropic hormones. He offered to measure blood samples taken from our patients over the implantation period using his new hCG-® assay. He telephoned: three or more of our patients previously undiagnosed had actually produced short-lived rises of hCG-® over this period. Everything changed with this information. We had established pregnancies after all, but they had aborted very early. We called them biochemical pregnancies, a term that still sticks today. It had taken us almost three years to identify the cause of our failure, and the finger of suspicion pointed straight at Primulot. I knew it was luteolytic, but it was apparently also an abortifacient, and our ethical decision to use it had caused much heartache, immense loss of work and time, and despair for some of our patients. The social pressures had been immense, with critics claiming our embryos were dud and our whole program was a waste of time; but we had come through it and now knew exactly what to do next.

We accordingly reduced the levels of Primulot depot, and utilized hCG and progesterone as luteal aids. Suspicions were also emerging that human embryos were very poor at implanting. We had replaced single embryos into most of our patients, rarely two. Increasingly we began to wonder whether more should be replaced, as when we replaced two in a program involving transfer of oocytes and spermatozoa into the ampulla so that fertilization could occur in vivo.

This procedure was later called gamete intrafallopian transfer (GIFT) by Ricardo Asch. We now suspected that single embryo transfers could produce a 15–20% chance of establishing pregnancy, just as our first clinical pregnancy arose after the transfer of a single blastocyst in a patient stimulated with hMG and hCG (32). Then came the fantastic news—a human embryo fertilized and grown in vitro had produced a pregnancy. Everything seemed fine, even with ultrasound images. My culture protocols were satisfactory after all. Patrick rang: he feared the pregnancy was ectopic and he had to remove it sometime after 10 gestational weeks. Every new approach we tested seemed to be ending in a disaster, yet we would not stop, since the work itself seemed highly ethical, and conceiving a child for our patients was perhaps the most wonderful thing anyone could do for them. In any case, ectopic pregnancies are now known to be a regular feature with assisted conception.

I sensed that we were entering the final phase of our Oldham work, seven years after it began. We had to speed up, partly because Patrick was close to retiring from the National Health Service. Four stimulation protocols were tested in an attempt to avoid problems with the luteal phase: hMG and hCG; clomiphene, hMG, and hCG to gain a better luteal phase; bromocriptine, hMG, and hCG because some patients had high prolactin concentrations; and hCG alone at mid-cycle. We also tested what came to be known as GIFT, calling it ORTI (oocyte recovery with tubal insemination, by transferring one or two eggs and spermatozoa to the ampulla) (Fig. I.5). Natural-cycle IVF was introduced, based on collections of urine samples at regular intervals eight times daily, to measure exactly the onset of the LH surge, using a modified HiGonavis assay (Fig. I.6). Cryopreservation was also introduced, by freezing oocytes and embryos that looked to be in good condition when thawed. A recipient was given a donor egg fertilized by her husband's spermatozoa, but pregnancy did not occur.

Lesley and John Brown came as the second entrants for natural-cycle IVF. Lesley had no oviducts. Her egg was aspirated in a few moments and inseminated simply and efficiently. The embryo grew beautifully and was

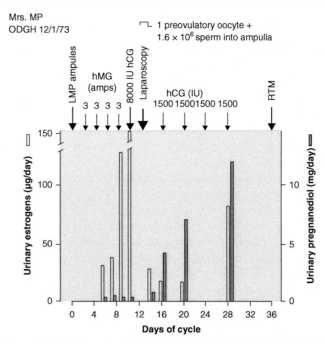

Figure I.5 The first attempts at gamete intrafallopian transfer (GIFT) were called oocyte recovery with tubal insemination (ORTI). In this treatment cycle, using human menopausal gonadotropin (hMG) and human chorionic gonadotropin (hCG), including additional injections of hCG for luteal support, a single preovulatory oocyte and 1.6 million sperm were transferred into the ampulla. *Abbreviations*: LMP, last menstrual period; ODGH, Oldham and District General Hospital return to menstruation (RTM) indicates stages of the menstrual cycle.

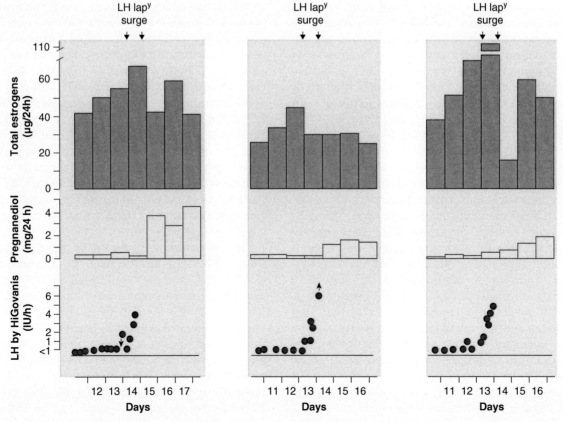

Figure I.6 Recording the progress of the human natural menstrual cycle for in vitro fertilization (IVF). Three patients are illustrated. All three displayed rising 24-hour urinary estrogen concentrations during the follicular phase and rising urinary pregnanediol concentrations in the luteal phase. Luteinizing hormone (LH) levels were measured several times daily and the data clearly reveal the exact time of onset of the LH surge.

transferred an hour or so after it became 8-cell. Their positive pregnancy test a few days after transfer was another milestone—surely nothing could now prevent their embryo developing to full term in a normal reproductive cycle, but those nine months lasted a very long time. Three more pregnancies were established using natural-cycle IVF as we abandoned the other approaches. A triploid embryo died in utero—more bad luck. A third pregnancy was lost through premature labor on a mountain walking holiday, two weeks after the mother's amniocentesis (32,33). It was a lovely, well-developed boy. Louise Brown's birth, and then Alistair's, proved to a waiting world that science and medicine had entered human conception. Our critics declared that the births were a fake, and advised against attending our presentation on the whole of the Oldham work at the Royal College of Obstetricians and Gynaecologists.

IVF WORLDWIDE

The Oldham period was over. Good facilities were now needed, with space for a large IVF clinic. Bourn Hall was an old Jacobean house in lovely grounds near Cambridge (Fig. I.7). Facilities on offer for IVF in Cambridge were far too small, so we purchased it mostly with venture capital. It was essential to conceive 100 or 1000 IVF babies to ensure that the method was safe and effective clinically. The immense delays in establishing Bourn Hall delayed our work by two years after Louise's birth. Finally, on minimal finance, Bourn Hall was opened in September 1980 on a shoestring, supported by our own cash and loans. The delay gave the rest of the world a chance to join in IVF. Alex Lopata delivered an IVF baby in Australia, and one or two others were born elsewhere. Natural-cycle IVF was chosen initially at Bourn Hall since it had proved successful in Oldham, and we became experts in it. Pregnancies flowed, at 15% per cycle. An Australian team of Alan Trounson and Carl Wood announced the establishment of several IVF pregnancies after stimulation by clomiphene and hCG and replacing two or three embryos (34), so they had moved ahead of us during the delayed opening of Bourn Hall. Our own effort now expanded prodigiously. Thousands of patients queued for IVF. Simon Fishel, Jacques Cohen, and Carol Fehilly joined the embryology team among younger trainees, and new clinicians joined Patrick and John Webster. Patients and pregnancies increased rapidly, and the world was left standing far behind. Howard and Georgeanna Jones began in Norfolk using gonadotropins for ovarian stimulation. Jean Cohen began in Paris, Wilfred Feichtinger and Peter Kemeter in Vienna, Klaus Diedrich and Hans van der Venn in Bonn, Lars Hamberger and Matts Wikland in Sweden, and Andre van Steirteghem and Paul Devroey in Brussels. IVF was now truly international.

The opening of Bourn Hall had not deterred our critics. They put up a fierce rearguard action against IVF, alongside LIFE, Society for the Unborn Child, individual gynecologists, and others.

Objections raised against IVF included low rates of pregnancy (no one mentioned the similar low rates of pregnancy with natural conception), the possibilities of oocyte and embryo donation, surrogate mothers, unmarried parents, one-sex parents, embryo cryopreservation, cloning, and endless other objections.

LIFE issued a legal action against me for the abortion of an embryo grown for 14 days and longer in vitro. Their action was rejected by the U.K. Attorney General since the laws of pregnancy began after implantation. We fully respected the intense ethical nature of our proceedings. We also recognized the need for research, and the necessity to protect or cryopreserve the best embryos for later replacement into their mothers. Those not replaced had to be used for research under strict controls, combined with open publication and discussion of our work.

Each year, 1000, rising to almost 2000, patients passed through Bourn Hall. Different stimulation regimens or new procedures could be tested in very little time.

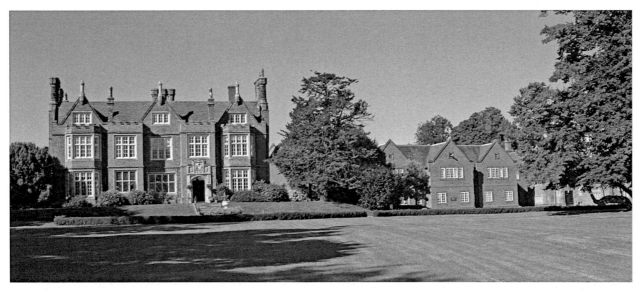

Figure I.7   Bourn Hall. *Source*: Courtesy of Dr P Brinsden.

Clomiphene/hMG was reintroduced. Bourn babies increased: 20, 50, 100 to 1000 after five to six years. This was far more than half of the world's entire IVF babies, including the first born in the United States, Germany, Italy, and many other countries. Detailed studies were performed on embryo culture, implantation, and abortion. We even tried aspirating epididymal spermatozoa for IVF, without achieving successful fertilization.

Among the immense numbers of patients, people with astonishingly varied conditions of infertility emerged. Some were poor responders in whom immense amounts of endocrine priming were essential, women with a natural menstrual cycle that was not as it should have been, previous misdiagnoses which had laid the cause of infertility on the wife when the husband had never even been investigated, and men bringing semen samples that we discovered had been obtained from a friend. The collaboration between nurses, clinicians, and scientists was remarkable. Yet trouble—ethical trouble—was never far away. I purchased a freezing machine to resume our Oldham work, but, unknown to me, Patrick talked to officers of the British Medical Association (BMA) and for some reason agreed to delay embryo cryopreservation. Apparently, the BMA felt it would be an unwelcome social development. I did not approve of these reservations: David Whittingham had shown how low-temperature cryostorage was successful with mouse embryos, without causing genetic damage. "Freezing and cloning" became a term of intense approbation at this time. I unwillingly curtailed our cryopreservation program.

One weekend, a major trouble erupted as a result of this difference between Patrick and me. My duties in Bourn Hall prevented me from attending a conference in London. Trying to be helpful, I telephoned my lecture to London. Reception at the other end was apparently so poor as to lead to misinterpretations of what I had said. Next morning, the press furore about my supposed practice of cryopreserving embryos after IVF was awful, so bad, indeed, that legal action had to be taken. Luckily, my lecture had been recorded, and listening to the tapes with a barrister revealed nothing contentious. I had said nothing improper in my lecture or during the question-answer session. That day, I issued seven libel actions against the cream of British society: the BMA and its secretary, the BBC, *The Times*, and other leading newspapers. There were seven in one day and another one later! If only one was lost, I could be ruined and disgraced. However, they were all won, even though it took several years with the BMA and its secretary. These legal actions had inhibited our research, the cryopreservation program being shut down for more than a year. Every single embryological note of mine from those days in Oldham and from Bourn Hall was examined in detail for my opponents by someone who was clearly an embryologist. Nothing was found to incriminate me.

That wretched period passed. The number of babies kept on growing, embryo cryopreservation was resumed, and Gerhard Dealmaker in The Netherlands beat us and the world to the first "ice" baby (35). Colin Howles and Mike McNamee joined us in endocrinology, and Mike Ashwood-Smith and Peter Holland's in embryology, as the old team faded away. Fascinating days had returned. Working with barristers, we designed consent forms which were far in advance of those used elsewhere. Oocyte donation and surrogacy by embryo transfer were introduced. The world's first paper on embryo stem cells appeared in *Science* in 1984, sent from Bourn Hall, and the world's first on human preimplantation diagnosis in 1987 appeared in *Human Reproduction*. However, embryo research faltered as all normal embryos were cryopreserved for their parents, so almost none were available for study. Alan Handyside, one of our Cambridge PhDs, joined Hammersmith Hospital in London to make major steps in introducing preimplantation genetic diagnosis (36). As we reached 1000 pregnancies, our data showed the babies to be as normal as those conceived in vivo.

Test-tube babies (an awful term) were no longer unique and were accepted worldwide, exactly as Patrick and I had hoped. Our work was being recognized (Fig. I.8). Clinics sprang up everywhere. Ultrasound was introduced to detect follicles for aspiration by the Scandinavians (37), making laparoscopy for oocyte recovery largely redundant. Artificial cycles were introduced in Australia and intracytoplasmic sperm injection (ICSI) in Belgium (38), and gonadotropin-releasing hormone agonists were used to inhibit the LH surge. Ian Craft in London showed how postmenopausal women aged 52 or more could establish pregnancies using oocyte donation and endocrine support. Women over 60 years of age conceived and delivered children. This breakthrough was especially welcome to me, since older women surely have the right to have children at ages almost the same as those possible for men.

Ethics continued side by side with advancing science and medicine. The U.K. governmental Warnock report recommended permitting embryo research and proposed a Licensing Authority for IVF. A year or so later, the U.K. House of Lords, in all its finery, responded with a 3:1 vote in favor, decisive support for all we had done in Mill

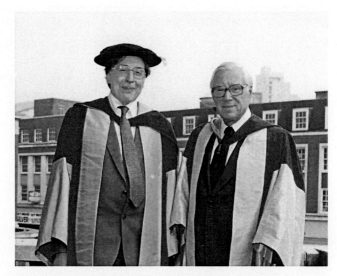

Figure I.8 A happy picture of Patrick and me, standing in our robes after being granted our Hon. DSc by Hull University.

Hill, Cambridge, and Oldham. What a wonderful day! The British House of Commons passed a liberal IVF law after intense debate, and so did the Spanish government, although elsewhere things were not so liberal. Ten years after the birth of Louise Brown, the British Parliament had therefore accepted IVF, research on human embryos until day 14, and establishing research embryos. Cloning and embryo stem cells still bothered the politicians in 1988, to re-emerge in 1998, gray shadows of my earlier times in Glasgow. IVF had also become fundamental to establish embryonic stem cells for organ repair, or cloning. During all this activity, tragedy struck all of us in Bourn Hall. Jean Purdy died in 1986 and Patrick Steptoe in 1988. They at least saw IVF come of age.

By the 1990s, burgeoning medical science was digging deeper into endless aspects of human conception in vitro. The intracytoplasmic injection of a single spermatozoon into an oocyte to achieve fertilization, ICSI, was one of the greatest advances since IVF was introduced. It transformed the treatment of male infertility, enabling severely oligozoospermic men to father their own children. It did not stop there, since epididymal spermatozoa and even those aspirated from the testis could be used for ICSI. Spermatids have also been used. ICSI became so simple that many clinics reduced IVF to fewer and fewer cases. New gonadotropin-releasing hormone antagonists introduced novel ways to control the cycle, enabling many oocytes to be stimulated by hMG and, subsequently, using recombinant human FSH. Treatment in the natural cycle could be improved, since these antagonists control LH levels and prevent premature LH surges. My own interests were returning to embryology, as the molecular biology revolution influenced our thinking. I am convinced that the oocyte and egg must be highly programmed, timewise, in embryonic polarities and integrating genetic systems such that the tight systems place every new gene product in its right place in the one-cell egg and cleaving embryo. This must be right; there can surely be no other explanations for the fabulous modification in embryonic growth in the first week or two of embryonic life. I have been delighted to work with Chris Hansis on identifying a gene (for hCG-®) in one blastomere of four- and eight-cell human embryos, providing evidence of blastomere differentiation at this early stage of embryogenesis (39).

This topic returns me to my scientific origins studying mouse embryos in the Institute of Animal Genetics in Edinburgh, where Waddington reported the amazing story of the gene *Aristapedia* in *Drosophila*, which he had induced to grow legs in place of eyes. These unusual flies then bred true, showing he had uncovered a gene that had been silenced for millions of years and how this could be an essential component of normal differentiation. He called it epigenesis, and we fear today that some aspects of IVF may lead to deleterious epigenetic changes in children such as Angelman or Beckwith–Wiedemann syndrome. Risks of epigenetic changes in cattle embryos and those of other species may be heightened by adding serum to media used to culture embryos to cause, for example large-calf syndrome. It would be wise to be well aware of these findings when practicing human IVF, for example by assessing the role of sera in human culture media.

IVF OUTLOOK

In one sense, opening up human conception in vitro was perhaps among the first examples of applied science in modern "hi tech." Human IVF has since spread throughout the world, with apparently more than 3.5 million babies born worldwide by 2008— yet Louise Brown is only just 30 years of age. The need for IVF and its derivatives is greater than ever, since up to 10% of couples may suffer from some form of infertility. Major advances in genetic technologies now identify hundreds of genes in a single cell, and diagnosing genetic disease in embryos promises to help avoid desperate genetic diseases in newborn children. Indeed, the ethics of this field have now become even more serious, since the typing of embryo genotypes provides detailed predictions of future life and health.

IVF has now combined closely with genetics to eliminate disease or disability genes, or lengthen the life span. But most of all, practicing IVF teaches a wider understanding of the desire and love for a child and a partner, the wonderful and ancient joys of parenthood, the pain of failure, the deep motivation needed in donating and receiving an urgently needed oocyte or a surrogate uterus. Parenthood is more responsible than ever before. Its complex choices are gathered before couples everywhere by the information revolution, placing family responsibilities on patients themselves, where it really matters. And IVF now reveals more and more about miracles preserved in embryogenesis from flies and frogs to humankind, over 600 million years of evolution.

The human genome project is now complete and will inevitably assist IVF since we will soon understand the genetic aspects of early embryo growth and how to detect abnormal genes in embryos. This textbook contains chapters which describe in detail the several advances and developments which have expanded the possibilities of treating diverse causes of human infertility as well as numerous genetic disorders.

Already it is clear that a staggering array of genes operates in preimplantation stages in mammalian including human embryos, and new methods are being introduced to deal with such highly multigenic embryonic systems. We are indeed enmeshed in a field embracing some of the most fundamental evolutionary stages of our existence as we pass from oocyte to blastocyst and to implantation.

REFERENCES

1. Pincus G, Saunders B. The comparative behavior of mammalian eggs in vivo and in vitro. VI. The maturation of human ovarian ova. Anat Rec 1939; 75: 537–45.
2. Menkin MF, Rock J. Am J Obstet Gynecol 1949; 55: 440.
3. Hayashi M. Seventh International Conference of the International Planned Parenthood Federation. Excerpta Medica, 1963: 505.

4. Austin CR. Adv Biosci 1969; 4: 5.
5. Chang M. Adv Biosci 1969; 4: 13.
6. Chang MC. The maturation of rabbit oocytes in culture and their maturation, activation, fertilization and subsequent development in the fallopian tubes. J Exp Zool 1955; 128: 379–405.
7. Runner M, Gates AH. Sterile, obese mothers. J Hered 1954; 45: 51–5.
8. Gates AH. Viability and developmental capacity of eggs from immature mice treated with gonadotrophins. Nature 1954; 177: 754–5.
9. Fowler RE, Edwards RG. Induction of superovulation and pregnancy in mature mice by gonadotrophins. J Endocrinol 1957; 15: 374–84.
10. Edwards RG, Gates AH. Timing of the stages of the maturation divisions, ovulation, fertilization and the first cleavage of eggs of adult mice treated with gonadotrophins. J Endocrinol 1959; 19: 292–304.
11. Edwards RG. Meiosis in ovarian oocytes of adult mammals. Nature (London) 1962; 196: 446–50.
12. Cole R, Edwards RG, Paul J. Cytodifferentiation and embryogenesis in cell colonies and tissue cultures derived from ova and blastocysts of the rabbit. Dev Biol 1966; 13: 385–407.
13. Edwards RG. Maturation in vitro of mouse, sheep, cow, pig, rhesus monkey and human ovarian oocytes. Nature 1965; 208: 349–51.
14. Edwards RG. Maturation in vitro of human ovarian oocytes. Lancet 1965; 2: 926–9.
15. Edwards RG, Donahue R, Baramki T, Jones H Jr. Preliminary attempts to fertilize human oocytesmatured in vivo. AmJ Obstet Gynecol 1966; 96: 192–200.
16. Yanagimachi R, Chang MC. J Exp Zool 1964; 156: 361–76.
17. Edwards RG, Talbert L, Israestam D, et al. Diffusion chamber for exposing spermatozoa to human uterine secretions. Am J Obstet Gynecol 1968; 102: 388–96.
18. Steptoe PC. Laparoscopy and ovulation. Lancet 1968; 2: 913.
19. Edwards RG, Bavister BD, Steptoe PC. Early stages of fertilisation in vitro of human oocytes matured in vitro. Nature (London) 1969; 221: 632–5.
20. Gardner RL, Edwards RG. Control of the sex ratio at full term in the rabbit by transferred sexed blastocysts. Nature (London) 1968; 218: 346–8.
21. Henderson SA, Edwards RG. Chiasma frequency and maternal age in mammals. Nature (London) 1968; 218: 22–8.
22. Edwards RG, Sharpe DJ. Social values and research in human embryology. Nature (London) 1971; 231: 81–91.
23. Palmer R. Acad Chir 1946; 72: 363.
24. Fragenheim H. Geburts Frauenheilkd 1964; 24: 740.
25. Steptoe PC. Laparoscopy in Gynaecology. Edinburgh: Livingstone, 1967.
26. Lunenfeld B. In: Inguilla W, Greenblatt RG, Thomas RB, eds. The Ovary. Springfield, IL: CC Thomas, 1969.
27. Steptoe PC, Edwards RG. Laparoscopic recovery of preovulatory human oocytes after priming of ovaries with gonadotrophins. Lancet 1970; 1: 683–9.
28. Edwards RG, Steptoe PC, Purdy JM. Fertilization and cleavage in vitro of preovulatory human oocytes. Nature (London) 1970; 227: 1307–9.
29. Steptoe PC, Edwards RG, Purdy JM. Human blastocysts grown in culture. Nature (London) 1971; 229: 132–3.
30. Edwards RG, Surani MAH. The primate blastocyst and its environment. Uppsala J Med Sci 1978; 22: 39–50.
31. Csapo AI, Pulkkinen MO, Kaihola HL. The relationship between the timing of luteectomy and the incidence of complete abortions. Am J Obstet Gycecol 1974; 118: 985–9.
32. Steptoe PC, Edwards RG. Reimplantation of a human embryo with subsequent tubal pregnancy. Lancet 1976; 1: 880–2.
33. Edwards RG, Steptoe PC, Purdy JM. Clinical aspects of pregnancies established with cleaving embryos grown in vivo. Br J Obstet Gynaecol 1980; 87: 757–68.
34. Trounson AO, Leeton JF, Wood C, et al. Pregnancies in humans by fertilization in vitro and embryo transfer in the controlled ovulatory cycle. Science 1981; 212: 681–2.
35. Zeilmaker GH, Alberda T, Gent I, et al. Two pregnancies following transfer of intact frozen–thawed embryos. Fertil Steril 1984; 42: 293–6.
36. Handyside A, Kontogianni EH, Hardy K, Winston RML. Pregnancies from biopsied human preimplantation embryos sexed by Y-specific DNA application. Nature (London) 1990; 344: 768–70.
37. Wikland M, Enk L, Hamberger L. Transvesical and transvaginal approaches for the aspiration of follicles by use of ultrasound. Ann NY Acad Sci 1985; 442: 182–94.
38. Palermo G, Joris H, Devroey P, et al. Pregnancies after intracytoplasmic injection of single spermatozoon into an oocyte. Lancet 1992; 340: 17–18.
39. Hansis C, Edwards RG. Cell differentiation in the preimplantation human embryo. Reprod BioMed Online 2003; 6: 215–20.

Robert Edwards: The path to IVF*

Martin H. Johnson

*This article is based on the research undertaken in preparation for the introductory lecture to the Nobel Symposium held in the Karolinska Institute, Stockholm, in December 2010 to celebrate the award of the Nobel Prize in Physiology or Medicine to Robert Geoffrey Edwards. An abbreviated account of the contents of this paper was published as "Robert Edwards: Nobel Laureate in Physiology and Medicine" in "Les Prix Nobel 2010," edited by Professor Karl Grandin, and published by the Nobel Foundation; this version is reproduced as published in Reproductive BioMedicine Online (2011) 23, 245–262, with the permission of the Editors and Publishers of Reproductive BioMedicine Online.

INTRODUCTION

Robert G Edwards was awarded the 2010 Nobel Prize for Physiology or Medicine "for the development of in vitro fertilization" (1). There is a variety of accounts of the events leading up to this discovery and its acceptance, most of them by participants (2), but historical scholarship is rarer. This account uses verifiable sources to produce a historical narrative of the path to in vitro fertilization (IVF) that differs in a number of places from the conventionally accepted version and adds further detail.

EDWARDS' LIFE HISTORY: SOURCES

Primary sources used were the publications by Edwards and Steptoe during the 1950s, 1960s, and 1970s; archives of the Royal Society of Medicine, Cambridge University, the Physiology Library at Cambridge, and the personal papers of RG Edwards (courtesy of Ruth Edwards); unpublished transcripts of interviews with RG Edwards, K Elder, and RL Gardner; personal recollections from the late 1970s by Edwards and Steptoe as recalled in interviews with Danny Abse for the autobiographical account "A Matter of Life" and on film with Peter Williams; members of RG Edwards' family and his colleagues and former students and staff members for clarificatory evidence about personal recollections by Edwards, for additional verifiable information and with whom to test some new interpretations.

CHILDHOOD BACKGROUND

Robert Geoffrey Edwards was born on September 27, 1925 in the small Yorkshire mill town of Batley, the year of the Batley deluge and "great flood." He arrived into a working-class family, and Edwards, who was known by his middle name of Geoff until he was 18, was the second of three brothers, with an older brother, Sammy and a younger one, Harry. These brothers he describes as competitive, "all determined to win or, if not to win, to go down fighting" (3). Sammy was named after his father, Samuel, who was frequently away from home working on the railways, maintaining the track in the Blea Moor tunnel on the Carlisle-Settle line. It was an unhealthy place to work, some 2600 m long and filled with coal-fired smoke that exacerbated Samuel's bronchitis, a consequence of being gassed in World War I. The one perk of working on the railways was the free rail pass for the family's annual holiday, which was regularly taken in far-away Southend-on-Sea, located near the mouth of the Thames and considered then to be a top-spot resort by working-class families.

Edwards' mother, Margaret, was a machinist in a local mill. She came originally from Manchester, to where the family relocated when Edwards was about five, having been offered the relative security of a council house at 25 Highgate Crescent in the suburb of Gorton. It was in Manchester that Edwards was to receive his education. In those days, bright working-class children could take a scholarship exam at age 10 or 11 to compete for the few coveted places at a grammar school: the potential pathway out of poverty and even to University. All three brothers passed the exam, but Sammy decided against grammar school, preferring to leave education as soon as he could to earn. His mother was reportedly furious at this wasted opportunity, and so when her two younger sons passed, there was no question that they would continue in education and it was with that that Geoff/Bob progressed in 1937 to Manchester Central Boy's High School (the building that now houses Shena Simon College in Whitworth Street), which also claims James Chadwick FRS (1891–1974) as an alumnus. Chadwick, like Edwards, was a Cambridge professor and the 1935 Nobel Laureate in Physics for discovering the neutron (4). The Edwards' summers were spent in the Yorkshire Dales, to where their mother took her sons to be closer to their father's place of work. There, Edwards labored on the farms and developed an enduring affection for the Dales.

These early experiences were formative. Edwards first became a life-long egalitarian, for five years a Labour Party Councillor (5), willing to listen to and talk with all and sundry, regardless of class, education, status, and background. Second, he developed an enduring curiosity about agricultural and natural history and especially the reproductive patterns among the Dales' sheep, pigs, and cattle. Finally, he claimed great pride in being a "Yorkshire man," traditionally having attributes of affability and generosity of spirit combined with no-nonsense blunt-speaking. Indeed, following his only meeting with Gregory Pincus [1903–1967; (6)] at a conference in Venice in May 1966, at which Edwards, the young pretender, clashed with the "father of the pill" over the timing of egg maturation in humans; he paid Pincus the biggest compliment he could imagine, saying "He would have made a fine Yorkshireman!" (3).

The intervention of World War II was to provide an unwelcome interruption to Edwards' education: when he left school in 1943, he was conscripted for war service into the British Army for almost four years (Fig. 1). To his surprise, as someone from a working-class family, he was identified as potential officer material and sent on an officer-training course, before being commissioned in 1946. However, his army experiences were broadly negative, the alien lifestyle of the officers' mess not being to his taste and reinforcing his socialist ideals. The one positive feature of his war service was the chance to travel overseas; particularly appreciated was his time in the Middle East. The years in the army were broken by nine months' compassionate leave back in the Yorkshire Dales, to which he was released to help and run a farm when his farmer friend there fell ill. So engaged did he become in farming life that, after discharge from the army in 1948, he returned home to Gorton, from where he applied to read agricultural sciences at the University College of North Wales at Bangor.

Having gained a place and a government grant to fund it, the six or so months that intervened were occupied in a government desk job in Salford, Greater Manchester, helping to organize the newly formed National Health Service. This office-work experience reinforced the anticipatory attractions of agricultural science. So his disappointment in the course offered at Bangor was acute. By that time, he was a relatively experienced 23-year-old, described by his impressionable 18-year-old public-school educated and self-described "unlikely" friend, John Slee (Fig. 2) (7), as being "both ambitious and flexible, and unusually confident in his own judgement." In Edwards' confident judgment, the course on offer was not "scientific," and he was bored through two tedious years of agricultural descriptions, after which he reported that his teachers were "glad to see the back of him" in Zoology for a year, a course much more to his style and led by the more intellectually challenging Rogers Brambell FRS [1901–1970; (8)]. However, that year was not enough to salvage his honors degree, and in 1951, aged 26 he gained a simple pass. Unbeknown to him at the time, he was not alone in this undistinguished academic embarrassment, as neither "Tibby" Marshall FRS [1878–1949; (9)], the founder of the Reproductive Sciences, nor Sir Alan Parkes FRS [1900–1990; (10)], the first Professor of Reproductive Sciences at Cambridge, who was later to recruit Edwards there, distinguished themselves as undergraduates. In 1951, however, Edwards "was disconsolate. It was a disaster. My grants were spent and I was in debt. Unlike some of the students I had no rich parents ... I could not write home, 'Dear Dad, please send me £100 as I did badly in the exams'" (3).

However, his low spirits did not last long. He learnt that John Slee had been accepted on a postgraduate diploma course in Animal Genetics at Edinburgh University under Conrad Waddington FRS [1905–1975; (11)], who had moved there in 1947 from Christ's College in Cambridge, home also to both Marshall and Parkes. Edwards applied, and, despite his pass degree and to his amazement, he was accepted. That summer, he worked in Yorkshire and

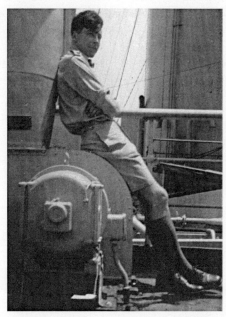

Figure 1 Edwards on National War Service in the1940s. *Source*: Courtesy of Ruth Edwards.

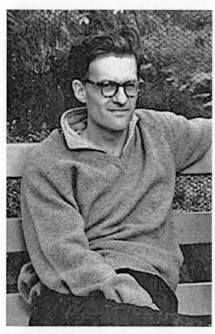

Figure 2 John Slee in the 1960s. *Source*: Courtesy of Ruth Edwards.

Wiltshire harvesting hay, as well as portering bananas and heaving sacks of flour in Manchester docks and taking a menial job with a newspaper, all to earn enough to pay his way in Edinburgh (3).

FAMILY LIFE

In Edinburgh, Edwards not only started to map out his scientific career, but importantly also met Ruth Fowler (Fig. 3), who was to become his life-long scientific collaborator and whom he was to marry in 1954, their five daughters arriving between 1959 and 1964: Caroline, Sarah, Jenny, and twins Anna and Meg. When they met, according to Edwards, in a statistics class, Ruth was studying for a genetics degree. Edwards claims that he was initially somewhat overwhelmed, even "intimidated" by Ruth's august family background. Her father, Sir Ralph Fowler FRS [1889–1944; (12)] and her maternal grandfather, Lord Ernest Rutherford FRS [1871–1937; (13)], were not only both "titled," but both also had the most impressive academic credentials imaginable: a world away from a working-class Northern family. Ralph Fowler was Plummer Professor of Mathematical Physics in Cambridge from 1932 to 1944. He was evidently an exceptionally talented mathematical physicist, a fine sportsman and "an inspirational teacher and leader of men" (12). Back in Cambridge in 1919 after World War I, he was stimulated to work with Rutherford, who had recently arrived there to take the chair of Experimental Physics. Rutherford was the first Nobel laureate in Ruth's family, having been awarded the 1908 Nobel Prize for Chemistry "for his investigations into the disintegration of the elements, and the chemistry of radioactive substances" (13).

Ralph Fowler not only worked under Rutherford, but in the course of doing so met his only daughter, Eileen, whom he married in 1921. They had four children, of whom Ruth was the last, born in December 1930. Tragically her mother died shortly afterwards and Ruth was to know only Mrs Phyllida Cook as her "mother"; both families moved into Cromwell House in Trumpington, Cambridge and were brought up together (12). Her father, although himself unwell, was to undertake grueling high security war work at the Ordnance Board and later at the Admiralty during World War II. His health deteriorated and he died at the relatively young age of 55 when Ruth was 13.

EDWARDS, THE RESEARCH SCIENTIST

The intellectual spirit of scientific enquiry that Edwards experienced in Edinburgh fitted his aptitudes well, for Waddington rewarded his Diploma year with a three-year PhD place (1952–55), followed by two years of postdoctoral research, and funded it to the princely sum of £240 per year (3). His chosen field of research was the developmental biology of the mouse. Edwards saw that to understand development involved engaging in an interdisciplinary mix, not just of embryology and reproduction, the conventional view at the time, but also of genetics. Given the scientific and social emphasis on genetics over the last 40 or so years, it is important to understand how advanced this view was in the 1950s, when genetic knowledge was still rudimentary and largely alien to the established developmental and reproductive biologists of the day, as Edwards himself was later to recall (14). For example, it was in the 1950s that DNA was established as the molecular carrier of genetic information (15–18), that it was first demonstrated that each cell of the body carried a full set of DNA/genes (19–21) and that genes were selectively expressed as mRNA to generate different cell phenotypes (22). Moreover, it was only by the late 1950s that cytogenetic studies led to the accepted human karyotype as 46 chromosomes (23,24), that agreement was reached on the Denver system of classification of human chromosomes (25) and that the chromosomal aneuploidies underlying developmental anomalies such as Down, Turner, and Klinefelter Syndromes were described (26–29).

The dates of these discoveries make Edwards' research between 1952 and 1957 all the more remarkable. Working under his supervisor Alan Beatty, he generated haploid, triploid, and aneuploid mouse embryos and studied their potential for development. In order to undertake what were, in effect, early attempts at "genetic engineering" in mammals, he needed to be able to manipulate the chromosomal composition of eggs, spermatozoa, and embryos. In mice, spermatozoa were abundant, and were studied in experiments mostly undertaken with a visiting Argentinean postdoc, Julio Sirlin (Fig. 4), whom Edwards describes as being "... the first man with whom I collaborated who was prepared to work at my pace" (3). Together they labeled spermatozoa radioactively in vivo in order to study the kinetics of spermatogenesis and then to follow the radioactive products post fertilization, thereby to demonstrate the fate of the male contributions to early development. They also exposed males and/or their spermatozoa to various agents, such as chemical mutagens and UV- or x-ray irradiation, and examined the effects on sperm-fertilizing capacity, and where it was shown to be present, how the treatment impacted on development. In some cases, sperm activation of the egg was evident, but in the absence of any functional sperm

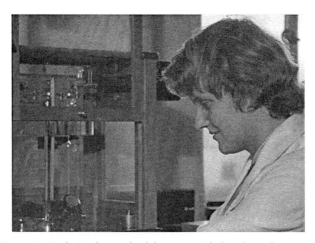

Figure 3 Ruth Fowler in the laboratory, Edinburgh in the 1950s.
Source: Courtesy of Ruth Edwards.

chromatin, and so gynogenetic embryos were formed. These experiments resulted in 14 papers, including four in *Nature*, between 1954 and 1959 (see ref. (30), for a full bibliographic record of Edwards).

Eggs and embryos were not as abundant as spermatozoa, and overcoming this problem led Edwards to two discoveries that proved to be of particular significance for his later IVF work. First, working with his wife Ruth, he devised ways of increasing the numbers of synchronized eggs recoverable from adult female mice through a series of papers, the first published in 1957 (31), on the control of ovulation induced by use of exogenous hormones. In doing so, they overturned the conventional wisdom that superovulation of adults was not possible. Second, working with an American postdoc, Alan Gates (Fig. 5) (32), Edwards described the remarkable timed sequence of egg chromosomal maturation events that led up to ovulation after injection of the ovulatory hormone, human chorionic gonadotropin.

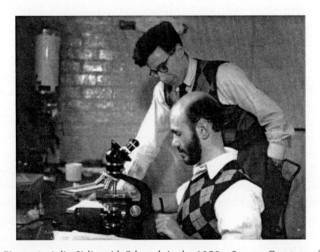

Figure 4   Julio Sirlin with Edwards in the 1950s. *Source*: Courtesy of Julio Sirlin.

His six years in Edinburgh, between 1951 and 1957, give an early taste of his prodigious energy, resulting in 38 papers (30). Indeed so productive was this period that the last of the Edinburgh-based papers did not appear in print until 1963. These papers firmly placed the young Edwards at the forefront of studies on the genetic manipulation of development and started to attract attention.

It was also in Edinburgh that Edwards' interest in ethics was first sparked by the interdisciplinary debates among scientists and theologians that Waddington organized, and, as a result, he went on what he describes as a "church crawl," trying the 10 or so variants of Christianity on offer in 1950s Edinburgh. He did not emerge from his consumer testing "God-intoxicated" (3), but convinced that man held his own future in his own hands. Edwards' humanist ethical sympathies and antipathy to the "revealed truths" of religion were to be developed further in all his later encounters (30).

AN AMERICAN DIVERSION

These 1950s studies in science and ethics were to form the platform on which Edwards' later IVF work was to be based, but before that his interests and life took a diversion to the California Institute of Technology for the year 1957–1958. He describes his year at Caltech as being "a bit of a holiday," but it was a holiday which with hindsight had both distracting and significant consequences. He went there to work with Albert Tyler [1906–1968; (33)], an influential elder statesman of American reproductive science, working on spermatozoon–egg interactions. Caltech was then a hot bed of developmental biology, and Tyler had clustered around him an exciting group of young scientists, which included that year a visit by the English doyen of fertilization, Lord Victor Rothschild FRS [1910–1990; (34)]. Rothschild was later to clash scientifically with Edwards over his IVF work (35), a clash in which the younger man triumphed again (36),

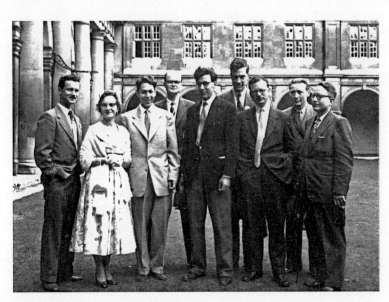

Figure 5   Edwards as "a very recent PhD student" (*centre*) and Alan Gates (*extreme left*) at a meeting in Trinity College Cambridge in the late 1950s. *Source*: Courtesy of Ruth Edwards.

just as he had with Pincus. Tyler was exploring the molecular specificity of egg–spermatozoon interactions and had turned for a model to immunology. Immunology was then at an exciting phase in its development, with the engaging Sir Peter Medawar FRS [1915–1987, Nobel Laureate in Physiology or Medicine, 1960; (37)], influentially for Bob, extending his ideas on immunological tolerance to the paradox of the "fetus as an allograft": a semi-paternal graft nonetheless somehow protected from maternal immune attack inside the mother's uterus (38). This confluence of reproduction and immunology excited Edwards' restless curiosity and hence the choice of Tyler. Significantly, the subject also offered funding possibilities via the Ford and Rockefeller Foundations and the Population Council, which were increasingly concerned about world population growth and the need for better methods to control fertility (39–41). Immunocontraception then seemed to offer tantalizingly specific possibilities, alas not much closer to being realized today (42).

So when Edwards returned to the United Kingdom from CalTech in 1958 at Alan Parkes' invitation to join him at the Medical Research Council (MRC) National Institute for Medical Research (NIMR) at Mill Hill in north London, it was to work on the science of immunocontraception (5). This period in the United States initiated a series of 23 papers on the immunology of reproduction between 1960 and 1976 (30). It also prompted Edwards' first involvement in founding an international society in 1967 in Varna Bulgaria, (Fig. 6) when the International Coordinating Committee for the Immunology of Reproduction was created (43). Immunoreproduction was, in retrospect, to prove a distracting diversion from what was to become Edwards' main work, albeit one that continued to enthuse and stimulate his imagination for many years. Indeed, it was his research into immunoreproduction that led serendipitously to his first meeting with Patrick Steptoe (see later). The period

at Mill Hill, between 1958 and 1962, seems to have been a period of increasing intellectual conflict for him. While being enthusiastic about the science underlying immunocontraception, his old interests in eggs, fertilization and, in particular, the genetics of development were gradually reasserting themselves. His day job was therefore increasingly supplemented by evening and weekend flirtations with egg maturation.

THE CRUCIAL EGG-MATURATION STUDIES

The stimulus that re-awakened Edwards' interest in eggs was provided by the then recent consensus about the number of human chromosomes and, more particularly the descriptions in 1959 of the pathologies in man that resulted from chromosomal anomalies. Thus, his 1962 *Nature* paper begins: "Many of the chromosomal anomalies in man and animals arise through non-disjunction or lagging chromosomes during meiosis in the oocyte. Investigation of the origin and primary incidence of such anomalies would be greatly facilitated if meiotic stages etc., were easily available" (44).

The idea that these aneuploidies in humans might result from errors in the complex chromosomal dance that he and Gates had observed in maturing mouse eggs drove his thinking. The possible clinical relevance of his work on egg maturation and aneuploidy in the mouse was becoming significant.

So Edwards resumed his experimenting with mice, trying to mimic in vitro the in-vivo maturation of eggs, one rationale being that this route would open the possibility of similar studies in humans, in which not even induced ovulation had then been described (45). He tried releasing the immature eggs from their ovarian follicles into culture medium containing the ovulatory hormone human chorionic gonadotropin, to explore whether he could simulate their in-vivo development.

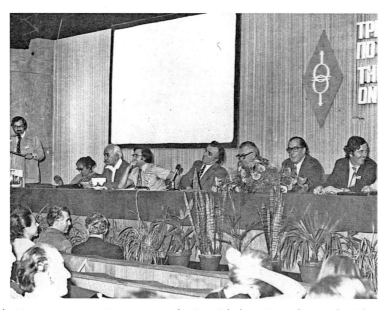

Figure 6 Edwards at one of the Varna meetings on Immunoreproduction; Schulman is speaking and to Edwards' left is Bratanov, and seated two to his right is Shanta Rao. *Source*: Courtesy Barbara Rankin.

Amazingly he found it worked first time; the eggs seemed to mature at the same rate as they had in vivo. However, they did so whether or not the hormone had been added. The eggs evidently were maturing spontaneously when released from their follicles. The same happened in rats and hamsters. If this also were to happen in humans, then the study of the chromosomal dance during human egg maturation was a realistic practical possibility, as was IVF and thereby studies on the genetics of early human development. Edwards' excitement at seeing eggs spontaneously maturing was temporarily blunted by his library discovery that Pincus in the 1930s (46,47) and M C Chang [1908–1991; (48,49)] earlier in the 1950s had been there before him, using both rabbit and, Pincus claimed, human eggs.

In order to pursue his cytogenetic studies on maturation, he needed a reliable supply of human ovarian tissue from which to retrieve and mature eggs. This requirement posed difficulties for a scientist with no medical qualification, given the elitist attitudes and lack of scientific awareness then prevalent amongst most of the U.K. gynecological profession (2,50,51). His first breakthrough came with Molly Rose, who was a gynecologist at the Edgeware General Hospital, northwest London, near Mill Hill. Edwards was introduced to her through John Humphrey FRS [1915–1997; (52)], who was the medically qualified Head of Immunology at Mill Hill. Humphrey, notwithstanding his more privileged social background, was a kindred spirit for Edwards, sharing his passion for science, its social application and utility, as well as his left-wing politics; indeed he had been a Marxist until 1940 and was for many years denied entry to the United States as a result. Edwards asked Humphrey if he knew anyone who might be helpful, and he not only suggested Rose, but also offered to arrange an introduction. Rose was to provide biopsied ovarian samples intermittently for the next 10 years.

Between 1960 and 1962, Edwards used human ovarian biopsies provided by Rose to try to repeat and extend Pincus' observations from the 1930s. Given the sporadic supply of human material, he also tried dog, monkey and baboon ovarian eggs, but in all cases with limited success compared with smaller rodents. In the 1962 *Nature* paper (44), he cautiously interprets the few maturing human (3/67), monkey (10/56) and baboon (13/90) eggs that he had observed as most likely arising from in-vivo stimulation and thus partially matured at the time of their recovery from the biopsy. He suggests that Pincus' observations on human eggs are also likely to be artifactual, the source of his Venice spat with Pincus some 4 years later (vide supra). This 1962 paper ends with the report of an ingenious experimental approach to try and persuade the reluctant human eggs to mature. Thus, the ovarian arteries of patients undergoing ovarian removal were cannulated and perfused with hormones post-removal, perhaps unsurprisingly in retrospect, without success.

However, by this time, his quest for human eggs, and his dreams of IVF and studying the genetics and development of early human embryos, had reached the ears of the then Director of the Institute, Sir Charles Harington

FRS [1897–1972; (53)], who banned any work on human IVF at NIMR (3). Alan Parkes was no longer able to defend Edwards, having left in 1961 to take up his chair in Cambridge and, although he had asked Edwards to join him there, funding was not available until 1963. So by the time Edwards left Mill Hill in 1962 for a year in Glasgow, he had encountered a taste of the opposition to come.

GLASGOW AND STEM CELLS

Edwards had accepted an invitation from John Paul to spend a year in the biochemistry department at Glasgow University. Paul was then the acknowledged master of tissue culture in the United Kingdom and had got wind of some experiments that Edwards had been doing on the side at NIMR attempting to generate stem cells from rabbit embryo cultures (14). The objective of this strategy was to use these stem cells to study early developmental mechanisms, either in vitro, or in vivo after their incorporation into embryos. Paul had proposed that they work together, with fellow Glasgow biochemist Robin Cole, to see what progress might be made. This must have been an attractive invitation, not simply because the challenge was scientifically interesting, but also because Edwards could learn more about culture media for his eggs and hopefully later embryos, then an uncertain prospect, successful mouse embryo culture only recently having been described (54). However, by this time, the Edwards family was growing, so Ruth remained in north London with their young daughters, while her husband commuted to Glasgow for the working week.

The collaboration was to result in two papers (55,56) remarkable for their prescience. They described the production of embryonic stem cells from both rabbit blastocysts and the inner cell masses dissected from them. The cells were capable of proliferating through over 100 generations and of differentiating into various cell types. These experiments were initiated some 20 years before Evans and Kaufman (57) described the derivation of embryonic stem cells from mice. That this work has largely been ignored by those in the stem cell field is probably mainly attributable to its being too far ahead of its time (58). Thus, reliable molecular markers for different types of cells were not available then, nor were appropriate techniques with which to critically test the developmental potential of the cultured cells.

THE MOVE TO CAMBRIDGE

Edwards arrived in Cambridge from Glasgow in 1963 as a Ford Foundation Research Fellow. He had previously visited Cambridge at least once, as "a recently graduated PhD" in the late 1950s for a conference on Reproduction held in Trinity College (Fig. 5), where he recalls meeting some of the big names in the subject, including John Hammond, Alan Parkes, MC Chang, Thaddeus Mann, Rene Moricard, Bunny Austin, and Charles Thibault (14). Although Edwards was to remain in Cambridge for the rest of his career, in 1963 his reactions to the place were mixed. He describes how he immediately reacted against the then extant "misogynist public-school traditions; the exclusivity," "the privileges given to the already privileged." But he set against that the "sheer beauty of the place," the concern with the truth and high seriousness," the ambience of scientific excellence… I was surrounded by so many talented young men and women" (3). He, Ruth, and his five daughters settled in a house in Gough Way, off the Barton Road.

Edwards worked in a cluster of seven smallish rooms at the top of the Physiological Laboratory backing onto Downing Place (Fig. 7). These were collectively known as the "Marshall laboratory" and were to be shared eventually with two other groups. One group was led initially by Sir Alan Parkes, the first Mary Marshall and Arthur Walton Professor of Reproductive Physiology at the University (10), who had arrived in 1961. His group included scientists with mainly zoological or comparative interests, such as his wife Ruth Deansley, Bunny Austin, and Dick Laws FRS, who with Parkes was often away "in the field" collecting material, especially in Uganda at the Nuffield Unit of Tropical Animal Ecology (10). Much of this material was examined histologically under the skilled eye of Frank Lemon, the senior technician. Research students included Martin Richards, CJ Dominic, Margaret Mitchell, and Barbara Weir (59). Parkes was also much involved at this time in writing and committee work, especially with the World Health Organization which was then becoming concerned about world population growth and ways to curb it (10). Parkes was also acting as an unpaid company secretary to the then fledgling *Journal of Reproduction and Fertility* [called *Reproduction* since 2001; (59–61)].

In 1967, Parkes retired. Edwards applied for his chair on January 6, 1966 (62), but was unsuccessful, the chair passing to Thaddeus Mann FRS [1908–1993; (63)], who worked on the biochemistry of semen. Mann decided not to relocate to the Physiology Laboratory from his Cambridge base at the Agricultural Research Council Unit of Reproductive Physiology and Biochemistry at Huntingdon Road, where he was Director. Neither was the leadership of the Marshall laboratory to pass to Edwards, as the University appointed as its head his more senior colleague and friend Colin "Bunny" Austin [1914–2004;

(64)], who had been in Cambridge intermittently since 1962 (Figs. 8 and 9). Austin was elected the first Charles Darwin Professor of Animal Embryology (1967–1981) and began attracting several upcoming reproductive biologists to the Marshall Laboratory, including John Marston, David Whittingham, and Matthew Kaufmann. In addition, a new group was formed in 1967, with the arrival from the Strangeways laboratory of Denis New (1929–2010), as university lecturer in histology (65). New built a group comprising initially research assistant Pat Coppola (to be followed later by Stephanie Ellington) and PhD students Chris Steele and David Cockroft, later joined by postdoc Frank Webb, and visiting scientists such as Joe Daniels Jr, on leave from the University of Colorado.

It was against this varied scientific background that Edwards, who was already 38 when he arrived in Cambridge, began for the first time to assemble his own group. Initially,

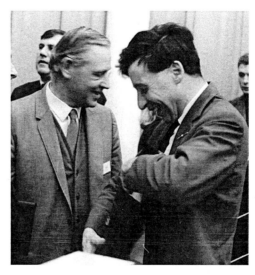

Figure 8 Edwards with "Bunny" Austin (1960s). *Source*: Courtesy of Ruth Edwards.

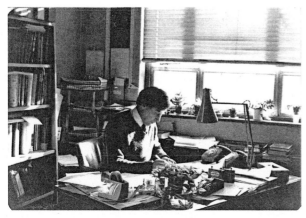

Figure 7 Edwards in his office backing onto Downing Place in the Marshall laboratory (1970s). *Source*: Courtesy of Barbara Rankin.

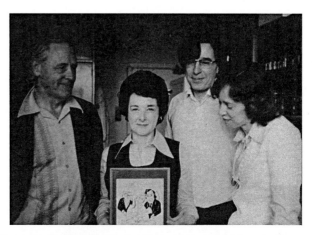

Figure 9 Barbara Rankin holding a cartoon of Edwards, Steptoe, and Purdy holding Lousie Brown drawn by Alan Handyside who also took the photograph. With Austin are (*left*) Edwards and Purdy (*right*) after the return of the latter two from Oldham and the birth of Louise Brown in 1978. *Source*: Courtesy of Barbara Rankin.

his technical assistance was provided by Clare Jackson and then Valerie Hunn, after whom he recruited Jean Purdy (Fig. 10) in 1968, one of her attractions being her nursing qualification, a sign of the increasing importance that his forays into use of clinical material was assuming. Purdy was to stay with him until her early death at age 39 in 1985 (66). Also joining him as a part-time secretary in 1969, Barbara Rankin (b. 1933; Fig. 9) was to remain with him until 1987. He also began recruiting his first graduate students. Initially, he helped co-supervise (with Alan Parkes) Anne Vickers (67), who sexed fixed whole-mouse blastocysts by karyotyping. This work led directly to his collaboration on preimplantation genetic diagnosis (PGD) (see later) with Richard Gardner, one half of his first pair of graduate students, the other being this author. The two students started PhD training with Edwards in 1966 (68,69). Gardner studied early mouse embryology from 1966 to 1971 and until 1973 as a postdoctoral worker, before moving to Zoology in Oxford. This author worked on immunoreproduction from 1966 to 1969, returning as a postdoc between 1971 and 1974 after two years in the United States before moving to the Anatomy Department in Cambridge.

From 1969 onwards, Edwards' group increased in size substantially as more accommodation was made available to the Marshall laboratory. David Griffin (now retired from the World Health Organization) was to join as Head Technician between 1970 and 1975, with junior technicians including Sheila Barton, Sally Fawcitt, Sylvia Jackson, Vinitha Dharawardena, and Brenda Dickstein, in addition to Jean Purdy. Early graduate students recruited included Roger Gosden (1970–1974), Carol Readhead (1972–1976), and Rob Gore-Langton (1973–1978), all working on follicle growth, Craig Howe (1971–1974) working on immunoreproduction, and Azim Surani (1975–1979) on implantation. A "third generation" of graduate students also arrived; for example, Janet Rossant (from 1972) studied with Gardner and Alan Handyside (from 1974) studied with Johnson. Postdoctoral

workers also arrived, including Ginny Papaioannou (1971–1974), Hester Pratt (1972–1974), and Frank Webb (1976–1977). Ruth Fowler-Edwards also resumed working in the laboratory, developing hormonal assays and studying the endocrine aspects of follicle development and early pregnancy. Thus, slowly until 1969, and more rapidly thereafter, Edwards built a lively group, its members working in diverse areas of reproductive science that reflected his own broad interests and knowledge. Moreover, Edwards encouraged a spirit of open communication and egalitarianism, which extended across all three groups, with sharing of resources, space, equipment, knowledge, and ideas, as well as social activities.

Through the 1960s, Edwards was funded by the Ford Foundation via grants first to Parkes and then to Austin to continue work on basic reproductive mechanisms, with an eye to developing new methods of fertility control. So he continued to pursue both the immunology of reproduction and egg maturation, for the latter collecting pig, cow, sheep, the odd monkey, and some human eggs. He showed that eggs of all these species would indeed mature in vitro, but that the eggs of larger animals simply needed a longer time than those of smaller ones, human eggs taking up to 36 hours rather than the 12 hours or less erroneously reported by Pincus. These cytogenetic studies were reported in two seminal papers in 1965 (70,71), both of which are primarily concerned with understanding the kinetics of the meiotic chromosomal events during egg maturation. In its discussion, the Lancet paper displays a breathtaking clarity of vision as Edwards sets out a program of research that predicted the events of the next 20 years and beyond (Table 1). Significantly, if not surprisingly given his research interests, the early study and detection of genetic disease is afforded a heavy focus compared with the slight emphasis on infertility alleviation.

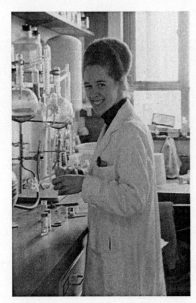

Figure 10 Jean Purdy (1946–1985). *Source*: Courtesy of Barbara Rankin.

Table 1 Key Points in the Program of Research Laid Out in the Discussion to Edwards' 1965 Lancet Paper

1. Studies on non-disjunction of meiotic chromosomes as a cause of aneuploidy in humans[a]
2. Studies on the effect of maternal age on non-disjunction in relation to the origins of trisomy 21[a]
3. Use of human eggs in IVF to study fertilization
4. Study of culture methods for human eggs fertilized in vitro
5. Use of priming hormones to increase the number of eggs per woman available for study/use
6. Study of early IVF embryos for evidence of ([ab]) normality – especially aneuploidies arising prior to or at fertilization[a]
7. Control of some of the genetic diseases in man[a]
8. Control of sex-linked disorders by sex detection at blastocyst stage and transfer of only female embryos[a]
9. Intracervical transfer of IVF embryos into the uterus
10. Use of IVF embryos to circumvent blocked tubes[b]
11. Avoidance of a multiple pregnancy (as observed after hormonal priming and in vivo insemination) by transfer of a single IVF embryo

[a]Five aims relating specifically to genetic disease.
[b]One aim relating specifically to infertility relief.

This genetic focus continues in his research papers over the next four years. Thus, within three years, working with a graduate student called Gardner, he provided proof of principle for PGD, in a paper on rabbit embryo sexing published in 1968 (72), a paper that was to anticipate the development of PGD clinically by some 22 years (73). Likewise, working with the Cambridge geneticist Alan Henderson, Edwards was to develop his "production line theory" of egg production to explain the origins of maternal aneuploidy in older women. Thus, the earliest eggs to enter meiosis in the fetal ovary were shown to have more chiasmata and to be ovulated earlier in adult life than those entering meiosis later in fetal life (Fig. 11) (74,75).

THE PROBLEM OF FERTILIZATION OF THE HUMAN EGG

Notwithstanding his broad range of scientific interests, Edwards' ambitions to achieve IVF in humans remained undiminished. In 1966, this was no trivial task, having been accomplished convincingly only in rabbit and hamster (76,77). In trying to achieve this aim, he was engaging in two struggles: the first being simply but critically the continuing practical difficulty in obtaining a regular supply of human ovarian tissue. Local Cambridge sources proved unreliable and Rose was now two to three hours' drive away in London; so, during the summer of 1965, Edwards turned to the United States for help and approached Victor McKusick, a leading American cytogeneticist at The Johns Hopkins University. There he initiated his longstanding contact with Howard and Georgeanna Jones in Obstetrics and Gynecology (78). The supply of American eggs they generated during his six-week stay allowed him to confirm the maturation timings that were published in 1965.

However, it was the second scientific struggle that was then occupying most of his attention, namely that in order to fertilize these in-vitro matured eggs, he had to "capacitate" the spermatozoa, a final maturation process which spermatozoa undergo physiologically in the uterus and that is essential for the acquisition of fertilizing competence. Failing to achieve this convincingly at

Johns Hopkins, he made a second transatlantic summer journey in 1966 to visit Luther Talbot and his colleagues at Chapel Hill. He tried a variety of ways (79) to overcome the problem of "sperm capacitation," one of the most ingenious of which was to construct a 2.5 cm-long chamber from a nylon tube, plugged at each end, and with holes drilled in the walls which were encased in panels made of Millipore membrane (80). The chamber, which had a short thread attached to it, fitted snugly inside the inserter tube of an intrauterine device and so could be placed into the volunteer woman's uterus intra-cervically at mid-cycle, where it sat for up to 11 hours before being recovered by gently pulling on the thread, exactly as was being done routinely for insertion and removal of intrauterine devices. By placing spermatozoa within the chamber, the membrane of which permitted equilibration of its contents with uterine fluid, he hoped to expose them to a capacitating environment. However, this ingenious approach, like the many others, failed in this case most probably because the chamber itself induced an inflammatory response or a local bleed. For all the ingenuity of his various experimental approaches to achieve capacitation, and despite the occasional evidence of early stages of fertilization using such spermatozoa, no reliable evidence for the completion of the process was forthcoming. Then in 1968 both struggles began to resolve.

THE MEETING WITH PATRICK STEPTOE

Patrick Steptoe (1913–1988; Fig. 12) had been a consultant obstetrician at Oldham General Hospital since 1951 (81), where for several years he had been pioneering the development and use of the laparoscope in gynecological surgery (81,82). Much to his frustration, his progress had fallen on the largely deaf ears of the conservative gynecological hierarchy, and indeed incited considerable

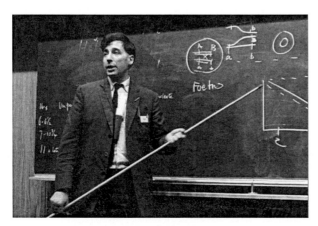

Figure 11 Edwards talks about his "production line" hypothesis (late 1960s). *Source*: Courtesy of Ruth Edwards.

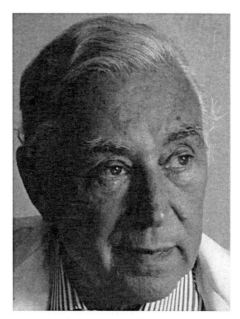

Figure 12 Patrick Steptoe (1913–1988). Source: Courtesy of Andrew Steptoe.

Table 2   Edited Record from the RSM Endocrinology Section: General Minutes, 1946–1975 (ref: RSM/J/19/4/1) p.365 (with permission)

A joint meeting of the SECTION OF ENDOCRINOLOGY of the Royal Society of Medicine with the SOCIETY FOR THE STUDY OF FERTILITY was held at 1 Wimpole Street, W.1., Wednesday, February 28, 1968, at 10.00 am.

The meeting was attended by approximately 127 Fellows, members, and guests and the program was as follows:

"FERTILITY AND INFERTILITY"

10.00: Chairman's opening remarks

10.10: Sperm capacitation. C.R. Austin, Department of Embryology, Cambridge

10.35: Immunological aspects of infertility. R.G. Edwards, Department of Physiology, Cambridge

11.00: Coffee

11.30: The rating of semen quality by chemical methods. Dr T Mann, Department of Physiology of Reproduction, Cambridge

11.55: Endocrine studies in women with secondary amenorrhea. Prof. Ivor H Mills and RJ Wilson, Department of Investigative Medicine, Cambridge

12.20: Some investigation in male hypogonadism. Prof. FTG Prunty, Department of Chemical Pathology, St Thomas's Hospital Medical School, London

12.45: Lunch

2.15: A gonadotropin stimulation test for ovarian responsiveness. GIM Sawyer, University College Hospital Medical School, London

2.40: Factors affecting the response to clomiphene therapy. D Ferriman, AW Purdie, and M Corns, North Middlesex Hospital, London

3.05: Comparison of clomiphene and FSH for treatment of anovulation. AD Tsapoulis and AC Crooke, Department of Clinical Endocrinology, Birmingham

3.30: Tea

4.00: Time cause of urinary oestrogen excretion after various schemes of Pergonal therapy. JK Butler, GD Searle and Co., High Wycombe, Bucks

4.25: Recent developments in the control of fertility. Sir Alan S Parkes, Cambridge

4.50: General discussion

[signed] CL Cope 26/6/1968 [pasted in] 26th June 1968

opposition and some outright hostility (83). Edwards' claim was that he was scanning the medical and scientific journals in the library and came across a paper by Steptoe describing his experiences with laparoscopy (3,81,84). Edwards goes on to describe how he rang Steptoe to discuss a possible collaboration, but was "warned off" Steptoe by London gynecological colleagues (85). This warning and the daunting prospect of collaboration in far-away Oldham, deterred him from following through. Finally, Edwards reported actually meeting Steptoe later at a meeting at the Royal Society of Medicine, at which, ironically, Edwards was talking about his work on immunoreproduction, not his attempts at IVF.

The Steptoe paper that Edwards found that day in the library was cited in his tributes to the then-deceased Steptoe (81,84) as being a Lancet paper entitled "Laparoscopy and ovulation" (86). However, these later recollections do not withstand scrutiny. Thus, the Lancet paper cited was published in October 1968, but their first meeting was in fact earlier that year, on Wednesday February 28, 1968 at a joint meeting of the Section of Endocrinology of the Royal Society of Medicine with the Society for the Study of Fertility held at 1 Wimpole Street (Table 2) (87). Moreover, according to Steptoe (88), they had already commenced collaborating prior to October 1968; indeed their first paper together was submitted for publication later that year in December 1968 (see next section). Clearly, the paper read by Edwards must have been another, earlier than October 1968, one that proceeded February 1968 by several months. Indeed, in an earlier account, Edwards describes the library "Eureka" moment as occurring in "one autumn day in 1967" (3). So which was the paper by Steptoe that Edwards saw and what about it attracted his

attention? Looking at Steptoe's possible publications in journals, there is none listed for 1967, but there are two 1967 conference reports and Steptoe's book on gynecological laparoscopy (82,89,90). Of the few journal papers, only two concern laparoscopy, one from January 1966 in the British Medical Journal (BMJ), and one from August 1965 in the Journal of Obstetrics and Gynaecology of the British Commonwealth (JOGBrC). Which of these five publications (Table 3) did Edwards read? The 1966 BMJ publication (91) is a letter entitled "The fifth freedom." It responds to a paper by Sir Dugald Baird on the "problem of excessive fertility in women." Steptoe concurs that there is a problem, but disagrees with the proposed contraceptive solution, advising laparoscopic sterilization for women as safer and more effective. He also discusses how laparoscopy can be used postoperatively to confirm that tubes were indeed blocked. The JOGBrC paper (92) is entitled "Gynaecological endoscopy – laparoscopy and culdoscopy" and reviews the history of endoscopy and Steptoe's experiences with it. It is in essence a very abbreviated version of his book (82), which was to be published in the following year. The two reports of the conference proceedings (89,90) are slightly more detailed accounts than the BMJ letter and are much abbreviated versions of the JOGBrC paper.

Of these five publications, the Sydney conference proceedings (90) can probably be dismissed as they only arrived in the Cambridge library in May 1968. The proceedings from Stockholm (89) are now no longer available in Cambridge, but evidence of their presence in the Physiology library in 1967 has been uncovered in an old catalog record, and so they would have been newly available to Edwards from November 1967 at the earliest. The BMJ letter (91) seems unlikely.

Table 3 Steptoe's Papers from 1967 and Earlier

Publication	Title	Type of publication	Location in Cambridge; date of arrival
Steptoe (82)	Laparoscopy in gynaecology	Book	University library; March 1967
Steptoe (89)	A new method of tubal sterilisation	Conference proceedings (Stockholm)	Physiology library; arrival date unknown, published in November 1967
Steptoe (90)	Laparoscopic studies of ovulation, its suppression and induction, and of ovarian dysfunction	Conference proceedings (Sydney)	University library; May 1968
Steptoe (91)	The fifth freedom	BMJ letter (22 January), 234	Physiology library; January 1966
Steptoe (92)	Gynaecological endoscopy – laparoscopy and culdoscopy	Paper in J Obstet Gynaecol Br Commonw 72, 535–543	University library; August 1965 (moved to Clinical School library after 1973)

Although Edwards was involved in contraceptive studies over this period through his work on immunore-production and was a member of the Royal Society Population Study Group at the time (10), and so may well have read this correspondence, it seems unlikely that the BMJ letter would have caught his eye to such dramatic effect and so long after its publication in January 1966, being readily available each week in the Physiology Library. The JOGBrC paper from 1965 was located in the University library, which was physically more remote from Physiology and not so immediately available to Edwards. However, it was in exactly the sort of clinical journal that he might then have been trawling retrospectively in his attempts to solve the problem of sperm capacitation. Thus, although in the more recent accounts of these events, Edwards (84,81) records his motivation for contacting Steptoe as being the potential value of the laparoscopic approach for egg collection, in 1967 eggs was not the foremost subject on his mind. Indeed in two earlier accounts, one written (3) and one spoken ((85); Supplementary video), Edwards claims he saw laparoscopy as a way of recovering capacitated spermatozoa from the oviduct by flushing with a small volume of medium: "a practical way ... of letting spermatozoa be in contact with the secretions of the female tract" (3). He says he actually rang Steptoe to ask whether this really was possible and was reassured by him that this was the case.

However, the only publication by Steptoe that explicitly lays out this possibility is his book (82). Thus, on page 27 he reports "By means of laparoscopy, Sjovall (1964) has carried out extended post-coital tests and has recovered spermatozoa from the fimbriated end of the tubes ..."; and on page 70, he writes "An extended post-coital test can be done by aspirating fluid from the tubal ostium ...". Moreover, Steptoe's book arrived in the University library in March 1967. However, against this conclusion sits Steptoe's recollection that Edwards had rung him just before his book was published, that is before March 1967 (3). This memory conflicts with both his and Edwards' memories elsewhere of the phone conversation being in the autumn of 1967, so the matter remains one for conjecture, but the book seems the most likely source. It is possible that Edwards' attention was drawn to the book by a review of it in the BMJ on November 11, 1967 (93).

THE FERTILIZATION OF THE HUMAN EGG RESOLVED

Despite the initiation of the collaboration with Steptoe, the actual solution to the capacitation problem existed nearer to home than Oldham, in the laboratories shared with Austin. In the early 1950s, Austin, and independently MC Chang, had discovered the requirement for sperm capacitation (94,95). After his appointment to the Cambridge chair, Austin's first graduate student (1967–1972) was Barry Bavister, who set to work to try and resolve the factors influencing the capacitation of hamster spermatozoa in vitro. In 1968, Bavister discovered a key role for pH, showing how higher rates of fertilization could be obtained by simply increasing the alkalinity of the medium (96). Edwards seized on this observation and co-opted Bavister to his project. That proved to do the trick, and in December 1968 Edwards, together with Bavister and Steptoe, submitted the paper to *Nature*, in which IVF in humans was described convincingly for the first time (97).

The 1969 *Nature* paper makes modest claims. Only 18 of 56 eggs assigned to the experimental group showed evidence of "fertilization in progress"; of which only two were described as having the two pronuclei to be expected if fertilization was occurring normally (Table 4). However, like Edwards' other papers, this one is a model of clarity, describing well-controlled experiments, cautiously interpreted. Despite the relatively small numbers, this paper convinced where previous claims had failed (98–103), precisely because the skilled hands and creative intellect that were behind it are so evident from its text.

The provenance of the eggs described in the 1969 paper is not immediately clear from the paper itself. All were obtained by in-vitro maturation after ovarian biopsy. In addition to Steptoe's coauthorship, four other gynecologists are thanked in the Acknowledgements section of the paper: Molly Rose, Norman Morris [1920–2008; Professor of Obstetrics and Gynecology at Charing Cross Hospital, London from 1958 to 1985; (104)], Janet Bottomley (1915–1995; Consultant Obstetrician and Gynecologist at Addenbrooke's Hospital, Cambridge from 1958 to 1976) and Sanford Markham (b. 1934; Chief of the Section of Obstetrics and Gynaecology at the U.S.

Egg characteristic	Experimental group	Control group
Assigned	56	17
Surviving	54/56	17/17
Matured to metaphase II	34/54	7/17
Some evidence of sperm penetration	18/34	
Spermatozoon within the zona pellucida	6/18	
Spermatozoon inside zona pellucida (c.7 hr post insemination)	5/18	
Evidence of pronuclei (c.11 hr post insemination)	7/18	0/7
No. with two pronuclei	2/18	

Table 4 Summary of Data from Ref. 97

Air Force Hospital, South Ruislip, to the north west of London from 1967 to 1972). Markham, now Professor of Obstetrics and Gynecology at Florida International University, Miami, writes:

"I believe that I met Bob by introduction from Dr. Roger Short at a Royal College of Medicine conference in London ... probably in early 1968 [possibly the Royal Society of Medicine's 28 February meeting at which Steptoe and Edwards first met?]. Bob mentioned that he was in need of ovarian tissue from reproductive aged women ... I offered to obtain tissue if we could work out a scheme to transport the tissue ... to Cambridge ... He provided the media and container and a driver that came to our hospital ... I remember three samples, however, there may have been others. In each case the whole wedge ... or ... ovary was sent (after sampling for pathology). In all cases the patients provided their consent for utilization of their tissue for research. They were not told what the research work involved. These samples were most likely sent in mid to late 1968 and possibly in early 1969. ... These ... were planned surgeries which were accomplished at specific times in their menstrual cycle. Unfortunately, I do not know if the tissues supplied were indeed the tissues used in data for his 1969 paper published in Nature."

It is possible that they were used, but unsuccessfully, not contributing to the 18 eggs showing fertilization. Thus, according to Edwards (3), Jean Purdy drove to Edgeware General Hospital to collect:

"the last piece of ovarian tissue that I was to obtain from the Edgware General Hospital. It yielded me 12 human eggs. Those eggs were soon ripening in mixtures of culture medium I had used over many years to which some of Barry [Bavister]'s fluid had been added. Thirty-six hours later we judged that they were ready for fertilization."

Nine of these were inseminated, leaving three as controls. Ten hours later, when Edwards and Bavister returned to the laboratory late at night:

"a spermatozoon was just passing into the first egg ... An hour later we looked at the second egg. Yes, there it was, the earliest stages of fertilization. A spermatozoon had entered the egg without any doubt – we had done it ... We examined other eggs and found more and more evidence. Some ova were in the early stages of fertilization with the sperm tails following the sperm heads into the depths of the egg; others were even more advanced with two nuclei – one from the sperm and one from the egg – as each gamete donated its genetic component to the embryo."

This (unverified) account suggests that Rose provided the first group of eggs to be fertilized in "Bavister's medium." Moreover, since only 18 of the eggs in the paper showed evidence of fertilization (Table 4), nine of those seem to have come from Rose, including presumptively the two described as having two pronuclei. Rose was invited to be a co-author, but she declined for reasons unknown. The source of the remaining nine eggs is unknown, but may have come from Oldham General Hospital. The Acknowledgements section thanks Drs C Abberley, G Garrett, and L Davies "for their help," all from Oldham General. John Webster, a later gynecological colleague of Steptoe, having consulted his colleague John Battie, writes of these:

"Cyril Adderley, not Abberley, was the Group Pathologist in Oldham. Geoff Garrett ... was also a pathologist there ... there was no L. Davies there but a John Davies, a haematologist, and a Vincent John Davies, a histologist ... and my money would go on V. J. as I think a histologist rather than a haematologist would have been of more help to him ...?"

The first two of these have elsewhere been described as helpful in setting up the embryology laboratory in Oldham, largely through the provision or loan of equipment required locally for egg maturation and fertilization, so their involvement in direct provision of eggs seems unlikely.

The Nature paper also supports Oldham as the source of the remaining eggs: "Some eggs were transported from Oldham to Cambridge" (97), and in his retrospective 1980 account of the events, Edwards says that at Oldham they began to repeat the experiment:

"Twelve women whose ovaries had to be removed [presumably laparoscopically] for serious medical conditions provided us with the necessary eggs over the next few months. We fertilized many more eggs and were able to make detailed examinations of the successive stages of fertilization (3)."

So it seems reasonable to conclude that those eggs described in the paper as "undergoing fertilization" were provided in roughly equal numbers by Rose and Steptoe.

However, with Steptoe on board, Rose no longer featured as a supplier of eggs (3). While the initial attraction of laparoscopy for Edwards had been the recovery of capacitated spermatozoa from the oviduct, once working with Steptoe he rapidly saw the wider possibilities for recovery of in-vivo matured eggs from the ovary (86). Indeed, the 1969 paper includes the following statement:

"Problems of embryonic development are likely to accompany the use of human oocytes matured and fertilized in vitro. When oocytes of the rabbit and other species were matured in vitro and fertilized in vivo, the pronuclear stages appeared normal but many of the resulting embryos had subnuclei in their blastomeres, and almost all of them died during the early cleavage stages ... When maturation of rabbit oocytes was started in vivo by injecting gonadotropins into the mother, and completed in the oviduct or in vitro, full term rabbit fetuses were obtained (97)."

The paper goes onto discuss how the use of hormonal priming to stimulate intrafollicular egg maturation might be achieved and reports: "Preliminary work using laparoscopy has shown that oocytes can be recovered from ovaries by puncturing ripening follicles in vivo. ..."

Through these preliminary collaborative studies, Edwards and Steptoe were already building a research partnership. Although both were very different personalities, and brought very different skills to the project, they shared energy, commitment, and vision. Each was also marginalized by his professional peers, a marginalization that also perhaps helped to cement their partnership (2).

With the paper's publication, announced to the media on St Valentine's day (105), all hell was let loose. The impossible tangle of TV cables and pushy reporters trying to force their way up the stairs to the fourth floor laboratories proved a major disruption to the Physiological laboratory in general and to the members of the Marshall laboratory in particular. It was something that was to recur episodically over the next 10 years.

THE BATTLES BEGIN

However, 1969 seemed to be a good year for Edwards. Not only did IVF succeed at long last, and his partnership with Steptoe seemed set to flourish, but also so impressed were the Ford Foundation with his work that in late 1968 they had established, at Austin's prompting (106), an endowment fund with the University of Cambridge to cover the salary cost of a Ford Foundation Readership [a half-way step to a professorship; (107)]. Elated by his promotion and their achievement, Edwards and Steptoe pressed on, the latter's laparoscopic skills coming to the fore, first in 1970 with the collection of in-vivo matured eggs from follicles after mild hormonal stimulation (108), and then achieving regular fertilization of these eggs and their early development through cleavage to the blastocyst stage (109,110). So well was the work going that in late 1970 and early 1971 they confidently applied to the U.K. Medical Research Council for funding.

However, any illusions that Edwards may have had that their achievements would prove a turning point in his fortunes were soon shattered. The hostility of much of the media coverage to his work in 1969 heralded the dominant pattern of scientific and medical responses for the next 10–15 years and resulted just two months later

in the MRC rejecting the grant application (2). The practical consequences of this rejection were profound – both psychologically and physically – not least that for the next seven years, Edwards and Purdy shuttled on the 12-hour round trip between Cambridge and Oldham, Greater Manchester, paradoxically just north of his schoolboy haunts of Gorton, where Steptoe and he set up a small laboratory and clinic in Dr Kershaw's cottage hospital, all the while leaving Ruth and his five daughters in Cambridge.

The professional attacks on Edwards and his work took a number of forms (2), and one must try to make a mental time trip back to the 1960s and 1970s to understand their basis. Despite the nature of the political and religious battles to come, his scientific and medical colleagues did not focus on the special status of the human embryo as an ethical issue. Ethical issues were raised professionally, but took quite a different form. It is perhaps difficult now to comprehend the complete absence of infertility from the consciousness of most gynecologists in the United Kingdom at the time, of whom Steptoe was a remarkable exception (81). Indeed, even Edwards' strong commitment to treating infertility came to the fore only after he had teamed up with Steptoe, his previous priority being the study and prevention of genetic and chromosomal disorders.

In the several reports from the Royal College of Obstetricians and Gynaecologists and the MRC during the 1960s examining the areas of gynecological ignorance that needed academic attention, infertility simply did not feature (50,51). Overpopulation and family planning were seen as dominant concerns and the infertile were ignored as, at best, a tiny and irrelevant minority and at worst as a positive contribution to population control. This was a values system that Edwards did not accept (111), and the many encouraging letters he received from infertile couples spurred him on and provided a major stimulus to his continued work later, despite so much professional and press antagonism. For his professional colleagues, however, the fact that infertility was not seen as a significant clinical issue meant that any research designed to alleviate it was viewed not as experimental treatment, but as using humans in experiments. Given the sensitivity to the relatively recent Nazi "medical experiments," the formal acceptance of the Helsinki Declaration (112,113) and the public reaction and disquiet surrounding the recent publication of "Human guinea-pigs" (114), this distinction was critical. The MRC, in rejecting the grant application, took the position that what was being proposed was human experimentation, and so were very cautious, emphasizing risks rather than benefits, of which they saw few if any (2).

Edwards and Steptoe were also attacked for their willingness to talk with the media. It is difficult nowadays, when the public communication of science is embedded institutionally, to understand how damaging to them this was. The massive press interest of the late 1960s was unabated in the ensuing years, and so Edwards was faced with a choice: either he could keep his head down and allow press fantasies and speculations to go unanswered and unchallenged, or he could engage, educate, and debate. For him this was no choice, regardless of the consequences professionally (30). His egalitarian spirit demanded that he trust common people's common sense. His radical political views demanded that he fought the corner of the infertile: the underdog with no voice. The Yorkshireman in him relished engagement in the debate and argument. In Edwards and Sharpe (111), he sets out his reasons for public engagement and acknowledges the risk to his own interests:

> "Scientists may have to make disclosures of their work and its consequences that run against their immediate interests; they may have to stir up public opinion, even lobby for laws before legislatures."

And risk it was. One of the scientific referees on their MRC grant application started his referee's report declaring the media exposure distasteful:

> "Dr. Edwards feels the need to publicise his work on radio and television, and in the press, so that he can change public attitudes. I do not feel that an ill-informed general public is capable of evaluating the work and seeing it in its proper perspective. This publicity has antagonised a large number of Dr. Edwards' scientific colleagues, of whom I am one (2)."

Edwards' pioneering role in the public communication of science proved to be disadvantageous to his work.

The Edwards and Sharpe (111) paper is a tour de force in its survey of the scientific benefits and risks of the science of IVF, in the legal and ethical issues raised by IVF, and in the pros and cons of the various regulatory responses to them. It sets out the issues succinctly and anticipates social responses that were some 13–19 years into the future. Edwards built on his strong commitment to social justice based on a social ethic in subsequent years, as he engaged at every opportunity with ethicists, lawyers and theologians, arguing, playing "devil's advocate" (literally, in the eyes of some), and engaging in what would now be called practical ethics as he hammered out his position and felt able to fully justify his instincts intellectually.

However, the establishment was, with few exceptions, unwilling to engage seriously in ethical debates (115,116) in advance of the final validation of IVF that was to come in 1978 with the birth of Louise Brown (Fig. 13) (117). Only then did the UK social, scientific, and medical hierarchies, such as the MRC, the British Medical Association, the Royal Society, and Government move gradually from their almost visceral reactions against IVF and its possibilities to serious engagement with the issues (118). Then, to their credit, both the MRC and the Thatcher Government of the time came on board, but it was not until 1989, 24 years after Bob's 1965 visionary paper in the Lancet, that the UK Parliament finally gave its stamp of approval to his vision, and then only after a fierce battle lasting some 11 years (118,119).

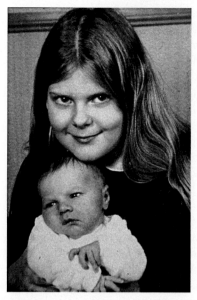

Figure 13 Louise Brown holding the 1000th Bourn Hall baby, 1987. *Source*: Courtesy of Bourn Hall Clinic.

DISCUSSION

This paper describes some of the early years of Edwards' life and work, in order to provide a context for the events leading up to the 1969 *Nature* paper describing IVF and the final validation of the claims made in that paper with the birth of Louise Brown in 1978. It is evident even from the earliest stages of his late entry into research that Edwards is a man of extraordinary energy and drive, qualities sustained throughout his long career, witnessing his prodigious output of papers between 1954 and 2008 (30). Indeed, several of the referees on the unsuccessful MRC grant application specifically criticized his "overenthusiasm," doubting that he could achieve the program he sets out therein as "too ambitious" (2). Tenacity of purpose comes through clearly in Edwards' work, a trait he is inclined to attribute to his Yorkshire origins, but which may also be fuelled by his working-class determination to show himself as good as the next (wo)man.

The influence of Waddington's Edinburgh Institute, of Waddington himself, and of his supervisor, Alan Beatty, on Edwards' interests and values is also clear from the dominant role that developmental genetics played in his thinking, especially until the time he met Steptoe. Indeed, from examination of Edwards' papers and interests, his passionate conversion to the cause of the infertile seems directly attributable to Steptoe's influence. Admittedly, Edwards' forays into immunoreproduction did involve consideration of immunological causes of infertility, but these were more usually of interest to him as models for developing new contraceptive agents. Indeed, Edwards was as captured as most reproductive biologists of the time by the 1960s' consensus on the need for better methods of world population control. This position was understandable given the reality of those concerns, as is demonstrated now in the problem of global warming that is attributable at least in part to a failure to control population growth. It is a measure of his imagination and empathy that he could grasp so rapidly Steptoe's understanding of the plight of the infertile and so flexibly incorporate this understanding into his plans. That empathy clearly reflects his underprivileged origins, his espousal of the cause of the junior, the disadvantaged, the ill-informed, and the underdog being a thread running through his career. Edwards can be very critical, but I have found no one who can remember him ever being nasty or vindictive. Even when he disagrees with someone passionately, he never loses his respect for them as people. That Steptoe tapped into this sentiment is clear.

The way in which Edwards met Steptoe has been absorbed into folklore, but an examination of the evidence seems to warrant some revision to commonly held later reminiscences. It remains uncertain exactly which publication(s) by Steptoe it was that Edwards read in 1967, but seems likely that he did read Steptoe's book. Thus, it was spermatozoa, not eggs, that were exercising Edwards in 1967, and it was the problem of sperm capacitation, not egg retrieval, to which Steptoe and his laparoscope seemed to offer a solution. The book is the only place that this issue is specifically addressed. Their actual meeting at the Royal Society of Medicine is also re-evaluated: Edwards was an invited speaker lecturing about his work on immunoreproduction; so paradoxically, what has been seen as a side track to his main work was, albeit serendipitously, the reason for their actual meeting.

The early collaboration between them involved the recovery of ovarian biopsies, just like those Rose and others had been providing. However, the attractions of pre-ovulatory follicular egg recovery were already clear to them both by the end of 1968, and became, with embryo replacement, the central planks of their partnership. Steptoe and Edwards were in many ways an unlikely partnership. Their personal styles were very different, and there are clear hints in his writings that Edwards found their early days together difficult. But like most successful partnerships, their differences were sunk in a mutual respect for the other's pioneering skills and willingness to take on the established conventions. In Jean Purdy, they also had a partner who smoothed the bumps on the path of their work together (Fig. 14).

However, it remains Edwards' extraordinary foresight that marks him out so distinctively. His combination of vision and intellectual rigor is evident not just in his work on stem cells, PGD and, with Steptoe, infertility, but also in his pioneering work in the public communication of science, in how ethical discourse about reproduction is conducted, and in consideration of regulatory issues. The epithet "the father of Assisted Reproductive Technique" is surely deservedly appropriate.

ACKNOWLEDGMENTS

I thank the Edwards' family for their help in writing this account, for which, however, I take full responsibility. I also thank Sandy Markham and John Webster for allowing me to quote our correspondence, Margaret Wilson for her help with locating books and periodicals, and Kay Elder, Ralph Robinson, and Sarah Franklin for their unfailing wisdom and help. I also thank Barry Bavister, Richard Gardner, Roger Gosden, David Griffin, Ginny Papaioannou, Barbara Rankin, Carol Readhead, Martin Richards, Janet Rossant, Pat Tate, and Frank Webb for contributing their own memories from their own papers and for correcting mine. I thank Ruth Edwards for permission to reproduce Figures 1–3, 5, 8, and 11, Barbara Rankin for permission to reproduce Figures 6, 7, 9, and 10, Andrew Steptoe for permission to reproduce Figure 12, Bourn Hall Clinic for permission to reproduce Figures 13 and 14, and Peter Williams for permission to include the movie clip in the Supplementary material. The research was supported by a grant from the Wellcome Trust (088708), which otherwise had no involvement in the research or its publication.

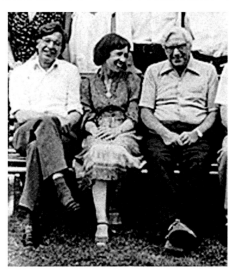

Figure 14   Edwards, Purdy, and Steptoe at Bourn Hall, 1981. *Source*: Courtesy of Bourn Hall Clinic.

REFERENCES

1. Nobel, 2010. [Available from: http://nobelprize.org/nobel_prizes/medicine/laureates/2010/announcement.html].
2. Johnson MH, Franklin SB, Cottingham M, Hopwood N. Why the medical research council refused Robert Edwards and Patrick Steptoe support for research on human conception in 1971. Hum Reprod 2010; 25: 2157–74.
3. Edwards RG, Steptoe PC. A Matter of Life: The Story of a Medical Breakthrough. London, UK: Hutchinson, 1980.
4. Massey H, Feather N. James Chadwick. 20 October 1891–24 July. Biogr Mems Fell R Soc 1974; 22: 10–70.
5. Ashwood-Smith M. Robert Edwards at 55. Reprod BioMed Online 2002; 4(Suppl 1): 2–3.
6. Ingle DJ. Gregory Goodwin Pincus. April 9, 1903-August 22, 1967. Biogr Mems Natl Acad Sci USA 1971: 229–270. [Available from: http://www.nap.edu/readingroom.php?book=biomemsandpage=ggpincus.html].
7. Slee J. RGE at 25 – personal reminiscences. Reprod BioMed Online 2002; 4(Suppl 1): 1.

8. Oakley CL. Francis William Rogers Brambell. 1901–1970. Biogr Mems Fell R Soc 1973; 19: 129–171.

9. Parkes AS. Francis Hugh Adam Marshall. 1878–1949. Biogr Mems Fell R Soc 1950; 7: 238–251.

10. Polge C. Sir Alan Sterling Parkes. 10 September 1900–17 July. Biogr Mems Fell R Soc 2006; 52, 263–283.

11. Robertson A. Conrad Hal Waddington. 8 November 1905–26 September. Biogr Mems Fell R Soc 1977; 23: 575–622.

12. Milne EA. Ralph Howard Fowler. 1889–1944. Biogr Mems Fell R Soc 1945; 5: 60–78.

13. Eve AS, Chadwick J. Lord Rutherford. 1871–1937. Biogr Mems Fell R Soc 1938; 2: 394–423.

14. Edwards RG. An astonishing journey into reproductive genetics since the 1950's. Reprod Nutr Dev 2005; 45: 299–306.

15. Watson JD, Crick FH. Genetical implications of the structure of deoxyribonucleic acid. Nature 1953a; 171: 964–7.

16. Watson JD, Crick FH. Molecular structure of nucleic acids: a structure for deoxyribose nucleic acid. Nature 1953b; 171: 737–8.

17. Franklin R, Gosling R. Molecular configuration in sodium thymonucleate. Nature 1953; 171: 740–1.

18. Wilkins MHF, Stokes AR, Wilson HR. Molecular structure of deoxypentose nucleic acids. Nature 1953; 171: 738–40.

19. Gurdon JB. The developmental capacity of nuclei taken from intestinal epithelium cells of feeding tadpoles. Development 1962a; 10: 622–40.

20. Gurdon JB. Adult frogs derived from the nuclei of single somatic cells. Dev Biol 1962b; 4: 256–73.

21. Gurdon JB, Elsdale TR, Fischberg M. Sexually mature individuals of Xenopus laevis from the transplantation of single somatic nuclei. Nature 1958; 182; 64–5.

22. Weinberg AM. Messenger RNA: origins of a discovery. Nature 2001; 414: 485.

23. Ford CE, Hamerton JL. The chromosomes of man. Nature 1956; 178: 1020–23.

24. Tjio JH, Levan A. The chromosome number of man. Hereditas 1956; 42: 1–6.

25. Conference, Denver. A proposed standard system of nomenclature of human mitotic chromosomes. Lancet 1960; 275: 1063–65.

26. Ford CE, Jones KW, Polani PE, De Almeida JC, Briggs JH. A sex-chromosome anomaly in a case of gonadal dysgenesis (Turner's syndrome). Lancet 1959a; 273: 711–13.

27. Ford CE, Polani PE, Briggs JH, Bishop PM. A presumptive human XXY/XX mosaic. Nature 1959b; 183: 1030–32.

28. Jacobs PA, Strong JA. A case of human intersexuality having a possible XXY sex-determining mechanism. Nature 1959; 183: 302–3.

29. Lejeune J, Gautier M, Turpin R. Etude des chromosomes somatiques de neuf enfants mongoliens. Comptes Rendus Hebd Seances Acad Sci 1959; 248: 1721–22.

30. Gardner RL, Johnson MH. Bob Edwards and the first decade of reproductive biomedicine. Online Reprod BioMed Online 2011; 22: 106–24.

31. Fowler RE, Edwards RG. Induction of superovulation and pregnancy in mature mice by gonadotrophins. J Endocr 1957; 15: 374–84.

32. Edwards RG, Gates AH. Timing of the stages of the maturation divisions, ovulation, fertilization and the first cleavage of eggs of adult mice treated with gonadotrophins. J Endocr 1959; 18: 292–304.

33. Horowitz NH, Metz CB, Piatigorsky J, Piko L, Spikes JD, Ycas M. Albert Tyler. Science 1969; 163: 424.

34. Reeve S. Nathaniel Mayer Victor Rothschild, G.B.E., G.M. Third Baron Rothschild. 31 October 1910–20 March. Biogr Mems Fell R Soc 1994; 39: 364–80.

35. Rothschild. Did fertilization occur? Nature 1969; 221: 981.

36. Edwards RG, Bavister BD, Steptoe PC. Early stages of fertilization in vitro of human oocytes matured in vitro. Nature 1969b; 221: 632–5.

37. Mitchison NA. Peter Brian Medawar. February 1915–2 October. Biogr Mems Fell R Soc 1990; 35: 282–301.

38. Medawar PB. Some immunological and endocrinological problems raised by the evolution of viviparity in.vertebrates. Symp Soc Exp Biol 1953; 7: 320–38.

39. Clarke AE. Disciplining Reproduction: Modernity, American Life Sciences, and the Problems of Sex. Berkeley, California, USA: University of California Press, 1998.

40. Connelly M. Fatal Misconception: The Struggle to Control World Population. Cambridge, USA: Harvard University Press, 2008.

41. Marks LV. Sexual Chemistry: A History of the Contraceptive Pill. New Haven, USA: Yale University Press, 2001.

42. Naz RK, Gupta SK, Gupta JC, Vyas HK, Talwar GP. Recent advances in contraceptive vaccine development: a mini-review. Hum Reprod 2005; 20: 3271–83.

43. Rukavina D. The history of reproductive immunology: my personal view. Am J Reprod Immunol 2008; 59: 446–50.

44. Edwards RG. Meiosis in ovarian oocytes of adult mammals. Nature 1962; 196: 446–50.

45. Gemzell CA. The induction of ovulation with human pituitary gonadotrophins. Fertil Steril 1962; 13: 153–68.

46. Pincus G, Enzmann EV. The comparative behavior of mammalian eggs in vivo and in vitro I. the activation of ovarian eggs. J Exp Med 1935; 62: 665–75.

47. Pincus G, Saunders B. The comparative behavior of mammalian eggs in vivo and in vitro VI. The maturation of human ovarian ova. Anat Rec 1939; 75: 537–45.

48. Greep RO. Min Chueh Chang. October 10, 1908–June 5, 1991. Biogr Mems Natl Acad Sci USA. 2010. [Available from: http://www.nap.edu/readingroom.php?book=biomemsandpage=mchang.html].

49. Chang MC. The maturation of rabbit oocytes in culture and their maturation, activation, fertilization and subsequent development in the Fallopian tubes. J Exp Zool 1955; 128: 379–405.

50. MRC. 1969. Research in Obstetrics and Gynaecology: Report to the Secretary of the Council by Section A1, General Clinical Medicine. National Archives, FD 7/912.

51. RCOG. Macafee Report. The Training of Obstetricians and Gynaecologists in Britain, and Matters Related Thereto: The Report of a Select Committee to the Council of the Royal College of Obstetricians and Gynaecologists. London, UK: RCOG, 1967.

52. Askonas BA. John Herbert Humphrey. 16 December 1915–25 December. Biogr Mems Fell R Soc 1990; 36: 274–300.

53. Himsworth H, Pitt-Rivers R. Charles Robert Harington. 1897–1972. Biogr Mems Fell R Soc 1972; 18, 266–308.

54. McLaren A, Biggers JD. Successful development and birth of mice cultivated in vitro as early embryos. Nature 1958; 182: 877–8.

55. Cole RJ, Edwards RG, Paul J. Cytodifferentiation in cell colonies and cell strains derived from cleaving ova and blastocysts of the rabbit. Exp Cell Res 1965; 37: 501–4.

56. Cole RJ, Edwards RG, Paul J. Cytodifferentiation and embryogenesis in cell colonies and tissue cultures derived from ova and blastocysts of the rabbit. Dev Biol 1966; 13: 385–407.

57. Evans MJ, Kaufman MH. Establishment in culture of pluripotential cells from mouse embryos. Nature 1981; 292: 154–6.

58. Edwards RG. IVF and the history of stem cells. Nature 2001; 413: 349–51.

59. Parkes AS. Off-beat Biologist. Cambridge, UK: The Galton Foundation, 1985.

60. Cook B. JRF – the first 100 volumes. Reproduction 1994; 100: 2–4.

61. Clarke J. The history of three scientific societies: the Society for the Study of Fertility (now the Society for Reproduction and Fertility) (Britain), the Societe 'Francaise pour l'Etude de la Fertilite', and the Society for the Study of Reproduction (USA). Stud Hist Phil Biol Biomed Sci 2007; 38: 340–57.

62. Edwards RG. Letter to Cambridge University Registrary, plus supporting documents, applying for the Mary Marshall and Arthur Walton Professorship of the Physiology of Reproduction. Edwards' papers, 6 Jan 1966. Uncatalogued, Churchill College Archive. 1966.

63. Polge C. 1993. Obituary: Professor Thaddeus Mann. The Independent, 9 December.

64. Short R. Colin Austin. Aust Acad Sci Newslett 2004; 60: 11.

65. Arechaga J. Technique as the basis of experiment in developmental biology: An interview with Denis A.T. New Int J Dev Biol 1997; 41: 139–52.

66. Edwards RG, Steptoe PC. Preface. In: Edwards RG, Purdy JM, Steptoe PC, eds. Implantation of the Human Embryo. London, UK: Academic Press, 1985: vii–viii.

67. Vickers AD. A direct measurement of the sex-ratio in mouse blastocysts. Reproduction 1967; 13: 375–6.

68. Gardner RL. Bob Edwards – 2010 nobel laureate in physiology or medicine. Physiology News 2011; 82: 18–22.

69. Gardner RL, Johnson MH. Robert Edwards. Hum Reprod 1991; 6: iii–iv.

70. Edwards RG. Maturation in vitro of human ovarian oocytes. Lancet 1965a; 286: 926–929.

71. Edwards RG. Maturation in vitro of mouse, sheep, cow, pig, rhesus monkey and human ovarian oocytes. Nature 1965b; 208: 349–51.

72. Gardner RL, Edwards RG. Control of the sex ratio at full term in the rabbit by transferring sexed blastocysts. Nature 1968; 218: 346–9.

73. Theodosiou AA, Johnson MH. The politics of human embryo research and the motivation to achieve PGD. Reprod BioMed Online 2011; 22: 457–71.

74. Edwards RG. Are oocytes formed and used sequentially in the mammalian ovary? Phil Trans R Soc B 1970; 259: 103–5.

75. Henderson SA, Edwards RG. Chiasma frequency and maternal age in mammals. Nature 1968; 218: 22–8.

76. Chang MC. Fertilization of rabbit ova in vitro. Nature 1959; 184: 466–7.

77. Yanagimachi R, Chang M.C. Fertilization of hamster eggs in vitro. Nature 1963; 200: 281–2.

78. Jones Jr HW. From reproductive immunology to Louise Brown. Reprod BioMed Online 2002; 4(Suppl 1): 6–7.

79. Edwards RG, Donahue RP, Baramki TA, Jones Jr HW. Preliminary attempts to fertlilize human oocytes matured in vitro. Am J Obstet Gynecol 1966; 96: 192–200.

80. Edwards RG, Talbert L, Israelstam D, Nino HN, Johnson MH. Diffusion chamber for exposing spermatozoa to human uterine secretions. Am J Obstet Gynecol 1968: 102: 388–396.

81. Edwards RG. Patrick Christopher Steptoe, C. B. E. 9 June 1913–22 March 1988. Biogr Mems Fell R Soc 1996; 42: 435–52.

82. Steptoe PC. Laparoscopy in Gynaecology. Edinburgh, UK: E and S. Livingstone, 1967a.

83. Philipp E. Obituary: P C Steptoe CBE, FRCSED, FRCOG, FRS. Br Med J 1988; 296: 1135.

84. Edwards RG. Tribute to Patrick Steptoe: beginnings of laparoscopy. Hum Reprod 1989; 4(Suppl): 1–9.

85. Edwards RG. Interviewed in: To Mrs. Brown a daughter. Peter Williams TV: The Studio, Boughton. Faversham, UK (see Supplementary Material), 1978.

86. Steptoe PC. Laparoscopy and ovulation. Lancet 1968; 292: 913.

87. Hunting P. The history of the royal society of medicine. London, UK: The Royal Society of Medicine Press Ltd, 2002.

88. Steptoe PC. Laparoscopy: diagnostic and therapeutic uses. Proc Roy Soc Med 1969; 62: 439–441.

89. Steptoe PC. A new method of tubal sterilisation. In: Westin B, Wiqvist N, eds. Amsterdam: Fertility and Sterility: Proc 5th World Congress June 16–22, 1966. Stockholm: International Congress Series no. 133, Excerpta Medica Foundation, 1967b: 1183–1184.

90. Steptoe PC. Laparoscopic studies of ovulation, its suppression and induction, and of ovarian dysfunction. In: Wood C, Walters WAW, eds. Fifth World Congress of Gynaecology and Obstetrics, held in Sydney, Australia, September, 1967. Butterworths, Sydney, Australia, 1967c: 364.

91. Steptoe PC. The fifth freedom. Br Med J 1966; 1: 234.

92. Steptoe PC. Gynaecological endoscopy–laparoscopy and culdoscopy. J Obstet Gynaecol Br Commonwealth 1965; 72: 535–43.

93. Morrison DL. Laparoscopy. BMJ 1967; 4: 34.

94. Austin CR. Observations of the penetration of sperm into the mammalian egg. Aust J Sci Res B 1951; 4: 581–96.

95. Chang MC. Fertilizing capacity of spermatozoa deposited into the fallopian tubes. Nature 1951; 168: 697–8.

96. Bavister BD. Environmental factors important for in vitro fertilization in the hamster. Reprod 1969; 18: 544–545.

97. Edwards RG, Bavister BD, Steptoe PC. Did fertilization occur? Nature 1969a; 221: 981–2.

98. Hayashi M. Fertilization in vitro using human ova. In: Proceedings of the 7th International Planned Parenthood Federation, Singapore. Excerpta Medica International Congress Series No. 72. Amsterdam, Netherlands, 1963.

99. Petrov GN. Fertilization and first stages of cleavage of human egg in vitro. Arkhiv Anatomii Gistologii i Embriologii 1958; 35: 88–91.

100. Petrucci D. Producing transplantable human tissue in the laboratory. Discovery 1961; 22: 278–83.

101. Rock J, Menkin M. In vitro fertilization and cleavage of human ovarian eggs. Science 1944; 100: 105–7.

102. Shettles LB. A morula stage of human ovum developed in vitro. Fertil Steril 1955; 9: 287–9.

103. Yang WH. The nature of human follicular ova and fertilization in vitro. J Jpn Obstet Gynecol Soc 1963; 15: 121–130.

104. Anon, 2008. Morris, Prof. Norman Frederick. In: Who Was Who 1920–1980. A & C Black and Oxford University Press. [Available from: http://www.ukwhoswho.com/view/article/oupww/whowaswho/U28190].

105. Anon, 1969. New step towards test-tube babies. Nature-Times News Service; The Times 14 February, 1.

106. Holmes RF. Letter to D Kellaway, (Sec Fac Board Biol. B), dated 21 May. University of Cambridge Archives, 1968; 731.020.

107. Hankinson GS. Letter (G.B.6812.534) from the General Board of the Faculties, the Old Schools, Cambridge to RG Edwards detailing some aspects of the Ford Foundation endowment fund, 20 December 1968. Edwards papers uncatalogued, Churchill College Archive.1968.

108. Steptoe PC, Edwards RG. Laparoscopic recovery of preovulatory human oocytes after priming of ovaries with gonadotrophins. Lancet 1970; 295: 683–9.

109. Edwards RG, Steptoe PC, Purdy JM. Fertilization and cleavage in vitro of preovulatory human oocytes. Nature 1970; 227: 1307–9.

110. Steptoe PC, Edwards RG, Purdy JM. Human blastocysts grown in culture. Nature 1971; 229: 132–3.

111. Edwards RG, Sharpe DJ. Social values and research in human embryology. Nature 1971; 231: 87–91.

112. Helsinki Declaration, Human Experimentation: Code of Ethics of World Medical Association. Br Med J 1964; 2: 177.

113. Hazelgrove J. The old faith and the new science. the Nuremberg Code and human experimentation ethics in Britain 1946–73. Soc Hist Med 2002; 15: 109–135.

114. Pappworth MH. Human Guinea-Pigs. London, UK: Routledge and Keegan Paul, 1967.

115. Edwards RG. Fertilization of human eggs in vitro: morals, ethics and the law. Q Rev Biol 1974; 49: 3–26.

116. Jones A, Bodmer WF. Our Future Inheritance: Choice or Chance? London, UK: Oxford University Press, 1974.

117. Edwards RG, Steptoe PC. Birth after the reimplantation of a human embryo. Lancet 1978; 312: 366.

118. Johnson MH, Theodosiou AA. PGD and the making of the genetic embryo as a political tool. In: McLean S, ed. Regulating PGD: A Comparative and Theoretical Analysis. London, UK: Routledge, 2011.

119. Mulkay M. The embryo research debate: science and the politics of reproduction. Cambridge, UK: Cambridge University Press, 1997.

Quality management in reproductive medicine

Christoph Keck, Cecilia Sjöblom, Robert Fischer, Vera Baukloh, and Michael Alper

INTRODUCTION

Although quality management (QM) in the healthcare industry is not a household term, quality management systems (QM systems) have become an integral management tool in many IVF centers around the world. The European Union Tissue Directive, issued in 2004, clearly demands a quality management system for any institution handling human gametes/embryos. The primary concern of any healthcare system is, and will continue to be, medical performance. However, if we regard healthcare systems as "corporations" dealing with patients, referring doctors, and employees, in addition to medical performance, then other qualities will have to be taken into consideration. More and more hospitals as well as independent medical practices will have to document the quality of their services to their patients and cost-bearers. This will mean that strict procedures for documentation of results will be needed and, furthermore, medical institutions will have to answer the question of whether or not they provide their services in a cost-effective way. Many rules (such as the measures for limiting the spread of infections and the statute on protection against radiation) are set by law. However, beyond these rules, many medical institutions currently develop their own internal standards. These standards are often only informally documented and, most of the time, are fragmentary. Although it is not always obvious, these standards can affect and direct the internal workings of the organization and the interaction of various areas within the company. They may also affect the interaction of the company with external partners. With internal systems such as these, enormous differences can exist from one system to another with respect to the importance and validity of various sections and procedures. The Joint Commission on Accreditation of Health Care Organizations calls these elements of quality management "functions." One can show that these "functions" differ from one institution to another, no matter whether or not they are applied in clinics or private practices, group or single provider practices, or government medical institutions. Essential elements are identifiable and applicable to every institution that aims at fulfilling the wishes and demands of its customers. It is not only patients who are considered "customers," but all communication partners, including the referring physicians, the company's suppliers, and the company's own employees are customers as well. The individual elements of a quality management system are developed to different degrees, always according to the tasks and the orientation of the particular institution. They exist in varied, yet always definable relationships, to one another. All of these elements and their interconnection as a whole enable a clinic or private practice to reach the expected and agreed results with the customer on a timely basis, and with an appropriate use of resources. The sum of directive elements and elements that transcend or relate to the process is called the "quality management system" of a clinic or a private practice. Of all the medical fields, reproductive medicine has led the way (in Europe) with the introduction of QM systems over the past several years. In this chapter, different QM systems are described, the instruments of these systems are discussed, and the question of how QM systems contribute to success in reproductive medicine is addressed.

DIFFERENT QUALITY MANAGEMENT SYSTEMS

In the past, a series of specific QM systems for various industries have come into existence worldwide. In 1964, the Good Production Practice [World Health Organization (WHO) directive] was developed for the pharmaceutical and food industries. The Good Laboratory Practice [Organization for Economic Cooperation and Development (OECD) directive] followed in 1978 and the Hazard Analysis of Critical Control Points (National Advisory Committee on Microbiological Criteria for Foods directive) in 1992. The EU with its "Global Concept" (1985) strongly promoted the development of QM systems and expanded them to production and services, which therefore covered the documentation of ecologically justifiable dealings in energy, material, and waste.

ISO 9001 Standards

The systems that followed – the manuals of the International Standardization Organization (ISO 9000 series) – became the most widespread, worldwide standard. In the 1980s, the ISO created regulations for QM systems with the standard series 9001 through 9004 developed for the production of goods and services. These manuals described the basic elements of the QM system in a relatively abstract manner. Medical institutions were required to adapt these standards to suit them and this required some interpretation and modification. The introduction of ISO 9000 states: "The demands of the organizations differ from each other; during the creation of quality management systems and putting them into practice, the special goals of the organization, its products and procedures and specific methods of acting must be taken into consideration unconditionally." This means that, for medical applications, the standards state which elements should be considered in the QM system, but the manner in which these elements should be realized in the specific medical organization have to be defined individually. The ISO standards have now been adapted to medicine, which is fortunate since there is no QM system specifically designed for hospitals or medical practices. ISO 9001 through 9003 standards contain the elements important for a quality system (Table 32.1). The criteria according to which QM systems are applied vary with the type of enterprise. For example, the 9001 standard is applicable to the manufacturing and complicated service companies including hospitals. On the other hand, the 9002 standard is more suitable for rehabilitation and foster-care institutions (1). The application of a certified QM system for hospitals can be performed on the basis of ISO 9001 or ISO 9004 (2). As mentioned earlier, in vitro fertilization (IVF) units occupy a special place within clinical medicine. It is a highly specialized area involving the interaction of staff in various areas, including the laboratory, ultrasound, administration, physicians, and

nurses. Treatment can only be successful when a structured interaction exists between the clinical and laboratory departments. ISO 9001:2000 (3) is very much concentrated on a process approach and directed to the outcome of the process; i.e., the products or services meet the previously determined requirements. Since this does not necessarily assure that a laboratory will be successful, or that it will achieve the highest level of care for the patients that it serves, assisted reproduction technique (ART) laboratories may also want to consider additional requirements, including standards concerning qualification and competence. Relevant standards are provided by the ISO/IEC 17025:1999 (4) (IEC being the International Electrotechnical Commission). This standard, entitled "General requirements for the competence of testing and calibration laboratories," replaces both the ISO/IEC Guide 25 (5) and the European standard EN 45001 (6). Compliance with the ISO 17025 standard can lead to accreditation (defined as "a procedure by which an authoritative body gives formal recognition that a body or person is competent to carry out specific tasks"), which exceeds certification (defined as "a procedure by which a third party gives written assurance that a product, process or service conforms to specific requirements"). ART laboratories should consider ISO 17025 accreditation (see chap. 3). However, one should realize that both ISO/IEC Guide 25 and EN 45001 are focused more on the technical aspects of competence, and do not cover all areas within clinical laboratories. It has already been stated that although the ISO standards are the most widely accepted standards in the world, there is no appropriate international standard for laboratories in the healthcare sector. To fill this "vacuum," several professional associations and laboratory organizations have also framed and published standards and guidelines, most of which are confined to a specific clinical laboratory discipline. Some specific and relevant examples of guidelines for ART laboratories commonly available are: (7–10).

1. Guidelines for human embryology and andrology laboratories, the American Fertility Society, 1992.
2. Guidelines for good practice in IVF laboratories, the European Society of Human Reproduction and Embryology (ESHRE), 2000.
3. Reproductive laboratory accreditation standards, College of American Pathology, 2002.
4. Accreditation standards and guidelines for IVF laboratories, the Association of Clinical Embryologists, 2000.

The above-mentioned guidelines and standards describe the specific requirements for reproductive laboratories, and include various aspects of the implementation of a QM system. These well-defined standards describe the minimum conditions that should be met by laboratories/clinics. Recently, the EU Tissue Directive (11) has been released, which demands a quality QM system for every medical institution dealing with human gametes or embryos.

Table 32.1   Elements/Criteria of the ISO Standard

Number	Quality element according to ISO 9000 ff.
1	Responsibility
2	Quality management system
3	Contract control
4	Design management
5	Document and data management
6	Measures
7	Management of products provided by customers
8	Designating and retrospective observation
9	Process management
10	Revision
11	Control of the revision resources
12	Evidence of revisions
13	Defective product management
14	Corrections and preventive measures
15	Handling, storage, packaging, conservation, distribution
16	Quality report management
17	Internal quality audits
18	Training
19	Maintenance
20	Statistical methods

TQM and EFQM

There is a wide range of quality management models and strategies based on continuous improvement. Two of the best-documented models/strategies are Total Quality Management (TQM) and the Excellence Model of the European Foundation for Quality Management (EFQM). Total Quality Management is an all-encompassing concept that integrates quality control, assurance, and improvement. It is more a philosophy than a model. The basics of this concept were developed after World War II by Deming. Both the TQM and the EFQM models incorporate the objective of continuously striving to improve every aspect of a service, and require continuous scrutiny of all components of the quality management system of an organization. Measurement and feedback are crucial elements in quality management. This can be illustrated by the so-called Deming cycle ("Plan–Do–Check–Act" cycle) (Fig. 32.1). Important elements of a TQM program are:

1. Appropriately educated and trained personnel with training records.
2. Complete listing of all technical procedures performed.
3. Housekeeping procedures: cleaning and decontamination procedures.
4. Correct operation, calibration, and maintenance of all instruments with manuals and logbook records.
5. Proper procedure policy and safety manuals.
6. Consistent and proper execution of appropriate techniques and methods.
7. Proper documentation, record keeping, and reporting of results.
8. Thorough description of specimen collection and handling, including verification procedures for patient identification and chain of custody.
9. Safety procedures, including appropriate storage of materials.
10. Infection control measures.
11. Documentation of suppliers and sources of chemicals and supplies, with dates of receipt/expiry.
12. System for appraisal of test performance correction of deficiencies and implementation of advances and improvements.
13. Quality materials, tested with bioassays when appropriate.
14. Quality assurance programs.

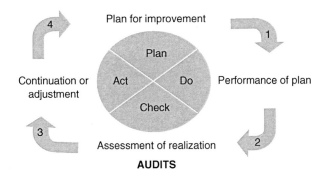

Figure 32.1 Total quality management (TQM): the Deming cycle.

QUALITY POLICY

One of the first steps for the implementation of a QM system in medical institutions is to define the quality policy. Quality policies are a group of principles that establish the workings of the institution. Although successful treatment of an existing disease or reduction of discomfort is certainly the highest priority for most medical institutions, it might be an important goal to achieve this in the most efficient manner possible. This means that structure is needed to assure that diagnostic and therapeutic procedures are performed using as little financial, organizational, personnel, or time resources as possible, while still striving for a high quality of treatment. After all, optimum quality is achieved by the "right" balance of cost with quality achievement. The quality policy of a medical institution cannot be defined by a single person (e.g., the owner or medical director), but should be developed as a consensus between management and employees. Only in this way will personnel identify with the quality policy of the institution. A quality policy should be formulated in an active manner and the formulation should also be short and simple so that every employee can repeat the quality policy at any time. The most important aspects of the quality policy should be posted in suitable and accessible areas of the institution for employees, patients, and visitors, to strengthen the employees' knowledge of common goals, improve their identification with their own fields of competence, and communicate these principles to others. It is important to state that quality policies should be reviewed periodically to make sure that the principles are still valid and that management and employees still agree with them. As an organization's perspectives and goals change, the quality policy needs to be modified accordingly.

MANAGEMENT'S RESPONSIBILITY

In spite of the fact that the responsibility of management (or the governing structure) can be defined differently in various medical institutions, according to ISO standards, certain generally valid aspects can be defined. The hierarchy of the institution has to be defined and outlined clearly. While, in most cases, hospitals are administered by an appointed director, the structure might be more difficult in private centers with multiple partners in equal positions. In such cases, an agreement that describes the division of responsibilities for particular fields among the partners must be in place and in these cases several possibilities are available. For example, it is possible to place specific responsibilities permanently under the authority of one of the partners (e.g., personnel development/ accounting/billing, etc.). However, for many privately held practices, a model of dividing these tasks on a rotational basis has been successful; i.e., dividing the responsibility for various fields equally among all of the partners (in leadership positions) so that all partners are familiar with the different responsibilities. The picture becomes far more complex if there are many administrative layers

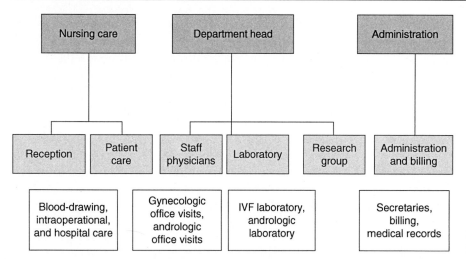

Figure 32.2 Organizational diagram. *Abbreviation*: IVF, in vitro fertilization.

to the organization and it is here that clear descriptions of authority for all positions within the organization are required and must be available to everyone within the organization. The more complex the hierarchic structures within a medical institution are, the more precisely these structures have to be defined for the system to work effectively and robustly at all times and under all (extraordinary) conditions. The "decision" of the head of the organization must be available at any time, even if he or she is absent. Therefore, this must be absolutely clear to everyone within the organization who has the competence and authority to make decisions. It is also important for all partners outside of the company to be aware of who the decision makers are for various tasks. There are various ways of making these structures as transparent as possible. One easy way is the development of an organizational diagram (Fig. 32.2). This organizational diagram can be placed in a suitable and accessible location, helping employees to understand everyone's roles and responsibilities. Furthermore, making the organizational diagram available to everyone strengthens trust, cooperation, and professionalism within the company. It is also important in communication with patients, interested parties, or cooperating departments. The organizational diagram should be updated frequently. Management should strongly support the quality policies for the company, and should take an active part in its development and implementation. It is important to lead by example.

MANAGEMENT OF PROCESSES

Processes are all the procedures that are necessary for the completion of tasks. For medical facilities, the most important processes are those of diagnostic and therapeutic procedures. In addition, many other processes are involved in the care of patients, such as the scheduling of patients for tests, communication, and anything else that may greatly affect the patient's (= customer's) perspective. Sometimes poor communication can ruin a patient's experience, despite the best diagnostic procedures within the organization. In fact, it is our observation that it is more likely that a patient will leave a medical facility

because of an organizational problem such as a substandard secretarial or administrative problem rather than a medical deficiency. Even with properly working medical treatment, poor communication with colleagues can endanger or directly destroy the positive result of the treatment. When establishing a QM system, it is necessary to precisely define and describe all relevant processes and to structure them according to QM guidelines. These descriptions are often best realized by flow diagrams that can overlap in various places. These areas of contact between two flow diagrams are called "boundaries, interferences, joints, or areas of juncture."

Documentation in a QM System

In addition to defining the processes relevant for the system, it is important for everything to be documented. The different levels of documentation are shown in Figure 32.3. One of the most important documents in a QM system is the quality manual. The main purpose of the quality manual is to outline the structure of the documentation used in the quality system (12). It should also include or refer to the standard operating procedures (SOPs). There should be clear definitions of the management's areas of responsibility, including its responsibility for ensuring compliance with the international standards on which the system is built. A simple overview of the quality system requirements and the position of the quality manual are shown in Figure 32.3. A good-quality manual should be precise and brief; it should be an easily navigable handbook for the whole quality system. The most important procedures are preferably included in the manual itself, but deeper descriptions should be referred to in the underlying documentation. An easy way to start building a system is to make up a table of contents for the quality manual and to decide which processes should be described in the manual and which should rather be described in the underlying documentation (e.g., SOPs). Whereas the quality manual contains more general information, the individual processes and procedures are described in a more detailed way in handbooks/job instructions or SOPs. These SOPs go through the processes step-by-step and

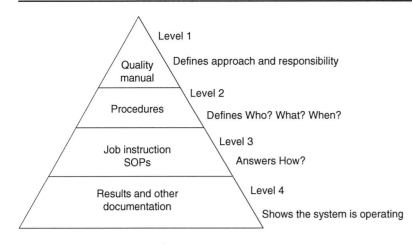

Figure 32.3 Levels of documentation. *Abbreviation*: SOP, standard operating procedure.

describe the materials and methods used and the way the process is performed precisely. Standard operating procedure manuals should be available to all personnel and every single procedure in these manuals must be fully documented with signature, date, and regular review.

Document Control

According to ISO 9001:2000 4.2.3, the clinic should establish and maintain procedures to control all documents that form part of its quality documentation. This includes both internally generated documentation such as SOPs and protocol sheets, and externally generated documentation such as law texts, standards, and instruction manuals for equipments. Document handling and control are an important part of the quality system and, if not designed properly, can become a heavy load for a smooth running system. Since it is something that touches every part of the system, it is important to sit down and think through how this system of paperwork shall be handled in your clinic and to ensure that the system you choose covers the demands of the standards. The identification of the documents should be logical, and it is a good suggestion to use numbers as unique identifiers. The same identification number could then be used for the file name within the computerized version. The issue number in parentheses or after a dash could follow this number. Pagination is important. If you choose not to use pagination, you must clearly mark where the document starts and ends. The dates of issue together with information on who wrote the document and who approved it (signature) are usually included in the document header. Questions that should have an answer in your document control system:

1. Is *all* documentation in the laboratory or clinic covered by your document control system?
2. Who writes or changes the document?
3. Who approves and has the authority to issue documents?
4. Does the document have
   a. A unique identification?
   b. Issue number and current revision status?
   c. Date of latest issue?
   d. Pagination?
5. Where can I find the document: physical location, level in the system, and on computer file?
6. Who assures that only the latest issue of the document is present in the system, removes outdated issues, and files them?
7. Are amendments to documents clearly marked, initialled, and dated?
8. How are changes in a document implemented with the personnel?

Documentation of Results

A very important level of documentation is that of the "results." This includes not only the results of treatment such as pregnancy rate per treatment cycle, but also all documents referring to:

1. Control of quality records,
2. Internal audits,
3. Control of nonconformity,
4. Corrective and preventive action.

Incubators are one of the most important pieces of equipment in the IVF laboratory and need to be controlled properly. Two markers of incubator performance are the temperature and the CO_2 level. These two parameters are documented on the control cards, and upper and lower limits of tolerance are defined to determine when corrective actions are needed (Fig. 32.4). It is useful to plot results of system checks on a graph, so that there is a clear visual image that can monitor:

1. Dispersion: Increased frequency of both high and low numbers.
2. Trend: Progressive drift of reported values from a prior mean.
3. Shift: An abrupt change from the established mean.

If nonconformity to the standard is diagnosed, it is important to collect data on:

1. When the problem was realized.
2. How often the problem could be identified.
3. How conformity to the standards could be reassured.

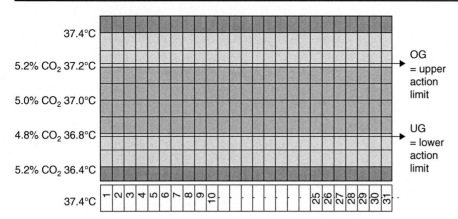

Figure 32.4 Monitoring temperature and CO_2 levels in an incubator.

Audits and Management Reviews

Audits are essential to ensure that a quality system is working. Audits can be internal, initiated by the organization itself, or external, initiated by a governing body, certification, or accreditation body. ISO 9001:2000 8.8.2 lays out the rules for internal audits and demands that the clinic undertakes internal audits at planned intervals to determine how well the system is functioning and if it is effectively implemented and maintained. Audits are tools for improving and keeping your system up to date with the standards and it is the quality manual that should include specific instructions covering both how and how often they shall be performed. The management usually chooses internal auditors, and they should be familiar with both the standards and the activities performed in the clinic. The manual should include a document describing the approach and the areas of responsibility for the internal auditors and have well-documented procedures for how internal auditors are trained. To achieve a certification according to ISO 9001:2000, the clinic needs to be audited externally by a certification body. Many organizations believe that having an audit and not finding any nonconformities is a proof of an outstanding performance. However, the other possibility is that it could be due to an inadequate audit procedure. If an audit is properly conducted, even in organizations with outstanding performance, areas for improvement will be found; therefore, people should put in a lot of effort to find the right certification body to undertake the audits. Some questions that might help to identify a good certification body are:

- Are they accredited to certify medical institutions?
- Have they previously certified IVF clinics and how many?
- Do they have IVF experts on their audit team?
- How much time do they allocate to the audit?

While to some it may seem obvious, it is important to mention, especially with respect to the factors above, that the cheapest certifying body is not necessarily the best.

Together with the audits, the management review is important for improvement of the system and for the long-term correction of errors and incidents that might occur. According to ISO 9007:2000 5.6, the management of the clinic with executive responsibility shall periodically conduct a review of the quality system and testing activities. The quality manual shall include a written agenda for these reviews, which should fulfill the demands in the standard.

INCIDENTS AND COMPLAINTS

All clinics should have a policy and procedure for the resolution of incidents and complaints received from patients, clients, and/or other parties. The routines of how these are filed and how corrective actions are taken should be documented in a clinic's quality manual. When applying a quality system it is important not to hide these incidents and complaints, but to use them as resources to improve the system. The management reviews should ensure that the incidents and complaints lead to long-term corrections and improvements in the quality of work.

STAFF MANAGEMENT

High-quality treatment can only be realized with qualified staff. Therefore, recruitment, training, and motivation of highly qualified people are the most important tasks for the management team of an organization. To make sure that a sufficient number of qualified people are working within the respective areas of the institution, a staff requirement plan should be developed. This can be organized in different ways:

1. Allocating people according to their abilities.
2. Allocating people according to different responsibility levels.
3. Allocating people according to the type of work that has to be done.

In most medical institutions it is recommended to define the levels for which the number of staff should be planned. Thus, the leading level (management) and other levels (which can be further divided according to qualification) are defined. The number of employees should be determined, for particular fields, according to their tasks and the range of treatments. This is why a regulation for the equalization of staff must be created. This system makes planning easier, and emphasizes the qualifications and, for instance, the procedure of substitution. The development of work descriptions is crucial for this system. They must be created for particular posts, and must state, among other things, at which post a given employee works, what his or her qualification is, and which qualification attributes are required. In addition to this formal information, the work description should also contain information about the employee's personal attributes. For various posts, different qualities are important:

1.   Social competence
2.   Organizing abilities
3.   Communication abilities, etc.

The staff requirement plan must be set up so that it is possible to react sufficiently to unexpected situations. Furthermore, it must consider staff absenteeism caused by holidays, illness, and further education. A minimal presence of employees must be determined for certain fields, which does not depend on the actual workload. For the development of a staff requirement plan for an IVF center, the medical as well as the nonmedical areas have to be defined and considered. The question of how many people are needed to do the job properly can be answered on the basis of calculating the "influence magnitudes." The type of services offered strongly influences the number of people required. Thus, the staff requirements are different in a center in which predominantly conservative treatments and intrauterine inseminations are performed, compared with a center in which predominantly IVF/intracytoplasmic sperm injection (ICSI) and cryopreservation cycles are performed.

Training of Employees

One of the most important principles for the management of a medical institution is: "Give your employees the chance to be the best." This means that if you expect your employees to do their work at the highest quality level possible, you should give them proper training. In principle, there are two different types of educational events:

1.   Internal events of further education
2.   External events of further education (i.e., conventions, conferences, workshops, etc.).

The advantage of internal events of further education is that they can be offered on a regular basis and are usually "low-budget projects," whereas external events need more organizational and financial input. However, when carefully planned, external educational events sometimes have a higher motivational aspect. So the management team should take care to offer a balanced program of internal and external educational events. To make it possible to use the clinics' resources adequately and to estimate and plan the potential of development with regard to the individual abilities of particular employees

or with regard to the abilities of the entire institution, educational activities should be evaluated and analyzed at regular intervals. For example, at the beginning of each year, the employee should decide which educational events he or she would like to visit or take part in. This helps the management to introduce new fields of activity, and also allows them to perform advance planning of the specialization. It is striking to see that, in most ART centers, detailed and prospective plans have been developed for the training of medical doctors, but far less attention has been paid to the training of nurses, technicians, etc. However, a well-trained nurse can significantly reduce the workload for the doctor and tremendously increase the patient's trust in the institution while also improving the referring doctor's satisfaction.

Therefore, besides training activities for the doctors, adequate educational events for nurses and technicians, etc., should be considered.

Interaction between Management and Employees

Success in reproductive medicine clearly depends on an optimal interaction between different professional groups: i.e., success can be achieved only if doctors communicate and work together with staff in the laboratory, nurses, receptionists, etc. The same is true for the interaction between management and employees. Communication and collaboration between different professional groups of the same hierarchic rank is called "horizontal" communication, whereas communication and collaboration between professional groups of different hierarchic ranks is called "vertical" communication. One of the most important instruments to optimize vertical communication is the "staff interview." The staff interviews should occur periodically. At these interviews the empolyees and their direct superiors discuss their collaboration and identify areas for improvement. The interview should take place in a structured way and a protocol should be written and signed by both sides, so that the content of the interview is assigned some kind of formal character. However, details of the interview can never be communicated with others without mutual consent. For the employee, the goals/opportunities of the interview are:

1.   To become familiar with the goals of the department,
2.   To realize weaknesses and strengths,
3.   To be able to discuss own experiences/opinions on the management style,
4.   To discuss further strategies for professional development,
5.   To participate in planning goals/strategies for the future.

For the superior, the goals/opportunities of the interview are:

1.   To discuss the coworker's performance,
2.   To focus the activities of the employee on future goals of the institution,

3. To increase mutual understanding in the event of problems,
4. To increase the employee's responsibility,
5. To get feedback on his/her management skills.

For the above-mentioned reasons, the staff interview is one of the most important and powerful tools in staff development, and should be widely used in the process of continuous improvement.

The EU Tissues and Cells Directive

The increase in use, donation, and storage of human tissue has led to the creation of directives from the European Council. In March 2004, the European parliament issued a new version of the directive on setting standards of quality and safety for the donation, procurement, testing, processing, preservation, storage, and distribution of human tissues and cells. When these directives were issued, there was a need to adapt the requirements to the actual setting of an IVF laboratory. However, in the meantime, these directives have been implemented by many IVF centers around the world and a position paper has been issued by the ESHRE outlining how these directives should be applied. Independent of this position, paper authorities in each country interpret the directive differently, which makes it difficult to share experiences between centers in different countries. Furthermore auditing processes need to be adapted from country to country.

The main differences between the countries concern requirements for (1) air quality (2) frequency of screening of patients, and (3) staff training.

However, the central part of the EU directive is very clear, concerning the demand for a quality system. Therefore the directive states that "Tissue establishments shall take all necessary measures to ensure that the quality system includes at least the following documentation: standard operating procedures, guidelines, training and reference manuals." Certainly by achieving accreditation to either ISO17025 or ISO15189 this demand will be fulfilled together with several other demands of the directive.

CONCLUSIONS

No internationally accepted standards exist for quality in the IVF laboratory and the IVF center as a whole. To assure high quality and continual improvement, it is recommended that all IVF centers striving for excellence should consider a QM system. Furthermore, legal guidelines and the recently released EU Tissue Directive clearly demand a QM system for medical institutions. A QM system allows the organization to gain control of its documents and procedures and to monitor the clinical and nonclinical outcomes. Furthermore, the issues of staff recruitment and staff development can be addressed systematically and thereby, again, the overall outcome will be improved. The ISO standards offer the medical facility access to an internationally endorsed and proven QM system. ART practitioners in particular have the unique opportunity to set the standard in medicine for quality management principles.

SUGGESTED READING

Alper MM, Brinsden PR, Fischer R, Wikland M. Is your IVF programme good? Hum Reprod 2002; 17: 8–10.

American Society for Reproductive Medicine. Revised minimum standards for in vitro fertilization, gamete intrafallopian transfer and related procedures. http://www.asrm.com/media/practice/revised.html (1998)

Bloor G. Organisational culture, organisational learning and total quality management: a literature review and synthesis. Aust Health Rev 1999; 22: 162–79.

Bron MS, Salmon JW. Infertility services and managed care. Am J Manag Care 1998; 4: 715–20.

Brown RW. Errors in medicine. J Qual Clin Pract 1997; 17: 21–5.

Carson BE, Alper MM, Keck C. Quality management systems for assisted reproductive technology. London: Taylor and Francis, 2004.

Clancy C. AHRQ: coordinating a quantity of quality. Healthplan 2003; 44: 42–6.

Collings J. An international survey of the health economics of IVF and ICSI. Hum Reprod Update 2002; 8: 265–77.

Colton D. The design of evaluations for continuous quality improvement. Eval Health Prof 1997; 20: 265–85.

Darr K. Risk management and quality improvement: together at last – Part. Hosp Top 1999; 77: 29–35.

Garceau L, Henderson J, Davis LJ, et al. Economic implications of assisted reproductive techniques: a systematic review. Hum Reprod 2002; 17: 3090–109.

Geraedts HP, Montenarie R, Van Rijk PP. The benefits of total quality management. Comput Med Imaging Graph 2001; 25: 217–20.

Glattacker M, Jackel WH. [Evaluation of quality assurance – current data and consequences for research]. Gesundheitswesen 2007; 69(5): 277–83.

Gondringer NS. Benchmarking: friend or foe. AANAJ 1997; 65: 335–6.

Greenberg L. Accreditation strengthens the disease management bridge over the quality chasm. Dis Manag 2003; 6: 3–8.

ISO/DIS 15189:2:2002. Medical Laboratories – Particular requirements for quality and competence. Geneva: International Standardization Organization, 2002.

Matson PL. Internal quality control and external quality assurance in the IVF laboratory. Hum Reprod 1998; 13(Suppl 4): 156–65.

Minkman M, Ahaus K, Huijsman R. Performance improvement based on integrated quality management models: what evidence do we have? A systematic literature review. Int J Qual Health Care 2007; 19(2): 90–104.

Sackett DL, Rosenberg WMC, Gray JAM, et al. Evidence based medicine: what it is and what it isn't. Br Med J 1996; 312: 71–6.

Sandle LN. The management of external quality assurance. J Clin Pathol 2005; 58(2): 141–4.

Sciacovelli L, Secchiero S, Zardo L, et al. Risk management in laboratory medicine: quality assurance programs and professional competence. Clin Chem Lab Med 2007; 45(6): 756–65.

Shaw CD. External quality mechanisms for health care: summary of the ExPeRT project on visitatie, accreditations, EFQM and ISO assessment in European Union countries. External Peer Review Techniques. European Foundation for Quality Management. International Organization for Standardization. Int J Qual Health Care 2000; 12: 169–75.

Varkey P, Reller MK, Resar RK. Basics of quality improvement in health care. Mayo Clin Proc 2007; 82(6): 735–9.

Vogelsang J. Quantitative research versus quality assurance, quality improvement total quality management and continuous quality improvement. J Perianesth Nurs 1999; 14: 78–81.

Warnes GM, Norman RJ. Quality management systems in ART: are they really needed? An Australian clinic's experience. Best Pract Res Clin Obstet Gynaecol 2007; 21(1): 41–55.

Yasin MM, Meacham KA, Alavi J. The status of TQM in healthcare. Health Mark Q 1998; 15: 61–84.

RELEVANT INTERNET ADDRESSES

http://www.agrbm.de
http://www.asrm.com
http://www.eshre.com
http://www.ferti.net
http://www.guideline.gov
http://www.iso.ch
http://www.isoeasy.org
http://www.ivf.net/ace
http://www.praxion.com

REFERENCES

1. Pinter E, Vitt KD. Umfassendes Qualitätsmanagement für das Krankenhaus – Perspektiven und Beispiele. Frankfurt: pmi-Verlag, 1996.
2. Viethen G. Qualität im Krankenhaus. Grundbegriffe und Modelle des Qualitätsmanagements. Stuttgart: Schattauer-Verlag, 1995.
3. ISO 9001:2000. Quality management systems – Requirements. Geneva: International Standardization Organization, 1987.
4. ISO/IEC 17025:1999. General requirements for the competence of testing and calibration laboratories. Geneva: International Standardization Organization, 1999.
5. ISO/IEC Guide 25:1990.General requirements for the competence of testing and calibration laboratories. Geneva: International Standardization Organization, 1990.
6. EN 45001:1991. General criteria for the operation of testing laboratories.
7. American Fertility Society. Guidelines for human andrology laboratories. Suppl 1: 1–16.
8. Gianaroli L, Plachot M, Van Kooij R, et al. Committee of the special interest group on embryology. ESHRE guidelines for good practice in IVF laboratories. Hum Reprod 2000; 15: 2241–6.
9. [Available from: http://www.cap.org/lap/rlap.html]
10. Association of Clinical Embryologists UK. Accreditation standards and guidelines for IVF laboratories, 2001. [Available from: http://www.ivf.net/ace/accred1.html]
11. Directive 2004/23/EC of the European Parliament and of the Council of 31 March, 2004 on setting standards of quality and safety for the donation, procurement, testing, processing, preservation, storage and distribution of human tissues and cells. Official Journal of the European Union, L 102, 7.4.2004, 48–58. [Available from: http://europa.eu.int/eur-lex/en/oj/]
12. Huismam W. Quality system in the medical laboratory: the role of a quality manual. Ann Biol Clin (Paris) 1994; 52: 457–61.

33

Lifestyle, periconception, and fertility

Robert J. Norman, Lisa J. Moran, and Sarah A. Robertson

INTRODUCTION

Reproductive health critically impacts a couple's well-being and functional capacity throughout their life. The reproductive system, with its controlling hormones and cyclical changes, governs physiological events at puberty, across the menstrual cycle, during pregnancy, and in parturition, lactation, and menopause. The majority of women experience some form of reproductive disorder over the course of life, and many chronic and severe reproductive disorders remain without preventative strategies, clear diagnostics, or successful treatment. Even "normal" pregnancy can reveal or precipitate underlying chronic metabolic disease. The direct cost of maternal and neonatal conditions is substantial (1).

Importantly, the reproductive health of a woman and of her partner is also the single greatest determinant of the health and well-being of their children. We now understand that the life potential of every individual is set in train in very early life, during the periconception period when the oocytes mature and embryos are formed. A less than optimal environment in utero predisposes an individual to diseases in adulthood including obesity, heart disease, diabetes, and stroke, to an extent comparable in magnitude to genetic predisposition and lifestyle factors such as obesity and smoking (2). Understanding early life events and how they contribute to health or resilience to disease is a fundamental component of intergenerational health, whereby the health of one generation affects that of the next.

Fundamental knowledge gaps that currently exist are:

1. What environmental and genetic factors determine the optimal function of sperm and eggs?
2. What are the critical biological events and pathways in the periconception period that promote or constrain developmental competence in the oocyte and embryo, to affect health and functional capacity in later life?
3. How do environmental conditions, genes, and maternal reproductive disorders influence developmental competence in the oocyte and embryo, and optimal growth in the fetus?
4. How do we best translate fundamental knowledge gains to better predict and diagnose reproductive disorders, improve periconception health, and maximize pregnancy outcome?
5. What is the role of male factors in determining health in the sperm, embryo, and fetus?

GOALS OF PRE-CONCEPTION HEALTH

Our goal should be to make important basic discoveries and to capitalize on these to prevent disease and disability and build resilience in our community through clinical and public health interventions targeting early stages in life. This will be best achieved by a cross-disciplinary approach spanning basic biomedical science, epidemiology, and translational research. Integration of cell and molecular biology, physiology, immunology, and new technologies (genomics and sensing) with clinical and epidemiological studies promise the best approach to new paradigms for appropriate health care. Preconception care is more than just improving fertility – it is also about optimal outcomes for children born as a result of both natural conception and after assisted reproductive technique (ART).

SOCIETAL IMPORTANCE

The global community recognizes the critical value of reproductive health and its necessity for health and resilience in our children. This is reflected in the Australian Federal Government's "Healthy Start to Life" National Research Priority. International commitment to reproductive health was declared at the 1994 International Conference on Population and Development in Cairo (3), reaffirmed at the 1995 Fourth World Conference on Women (4), and reinforced in 2000, when the UN Millennium Declaration specified the 5th Millennium Development Goal to "Improve maternal health," with a focus on sexual and reproductive health (5). While the quality of reproductive health in first world countries is clearly higher than in developing countries, major opportunity for health gains exist there also for women and future generations, particularly in economically disadvantaged or rural communities.

A GROWING UNDERSTANDING OF PRECONCEPTION CARE

Exposure to teratogens and nutrient deficiency were linked to congenital defects during the last century and these concepts dominated maternal–fetal research. In the 21st century, the greatest health gains stand to be made from research addressing more cryptic but pervasive ill-health outcomes with long latencies that are functional rather than structural, which emerge through interactions between the individual and the environment, and which have effects that endure across generations.

There are multiple points of vulnerability throughout the pre-birth and post-birth phases of life that are prone to the positive or negative impact of internal and external influences. We and others have shown that the very earliest stages of embryogenesis are most susceptible. At this time the organism is rapidly developing and must exhibit great plasticity to best survive the number and scale of critical transitions from zygote to fetus (6).

The earliest determinant of life potential is the oocyte, the developmental competence of which is influenced by the local hormonal, growth factor, and cellular environment of the ovarian follicle in which it grows (7,8). After fertilization, developmental plasticity is desirable so that the early embryo can respond to the demands and opportunities of the outside world by adaptation, rather than by adhering to a standard fixed phenotype that may be inappropriate to the changing external environment. Plasticity can be exerted at the cellular level by adjustment of cell numbers and fate, and at the molecular level by changes in gene expression pathways or the more permanent effects of epigenetics (9–11). Together these processes exert modifications through which the periconception environment can modulate the phenotype to "best suit" the prevailing or predicted afterbirth environment. Cytokines and growth factors secreted by maternal tract cells, as well as metabolic substrates and other physiochemical agents, are implicated as signals through which the embryo senses its local environment (12).

From the mother's perspective, imposing constraints and selection pressures upon the conceptus is necessary to avoid unfavorable investment of reproductive resources and to maximize offspring health. The mammalian female has limited opportunities for pregnancy during her reproductive life span and each pregnancy costs resources and poses a risk to her own health. The majority of early embryos fail to survive and only ~60% of embryos that implant persist beyond the second week. There are evolutionary advantages associated with active female-controlled processes for discerning the suitability of male gametes and embryos (13). The female immune response is "aware" of fetal transplantation antigens and is competent to discriminate the reproductive fitness and compatibility of the male partner and the integrity and developmental competence of the conceptus tissue (14,15). Since the immune response is modulated by the individual's infectious, inflammatory, stress, nutritional, and metabolic status, immune influence on progression or disruption of pregnancy may be further influenced by environmental stressors and resource availability. Emerging evidence suggests that the immune system can integrate these signals to exert executive quality control to either accommodate or reject the conceptus. "Immune-mediated quality control" facilitates optimal female

reproductive investment and explains the evolutionary advantage of engaging the immune system in the events of reproduction (16).

With plasticity and maternal selection comes the risk of poor outcomes – when embryo sensing of the external environment fails to properly indicate and match the reality, where compromises made to favor immediate survival are suboptimal for longevity of life after birth – or when maternal quality control systems are inappropriately executed or otherwise faulty. In broad terms it seems that extreme adaptation causes loss of functional capacity and resistance to future stressors, while maintenance of capacity in early intrauterine life improves the likelihood of subsequent health and resilience in adulthood (17). If capacity is lost in early embryonic and fetal development, the possibility of dysfunction in later life becomes higher (Fig. 33.1).

The permanent effects of exerting early plasticity are often not readily observable until later in fetal or postnatal life. Changes in cell numbers and lineage allocation, or in gene or protein expression in blastocysts due to perturbation in the local physiochemical or cytokine environment (18–20) cause differences in placental structure and nutrient transport function, which is the key limiting factor in fetal growth (21,22).

Experimental perturbations at various stages of pregnancy implicate the first days of life as the most susceptible period for later fetal and postnatal growth impairment (23). Altered embryo development, or insufficient maternal support of the conceptus at implantation can lead to later miscarriage, or "shallow" placental development resulting in preeclampsia, fetal growth restriction, and/or preterm delivery (24,25). In turn these conditions affect growth after birth and impart a "thrifty" phenotype that leads to metabolic disorder and onset of chronic disease. Thus maternal stress in the periconception period due to nutritional, metabolic, immunological, infectious, pharmacological, or

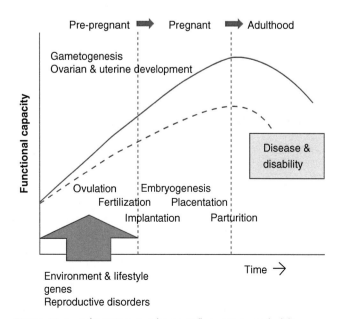

Figure 33.1 Adaptation to adverse influences in early life causes loss of functional capacity after birth.

psychosocial perturbations can exert subtle but permanent alterations in the life-course trajectory of the offspring (Fig. 33.2).

Epidemiological evidence in humans is consistent with the animal data showing that environment before birth sets in train either good health or disease in later life, and that early pregnancy is the most vulnerable period (18,26,27). Vulnerability to pathologies of pregnancy that precipitate poor perinatal outcome is further influenced by maternal, paternal, and fetal genotype (28). Low birth weight for gestational age predisposes to later incidence of cardiovascular disease, impaired glucose tolerance, hypertension, and hyperlipidemia, particularly when there is postnatal catch-up growth due to overnutrition (29–33). The association between perinatal parameters and adult health is evident even after adjusting for lifestyle factors, occupation, income, diet, and socioeconomic status.

Maternal reproductive disorders such as polycystic ovary syndrome (PCOS), endometriosis, and ovulation disorders influence periconception events, alter endometrial receptivity, and quality control sensing, and impart stress on the gametes and embryo (Fig. 33.2) (34,35). Chronic sexually transmitted infection is another key factor that influences the maternal environment. All of these conditions may exert their effects through altering the cytokine environment and local inflammatory mediators, as well as through effects on reproductive tissue structural integrity and function. ART, which is now the method of conception for 3% of Australian children (36), also inflicts substantial stress on the embryo (37). We now recognise that in vitro embryo culture in media deficient in maternal signaling factors, as well as the gonadotropin-induced altered hormone environment imposed on the oocyte prior to conception, predispose to growth restriction and attendant life-long effects on children (37–39). There is evidence that transgenerational programming is a key factor in PCOS and that other forms of reproductive dysfunction can be programmed in utero (40–42). Competition in the womb through twinning or higher order multiple pregnancy, irrespective of ART or spontaneous occurrence, also causes fetal growth impairment and can bring adverse life-long consequences (43).

FACTORS THAT AFFECT FERTILITY

Weight, Exercise, and Nutrition

The prevalence of overweight young couples in the reproductive age of life is steadily increasing (44) and there is now abundant evidence that female weight disorders, both under- and overweight, impair spontaneous fertility (45,46). There is also emerging evidence to implicate male weight disorders with subfertility (47). The data for the effect of weight on fertility after IVF is not as clear for both males and females. Initial data on the adverse effect of female infertility was compelling and has been sustained (48–50), although the degree of impact has been tempered by improved culture media and conditions reflected in the reduced differential between obese and nonobese pregnancy rates in recent publications. It is reasonable to assume ongoing pregnancy rates are less after IVF in obese women with a higher risk of miscarriage, congenital abnormality, gestational diabetes, preeclampsia, and complications of delivery and in the puerperium. Male obesity also impairs fertility after IVF, although the impact is not as marked (51). Recent data also suggests a non-genomic transfer of metabolic disorders via sperm and if confirmed, this implies much more attention needs to be paid to optimization of male and female health and nutrition prior to pregnancy (52).

Diet

There are a number of dietary factors that have an impact on reproduction:

- Vitamins. While there is little conclusive evidence on the effect of vitamins on fertility, more substantive evidence, particularly on folic acid, is published on their effect on reducing congenital abnormalities (53). It is therefore advised that women take up to 400 ug of folate for several weeks prior to conception and, where there is a higher risk of abnormality, 5 mg. It is recommended women avoid vitamin A and foods containing this vitamin while considering consuming vitamin D, given the alleged deficiency in many populations (54–57).
- Iodine. Many women seeking pregnancy are iodine deficient and iodine is often added to prenatal supplements or foods (58,59).
- Male antioxidants. Oxidative stress is frequently described in infertile males and the role of antioxidants has been debated (60). While several commercial

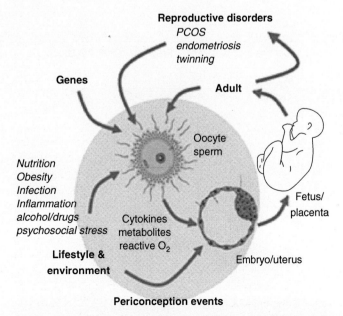

Figure 33.2 Periconception events are influenced by genes, a range of lifestyle/environmental factors, and maternal factors including reproductive disorders to impact fetal development and adult outcome.

preparations exist, attention to increased fruit and vegetables in the diet and avoidance of adverse lifestyle factors including environmental chemical exposure should be the first step (61).

- Alcohol. It remains unclear regarding the level of alcohol consumption allowable in the periconception period and several official bodies recommend complete abstinence (57). A large European study of more than 4000 couples linked high alcohol use (≥8 drinks/week) to reduced fertility (62) and the role of alcohol in the fetal alcohol syndrome is well-known (63).
- Caffeine. Caffeine is the most popular neurostimulant and is found in drinks and foods across all cultures. A high consumption of caffeine may be associated with impaired fecundity although the evidence is not conclusive (57,64–69). While a safe level of caffeine has not been defined, it seems reasonable to keep this below 200–300 mg per day (less than 2 cups of coffee per day) (68–71).
- Methyl mercury. Certain types of fish high in mercury should be avoided while acknowledging that a high polyunsaturated diet as given by fish is desirable (54,55,72).

Smoking

Meta-analysis of the literature indicates that smoking is a very significant risk factor for male and female infertility and that it negatively affects the outcomes of IVF cycles (73–75). For female smokers this can be as high an odds ratio for infertility as 1.6 (1.34–1.91) (74). Sperm studies have shown increased oxidative stress, a lower sperm count, and abnormal sperm fertilizing capacity, with a significantly reduced chance of pregnancy in a female partner (76,77). Passive smoking is also important in increasing complications in pregnancy as well as in IVF cycles (78–80).

Illicit Drugs

Marijuana increases female infertility (81) and significantly affects sperm function and form (82). Cocaine impairs ovarian responsiveness and alters sperm function (83,84) while heroin and methadone also have significant effects (45,85). Anabolic steroids can reduce testicular sperm production, while the role of other lifestyle drugs is still to be explored (86).

Other Prescription Drugs

There are many drugs that appear to affect fertility and alter reproductive outcomes (57,87). These should be assessed during initial consultations and the patient should be recommended to seek alternatives if actively trying to become pregnant.

Stress

There is growing evidence that stress is associated with negative reproductive outcomes, including IVF therapies (88–92). Appropriate counseling and lifestyle adjustments may ameliorate these effects.

Environmental Pollutants

While there is a vast and controversial literature on this subject, some environmental agents may adversely affect outcomes of reproductive interventions (72,93–95). It would seem prudent to ask all patients for their occupational and environmental exposures to endocrine disrupting chemicals such as phthalates and other potentially dangerous products (54–56,72,93,95–98).

Vaccinations

There is little data on the impact of vaccinations on fertility but the consequences of becoming infected with rubella, herpes zoster, varicella zoster, and influenza would suggest that immunization prior to pregnancy would be appropriate (54,99,100).

Sexually Transmitted Diseases

It is increasingly evident that bacterial and viral infections of the reproductive tissues can alter immune and inflammatory parameters in such a way as to impede periconception events and reduce fertility. The recommendation is that couples should seek advice from their clinical care provider regarding detection and treatment of any infection of the reproductive tract, remembering that many (such as Chlamydia) are widespread in the community and may not necessarily result in signs or symptoms.

PREPREGNANCY PREPARATION

Given the theoretical and practical background to preconception health, the desire of infertile couples to seek specialist treatment and the opportunity to favorably influence outcomes of fertility treatment, all clinics should have a program to assess adverse genetic and lifestyle influences on reproduction and an intervention protocol to minimise their detrimental effects. This is best achieved at the first interview with the doctor or nurse. Action can then be advised while there is time for an effective plan to be instituted by the clinic and couple (Fig. 33.3). This may be as simple as taking folic acid and changing diet to optimize the periconception environment through to active weight loss programs, smoking cessation interventions, and elimination of inappropriate alcohol and drug use. There is currently no evidence assessing this approach and a recent Cochrane review was unable to come up with any randomised trials on intervention for lifestyle in infertile couples (101). There is more research on weight management and fertility. Several groups have described programs for weight loss in the context of a fertility clinic with the best known being that by Clark from Adelaide (Fertility Fitness) (102,103). In this program, 5% weight loss was associated with a dramatic improvement in spontaneous and IVF pregnancy rates. Other popular community or expert-based facilities are available in the general community to improve lifestyle prior to pregnancy or while actively intervening.

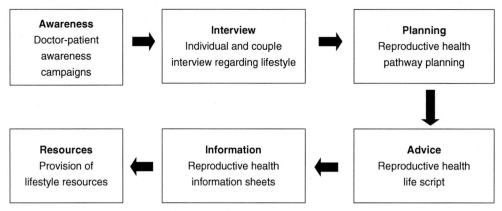

Figure 33.3 An approach to assessing and managing lifestyle in a clinical setting.

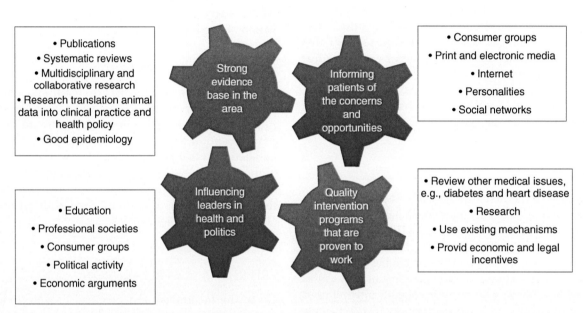

Figure 33.4 A society-wide approach to achieving lifestyle changes.

There is a responsibility on governments to facilitate and encourage various aspects of preconception care including promoting vaccination, controlling alcohol and smoking use, providing a safe workplace, and giving general reproductive education (Fig. 33.4). The clinic and individual, however, have an even greater role in safeguarding reproductive security by ensuring any pregnancy is conceived with gametes and embryos that have had the best chance to achieve their full genetic potential.

SUMMARY

In summary, there is compelling evidence that external and endogenous events impact preconception and very early pregnancy to benefit or constrain the later health of the neonate, child, and adult. Events in the pre- and peri-implantation period, spanning gametogenesis, conception, and early placental morphogenesis, have the power to impart long-term susceptibility or resilience in our children and community.

Defining the nature and actions of these external and endogenous events is now within reach. We know several of the key interlocutory signals between the oocyte and follicle, the sperm and oocyte, and the conceptus and uterus, but their full identity and interaction with environmental factors, reproductive disorders, and genetic background remains to be elucidated. Some of the most potent stressors for embryos and gametes are lifestyle factors – very young or older age, obesity, sexually transmitted infection, drugs, alcohol, diet, vitamin deficiency, and psychosocial stress. Understanding how these factors affect periconception biology will inform how public health initiatives can be targeted to modify behaviors and educate prospective parents. Similarly, the maternal reproductive disorders that impact early development are amenable to better diagnosis and clinical treatments. Defining their effects on the ovary and uterus, gametes, embryo and placenta, and their interactions with environmental factors in the context of different genetic settings, is required to focus and prioritize clinical interventions. Despite the complexity in these interactions, we postulate that several stressors converge through a few key common inflammatory and metabolic pathways. Therefore, the prospect of identifying drug targets or interventions to minimise, reverse, or protect against adverse early environments may also be achievable.

REFERENCES

1. Australia's Health 2008 Cat. no. AUS 99. Canberra: Australian Institute of Health and Welfare, 2008.
2. Barker DJ, Clark PM. Fetal undernutrition and disease in later life. RevReprod 1997; 2: 105–12.
3. United Nations International Conference on Population and Development (ICPD). Programme of Action of the United Nations International Conference on Population & Development. Egypt, Cairo: Reproductive Rights and Reproductive Health, 1994.
4. Mongella G. The United Nations: Report of the Fourth World Conference on Women. Beijing, China, 1996.
5. Sachs JD. Investing in Development: A Practical Plan to Achieve the Millennium Development Goals. 2005.
6. Thompson JG, Lane M, Robertson SA. Adaptive responses of embryos to their microenvironment and consequences for post-implantation development. In: Owens JS, Wintour M, eds. Early life origins of health and disease. Landes Bioscience, 2005: 58–69.
7. Sutton ML, Gilchrist RB, Thompson JG. Effects of in-vivo and in-vitro environments on the metabolism of the cumulus-oocyte complex and its influence on oocyte developmental capacity. Hum Reprod Update 2003; 9: 35–48.
8. Mtango NR, Potireddy S, Latham KE. Oocyte quality and maternal control of development. Int Rev Cell Mol Biol 2008; 268: 223–90.
9. Young LE. Imprinting of genes and the Barker hypothesis. Twin Res 2001; 4: 307–17.
10. Morgan HD, Santos F, Green K, Dean W, Reik W. Epigenetic reprogramming in mammals. Hum Mol Genet 2005; 14:R47–58.
11. Kaminsky ZA, Tang T, Wang SC, et al. DNA methylation profiles in monozygotic and dizygotic twins. Nat Genet 2009; 41: 240–5.
12. Robertson SA, Chin PY, Glynn DJ, Thompson JG. periconception cytokines – setting the trajectory for embryo implantation, pregnancy and beyond. Am J Reprod Immunol 2011; 66(Suppl 1): 2–10.
13. Eberhard WG. Postcopulatory sexual selection: Darwin's omission and its consequences. Proc Natl Acad Sci USA 2009; 106(Suppl 1): 10025–32.
14. Robertson SA, Guerin LR, Moldenhauer LM, Hayball JD. Activating T regulatory cells for tolerance in early pregnancy - the contribution of seminal fluid. J Reprod Immunol 2009; 83: 109–16.
15. Trowsdale J, Betz AG. Mother's little helpers: mechanisms of maternal-fetal tolerance. Nat Immunol 2006; 7: 241–6.
16. Robertson SA. Immune regulation of conception and embryo implantation-all about quality control? J Reprod Immunol 2010; 85: 51–7.
17. Watkins AJ, Papenbrock T, Fleming TP. The preimplantation embryo: handle with care. Semin Reprod Med 2008; 26: 175–85.
18. Kwong WY, Wild AE, Roberts P, Willis AC, Fleming TP. Maternal undernutrition during the preimplantation period of rat development causes blastocyst abnormalities and programming of postnatal hypertension. Development 2000; 127: 4195–202.
19. Lane M, Gardner DK. Differential regulation of mouse embryo development and viability by amino acids. J Reprod Fertil 1997; 109: 153–64.
20. Sjoblom C, Roberts CT, Wikland M, Robertson SA. Granulocyte-macrophage colony-stimulating factor alleviates adverse consequences of embryo culture on fetal growth trajectory and placental morphogenesis. Endocrinology 2005; 146: 2142–53.
21. Tam PP. Postimplantation development of mitomycin C-treated mouse blastocysts. Teratology 1988; 37: 205–12.
22. Godfrey KM. The role of the placenta in fetal programming-a review. Placenta 2002; 23(Suppl A): S20–7.
23. Hoet JJ, Ozanne S, Reusens B. Influences of pre- and postnatal nutritional exposures on vascular/endocrine systems in animals. Environ Health Perspect 2000; 108(Suppl 3): 563–8.
24. Fowden AL, Forhead AJ, Coan PM, Burton GJ. The placenta and intrauterine programming. J Neuroendocrinol 2008; 20: 439–50.
25. Maltepe E, Bakardjiev AI, Fisher SJ. The placenta: transcriptional, epigenetic, and physiological integration during development. J Clin Invest 2010; 120: 1016–25.
26. Barker DJ, Gluckman PD, Robinson JS. Conference report: fetal origins of adult disease–report of the First International Study Group, Sydney, 29–30 October 1994. Placenta 1995; 16: 317–20.
27. Stein AD, Lumey LH. The relationship between maternal and offspring birth weights after maternal prenatal famine exposure: the Dutch Famine Birth Cohort Study. Hum Biol 2000; 72: 641–54.
28. van Dijk M, Mulders J, Poutsma A, et al. Maternal segregation of the Dutch preeclampsia locus at 10q22 with a new member of the winged helix gene family. Nat Genet 2005; 37: 514–19.
29. Vickers MH, Breier BH, Cutfield WS, Hofman PL, Gluckman PD. Fetal origins of hyperphagia, obesity, and hypertension and postnatal amplification by hypercaloric nutrition. Am J Physiol Endocrinol Metab 2000; 279: E83–7.
30. Eriksson JG, Forsen T, Tuomilehto J, et al. Catch-up growth in childhood and death from coronary heart disease: longitudinal study. BMJ 1999; 318: 427–31.
31. Ong KK, Ahmed ML, Emmett PM, Preece MA, Dunger DB. Association between postnatal catch-up growth and obesity in childhood: prospective cohort study. BMJ 2000; 320: 967–71.
32. Veening MA, Van Weissenbruch MM, Delemarre-Van De Waal HA. Glucose tolerance, insulin sensitivity, and insulin secretion in children born small for gestational age. J Clin Endocrinol Metab 2002; 87: 4657–61.
33. Parker L, Lamont DW, Unwin N, et al. A lifecourse study of risk for hyperinsulinaemia, dyslipidaemia and obesity (the central metabolic syndrome) at age 49–51 years. Diabet Med 2003; 20: 406–15.
34. Davies MJ, Norman RJ. Programming and reproductive functioning. Trends Endocrinol Metab 2002; 13: 386–92.
35. Lord JM, Norman R. Obesity, polycystic ovary syndrome, infertility treatment: lifestyle modification is paramount. BMJ 2006; 332: 609.
36. Laws PJ, Abeywardana S, Walker J, Sullivan EA. Australia's mothers and babies 2006. AIHW cat no PER 46 Sydney: AIHW National Perinatal Statistics Unit. 2008; Perinatal statistics series(no. 22).
37. Thompson JG, Kind KL, Roberts CT, Robertson SA, Robinson JS. Epigenetic risks related to assisted

reproductive technologies: short- and long-term consequences for the health of children conceived through assisted reproduction technology: more reason for caution? Hum Reprod 2002; 17: 2783–6.

38. De Rycke M, Liebaers I, Van Steirteghem A. Epigenetic risks related to assisted reproductive technologies: risk analysis and epigenetic inheritance. Hum Reprod 2002; 17: 2487–94.

39. Basatemur E, Sutcliffe A. Follow-up of children born after ART. Placenta 2008; 29&Suppl B): 135–40.

40. Dumesic DA, Abbott DH, Padmanabhan V. Polycystic ovary syndrome and its developmental origins. Rev Endocr Metab Disord 2007; 8: 127–41.

41. Rhind SM, Rae MT, Brooks AN. Effects of nutrition and environmental factors on the fetal programming of the reproductive axis. Reproduction 2001; 122: 205–14.

42. Norman RJ, Hicket T, Moran L. Genetic/epigenetic and environmental origins of PCOS. Early Hum Dev 2007; 83: S43–S4.

43. Davies MJ. Fetal programming: the perspective of single and twin pregnancies. Reprod Fertil Dev 2005; 17: 379–86.

44. Cameron AJ, Welborn TA, Zimmet PZ, et al. Overweight and obesity in Australia: the 1999-2000 Australian Diabetes, Obesity and Lifestyle Study (AusDiab). Med J Aust 2003; 178: 427–32.

45. Ramlau-Hansen CH, Thulstrup AM, Nohr EA, et al. Subfecundity in overweight and obese couples. Hum Reprod 2007; 22: 1634–7.

46. Hassan MA, Killick SR. Negative lifestyle is associated with a significant reduction in fecundity. Fertil Steril 2004; 81: 384–92.

47. Hammoud AO, Gibson M, Peterson CM, Meikle AW, Carrell DT. Impact of male obesity on infertility: a critical review of the current literature. Fertil Steril 2008; 90: 897–904.

48. Maheshwari A, Stofberg L, Bhattacharya S. Effect of overweight and obesity on assisted reproductive technology–a systematic review. Hum Reprod Update 2007; 13: 433–44.

49. Wang JX, Davies M, Norman RJ. Body mass and probability of pregnancy during assisted reproduction treatment: retrospective study. BMJ 2000; 321: 1320–1.

50. Nichols JE, Crane MM, Higdon HL, Miller PB, Boone WR. Extremes of body mass index reduce in vitro fertilization pregnancy rates. Fertil Steril 2003; 79: 645–7.

51. Bakos HW, Henshaw RC, Mitchell M, Lane M. Paternal body mass index is associated with decreased blastocyst development and reduced live birth rates following assisted reproductive technology. Fertil Steril 2011; 95: 1700–4.

52. Ng SF, Lin RC, Laybutt DR, et al. Chronic high-fat diet in fathers programs beta-cell dysfunction in female rat offspring. Nature 2010; 467: 963–6.

53. MRC Vitamin Study Research Group. Prevention of neural tube defects: results of the Medical Research Council Vitamin Study. Lancet 1991; 338: 131–7.

54. Harris M, Bennett J, Del Mar C, et al. Guidelines for preventive activities in general practice, 7th edn. In: Practitioners TRACoG, ed Victoria, Australia: The Royal Australian College of General Practitioners, 2009.

55. Government of South Australia Department of Health. South Australian Perinatal Practice Guidelines. In: AfU. editor 2009. [Available from: http://www.health.sa.gov.au/PPG/Default.aspx?tabid = 222/]

56. Health Council of the Netherlands. Preconception Care: A Good Beginning. The Hague: Health Council of the Netherlands, 2007.

57. Anderson K, Nisenblat V, Norman R. Lifestyle factors in people seeking infertility treatment – A review. Aust NZ J Obstet Gynaecol 2010; 50: 8–20.

58. Zimmermann M, Delange F. Iodine supplementation of pregnant women in Europe: a review and recommendations. Eur J Clin Nutr 2004; 58: 979–84.

59. Food Standards Australia and New Zealand. Proposal P1003 Mandatory Iodine Fortification for Australia Assessment Report. In:; AfU. editor 2008. [Available from: http://fedlaw.gov.au/ComLaw/Legislation/LegislativeInstrument1.nsf/framelodgmentattachments/19ADA6A8E2826419CA2574DC00012A07]

60. Tremellen K. Oxidative stress and male infertility–a clinical perspective. Hum Reprod Update 2008; 14: 243–58.

61. Gharagozloo P, Aitken RJ. The role of sperm oxidative stress in male infertility and the significance of oral antioxidant therapy. Hum Reprod 2011; 26: 1628–40.

62. Olsen J, Bolumar F, Boldsen J, Bisanti L. Does moderate alcohol intake reduce fecundability? A European multicenter study on infertility and subfecundity. European Study Group on Infertility and Subfecundity. Alcohol Clin Exp Res 1997; 21: 206–12.

63. Mukherjee RA, Hollins S, Abou-Saleh MT, Turk J. Low level alcohol consumption and the fetus. BMJ 2005; 330: 375–6.

64. Bolumar F, Olsen J, Rebagliato M, Bisanti L. Caffeine intake and delayed conception: a European multicenter study on infertility and subfecundity. European Study Group on Infertility Subfecundity. Am J Epidemiol 1997; 145: 324–34.

65. Hatch EE, Bracken MB. Association of delayed conception with caffeine consumption. Am J Epidemiol 1993; 138: 1082–92.

66. Stanton CK, Gray RH. Effects of caffeine consumption on delayed conception. Am J Epidemiol 1995; 142: 1322–9.

67. Wilcox A, Weinberg C, Baird D. Caffeinated beverages and decreased fertility. Lancet 1988; 2: 1453–6.

68. Leviton A, Cowan L. A review of the literature relating caffeine consumption by women to their risk of reproductive hazards. Food Chem Toxicol 2002; 40: 1271–310.

69. Nawrot P, Jordan S, Eastwood J, et al. Effects of caffeine on human health. Food Addit Contam 2003; 20: 1–30.

70. Higdon JV, Frei B. Coffee and health: a review of recent human research. Crit Rev Food Sci Nutr 2006; 46: 101–23.

71. Signorello LB, McLaughlin JK. Maternal caffeine consumption and spontaneous abortion: a review of the epidemiologic evidence. Epidemiology 2004; 15: 229–39.

72. McDiarmid MA, Gardiner PM, Jack BW. The clinical content of preconception care: environmental exposures. Am J Obstet Gynecol 2008; 199(6 Suppl 2): S357–61.

73. Waylen AL, Metwally M, Jones GL, Wilkinson AJ, Ledger WL. Effects of cigarette smoking upon clinical outcomes of assisted reproduction: a meta-analysis. Hum Reprod Update 2009; 15: 31–44.

74. Augood C, Duckitt K, Templeton AA. Smoking and female infertility: a systematic review and meta-analysis. Hum Reprod 1998; 13: 1532–9.

75. Feichtinger W, Papalambrou K, Poehl M, Krischker U, Neumann K. Smoking and in vitro fertilization: a meta-analysis. J Assist Reprod Genet 1997; 14: 596–9.

76. Frey KA, Navarro SM, Kotelchuck M, Lu MC. The clinical content of preconception care: preconception care for men. Am J Obstet Gynecol 2008; 199(6 Suppl 2): S389–95.

77. Zitzmann M, Rolf C, Nordhoff V, et al. Male smokers have a decreased success rate for in vitro fertilization and intracytoplasmic sperm injection. Fertil Steril 2003; 79(Suppl 3): 1550–4.

78. Lindbohm ML, Sallmen M, Taskinen H. Effects of exposure to environmental tobacco smoke on reproductive health. Scand J Work Environ Health 2002; 28(Suppl 2): 84–96.

79. Castles A, Adams EK, Melvin CL, Kelsch C, Boulton ML. Effects of smoking during pregnancy. Five meta-analyses. Am J Prev Med 1999; 16: 208–15.

80. Neal MS, Hughes EG, Holloway AC, Foster WG. Side-stream smoking is equally as damaging as mainstream smoking on IVF outcomes. Hum Reprod 2005; 20: 2531–5.

81. Mueller BA, Daling JR, Weiss NS, Moore DE. Recreational drug use and the risk of primary infertility. Epidemiology 1990; 1: 195–200.

82. Battista N, Pasquariello N, Di Tommaso M, Maccarrone M. Interplay between endocannabinoids, steroids and cytokines in the control of human reproduction. J Neuroendocrinol 2008; 20(Suppl 1): 82–9.

83. Thyer AC, King TS, Moreno AC, et al. Cocaine impairs ovarian response to exogenous gonadotropins in nonhuman primates. J Soc Gynecol Investig 2001; 8: 358–62.

84. George VK, Li H, Teloken C, et al. Effects of long-term cocaine exposure on spermatogenesis and fertility in peripubertal male rats. J Urol 1996; 155: 327–31.

85. Ragni G, De Lauretis L, Bestetti O, Sghedoni D, Gambaro V. Gonadal function in male heroin and methadone addicts. Int J Androl 1988; 11: 93–100.

86. Pasqualotto FF, Lucon AM, Sobreiro BP, Pasqualotto EB, Arap S. Effects of medical therapy, alcohol, smoking, and endocrine disruptors on male infertility. Rev Hosp Clin Fac Med Sao Paulo 2004; 59: 375–82.

87. Pandiyan N. Medical drugs impairing fertility. In: Nicolopolou-Stamati P, Hens L, Howard CV, eds. Reproductive Health and the Environment. Dordrecht, The Netherlands: Springer, 2007: 187–205.

88. Nakamura K, Sheps S, Arck PC. Stress and reproductive failure: past notions, present insights and future directions. J Assist Reprod Genet 2008; 25: 47–62.

89. Barzilai-Pesach V, Sheiner EK, Sheiner E, Potashnik G, Shoham-Vardi I. The effect of women's occupational psychologic stress on outcome of fertility treatments. J Occup Environ Med 2006; 48: 56–62.

90. Smeenk JM, Verhaak CM, Vingerhoets AJ, et al. Stress and outcome success in IVF: the role of self-reports and endocrine variables. Hum Reprod 2005; 20: 991–6.

91. Klonoff-Cohen H, Natarajan L. The concerns during assisted reproductive technologies (CART) scale and pregnancy outcomes. Fertil Steril 2004; 81: 982–8.

92. Zorn B, Auger J, Velikonja V, Kolbezen M, Meden-Vrtovec H. Psychological factors in male partners of infertile couples: relationship with semen quality and early miscarriage. Int J Androl 2008; 31: 557–64.

93. Homan GF, Davies M, Norman R. The impact of lifestyle factors on reproductive performance in the general population and those undergoing infertility treatment: a review. Hum Reprod Update 2007; 13: 209–23.

94. Foster WG, Neal MS, Han MS, Dominguez MM. Environmental contaminants and human infertility: hypothesis or cause for concern? J Toxicol Environ Health B Crit Rev 2008; 11: 162–76.

95. Mendola P, Messer LC, Rappazzo K. Science linking environmental contaminant exposures with fertility and reproductive health impacts in the adult female. Fertil Steril 2008; 89(Suppl 2): e81–94.

96. Fei C, McLaughlin JK, Lipworth L, Olsen J. Maternal levels of perfluorinated chemicals and subfecundity. Hum Reprod 2009; 24: 1200–5.

97. Wong WY, Zielhuis GA, Thomas CM, Merkus HM, Steegers-Theunissen RP. New evidence of the influence of exogenous and endogenous factors on sperm count in man. Eur J Obstet Gynecol Reprod Biol 2003; 110: 49–54.

98. Ford JH, MacCormac L, Hiller J. PALS (pregnancy and lifestyle study): association between occupational and environmental exposure to chemicals and reproductive outcome. Mutat Res 1994; 313: 153–64.

99. Australian Technical Advisory Group on Immunisation of the Australian Government Department of Health and Ageing (ATAGI). The Australian Immunisation Handbook. 9th edn. Australian Government: Canberra, 2008.

100. Practice Committee of American Society for Reproductive Medicine. Vaccination guidelines for female infertility patients. Fertil Steril 2008; 90(Suppl 5): S169–71.

101. Anderson K, Norman RJ, Middleton P. Preconception lifestyle advice for people with subfertility. Cochrane Database Syst Rev 2010:CD008189.

102. Clark AM, Ledger W, Galletly C, et al. Weight loss results in significant improvement in pregnancy and ovulation rates in anovulatory obese women. Hum Reprod 1995; 10: 2705–12.

103. Clark AM, Thornley B, Tomlinson L, Galletley C, Norman RJ. Weight loss in obese infertile women results in improvement in reproductive outcome for all forms of fertility treatment. Hum Reprod 1998; 13: 1502–5.

Indications for IVF treatment: From diagnosis to prognosis

Ido Ben-Ami, Arie Raziel, Shevach Friedler, Yariv Gidoni, Raphael Ron-El, and Bart C. J. M. Fauser

INTRODUCTION

Since the birth of the first IVF baby almost 30 years ago, dramatic developments have occurred in the field of in vitro fertilization (IVF). IVF was initially designed to overcome the problem of tubal infertility but is now widely held to represent the treatment of choice for unexplained infertility, male factor, endometriosis, and ovarian dysfunction resistant to ovulation induction (1,2). The introduction of intracytoplasmic sperm injection (ICSI) has rendered severe forms of male infertility amenable to treatment and further widened the scope of IVF. High profile publicity given to the latest achievements with IVF has led to its perception as a panacea for all those having difficulty in conceiving a pregnancy. This has been reflected in the rapid expansion of indications for IVF (for the estimated annual IVF cycles in the EU, for example, see reference (3)). The degree to which IVF merits this growth in application remains unclear however, since prospective randomized trials comparing the effectiveness of IVF with simpler fertility treatments remain scarce.

In recent years, increasing attention has been given to the balance between benefits, burdens, and risks of IVF treatment, and the concept of achieving pregnancy at all costs is increasingly rejected (4). The level of provision of IVF treatment varies greatly from country to country, and few provide access to IVF treatment to all those who may benefit (5). The challenge is therefore twofold: First, to identify those couples for whom the potential benefits of IVF treatment merit the associated risks and costs, and second, to improve the risk/benefit balance in favor of the latter. In recent years, progress has been made on both counts. New studies focusing on IVF outcomes have further clarified those factors that determine outcome and offer the prospect of individualizing ovarian stimulation protocols and embryo transfer policies. The concept of considering indications for IVF has become more sophisticated than simply identifying a cause for infertility that might be amenable to IVF.

CONVENTIONAL APPROACH: DIAGNOSIS AS THE INDICATION FOR IVF

The original indication for IVF, tubal disease, remains an important medical indication for IVF, but in terms of numbers of patients treated, other indications have become more important. National guidelines for IVF continue to focus primarily on underlying diagnoses when determining indications for IVF (Table 34.1). Over the years, a consensus has grown as to what constitute the primary medical indications (Fig. 34.1). This is reflected in the similar frequency of indications revealed by independent databases. Variations between databases may simply reflect differences in definition or population. Patients with low-grade endometriosis may, for instance, be considered as having either a tubal or an idiopathic indication. Depending on inclusion and exclusion criteria, infertility is categorized as idiopathic in 10% to more than 30% of cases.

The extent to which the underlying pathology itself can impact on the chance of success has been the subject of considerable study. Initial reports indicated certain causes of infertility to be associated with a lower chance of success than other causes. However, large published studies on the effect of the cause of female infertility have shown no significant effect on outcome of IVF (2,6) (Table 34.2, Fig. 34 2). Instead, pregnancy chances were again determined by female age, duration of infertility, and previous pregnancy (2). In recent years, the impact of certain underlying causes of infertility on IVF outcome has become clearer.

Endometriosis

Early reports from major IVF centers indicated that IVF success rates in women were not adversely affected by endometriosis (7,8). These were followed by a number of studies that reported a significant decrease in the fertilization rate in vitro in women with endometriosis (9,10). Endometriosis may cause infertility by distorting adnexal anatomy, interfering with oocyte capture,

Table 34.1   IVF Indications as Recommended by the Dutch Society of Obstetrics & Gynaecology

1. Tubal pathology
   - If tubal surgery is not a realistic option, IVF is the method of choice.
   - In case of impaired tubal function but no occlusion is present, or following tubal surgery, IVF is the method of choice after an infertility duration of 2 years or longer. Depending on the female age, IVF can be done after a shorter duration of infertility.
2. Unexplained infertility (idiopathic)[a]
   - In case of idiopathic infertility, IVF is indicated if the duration is 3 years or longer. If the woman is older than 36 years, IVF may be considered earlier.
3. Male infertility
   - Total motile sperm count (TMC) <1 million: First treatment of choice is ICSI
   - TMC >1 and <10 million: IVF can be performed if infertility duration is 2 years or longer[a]
   - TMC >10 million: Treat as unexplained infertility
4. Endometriosis
   - In case of mild or moderate endometriosis, treat as unexplained infertility.
   - In case of severe endometriosis policy treat as tubal pathology
5. Cervical factor / immunological infertility[a]
   - After an infertility duration of 2 years, IVF is indicated. This may considered sooner if the woman is over 36 years of age.
6. Hormonal disturbances[a]
   - Anovulatory cycle abnormalities are an indication for IVF if 12 cycles of treat ment with ovulation induction have been unsuccessful.

[a]In these situations intrauterine insemination treatment merits consideration before proceeding to IVF.

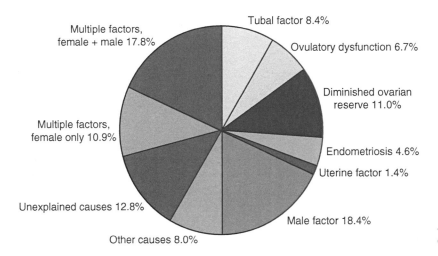

Figure 34.1 Relative frequency of indication for assisted reproductive techniques reported by US IVF Centers (CDC 2008).

Table 34.2   Impact of Cause of Infertility on Live Birth Rate from IVF

Cause of infertility	Number of cycles	Live birth rate (%) (95% CI)		
		Per treatment cycle	Per egg collection	Per embryo transfer
Tubal disease	19096	13.6 (13.0–14.0)	15.0 (14.5–15.6)	16.5 (15.9–17.1)
Endometriosis	4117	14.2 (13.2–15.3)	15.9 (14.7–17.0)	17.9 (16.6–19.3)
Unexplained	12340	13.4 (12.9–14.1)	15.2 (14.6–15.9)	19.7 (18.8–20.5)
Cervical	4232	14.2 (13.2–15.3)	16.2 (15.1–17.4)	18.8 (17.5–20.2)

Source: Adapted from Ref. 2.

impairing oocyte development, early embryogenesis, or endometrial receptivity (11,12). In a meta-analysis studying the effect of endometriosis on IVF, significantly lower fertilization, implantation, and pregnancy rates were observed in endometriosis when compared to tubal factor controls (13). Moreover, stronger negative associations were consistently observed in women with severe disease. However, none of the studies included were randomized controlled trials, limiting the conclusions that could be drawn. Data, mostly uncontrolled, indicate that surgery at any stage of endometriosis enhances the chances of natural conception (14). The

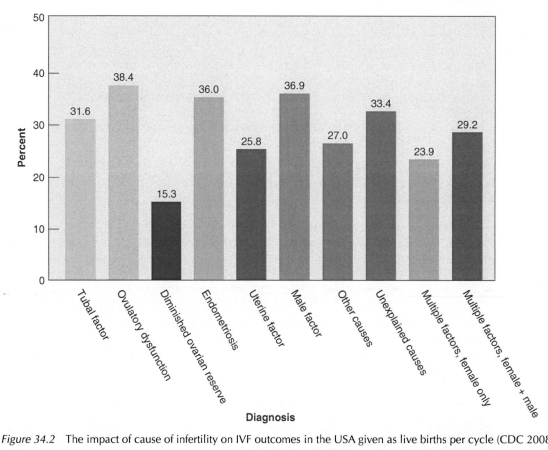

Figure 34.2   The impact of cause of infertility on IVF outcomes in the USA given as live births per cycle (CDC 2008).

risk of compromised ovarian function following surgery due to excision of excessive tissue or damage to hilar vessels sparked a rule of no surgery before IVF. Exceptions to this guidance are pain, hydrosalpinges, and very large endometriomas. Medical treatment – e.g., 3–6 months of gonadotropin-releasing hormone (GnRH) analogues – improves the outcome of IVF. When age, ovarian reserve, and male and tubal status permit, surgery should be considered immediately, so that time is dedicated to attempts to conceive naturally. In other cases, the preference is for administration of GnRH analogues before IVF, and no surgery beforehand (15).

Tubal Dysfunction

No randomized control studies have been performed comparing tubal surgery and IVF in patients with tubal damage or dysfunction. The decision to carry out IVF rather than tubal surgery has therefore a large subjective element, and tends to be based on a clinical assessment of the severity of tubal damage, the age of the patient, and the availability of specialized surgical services and IVF.

The impact of tubal dysfunction on IVF outcome is similarly controversial (16,17). Although tubal disease in general is not associated with poor outcome from IVF, there is a substantial body of evidence that distal tubal disease associated with hydrosalpinx may affect the chances of success from IVF treatment. Several retrospective studies have indicated that hydrosalpinges negatively

influence the chance of success with IVF by decreasing implantation rates or toxic effects on the embryo or endometrium (18–20). In a meta-analysis evaluating differences in pregnancy rates after IVF in tubal infertility with and without hydrosalpinx, pregnancy rates of 31.2% were observed in the absence of hydrosalpinx and 19.7% in the presence of hydrosalpinx (OR = 0.64, 95% confidence interval: 0.56–0.74) (21). A recent systematic review including five randomized trials observed that the odds of achieving an ongoing pregnancy were twice as great after laparoscopic salpingectomy for hydrosalpinges before IVF (OR = 2.14, CI = 1.23–3.73) (22). In a randomized study, proximal tube occlusion was shown to be as effective as salpingectomy in improving implantation rates when compared to no intervention (23). Any discussion of the potential risks and benefits should also highlight the potential effect of delaying IVF treatment, especially in older patients where other factors may play the determining role.

Anovulation

Chronic anovulation is a common cause of infertility. Most anovulatory women have irregular menstrual cycles and normal serum FSH concentrations (World Health Organization (WHO) group 2) (24,25). Depending on the criteria used, polycystic ovary syndrome (PCOS) is diagnosed in approximately 60–70% of these women (26,27). Cumulative singleton live birth rates of up to 71% in two years can be achieved in this group of patients with classical induction of ovulation applying clomiphene citrate as first line and exogenous gonadotropins as second line treatment (28). Alternative treatment options such as IVF should therefore be avoided as first line therapy in these patients, except for subgroups with a poor prognosis. Those women who may benefit from IVF as first line therapy can be identified by older age, longer duration of infertility, and higher insulin:glucose ratio (28). When classical ovulation induction fails, IVF is a feasible therapeutic option (29). Although PCOS patients are typically characterized by producing an increased number of oocytes, they are often of poor quality, leading to lower fertilization, cleavage and implantation rates, and a higher miscarriage rate (30). Despite reduced overall fertilization, IVF pregnancy rates in PCOS patients appeared to be comparable to ovulatory women (31–33). In a meta-analysis of IVF outcome in women diagnosed with PCOS on the basis of the Rotterdam criteria (34), it was shown that the cycle cancellation rate was significantly increased in patients with PCOS (12.8% versus 4.1%; OR 0.5; 95% CI, 0.2–1.0). Duration of stimulation was significantly longer in patients with PCOS (1.2 days; 95% CI, 0.9–1.5), even when the daily dose of FSH was similar to that of women without PCOS. Although PCOS subjects produced more oocytes, a lower fertilization rate was observed (29).

In a study in which IVF outcome was compared between a carefully defined group of women with WHO 2 anovulatory infertility and matched control group of women with tubal infertility, (35) obese women suffering from WHO 2 anovulatory infertility were at an increased risk of having their IVF cycle cancelled due to insufficient response. However, once oocyte retrieval was achieved, live birth rates were comparable with controls.

Male Factor Infertility

Poor semen quality is the single cause of infertility in approximately 20% of infertile couples, and an important contributing factor in another 20–40% of them (36). Fortunately, high female fecundity can often compensate for the presence of low sperm concentrations (37). In those couples presenting with male factor infertility, intrauterine insemination (IUI) with washed and prepared sperm can be an effective treatment (38). The additional value of ovarian stimulation to IUI in this context remains a topic of debate (39,40). Whereas ovarian stimulation with clomiphene citrate does not appear to increase the efficacy of IUI (41,42), or when the female partner is over the age of 35 years, the addition of gonadotropin ovarian hyperstimulation does appear to increase pregnancy rates, but at the expense of higher incidence of multiple pregnancy (39).

Best results with IUI are achieved when the total motile sperm count in the insemination specimen exceeds a threshold of approximately 10 million and 14% or more of sperm have normal morphology (strict criteria; WHO III standard) (43,44). Higher counts do not further increase the likelihood for success and IUI is

---

Table 34.3 Indications for ICSI

- Total motile sperm count (TMC) <1 million
- <4% normal morphology and TMC <5 million
- No or poor fertilization in the first IVF cycle when TMC <10 million
- No or poor fertilization in two IVF cycles when TMC >10 million
- Epididymal or testicular spermatozoa

---

seldom successful if fewer than 1 million total motile sperm are present (44).

The results of IVF in the treatment of male factor infertility are determined primarily by the age of the woman (45), the degree of sperm motility, and sperm morphology (46–48). Many studies have reported a strong correlation between impaired semen parameters and fertilization capacity in IVF, and when severe male factor infertility is present, total fertilization failure (TFF) may occur. In many centers, a post-wash total motile sperm count of less than 500,000 is considered to indicate ICSI treatment, (49) while others apply a cut off value of 1 million (Table 34.3). These values remain largely arbitrary, since few reliable data are available that enable the prediction of the chance of TFF in a given couple (48).

Although ICSI has transformed the fertility prognosis for couples with severe male factor infertility (including those where TFF occurs during IVF), the appropriate indications for ICSI remain controversial (50). While in some countries ICSI tends to be restricted to treating severe oligoasthenospermia and TFF, other European and US centers apply a more liberal policy to the use of ICSI, reflecting primarily differences in national or local funding policy. However, absolute indications for ICSI are agreed to include the use of microsurgical (epididymal or testicular) aspirated spermatozoa (Table 34.3). While many clinics have a lower clinical threshold for applying ICSI, and some apply it to all cases of IVF, this approach is not supported by well-designed prospective studies. In one study comparing IVF to ICSI in couples with tubal infertility but with normozoospermic semen, no differences in fertilization rates were observed (51). There is some evidence that ICSI may have detrimental effects, leading to poorer embryo development compared to IVF (52,53). In a multicenter randomized study comparing ICSI to IVF in the treatment of unexplained infertility, no benefit of ICSI was demonstrated (54). However, ICSI may yield higher fertilization rates for oocytes matured in vitro (55) and cryopreserved (56) oocytes that often exhibit a hardened zona (57).

Unexplained Infertility

The incidence of unexplained infertility ranges between 10% and as high as 30% among infertile populations, depending on diagnostic criteria (58). Spontaneous pregnancy chances in these untreated couples vary from 30% to 70% within two years (59). In the absence of a specific medical cause, a specific treatment for unexplained infertility is lacking (60). These couples are exposed to several empirical treatments, such as clomiphene citrate (61), controlled ovarian hyperstimulation combined with IUI (COH/IUI), and/or IVF with or without ICSI (60). In general, IUI has been shown to result in pregnancy rates varying between 2% and 4% per cycle. However, when combined with vigorous ovarian stimulation, complication rates (especially high order multiple pregnancies) are unacceptably high (62).

Steures et al. demonstrated in a randomized controlled trial (RCT) that in couples with a spontaneous pregnancy prognosis between 30% and 40%, six months of COH/IUI led to the same percentage of pregnancies as six months of expectant management (63). Whether treatment in couples with a poorer prognosis is superior to expectant management is, unfortunately, not yet sufficiently investigated in RCTs. Likewise, in a randomized comparison of 250 couples between a single IVF cycle and six months expectant management, no difference in pregnancy rates was observed when bilateral tubal occlusion was excluded (64). For the group of patients with more subtle abnormalities (such as endometriosis, minor tubal disease, oligozoospermia, or unexplained infertility) proper management should focus on prognosis rather than diagnosis. The prognosis of a given couple for spontaneous pregnancy should be weighed against pregnancy chances after more invasive treatment strategies such as IUI (with or without ovarian stimulation) or IVF.

A recent randomized controlled study compared the time to pregnancy and health care costs (i.e., costs related to treatment, pregnancy, and newborn care), as well as the efficacy and adverse events, of two infertility treatment strategies for couples with unexplained infertility who were candidates for ovulation induction with IUI as their initial treatment. Compared with conventional infertility treatment and when the woman was younger than 40 years, an accelerated approach to IVF that started with clomiphene citrate (CC)/IUI, but eliminated gonadotropin/IUI, resulted in a shorter time to pregnancy, with fewer treatment cycles, and at suggested cost savings (65).

In conclusion, a true cause for infertility cannot be found in many couples presenting with fertility problems. Therefore, causal therapy is only possible in a small proportion of patients. For the remaining couples a pragmatic prognosis-oriented approach should be applied. Most importantly, chances for spontaneous pregnancy should be assessed for each given couple. Evidence is accumulating that female age is by far the most crucial factor in determining chances for pregnancy, either spontaneously or after fertility therapy. This becomes even more predominant over the years, since women in the western world tend to delay their wish to conceive. Increasing attention is now focusing on the identification of prognostic factors capable of determining the chance of spontaneous conception and of successful outcome to infertility treatment in individual couples. When considering treatment options for couples with unexplained infertility, it is prudent to consider simple treatment before complex treatment and to balance what is known about effectiveness against the cost and adverse effects of different treatments.

OTHER INDICATIONS FOR IVF AND ASSOCIATED TECHNOLOGIES

Fertility Preservation

Women with malignancy or other illnesses who require treatments that pose a negative effect to future fertility (i.e., chemotherapy, radiation therapy) may be candidates for urgent IVF and cryopreservation of embryos before the initiation of the treatment, if time and health allow (66). Oocyte cryopreservation is a viable option for women having no male partner (67) who ask for fertility preservation because of either severe malady or an emerging premature ovarian failure (68), and also for healthy aging women and those who anticipate delayed childbearing (67,68).

Gestational Surrogacy

For women with no functional uterus, either due to developmental anomaly (e.g., Mayer-Rokitansky-Küster-Hauser syndrome), advanced disease (multiple myomas, severe intrauterine adhesions), or previous hysterectomy, and for women suffering from severe medical conditions that preclude pregnancy, gestational surrogacy offers the opportunity to have their own genetic offspring (69).

Preimplantation genetic diagnosis and screening

Preimplantation genetic diagnosis (PGD) has been developed for patients at high risk of transmitting a genetic abnormality to their children, which includes all monogenic defects (autosomal recessive, autosomal dominant, and X-linked disorders) (70). More recently, DNA amplification-based PGD applications have broadened and include sibling--donor selection through HLA-matching (71), and the analysis of familial chromosomal rearrangements (72). Preimplantation genetic screening (PGS) applies the same technology in couples having no known chromosomal or genetic abnormality in efforts to identify and exclude aneuploid embryos. The beneficial effect of PGS was expected to be greatest in women of advanced maternal age, since aneuploidies in clinically recognized pregnancies occur more frequently when a woman passes 35 years of age (73) and it is in these women that pregnancy chances decline sharply both in normal conception and after IVF (74). Next to women of advanced maternal age, PGS has been offered to women with a history of recurrent miscarriage, women with a history of repeated implantation failure (i.e., several failed IVF cycles), and women with a partner with low sperm quality (severe male factor), mainly since high percentages of aneuploidies have been found in the embryos of these women. However, recent systematic review and meta-analysis of randomized controlled trials found that there was no evidence of a beneficial effect of PGS as currently applied on the live birth rate after IVF. On the contrary, for women of advanced maternal age

PGS significantly lowered the live birth rate. It was concluded that new approaches in the application of PGS should be evaluated carefully before their introduction into clinical practice (75).

From Diagnosis to Prognosis

Infertility is defined as the inability of a couple to conceive within one year of regular intercourse. These infertile couples can be separated into two groups; those who are unable to conceive without therapy (i.e., absolute infertility), and those with reduced fertility chances who still have a considerable chance to conceive spontaneously with time. Disease states underlying the inability to conceive spontaneously include anovulation, complete tubal occlusion, and azoospermia. Hence, an underlying cause for the infertility can be diagnosed conclusively in these conditions. A regular fertility work up – including tests to evaluate ovulation, sperm analysis, and tests for tubal patency – can easily identify these problems.

In couples with decreased fertility, conditions such as endometriosis, oligozoospermia, or luteal phase insufficiency may be found, but it remains uncertain to what extent they contribute to the reduced fertility. Hence, in a large number of couples attending a physician for fertility problems, a clear diagnosis explaining their decreased or absent fertility cannot be found (also referred to as unexplained subfertility). Indeed, success rates per cycle of a given treatment should be weighed against costs, side effects, and inconvenience for the patient, and the chances of complications for mother and child. Risks for finance driven overtreatment remain substantial.

Many endogenous factors play a role in determining how an individual woman will respond to IVF treatment. However, any individual approach to infertility treatment must begin with an assessment of a given couple's chance of conceiving spontaneously. The chance of achieving a spontaneous pregnancy is frequently underestimated by couples and their physicians (76). The increasing tendency to delay childbearing for career, social, or other reasons is putting physicians under greater pressure to intervene when spontaneous conception does not occur quickly. Time is increasingly an issue for couples seeking to conceive. Yet patience can pay dividends for many who are now subject to premature and unnecessary intervention. Most couples seeking help will present with subfertility rather than absolute infertility. On the basis of a modest range of investigations and certain individual characteristics, the chances of an individual couple conceiving spontaneously over a given period of time can be calculated.

Several studies developed prediction models for calculating individual chances of spontaneous conception in subfertile couples (37,77,78). On the basis of the results of a number of fertility investigations and patient parameters such as age and duration of infertility, the chance of conception over a given time frame can be calculated. For instance, after three years of failure to conceive, the residual likelihood of spontaneous pregnancy in untreated couples with unexplained infertility falls to 40% and after five years to 20% (76,79).

When considering the appropriate moment for therapeutic intervention for couples with unexplained infertility, prognostic models may aid the clinician. Caution is, however, required when applying a prediction model developed elsewhere to one's own patient population. Before a prediction model can be introduced into everyday clinical practice, prospective external validation is required. Furthermore, knowledge of the development cohort is important when selecting a model for application in one's own setting. Few prediction models have been subject to validation on a different population to that on which the model was developed (80). For example, the discriminative ability and reliability of the Eimers model for predicting spontaneous pregnancy among subfertile women was measured on an independent Canadian data set (81). The model which was developed in Dutch population in 1994 was found to have a moderate predictive power in the Canadian population in which the birth rate was generally lower. With adjustment for the average live birth rate, the Eimers model gave reliable spontaneous pregnancy predictions. In a prospective evaluation of the performance of the Eimers model in a tertiary care center, the expected and observed incidence of spontaneous pregnancy in the different risk groups correlated well (82). More recently, the Hunault synthesis model was shown in a prospective study to accurately predict spontaneous pregnancy in subfertile couples (83).

In those with a poor chance of conceiving spontaneously, or with other fertility treatments, consideration of a number of factors will aid in assessing the likely outcome of IVF. While duration of infertility has been shown to be associated with the chance of spontaneous pregnancy (84), its impact on the chance of success with IVF treatment has been less clear (85). In a large retrospective analysis of factors affecting outcomes in IVF, there was a significant decrease in age-adjusted live birth rates with increasing duration of infertility (2). Previous pregnancy had a significantly positive impact on the chance of success with IVF with the effect being stronger for pregnancies resulting in a live birth. This positive association with previous live birth was even stronger if it had followed IVF pregnancy. The same authors calculated a previous live birth to be associated with a live birth rate per IVF treatment cycle of 23.2% compared with 12.5% when no previous pregnancy had occurred. This association with previous pregnancy and successful outcome has since been confirmed by other studies (7,86). In a recent review and meta-analysis that aimed to identify the most relevant predictors for success in IVF, it was found that female age, duration of subfertility, basal FSH, and number of oocytes, all reflecting ovarian function, were predictors of pregnancy after IVF (87).

Ovarian Aging

The most prominent determining factor for IVF outcome is the individual variability in ovarian response to stimulation. Rather than exhibiting the desired response, women can present with either a hypo-response or a hyper-response to stimulation. While hyper-response to gonadotropin stimulation can usually be prevented by modification of the stimulation regimen, a poor response to ovarian stimulation is highly resistant to therapeutic intervention (88). Strategies for stimulating "low responders" include varying the dose or day of the cycle for initiating stimulation with gonadotropins. Studies undertaken so far have been unable to demonstrate a beneficial effect of gonadotropin dose increase in patients who exhibit a poor response to standard dose regimens (88,89). Alternative approaches include early cessation or micro-dose GnRH agonist protocols, and the adjunctive use of aromatase inhibitors, growth hormone, GnRH antagonists (90,) and dehydroepiandrosterone (DHEA) (91). Initial small studies focusing on surrogate outcomes such as number of cancelled cycles rather than ongoing pregnancy could produce encouraging results. However, at present, no therapeutic intervention has been shown in large randomized studies to offer a solution to poor response to ovarian stimulation in IVF. It might indeed be argued that therapeutic interventions aimed at increasing the chance of meeting criteria for oocyte pick-up are unethical unless ongoing pregnancy rates can also be shown to improve.

Poor response to ovarian stimulation for IVF is clearly associated with chronological aging. Maternal age is the most important factor in determining the likelihood of success with IVF. An age-related decline in response to stimulation with gonadotropins and a reduction in the number of oocytes (92), oocyte quality (93), fertilization rates (94,95), and ultimately embryos (96,97) have been well documented. Many studies point to the age of 40 years as being a significant cut-off line for the effectiveness of IVF (98–101). This age-related effect on pregnancy rates is similar to that reported in donor sperm programs (102) and chances for spontaneous pregnancy. A multiple regression analysis of factors influencing IVF outcomes, revealed a predicted live birth rate of 17% per cycle at the age of 30 years, falling to just 7% at 40 years and 2% at 45 years (2). Although age is an important predictor of IVF outcome (103), chronological age is poorly correlated with ovarian aging. The association between cycle cancellation and poor success rates and poor ovarian response due to diminished ovarian reserve is well established (104,105). A major individual variability exists in follicle pool depletion within the normal range of menopausal age, as complete follicle pool exhaustion may occur between 40 and 60 years. The quantity and quality of the primordial follicle pool diminishes with age, reducing ovarian reserve (106). This results in a decline in both therapy-induced and spontaneous pregnancies (107). However, while some women above 40 years of age will show a good response to ovarian stimulation, and subsequently conceive with IVF, other women under 40 years may fail to respond, as a result of accelerated ovarian aging (108). The concept of poor response as a feature of chronological and ovarian aging has been further supported by studies linking poor response to ovarian hyperstimulation to subsequent early

menopause (109–111). Indeed, the response of a woman to ovarian hyperstimulation for IVF can be considered as an extended challenge test of ovarian function. In recent years attention has been given to the identification of sensitive and specific markers of ovarian aging which may enable prediction of poor or good response to ovarian hyperstimulation. This would open the way to improved counseling and patient selection for IVF.

The value of FSH and other prognostic markers in predicting ovarian response to hyperstimulation in IVF treatment is dealt with further in chapter 36.

Clearly related to the ovarian response to stimulation, the number of embryos available for transfer appears to be a crucial factor in determining the chance of success with IVF (109) and this is of equal importance in older women (112). Two studies reported on the number of embryos transferred and IVF success (113,114). One study categorized the number to more than two and two or less embryos transferred. Women where more than two embryos were transferred had significantly higher pregnancy chances (113). The second study showed higher, though not statistically significant, chances of pregnancy when transferring more embryos (114).These data suggest uterine senescence to be less important than embryo quality in determining IVF outcome in older women. Further support for this comes from the observed success of oocyte donation programs in women over the age of 40 years (115).

LIFESTYLE AND CONCURRENT MEDICAL CONDITIONS

There is now a substantial amount of evidence showing that environmental and lifestyle factors influence the success rates of assisted reproductive techniques (116–118) and it is therefore important that serious attempts are made to provide adequate preconceptional screening counseling and interventions to optimize health prior to starting IVF. The importance of full medical assessment prior to IVF treatment is increasing as the average age of the patients continues to rise. A greater proportion of infertility patients may now also present with concurrent medical conditions that may have an impact on the safety and management of the IVF treatment as well as pregnancy. The appropriate management of the medically complicated patients presenting for IVF can be complex and often requires an interdisciplinary approach.

The most important lifestyle factor impacting on fertility outcomes is tobacco smoking. Cigarette smoke contains several thousand components (e.g., nicotine, polycyclic aromatic hydrocarbons, and cadmium) with diverse effects. Each stage of reproductive function, folliculogenesis, steroidogenesis, embryo transport, endometrial receptivity, endometrial angiogenesis, uterine blood flow, and uterine myometrium is a target for cigarette smoke components (119,122,123). Reports have appeared linking smoking to damage of the meiotic spindle in oocytes, increasing the risk of chromosomal errors (120). In men who smoke, all parameters of sperm quality are reduced (117). Smoking in men and passive smoking in women has been associated with a longer time to achieve a pregnancy (117). The effects of cigarette smoke are dose-dependent and are influenced by the presence of other toxic substances and hormonal status. Individual sensitivity, dose, time, and type of exposure also play a role in the impact of smoke constituents on human fertility (119). Furthermore, smoking during pregnancy has long been known to increase the risk of a number of adverse obstetric and fetal outcomes such as miscarriage, placenta praevia, preterm birth, and low birth weight (117). The effects of smoking on live birth rate among women who undergo IVF are similar in magnitude to the effect of an increase in female age of more than 10 years (116). As a result, smokers require twice as many IVF cycles to become pregnant as nonsmokers (116). The American Society for Reproductive Medicine Practice Committee publication on smoking and infertility has highlighted the considerable contribution of smoking to infertility and treatment outcomes and the need for a more proactive approach to stop smoking prior to fertility treatment (121).

Epidemiological evidence clearly shows that being overweight contributes to menstrual disorders, infertility, miscarriage, poor pregnancy outcome, impaired fetal well-being, and diabetes mellitus (124). Compared with women with a BMI of 25 kg/m^2 or less, women with a BMI $\geq$ 25 kg/m^2 have a lower chance of pregnancy following IVF (odds ratio (OR) 0.71, 95% CI: 0.62, 0.81), require higher dose of gonadotropins (weighed mean differences 210.08, 95% CI: 149.12, 271.05) and have an increased miscarriage rate (OR 1.33, 95% CI: 1.06, 1.68) (125). In men, a BMI <20 kg/m^2 or >25 kg/m^2 is associated with reduced sperm quality (117). A number of studies have shown that weight loss can improve fecundity in overweight women, and many centers include weight loss programs as part of their fertility treatment. However, little data is available regarding the impact of type of diet on IVF outcomes.

Recent studies have highlighted the importance of certain nutritional factors for healthy gamete development and hence embryo quality. Folic acid supplementation was shown to alter the vitamin microenvironment of the oocyte (126), while seminal plasma cobalamin levels were demonstrated to effect sperm concentration (127). Concerns that folate supplementation may increase twinning rates in IVF are better addressed by practicing single embryo transfer, rather than withholding folate supplementation (128). Women with higher vitamin D level in their serum and follicular fluid were significantly more likely to achieve clinical pregnancy following IVF (129).

It is becoming clear that preconceptional care aimed at optimizing medical, lifestyle, and nutritional factors should be an integral part of fertility therapies; and in our center, all IVF patients attend a preconceptional clinic before commencing treatment.

DEFINING SUCCESS IN IVF

The approach of maximizing pregnancy rates per cycle has led to very complex and costly ovarian hyperstimulation protocols with considerable risk of side effects and complications. In fact, many couples do not consider a second IVF attempt, even if they can afford one, because of the stress associated with the first treatment cycle (130). Research on less complex, more patient-friendly stimulation protocols, along with transfer of a reduced number (preferably one) of embryos, will only prosper in an environment in which singleton healthy birth is regarded as the most appropriate endpoint of infertility treatment. This primary outcome should be judged in the context of the risk of adverse effects, complications, and costs per treatment (which might include multiple cycles) or during a given treatment period. In a recent randomized study, the cumulative live singleton birthrate achieved at one year after commencing treatment was measured after two treatment strategies (130). The "conventional" strategy consisted of three cycles in which the conventional "long protocol" was applied and two embryos per cycle transferred. The mild strategy comprised of four cycles in which a mild stimulation protocol was combined with the transfer of just one embryo. After one year of treatment, cumulative singleton rates were equivalent, but those treated with the mild strategy had incurred lower costs, far fewer multiple pregnancies, and lower dropout rates (130) (Fig. 34.3). If IVF outcomes are expressed in terms of live singleton birth per period of treatment, milder regimens with fewer risks and complications will be more readily adopted into clinical practice, improving the prognosis of a complication free successful IVF treatment (131).

THE FUTURE

As our knowledge of factors influencing outcome following fertility therapies increases, treatment will become more individualized, maximizing cost effectiveness and minimizing inconvenience and risk for the patient. Prognostic models based on individual factors are likely to predominate over population cost-effectiveness considerations when deciding, for instance, who receives IUI rather than IVF for the treatment of unexplained infertility. In addition, the developments of mild hyperstimulation IVF and the prospect of improving implantation rates by optimizing embryo culture conditions and the provision of preimplantation genetic screening will demand continuing reassessment of the cost–benefit issues. This degree of individualization requires the development and application of sophisticated, accurate, and prospectively validated prediction models. An individual approach to IVF may have an impact on one of the major problems still facing IVF, that of multiple pregnancy.

A major limit on the indications for IVF is the process of ovarian aging. Apart from donation, there appears to be little sign of a therapeutic intervention capable of circumventing this phenomenon. While the ongoing tendency to delay childbirth will increase the need for assisted conception services, the negative impact of aging on IVF outcome is likely to increase.

In the future, IVF will be increasingly applied for indications other than infertility. The growing applications

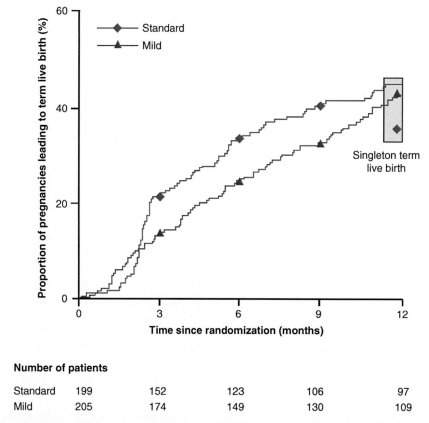

Figure 34.3 Proportions of pregnancies leading to cumulative term live births within 12 months after starting IVF Mild: Mild ovarian stimulation with GnRH antagonist and single embryo transfer Standard: Standard ovarian stimulation with GnRH antagonist and dual embryo transfer. The shaded area represents the singleton live birth rate after 12 months (113).

for PGD are producing a new range of indications for IVF. IVF is becoming simply a tool to enable PGD, and thus prevention of hereditary disorders in normally fertile couples at risk of having children with serious medical conditions. In addition, IVF allows the creation of "designer babies" capable of donating HLA matching tissue to treat a sick sibling. While these indications for IVF remain under close scrutiny by national regulators of IVF, they are likely to become established in the near future. The theoretical possibilities for medical therapies based on the in vitro culture and selective differentiation of embryonic stem cells are likely to be translated into therapeutic reality before long. The treatment of infertility may very soon be but a minor indication for IVF.

SUMMARY

At the time of its introduction into clinical practice, the principal indication for IVF was tubal infertility. Since then the indications have multiplied, and IVF now has a central place in the treatment of female and male factor infertility, as well as the infertile couple with no clear underlying cause. The underlying indication for treatment has a limited impact on the probability of success. More important determining factors are patient age and duration of infertility. With increasing knowledge of the factors that influence a given couple's chance of conceiving either spontaneously or following fertility treatment, the emphasis is shifting from

diagnosis to prognosis. The most important variable with respect to IVF is the response of the patient to ovarian stimulation. In recent years, the link between poor response to ovarian stimulation and ovarian ageing has become clear, but effective remedial therapies remain elusive. Certain lifestyle factors such as smoking and obesity have also been shown to impact negatively on fertility and IVF outcomes. These factors are amenable to intervention and due attention should be given by both clinicians and their patients to optimizing preconceptional conditions for a successful treatment and pregnancy.

REFERENCES

1. Steptoe PC, Edwards RG, Purdy JM. Clinical aspects of pregnancies established with cleaving embryos grown in vitro. Br J Obstet Gynaecol 1980; 87: 757–68.
2. Templeton A, Morris JK, Parslow W. Factors that affect outcome of in-vitro fertilisation treatment. Lancet 1996; 348: 1402–6.
3. de Mouzon J, Goossens V, Bhattacharya S, et al. Assisted reproductive technology in Europe, 2006: results generated from European registers by ESHRE. Hum Reprod 2010; 25: 1851–62.
4. Fauser BC, Devroey P, Yen SS, et al. Minimal ovarian stimulation for IVF: appraisal of potential benefits and drawbacks. Hum Reprod 1999; 14: 2681–6.
5. Nachtigall RD. International disparities in access to infertility services. Fertil Steril 2006; 85: 871–5.

6. Hull MG, Eddowes HA, Fahy U, et al. Expectations of assisted conception for infertility. BMJ 1992; 304: 1465–9.

7. Mahadevan MM, Trounson AO, Leeton JF. The relationship of tubal blockage, infertility of unknown cause, suspected male infertility, and endometriosis to success of in vitro fertilization and embryo transfer. Fertil Steril 1983; 40: 755–62.

8. Jones HW Jr, Acosta AA, Andrews MC, et al. Three years of in vitro fertilization at Norfolk. Fertil Steril 1984; 42: 826–34.

9. Wardle PG, Mitchell JD, McLaughlin EA, et al. Endometriosis and ovulatory disorder: reduced fertilisation in vitro compared with tubal and unexplained infertility. Lancet 1985; 2: 236–9.

10. Simon C, Gutierrez A, Vidal A, et al. Outcome of patients with endometriosis in assisted reproduction: results from in-vitro fertilization and oocyte donation. Hum Reprod 1994; 9: 725–9.

11. Dmowski WP, Rana N, Michalowska J, et al. The effect of endometriosis, its stage and activity, and of autoantibodies on in vitro fertilization and embryo transfer success rates. Fertil Steril 1995; 63: 555–62.

12. Gupta S, Goldberg JM, Aziz N, et al. Pathogenic mechanisms in endometriosis-associated infertility. Fertil Steril 2008; 90: 247–57.

13. Barnhart K, Dunsmoor-Su R, Coutifaris C. Effect of endometriosis on in vitro fertilization. Fertil Steril 2002; 77: 1148–55.

14. Vercellini P, Somigliana E, Vigano P, et al. Endometriosis: current therapies and new pharmacological developments. Drugs 2009; 69: 649–75.

15. de Ziegler D, Borghese B, Chapron C. Endometriosis and infertility: pathophysiology and management. Lancet 2010; 376: 730–8.

16. Check JH, Lurie D, Callan C, Baker A, Benfer K. Comparison of the cumulative probability of pregnancy after in vitro fertilization-embryo transfer by infertility factor and age. Fertil Steril 1994; 61: 257–61.

17. Dor J, Seidman DS, Ben-Shlomo I, et al. Cumulative pregnancy rate following in-vitro fertilization: the significance of age and infertility aetiology. Hum Reprod 1996; 11: 425–8.

18. Barmat LI, Rauch E, Spandorfer S, et al. The effect of hydrosalpinges on IVF-ET outcome. J Assist Reprod Genet 1999; 16: 350–4.

19. Cohen MA, Lindheim SR, Sauer MV. Hydrosalpinges adversely affect implantation in donor oocyte cycles. Hum Reprod 1999; 14: 1087–9.

20. de Wit W, Gowrising CJ, Kuik DJ, Lens JW, Schats R. Only hydrosalpinges visible on ultrasound are associated with reduced implantation and pregnancy rates after in-vitro fertilization. Hum Reprod 1998; 13: 1696–701.

21. Aboulghar MA, Mansour RT, Serour GI. Controversies in the modern management of hydrosalpinx. Hum Reprod Update 1998; 4: 882–90.

22. Johnson N, van Voorst S, Sowter MC, Strandell A, Mol BW. Surgical treatment for tubal disease in women due to undergo in vitro fertilisation. Cochrane Database Syst Rev 2010; CD002125.

23. Kontoravdis A, Makrakis E, Pantos K, et al. Proximal tubal occlusion and salpingectomy result in similar improvement in in vitro fertilization outcome in patients with hydrosalpinx. Fertil Steril 2006; 86: 1642–9.

24. The ESHRE Capri Workshop Group. Anovulatory infertility. Hum Reprod 1995; 10: 1549–53.

25. Rowe PJ. World Health Organization. WHO Manual for the Standardized Investigation and Diagnosis of the Infertile Couple. Cambridge, New York: Published on behalf of the World Health Organization by Cambridge University Press, 1993.

26. van Santbrink EJ, Hop WC, Fauser BC. Classification of normogonadotropic infertility: polycystic ovaries diagnosed by ultrasound versus endocrine characteristics of polycystic ovary syndrome. Fertil Steril 1997; 67: 452–8.

27. Laven JS, Imani B, Eijkemans MJ, Fauser BC. New approach to polycystic ovary syndrome and other forms of anovulatory infertility. Obstet Gynecol Surv 2002; 57: 755–67.

28. Eijkemans MJ, Imani B, Mulders AG, Habbema JD, Fauser BC. High singleton live birth rate following classical ovulation induction in normogonadotrophic anovulatory infertility (WHO 2). Hum Reprod 2003; 18: 2357–62.

29. Heijnen EM, Eijkemans MJ, Hughes EG, et al. A metaanalysis of outcomes of conventional IVF in women with polycystic ovary syndrome. Hum Reprod Update 2006; 12: 13–21.

30. Qiao J, Feng HL. Extra- and intra-ovarian factors in polycystic ovary syndrome: impact on oocyte maturation and embryo developmental competence. Hum Reprod Update 2011; 17: 17–33.

31. Dor J, Shulman A, Levran D, et al. The treatment of patients with polycystic ovarian syndrome by in-vitro fertilization and embryo transfer: a comparison of results with those of patients with tubal infertility. Hum Reprod 1990; 5: 816–18.

32. Urman B, Fluker MR, Yuen BH, et al. The outcome of in vitro fertilization and embryo transfer in women with polycystic ovary syndrome failing to conceive after ovulation induction with exogenous gonadotropins. Fertil Steril 1992; 57: 1269–73.

33. Homburg R, Berkowitz D, Levy T, et al. In vitro fertilization and embryo transfer for the treatment of infertility associated with polycystic ovary syndrome. Fertil Steril 1993; 60: 858–63.

34. Rotterdam ESHRE/ASRM-Sponsored PCOS Consensus Workshop Group. Revised 2003 consensus on diagnostic criteria and long-term health risks related to polycystic ovary syndrome. Fertil Steril 2004; 81: 19–25.

35. Mulders AG, Laven JS, Imani B, Eijkemans MJ, Fauser BC. IVF outcome in anovulatory infertility (WHO group 2)–including polycystic ovary syndrome–following previous unsuccessful ovulation induction. Reprod Biomed Online 2003; 7: 50–8.

36. Schlegel PN, Girardi SK. Clinical review 87: In vitro fertilization for male factor infertility. J Clin Endocrinol Metab 1997; 82: 709–16.

37. Collins JA, Burrows EA, Wilan AR. The prognosis for live birth among untreated infertile couples. Fertil Steril 1995; 64: 22–8.

38. Cohlen BJ, Vandekerckhove P, te Velde ER, Habbema JD. Timed intercourse versus intra-uterine insemination with or without ovarian hyperstimulation for subfertility in men. Cochrane Database Syst Rev 2000; CD000360.

39. Fauser BC, Devroey P, Macklon NS. Multiple birth resulting from ovarian stimulation for subfertility treatment. Lancet 2005; 365: 1807–16.

40. Cohlen B, Cantineau A, D'Hooghe T, te Velde E. Multiple pregnancy after assisted reproduction. Lancet 2005; 366: 452–3; author reply 453–454.

41. Martinez AR, Bernardus RE, Voorhorst FJ, Vermeiden JP, Schoemaker J. Intrauterine insemination does and clomiphene citrate does not improve fecundity in couples with infertility due to male or idiopathic factors: a prospective, randomized, controlled study. Fertil Steril 1990; 53: 847–53.

42. Arici A, Byrd W, Bradshaw K, et al. Evaluation of clomiphene citrate and human chorionic gonadotropin treatment: a prospective, randomized, crossover study during intrauterine insemination cycles. Fertil Steril 1994; 61: 314–18.

43. Van Voorhis BJ, Barnett M, Sparks AE, et al. Effect of the total motile sperm count on the efficacy and cost-effectiveness of intrauterine insemination and in vitro fertilization. Fertil Steril 2001; 75: 661–8.

44. van der Westerlaken LA, Naaktgeboren N, Helmerhorst FM. Evaluation of pregnancy rates after intrauterine insemination according to indication, age, and sperm parameters. J Assist Reprod Genet 1998; 15: 359–64.

45. Forti G, Krausz C. Clinical review 100: Evaluation and treatment of the infertile couple. J Clin Endocrinol Metab 1998; 83: 4177–88.

46. Van Uem JF, Acosta AA, Swanson RJ, et al. Male factor evaluation in in vitro fertilization: Norfolk experience. Fertil Steril 1985; 44: 375–83.

47. Donnelly ET, Lewis SE, McNally JA, Thompson W. In vitro fertilization and pregnancy rates: the influence of sperm motility and morphology on IVF outcome. Fertil Steril 1998; 70: 305–14.

48. Repping S, van Weert JM, Mol BW, de Vries JW, van der Veen F. Use of the total motile sperm count to predict total fertilization failure in in vitro fertilization. Fertil Steril 2002; 78: 22–8.

49. Devroey P, Vandervorst M, Nagy P, Van Steirteghem A. Do we treat the male or his gamete? Hum Reprod 1998; 13(Suppl 1): 178–85.

50. Devroey P, Van Steirteghem A. A review of ten years experience of ICSI. Hum Reprod Update 2004; 10: 19–28.

51. Staessen C, Camus M, Clasen K, De Vos A, Van Steirteghem A. Conventional in-vitro fertilization versus intracytoplasmic sperm injection in sibling oocytes from couples with tubal infertility and normozoospermic semen. Hum Reprod 1999; 14: 2474–9.

52. Ola B, Afnan M, Sharif K, et al. Should ICSI be the treatment of choice for all cases of in-vitro conception? Considerations of fertilization and embryo development, cost effectiveness and safety. Hum Reprod 2001; 16: 2485–90.

53. Verpoest W, Tournaye H. ICSI: hype or hazard? Hum Fertil (Camb) 2006; 9: 81–92.

54. Bhattacharya S, Hamilton MP, Shaaban M, et al. Conventional in-vitro fertilisation versus intracytoplasmic sperm injection for the treatment of non-male-factor infertility: a randomised controlled trial. Lancet 2001; 357: 2075–9.

55. Barnes FL, Crombie A, Gardner DK, et al. Blastocyst development and birth after in-vitro maturation of human primary oocytes, intracytoplasmic sperm injection and assisted hatching. Hum Reprod 1995; 10: 3243–7.

56. Kuleshova L, Gianaroli L, Magli C, Ferraretti A, Trounson A. Birth following vitrification of a small number of human oocytes: case report. Hum Reprod 1999; 14: 3077–9.

57. Zhang X, Rutledge J, Armstrong DT. Studies on zona hardening in rat oocytes that are matured in vitro in a serum-free medium. Mol Reprod Dev 1991; 28: 292–6.

58. Aboulghar MA, Mansour RT, Serour GI, Al-Inany HG. Diagnosis and management of unexplained infertility: an update. Arch Gynecol Obstet 2003; 267: 177–88.

59. Smeenk JM, Braat DD, Stolwijk AM, Kremer JA. Pregnancy is predictable: a large-scale prospective external validation of the prediction of spontaneous pregnancy in subfertile couples. Hum Reprod 2007; 22: 2344–5; author reply 2345–2346.

60. Brandes M, Hamilton CJ, van der Steen JO, et al. Unexplained infertility: overall ongoing pregnancy rate and mode of conception. Hum Reprod 2011; 26: 360–8.

61. Hughes E, Brown J, Collins JJ, Vanderkerchove P. Clomiphene citrate for unexplained subfertility in women. Cochrane Database Syst Rev 2010; CD000057.

62. Guzick DS, Carson SA, Coutifaris C, et al. Efficacy of superovulation and intrauterine insemination in the treatment of infertility. National Cooperative Reproductive Medicine Network. N Engl J Med 1999; 340: 177–83.

63. Steures P, van der Steeg JW, Hompes PG, et al. Intrauterine insemination with controlled ovarian hyperstimulation versus expectant management for couples with unexplained subfertility and an intermediate prognosis: a randomised clinical trial. Lancet 2006; 368: 216–21.

64. Soliman S, Daya S, Collins J, Jarrell J. A randomized trial of in vitro fertilization versus conventional treatment for infertility. Fertil Steril 1993; 59: 1239–44.

65. Reindollar RH, Regan MM, Neumann PJ, et al. A randomized clinical trial to evaluate optimal treatment for unexplained infertility: the fast track and standard treatment (FASTT) trial. Fertil Steril 2010; 94: 888–99.

66. Oktay K, Rodriguez-Wallberg K, Schover L. Preservation of fertility in patients with cancer. N Engl J Med 2009; 360: 2682–3; author reply.

67. Grifo JA, Noyes N. Delivery rate using cryopreserved oocytes is comparable to conventional in vitro fertilization using fresh oocytes: potential fertility preservation for female cancer patients. Fertil Steril 2010; 93: 391–6.

68. Oktay K, Rodriguez-Wallberg KA, Sahin G. Fertility preservation by ovarian stimulation and oocyte cryopreservation in a 14-year-old adolescent with Turner syndrome mosaicism and impending premature ovarian failure. Fertil Steril 2010; 94: 753.e715–59.

69. Brinsden PR. Gestational surrogacy. Hum Reprod Update 2003; 9: 483–91.

70. Harton GL, De Rycke M, Fiorentino F, et al. ESHRE PGD consortium best practice guidelines for amplification-based PGD. Hum Reprod 2011; 26: 33–40.

71. Van de Velde H, De Rycke M, De Man C, et al. The experience of two European preimplantation genetic diagnosis centres on human leukocyte antigen typing. Hum Reprod 2009; 24: 732–40.

72. Fiorentino F, Kokkali G, Biricik A, et al. Polymerase chain reaction-based detection of chromosomal imbalances on embryos: the evolution of preimplantation

genetic diagnosis for chromosomal translocations. Fertil Steril 2010; 94: 2001–11; 2011.e2001–2006.

73. Hassold T, Hunt P. To err (meiotically) is human: the genesis of human aneuploidy. Nat Rev Genet 2001; 2: 280–91.

74. Lintsen AM, Eijkemans MJ, Hunault CC, et al. Predicting ongoing pregnancy chances after IVF and ICSI: a national prospective study. Hum Reprod 2007; 22: 2455–62.

75. Mastenbroek S, Twisk M, van der Veen F, Repping S. Preimplantation genetic screening: a systematic review and meta-analysis of RCTs. Hum Reprod Update 2011; 17: 454–66.

76. Evers JL. Female subfertility. Lancet 2002; 360: 151–9.

77. Eimers JM, te Velde ER, Gerritse R, et al. The prediction of the chance to conceive in subfertile couples. Fertil Steril 1994; 61: 44–52.

78. Snick HK, Snick TS, Evers JL, Collins JA. The spontaneous pregnancy prognosis in untreated subfertile couples: the Walcheren primary care study. Hum Reprod 1997; 12: 1582–8.

79. Collins JA, Rowe TC. Age of the female partner is a prognostic factor in prolonged unexplained infertility: a multicenter study. Fertil Steril 1989; 52: 15–20.

80. Stolwijk AM, Straatman H, Zielhuis GA, et al. External validation of prognostic models for ongoing pregnancy after in-vitro fertilization. Hum Reprod 1998; 13: 3542–9.

81. Hunault CC, Eijkemans MJ, te Velde ER, Collins JA, Habbema JD. Validation of a model predicting spontaneous pregnancy among subfertile untreated couples. Fertil Steril 2002; 78: 500–6.

82. Collins JA, Milner RA, Rowe TC. The effect of treatment on pregnancy among couples with unexplained infertility. Int J Fertil 1991; 36: 140–1; 145–152.

83. van der Steeg JW, Steures P, Eijkemans MJ, et al. Pregnancy is predictable: a large-scale prospective external validation of the prediction of spontaneous pregnancy in subfertile couples. Hum Reprod 2007; 22: 536–42.

84. Salat-Baroux J, Alvarez S, Antoine JM, et al. Results of IVF in the treatment of polycystic ovary disease. Hum Reprod 1988; 3: 331–5.

85. Goverde AJ, McDonnell J, Vermeiden JP, et al. Intrauterine insemination or in-vitro fertilisation in idiopathic subfertility and male subfertility: a randomised trial and cost-effectiveness analysis. Lancet 2000; 355: 13–18.

86. Croucher CA, Lass A, Margara R, Winston RM. Predictive value of the results of a first in-vitro fertilization cycle on the outcome of subsequent cycles. Hum Reprod 1998; 13: 403–8.

87. van Loendersloot LL, van Wely M, Limpens J, et al. Predictive factors in in vitro fertilization (IVF): a systematic review and meta-analysis. Hum Reprod Update 2010; 16: 577–89.

88. Tarlatzis BC, Zepiridis L, Grimbizis G, Bontis J. Clinical management of low ovarian response to stimulation for IVF: a systematic review. Hum Reprod Update 2003; 9: 61–76.

89. van Hooff MH, Alberda AT, Huisman GJ, Zeilmaker GH, Leerentveld RA. Doubling the human menopausal gonadotrophin dose in the course of an in-vitro fertilization treatment cycle in low responders: a randomized study. Hum Reprod 1993; 8: 369–73.

90. Karande VC. Managing and predicting low response to standard in vitro fertilization therapy: a review of the options. Treat Endocrinol 2003; 2: 257–72.

91. Wiser A, Gonen O, Ghetler Y, et al. Addition of dehydroepiandrosterone (DHEA) for poor-responder patients before and during IVF treatment improves the pregnancy rate: a randomized prospective study. Hum Reprod 2010; 25: 2496–500.

92. Piette C, de Mouzon J, Bachelot A, Spira A. In-vitro fertilization: influence of women's age on pregnancy rates. Hum Reprod 1990; 5: 56–9.

93. Tucker MJ, Morton PC, Wright G, et al. Factors affecting success with intracytoplasmic sperm injection. Reprod Fertil Dev 1995; 7: 229–36.

94. Ashkenazi J, Orvieto R, Gold-Deutch R, et al. The impact of woman's age and sperm parameters on fertilization rates in IVF cycles. Eur J Obstet Gynecol Reprod Biol 1996; 66: 155–9.

95. Yie SM, Collins JA, Daya S, et al. Polyploidy and failed fertilization in in-vitro fertilization are related to patient's age and gamete quality. Hum Reprod 1996; 11: 614–17.

96. Hull MG, Fleming CF, Hughes AO, McDermott A. The age-related decline in female fecundity: a quantitative controlled study of implanting capacity and survival of individual embryos after in vitro fertilization. Fertil Steril 1996; 65: 783–90.

97. Sharif K, Elgendy M, Lashen H, Afnan M. Age and basal follicle stimulating hormone as predictors of in vitro fertilisation outcome. Br J Obstet Gynaecol 1998; 105: 107–12.

98. Yaron Y, Botchan A, Amit A, et al. Endometrial receptivity: the age-related decline in pregnancy rates and the effect of ovarian function. Fertil Steril 1993; 60: 314–18.

99. Roest J, van Heusden AM, Mous H, Zeilmaker GH, Verhoeff A. The ovarian response as a predictor for successful in vitro fertilization treatment after the age of 40 years. Fertil Steril 1996; 66: 969–73.

100. Legro RS, Shackleford DP, Moessner JM, Gnatuk CL, Dodson WC. ART in women 40 and over. Is the cost worth it? J Reprod Med 1997; 42: 76–82.

101. Malizia BA, Hacker MR, Penzias AS. Cumulative live-birth rates after in vitro fertilization. N Engl J Med 2009; 360: 236–43.

102. van Noord-Zaadstra BM, Looman CW, Alsbach H, et al. Delaying childbearing: effect of age on fecundity and outcome of pregnancy. BMJ 1991; 302: 1361–5.

103. Chuang CC, Chen CD, Chao KH, et al. Age is a better predictor of pregnancy potential than basal follicle-stimulating hormone levels in women undergoing in vitro fertilization. Fertil Steril 2003; 79: 63–8.

104. Pellicer A, Lightman A, Diamond MP, Russell JB, DeCherney AH. Outcome of in vitro fertilization in women with low response to ovarian stimulation. Fertil Steril 1987; 47: 812–15.

105. Jenkins JM, Davies DW, Devonport H, et al. Comparison of 'poor' responders with 'good' responders using a standard buserelin/human menopausal gonadotrophin regime for in-vitro fertilization. Hum Reprod 1991; 6: 918–21.

106. te Velde ER, Pearson PL. The variability of female reproductive ageing. Hum Reprod Update 2002; 8: 141–54.

107. Scott RT, Opsahl MS, Leonardi MR, et al. Life table analysis of pregnancy rates in a general infertility

population relative to ovarian reserve and patient age. Hum Reprod 1995; 10: 1706–10.

108. Beckers NG, Macklon NS, Eijkemans MJ, Fauser BC. Women with regular menstrual cycles and a poor response to ovarian hyperstimulation for in vitro fertilization exhibit follicular phase characteristics suggestive of ovarian aging. Fertil Steril 2002; 78: 291–7.

109. de Boer EJ, den Tonkelaar I, te Velde ER, et al. A low number of retrieved oocytes at in vitro fertilization treatment is predictive of early menopause. Fertil Steril 2002; 77: 978–85.

110. Nikolaou D, Lavery S, Turner C, Margara R, Trew G. Is there a link between an extremely poor response to ovarian hyperstimulation and early ovarian failure? Hum Reprod 2002; 17: 1106–11.

111. Lawson R, El-Toukhy T, Kassab A, et al. Poor response to ovulation induction is a stronger predictor of early menopause than elevated basal FSH: a life table analysis. Hum Reprod 2003; 18: 527–33.

112. van Kooij RJ, Looman CW, Habbema JD, Dorland M, te Velde ER. Age-dependent decrease in embryo implantation rate after in vitro fertilization. Fertil Steril 1996; 66: 769–75.

113. Sharma V, Allgar V, Rajkhowa M. Factors influencing the cumulative conception rate and discontinuation of in vitro fertilization treatment for infertility. Fertil Steril 2002; 78: 40–6.

114. Hauzman E, Fedorcsak P, Klinga K, et al. Use of serum inhibin A and human chorionic gonadotropin measurements to predict the outcome of in vitro fertilization pregnancies. Fertil Steril 2004; 81: 66–72.

115. Abdalla HI, Burton G, Kirkland A, et al. Age, pregnancy and miscarriage: uterine versus ovarian factors. Hum Reprod 1993; 8: 1512–17.

116. Lintsen AM, Pasker-de Jong PC, de Boer EJ, et al. Effects of subfertility cause, smoking and body weight on the success rate of IVF. Hum Reprod 2005; 20: 1867–75.

117. Younglai EV, Holloway AC, Foster WG. Environmental and occupational factors affecting fertility and IVF success. Hum Reprod Update 2005; 11: 43–57.

118. Homan GF, Davies M, Norman R. The impact of lifestyle factors on reproductive performance in the general population and those undergoing infertility treatment: a review. Hum Reprod Update 2007; 13: 209–23.

119. Dechanet C, Anahory T, Mathieu Daude JC, et al. Effects of cigarette smoking on reproduction. Hum Reprod Update 2011; 17: 76–95.

120. Zenzes MT, Wang P, Casper RF. Cigarette smoking may affect meiotic maturation of human oocytes. Hum Reprod 1995; 10: 3213–17.

121. Practice Committee of the American Society for Reproductive Medicine. Smoking and Fertility. Fertil Steril 2006; 86: S172–7.

122. Zenzes MT, Krishnan S, Krishnan B, Zhang H, Casper RF. Cadmium accumulation in follicular fluid of women in in vitro fertilization-embryo transfer is higher in smokers. Fertil Steril 1995; 64: 599–603.

123. Paszkowski T, Clarke RN, Hornstein MD. Smoking induces oxidative stress inside the Graafian follicle. Hum Reprod 2002; 17: 921–5.

124. Norman RJ, Clark AM. Obesity and reproductive disorders: a review. Reprod Fertil Dev 1998; 10: 55–63.

125. Maheshwari A, Stofberg L, Bhattacharya S. Effect of overweight and obesity on assisted reproductive technology–a systematic review. Hum Reprod Update 2007; 13: 433–44.

126. Boxmeer JC, Brouns RM, Lindemans J, et al. Preconception folic acid treatment affects the microenvironment of the maturing oocyte in humans. Fertil Steril 2008; 89: 1766–70.

127. Boxmeer JC, Smit M, Weber RF, et al. Seminal plasma cobalamin significantly correlates with sperm concentration in men undergoing IVF or ICSI procedures. J Androl 2007; 28: 521–7.

128. Boxmeer JC, Fauser BC, Macklon NS. Effect of B vitamins and genetics on success of in-vitro fertilisation. Lancet 2006; 368: 200.

129. Ozkan S, Jindal S, Greenseid K, et al. Replete vitamin D stores predict reproductive success following in vitro fertilization. Fertil Steril 2010; 94: 1314–19.

130. Heijnen EM, Eijkemans MJ, De Klerk C, et al. A mild treatment strategy for in-vitro fertilisation: a randomised non-inferiority trial. Lancet 2007; 369: 743–9.

131. Heijnen EM, Macklon NS, Fauser BC. What is the most relevant standard of success in assisted reproduction? The next step to improving outcomes of IVF: consider the whole treatment. Hum Reprod 2004; 19: 1936–8.

35

Initial investigation of the infertile couple

Isabelle Roux, Togas Tulandi, Peter Chan, and Hananel Holzer

INTRODUCTION

Infertility affects one in six to seven couples. After one year of unprotected intercourse, 85% to 90% of the couples will succeed to conceive. Among the remaining couples, 5% will conceive during the second year. Infertility is defined as failure to conceive after 12 months of unprotected intercourse (1).

In general, infertility investigations are conducted after 12 months of exposure. However, some cases including those with oligo/amenorrhea, history of pelvic surgery, tubal infection, or chemotherapy require earlier investigations. For women older than 35 years, investigations should be started after six months of attempts. This is due to age-related fertility decline in both spontaneous pregnancies and ART-induced pregnancies (2).

Infertility is related to female factor in 33%, male factor in 20%, both male and female factor in 39%, and is unexplained in 8% of cases (3). Treatment is based on the diagnosis of infertility.

The purpose of our review is to provide an overview of investigation of the infertile couple.

General and Couple Assessment

History taking is a crucial part of infertility investigations (4). Taking a history is an integral part in the evaluation of infertile couples that could not be replaced by a questionnaire. This includes sexual history such as frequency and timing of sexual intercourse and a possibility of sexual dysfunction, history of genetic disease, consanguinity, current and past medications, previous treatment, and lifestyle including smoking (5,6). Cessation of smoking is essential not only for general health but also to increase fertility. In our institution, we also evaluate the patient's rubella titer and diabetes screening for women with polycystic ovarian syndrome (PCOS) or obesity. Both couples will be tested for their HIV status and hepatitis B and C serology. We advise regular intake of folic acid.

Female Investigation

Female factors of infertility include ovulation disorders (32%) and tubal damage (26%) (3). Uterine cavity abnormalities can be a contributing factor to infertility with an increased prevalence in infertile patients (7).

Clinical History

In addition to history taking for both partners, gynecological history is essential. This includes menstrual history, previous pregnancy and outcome, history of sexually transmitted disease, and previous methods of contraception. Pelvic surgeries potentially leading to adhesions or impairing tubal and ovarian function should be noted.

Menstrual history provides an indication of the ovulation status. For example, a history of regular 24 to 35 day menses is consistent with ovulation in 97% of cases (8). History of oligomenorrhea or amenorrhea is strongly predictive of anovulation. General history should focus on weight changes and on endocrine diseases that could interfere with the gonadal function like hypothyroidism.

Physical Examination

Physical examination should include the patient's weight and height, identification of thyroid abnormalities, breast secretion, hirsutism, and other signs of hyperandrogenism. This is followed by pelvic examination.

Tests

Female tests are performed to evaluate three principles axes: ovaries, tubes, and uterus. Initial infertility tests are summarized in Figure 35.1.

Ovaries

Ovarian function and reserve are examined by hormonal tests and ultrasonography.

Ovarian Function Ovulation was historically assessed by basal body temperature (BBT) measurement. Although a biphasic BBT provides presumptive evidence of ovulation, monophasic or uninterpretable BBT are also common in ovulatory patients. In fact, BBT cannot accurately predict ovulation and its timing (9,10).

Other tests such as urinary luteinizing hormone (LH) and serum mid-luteal progesterone can be used to diagnose ovulation. Commercially available urinary LH kit identifies mid-cycle LH surge as an indirect sign of ovulation. Urinary LH helps to determine the fertile period.

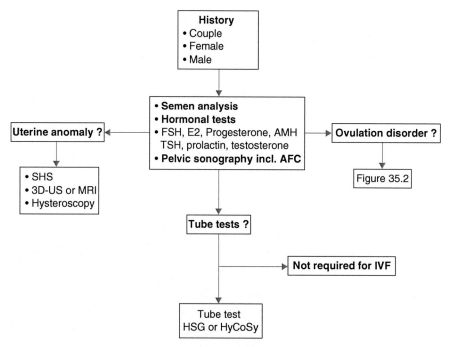

Figure 35.1 Initial infertility tests.

However, false–positive LH test could occur in 7% of cases (11) and repetitive use could be expensive and frustrating. Mid-luteal serum progesterone seems to be an easy method to retrospectively confirm ovulation. Yet, progesterone concentration fluctuations are wide even among normal women impairing interpretation. Values greater than 3.0 ng/ml might be presumptive of ovulation (12). Some authors reported that serum progesterone levels greater than 10 ng/ml correlated with a normal "in phase" endometrial histology (13). Whether it is correlated with luteal function is unclear.

Endometrial biopsy and dating is another test to evaluate ovulation. However, the results are not clearly related to the fertility status and its clinical use is limited (14). Accordingly, many authors advocated to abandon endometrial biopsy as a routine test (15,16). Today, the most commonly used test for ovulation is still mid-luteal phase serum luteal progesterone measurement.

Other Endocrine Evaluations Hormonal disturbances impairing hypothalamic–pituitary–ovarian axis such as thyroid dysfunction or hyperprolactinemia should be evaluated. Serum thyroid-stimulating hormone (TSH) and prolactin determinations can identify thyroid disorders and/or hyperprolactinemia that may require a specific treatment. Clinical significance of TSH tests seems to be limited to patients with ovulatory cycles (17). These tests are usually performed as part of screening tests. They certainly should be done in women suspected to have thyroid dysfunction or hyperprolactinemia.

Clinical hyperandrogenism should be confirmed by serum androgen measurements including serum free testosterone, delta-4-androstenedione, or dehydroepiandrosterone sulfate. Biological hyperandrogenism requires further investigations to rule out the presence of nonclassical congenital adrenal hyperplasia (serum 17-hydroxy-progesterone measurement), Cushing syndrome, or androgen-producing tumor.

Postcoital Test Postcoital Test (PCT) evaluates the adequacy of cervical mucus at late follicular phase and its interaction with sperm. It was a traditional method for identifying cervical factor and indirectly a male factor. This test has a poor interobserver and intra-observer reproducibility (18). Since there is no universal definition of cervical infertility and the current treatments for unexplained infertility (such as ovulation induction and intrauterine insemination) could overcome cervical factors, PCT should not be part of the routine fertility evaluation. (12). More importantly, routine use of PCT has no effect on pregnancy rate (19).

Women with regular cycles ovulate most probably each month. Infertile women require investigations for ovarian function and ovarian reserve. Figure 35.2 demonstrates tests for ovulation functions.

Ovarian Reserve Serum measurements of follicle stimulating hormone (FSH) and estradiol (E2) are performed in the early follicular phase – from day 2 to 5 of the cycle. FSH is an indirect marker of ovarian reserve. It predicts ovarian response to FSH stimulation (20). FSH is downregulated by E2. Accordingly, low FSH value could be encountered when the level of E2 is high. Both hormones should be evaluated together. The upper threshold of FSH varies between 10 and 25 IU/L (20,21). The accuracy of FSH to predict poor response is more accurate at very high threshold levels (22).

Another marker for ovarian reserve is serum anti-Mullerian hormone (AMH). It is a dimeric glycoprotein member of the TGF-β superfamily produced only by the

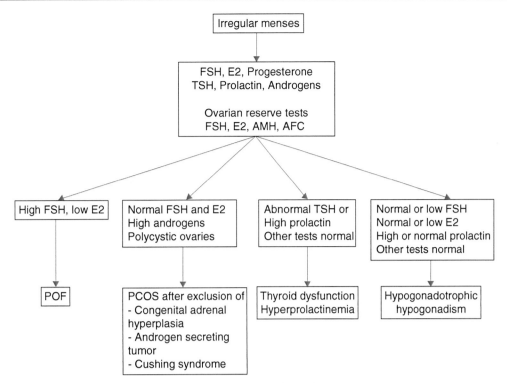

Figure 35.2   Tests for ovulation function.

ovaries in women. AMH expression is absent in primordial follicles and appears in granulosa cells of primary follicles. The strongest staining of AMH is observed in pre-antral and small antral follicles. AMH is found in growing follicles until they become dominant (23). Thus, AMH is a direct ovarian reserve marker representing different stages of growing follicles.

AMH is undetectable after menopause (24) and it does not seem to be regulated by FSH (25). Since cyclic variation of AMH is minimal (26), this test can be done at any time of the cycle. Normal values of AMH are described by a few normograms (27,28). For evaluation of ovarian reserve, AMH seems to be more sensitive than other ovarian markers (29). Low AMH value predicts poor ovarian response to ovarian stimulation. Some authors have advocated the use of AMH as diagnostic criteria for PCOS (30).

Pelvic transvaginal ultrasonography has become a mandatory tool in the investigation of infertility. It provides information about the uterus, the ovaries, and to a certain extent the fallopian tubes such as the presence of hydrosalpinx. Measurement of antral follicle count (AFC) in early follicular phase indicates the patient's ovarian reserve. Similar to AMH, AFC is a direct ovarian reserve marker. Antral follicles of 2–6 mm are more predictive of the ovarian response than those measuring 7–10 mm (31). In general, the low range for AFC is comprised between 3 and 10 follicles (22). Low AFC indicates low ovarian reserve.

Ultrasound (US) appearance of the ovaries is included in the Rotterdam criteria of PCOS (32). Either 12 or more follicles measuring 2–9 mm in diameter per ovary, or increased ovarian volume (>10 cm³) is one of the three diagnostic criteria of PCOS (33).

Serum inhibin B measurement has been used as an indicator of ovarian reserve. It is a glycoprotein produced by growing follicles in the early and mid-follicular phase. However, due to its lack of accuracy, it is not done routinely anymore (22,34). Other tests that have gone into disfavor are dynamic ovarian reserve tests including clomiphene citrate challenge test (CCCT) (35) and exogenous FSH ovarian reserve test (EFORT) (36). They are time consuming and their predictive values are inferior to other ovarian markers (34).

The two best predictive tests of ovarian reserve and ovarian response to stimulation are serum AMH and AFC (22,37). They are also good prognostic factors for ovarian hyperstimulation syndrome (38). However, ovarian reserve markers, even AMH and AFC, are not good prognostic factors for pregnancy rate, suggesting that they are quantitative but not qualitative markers (37,39).

FSH is a less sensitive marker than AMH and AFC. Yet, high FSH level indicates ovarian failure. Premature ovarian failure (POF) consists of amenorrhea with high serum FSH and low E2 (40,41) in women below the age of 40 years. The prevalence of POF is estimated to be from 1% to 3% (42). It could be due to chemotherapy, pelvic radiation, or surgery, but 90% of POF is unexplained (40). Women with POF should be further investigated with chromosomal analysis to evaluate the presence of X-chromosome abnormalities. Karyotype will look for Turner syndrome. Premutation of FMR1 gene is associated with POF. Mutation of FMR1 gene is responsible of fragile X syndrome that is the most common cause of familial mental retardation. Since autoimmune oophoritis may lead to POF and can be associated with Addison disease, autoimmune context including adrenal antibodies should be examined (40).

Fallopian Tubes

Tubal assessment is required to diagnose tubal infertility. When IVF is indicated (severe sperm abnormality, known severe endometriosis, women of advanced maternal age), tubal patency does not need to be verified. Different methods to assess tubal patency are hysterosalpingography (HSG), hysterosalpingo-contrast-sonography (HyCoSy), and laparoscopy with chromotubation.

HSG HSG is the radiographic evaluation of the fallopian tubes. Radiography images are obtained intermittently after injection of oil-based or water-soluble contrast media. The contraindications to HSG are contrast allergy, pregnancy, and active pelvic infection. Uterine cavity, Fallopian tube architecture, hydrosalpinx, tubal phimosis, and peritoneal spillage are assessed. HSG should be performed between menstrual day–6 to 11 to ensure the absence of pregnancy and facilitate maximum uterine visibility with a thin proliferative phase endometrium. Some patients can experience pain that leads to the termination of the procedure. Post-HSG infection can occur in 0.3% to 3.1% of cases, particularly when HSG findings are abnormal (43). Prophylactic antibiotics including doxycycline are commonly prescribed to reduce this risk (44).

"Proximal tubal occlusion" is usually due to tubal spasm or collection of debris or minimal adhesions. This finding should be followed by selective tubal catheterization. HSG sensitivity and specificity are 65% and 83% respectively (45). HSG is more specific for detecting distal as opposed to proximal occlusion (45), and it has a high correlation (94%) with laparoscopy findings (46).

Chlamydia trachomatis serology detecting immunoglobulin-G has been advocated for screening patients at high risk for tubal damage and to increase the prediction of tubal disease in conjunction with HSG. Negative serology and normal HSG indicates low probability of tubal disease on laparoscopy examination (<5%) (47). On the other hand, patients with positive serology have a high risk for tubal pathology and complications after HSG (48). This test is not widely used.

HyCoSy HyCoSy is ultrasonography combined with uterine instillation of saline or contrast media. The presence of fluid in the cul-de-sac after uterine instillation implies at least one patent tube (49). Tubal patency can also be distinguished by visualization of intratubal flow. Pain induced by HyCoSy and its complications are comparable to HSG (50). Although HyCoSy might have been considered inferior to HSG for evaluating tubal patency (46,51), other comparative studies showed that HyCoSy is as reliable as HSG (52).

Laparoscopy Laparoscopy with chromopertubation has been considered as the "gold standard" for evaluating tubal patency. Its advantages include the possibility of evaluating the abdominal cavity and the presence of endometriosis, of treating endometriosis, adhesions, or of repairing tubes. Hysteroscopy can also be performed at the same time. On the other hand, laparoscopy is an invasive test that requires general anesthesia. The risk of major complications is low (<5%) (53). Laparoscopy is indicated when there is evidence or strong suspicion of endometriosis, pelvic/adnexal adhesions, or significant tubal disease requiring treatment (12). Laparoscopic examination will confirm the US findings of a hydrosalpinx. The specificity of ultrasonographic detection of hydrosalpinx is over 99% (54).

HSG and HyCoSy are the first line tests to evaluate the Fallopian tubes in infertile women. They are generally well tolerated, inexpensive, and capable of demonstrating tubal patency at rates as high as 80% (52). The choice between these two techniques depends on the patient's allergy, availability, and the operator's experience. With the availability of minimally invasive tests, diagnostic laparoscopy is rarely required.

Uterus

Intrauterine lesions including endometrial polyps, submucosal myomas, adhesions, or uterine septum can interfere with spontaneous fertility and compromise pregnancy rates in assisted reproduction.

Two-dimension transvaginal US is an inexpensive, easy, and well-tolerated procedure. Its sensitivity to detect intrauterine lesion ranges from 56% to 89% (55,56). However, it may be difficult to detect the presence of submucosal fibroids in the presence of multiple fibroids, endometrial polyp in the presence of thick endometrium, and to diagnose synechia or uterine malformations.

Besides evaluating tubal patency, HSG can also provide assessment of the uterine cavity. However, the findings of intrauterine filling defects could also be due to air bubbles, mucus, and menstrual debris. False negative findings can result from excessive amount of contrast media obliterating shadows caused by small lesions. Compared to hysteroscopy, HSG has a sensitivity of 60% to 98% and a low specificity from 15% to 80% with high rates of false positive and false negative (57,58). HSG provides an idea of the uterine cavity but it should not be used specifically to evaluate the uterine cavity.

Saline hysterosonography (SHS) is US combined with saline infusion of the uterine cavity. This method improves the delineation of the cavity. SHS has a high sensitivity from 78% to 100% and a high specificity from 71% to 91% (56,59,60). SHS is more efficient for diagnosing polyp or submucosal fibroid than endometrial hyperplasia and structural abnormalities (56,59,60). It is also more accurate than US and HSG. However, hysteroscopy remains the most accurate test for evaluation of the uterine cavity (56,59,60). Following examination of the uterine cavity, the procedure could be extended to assess the integrity of the fallopian tubes (HyCoSy). Three-dimensional SHS (3D-SHS) could also be performed. 3D-SHS is superior to SHS and seems to be comparable with hysteroscopy for diagnosing intrauterine lesions (61,62).

Hysteroscopy allows visualization of the uterine cavity but not the tissue surrounding the cavity. As expected, the presence of a rudimentary horn will be missed. Accordingly, uterine anomaly should be investigated by MRI, three-dimensional ultrasonography (3D-US), or a combination of laparoscopy and hysteroscopy. MRI is an accurate and noninvasive test but it is costly. Laparoscopy is accurate but invasive. 3D-US seems to be a good compromise. 3D-US is accurate for diagnosing congenital Mullerian anomalies, highly correlated with the results of MRI, laparoscopy, or hysteroscopy, particularly when performed during the luteal phase (63).

The use of small diameter hysteroscope allows hysteroscopy to be conducted in the office setting. Polypectomy or adhesiolysis can also be performed (64,65). Hysteroscopy is not a part of routine infertility investigations, but it is a useful test to evaluate and confirm a suspected intrauterine abnormality (66).

Two-dimensional US is the first test to screen a suspected intrauterine abnormality. Other tests include SHS for polyp or intrauterine myoma assessment and 3D-US or MRI for Mullerian anomalies. Hysteroscopy remains the gold standard for evaluation of the uterine cavity.

Male Investigation

The basic male investigation begins with a detailed history and physical examination. Semen analysis and serum hormonal profile represent the first line laboratory investigation. The goal of these investigations is to identify the underlying causes of male factor that can be corrected to enhance the fertility status. More importantly, a thorough male fertility evaluation may reveal serious associated conditions including testis cancer, osteoporosis/osteopenia, genetic and hormone disorders that can have significant health consequences or even be life threatening.

Clinical History

A general history should include the developmental history such as congenital malformation of the genitalia, cryptorchidism, and delayed onset of puberty. Previous history of herniorrhaphy, particularly in childhood, may result in inadvertent damage to the vas deferens that is unrecognized. History of mumps orchitis, particularly in adolescence, sexually transmitted infections, genitourinary surgeries, instrumentation, or trauma should be enquired. Symptoms of the lower urinary tract, erectile and ejaculatory functions should also be carefully reviewed.

A thorough review of related organ system function such as pulmonary disease and upper respiratory infections may suggest genetic conditions such as Young's syndrome, Kartagener's syndrome (immotile cilia syndrome; primary ciliary dyskinesia), or cystic fibrosis. A history of a metabolic or neurological condition may be related to impaired erectile and ejaculatory function. History of gonadotoxic treatment should also be recorded. Use of medication, alcohol, drugs, and occupational and environmental exposure of toxins such as heat and other chemicals that can act as endocrine disruptors are elements to be recorded as well.

Physical Examination

A thorough physical examination should focus on general signs such as secondary sex characteristics that reflect normal androgenization (hair distribution, absence of gynecomastia, skeletal muscle development) and on the genitalia.

Genital examination includes localization of the penile urethral meatus and palpation of the testes for their size and consistency. Testis cancer risks increased significantly among men with infertility and can be diagnosed by proper testicular examination. Testicular size can be assessed by using testis-shaped models of defined sizes (Prader orchidometer) and may be indicative of spermatogenesis. The normal range is 12–30ml (67). Small testes are related to testicular dysfunction or hypogonadism.

Size, texture, position, and orientation of the epididymides and the bilateral presence of the vasa should also be carefully examined. Congenital bilateral absence of vas deferens (CBAVD) suggests the presence of mutation of the cystic fibrosis transmembrane conductance regular gene (CFTR). Cysts or nodularity of the epididymis suggest congenital or inflammatory changes that can lead to obstruction.

Examination of the spermatic cord in the upright position is important to evaluate the presence of varicoceles. Varicocele is classified into three grades: I – palpable only with Valsalva maneuver; II – palpable even without Valsalva maneuver; and III – detectable by visual inspection. Digital rectal examination can detect cysts in the seminal vesicles and prostatic adenoma and neoplasia.

Laboratory Investigations

The first line laboratory investigation for male infertility includes semen analysis. There are inter-laboratory and intraindividual variations in semen analysis (68). Thus, abnormal semen analysis results should be repeated at least one month later to confirm the diagnosis (69).

According to the WHO, semen sample should be collected by masturbation after 2–7 days of abstinence. In exceptional circumstances, semen may be produced at home or during sexual intercourse using a special condom. How the sample was produced, difficulties in semen production, and any loss of any fraction of the sample should be reported.

Aspermia is the absence of semen that can be related to retrograde ejaculation or anejaculation due to psychological or neurological causes. In case of retrograde ejaculation, a post-orgasm urine analysis may be performed with specific preparation (such as alkalinization of urine) to evaluate sperm quality.

Semen analysis assesses such parameters as volume, pH, sperm concentration, vitality, motility, and morphology. The main reference values of semen analysis according to the WHO are summarized in Table 35.1.

The bulk of semen volume is made up of secretions from the male accessory gland in the reproductive tract, mainly seminal vesicles and prostate. Low semen volume may be associated with the absence or blockade of

Table 35.1 Reference Values of Semen Analysis According to WHO

Criteria	Reference value
Volume	≥1.5 mL
Total sperm number	≥39 millions/ejaculate
Sperm concentration	≥15 millions/mL
Total motility	≥40%
Progressive motility	≥32%
Normal morphology	≥4%
Vitality	≥58%

the seminal vesicles or the ejaculatory duct in the prostate. In men with CBAVD, low semen volume is often seen due to the poor development of the seminal vesicles. Low semen volume can also be the result of collection problem, androgen deficiency, or partial retrograde ejaculation. High semen volume may reflect active exudation in cases of active inflammation of the accessory organs.

The pH of semen reflects the balance of the pH values of the secretions from various accessory glands, with the secretion of the seminal vesicles being alkaline and prostate acidic. A pH less than 7 in a sample with low volume and azoospermia strongly suggests ejaculatory duct obstruction or CBAVD.

In the absence of obstruction in the excurrent ductal system, the total number of spermatozoa per ejaculate and spermatozoa concentration in semen can both reflect testicular capacity in sperm production. Technically, the number of spermatozoa in the ejaculate is calculated from the concentration of spermatozoa. The total number of spermatozoa per ejaculate may be affected by the completeness of semen collection or accidental spillage of the sample while the concentration of spermatozoa in semen is influenced by the volume of the secretions from accessory glands. The total numbers of spermatozoa per ejaculate and the sperm concentration have been shown to correlate to both time to pregnancy (TTP) and pregnancy rate (70).

Although there is no agreed definition of severe oligozoospermia, the limit of 5 millions/ml is generally accepted. Azoospermia is defined by the absence of spermatozoa identified in the sample and cryptozoospermia by the identification of spermatozoa only in the sediment of the semen post-centrifugation. Azoospermia is classified based on its etiology as obstructive azoospermia (OA) or nonobstructive azoospermia (NOA).

Biochemical assays of semen may reflect function or blockade of the accessory sex organs and excurrent ductal system.

There are specific markers for each accessory gland that we are not going to develop here because they are not used widely. For example, seminal level of fructose, which is produced by seminal vesicles will be low in cases of ejaculatory duct obstruction and seminal vesicles agenesis or dysfunction. Sperm motility is graded as (1) progressive motility (PR: Spermatozoa moving actively regardless of the speed); (2) nonprogressive

motility (NP: Motility with an absence of progression); and (3) immotile. Previous categorization of sperm progressive motility as rapid or slow is no longer used because of the difficulties to objectively define the speed of forward progression (71). However, when discussing sperm motility, it is important to specify total motility (PR+NP) or progressive motility (PR). Sperm vitality is an important variable, especially for samples with less than 40% progressively motile spermatozoa. The percentage of dead spermatozoa cannot exceed the percentage of immotile spermatozoa.

Morphological anomalies in spermatozoa could be identified in the head, neck and mid-piece, and tail. Morphological anomalies are commonly found in more than one part of a spermatozoon. Defective spermatogenesis and some epididymal pathologies may contribute to an increased percentage of abnormal morphology of spermatozoa. Spermatozoa with abnormal morphology generally have a lower fertilizing potential, depending on the types of anomalies, and may also have abnormal DNA. Unfortunately, assessment of sperm morphology is associated with a number of technical difficulties related to variation in interpretation or poor performance in external quality control assessments.

Identification of non-sperm cells, such as epithelial cells or rounds cells (germ cells or leukocytes), may be indicative of a pathology of the efferent ducts (ciliary tufts), testicular damage (immature germ cells), or inflammation of the accessory glands (leucocytes). If the estimate of round cell concentration exceeds 10^6 per ml, their nature should be assessed (71). Special staining assessing their peroxidase activities could indicate that the round cells are leukocytes. Excessive numbers of leukocytes in the ejaculate may be associated with inflammation or infection. Leukocytes can impair sperm motility and DNA integrity through oxidative stress.

The WHO semen reference values were revised in 2010 (71). It is interesting to understand how these criteria were chosen. To begin with, the study population from whom the reference values are derived may not necessarily be an ideal representative sample of the whole population because of selection bias due to the embarrassing nature of reproductive studies (72–74). The subset of fertile men with TTP less than 12 months was selected to provide reference values for human semen, since infertility is currently defined as a failure to conceive after at least 12 months of unprotected intercourse. Data from 1953 semen samples from five studies done in eight countries in three continents in accordance to the WHO criteria were combined and analysed (75). Since there is no reason to believe that high sperm numbers or percentages of progressively motile or morphologically normal spermatozoa are harmful to fertility (76) and that "too high" values appear to be clinically irrelevant, one-sided lower reference limits seems appropriate for the various semen parameters.

Many lower reference limits for semen variables have been proposed but it is widely accepted that 95% of the data should be included in the reference interval when establishing the reference limits. Hence, a one-sided distribution at reference limit of fifth percentiles (with 95% confidence intervals) was chosen for all semen parameters. Interpretation of semen parameters should be done with caution. First, all males from the reference population, even under the fifth centiles were fertile with TTP <12 months. Thus not all men with semen parameters below the reference values can be labelled with certainty to be "infertile." Second, the measurements made on the whole population of ejaculated spermatozoa cannot define the fertilizing capacity of the few that reach the site of fertilization. Thus, one should not use semen parameters to "predict" success of fertility even in the setting of assisted reproduction. Nevertheless, semen analysis provides essential information that can guide clinicians to additional investigations and management aiming at improving the fertility status of couples experiencing difficulty to conceive.

Antisperm autoantibodies can be suspected when urological history is suggestive (hernia or testicular surgery, testicular trauma, genitalia infection, or vasectomy) or when agglutination of sperm (motile spermatozoa sticking to each other) is noted in semen analysis. Antisperm antibodies (ASA) are more frequent among infertile males and may impair sperm penetration of cervical mucus (77), zona pellucida interaction, and oocyte fusion. Autoimmune infertility is a controversial issue and the standard for clinical interpretation of the presence of ASA is not established (77,78). Thus, ASA tests should not be part of the routine male fertility evaluation.

Sperm DNA can be modified through various mechanisms responsible for DNA fragmentation occurring during spermatogenesis and transport through the reproductive tract (79). Although high levels of DNA damage often correlate to poor semen parameters and infertile men, DNA damage is also found in men with normal semen parameters (80). Low DNA fragmentation is significantly associated with pregnancy in vivo and after IUI (81) but this association is not strong enough after IVF or intracytoplasmic sperm injection (ICSI) (82) to provide a clinical indication for routine use of this test (79).

Ultrasonography can be done scrotally to evaluate scrotal and inguinal pathologies (e.g., varicoceles and testicular mass) or transrectally to assess the prostate and ejaculatory ducts (for cystic lesions or obstruction). US is not done routinely in male fertility evaluation. Its goal is to confirm a pathology that was suspected during physical examination or suggested based on semen and hormonal analysis.

If the semen analysis is abnormal, further tests are requested to discriminate pituitary–hypothalamic axis from testicular dysfunction and genitalia obstruction. Serum FSH and total testosterone measurements should be performed in all cases of oligospermia. Additional hormonal evaluation such as LH, prolactin, and TSH should be requested if the clinical findings suggest a specific pathology (69).

Low levels of FSH, LH (<2 IU/L), and testosterone in the context of low sperm concentration suggest hypogonadotropic hypogonadism. Though it is not a common cause of male infertility, this endocrinopathy may be a result of Kallmann's syndrome or acquired causes as hyperprolactinemia and hemochromatosis.

In case of low sperm concentration due to primary testicular failure, the testosterone will be low while FSH and LH will be high (>8 IU/L). However, if testicular failure impairs mainly the spermatogenesis and not endocrine function, testosterone and LH levels may be within the normal ranges.

Genetic Testing

In case of testicular failure, genetic testing including karyotype analysis and Y-chromosome microdeletion should performed. A karyotype analysis can diagnose numeric chromosomal abnormalities [e.g., Klinefelter' syndrome (KS)] or other chromosomal structure abnormalities (e.g., Robertsonian or reciprocal translocations). KS is the most common chromosomal abnormality: Non-mosaic KS accounts for 11% of azoospermia cases and mosaic KS accounts for 0.5% of severe oligospermia cases (83). In about half of azoospermic men with KS, testicular sperm extraction may allow sperm retrieved for ICSI. However, due to the increased risks of sperm chromosomal aneuploidy, genetic counseling including preimplantation genetic diagnosis (PGD) should be discussed with the couples prior to assisted reproduction.

The short arm (Yp) of the Y chromosome contains sex determination genes (SRY), and the long arm (Yq) contains genes that are important for spermatogenesis. Y chromosome microdeletions in three specific regions of the Yq, termed AZFa, AZFb, and AZFc (AZF – "azoospermic factor") can severely impair spermatogenesis. AZFa is located on proximal Yq11 (Yq11.21) while AZFb and AZFc are located on distal Yq11 (q11.23) (84). The approximate prevalence of AZF microdeletions in men with azoospermia is 7% (85). The vast majority of the AZF mutations arise de novo. AZFc is the most common deletion, seen in 60% of all Y chromosome microdeletions. About a third of men with a microdeletion in only the AZFc region may have severe oligozoospermia, while the majority are azoospermic. Testicular sperm extraction in more than half of azoospermic men with AZFc deletion may have sperm recovered for ICSI (86). If sperm is extracted and ICSI performed, vertical transmission of the mutation and likely infertility in male offspring are inevitable. Thus genetic counseling is important for these men.

Deletions involving AZFa or the entire region of AZFb are generally azoospermic (86). The histological findings in AZFa deletion men is usually Sertoli cell-only syndrome, while those with AZFb deletion tend to have germ cell arrest at the primary spermatocyte stage. The prognosis for sperm recovery by TESE is extremely poor and other options such as the use of donor sperm or adoption, if appropriate, should be discussed.

CBAVD is a common cause of primary obstructive azoospermia in healthy men with no prior history of genitourinary disorders. Of these men with CBAVD, more than 50% are heterozygous for the CFTR gene mutation or carry compound heterozygous mutations including milder coding mutations for the CFTR gene (87). Cystic fibrosis is a serious autosomal recessive condition. The cumulative carrier frequency varies according to the ethnic races. A carrier frequency as high as one in 25 is seen in men who are Northern European descendents or Ashkenazi Jews. CBAVD can be viewed as the mildest phenotype within the CFTR gene mutation spectrum. The clinical phenotype includes variants but obstructive azoospermia is consistent. Concerning the genitalia fibrous cord-like vas may be palpable, only the seminal vesicles and proximal vas may be missing, or asymmetry may be apparent (85). Renal tract anomalies (hypoplasia/ agenesis) affect about 10% of CBAVD patients, indicating the need for renal tract evaluation (88). History of non-severe pulmonary diseases or asthma may or may not be present.

CFTR mutation should be tested in all OA patients. More than 1200 mutations have been detected but only a few dozen prevalent CF-associated mutations are routinely screened. This means that a negative result does not exclude an unknown mutation. When a mutation is detected in the male, CFTR screening of the female partner is essential, but even then a negative result leaves a small residual risk of a CF affected offspring. Where CFTR mutations are found in both partners, preimplantation genetic diagnosis may be proposed to the couple to prevent the birth of a child with cystic fibrosis.

CONCLUSION

Infertility is a difficult situation for a couple. Basic investigations are the first step of infertility management, providing a diagnosis and a prognosis. Each member of the couple should undergo basic infertility investigations including evaluation of the uterine cavity, the Fallopian tubes, ovarian function and reserve, and semen analysis. These investigations could create anxiety. Our goal as physicians is to provide education and assistance including emotional support during the initial investigations and later during the treatment.

REFERENCES

1. The Practice Committee of the American Society for Reproductive Medicine. Definitions of infertility and recurrent pregnancy loss. Fertil Steril 2008; 90(Suppl 5): S60.
2. The Committee on Gynecologic Practice of the American College of Obstetricians and Gynecologists and the Practice Committee of the American Society for Reproductive Medicine. Age-related fertility decline: a committee opinion. Fertil Steril 2008; 90(Suppl 5): S154–5.
3. Thonneau P, Marchand S, Tallec A, et al. Incidence and main causes of infertility in a resident population (1,850,000) of three French regions (1988–1989). Hum Reprod 1991; 6: 811–16.
4. Tulandi T, Platt R. The art of taking a history. Fertil Steril 2004; 81: 11–12; discussion 8.
5. Augood C, Duckitt K, Templeton AA. Smoking and female infertility: a systematic review and meta-analysis. Hum Reprod 1998; 13: 1532–9.
6. Waylen AL, Metwally M, Jones GL, Wilkinson AJ, Ledger WL. Effects of cigarette smoking upon clinical outcomes of assisted reproduction: a meta-analysis. Hum Reprod Update 2009; 15: 31–44.
7. Chan YY, Jayaprakasan K, Zamora J, et al. The prevalence of congenital uterine anomalies in unselected and high-risk populations: a systematic review. Hum Reprod Update 2011; 17: 761–71.
8. Magyar DM, Boyers SP, Marshall JR, Abraham GE. Regular menstrual cycles and premenstrual molimina as indicators of ovulation. Obstet Gynecol 1979; 53: 411–14.
9. Guermandi E, Vegetti W, Bianchi MM, et al. Reliability of ovulation tests in infertile women. Obstet Gynecol 2001; 97: 92–6.
10. Luciano AA, Peluso J, Koch EI, et al. Temporal relationship and reliability of the clinical, hormonal, and ultrasonographic indices of ovulation in infertile women. Obstet Gynecol 1990; 75(3 Pt 1): 412–16.
11. McGovern PG, Myers ER, Silva S, et al. Absence of secretory endometrium after false-positive home urine luteinizing hormone testing. Fertil Steril 2004; 82: 1273–7.
12. The Practice Committee of the American Society for Reproductive Medicine. Optimal evaluation of the infertile female. Fertil Steril 2006; 86(5 Suppl 1): S264–7.
13. Jordan J, Craig K, Clifton DK, Soules MR. Luteal phase defect: the sensitivity and specificity of diagnostic methods in common clinical use. Fertil Steril 1994; 62: 54–62.
14. Coutifaris C, Myers ER, Guzick DS, et al. Histological dating of timed endometrial biopsy tissue is not related to fertility status. Fertil Steril 2004; 82: 1264–72.
15. Garcia JE. Endometrial biopsy: a test whose time has come. Fertil Steril 2004; 82: 1293–4; discussion 9–302.
16. Kazer RR. Endometrial biopsy should be abandoned as a routine component of the infertility evaluation. Fertil Steril 2004; 82: 1297–8; discussion 300–2.
17. Lincoln SR, Ke RW, Kutteh WH. Screening for hypothyroidism in infertile women. J Reprod Med 1999; 44: 455–7.
18. Jette NT, Glass RH. Prognostic value of the postcoital test. Fertil Steril 1972; 23: 29–32.
19. Oei SG, Helmerhorst FM, Bloemenkamp KW, et al. Effectiveness of the postcoital test: randomised controlled trial. BMJ 1998; 317: 502–5.
20. Scott RT, Toner JP, Muasher SJ, et al. Follicle-stimulating hormone levels on cycle day 3 are predictive of in vitro fertilization outcome. Fertil Steril 1989; 51: 651–4.
21. Muasher SJ, Oehninger S, Simonetti S, et al. The value of basal and/or stimulated serum gonadotropin levels in prediction of stimulation response and in vitro fertilization outcome. Fertil Steril 1988; 50: 298–307.
22. Broekmans FJ, Kwee J, Hendriks DJ, Mol BW, Lambalk CB. A systematic review of tests predicting ovarian reserve and IVF outcome. Hum Reprod Update 2006; 12: 685–718.
23. Weenen C, Laven JS, Von Bergh AR, et al. Anti-Mullerian hormone expression pattern in the human ovary: potential implications for initial and cyclic follicle recruitment. Mol Hum Reprod 2004; 10: 77–83.
24. La Marca A, Sighinolfi G, Radi D, et al. Anti-Mullerian hormone (AMH) as a predictive marker in assisted reproductive technology (ART). Hum Reprod Update 2010; 16: 113–30.

25. Bath LE, Wallace WH, Shaw MP, Fitzpatrick C, Anderson RA. Depletion of ovarian reserve in young women after treatment for cancer in childhood: detection by anti-Mullerian hormone, inhibin B and ovarian ultrasound. Hum Reprod 2003; 18: 2368–74.

26. Tsepelidis S, Devreker F, Demeestere I, et al. Stable serum levels of anti-Mullerian hormone during the menstrual cycle: a prospective study in normo-ovulatory women. Hum Reprod 2007; 22: 1837–40.

27. Nelson SM, Messow MC, McConnachie A, et al. External validation of nomogram for the decline in serum anti-Mullerian hormone in women: a population study of 15,834 infertility patients. Reprod Biomed Online 2011; 23: 204–6.

28. Almog B, Shehata F, Suissa S, et al. Age-related normograms of serum antimullerian hormone levels in a population of infertile women: a multicenter study. Fertil Steril 2011; 95: 2359–63; 63 e1.

29. de Vet A, Laven JS, de Jong FH, Themmen AP, Fauser BC. Antimullerian hormone serum levels: a putative marker for ovarian aging. Fertil Steril 2002; 77: 357–62.

30. Pigny P, Jonard S, Robert Y, Dewailly D. Serum anti-Mullerian hormone as a surrogate for antral follicle count for definition of the polycystic ovary syndrome. J Clin Endocrinol Metab 2006; 91: 941–5.

31. Haadsma ML, Bukman A, Groen H, et al. The number of small antral follicles (2–6 mm) determines the outcome of endocrine ovarian reserve tests in a subfertile population. Hum Reprod 2007; 22: 1925–31.

32. The Rotterdam ESHRE/ASRM-sponsored PCOS consensus workshop group. Revised 2003 consensus on diagnostic criteria and long-term health risks related to polycystic ovary syndrome (PCOS). Hum Reprod 2004; 19: 41–7.

33. Balen AH, Laven JS, Tan SL, Dewailly D. Ultrasound assessment of the polycystic ovary: international consensus definitions. Hum Reprod Update 2003; 9: 505–14.

34. Sills ES, Alper MM, Walsh AP. Ovarian reserve screening in infertility: practical applications and theoretical directions for research. Eur J Obstet Gynecol Reprod Biol 2009; 146: 30–6.

35. Navot D, Rosenwaks Z, Margalioth EJ. Prognostic assessment of female fecundity. Lancet 1987; 2: 645–7.

36. Fanchin R, de Ziegler D, Olivennes F, et al. Exogenous follicle stimulating hormone ovarian reserve test (EFORT): a simple and reliable screening test for detecting 'poor responders' in in-vitro fertilization. Hum Reprod 1994; 9: 1607–11.

37. van Rooij IA, Broekmans FJ, te Velde ER, et al. Serum anti-Mullerian hormone levels: a novel measure of ovarian reserve. Hum Reprod 2002; 17: 3065–71.

38. Broer SL, Dolleman M, Opmeer BC, et al. AMH and AFC as predictors of excessive response in controlled ovarian hyperstimulation: a meta-analysis. Hum Reprod Update 2011; 17: 46–54.

39. Broer SL, Mol BW, Hendriks D, Broekmans FJ. The role of antimullerian hormone in prediction of outcome after IVF: comparison with the antral follicle count. Fertil Steril 2009; 91: 705–14.

40. Nelson LM, Covington SN, Rebar RW. An update: spontaneous premature ovarian failure is not an early menopause. Fertil Steril 2005; 83: 1327–32.

41. de Moraes-Ruehsen M, Jones GS. Premature ovarian failure. Fertil Steril 1967; 18: 440–61.

42. Aiman J, Smentek C. Premature ovarian failure. Obstet Gynecol 1985; 66: 9–14.

43. Stumpf PG, March CM. Febrile morbidity following hysterosalpingography: identification of risk factors and recommendations for prophylaxis. Fertil Steril 1980; 33: 487–92.

44. ACOG Committee on Practice Bulletins—Gynecology. ACOG practice bulletin No. 104: antibiotic prophylaxis for gynecologic procedures. Obstet Gynecol 2009; 113: 1180–9.

45. Swart P, Mol BW, van der Veen F, et al. The accuracy of hysterosalpingography in the diagnosis of tubal pathology: a meta-analysis. Fertil Steril 1995; 64: 486–91.

46. Darwish AM, Youssef AA. Screening sonohysterography in infertility. Gynecol Obstet Invest 1999; 48: 43–7.

47. Meikle SF, Zhang X, Marine WM, et al. Chlamydia trachomatis antibody titers and hysterosalpingography in predicting tubal disease in infertility patients. Fertil Steril 1994; 62: 305–12.

48. den Hartog JE, Lardenoije CM, Severens JL, et al. Screening strategies for tubal factor subfertility. Hum Reprod 2008; 23: 1840–8.

49. Habibaj J, Kosova H, Bilali S, Bilali V, Qama D. Comparison between transvaginal sonography after diagnostic hysteroscopy and laparoscopic chromopertubation for the assessment of tubal patency in infertile women. J Clin Ultrasound 2011.

50. Ayida G, Kennedy S, Barlow D, Chamberlain P. A comparison of patient tolerance of hysterosalpingo-contrast sonography (HyCoSy) with Echovist-200 and X-ray hysterosalpingography for outpatient investigation of infertile women. Ultrasound Obstet Gynecol 1996; 7: 201–4.

51. Fleischer AC, Vasquez JM, Cullinan JA, Eisenberg E. Sonohysterography combined with sonosalpingography: correlation with endoscopic findings in infertility patients. J Ultrasound Med 1997; 16: 381–4; quiz 5–6.

52. Saunders RD, Shwayder JM, Nakajima ST. Current methods of tubal patency assessment. Fertil Steril 2011; 95: 2171–9.

53. Tian YF, Lin YS, Lu CL, et al. Major complications of operative gynecologic laparoscopy in southern Taiwan: a follow-up study. J Minim Invasive Gynecol 2007; 14: 284–92.

54. Guerriero S, Ajossa S, Lai MP, et al. Transvaginal ultrasonography associated with colour Doppler energy in the diagnosis of hydrosalpinx. Hum Reprod 2000; 15: 1568–72.

55. Bonnamy L, Marret H, Perrotin F, et al. Sonohysterography: a prospective survey of results and complications in 81 patients. Eur J Obstet Gynecol Reprod Biol 2002; 102: 42–7.

56. Grimbizis GF, Tsolakidis D, Mikos T, et al. A prospective comparison of transvaginal ultrasound, saline infusion sonohysterography, and diagnostic hysteroscopy in the evaluation of endometrial pathology. Fertil Steril 2010; 94: 2720–5.

57. Roma Dalfo A, Ubeda B, Ubeda A, et al. Diagnostic value of hysterosalpingography in the detection of intrauterine abnormalities: a comparison with hysteroscopy. AJR Am J Roentgenol 2004; 183: 1405–9.

58. Gaglione R, Valentini AL, Pistilli E, Nuzzi NP. A comparison of hysteroscopy and hysterosalpingography. Int J Gynaecol Obstet 1996; 52: 151–3.

59. Bingol B, Gunenc Z, Gedikbasi A, et al. Comparison of diagnostic accuracy of saline infusion sonohysterography, transvaginal sonography and hysteroscopy. J Obstet Gynaecol 2011; 31: 54–8.

60. Soares SR, Barbosa dos Reis MM, Camargos AF. Diagnostic accuracy of sonohysterography, transvaginal sonography, and hysterosalpingography in patients with uterine cavity diseases. Fertil Steril 2000; 73: 406–11.

61. Makris N, Kalmantis K, Skartados N, et al. Three-dimensional hysterosonography versus hysteroscopy for the detection of intracavitary uterine abnormalities. Int J Gynaecol Obstet 2007; 97: 6–9.

62. Abou-Salem N, Elmazny A, El-Sherbiny W. Value of 3-dimensional sonohysterography for detection of intra-uterine lesions in women with abnormal uterine bleeding. J Minim Invasive Gynecol 2010; 17: 200–4.

63. Caliskan E, Ozkan S, Cakiroglu Y, et al. Diagnostic accuracy of real-time 3D sonography in the diagnosis of congenital Mullerian anomalies in high-risk patients with respect to the phase of the menstrual cycle. J Clin Ultrasound 2010; 38: 123–7.

64. Bettocchi S, Nappi L, Ceci O, Selvaggi L. Office hysteroscopy. Obstet Gynecol Clin North Am 2004; 31: 641–54, xi.

65. Pundir J, El Toukhy T. Uterine cavity assessment prior to IVF. Women's health (London, England) 2010; 6: 841–7; quiz 7–8.

66. Crosignani PG, Rubin BL. Optimal use of infertility diagnostic tests and treatments. The ESHRE Capri Workshop Group. Hum Reprod 2000; 15: 723–32.

67. Lanfranco F, Kamischke A, Zitzmann M, Nieschlag E. Klinefelter's syndrome. Lancet 2004; 364: 273–83.

68. Alvarez C, Castilla JA, Martinez L, et al. Biological variation of seminal parameters in healthy subjects. Hum Reprod 2003; 18: 2082–8.

69. The Male Infertility Best Practice Policy Committee of the American Urological Association and The Practice Committee of the American Society for Reproductive Medicine. Report on optimal evaluation of the infertile male. Fertil Steril 2006; 86(5 Suppl 1): S202–9.

70. Slama R, Eustache F, Ducot B, et al. Time to pregnancy and semen parameters: a cross-sectional study among fertile couples from four European cities. Hum Reprod 2002; 17: 503–15.

71. World Health Organization. WHO Laboratory Manual for the Examination and Processing of Human Semen, 5th edn. Cambridge: Cambridge University Press, 2010.

72. Handelsman DJ, Dunn SM, Conway AJ, Boylan LM, Jansen RP. Psychological and attitudinal profiles in donors for artificial insemination. Fertil Steril 1985; 43: 95–101.

73. Tielemans E, Burdorf A, te Velde E, et al. Sources of bias in studies among infertility clients. Am J Epidemiol 2002; 156: 86–92.

74. Handelsman DJ. Sperm output of healthy men in Australia: magnitude of bias due to self-selected volunteers. Hum Reprod 1997; 12: 2701–5.

75. Cooper TG, Noonan E, von Eckardstein S, et al. World Health Organization reference values for human semen characteristics. Hum Reprod Update 16: 231–45.

76. Tournaye H, Staessen C, Camus M, et al. No evidence for a decreased fertilizing potential after in-vitro fertilization using spermatozoa from polyzoospermic men. Hum Reprod 1997; 12: 2183–5.

77. Francavilla F, Santucci R, Barbonetti A, Francavilla S. Naturally-occurring antisperm antibodies in men: interference with fertility and clinical implications. An update. Front Biosci 2007; 12: 2890–911.

78. Zini A, Fahmy N, Belzile E, et al. Antisperm antibodies are not associated with pregnancy rates after IVF and ICSI: systematic review and meta-analysis. Hum Reprod 2011; 26: 1288–95.

79. Sakkas D, Alvarez JG. Sperm DNA fragmentation: mechanisms of origin, impact on reproductive outcome, and analysis. Fertil Steril 2010; 93: 1027–36.

80. Schulte RT, Ohl DA, Sigman M, Smith GD. Sperm DNA damage in male infertility: etiologies, assays, and outcomes. J Assist Reprod Genet 2010; 27: 3–12.

81. Evenson D, Wixon R. Meta-analysis of sperm DNA fragmentation using the sperm chromatin structure assay. Reprod Biomed Online 2006; 12: 466–72.

82. Collins JA, Barnhart KT, Schlegel PN. Do sperm DNA integrity tests predict pregnancy with in vitro fertilization? Fertil Steril 2008; 89: 823–31.

83. Van Assche E, Bonduelle M, Tournaye H, et al. Cytogenetics of infertile men. Hum Reprod 1996; 11(Suppl 4): 1–24; discussion 5–6.

84. Vogt PH, Edelmann A, Kirsch S, et al. Human Y chromosome azoospermia factors (AZF) mapped to different subregions in Yq11. Hum Mol Genet 1996; 5: 933–43.

85. McLachlan RI, O'Bryan MK. Clinical Review#: State of the art for genetic testing of infertile men. J Clin Endocrinol Metab 95: 1013–24.

86. Hopps CV, Mielnik A, Goldstein M, et al. Detection of sperm in men with Y chromosome microdeletions of the AZFa, AZFb and AZFc regions. Hum Reprod 2003; 18: 1660–5.

87. Dork T, Dworniczak B, Aulehla-Scholz C, et al. Distinct spectrum of CFTR gene mutations in congenital absence of vas deferens. Hum Genet 1997; 100: 365–77.

88. Schlegel PN, Shin D, Goldstein M. Urogenital anomalies in men with congenital absence of the vas deferens. J Urol 1996; 155: 1644–8.

36

Prognostic testing for ovarian reserve

Frank J. Broekmans, Simone L. Broer, Bart C. J. M. Fauser, and Nick S. Macklon

FEMALE REPRODUCTIVE AGEING

Age-Related Subfertility and Ovarian Reserve

With the postponement of childbearing in Western societies, rates of subfertility related to female age have increased considerably (1). An increasing proportion of couples therefore depend on assisted reproductive technique (ART) to achieve a pregnancy. The increase of subfertility with increasing female age is mainly based on changes in ovarian function referred to as decreasing ovarian reserve. Ovarian reserve can be defined as the number and quality of the remaining follicles and oocytes in both ovaries at a given age. Decline in follicle numbers dictates the occurrence of irregular cycles and menopause, while quality decay results in decreasing fertility, defined as the capacity to conceive and give birth to a child (Fig. 36.1) (2).

Variability of Reproductive Ageing

There is substantial individual variation in the onset of menopause, varying roughly between 40 and 60 years, with a mean age of 51 years. This variation has shown to be rather constant over time and populations worldwide (3,4). Female fecundity is believed to decrease after the age of 31 years, a decrease that may accelerate after age 37 years leading to sterility at a mean age of 41 (5). As with menopause, the rate of decline in fertility may vary considerably between women of the same age. This implies that a woman at the age of 35 years either may be close to natural sterility or have a normal fertility comparable to a 25-year-old. The decrease of female fertility is believed to exhibit the same range of variation as for the occurrence of menopause (6). This implies that age at menopause, which is determined by the remaining follicle numbers, is considered a proxy variable for age at loss of natural fertility, with a fixed time period of 10 years in between. The correct prediction of menopause in an individual woman would therefore provide valuable information regarding a woman's fertile life span and hence aid in preventing future subfertility. At present, however, reliable means of prediction remain elusive (Fig. 36.2).

Natural and Assisted Fertility Decline

The human species can be considered as relatively subfertile compared to animals (7,8). The average monthly fecundity rate of about 20% implies that among human couples trying to conceive, many exposure months may be needed to achieve their goal, especially if monthly fecundity has dropped with increasing female age (9). The proportion of subfertile couples (failing to achieve a vital pregnancy within one year) will amount to 10–20% in the age group of women over 35 years, compared to only 4% for women in their 20s. These subfertility rates may rise to 30–50% for only moderately fecund women of age 35 years and over who have tried to conceive for several years (9,10). The maintenance of regular menstrual cycles until an age when natural fecundity has already been reduced to zero means that women are largely unaware that this process is taking place.

The age-related decline in female fertility has also been shown in numerous reports concerning ART [i.e., in vitro fertilization (IVF)] programs. After a mean female age of ~ 34 years the chance of producing a live birth in ART programs decreases steadily and reduces to less than 10% per cycle in women over 40 years of age (Fig. 36.3). The effect of female age has also been shown for the chance of an IVF embryo to implant after IVF (11). A poor response to ovarian hyperstimulation for IVF, especially in those with abnormal ovarian reserve test (ORT) results, is a strong predictor of poor prospects of becoming pregnant, and also of clearly reduced spontaneous fecundity and early menopause (12–14).

Ovarian Reserve Prediction

The knowledge and insights into the process of ovarian ageing imply that for ovarian reserve testing prior to ART, female age remains the predictor of first choice. The availability of a test capable of providing reliable information regarding a woman's individual ovarian reserve within a certain age category would enable the clinician to provide an individually tailored treatment plan. For instance, in older women the finding of a high ovarian reserve may justify the decision to allow ART treatment, while in young women with exhausted reserve

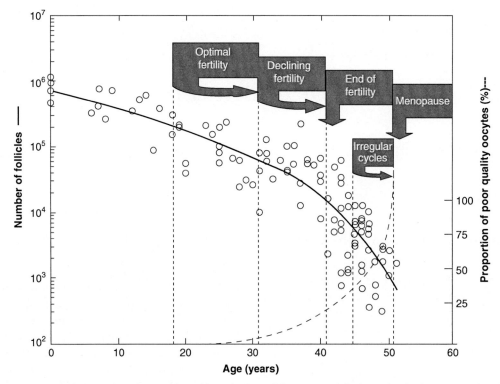

Figure 36.1   Quantitative (solid line) and qualitative (dotted line) decline of the ovarian follicle pool, which is assumed to dictate the onset of the important reproductive events. *Source*: Adapted from Ref. 60.

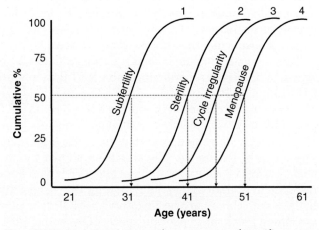

Figure 36.2   Variations in age at the occurrence of specific stages of ovarian ageing. For explanation of the background of data, see te Velde and Pearson (2). *Source*: From Ref. 2.

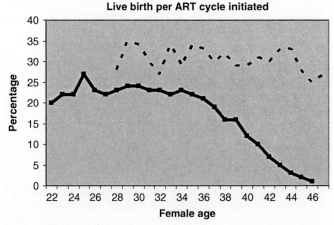

Figure 36.3   Effect upon average singleton live birth rates of female age, showing a steady decrease after the age of 34 years. The dotted line represents the average singleton live birth rate after oocyte donation as a function of the recipient age. It underlines the potential of oocyte donation in the treatment of women who remained unsuccessful in the previous IVF treatment. Data were drawn from the 2003 CDC ART report (http://www.cdc.gov/art/). *Abbreviations*: ART, assisted reproductive technique.

either early application or even refusal of ART could be the consequence. Ultimately, the response to maximal ovarian stimulation may provide further information on the reserve capacity of the ovaries. In the following two sections the biological rationale behind ovarian reserve testing and the accuracy and clinical value of several of these tests will be discussed.

THE PHYSIOLOGICAL BACKGROUND TO OVARIAN RESERVE TESTING

Follicle Quantity

Ovarian reserve can be considered normal in conditions where stimulation with the use of exogenous gonadotropins

will result in the development of some 5–13 follicles and the retrieval of a corresponding number of healthy oocytes at follicle puncture (15,16). With such a yield the chances of producing a live birth through IVF are considered optimal (17). In addition to the number of recruitable follicles that determines the ovarian reserve status, follicle sensitivity to follicle-stimulating hormone (FSH) and the pharmacodynamics of FSH also determine a woman's extent of ovarian response to stimulation. The dose of FSH used may be another factor although the therapeutic range is generally considered as quite narrow. Higher doses of FSH may lead to higher numbers of oocytes retrieved in younger patients (18), but not in all cohorts (19). Such an approach will certainly fail in older women (20) or in women expected to have a poor response to stimulation based on an abnormal ORT (21).

Female Age

In general, as outlined before, age of the woman is a simple way of obtaining information on the extent of her ovarian reserve, both regarding quantity as well as quality (22). However, in view of the substantial variation in the decay of reproductive capacity with age the need exists to identify women with clearly accelerated ovarian ageing at a relatively young age. In addition, it would also be useful to identify women around the mean age at which natural fertility on average is lost (41 years) with still adequate ovarian reserve. In clinical terms the aim should be to identify women with a high risk of producing a poor response to ovarian hyperstimulation and/or a very low probability of becoming pregnant through IVF, as well as those who still produce enough oocytes and are likely to become pregnant even if female age is advanced. If it is going to be possible to identify such women, fertility management could be effectively individualized. For instance, stimulation dose or treatment scheme could be adjusted (23), counseling against initiation of IVF treatment or pertinent refusal could be effected, or treatment could be initiated early before the reserve has diminished too far.

Tests and their Valuation

Most tests examined in the literature are evaluated by their capacity to predict some defined outcome related to ovarian reserve. The preferred or gold standard outcome of prediction studies would be live birth after a series of ART exposure cycles, but other outcomes (especially oocyte yield or follicle number and pregnancy after one IVF/ICSI cycle) are in fact the most common. As the occurrence of pregnancy in a single exposure to IVF and embryo transfer will be dependent on many other factors besides ovarian reserve, like laboratory performance and transfer technique, focus has been mostly upon the capacity of these tests to predict the ovarian response. Indeed, most if not all ORTs relate to the size of the follicle cohort that is at any time responsive to FSH. The antral follicle count (AFC) assessed by transvaginal ultrasonography provides direct visual assessment of the cohort (24). The endocrine marker anti-Müllerian hormone (AMH) which is produced by the granulosa cells surrounding the antral follicles, provides a novel direct marker of quantity (25,26). Basal FSH, extensively studied in the past decades, provides the most indirect marker. FSH levels will become increased with advancing age, by a reduction in the release of inhibin B, thereby reducing the

negative feedback on FSH release from the pituitary (27). High FSH levels therefore represent small cohort size. Endocrine challenge tests in which the growth of antral follicles is stimulated by endogenous or exogenous FSH and response is assessed in terms of output of estradiol or inhibin B are also principally related to cohort size (25). However, they are considered as too laborious for screening purposes and do not add much predictive value compared to static tests like AMH or the AFC (28,29). The same may be true for the clomiphene citrate (CC) challenge test, in which a CC-induced rise in FSH levels is counteracted by release of estradiol and inhibin B from growing antral follicles. The size of the antral follicle cohort will determine the degree of subsequent FSH suppression. Like the other challenge tests, the CC challenge test does not provide much additional information compared to basal FSH (Fig. 36.4) (30,31).

Accuracy and Clinical Value

Ovarian reserve test evaluation using response and/or pregnancy as reference or outcome variables should imply the assessment of predictive accuracy and clinical value of the test. *Predictive accuracy* refers to the degree by which the outcome condition is predicted correctly. Summary statistics of accuracy include sensitivity (rate of correct identification of cases with, e.g., poor response), specificity (rate of correct identification of cases without poor response), and the likelihood ratio (how many times more likely particular test results are in patients with poor response compared to those without poor response) (32,33). Using the calculated sensitivity and specificity for each cut off level, a receiver operating characteristic (ROC) curve can be drawn and area under this curve calculated to represent the overall predictive accuracy of the test. Values of 1.0 imply perfect and 0.5 indicate completely absent discrimination.

If a test is to identify all cases that will respond poorly to stimulation without falsely labeling normal responders, the test must have high sensitivity and high specificity. Positive likelihood ratios above 10 and negative likelihood ratios below 0.1 are considered as indicators of an adequate diagnostic test, while values between 5 and 10 and below 0.2 are considered to indicate a moderate test. As such the likelihood ratio can be considered a clinically useful tool to help judge upon the performance of the test as the value will change when the cut off for an abnormal test is shifted.

Clinical value incorporates the question if application of the test at a certain cut off will really change management or costs or safety or success rates on a population basis. Assessment of the clinical value is a complex process in which the applicability in daily practice should become clear. The overall accuracy represented by the ROC curve, the choice of a cut off for abnormality, the rate of abnormal tests at that cut off, the posttest probability of disease (i.e., poor response or non-pregnancy), the valuation of false–positive and false–negative test results, and the consequence for patient management of an

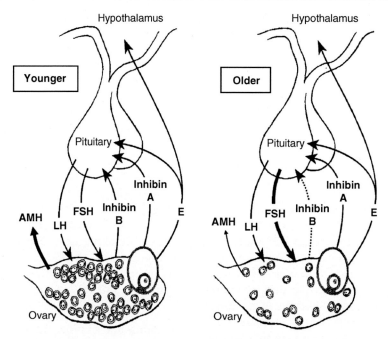

Figure 36.4   Illustration of the changes in follicle reserve with increasing female age and the effect of these quantitative changes upon several endocrine factors. *Abbreviations*: AMH, anti-Müllerian hormone; LH, luteinizing hormone; FSH, follicle-stimulating hormone. *Source*: Adapted from Ref. 61.

abnormal test will all contribute to the process of deciding whether a test is useful or not. The cost of carrying out the test as a routine measure and the burden to the patient balanced against the reduction in costs by excluding cases with low pregnancy prospects need to be incorporated in the decision process. Finally, clinical value may also be influenced by valuation from patients and health insurance preference regarding the consequences that should be drawn from abnormal tests (34).

Studies on the predictive accuracy and clinical value of ovarian reserve tests (ORT) should preferably be prospective in design. Moreover, they should examine cohorts of patients in IVF settings without exclusion of cases with signs of diminished ovarian reserve and patient management should not be influenced by the test under study (verification bias). Also, evaluation should be equally weighted for every case, thus every case should contribute the same amount of cycles to the analysis. In most studies only one IVF cycle is studied. A case control design for the purpose of OR testing bears the disadvantage of retrospection and the absence of a reliable estimate of the disease prevalence. The tests under study should in principle be reproducible, both at the laboratory (hormone assays) as well as at the operator level (ultrasound examination). Also, the outcome of treatment (response and pregnancy), serving as the reference for ovarian reserve, should be clearly defined.

Screening or Diagnosis

One aspect of clinical value deserves special attention. Ovarian reserve tests (ORTs) are mostly used as a diagnostic test, indicating that in case of an abnormal test result the diagnosis of diminished ovarian reserve is made (35,36). For the valuation of the test only proxy

variables of true ovarian reserve (poor ovarian response and non-pregnancy) are used. Also, false–positive test results may eliminate couples from the IVF trail that do have adequate prospects. Therefore, ORTs may better be considered as screening tests, where an abnormal test necessitates confirmation by another test. This other test may for instance be a first IVF attempt where ovarian response is the additional test. Alternatively, combinations of independently predictive tests or repeating of the initial test could improve the diagnostic performance of the single test, but existing literature shows a limited benefit of such approach (16,37–42).

THE VALUE OF OVARIAN RESERVE TESTING

Systematic Review

In recent reviews the predictive performance of ORTs was analysed by using the approach of the systematic review and meta-analysis (6,25,43,44). A strict approach was followed, where the accuracy of the prediction of two distinct outcomes in IVF treatment was presented and the clinical value was assessed. Also, the role of the test result in the choice of management options for the couple was included in the final judgment of the test. For example, a test identifying couples with a very poor prognosis leading to denial of treatment is certainly more valuable than the same test used only for counseling of the couple without strict consequences.

Poor-Response Prediction

From the extensive analysis in the review it appeared that the AFC and AMH are superior over the other ORTs, especially basal FSH. AMH and AFC are adequate

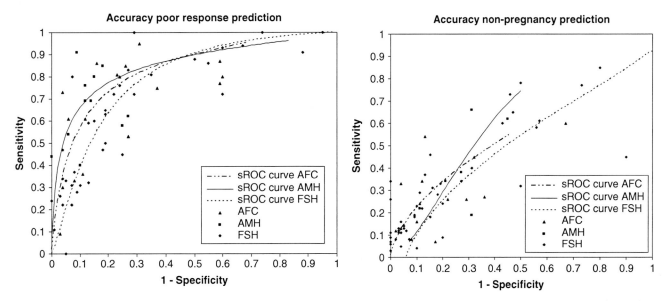

Figure 36.5 Ovarian reserve test performance (AFC, AMH, and FSH) showing receiver operator characteristic (ROC) curves for the prediction of poor response (*left panel*) and non-pregnancy (*right panel*) in IVF. Data were based on meta-analysis on ovarian reserve tests (25). *Abbreviations*: AFC, antral follicle count; AMH, anti-Müllerian hormone; FSH, follicle-stimulating hormone.

Table 36.1 The Clinical Value of Several Ovarian Reserve Tests for Outcome Prediction in IVF

Test	Prediction of poor response in IVF (pretest probability = 20%)		Prediction of non-pregnancy after IVF (pretest probability = 80%)	
	Positive test rate (for the pLR value ≥8)	Posttest probability (of *poor response*)	Positive test rate (for the pLR value ≥8)	Posttest probability (of *Non-pregnancy*)
FSH	5%	>60%	3%	>96%
AMH	13%	>67%	0%	>97%
AFC	12%	>67%	0%	>97%

predictors of a poor ovarian response to ovarian hyperstimulation in IVF, with the areas under the receiver operator characteristic curve (AUC–ROC) approaching 0.90 (Fig. 36.5). From the clinical value analysis it was suggested that AMH performs slightly better than the AFC and had the best sensitivity and specificity combination for predicting poor ovarian response (44). For instance, if the prevalence of poor response was set at 20% and the cut off chosen implied a positive likelihood ratio higher than 8, an abnormal AMH would indicate a posttest probability of poor ovarian response of around 65%. This would make the AMH test a clinically valuable test, especially as an abnormal test result would be found in 13% of patients (Table 36.1).

If poor response was to be the endpoint of interest then the clinical value of these tests would be satisfactory. Unfortunately though, no proven strategy to prevent the occurrence of poor response is currently known. Also, a poor response may not always imply a poor prognosis, especially in younger women (45). The same may be true for "poor responders'" after the application of mild stimulation protocols (46). In poor responders, in a first IVF cycle, it has become increasingly clear that any adaptation in the treatment protocol in a second cycle will improve neither the subsequent response nor the prognosis for pregnancy if randomized trials are concerned. However, some new expectations may emerge from the use of androgens or growth hormone, although larger studies may be needed here (47,48). All this may indicate that in predicted poor responders prior to starting IVF, the expectations of adapted management may also be marginal.

Only few studies exist on the effect of adapting the dosage of FSH based on prior ORTs to obtain an optimal number of oocytes and improve prospects for pregnancy. Klinkert et al. (49) have shown that predicted poor responders, based on an AFC of below 5, did not benefit from a higher starting dosage of gonadotropins in the first IVF treatment cycle. Also, Lekamge et al., (50), in a pseudo randomized design, has demonstrated that there is no proven clinical value of increasing the dosage FSH in patients with predicted low ovarian reserve. In contrast, in a study by Popovic-Todorovic et al., (40) an individualized dose regimen in IVF cases with normal basal FSH levels did increase the proportion of appropriate ovarian responses during controlled ovarian hyperstimulation. Even a higher ongoing pregnancy rate in the individualized dose group was reported. These findings

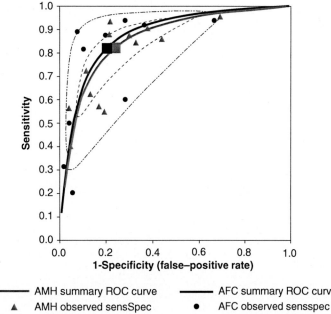

AMH summary ROC curve ——— AFC summary ROC curve
▲ AMH observed sensSpec ● AFC observed sensspec
■ AMH summary point estimate ■ AFC summary point estimate
------ AMH point estimate 95% CI ---·---· AFC point estimate 95% CI

Figure 36.6   Performance of AFC and AMH in the prediction of excessive response to ovarian hyperstimulation for IVF, demonstrated from the receiver operator characteristic (ROC) curve. Data were based on a recent meta-analysis (43). *Abbreviations*: AMH, anti-Müllerian hormone; AFC, antral follicle count.

together implicate the need for larger studies providing the final answer to the question whether a predicted poor responder will or will not benefit from the use of higher dosages of FSH.

This implies that a prior prediction of poor response is to be considered useless, unless this prediction would identify cases with a poor response due to FSH under dosing related to obesity or FSH receptor polymorphisms.

Excessive Response Prediction

Due to the promising results of poor response prediction, the possibility of excessive response prediction has become an area of study, especially since excessive responders may be in jeopardy due to high patient discomfort, reduced pregnancy rates, and ovarian hyper stimulation syndrome (OHSS) risks (51,52). In view of these drawbacks, elimination of exaggerated ovarian response in stimulation protocols will improve safety, success, and cost factors of ART programs.

A recent systematic review showed that both AMH and AFC are accurate predictors of excessive response to ovarian hyperstimulation (43). Summary estimates of sensitivity and specificity for AMH were 82% and 76%, respectively, and 82% and 80%, respectively, for AFC (Fig. 36.6). Abnormal test rates for AMH and AFC amounted up to ~14% and 16%, respectively, at cutoff levels where test performance is optimal (LR+ >8), with a posttest probability of ±70%.

The clinical value of excessive response prediction will depend on the consequences made to this prediction. To date, excessive responders in a first cycle may benefit from dose adaptation in a subsequent cycle, but there exist no comparative trials on this issue. The effect of individualized dose regimens on prior predicted excessive respond-

ers has been demonstrated by the results of the CONSORT study (53). Based on an algorithm for individualizing the FSH dosage using FSH, BMI, age, and the AFC, excessive responses could be clearly prevented, without an obvious reduction in pregnancy prospects.

Pregnancy Prediction

From the meta-analysis of the various reserve tests, the predictive ability toward the occurrence of pregnancy after one IVF cycle was shown to be only marginal, as only very small proportions of the nonpregnant cases will be predicted correctly and false positives remained even with extreme cut offs for an abnormal test (Fig. 36.5, Table 36.1). This finding should not be regarded as a surprise, as most tests relate to the quantitative aspects of the ovarian reserve that are constantly present (i.e., antral follicle cohort size), while the quality perspective is only tested against a single exposure which certainly will not be a good expression of a couple's fertility potential (only tested properly in a series of ART cycles). However, a recent study showed that although ovarian reserve markers may not predict pregnancy, they can be used to make a moderate distinction between patients with a good and poor prognosis. The success of IVF was found to mainly depend on maternal age and serum AMH concentrations (Table 36.2) (54).

First Cycle Poor Response

Testing for ovarian reserve may also be possible by using the quantity of the ovarian response to maximal ovarian stimulation in the first ART cycle. A poor response to stimulation, defined as a low number of mature follicles developed or oocytes obtained after a

Table 36.2   Probability of Live Birth after IVF According to Age and AMH as Calculated by La Marca et al. (54)

Age (years)	AMH (ng/ml)		
	<0.4	0.4–<2.8	≥2.8
<31	0.13 (0.04–0.36)	0.38 (0.26–0.51)	0.52 (0.38–0.67)
31–37	0.09 (0.02–0.24)	0.27 (0.21–0.35)	0.40 (0.28–0.54)
>37	0.05 (0.01–0.16)	0.18 (0.12–0.26)	0.29 (0.17–0.44)

Shown is the occurrence of abnormal ovarian test results, given a positive likelihood ratio (pLR) value of ≥6, and the concomitant posttest probabilities of poor response and non-pregnancy, given a prevalence of poor response of 20% and non-pregnancy of 80%. Data were based on a recent meta-analyses on ovarian reserve tests (25,62).

In poor response prediction only for the AFC a reasonable proportion of positive tests is observed at cutoff levels with a moderate to good levels of the pLR, leading to a substantial change in the chance of producing a poor response in IVF.

For non-pregnancy prediction the abnormal test rate is clearly low at the cutoff levels that leads to an appropriate overall test performance and probability of non-pregnancy shifts moderately in case of such test results.

Abbreviations: AMH, anti-Müllerian hormone.

conventional long GnRH agonist suppression protocol, will generally be interpreted as a proof of diminished ovarian reserve and reduced prognosis for pregnancy. Also, poor responders in IVF/ICSI treatment experience an earlier transition into menopause compared to normal responders, confirming the relation between response and fertility potential. Still, a poor response may also be caused by conditions like submaximal stimulation in obese women or carriers of an FSH receptor polymorphism or simply by chance. In such poor responders, prospects in the actual and subsequent cycles are not so unfavorable that refusal of treatment is justified. Only if a poor response occurs in cases with an unfavorable additional profile (female age over 38 years, abnormal ORT, repeated poor response) does prognosis for subsequent cycles become cumbersome enough for further denial of treatment (12,13,55,56). If the policy would be to allow any couple with female age under the age of 40 years to proceed to ART then a poor response combined with an appropriate ORT may be the best policy to direct further management.

Test Combinations

Improvement of ORT performance in the identification of women with a reduced quantitative ovarian reserve for their age category may come from combining endocrine and imaging tests. Combination of several endocrine and imaging tests into predictive models has shown to improve the accuracy of poor response prediction in single studies (25). In a meta-analysis on several models combining various single tests no clear improvement compared to the AFC and basal FSH could be found.

Currently the IMPORT and EXPORT study group is conducting an individual patient data meta-analysis. This international collaboration assesses the added value of ovarian reserve testing on simple patient characteristics, especially female age, and the value of the combination of ORTs in prediction ovarian response and pregnancy after

IVF. From the large body of data (n = 5058 cases) it is demonstrated that for the prediction of ovarian response, ORTs have added value on female age. Since the predictive value of female age alone is quite limited, tests like the AFC and AMH are sufficiently accurate to identify a poor responder, even without knowing the age of the patient. However, in the prediction of ongoing pregnancy after IVF not a single ORT or combinations of tests have added value to female age (57).

Female age is highly related to the prospects for pregnancy, yet highly insufficient in correctly predicting who will become pregnant and who will not. Age can obviously be used to build prognostic categories for individual patients, and from the IMPORT database it was made clear that ORTs like AMH and AFC aid in fine-tuning this prognosis, albeit with a certain level of imprecision. As described earlier this has also been demonstrated by La Marca et al., who showed that age and AMH can be used to place women in prognostic categories (see Table 36.2) (54).

Applicability of Ovarian Reserve Tests in ART Practice

To date it has been demonstrated that ORTs are adequate predictors of a poor and excessive response. However, the clinical applicability will rely on future studies that demonstrate if adjustment of clinical management can be justified based on these predictions and whether these adjustments would be cost-effective.

Moreover, ORTs do not predict pregnancy after ART and cannot be used for this objective. However, counseling on the basis of prognosis level from age and AMH/AFC is interesting, although much of the information comes from age and adding test could only be useful for counseling in certain subgroups, like older women.

The true challenge for ORTs lies in the possibility of identifying women with a reduced reproductive lifespan at such a stage in their lives that adequate action can be taken. In such test the preferable outcome variable to judge the test upon is the age at which a woman will become menopausal. The relation between menopausal age and the end of natural fertility has been hypothesized to be fixed (6) (Fig. 36.2). In a recent study the potential of AMH to predict menopause and thereby a woman's reproductive lifespan has become established. Using an age-specific AMH level, the age range in which menopause will occur can be individually calculated (58,59). This could open avenues for individualized prevention of age-related infertility.

RESUME

Age-related fertility decline varies considerably among women. Therefore, chronological female age, though informative on pregnancy prospects in assisted reproduction, will not always correctly express a woman's reproductive potential. Currently ORTs have shown to be accurate predictors of the quantitative aspects of the ovarian reserve and thereby of the response to ovarian hyperstimulation. However, they are not accurate predictors of the qualitative aspect of the ovarian reserve and thus are not good predictors of pregnancy after IVF.

REFERENCES

1. Stephen EH, Chandra A. Declining estimates of infertility in the United States: 1982–2002. Fertil Steril 2006; 86: 516–23.
2. Te Velde ER, Pearson PL. The variability of female reproductive aging. Hum Reprod Update 2002; 8: 141–54.
3. Morabia A, Costanza MC. International variability in ages at menarche, first livebirth, and menopause. World Health Organization Collaborative Study of Neoplasia and Steroid Contraceptives. Am J Epidemiol 1998; 148: 1195–205.
4. Thomas F, Renaud F, Benefice E, de Meeus T, Guegan JF. International variability of ages at menarche and menopause: patterns and main determinants. Hum Biol 2001; 73: 271–90.
5. van Noord-Zaadstra BM, Looman CWN, Alsbach H, et al. Delaying childbearing: effect of age on fecundity and outcome of pregnancy. BMJ 1991; 302: 1361–5.
6. Broekmans FJ, Soules MR, Fauser BC. Ovarian aging: mechanisms and clinical consequences. Endocr Rev 2009; 30: 465–93.
7. Viudes-de-Castro MP, Vicente JS. Effect of sperm count on the fertility and prolificity rates of meat rabbits. Anim Reprod Sci 1997; 46: 313–19.
8. Moce E, Lavara R, Vicente JS. Influence of the donor male on the fertility of frozen-thawed rabbit sperm after artificial insemination of females of different genotypes. Reprod Domest Anim 2005; 40: 516–21.
9. Evers JL. Female subfertility. Lancet 2002; 360: 151–9.
10. Menken J, Trussell J, Larsen U. Age and infertility. Science 1986; 233: 1389–94.
11. van Kooij RJ, Looman CW, Habbema JD, Dorland M, Te Velde ER. Age-dependent decrease in embryo implantation rate after in vitro fertilization. Fertil Steril 1996; 66: 769–75.
12. de Boer EJ, den TI, Te Velde ER, Burger CW, van Leeuwen FE. Increased risk of early menopausal transition and

natural menopause after poor response at first IVF treatment. Hum Reprod 2003; 18: 1544–52.
13. Lawson R, El Toukhy T, Kassab A, et al. Poor response to ovulation induction is a stronger predictor of early menopause than elevated basal FSH: a life table analysis. Hum Reprod 2003; 18: 527–33.
14. Klinkert ER, Broekmans FJ, Looman CW, Te Velde ER. A poor response in the first in vitro fertilization cycle is not necessarily related to a poor prognosis in subsequent cycles. Fertil Steril 2004; 81: 1247–53.
15. Fasouliotis SJ, Simon A, Laufer N. Evaluation and treatment of low responders in assisted reproductive technique: a challenge to meet. J Assist Reprod Genet 2000; 17: 357–73.
16. Popovic-Todorovic B, Loft A, Lindhard A, et al. A prospective study of predictive factors of ovarian response in 'standard' IVF/ICSI patients treated with recombinant FSH. A suggestion for a recombinant FSH dosage normogram. Hum Reprod 2003; 18: 781–7.
17. van der Gaast MH, Eijkemans MJ, van der Net JB, et al. Optimum number of oocytes for a successful first IVF treatment cycle. Reprod Biomed Online 2006; 13: 476–80.
18. Out HJ, David I, Ron-El R, et al. A randomized, double-blind clinical trial using fixed daily doses of 100 or 200 IU of recombinant FSH in ICSI cycles. Hum Reprod 2001; 16: 1104–9.
19. Harrison RF, Jacob S, Spillane H, Mallon E, Hennelly B. A prospective randomized clinical trial of differing starter doses of recombinant follicle-stimulating hormone (follitropin-beta) for first time in vitro fertilization and intracytoplasmic sperm injection treatment cycles. Fertil Steril 2001; 75: 23–31.
20. Yong PY, Brett S, Baird DT, Thong KJ. A prospective randomized clinical trial comparing 150 IU and 225 IU of recombinant follicle-stimulating hormone (Gonal-F*) in a fixed-dose regimen for controlled ovarian stimulation in in vitro fertilization treatment. Fertil Steril 2003; 79: 308–15.
21. Klinkert ER. Clinical Significance and Management of Poor Response in IVF. Utrecht: Academic Thesis, 2005.
22. Templeton A, Morris JK, Parslow W. Factors that affect outcome of in-vitro fertilisation treatment. Lancet 1996; 348: 1402–6.
23. Tarlatzis BC, Zepiridis L, Grimbizis G, Bontis J. Clinical management of low ovarian response to stimulation for IVF: a systematic review. Hum Reprod Update 2003; 9: 61–76.
24. Hendriks DJ, Mol BW, Bancsi LF, te Velde ER, Broekmans FJ. Antral follicle count in the prediction of poor ovarian response and pregnancy after in vitro fertilization: a meta-analysis and comparison with basal follicle-stimulating hormone level. Fertil Steril 2005; 83: 291–301.
25. Broekmans FJ, Kwee J, Hendriks DJ, Mol BW, Lambalk CB. A systematic review of tests predicting ovarian reserve and IVF outcome. Hum Reprod Update 2006; 12: 685–718.
26. Seifer DB, MacLaughlin DT, Christian BP, Feng B, Shelden RM. Early follicular serum mullerian-inhibiting substance levels are associated with ovarian response during assisted reproductive technique cycles. Fertil Steril 2002; 77: 468–71.
27. Klein NA, Houmard BS, Hansen KR, et al. Age-related analysis of inhibin A, inhibin B, and activin a relative

to the intercycle monotropic follicle-stimulating hormone rise in normal ovulatory women. J Clin Endocrinol Metab 2004; 89: 2977–81.

28. Hendriks DJ, Broekmans FJ, Bancsi LF, et al. Single and repeated GnRH agonist stimulation tests compared with basal markers of ovarian reserve in the prediction of outcome in IVF. J Assist Reprod Genet 2005; 22: 65–73.

29. Kwee J, Elting MW, Schats R, et al. Comparison of endocrine tests with respect to their predictive value on the outcome of ovarian hyperstimulation in IVF treatment: results of a prospective randomized study. Hum Reprod 2003; 18: 1422–7.

30. Hendriks DJ, Mol BW, Bancsi LF, Te Velde ER, Broekmans FJ. The clomiphene citrate challenge test for the prediction of poor ovarian response and nonpregnancy in patients undergoing in vitro fertilization: a systematic review.. Fertil Steril 2006; 86: 807–18.

31. Jain T, Soules MR, Collins JA. Comparison of basal follicle-stimulating hormone versus the clomiphene citrate challenge test for ovarian reserve screening. Fertil Steril 2004; 82: 180–5.

32. Deeks JJ. Systematic reviews in health care: Systematic reviews of evaluations of diagnostic and screening tests. BMJ 2001; 323: 157–62.

33. Grimes DA, Schulz KF. Refining clinical diagnosis with likelihood ratios. Lancet 2005; 365: 1500–5.

34. Mol BW, Verhagen TE, Hendriks DJ, et al. Value of ovarian reserve testing before IVF: a clinical decision analysis. Hum Reprod 2006; 21: 1816–23.

35. Levi AJ, Raynault MF, Bergh PA, et al. Reproductive outcome in patients with diminished ovarian reserve. Fertil Steril 2001; 76: 666–9.

36. Scott RT Jr. Hofmann GE. Prognostic assessment of ovarian reserve [see comments]. Fertil Steril 1995; 63: 1–11.

37. Bancsi LF, Broekmans FJ, Looman CW, Habbema JD, Te Velde ER. Impact of repeated antral follicle counts on the prediction of poor ovarian response in women undergoing in vitro fertilization. Fertil Steril 2004; 81: 35–41.

38. Bancsi LF, Broekmans FJ, Looman CW, Habbema JD, Te Velde ER. Predicting poor ovarian response in IVF: use of repeat basal FSH measurement. J Reprod Med 2004; 49: 187–94.

39. Bancsi LF, Broekmans FJ, Eijkemans MJ, et al. Predictors of poor ovarian response in in vitro fertilization: a prospective study comparing basal markers of ovarian reserve. Fertil Steril 2002; 77: 328–36.

40. Popovic-Todorovic B, Loft A, Bredkjaeer HE, et al. A prospective randomized clinical trial comparing an individual dose of recombinant FSH based on predictive factors versus a 'standard' dose of 150 IU/day in 'standard' patients undergoing IVF/ICSI treatment. Hum Reprod 2003; 18: 2275–82.

41. van Rooij IAJ, de Jong E, Broekmans FJM, Looman CWN, Habbema JDF. High follicle stimulating hormone levels should not necessarily lead to the exclusion of subfertile patients from treatment. Fertil Steril 2004; 81: 1478–85

42. Ng EH, Chan CC, Tang OS, Ho PC. Antral follicle count and FSH concentration after clomiphene citrate challenge test in the prediction of ovarian response during IVF treatment. Hum Reprod 2005; 20: 1647–54.

43. Broer SL, Dolleman M, Opmeer BC, et al. AMH and AFC as predictors of excessive response in controlled ovarian hyperstimulation: a meta-analysis. Human Reprod Update 2011; 17: 46–54.

44. Broer SL, Mol BW, Hendriks D, Broekmans FJ. The role of antimullerian hormone in prediction of outcome after IVF: comparison with the antral follicle count. Fertil Steril 2008; 91: 705–14.

45. Lashen H, Ledger W, Lopez-Bernal A, Barlow D. Poor responders to ovulation induction: is proceeding to in-vitro fertilization worthwhile? Hum Reprod 1999; 14: 964–9.

46. Verberg MF, Eijkemans MJ, Macklon NS, et al. Predictors of low response to mild ovarian stimulation initiated on cycle day 5 for IVF. Hum Reprod 2007; 22: 1919–24.

47. Kyrou D, Kolibianakis EM, Venetis CA, et al. How to improve the probability of pregnancy in poor responders undergoing in vitro fertilization: a systematic review and meta-analysis. Fertil Steril 2009; 91: 749–66.

48. Mochtar MH, van dV, Ziech M, van WM. Recombinant Luteinizing Hormone (rLH) for controlled ovarian hyperstimulation in assisted reproductive cycles. Cochrane Database Syst Rev 2007; CD005070.

49. Klinkert ER, Broekmans FJ, Looman CW, Habbema JD, Te Velde ER. Expected poor responders on the basis of an antral follicle count do not benefit from a higher starting dose of gonadotrophins in IVF treatment: a randomized controlled trial. Hum Reprod 2005; 20: 611–15.

50. Lekamge DN, Lane M, Gilchrist RB, Tremellen KP. Increased gonadotrophin stimulation does not improve IVF outcomes in patients with predicted poor ovarian reserve. J Assist Reprod Genet 2008; 25: 515–21.

51. Fauser BC, Diedrich K, Devroey P. Predictors of ovarian response: progress towards individualized treatment in ovulation induction and ovarian stimulation. Hum Reprod Update 2008; 14: 1–14.

52. Sunkara SK, Rittenberg V, Raine-Fenning N, et al. Association between the number of eggs and live birth in IVF treatment: an analysis of 400 135 treatment cycles. Hum Reprod 2011; 26: 1768–74.

53. Olivennes F, Howles CM, Borini A, et al. Individualizing FSH dose for assisted reproduction using a novel algorithm: the CONSORT study. Reprod Biomed Online 2009; 18: 195–204.

54. La Marca A, Nelson SM, Sighinolfi G, et al. Anti-Mullerian hormone-based prediction model for a live birth in assisted reproduction. Reprod Biomed Online 2011; 22: 341–9.

55. Hendriks DJ, Te Velde ER, Looman CW, Bancsi LF, Broekmans FJ. Expected poor ovarian response in predicting cumulative pregnancy rates: a powerful tool. Reprod Biomed Online 2008; 17: 727–36.

56. Oudendijk JF, Yarde F, Eijkemans MJ, Broekmans FJ, Broer SL. The poor responder in IVF: is the prognosis always poor? A systematic review. Human Reprod Update 2012; 18: 1–11.

57. Broer SL. On behalf of IMPORT study group. Assessment of Current and Future Ovarian Reserve Status. Academic Thesis. The Netherlands: University Utrecht, 2011.

58. Broer SL, Eijkemans MJ, Scheffer GJ, et al. Anti-mullerian hormone predicts menopause: a long-term follow-up study in normoovulatory women. J Clin Endocrinol Metab 2011; 96: 2532–9.

59. Tehrani FR, Shakeri N, Solaymani-Dodaran M, Azizi F. Predicting age at menopause from serum antimullerian hormone concentration. Menopause 2011; 18: 766–70.

60. de Bruin JP, te Velde ER. Female reproductive aging: concepts and consequences. In: Tulandi T, Gosden RG. ed. Preservation of Fertility. London, UK: Taylor & Francis, 2004: 3.

61. Soules MR, Battaglia DE, Klein NA. Inhibin and reproductive aging in women. Am J Human Biol 1998; 30: 193–204.

62. Broer SL, Mol BW, Hendriks D, Broekmans FJ. The role of antimullerian hormone in prediction of outcome after IVF: comparison with the antral follicle count. Fertil Steril 2009; 91: 705–14.

37

Drugs used for ovarian stimulation: Clomiphene citrate, aromatase inhibitors, metformin, gonadotropins, gonadotropin-releasing hormone analogs, and recombinant gonadotropins

Zeev Shoham and Colin M. Howles

INTRODUCTION

Infertility treatment became available owing to developments in the characterization and purification of hormones. Treatment with gonadotropins and clomiphene citrate (CC) became available in 1961. The purpose of this chapter is to overview the development, structure, and mode of action of treatments for ovulation induction (OI) and controlled ovarian stimulation (COS) for assisted reproductive techniques (ARTs).

CLOMIPHENE CITRATE

Drug Description

Clomiphene citrate was synthesized in 1956, and an indisputable therapeutic breakthrough occurred in 1961 when Greenblatt and his group discovered that CC, a nonsteroidal analog of estradiol, exerts a stimulatory effect on ovarian function in women with anovulatory infertility (1). The drug was approved for infertility treatment by the U. S. Food and Drug Administration in 1967.

Clomiphene citrate is a triphenylchloroethylene derivative in which the four hydrogen atoms of the ethylene core have been substituted with three phenyl rings and a chloride anion. One of the three phenyl rings bears an aminoalkoxy [OCH_2-CH_2-$N(C_2 K_2)_2$] side-chain, but the importance of its action on CC remains uncertain. The dihydrogen citrate moiety ($C_6H_8O_7$) accounts for the fact that commercially available preparations represent the dihydrogen citrate salt form of CC. Clomiphene citrate is a white or pale yellow, odorless powder, unstable in air and light, with a melting point of 116–118°C. It is a triarylethylene compound (1-p-diethyl aminoethoxyphenyl-1,2-diphenyl- 2-chloro-ethylene citrate), with a molecular weight of 598.09) chemically related to chlorotrianisene, which is a weak estrogen. Structurally, CC is related to diethylstilbestrol, a potent synthetic estrogen. Although this compound is not a steroid, but a triphenylchloroethylene, its steroic configuration bears a remarkable structural similarity to estradiol, and consequently facilitates binding to estrogen receptors (ERs).

Clomiphene citrate is available as a racemic mixture of two stereochemical isomers referred to as (cis) Zu-clomiphene or the (trans) En-clomiphene configuration (Fig. 37.1A, B), the former being significantly more potent. In the commercially available preparations, the isomers are in the ratio of 38% Zu and 62% En-clomiphene. Limited experience suggests that the clinical utility of CC may indeed be due to its cis isomer (2,3). However, it remains uncertain whether cis-CC is more effective than CC proper in terms of ovulation and conception rates (4–7). Following the development of a reverse-phase high-performance liquid chromatography (HPLC) assay, (8) it was apparent that each isomer exhibited its own characteristic pharmacokinetic profile, the En isomer being absorbed faster and eliminated more completely than the Zu isomer. Although CC tablets contain 62% En isomer and 38% Zu isomer, the observed plasma concentrations of the Zu isomer were much higher than those of the En isomer. Because the Zu isomer is considered more estrogenic than the En isomer, response of the target tissues should vary according to both the relative affinity and the concentrations of each isomer interacting with the relevant ER. Tracer studies of CC with radioactive carbon labeling have shown that the main route of excretion is via the feces, although small amounts are also excreted in the urine. After administration of CC for five consecutive days at a dose of 100 mg daily, the drug could be detected in serum for up to 30 days.

Mechanism of Action

Administration of CC is followed in short sequence by enhanced release of pituitary gonadotropins, resulting in follicular recruitment, selection, assertion of dominance, and rupture.

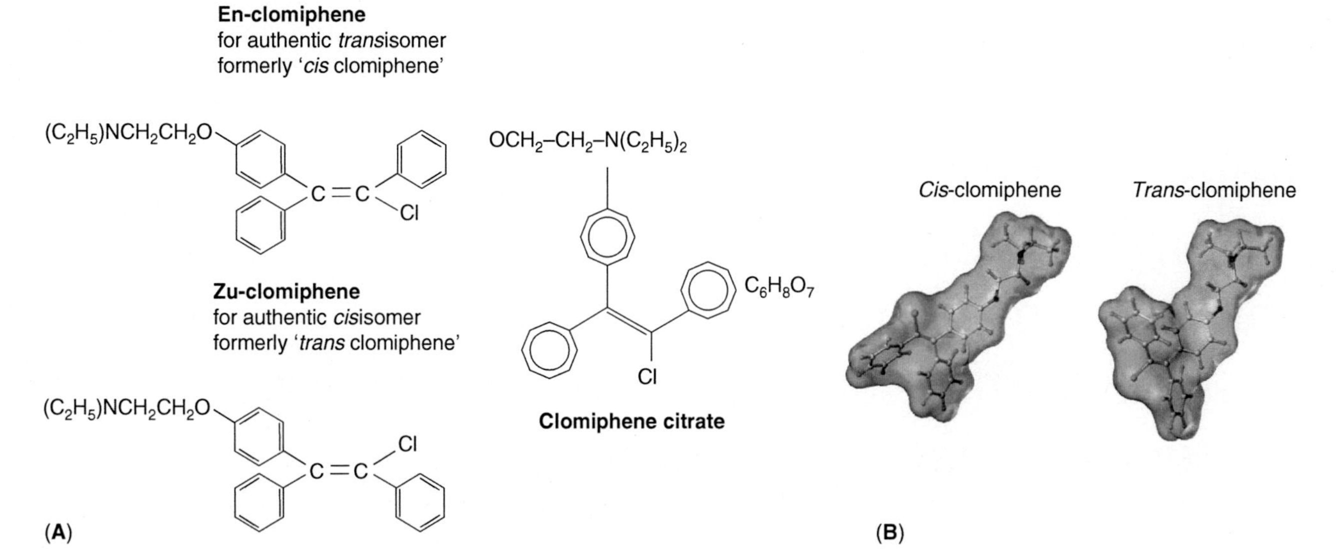

Figure 37.1 (**A**) Clomiphene citrate is available as a racemic mixture of two stereochemical isomers referred to as (*cis*) Zu-clomiphene or the (*trans*) En-clomiphene configuration, the former being significantly more potent. In the preparations commercially available, the isomers are in the ratio of 38% Zu- and 62% En-clomiphene. (**B**) The isomeric models in a different configuration.

The principal mechanism of CC action is a reduction in the negative feedback of endogenous estrogens due to prolonged depletion of hypothalamic and pituitary ER (9,10). This action consequently leads to an increase in the release of gonadotropin-releasing hormone (GnRH) from the hypothalamus into the hypothalamic-pituitary portal circulation, engendering an increase in the release of pituitary gonadotropins. Administration of a moderate gonadotropin stimulus to the ovary overcomes the ovulation disturbances and increases the cohort of follicles reaching ovulation (11,12). A marked increase in serum concentrations of luteinizing hormone (LH) in proportion to follicle-stimulating hormone (FSH) may sometimes occur, (13) and this temporary change in the ratio of LH:FSH appears to bring about some impairment of follicular maturation, resulting in delayed ovulation. Shortly after discontinuation of CC, both gonadotropins gradually decline to the preovulatory nadir, only to surge again at mid-cycle.

The drug interacts with ER-binding proteins similar to native estrogens and behaves as a competitive ER antagonist (14,15). Of importance, CC does not display progestational, corticotropic, androgenic, or antiandrogenic properties.

Indications and Contraindications for Treatment

Anovulatory infertility is the most important indication for CC treatment. In addition, treatment is indicated for women with oligomenorrhea, or amenorrhea, who responded to progesterone (P) treatment with withdrawal bleeding. Treatment is ineffective in women with hypogonadotropic hypogonadism (HH; WHO group I). Other controversial indications include luteal-phase defect, unexplained infertility, and women undergoing in vitro fertilization (IVF) when multiple follicle development is required. Contraindications to CC administration include preexisting ovarian cysts, with suspected malignancy, and liver disease.

Duration of Treatment

CC increases secretion of FSH and LH and is administered for a period of five days. In women with normal cycles, administration of CC for more than five days resulted in an initial increase of serum FSH concentration that lasted for 5–6 days, followed by a decline in serum FSH levels, despite continuation of the drug, whereas LH levels remained high throughout the entire treatment period (16,17).

Clomiphene citrate is usually administered on day 5 of spontaneous or induced menstruation. This is based on the theory that on day 5 the physiologic decrease in serum FSH concentration provides the means for selection of the dominant follicle. Initiation of the drug on day 2 induces earlier ovulation, which is analogous to the physiologic events of the normal menstrual cycle. The starting dose is usually 50 mg/day, owing to the observation that 50% of pregnancies occur with the 50 mg dose (18). To obtain good results, CC therapy should be carefully monitored. Obviously, serial measurements of LH, FSH, estradiol, and P and ultrasound measurements provide the most detailed information on the patient's response to treatment.

Results of Treatment

Clomiphene citrate induces ovulation in the majority of women. The ovulation rate ranges between 70% and 92%; however, the pregnancy rate is much lower. The discrepancy between the high ovulation rates and relatively low pregnancy rates may be due to the following factors:

1. Antiestrogen effects on the endometrium
2. Antiestrogen effects on the cervical mucus
3. Decrease of uterine blood flow
4. Impaired placental protein 14 synthesis
5. Subclinical pregnancy loss

6. Effect on tubal transport
7. Detrimental effects on the oocytes (19).

The Cochrane review (20) of clinical data regarding the use of CC for unexplained subfertility in women, based on five randomized trials of CC (doses ranging from 50 to 250 mg/day for up to 10 days) compared with placebo, or no treatment, showed that the odds ratio (OR) for pregnancy per patient was 2.38 [95% confidence interval (CI) 1.22–4.62]. The OR for pregnancy per cycle was 2.5 (95% CI 1.35–4.62). It was concluded from this review that CC appeared to improve pregnancy rates modestly in women with unexplained subfertility.

Side Effects and Safety

The most common side effects are hot flushes (10%), abdominal distention, bloating or discomfort (5%), breast discomfort (2%), nausea and vomiting (2%), visual symptoms, and headache (1.5%). A rise in basal body temperature may be noted during the five-day period of CC administration. Visual symptoms include spots (floaters), flashes, or abnormal perception. These symptoms are rare, universally disappear upon cessation of CC therapy, and have no permanent effect. The multiple pregnancy rate is approximately 5% and almost exclusively due to twins.

Several reports have associated long-term (>12 months) CC therapy with a slight increase in future risk of ovarian cancer [relative risk (RR) = 1.5–2.5] (21). Owing to these initial reports, the Committee on Safety of Medicines in the United Kingdom advised doctors to adhere to the manufacturers' recommendations of limiting treatment to a maximum of six months. However, this increased risk has not been confirmed by subsequent reports. Several case reports have linked CC with congenital malformations, especially neural tube defects (22–28). Data available on 3751 births after CC treatment included 122 children born with congenital malformations (major and minor), representing an incidence of 32.5/1000 births (29). This figure is within the range found among the normal population (30).

Summary

Clomiphene citrate is one of the most popular drugs for OI because it is easy to administer, highly effective, is considered safe, and the cost is minimal.

AROMATASE INHIBITORS

Aromatase, a cytochrome P450-dependent enzyme, acts as the ultimate step in the synthesis of estrogen, catalyzing the conversion of androgens to estrogens (31). The conversion of androgens to estrogens occurs also at peripheral sites, such as in muscle, fat, and the liver (32). Recently, a group of new, highly selective aromatase inhibitors has been approved to suppress estrogen production in postmenopausal women with breast cancer. Aromatase inhibitor is a competitive inhibitor of the

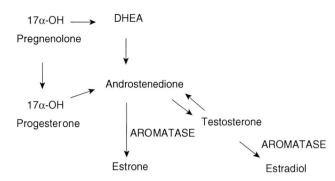

Figure 37.2 Aromatase inhibitor. Aromatase, an enzyme found in the liver, is responsible for the conversion of androgens – androstenedione and testosterone – into estrogens – estrone and estradiol. By inhibiting aromatase the body produces less estrogen and maintains a higher testosterone state. *Abbreviation*: DHEA, dehydroepiandrosterone sulfate.

Table 37.1 The Different Types and Generations of Aromatase Inhibitors

Generation	Type I	Type II
First	None	Aminoglutethimide
Second	Formestane	Fadrozole
		Rogletimide
Third	Exemestane	Anastrozole
		Letrozole
		Vorozole

aromatase enzyme system, and inhibits the conversion of androgens to estrogens. It inhibits the aromatase enzyme by competitively binding to the heme of the aromatase-cytochrome P450 subunit of the enzyme, resulting in a reduction of estrogen biosynthesis in all tissues where it is present (Fig. 37.2). Treatment significantly lowers serum estrone, estradiol, and estrone sulfate, and has not been shown significantly to affect adrenal corticosteroid synthesis, aldosterone synthesis, or synthesis of thyroid hormones. Maximum suppression is achieved within 48–78 hours. The first aromatase inhibitor to be developed was aminoglutethimide, but its usage was stopped owing to side effects, one of which was adrenal insufficiency (33). However, this development stimulated the formulation of numerous other aromatase inhibitors that were described as first-, second-, and third-generation inhibitors according to chronologic development. They were further classified as type I (steroid analogs of androstenedione) and type II (nonsteroidal) (Table 37.1).

Pharmacokinetics

Third-generation aromatase inhibitors are administered orally, and have a half-life of approximately 48 hours, which allows once-daily dosing (34,35). These drugs metabolize mainly in the liver, and are excreted through the biliary (85%) and the urinary (11%) systems.

Side Effects and Safety

Reported side effects are bone pain (20%), hot flushes (18%), back pain (17%), nausea (15%), and dyspnea (14%). These side effects are typically observed after long-term administration.

One major concern is the use of letrozole in OI or COS because of its possible teragenicity as observed in animal models. There was one concerning report (published as an abstract only – Biljan et al. (36)) of an increase in cardiac and bone malformations in letrozole-treated pregnancies. Following the publication of the abstract, the manufacturer, Novartis, wrote to clinicians in the United States and Canada stating that letrozole was not safe for use in women who were either desiring pregnancy or pregnant. Since this notification, there have been a series of published studies, including a multicenter retrospective analysis of 911 newborns conceived after CC or letrozole treatment (37). This did not show any teratogenic effect of letrozole, and they reported a similar rate of congenital malformation to that seen in women conceiving after treatment with CC. In the most recent paper by Badawy et al. (38) authors also stated that there was no observed increase in congenital malformations following the use of letrozole.

Drugs Available

Letrozole

This is chemically described as 4,4'-(1H- 1,2,4-triazole-1-ylmethylene) dibenzonitrile, with a molecular weight of 285.31 and empirical formula $C_{17}H_{11}N_5$.

Anastrozole

The molecular formula is $C_{17}H_{19}N_5$ with a molecular weight of 293.4.

Both drugs are approved for the treatment of breast cancer in postmenopausal women.

The first clinical study using an aromatase inhibitor (letrozole: AstraZeneca) for OI was published by Mitwally and Casper in 2001 (39). With letrozole treatment in patients with polycystic ovary syndrome (PCOS), ovulation occurred in 75% and pregnancy was achieved in 25%. Letrozole appears to prevent unfavorable effects on the endometrium that are frequently observed with antiestrogen use for OI. Since the initial observation, several studies have been published on the use of aromatase inhibitors in the treatment of infertile patients (40–42). The same investigators (43) showed that the use of an aromatase inhibitor reduced the FSH dose required for ovarian stimulation, without the undesirable antiestrogenic effects occasionally noted with CC.

A recent meta-analysis of six randomized controlled trials (RCTs) involving 841 patients with PCOS showed no significant differences in pregnancy, abortion, or multiple pregnancy rates between CC and letrozole (44). The authors concluded that letrozole may be as effective as CC for OI in patients with PCOS (44). It is now 10 years since the first successful report of the use of aromatase

inhibitors in OI. However, aromatase inhibitors have not been introduced into routine clinical practice (45,46). This may be either because they do not appear to significantly improve pregnancy rates versus current treatment options or simply due to the lack of large, well-designed randomized trials with positive results (45,46).

Two randomized studies have also compared the efficacy and safety of single-dose and multidose anastrozole with CC in infertile women with ovulatory dysfunction (47,48). Anastrozole was found to be less effective than CC in inducing ovulation in both studies. Anastrozole has also been shown to have a weaker effect on follicular growth than CC (49).

Aromatase inhibitors have also been investigated for use in ART. Four randomized trials have been published with letrozole in a total of 235 patients with poor ovarian response (50–53). When letrozole was combined with FSH, the gonadotropin dose required was consistently lower than when gonadotropins were used alone. In three trials, pregnancy rates were comparable in the treatment arms (51–53) and in one trial, pregnancy rates were lower in the letrozole arm than in the control arm (50). Only one randomized trial with letrozole has been reported in patients with normal ovarian response undergoing IVF or intracytoplasmic sperm injection (ICSI) (54). This was a pilot study involving 20 patients and showed an increased number of oocytes retrieved, and increased implantation and clinical pregnancy rates when letrozole was added to recombinant human (r-h)FSH (54). However, no significant difference between groups was shown, possibly owing to the small study population.

METFORMIN

The biguanide metformin (dimethylbiguanide) is an oral antihyperglycemic agent widely used in the management of noninsulin-dependent diabetes mellitus. It is an insulin sensitizer that reduces insulin resistance and insulin secretion. Over the last few years there has been increased interest in the use of metformin (at doses of 1500–2500 mg/day) to increase ovulatory frequency, particularly in women described as having PCOS.

There is, however, some recent conflicting evidence regarding the usefulness of metformin in PCOS patients. In a Cochrane systematic review, (55) metformin was concluded to be an effective treatment for anovulation in women with PCOS, with it being recommended to be a first-line treatment, and with some evidence of benefit on parameters of the metabolic syndrome. Ovulation rates were higher when combined with clomiphene (76% vs. 46% when used alone). Finally, the authors recommended that it should be used as an adjuvant to general lifestyle improvements, and not as a replacement for increased exercise and improved diet.

Subsequently, both the American Society for Reproductive Medicine Practice Committee (US) (56) and the National Institute for Clinical Excellence (UK) (57) have made recommendations for its use in treating anovulatory PCOS. In previously untreated women with PCOS, no superiority of the combination of CC and metformin, rather than CC alone, was demonstrated in a large, Dutch multicenter study (58). In a "head-to-head" study comparing CC with metformin as first-line treatment, although ovulation and pregnancy rates were similar, significantly fewer miscarriages and, therefore, more live births, were achieved with metformin (59). In a meta-analysis of randomized trials in PCOS patients undergoing OI or IVF/embryo transfer (ET), (60) coadministration of metformin to gonadotropins did not significantly improve ovulation (OR = 3.27, 95% CI 0.31–34.72) or pregnancy (OR = 3.46, 95% CI 0.98–12.2) rates. Metformin coadministration in an IVF treatment did not improve the pregnancy rate (OR = 1.29, 95% CI 0.84–1.98) but was associated with a reduction in the risk of ovarian hyperstimulation syndrome (OHSS) (OR = 0.21, 95% CI 0.11–0.41) (60). However, the authors concluded that the review was inconclusive in terms of not being able to exclude an important clinical treatment effect because of the small number of trials and small sample sizes of the individual trials limiting the power of the meta-analysis.

Neveu et al. (61) carried out an observational comparative study to determine which first-line medication (CC or metformin) was more effective in PCOS patients undergoing OI and to verify whether any patient characteristic was associated with a better response to therapy. The authors included "154 patients who had never been treated for OI to avoid confounding effects of a previous fertility treatment." Patients receiving metformin alone had an increased ovulation rate compared with those receiving CC alone (75.4% vs. 50%). Patients on metformin had similar ovulation rates compared with those in the combination group (75.4% vs. 63.4%). Pregnancy rates were equivalent in the three groups. Response to metformin was independent of body weight and dose. Finally, nonsmoking predicted better overall ovulatory response in addition to lower fasting glucose for CC, and lower androgens for metformin.

A recent literature review (62) was carried out to establish if metformin was efficacious when given to CC-resistant PCOS patients (the Medline database was searched from January 1, 1980 to January 1, 2005). When the data from four prospective double-blind placebo controlled trials were pooled, the overall effect of the addition of metformin in the CC patient was $p = 0.0006$ with a 95% CI of OR of 1.81–8.84. In only two trials the randomization was prospective; when the data of these two trials were pooled, the overall effect of the addition of metformin in the CC-resistant patient was $p < 0.0001$, with a 95% CI of OR of 6.24–70.27. Combining all data gave an overall positive effect of $p < 0.0001$, with a 95% CI of OR of 3.59–12.96. The authors concluded that the addition of metformin in the CC-resistant patient is highly effective in achieving OI. In the largest study to date, Legro and colleagues (63) randomized 626 subfertile women with PCOS who had received previous fertility therapy but were not known to be CC resistant, to have CC + placebo, extended-release metformin + placebo, or a combination of metformin + CC for up to six months. The dose of extended-release metformin was gradually increased until a maximum

dose of 2000 mg/day. Medication was discontinued when pregnancy was confirmed, and subjects were followed until delivery. The primary endpoint of the study was live birth rate. The live birth rate was 22.5% (47 of 209 subjects) in the CC group, 7.2% (15 of 208) in the metformin group, and 26.8% (56 of 209) in the combination therapy group ($p < 0.001$ for metformin vs. both CC and combination therapy; $p = 0.31$ for CC vs. combination therapy). Among pregnancies, the rate of multiple pregnancies was 6% in the CC group, 0% in the metformin group, and 3.1% in the combination therapy group. The rates of first trimester pregnancy loss did not differ significantly among the groups. However, the conception rate among subjects who ovulated was significantly lower in the metformin group (21.7%) than in either the CC group (39.5%, $p = 0.002$) or the combination therapy group (46%, $p < 0.001$). With the exception of pregnancy complications, adverse-event rates were similar in all groups, though gastrointestinal side effects were more frequent and vasomotor and ovulatory symptoms less frequent, in the metformin group than in the CC group. They concluded that CC was superior to metformin in achieving live birth in women with PCOS, although multiple births are a complication.

In spite of the nonsignificant difference in live birth rates, between CC and combination therapy, the latter group had superior ovulation rates versus CC or metformin alone (60.4 vs. 49.0 vs. 29.0%; Fig. 37.3) and a trend to an improvement in the pregnancy rate (absolute difference = 7.2%) following use of CC + metformin versus CC. There were some important reductions in body mass index (BMI) testosterone, insulin, and insulin resistance in patients treated with the combination versus CC alone.

Some of the differences in results reported in Legro et al. (63) compared with Palomba (59) may have been due to the inclusion of a large percentage of patients with a BMI >30 kg/m². However in a post hoc analysis, the largest differences in pregnancy rate and live birth rate in the CC versus CC +metformin groups were found in women with a BMI > 34 kg/m².

To conclude, whereas the adverse features of PCOS can be ameliorated with lifestyle intervention, such as diet and exercise, some further short-term benefits related to ovulation may be derived from medication with metformin. Further studies are warranted to examine the role of metformin in managing the long-term metabolic implications of PCOS.

Pharmacokinetics

Metformin is administered orally and has an absolute bioavailability of 50–60%, and gastrointestinal absorption is apparently complete within six hours of ingestion. Metformin is rapidly distributed following absorption and does not bind to plasma proteins. No metabolites or conjugates of metformin have been identified. Metformin undergoes renal excretion and has a mean plasma elimination half-life after oral administration of between four and 8.7 hours. Food decreases the extent of and slightly delays the absorption of metformin.

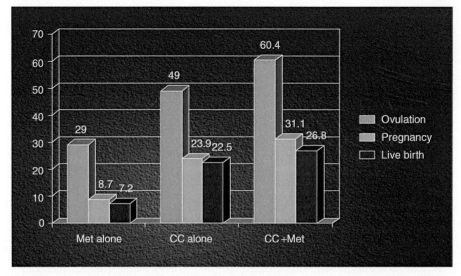

Figure 37.3   Ovulation, pregnancy, and live birth rates (%) in PCOS patients treated with Metformin (MET) alone, CC alone, or Metformin +CC. *Source*: Reproduced from Ref. 155 with permission. *Abbreviations*: PCOS, polycystic ovary syndrome; CC, clomiphene citrate.

Side Effects and Safety

In one U.S. double-blind clinical study of metformin in patients with type 2 diabetes, the most reported adverse reactions (reported in >5% patients) following metformin use were diarrhea (53%), nausea/vomiting (25.5%), flatulence (12.1%), asthenia (9.2%), indigestion (7.1%), abdominal discomfort (6.4%), and headache (5.7%).

Metformin use in women of reproductive age has an assured safety record (64).

GONADOTROPINS

Human Chorionic Gonadotropin: The Luteinizing Hormone Surge Surrogate

Owing to inconsistency of the spontaneous LH surge, in COS, and its inefficacy in patients being treated with GnRH agonists, human chorionic gonadotropin (hCG) has been uniformly adopted by all successful ovarian stimulation programs to effect the final triggering of ovulation. When preovulatory follicles are present, administration of hCG is followed by granulosa cell luteinization, a switch from estradiol to P synthesis, resumption of meiosis and oocyte maturation, and subsequent follicular rupture 36–40 hours later. These processes will occur only if the follicle is of appropriate size and granulosa and theca cell receptivity is adequate, depending on LH receptor status.

Human chorionic gonadotropin has been used as a surrogate LH surge because of the degree of homology between the two hormones. Both LH and hCG are glycoproteins with a molecular weight of approximately 30 kDa, and both have almost identical alfa subunits and a high cystine content (Fig. 37.4). Most important, they have the same natural function, that is, to induce luteinization and support lutein cells. Major differences include the sequence of the beta subunit, the regulation of secretion of both hormones, and the pharmacokinetics of clearance of hCG as opposed to LH (Table 37.2).

The plasma metabolic clearance rate of hCG is slower than that of LH; that is, a rapid disappearance phase in the

first five to nine hours after intramuscular (IM) injection, and a slower clearance rate in the 1–1.3 days after administration (Fig. 37.5). The calculated initial and terminal half-life of recombinant hCG is 5.5 + 1.3 and 3.1 + 3.0 hours, respectively, as opposed to 1.2 + 0.2 and 10.5 + 7.9 hours, respectively, for r-hLH, as determined after intravenous (IV) administration of the drugs (65). By day 10 after administration, <10% of the originally administered hCG was measurable (66). Some authors have advocated the presence of a serum factor directed against hCG preparations, which significantly prolongs the half-life of hCG administration to women who have received repeated courses of gonadotropins (67). Others have not found such a correlation (66). Ludwig et al. suggested that the main differences between LH and hCG lie within the N-linked oligosaccharides and the C-terminal sequence, in which the latter, and especially the O-linked oligosaccharides in this peptide, are responsible for the longer half-life of hCG compared with LH (68).

It is of interest that hCG does not inhibit the subsequent spontaneous LH surge by the intact pituitary, confirming that an ultrashort loop feedback of LH (here hCG) with its own secretion is not functional (69–71).

It has been found that elevated P levels immediately after hCG administration subsequently induce pituitary LH surges in CC/hMG (human menopausal gonadotropin) cycles (69).

The long serum half-life of hCG is likely to be an undesirable characteristic in clinical practice. Residual hCG may be mistaken for early detection of de novo synthesis of hCG by a newly implanted pregnancy. Additional consequences of hCG administration are the sustained luteotropic effect, development of multiple corpora lutea, and supraphysiologic levels of estradiol and P synthesis. Sustained high-level stimulation of the corpora lutea may lead to OHSS, a major complication of gonadotropin therapy (72). Administration of hCG results in an increase in LH-like activity, but does not reconstitute the mid-cycle physiologic FSH surge. Another disadvantage of hCG versus the physiologic LH surge is that of higher luteal-phase levels of estradiol and P induced by supraphysiologic

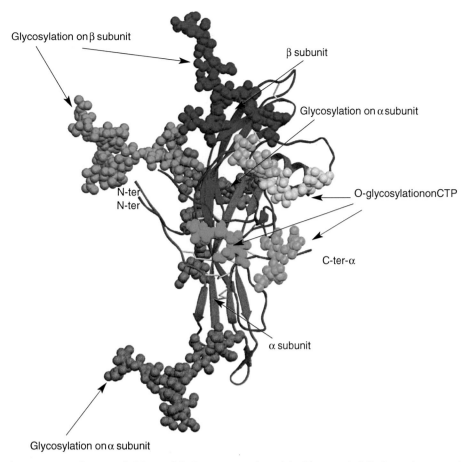

Glycosylation on β subunit

β subunit

Glycosylation on α subunit

O-glycosylation on CTP

N-ter
N-ter

C-ter-α

α subunit

Glycosylation on α subunit

Figure 37.4 Human chorionic gonadotropin (hCG) model. Computerized model of hCG with full glycosylation and cytidine triphosphate (CTP). (This model was created and provided by the scientific department of Serono Laboratories, USA.)

Table 37.2 Luteinizing Hormone (LH) and Human Chorionic Gonadotropin (hCG) Pharmacokinetics and Characteristics. Pharmacokinetics of Recombinant Human LH (r-hLH), Urinary Human Menopausal Gonadotropin (u-hMG), Urinary hCG (u-hCG), and Recombinant hCG(r-hCG). Results are Expressed as Mean ± SD.

Test drug	rhLH	uhMG	uhCG	rhCG
Subjects (*n*)	12	12	12	12
Route	IV	IV	IV	IV
Dose (IU)	300	300	5000	5000
C_{max} [a] (IU/l)	32.1 ± 5.0	24.0 ± 4.2	906 ± 209	1399 ± 317
$t_{1/2}$(1) [a] (hr)	0.8 ± 0.2	0.7 ± 0.2	5.5 ± 1.3	4.7 ± 0.8
$t_{1/2}$ [a] (hr)	10.5 ± 7.9	12.4 ± 12.3	31 ± 3	28 ± 3

[a]Based on serum concentrations measured with immunoradiometric assay (mean ± SD).
Abbreviations: IV, intravenous; C_{max}, maximum concentration; $t_{1/2}$ (1), initial half-life; $t_{1/2}$, terminal half-life.
Source: Adapted from Refs. 50 and 222.

hCG concentrations. Excessive levels of circulating estradiol have been implicated in the relatively high rates of implantation failure and early pregnancy loss observed in ovarian stimulation programs (73,74). Another possible disadvantage of the prolonged activity of hCG is that of small-follicle, delayed ovulation, which could be the cause of the development of multiple pregnancies.

Almost universal use of GnRH agonists and pituitary desensitization protocols has made the fear of untimely LH surges relatively obsolete; hence hCG, the timing of the LH-like stimulus, has been given greater flexibility.

Tan et al. (75) actually showed that there was no difference in cycle outcome with random timing of hCG administration over a three-day period. Unfortunately, invalidation of the pituitary mechanism that releases us from an inappropriate LH surge has also made us completely dependent on hCG, with all its inherent problems, for the final stage of ovulation triggering.

Another issue requiring clarification is the minimal effective dose of hCG to trigger oocyte maturation and ovulation. In a study examining the minimal effective dose of hCG in IVF, (76) dosages of 2000, 5000, and

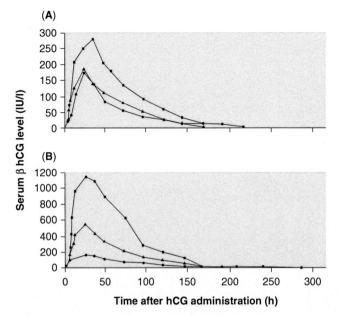

Figure 37.5 Pharmacokinetics of serum beta hCG in two hypogonadotropic women; (**A**) the first woman; (**B**) the second woman. Three regimens of human chorionic gonadotropin (hCG) injections were applied in each woman: 10,000 IU administered subcutaneously, or intramuscularly, and 5000 IU administered intramuscularly. *Source*: Modified from Ref. 221.

10,000 IU of urinary hCG (u-hCG) were administered to 88, 110, and 104 women, respectively. No differences in oocyte recovery were noted when comparing the groups that received 5000 and 10,000 IU. However, a significantly lower number of oocytes were aspirated in the 2000-IU group, compared with the 5000- and 10,000-IU groups.

With the development of recombinant technology, r-hCG became available for clinical use, and is as efficacious as u-hCG with the benefit of improved local tolerance (66,77,78). A study in IVF (78) showed that r-hCG 250 mcg is at least as effective as 5000 IU of u-hCG. The use of a higher dose of r-hCG, such as 500 mcg, resulted in the retrieval of more oocytes but also a threefold increase of OHSS. The local reaction at the injection site was significantly better than to the urinary product of equal dose (68). A total of 33 different non-gonadotropin proteins have been recently identified (using classical proteomic analyses) as contaminants in two commercially available preparations of u-hCG (79). Moreover, human prion peptides were detected in u-hCG (but were not identified in r-hCG) (79).

Gonadotropins: Historical Overview

In 1927, Aschheim and Zondek discovered a substance in the urine of pregnant women with the same action as the gonadotropic factor in the anterior pituitary (80). They called this substance gonadotropin or "prolan." Furthermore, they believed that there were two distinct hormones, prolan A and prolan B. They subsequently used their findings to develop the pregnancy test that carried their names. In 1930, Zondek reported that gonadotropins were also present in the urine of postmenopausal women, (81) and in the same year, Cole and Hart found gonadotropins in

Table 37.3	Milestones of Development in Infertility Treatment
1927	The discovery of pituitary hormone controlling ovarian function
1959	Purification and clinical use of pituitary and urine gonadotropins
1960	Clinical use of clomiphene citrate
1966	Use of clomiphene citrate and gonadotropin becomes common practice
1970	Development of radioimmunoassay for measuring hormone levels
1978	Ultrasound imaging of ovarian follicles
1984	Use of gonadotropin-releasing hormone (GnRH) agonists in infertility treatment
1985	Further purification of urinary gonadotropins
1990	Use of recombinant gonadotropins

the serum of pregnant mares (82). This hormone, pregnant mare serum gonadotropin, was found to have a potent gonadotropic effect in animals. However, it was only in 1937 that Cartland and Nelson were able to produce a purified extract of this hormone (83). It was not until 1948, as a result of the work of Stewart, Sano, and Montgomery, that gonadotropins in the urine of pregnant women were shown to originate from the chorionic villi of the placenta, rather than the pituitary. It was subsequently designated "chorionic gonadotropin" (84). After years of experiment, it gradually became apparent that the pituitary factor was needed for the production of mature follicles, and that chorionic gonadotropin could induce ovulation only when mature follicles were present (85). Within years, it became apparent that the use of gonadotropin extracts from non-primate sources was of limited clinical value owing to the development of antibodies that neutralized their therapeutic effect. In 1947, Piero Donini, a chemist at the Pharmaceutical Institute, Serono, in Rome tried to purify hMG from postmenopausal urine. This purification method was based on a method used by Katzman et al., published in 1943 (86). The first urine extract of gonadotropin contained LH and FSH and was named Pergonal, inspired by the Italian words "per gonadi" (for the gonads) (87). The approval to sell Pergonal was first granted by the Italian authorities in 1950 (Table 37.3). Only in 1961, with Pergonal treatment, was the first pregnancy achieved in a patient with secondary amenorrhea, which resulted with the birth (in 1962 in Israel) of the first normal baby girl (88). Urinary FSH (Metrodin) and highly purified FSH became available with the development of new technologies using specific monoclonal antibodies to bind the FSH and LH molecules in the hMG material in such a way that unknown urinary proteins could be removed. Metrodin has a specific activity of 100–200 IU of FSH/mg of protein, whereas Metrodin-HP highly purified has an activity of approximately 9000 IU/mg of protein.

HUMAN MENOPAUSAL GONADOTROPIN

Human menopausal gonadotropin contains an equivalent amount of 75 IU FSH and 75 IU LH in vivo bioactivity. Cook et al. (89) demonstrated that hMG preparations also contain up to five different FSH isohormones and up to nine LH species. These differences may cause discrepancies in patients' responses occasionally observed when using various lots of the same preparation.

Follicle-stimulating hormone, which is the major active agent, accounts for <5% of the local protein content in extracted urinary gonadotropin products (90). The specific activity of these products does not usually exceed 150 IU/ mg protein. The different proteins found in various hMG preparations include tumor necrosis factor binding protein I, transferrin, urokinase, Tamm-Horsfall glycoprotein, epidermal growth factor, and immunoglobulin-related proteins (91). Local side effects, such as pain and allergic reactions, have been reported and attributed to immune reactions related to non-gonadotropin proteins (92).

Technological improvements in recent years have resulted in the introduction of highly purified (HP) hMG, which can be administered subcutaneously (SC). Highly purified hMG contains more hCG and less LH than does traditional hMG (93). Accordingly, hMG and HP-hMG induce different follicular development profiles (93). A total of 34 co-purified proteins were recently identified in HP-hMG products (79). Importantly, human prion peptides were also detected in hMG and HP-hMG (79,94). The identification of human prion proteins in commercially available formulations has prompted careful examination of the risk of transmission of prion disease by urinary gonadotropins (79).

Information is scarce regarding the metabolism of gonadotropin hormones. It was shown that purified preparations of hFSH, hLH, and hCG injected (IV) in humans had serum half-lives (as determined by bioassays) of 180–240 minutes, 38–60 minutes, and 6–8 hours, respectively.

Measuring levels of gonadotropins by in vivo bioassays serves to compare biologic effects of gonadotropin preparations in a quantitative manner in animals. In the extensively used Steelman-Pohley assay, (95) 21-day-old female Sprague-Dawley rats are injected subcutaneously for three days and their ovaries weighed on the fourth day. Disadvantages of this assay are that its sensitivity is too low to detect small amounts of FSH in the serum, reproducibility is poor (+20% variation), and the procedure is cumbersome. The reliance on this assay, in effect, signifies that an ampoule of hMG, which appears to have 75 IU of FSH, may actually contain between 60 and 90 IU. Circulating levels of the gonadotropins measured at any given moment represent the balance between pituitary release and metabolic clearance. After IV injection, the initial half-life of urinary FSH was demonstrated to be approximately two hours, (96) and the true terminal (elimination) half-life appeared to be 17 + 5 hours. After IM injection of urinary FSH preparations, the half-life was estimated to be approximately 35 hours (66).

PURIFIED FOLLICLE-STIMULATING HORMONE

Further purification of hMG substantially decreased LH-like activity, leading to a commercial purified FSH (pFSH) preparation. Metrodin was introduced in the mid-1980s and is a product from the same source as

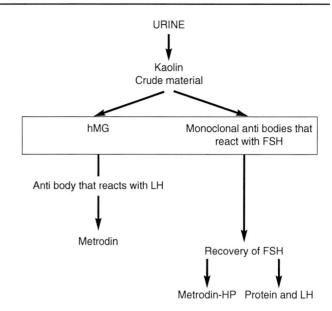

Figure 37.6 Schematic presentation of the production of human menopausal gonadotropin (hMG) and purification of urinary follicle-stimulating hormone (uFSH) and high-purity (HP)-FSH. Abbreviation: LH, luteinizing hormone.

hMG, but the LH component has been removed by immunoaffinity chromatography (Fig. 37.6).

Apart from obtaining a more purified product, the rationale of developing a pFSH preparation was that OI using gonadotropins in patients with elevated endogenous LH serum levels could, theoretically, preferably be performed without exogenously administered LH. It was also suggested that FSH alone could increase folliculogenesis (97). Furthermore, it was speculated that LH in gonadotropin preparations could be responsible for the high incidence of complications in patients with elevated serum LH levels (98,99). However, other studies (100,101) have indicated that the effectiveness of gonadotropin preparations and the occurrence of OHSS were not dependent on the LH:FSH ratio, (66) albeit the administration of pFSH to patients with PCOS did result in decreased LH levels, compared with hMG (102).

The desirable goal of having an FSH preparation of high purity led to the development of an immunopurified product (Metrodin-HP) of >95% purity (103).

RECOMBINANT HUMAN GONADOTROPINS (FOLLICLE-STIMULATING HORMONE, LUTEINIZING HORMONE, AND CHORIONIC GONADOTROPIN)

Following the development of highly purified urinary FSH, considerable improvements have facilitated both separation of FSH from hLH and its production using recombinant technology. Early technology focused on the production of biological molecules in bacterial cells (usually Escherichia coli). However, the structural complexity of human gonadotropins such as FSH and the need for posttranslational modification of the molecule by protein folding and glycosylation, made functional protein production impossible in prokaryotes. Thus, a mammalian cell culture system was employed with functional molecules being produced in Chinese hamster ovary (CHO) cells.

The world's first r-hFSH (follitropin alfa) preparation for clinical use was produced by Serono Laboratories in 1988, and was licensed for marketing in the European Union as GONAL-f in 1995. An r-hFSH (follitropin beta; Puregon) product was also licensed by Organon Laboratories in 1996. The genes for the other gonadotropins have also been transfected into mammalian cell lines, and r-hLH and r-hCG are now commercially available (r-hLH as Luveris, Merck Serono International, Switzerland; r-hCG as Ovidrel/Ovitrelle, Merck Serono International; and r-hFSH and r-hLH in a 2:1 ratio, Pergoveris, Merck Serono International). However, the following description of manufacturing techniques and physicochemical properties will focus on r-hFSH (follitropin alfa).

The production of hFSH by recombinant technology required isolation and cloning of genes for two subunits, the alfa subunit – which is also common to hLH and hCG – and a hormone-specific beta subunit. Appropriate vectors were prepared and transfected into suitable immortalized mammalian cell lines. The cell line originally chosen by Serono Laboratories was well-established (CHO-DUKX), and already being used to produce proteins such as recombinant human erythropoietin. These cells are normally dihydrofolate reductase deficient, and therefore sensitive to tetrahydrofolate analogs such as methotrexate. Cells were co-transfected with the human alfa and beta FSH genes and then treated with methotrexate, to select successfully transfected cells which could express the newly introduced genes.

A stable line of transformed cells was selected, which secreted high quantities of r-hFSH. These cell lines were used to establish a master cell bank (MCB), which now serves as the source of working cell banks (WCBs). The MCB consists of individual vials containing identical cells, which are cryopreserved until required. Thus, a continuous supply of r-hFSH with guaranteed consistency from WCB to WCB is now available by expansion of cells recovered from a single vial of the MCB (104). MCBs and WCBs are routinely tested for sterility, mycoplasma, and viral contamination.

Quantifying and Standardizing Gonadotropin Content

Traditionally, quantification of hFSH, LH, and hCG for clinical use has involved the use of in vivo bioassays. For hFSH, a number of bioassays have been assessed for this purpose, but one of the most robust and specific remains the Steelman-Pohley in vivo assay, first developed in the 1950s (95). FSH activity is quantified by rat ovarian weight gain and FSH vials or ampoules are subsequently filled according to the desired bioactivity, measured in IUs. However, the assay has a number of limitations: It is time consuming, cumbersome, uses large numbers of rats (which is of ethical concern), and is limited in its precision – the European Pharmacopoeia defines an activity range (80–125% of the target value) within which an FSH batch is acceptable for clinical use.

Recent advances in the manufacturing process for the r-hFSH follitropin alfa, however, enable high batch-to-batch consistency in both isoform profile and glycan species distribution (105,106). The most significant advantage of this over other commercially available gonadotropins is that it permits FSH to be quantified reliably by protein content (mass in mcg) rather than by biologic activity.

The coefficient of variation for an in vivo bioassay is typically ± 20%, compared with less than 2% for physicochemical analytic techniques, such as size exclusion HPLC (SE-HPLC) (105–107). As a result, Merck Serono International now quantify their r-hFSH (GONAL-f), r-hLH, and r-hCG protein by SE-HPLC, a precise and robust assay that results in a significant improvement in batch-to-batch consistency (108).

Physicochemical Consistency of R-hFSH: Glycan Mapping and Isoelectric Focusing

Glycan mapping provides a fingerprint of the glycan species of r-hFSH and an estimation of the degree of sialylation of the oligosaccharide chains. For each r-hFSH batch, intact glycan species are released by hydrazinolysis and labeled with a fluorescent derivative. As each glycan molecule is labeled with a single molecule of the dye, the response coefficient is the same for all glycan species, which are separated and detected by anion exchange chromatography and fluorimetry. Results are expressed as the relative percentage of the glycan species grouped as a function of their charge, which is related to the number of sialic acids they carry. The hypothetical charge number, Z, is defined as the sum of the percent areas under the curve in the neutral, mono-, di-, tri-, and tetrasialylated glycan regions, multiplied by their corresponding charge (108). The Z number was demonstrated to be a very precise estimate of the degree of sialylation, with a coefficient of variation of 2% or better.

Evaluation of GONAL-f batch data over time has demonstrated a highly consistent glycoform distribution, which reflects the high consistency of its molecular profile (105,106,109). The second physicochemical technique, isoelectric focusing, is performed in a gel matrix across a pH range of 3.5–7.0. After scanning the gel, the PI values and band intensities of the sample isoforms are compared with the reference standard. The distribution of the main bands from GONAL-f has remained similar to the reference standard over time, indicating a high consistency of isoform distribution (105).

Follitropin Alfa Filled by Mass

Between-batch analysis of the ratio of GONAL-f bioactivity, measured in IU using the Steelman-Pohley assay, and protein content, measured in mcg by SE-HPLC, has demonstrated a stable, normal distribution of specific activity with no bioreactor run effect (105). Similarly, drug substance production data over time also confirmed the well-controlled behavior and consistency of the GONAL-f manufacturing process (105,106). The highly consistent physicochemical and biologic properties of the product now permit FSH quantification by SE-HPLC, and vials or ampoules can be filled by mass (FbM) rather than by specific bioactivity. This product is referred to as GONAL-f FbM (Merck Serono International, Switzerland).

Once the physicochemical consistency of GONAL-f FbM had been demonstrated, the clinical relevance of the improved manufacturing process was assessed. A total of 131 women were enrolled into a multicenter, double-blind, randomized, parallel-group study comparing the efficacy and safety of four batches each of GONAL-f FbM and GONAL-f filled and released by IU (FbIU) in stimulating multiple follicular development prior to IVF (110). Adequate levels of ovarian stimulation were achieved with both preparations, resulting in a large number of embryos. The clinical pregnancy rate per treated cycle was 30.3% with the FbM preparation compared with 26.2% with FbIU. Both preparations showed similar levels of adverse events. However, it is the consistency of clinical response between batches that is of particular importance to physicians. The study demonstrated that the improved manufacturing process for the FbM over the FbIU preparation was associated with an improvement in the consistency of ovarian response ($p < 0.039$), including significantly improved between-batch consistency in the clinical pregnancy rate ($p < 0.001$). Compared with GONAL-f FbIU, the FbM preparation reduced the between-batch variability in clinical outcome.

Similar results were also demonstrated in larger studies in ART and OI of GONAL-f FbM versus FbIU (111–115). In a retrospective study by Balasch et al. (111) the clinical results during the introduction of GONAL-f FbM were compared with standard GONAL-f FbIU. The study included the last 125 patients treated with GONAL-f FbIU and the first 125 patients receiving GONAL-f FbM for ART ovarian stimulation. The patient demographics, oocyte yield, the number of metaphase II oocytes, and the fertilization rates were similar in both groups of patients. However, embryo quality as assessed on day 2 and implantation rates were significantly higher (18.6% vs. 28.6%, $p = 0.008$) in the r-hFSH FbM group. Accordingly, in spite of the mean number of embryos transferred being significantly lower in the r-hFSH FbM group, there was a trend for higher clinical pregnancy rates (44% vs. 35.2%) in this group of patients. In a large U.K. multicenter observational study carried out using GONAL-f FbM in 1427 ART patients, (112) the safety and efficacy of GONAL-f FbM was confirmed in routine clinical practice. The patients' mean age was 34.3 years and an average of 10.3 oocytes was retrieved. Only 2.7% of the patients who started FSH therapy did not receive hCG. The incidence of severe OHSS was 0.4% and the clinical pregnancy rate per cycle was 29.2%.

In the OI study, (113) following the use of GONAL-f FbM versus FbIU, fewer patients required an adjustment in the FSH dose (37% vs. 60%) and there were fewer canceled cycles (13% vs. 21%) during treatment using a chronic low-dose protocol. Hence, the quality of gonadotropin preparation may play an important role in the

consistency of the clinical response, including a reduction in the cycle cancellation (115).

Corifollitropin Alfa

The range of recombinant gonadotropins available for the treatment of subfertility has been expanded through protein engineering. An FSH molecule has been engineered to possess an extended half-life and duration of therapeutic action. This long-acting protein, designated FSH-C-terminal peptide (FSH-CTP, corifollitropin alfa) was first described by Bouloux and colleagues in 2001 (116). FSH-CTP consists of the alfa subunit of r-hFSH together with a hybrid beta subunit made up of the beta subunit of hFSH and the C-terminal part of the beta subunit of hCG. FSH-CTP has a longer half-life than standard r-hFSH. FSH-CTP initiates and sustains follicular growth for one week so one dose can replace the first seven daily injections of gonadotropin in COS. A single dose of FSH-CTP induces multifollicular growth accompanied by a dose-dependent rise in serum inhibin-B (117). The first live birth resulting from a stimulation cycle with FSH-CTP was reported in 2003 (118) and further studies have been carried out in subfertile patients undergoing ART and OI (119–124). FSH-CTP is now approved for use in Europe in ART cycles in combination with a GnRH antagonist.

Two large studies were conducted to demonstrate the noninferiority of FSH-CTP to r-hFSH (follitropin beta) (122,123). A multicenter, randomized, double blind, double-dummy clinical trial involving 34 centers and 1506 patients of 60–90 kg was initially performed (ENGAGE study) (123). Patients undergoing ART in a standard GnRH antagonist protocol received a single dose of FSH-CTP 150 mcg or daily doses of r-hFSH 200 IU during the first week of stimulation. Ongoing pregnancy rates per cycle initiated were not significantly different for FSH-CTP or r-hFSH (38.9% vs. 38.1%, respectively; estimated difference 0.9; $p = 0.71$). The reported incidence of moderate/severe OHSS was 4.1% with corifollitropin alfa versus 2.7% with follitropin beta (123).

A further study was conducted to evaluate the efficacy and safety of FSH-CTP in women with low body weight. The ENSURE study was a multicenter, randomized, double blind, double-dummy clinical trial involving 19 centers and 396 patients weighing <60 kg undergoing ART (122). Patients undergoing ART in a standard GnRH antagonist protocol received a single dose of FSH-CTP 100 mcg or daily doses of r-hFSH 150 IU during the first week of stimulation. The primary endpoint, the mean [standard deviation (SD)] number of oocytes retrieved per started cycle, was 13.3 (7.3) with FSH-CTP compared with 10.6 (5.9), which was within the predefined equivalence range (−3 to + 5 oocytes). The reported incidence of moderate or severe OHSS was 3.4% for corifollitropin alfa and 1.6% for follitropin beta (122).

FSH-CTP was developed with the aim of simplifying ART treatment regimens. However, there are concerns regarding the high incidence of OHSS associated with FSH-CTP in published studies and in clinical practice (122,123). Investigators of the multicenter, open-label,

Phase III TRUST study (designed to assess the immunogenicity of repeated exposure to FSH-CTP) raised concerns of the high rate of severe OHSS among their patients (125). Six of nine patients who received corifollitropin alfa at a single center developed severe OHSS 3–5 days after hCG administration (125). Three patients were hospitalized for several days and one experienced a pulmonary embolism despite appropriate therapy (125). In the TRUST study, 25 patients discontinued treatment after the first or second cycle because of an excessive response to COS or signs or symptoms of OHSS (124). The overall rate of moderate/severe OHSS in the study was 1.8% in Cycle 1, 1.0% in Cycle 2, and 0% in Cycle 3 (124). The effects of FSH-CTP cannot be adjusted to individual patient requirements, (125) therefore careful assessment of patient suitability is required before treatment is commenced.

OPTIMIZING OUTCOMES OF OVARIAN STIMULATION

Safety Profile of Gonadotropins

Accumulation of data on 1160 babies born after induction of ovulation with gonadotropins (29) revealed that major and minor malformations were found in 63 infants, representing an overall incidence of 54.3/1000 (major malformations 21.6/1000; minor malformations 32.7/1000). This rate of malformation is not significantly different from that of the general population.

Outcomes Achieved with r-hFSH Versus hMG

r-hFSH and hMG are the gonadotropins that are most frequently used for COS for IVF/ICSI. Outcomes achieved using these gonadotropins have been compared over many years in numerous retrospective studies, RCTs, and meta-analyses. Accumulating data suggest that all commercially available gonadotropins have similar efficacy and safety profiles (126). Indeed, there appears to be little overall difference between r-hFSH and hMG in outcomes of fresh ART cycles.

In 2003, Al-Inany et al. published a meta-analysis that compared r-hFSH with urinary FSH products (hMG, pFSH, and FSH-HP) in IVF/ICSI cycles using a long GnRH agonist protocol (127). Four of the 20 studies compared hMG with r-hFSH and showed no significant difference between hMG (n = 603 cycles) and r-hFSH (n = 611 cycles) in terms of clinical pregnancy rate per cycle initiated (OR = 0.81, 95% CI 0.63–1.05; $p = 0.11$) (128–131). A different meta-analysis from 2003 included six RCTs (n = 2030) of women undergoing COS for IVF/ICSI (132). Pooling of data from five RCTs that used a long GnRH agonist protocol showed that hMG resulted in significantly higher clinical pregnancy rates versus r-hFSH (RR = 1.22, 95% CI 1.03–1.44). However, there was no difference between groups in ongoing pregnancy rates or live births (RR = 1.20, 95% CI 0.99–1.45). A related Cochrane systematic review from 2003 also showed no difference in pooled data from four true RCTs in ongoing pregnancy/live birth rate per woman (OR = 1.27, 95% CI 0.98–1.64) (133).

In 2005, Al-Inany published an updated meta-analysis involving eight RCTs and 2031 participants. They showed no significant differences between hMG and r-hFSH in rates of ongoing pregnancy/live birth rate, clinical pregnancy, miscarriage, multiple pregnancy, or moderate/severe OHSS (134). This group published a third meta-analyses in 2008 including 12 trials involving 1453 hMG cycles and 1484 r-hFSH cycles. They showed a significantly higher live birth rate with hMG versus r-hFSH (OR = 1.2, 95% CI 1.01–1.42; $p = 0.04$) and similar rates of OHSS in each group (OR = 1.21, 95% CI 0.78–1.86; $p = 0.39$) (135). Also in 2008, Coomarasamy selected seven RCTs that used a long GnRH agonist protocol (136). A significant increase in live birth per woman randomized was found in favor of hMG versus r-hFSH (RR = 1.18, 95% CI 1.02–1.38; $p = 0.03$) (136). In 2009, Al-Inany et al. published a meta-analysis of six trials involving 2371 participants comparing HP-hMG and r-hFSH in women undergoing IVF/ICSI 93. No significant difference in the overall ongoing pregnancy/live birth rate was found between groups. However, when IVF cycles were analyzed alone, a significantly higher ongoing pregnancy/live birth rate was found in favor of HP-hMG (OR = 1.31, 95% CI 1.02–1.68; $p = 0.03$) (93).

The largest meta-analysis of r-hFSH and hMG to date was published in 2010, and included data from 16 RCTs involving 4040 patients undergoing fresh ART cycles (137). The primary endpoint of this analysis was the number of oocytes retrieved, which was selected to estimate directly the gonadotropin effects during COS. A recent study of more than 400,000 IVF cycles has confirmed that the number of oocytes retrieved is a robust surrogate outcome for clinical success (138). This large meta-analysis showed that r-hFSH resulted in the retrieval of significantly more oocytes versus hMG ($p < 0.001$), and a significantly lower dose of r-hFSH versus hMG was required ($p = 0.01$) (137). No significant difference was observed in baseline adjusted pregnancy rates (RR = 1.04; $p = 0.49$) or in OHSS (RR = 1.47; $p = 0.12$).

Individualization of Ovarian Stimulation

The objective of fertility treatment is the same for all women – optimization of outcomes with minimization of risks. It has become clear that the "one size fits all" approach to fertility treatment is too simplistic as each woman's ovarian response to stimulation is highly variable (139). Indeed, the use of flexible gonadotropin dosing during ovarian stimulation is now believed to be essential to optimizing cycle outcomes (139).

Accurate prediction of extremes of ovarian response prior to COS would allow tailoring of treatment in the first treatment cycle (139,140). Numerous biomarkers predictive of ovarian reserve and response to treatment have been proposed (140–142). Moreover, various algorithms have been developed to calculate the optimum FSH starting dose (140,143). The CONSORT treatment algorithm attempted to predict the optimum dose of r-hFSH (follitropin alfa) for ART based on individual patient characteristics: age, BMI, basal FSH, and antral follicle count (AFC). This algorithm resulted in an adequate oocyte yield, good pregnancy rate, and low incidence of OHSS. However, cycle cancellation due to an inadequate response occurred frequently in the lowest evaluable dose group (75 IU/day) (140).

Other factors that have been studied as potential predictors for ovarian response to COS include basal FSH, inhibin-B, estradiol, ovarian volume and vascular flow, and anti-Müllerian hormone (AMH). A number of studies have demonstrated the value of AMH, a marker of the total developing follicular cohort and growth of small follicles in the ovary, in predicting ovarian response (144–148). AMH has been shown to correlate significantly with oocyte yield and live birth, (146) and has also been shown to predict excessive response to controlled ovarian stimulation (145). A nomogram for the decline in serum AMH with age has been constructed and will facilitate counseling of patients regarding reproductive potential (149,150). Assessment of ovarian reserve by AMH before the first cycle of COS may provide a useful approach to individualize treatment (See Figure 42.1).

Efforts have also been made to identify markers that accurately predict response to the OI regimen to improve the safety, efficiency, and convenience of treatment for women with WHO group II anovulatory infertility (151,152). The selection of an appropriate starting dose of r-hFSH would allow physicians to individualize established treatment protocols (151). This could potentially shorten the time taken to reach the ovulation-triggering threshold and reduce the risk of cycle cancellation because of extreme responses to gonadotropins (151). However, attempts to identify factors predictive of response to OI have had limited success (152,153). A number of investigators have identified BMI as a marker of response to exogenous FSH and ovulation rates (152,154). The importance of BMI as a major determinant of successful ovulation was confirmed in a recent analysis of data from normogonadotropic, oligo-, or anovulatory women undergoing an OI using chronic low-dose, step-up treatment regimen (151). In addition, AFC and basal serum FSH concentration were shown to be associated with the response to treatment (151).

An individualized approach to ovarian stimulation is likely to result in optimal treatment outcomes (139). Determination of the most appropriate single or combination of drugs for ovarian stimulation, the daily dose, and duration of treatment is expected to enhance safety and cost-efficacy (139). Indeed, the identification of groups of patients who are likely to benefit from each available management strategy is essential (139). Such an approach would incorporate a wide variety of options based on the anticipated ovarian response.

Adjunctive Therapies

Supplementation of FSH with LH, growth hormone, or androgens may also help to improve the ovarian response and this is discussed in depth in Chapter 44. The use of supplementary LH has attracted the most interest in recent years. The classic "two cell–two gonadotropin"

model proposed that both FSH and LH are required for estradiol synthesis. LH binds to theca cells to induce synthesis of androgens, which diffuse out into the circulation and into the granulosa cells where, through the FSH-stimulated action of aromatase, they are converted to estrogen (155). Thus, LH regulates and integrates both granulosa and theca cell function during late preovulatory development. At this stage, FSH and LH work together to induce local production of growth factors needed for the paracrine regulation of follicular maturation.

LH supplementation is needed for healthy follicular development and oocyte maturation in patients with HH. In patients with HH, stimulation with FSH alone was significantly less effective than stimulation with FSH plus LH in a study by the European Recombinant Human LH Study Group (156). Based on these results, a product containing a fixed combination of r-hFSH and r-hLH in a 2:1 ratio [Pergoveris, Merck Serono S.A. – Geneva, Switzerland (an affiliate of Merck KGaA, Darmstadt, Germany)] was developed for follicular maturation in women with severe gonadotropin deficiency (157).

The use of GnRH agonists for pituitary downregulation in normogonadotropic women undergoing COS may result in LH levels below those that characterize HH. LH-like activity may be provided using hMG. Studies comparing r-hFSH and hMG have been reported earlier in this chapter and generally show little difference in outcomes. Two meta-analyses of studies comparing outcomes in women receiving supplementary r-hLH with those receiving only r-hFSH also showed no differences between treatment groups (158,159). Thus, it is generally accepted that LH supplementation has no benefit in normal responders undergoing COS.

There is, however, some evidence to suggest that LH has benefits in women aged above 35 years, and in poor or suboptimal responders to COS (160). A number of studies have suggested that LH supplementation may improve outcomes in cases of advanced maternal age (161–164). However, conflicting data has been reported from other studies (165). LH supplementation may also have benefits for women with a suboptimal response to stimulation, which is characterized by normal follicular development up to cycle days 5–7 followed by a plateau of this response on days 8–10. Suboptimal response may be due to LH-beta variant polymorphism, (166) or polymorphic variants of the FSH receptor (167,168). A significant improvement in fertilization and clinical pregnancy rates has been shown with the addition of r-hLH to r-hFSH in women who required high doses of r-hFSH in previous cycles (169). A number of other studies have also shown evidence of the benefit of LH supplementation in patients with suboptimal response to FSH (170–172).

GONADOTROPIN-RELEASING HORMONE

Introduction

Control of gonadotropin secretion is exerted by hypothalamic release of GnRH, initially known as LH-releasing hormone, but the lack of evidence for a specific

FSH-releasing hormone prompted a change in terminology. Gonadotropin-releasing hormone is produced and released from a group of loosely connected neurons located in the medial basal hypothalamus, primarily within the arcuate nucleus, and in the preoptic area of the ventral hypothalamus. It is synthesized in the cell body, transported along the axons to the synapse, and released in a pulsatile fashion into the complex capillary net of the portal system of the pituitary gland (173).

Gonadotropin-releasing hormone was first isolated, characterized, and synthesized independently in 1971 by Andrew Schally and Roger Guillemin, who were subsequently awarded the Nobel Prize for their achievement (174,175). Gonadotropin-releasing hormone is a decapeptide that, similar to several other brain peptides, is synthesized as part of a much larger precursor peptide, the GnRH-associated peptide, that has a 56 amino acid sequence. The structure of GnRH is common to all mammals, including humans, and its action is similar in both males and females. Gonadotropin-releasing hormone is a single-chain peptide comprising 10 amino acids with crucial functions at positions 1, 2, 3, 6, and 10. Position 6 is involved in enzymatic cleavage, positions 2 and 3 in gonadotropin release, and positions 1, 6, and 10 are important for the three-dimensional structure (Fig. 37.7).

In humans, the critical spectrum of pulsatile release frequencies ranges from the shortest interpulse frequency of approximately 71 minutes in the late follicular phase to an interval of 216 minutes in the late luteal phase (176,177).

GONADOTROPIN-RELEASING HORMONE AGONIST

Mechanism of Action

Although the exact cellular basis for desensitization of the gonadotroph has not been fully delineated, the extensive use of GnRH agonistic analogs in research facilitated an explosive augmentation of information and knowledge. Acute administration of GnRH agonist analogs increases gonadotropin secretion (the flare-up effect) and usually requires 7–14 days to achieve a state of pituitary suppression. Prolonged administration of GnRH agonistic analogs leads to downregulation of GnRH receptors. This phenomenon was first shown in 1978, when Knobil and coworkers published their classic paper demonstrating downregulation of gonadotropin secretion by sustained stimulation of the pituitary with GnRH (178). The agonist-bound receptor is internalized via receptor-mediated endocytosis, (179) with kinetics determined by the potency of the analog. The internalized complex subsequently undergoes dissociation, followed by degradation of the ligand and partial recycling of the receptors (180).

Biosynthesis

Native GnRH has a short plasma half-life and is rapidly inactivated by enzymatic cleavage. The initial concept was to create substances that prolong the stimulation of gonadotropin secretion. Analogs with longer half-life and higher receptor activities were created by a structural change at the position of enzymatic breakdown of GnRH.

The first major step in increasing the potency of GnRH was the substitution of glycine number 10 at the C-terminus. While 90% of the biologic activity is lost with splitting of the 10th glycine, it is predominantly restored with the attachment of NH_2-ethylamide to the proline at position 9 (181). The second major modification was the replacement of the glycine at position 6 by D-amino acids, which decreases enzymatic degradation (Fig. 37.7). The combination of these two modifications was found to have synergistic biologic activity. Agonistic analogs with D-amino acids at position 6, and NH2-ethylamide substituting the Gly10-amide, are

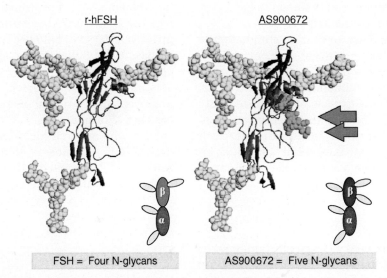

r-hFSH · AS900672

FSH = Four N-glycans · AS900672 = Five N-glycans

Figure 37.7 Gonadotropin-releasing hormone (GnRH) analog structure. A schematic illustration of native GnRH, GnRH agonist, and GnRH antagonist. Position 6 is involved in enzymatic cleavage, positions 2 and 3 in gonadotropin release, and positions 1, 6, and 10 are important for the three-dimensional structure. *Abbreviation*: FSH, follicle-stimulating hormone.

not only better protected against enzymatic degradation but also exhibit a higher receptor binding affinity. The affinity could be further increased by introduction of larger, hydrophobic, and more lipophilic amino acids at position number 6 (Table 37.4). The increased lipophilicity of the agonist is associated with a prolonged half-life, which may be attributed to reduced renal excretion through increased plasma protein binding, or fat tissue storage of nonionized fat-soluble compounds (181).

Thus, in all analogs, position 6 is substituted with a D-amino acid or a D-amino acid with different radicals. Insertion of D-amino acid blocks degradation and thus renders more stability and higher receptor affinity (182) (Table 37.4). The agonists leuprolide (D-Leu6,Pr9- NHEt) and buserelin [D-Ser(OtBu)6, Pr9-NHEt] contain an ethylamide, and goserelin [D-Ser(OtBu)6,Pro9- AzaGlyNH2] and histrelin (Nt-Bzl-D-His6,Pro9- AzaGlyNH2) contain azaglycine at position 10 and are, therefore, nonapeptides. Nafarelin [D-Nal(2)6] and triptorelin (D-Trp6) contain the original Gly10-amide, and are, therefore, decapeptides.

More than 1000 GnRH analogs have been synthesized and tested, but only a few have been introduced into clinical practice. Differences between analogs are mainly related to methods of administration and potency. The available data usually describe the relative potency of a certain GnRH agonist compared with native GnRH (Table 37.5). Direct comparison between the clinically available GnRH agonists under identical conditions has never been undertaken. Therefore, translation of data from these models to humans should be performed with caution.

All GnRH agonistic analogs are small polypeptide molecules that need to be administered parenterally, as they would otherwise be susceptible to gastrointestinal proteolysis. The oral and rectal administration of analogs is associated with very low biopotency (0.0–1% vs. parenteral administration). Intranasal spray is extremely effective, but the bioavailability is only 3–5%, and the relatively fast elimination kinetics requires frequent dosing (2–6 times/day) to obtain continuous stimulation and downregulation (183). For long-term treatment a depot formulation is available. The drug is formulated as

Table 37.4 The Structure of Gonadotropin-Releasing Hormone (GnRH) and GnRH Agonistic Analogs

Compound						6th position				10th position
Amino acid (no)	1	2	3	4	5	6	7	8	9	10
Native GnRH	Glu	His	Trp	Ser	Tyr	Gly	Leu	Arg	Pro	GlyNH$_2$
Nonapeptides										
Leuprolide						Leu				NHEt
Buserelin						Ser(OtBu)				NHEt
Goserelin						Ser(OtBu)				AzaGlyNH$_2$
Histrelin						DHis(Bzl)				AzaGlyNH$_2$
Decapeptides										
Nafarelin						2Nal				GlyNH$_2$
Triptorelin						Trp				GlyNH$_2$

Table 37.5 Trade Names, Plasmatic Half-Life, Relative Potency, Route of Administration, and Recommended Dose for the Clinically Available Gonadotropin-Releasing Hormone Analogs (GnRH-a)

Generic Name	Trade Name	Half-Life	Relative Potency	Administration Route	Recommended Dose
Native GnRH			1	IV SC	
Nonapeptides					
Leuprolide	Lupron	90 min	50–80	SC	500–1000 µg/day
			20–30	IM depot	3.75–7.5 mg/mo
Buserelin	Superfact, Supercur	80 min	20–40	SC	200–500 µg/day
				Intranasal	300–400 × 3–4/day
Histrelin	Supprelin	< 60 min	100	SC	100 µg/day
Goserelin	Zoladex	4.5 hr	50–100	SC implant	3.6 mg/mo
Decapeptides					
Nafarelin	Synarel	3–4 hr	200	Intranasal	200–400 × 2/day
Triptorelin	Decapeptyl	3–4.2 hr	36–144	SC	100–500 µg/day
				IM depot	3.75 mg/mo

controlled release depot preparations with the active substance dissolved, or encapsulated, in biodegradable material. Intramuscular injections provide maintained therapeutic levels for 28–35 days. Thus, monthly injections are sufficient for maintaining downregulation.

Side Effects

Side effects of GnRH agonist therapy are related to the fall in sex hormone serum concentration. As GnRH agonist interacts with GnRH receptors, which are mainly present in the pituitary, no systemic effects are common. The main symptoms of low serum concentrations of estrogen are flushes, decreased libido, impotence, vaginal dryness, reduced breast size, and emotional instability. One of the matters of concern is the effect of estrogen depletion on bone mineral density, as estrogen is of major importance in preventing the development of osteoporosis. A summary of data from different trials (184) showed that GnRH analog therapy caused significant but reversible bone loss. The mechanism appears to be similar to the development of postmenopausal osteoporosis; i.e., high bone turnover with elevated alkaline phosphatase and osteocalcin levels.

Teratogenic Effects

There does not appear to be an increased risk of birth defects, or pregnancy wastage in human pregnancies exposed to daily low-dose GnRH agonist therapy in the first weeks of gestation. Although placental transfer of GnRH agonists in pregnant rhesus monkeys was demonstrated, no deleterious effects were observed (185). From their toxicology studies in animals, no toxic effects were reported by the drug manufacturers (186). Although several authors claimed a normal outcome of pregnancy following inadvertent administration of a GnRH agonist during early pregnancy, (187–189) Ron-El et al. (190) reported the birth of a newborn with a small soft cleft palate. Lahat et al. reported a high incidence of attention deficit hyperactivity disorder in long-term follow up of children inadvertently exposed to GnRH agonists in early pregnancy (191). Therefore, as this complication is purely iatrogenic, it should best be avoided.

GONADOTROPIN-RELEASING HORMONE ANTAGONIST

Mechanism of Action

Antagonist analogs of GnRH have a direct inhibitory, reversible suppressive effect on gonadotropin secretion. Antagonistic molecules compete for and occupy pituitary GnRH receptors, thus competitively blocking the access of endogenous GnRH and precluding substantial receptor occupation and stimulation. Suppression attained by GnRH antagonists is immediate (no flare-up effect), and, as receptor loss does not occur, a constant supply of antagonists to the gonadotroph is required to ensure that all GnRH receptors are continuously

Table 37.6 Comparing Mechanisms of Action of Gonadotropin-Releasing Hormone (GnRH) Agonists and Antagonists

GnRH antagonist	GnRH agonist
Receptor blockage without receptor activation	Receptor downregulation
Competitive inhibition	Pituitary desensitization
Immediate and dose-dependent suppression	Initial flare-up
Rapid reversibility	Slow reversibility

occupied. Consequently, compared with agonistic analogs, a higher dose range of antagonists is required for effective pituitary suppression (Table 37.6).

Synthesis of GnRH Antagonists

Over the past three decades, thousands of GnRH analogs, both agonists and antagonists, have been synthesized. The first generations of antagonistic analogs were hydrophilic, and contained replacements for His at position 2 and for Trp at position 3. Inhibitory activity increased after incorporation of a D-amino acid at position 6. However, histamine release also increased, resulting in anaphylactic reactions that prevented their clinical use. In third-generation antagonistic analogs, the undesirable risk of anaphylaxis and edema was eliminated by replacing the D-Arg at position 6 by neutral D-ureidoalkyl amino acids, to produce compounds such as cetrorelix, iturelix, azaline B, ganirelix, abarelix, and antarelix (Table 37.7) (192–198).

Safety and Tolerability Studies

The introduction of GnRH antagonists in clinical use was delayed owing to the property of the first generation of antagonists to induce systemic histamine release and a subsequent general edematogenic state. Studies in rat mast cells confirmed that incorporation of D-Cit at position 6 of antagonists results in reduced histamine release (199,200). This characteristic of cetrorelix was first assessed in in vitro assays that demonstrated effective plasma concentrations to be significantly lower ($<10^3$) than the median effective dose for systemic histamine secretion, and, therefore, could confidently be regarded as insignificant. Owing to large disparities in such assays, cetrorelix safety was further tested in in vivo settings.

Cetrorelix injected at doses of 1.5 mg/kg subcutaneously and 1 and 4 mg/kg intravenously into rats caused no systemic adverse effects, such as edema, respiratory dysfunction, or cardiovascular compromise. In these animal studies no teratogenic effects, or detrimental influence on implantation rates or on embryonic development, were noted when administered in the periconceptional period. Several thousand human patients have been treated with third-generation GnRH antagonists (i.e., ganirelix, cetrorelix, or abarelix) without evidence of systemic, or major local skin reactions, and no cessation of

Table 37.7   Structure Formulation of Native Gonadotropin-Releasing Hormone (GnRH) and GnRH Antagonists

Name	Amino Acid Sequence
GnRH	pGlu-His-Trp-Ser-Tyr-Gly-Leu-Arg-Pro-Gly-NH$_2$
First Generation	
4F Ant	NAc⊗1, 1Pro-D4FPhe-DTrp-Ser-Tyr-DTrp-Leu-Arg-Pro-GlyNH$_2$
Second Generation	
NalArg	NACD2Nal-D4lFPhe-pTrp-Ser-Tyr-DArg-Leu-Arg-Pro-GlyNH$_2$
Detirelix	NACD2Nal-D4ClPhe-pTrp-Ser-Tyr-DHarg(Et2)-Leu-Arg-Pro-DAlaNH$_2$
Third Generation	
NalGlu	NACD2Nal-D4C7Phe-D3Pal-Ser-Arg-DGlut(AA)-Leu-Arg-Pro-DAlaNH$_2$
Antide	NACD2Nal-D4ClPhe-D3Pal-Ser-Lys(Nic)-DDLys(Nic)-Leu-Lys(Isp)Pro-DAlaNH$_2$
Org30850	NACD4ClPhe-D4ClPhe-DBal-Ser-Tyr-DLys-Leu-Arg-Pro-DAlaNH$_2$
Ramorelix	NACD2Nal-D4ClPhe-DTrp-Ser-Tyr-DSet(Rha)-Leu-Arg-Pro-AzaglyNH$_2$
Cetrorelix	NACD2Nal-D4ClPhe-D3Pal-Ser-Tyr-DCit-Leu-Arg-Pro-DAlaNH$_2$
Ganirelix	NACD2Nal-D4ClPhe-D3Pal-Ser-Tyr-DHarg(Et2)-Leu-Harg(Et2)-Pro-DAlaNH$_2$
A-75998	NACD2Nal-D4ClPhe-D3Pal-Ser-NMeTyr-DLys(Nic)-Leu-Lys(Isp)-Pro-DAlaNH$_2$
Azaline B	NACD2Nal-D4ClPhe-D3Pal-Ser-Aph(atz)-DAph(atz)-Leu-Lys(Isp)-Pro-DAlaNH$_2$
Antarelix	NACD2Nal-D4ClPhe-D3Pal-Ser-Tyr-DHcit-Leu-Lys(Isp)-Pro-DAlaNH$_2$

therapy was warranted due to side effects (199,201–205). The common side effects observed were injection-site reactions and possibly nausea, headache, fatigue, and malaise. No drug interactions were demonstrated in vitro with medications metabolized through the cytochrome P450 pathway.

It was suggested that GnRH antagonists may adversely affect oocyte or embryo quality, or the endometrium (206–211). However, the most recent evidence suggests that GnRH antagonists do not diminish oocyte or embryo quality or endometrial receptivity (212–214).

Advantages of GnRH Antagonists

The use of GnRH antagonists offers a number of potential advantages over agonists (215). Prolonged pretreatment to achieve pituitary downregulation is not required (216). GnRH antagonists are usually administered only when there is a risk of premature LH surge (usually from day 5 to 7 of stimulation) so symptoms of hypoestrogenemia are rare (215). Furthermore, lower total doses and fewer days of exogenous gonadotropin stimulation are required versus agonists (217). Consequently, the total cycle duration is shorter and subsequent cycles can be initiated rapidly (218).

A meta-analysis including 45 RCTs and 7511 women to compare GnRH antagonist and long GnRH agonist protocols for COS in ART showed no significant difference in the live birth or ongoing pregnancy rates, but a significantly lower incidence of OHSS with GnRH antagonists (218). Interestingly, the pituitary remains responsive to GnRH stimulation during antagonist co-treatment so a bolus dose of agonist can be administered (instead of hCG) to trigger final oocyte maturation. This approach may have the potential to reduce further the incidence of OHSS for those at high risk but requires further study (219,220).

It has been proposed that GnRH antagonist protocols may have particular benefit for patients at the anticipated extremes of ovarian response (147). A prospective cohort study of 538 patients was conducted to compare outcomes of GnRH agonist versus antagonist protocols in an attempt to individualize treatment based on baseline AMH level (147). GnRH antagonist co-treatment (vs. agonist co-treatment) resulted in a reduced cycle cancellation rate and treatment burden for poor responders (AMH 1 to <5 pmol/l) (147). However, GnRH antagonists were found to be most advantageous in high responders (AMH ≥15.0 pmol/l) (147). A higher fresh clinical pregnancy rate per oocyte retrieval ($p < 0.0010$) was achieved by a profound reduction in excessive response to COS and an increased proportion of fresh ET (vs. agonist co-treatment) (147).

The reduction in treatment burden (in terms of cycle duration and side effects) and a lower risk of OHSS compared with long agonist protocols means that GnRH antagonists are considered to be "patient-friendly" therapies. Although GnRH antagonists are being used with increasing frequency in COS protocols, GnRH agonists have been commercially available for much longer and there is a greater depth of knowledge on the use of these agents.

REFERENCES

1. Greenblatt RB, Barfield WE, Jungck EC, Ray AW. Induction of ovulation with MRL/41: preliminary report. J Am Med Assoc 1961; 178: 101–4.
2. Charles D, Klein T, Lunn SF, Loraine JA. Clinical and endocrinological studies with the isomeric components of clomiphene citrate. J Obstet Gynaecol Br Commonw 1969; 76: 1100–10.
3. Pandya G, Cohen MR. The effect of cis-isomer of clomiphene citrate (cis-clomiphene) on cervical mucus and vaginal cytology. J Reprod Med 1972; 8: 133–8.
4. MacLeod SC, Mitton DM, Parker AS, Tupper WR. Experience with induction of ovulation. Am J Obstet Gynecol 1970; 108: 814–24.
5. Murthy YS, Parakh MC, Arronet GH. Experience with clomiphene and cisclomiphene. Int J Fertil 1971; 16: 66–74.

6. Van Campenhout J, Borreman E, Wyman H, Antaki A. Induction of ovulation with cisclomiphene. Am J Obstet Gynecol 1973; 115: 321–7.

7. Connaughton JF Jr, Garcia CR, Wallach EE. Induction of ovulation with cisclomiphene and a placebo. Obstet Gynecol 1974; 43: 697–701.

8. Mikkelson TJ, Kroboth PD, Cameron WJ, et al. Single-dose pharmacokinetics of clomiphene citrate in normal volunteers. Fertil Steril 1986; 46: 392–6.

9. Kahwanago I, Heinrichs WL, Herrmann WL. Estradiol "receptors" in hypothalamus and anterior pituitary gland: inhibition of estradiol binding by SH-group blocking agents and clomiphene citrate. Endocrinology 1970; 86: 1319–26.

10. Etgen AM. Antiestrogens: effects of tamoxifen, nafoxidine, and CI-628 on sexual behavior, cytoplasmic receptors, and nuclear binding of estrogen. Horm Behav 1979; 13: 97–112.

11. Dickey RP, Holtkamp DE. Development, pharmacology and clinical experience with clomiphene citrate. Hum Reprod Update 1996; 2: 483–506.

12. Kousta E, White DM, Franks S. Modern use of clomiphene citrate in induction of ovulation. Hum Reprod Update 1997; 3: 359–65.

13. Vandenberg G, Yen SS. Effect of anti-estrogenic action of clomiphene during the menstrual cycle: evidence for a change in the feedback sensitivity. J Clin Endocrinol Metab 1973; 37: 356–65.

14. Clark JH, Markaverich BM. The agonistic-antagonistic properties of clomiphene: a review. Pharmacol Ther 1981; 15: 467–519.

15. Clark JH, Peck EJ Jr, Anderson JN. Oestrogen receptors and antagonism of steroid hormone action. Nature (London) 1974; 251: 446–8.

16. Adashi EY. Clomiphene citrate: mechanism(s) and site(s) of action – a hypothesis revisited. Fertil Steril 1984; 42: 331–44.

17. Messinis IE, Milingos SD. Future use of clomi - phene in ovarian stimulation. Clomiphene in the 21st century. Hum Reprod 1998; 13: 2362–5.

18. Messinis IE, Milingos SD. Current and future status of ovulation induction in polycystic ovary syndrome. Hum Reprod Update 1997; 3: 235–53.

19. Out HJ, Coelingh Bennink HJ. Clomiphene citrate or gonadotrophins for induction of ovulation?. Hum Reprod 1998; 13: 2358–61.

20. Hughes E, Collins J, Vandekerckhove P. Clomi phene citrate for unexplained subfertility in women. Cochrane Database Syst Rev 2000; CD000057.

21. Rossing MA, Daling JR, Weiss NS, et al. Ovarian tumors in a cohort of infertile women. N Engl J Med 1994; 331: 771–6.

22. Anencephaly, ovulation stimulation, subfertility, and illegitimacy [Letter]. Lancet 1973; 2: 916–17.

23. Singh M, Singhi S. Possible relationship between clomiphene and neural tube defects. J Pediatr 1978; 93: 152.

24. Dyson JL, Kohler HG. Anencephaly and ovulation stimulation. Lancet 1973; 1: 1256–7.

25. Sandler B. Anencephaly and ovulation stimulation. Lancet 1973; 2: 379.

26. Field B, Kerr C. Ovulation stimulation and defects of neural-tube closure [Letter]. Lancet 1974; 2: 1511.

27. Berman P. Congenital abnormalities associated with maternal clomiphene ingestion [Letter]. Lancet 1975; 2: 878.

28. James WH. Anencephaly, ovulation stimulation, and subfertility [Letter]. Lancet 1974; 1: 1353.

29. Shoham Z, Zosmer A, Insler V. Early miscarriage and fetal malformations after induction of ovulation (by clomiphene citrate and/or human meno tropins), in vitro fertilization, and gamete intra fallopian transfer. Fertil Steril 1991; 55: 1–11.

30. Harlap S. Ovulation induction and congenital malformations. Lancet 1976; 2: 961.

31. Goss PE, Gwyn KM. Current perspectives on aromatase inhibitors in breast cancer. J Clin Oncol 1994; 12: 2460–70.

32. Harvey HA. Aromatase inhibitors in clinical practice: current status and a look to the future. Semin Oncol 1996; 23: 33–8.

33. Smith IE, Fitzharris BM, McKinna JA, et al. Aminoglutethimide in treatment of metastatic breast carcinoma. Lancet 1978; 2: 646–9.

34. Lamb HM, Adkins JC. Letrozole. A review of its use in postmenopausal women with advanced breast cancer. Drugs 1998; 56: 1125–40.

35. Wiseman LR, Adkins JC. Anastrozole. A review of its use in the management of postmenopausal women with advanced breast cancer. Drugs Aging 1998; 13: 321–32.

36. Biljan MM, Hcmmings R, Brassard N. The outcome of 150 babies following the treatment wilh letrozole or lelrozole and gonadotrophins. Fertil Steril 2005; 84(Suppl): 1033.

37. Tulandi T, Martin J, Al-Fadhli R, et al. Congenital malformations among 911 newborns conceived after infertility treatment with letrozole or clomiphene citrate. Fertil Steril 2006; 85: 1761–5.

38. Badawy A, Shokeir T, Allam AF, et al. Pregnancy outcome after ovulation induction with aromatase inhibitors or clomiphene citrate in unexplained infertility. Acta Obstet Gynecol Scand 2009; 88: 187–91.

39. Mitwally MF, Casper RF. Use of an aromatase inhibitor for induction of ovulation in patients with an inadequate response to clomiphene citrate. Fertil Steril 2001; 75: 305–9.

40. Mitwally MF, Casper RF. Aromatase inhibition improves ovarian response to follicle-stimulating hormone in poor responders. Fertil Steril 2002; 77: 776–80.

41. Mitwally MF, Casper RF. Aromatase inhibition for ovarian stimulation: future avenues for infertility management. Curr Opin Obstet Gynecol 2002; 14: 255–63.

42. Fisher SA, Reid RL, Van Vugt DA, Casper RF. A randomized double-blind comparison of the effects of clomiphene citrate and the aromatase inhibitor letrozole on ovulatory function in normal women. Fertil Steril 2002; 78: 280–5.

43. Mitwally MF, Casper RF. Aromatase inhibition reduces gonadotrophin dose required for controlled ovarian stimulation in women with unexplained infertility. Hum Reprod 2003; 18: 1588–97.

44. He D, Jiang F. Meta-analysis of letrozole versus clomiphene citrate in polycystic ovary syndrome. Reprod Biomed Online 2011; 23: 91–6.

45. Papanikolaou EG, Polyzos NP, Humaidan P, et al. Aromatase inhibitors in stimulated IVF cycles. Reprod Biol Endocrinol 2011; 9: 85.

46. Polyzos NP, Mauri D, Tzioras S. Letrozole in ovulation induction: time to make decisions. Hum Reprod Update 2009; 15: 263–4.

47. Tredway D, Schertz JC, Bock D, et al. Anastrozole vs. clomiphene citrate in infertile women with ovulatory dysfunction: a phase II, randomized, dose-finding study. Fertil Steril 2011; 95: 1720–4.

48. Tredway D, Schertz JC, Bock D, et al. Anastrozole single-dose protocol in women with oligo- or anovulatory infertility: results of a randomized phase II dose-response study. Fertil Steril 2011; 95: 1725–9.

49. Griesinger G, von OS, Schultze-Mosgau A, et al. Follicular and endocrine response to anastrozole versus clomiphene citrate administered in follicular phase to normoovulatory women: a randomized comparison. Fertil Steril 2009; 91: 1831–6.

50. Davar R, Oskouian H, Ahmadi S, Firouzabadi RD. GnRH antagonist/letrozole versus microdose GnRH agonist flare protocol in poor responders undergoing in vitro fertilization. Taiwan J Obstet Gynecol 2010; 49: 297–301.

51. Garcia-Velasco JA, Moreno L, Pacheco A, et al. The aromatase inhibitor letrozole increases the concentration of intraovarian androgens and improves in vitro fertilization outcome in low responder patients: a pilot study. Fertil Steril 2005; 84: 82–7.

52. Goswami SK, Das T, Chattopadhyay R, et al. A randomized single-blind controlled trial of letrozole as a low-cost IVF protocol in women with poor ovarian response: a preliminary report. Hum Reprod 2004; 19: 2031–5.

53. Ozmen B, Sonmezer M, Atabekoglu CS, Olmus H. Use of aromatase inhibitors in poor-responder patients receiving GnRH antagonist protocols. Reprod Biomed Online 2009; 19: 478–85.

54. Verpoest WM, Kolibianakis E, Papanikolaou E, et al. Aromatase inhibitors in ovarian stimulation for IVF/ICSI: a pilot study. Reprod Biomed Online 2006; 13: 166–72.

55. Lord JM, Flight IH, Norman RJ. Insulin-sensitising drugs (metformin, troglitazone, rosiglitazone, pioglitazone, D-chiro-inositol) for polycystic ovary syndrome. Cochrane Database Syst Rev 2003: CD003053.

56. ASRM. Practice Committee Guidelines. Fertil Steril 2006; 86(Suppl 4): S221–3.

57. UK National Collaborating Centre for Women's and Children's Health. Fertility: Assessment and treatment for people with fertility problems. Clinical Guideline 11. UK: National Institute for Clinical Excellence, 2004.

58. Moll E, Bossuyt PM, Korevaar JC, Lambalk CB, van der Veen F. Effect of clomifene citrate plus metformin and clomifene citrate plus placebo on induction of ovulation in women with newly diagnosed polycystic ovary syndrome: randomised double blind clinical trial. BMJ 2006; 332: 1485.

59. Palomba S, Orio F Jr, Falbo A, et al. Prospective parallel randomized, double-blind, double-dummy controlled clinical trial comparing clomiphene citrate and metformin as the first-line treatment for ovulation induction in nonobese anovulatory women with polycystic ovary syndrome. J Clin Endocrinol Metab 2005; 90: 4068–74.

60. Costello MF, Chapman M, Conway U. A systematic review and meta-analysis of randomized controlled trials on metformin co-administration during gonadotrophin ovulation induction or IVF in women with polycystic ovary syndrome. Hum Reprod 2006; 21: 1387–99.

61. Neveu N, Granger L, St-Michel P, Lavoie HB. Comparison of clomiphene citrate, metformin, or the combination of both for first-line ovulation induction and achievement of pregnancy in 154 women with polycystic ovary syndrome. Fertil Steril 2007; 87: 113–20.

62. Siebert TI, Kruger TF, Steyn DW, Nosarka S. Is the addition of metformin efficacious in the treatment of clomiphene citrate-resistant patients with polycystic ovary syndrome? A structured literature review. Fertil Steril 2006; 86: 1432–7.

63. Legro RS, Barnhart HX, Schlaff WD, et al. Cooperative Multicenter Reproductive Medicine Network. Clomiphene, metformin, or both for infertility in the polycystic ovary syndrome. N Engl J Med 2007; 356: 551–66.

64. Franks S. When should an insulin sensitizing agent be used in the treatment of polycystic ovary syndrome? Clin Endocrinol (Oxf) 2011; 74: 148–51.

65. le Cotonnec JY, Porchet HC, Beltrami V, Munafo A. Clinical pharmacology of recombinant human luteinizing hormone: part I. Pharmacokinetics after intravenous administration to healthy female volunteers and comparison with urinary human luteinizing hormone. Fertil Steril 1998; 69: 189–94.

66. Diczfalusy E, Harlin J. Clinical-pharmacological studies on human menopausal gonadotrophin. Hum Reprod 1988; 3: 21–7.

67. Braunstein GD, Bloch SK, Rasor JL, Winikoff J. Characterization of antihuman chorionic gonado - tropin serum antibody appearing after ovulation induction. J Clin Endocrinol Metab 1983; 57: 1164–72.

68. Ludwig M, Doody KJ, Doody KM. Use of recombinant human chorionic gonadotropin in ovulation induction. Fertil Steril 2003; 79: 1051–9.

69. Kyle CV, Griffin J, Jarrett A, Odell WD. Inability to demonstrate an ultrashort loop feedback mechanism for luteinizing hormone in humans. J Clin Endocrinol Metab 1989; 69: 170–6.

70. Nader S, Berkowitz AS. Endogenous luteinizing hormone surges following administration of human chorionic gonadotropin: further evidence for lack of loop feedback in humans. J Assist Reprod Genet 1992; 9: 124–7.

71. Demoulin A, Dubois M, Gerday C, et al. Variations of luteinizing hormone serum concentrations after exogenous human chorionic gonadotropin administration during ovarian hyperstimulation. Fertil Steril 1991; 55: 797–804.

72. Golan A, Ron-El R, Herman A, et al. Ovarian hyperstimulation syndrome: an update review. Obstet Gynecol Surv 1989; 44: 430–40.

73. Gidley-Baird AA, O'Neill C, Sinosich MJ, et al. Failure of implantation in human in vitro fertilization and embryo transfer patients: the effects of altered progesterone/estrogen ratios in humans and mice. Fertil Steril 1986; 45: 69–74.

74. Forman R, Fries N, Testart J, et al. Evidence for an adverse effect of elevated serum estradiol concentrations on embryo implantation. Fertil Steril 1988; 49: 118–22.

75. Tan SL, Balen A, el Hussein E, et al. A prospective randomized study of the optimum timing of human chorionic gonadotropin administration after pituitary desensitization in in vitro fertilization. Fertil Steril 1992; 57: 1259–64.

76. Abdalla HI, Ah-Moye M, Brinsden P, et al. The effect of the dose of human chorionic gonadotropin and the type of gonadotropin stimulation on oocyte recovery

rates in an in vitro fertilization program. Fertil Steril 1987; 48: 958–63.

77. Lathi RB, Milki AA. Recombinant gonadotropins. Curr Womens Health Rep 2001; 1: 157–63.

78. The European Recombinant Human Chorionic Gonadotrophin Study Group. Induction of final follicular maturation and early luteinization in women undergoing ovulation induction for assisted reproduction treatment – recombinant hCG versus urinary hCG. Hum Reprod 2000; 15: 1446–51.

79. Van Dorsselaer A, Carapito C, Delalande F, et al. Detection of prion protein in urine-derived injectable fertility products by a targeted proteomic approach. PLos ONE 2011; 6: e17815.

80. Aschheim S, Zondek B. Die schwangerschaftsdiagnose aus dem harn durch nachweis des hypophysenvorderlappenhormons. Klin Wochenschr 1928; 7: 8–9.

81. Zondek B. Über die Hormone des Hypophysenvorderlappens. II. Follikelreifungshormon Prolan A-Klimakterium-Kastration. Klin Wochenschr 1930; 9: 393–6.

82. Cole H, Hart GH. Am J Physiol 1931; 93: 57–68.

83. Stewart HL, Sano ME, Montgomery TL. Hormone secretion by human placenta grown in tissue culture. J Clin Endocrinol 1948; 8: 175–88.

84. Kotz HL, Hermann W. A review of the endocrine induction of human ovulation. Fertil Steril 1961; 12: 375–94.

85. Knobil E, Kostyo J, Greep R. Lack of competitive inhibition between beef and monkey growth hormones in rhesus monkeys. Fed Proc 1958; 17: 88.

86. Katzman PA, Godfrid M, Cain CK, Doisy EA. J Biol Chem 1943; 148: 501–7.

87. Donini P, Montezemolo R. Rassegna di Clinica, Terapia e Scienze Affini. A publication of the Biologic Laboratories of the Instituto Serono, 1949: 48: 3–28.

88. Lunenfeld B, Sulimovici S, Rabau E, Eshkol A. L'Induction de l'ovulation dans les amenorhées hypophysaires par un traîtment de gonado trophines urinaries menopausiques et de gonado trophines chroniques. C R Soc Française de Gynecol 1973; 5: 1–6.

89. Cook AS, Webster BW, Terranova PF, Keel BA. Variation in the biologic and biochemical characteristics of human menopausal gonadotropin. Fertil Steril 1988; 49: 704–12.

90. Howles CM, Loumaye E, Giroud D, Luyet G. Multiple follicular development and ovarian steroidogenesis following subcutaneous administration of a highly purified urinary FSH preparation in pituitary desensitized women undergoing IVF: a multicentre European phase III study. Hum Reprod 1994; 9: 424–30.

91. Giudice E, Crisci C, Eshkol A, Papoian R. Composition of commercial gonadotrophin preparations extracted from human post-menopausal urine: characterization of non-gonadotrophin proteins. Hum Reprod 1994; 9: 2291–9.

92. Li TC, Hindle JE. Adverse local reaction to intramuscular injections of urinary-derived gonadotrophins. Hum Reprod 1993; 8: 1835–6.

93. Al-Inany HG, bou-Setta AM, Aboulghar MA, et al. Highly purified hMG achieves better pregnancy rates in IVF cycles but not ICSI cycles compared with recombinant FSH: a meta-analysis. Gynecol Endocrinol 2009; 25: 372–8.

94. Kuwabara Y, Mine K, Katayama A, et al. Proteomic analyses of recombinant human follicle-stimulating hormone and urinary-derived gonadotropin preparations. J Reprod Med 2009; 54: 459–66.

95. Steelman SL, Pohley FM. Assay of the follicle stimulating hormone based on the augmentation with human chorionic gonadotropin. Endocrinology 1953; 53: 604–16.

96. le Cotonnec JY, Porchet HC, Beltrami V, et al. Clinical pharmacology of recombinant human follicle-stimulating hormone (FSH). Comparative pharmacokinetics with urinary human FSH. Fertil Steril 1994; 61: 669–78.

97. Schoemaker J, Wentz AC, Jones GS, et al. Stimulation of follicular growth with "pure" FSH in patients with anovulation and elevated LH levels. Obstet Gynecol 1978; 51: 270–7.

98. Raj SG, Berger MJ, Grimes EM, Taymor ML. The use of gonadotropins for the induction of ovulation in women with polycystic ovarian disease. Fertil Steril 1977; 28: 1280–4.

99. McFaul PB, Traub AI, Thompson W. Treatment of clomiphene citrate-resistant polycystic ovarian syndrome with pure follicle-stimulating hormone or human menopausal gonadotropin. Fertil Steril 1990; 53: 792–7.

100. Jacobson A, Marshall JR. Ovulatory response rate with human menopausal gonadotropins of varying FSH-LH ratios. Fertil Steril 1969; 20: 171–5.

101. Louwerens B. The clinical significance of the FSH- LH ratio in gonadotropin preparations of human origin. A review. Acta Obstet Gynecol Scand 1969; 48(Suppl 1): 31–40.

102. Anderson RE, Cragun JM, Chang RJ, et al. A pharmacodynamic comparison of human urinary follicle-stimulating hormone and human meno – pausal gonadotropin in normal women and polycystic ovary syndrome. Fertil Steril 1989; 52: 216–20.

103. le Cotonnec JY, Porchet HC, Beltrami V, Howles C. Comparative pharmacokinetics of two urinary human follicle stimulating hormone preparations in healthy female and male volunteers. Hum Reprod 1993; 8: 1604–11.

104. Howles CM. Genetic engineering of human FSH (Gonal-F). Hum Reprod Update 1996; 2: 172–91.

105. Driebergen R, Baer G. Quantification of follicle stimulating hormone (follitropin alfa): is the in vivo bioassay still relevant in the recombinant age?. Curr Med Res Opin 2003; 19: 1–6.

106. Bassett RM, Driebergen R. Continued impro vements in the quality and consistency of follitropin alfa, recombinant human FSH. Reprod Biomed Online 2005; 10: 169–77.

107. Driebergen R, Basset R, Baer G, et al. Improvements in quantification of r-hFSH activity: SE-HPLC vs the in vitro rat bioassay. Hum Reprod 2002; 17: 80. 486.

108. Hermentin P, Witzel R, Kanzy EJ, et al. The hypothetical N-glycan charge: a number that characterizes protein glycosylation. Glycobiology 1996; 6: 217–30.

109. Gervais A, Hammel YA, Pelloux S, et al. Glycosylation of human recombinant gonadotropins: characterization and batch-to-batch consistency. Glycobiology 2003; 13: 179–89.

110. Hugues JN, Barlow DH, Rosenwaks Z, et al. Improvement in consistency of response to ovarian stimulation with recombinant human follicle stimulating hormone resulting from a new method for calibrating the therapeutic preparation. Reprod BioMed Online 2003; 6: 185–90.

111. Balasch J, Fabregues F, Penarrubia J, et al. Outcome from consecutive assisted reproduction cycles in

patients treated with recombinant follitropin alfa filled-by-bioassay and those treated with recombinant follitropin alfa filled-by-mass. Reprod Biomed Online 2004; 8: 408–13.

112. Lass A, McVeigh E. UK Gonal-f FbM PMS Group. Routine use of r-hFSH follitropin alfa filled-bymass for follicular development for IVF: a large multicentre observational study in the UK. Reprod Biomed Online 2004; 9: 604–10.

113. Martinez G, Sanguineti F, Sepulveda J, et al. A comparison between follitropin alpha filled by mass and follitropin alpha filled by bioassay in the same egg donors. Reprod Biomed Online 2007; 14: 26–8.

114. Carizza C, Alam V, Yeko T, et al. Gonal-F® filled by mass in ovulation induction. Hum Reprod Suppl 2003; 18: O117.

115. Wikland M, Hugues JN, Howles C. Improving the consistency of ovarian stimulation: follitropin alfa filled-by-mass. Reprod Biomed Online 2006; 12: 663–8.

116. Bouloux PM, Handelsman DJ, Jockenhovel F, et al. First human exposure to FSH-CPT in hypogonadotrophic hypogonadal males. Hum Reprod 2001; 16: 1592–7.

117. Duijkers IJ, Klipping C, Boerrigter PJ, et al. Single dose pharmacokinetics and effects on follicular growth and serum hormones of a long acting recombinant FSH preparation (FSH-CTP) in healthy pituitary- suppressed females. Hum Reprod 2002; 17: 1987–93.

118. Beckers NG, Macklon NS, Devroey P, et al. First live birth after ovarian stimulation using a chimeric long-acting human recombinant follicle-stimulating hormone (FSH) agonist (recFSH-CTP) for in vitro fertilization. Fertil Steril 2003; 79: 621–3.

119. Balen AH, Mulders AG, Fauser BC, et al. Pharmacodynamics of a single low dose of longacting recombinant follicle-stimulating hormone (FSH-carboxy terminal peptide, corifollitropin alfa) in women with World Health Organization group II anovulatory infertility. J Clin Endocrinol Metab 2004; 89: 6297–304.

120. Devroey P, Fauser BC, Platteau P, et al. Induction of multiple follicular development by a single dose of long-acting recombinant follicle-stimulating hormone (FSH-CTP, corifollitropin alfa) for controlled ovarian stimulation before in vitro fertilization. J Clin Endocrinol Metab 2004; 89: 2062–70.

121. Corifollitropin Alfa Dose-finding Study Group. A randomized dose-response trial of a single injection of corifollitropin alfa to sustain multifollicular growth during controlled ovarian stimulation. Hum Reprod 2008; 23: 2484–92.

122. Corifollitropin alfa Ensure Study Group. Corifollitropin alfa for ovarian stimulation in IVF: a randomized trial in lower-body-weight women. Reprod Biomed Online 2010; 21: 66–76.

123. Devroey P, Boostanfar R, Koper NP, et al. A double-blind, non-inferiority RCT comparing corifollitropin alfa and recombinant FSH during the first seven days of ovarian stimulation using a GnRH antagonist protocol. Hum Reprod 2009; 24: 3063–72.

124. Norman RJ, Zegers-Hochschild F, Salle BS, et al. Repeated ovarian stimulation with corifollitropin alfa in patients in a GnRH antagonist protocol: no concern for immunogenicity. Hum Reprod 2011; 26: 2200–8.

125. Santjohanser C. Letter to the editor 'Long-acting-FSH (FSH-CTP) in reproductive medicine.' Gynakol Endocrinol 2009; 3: 183.

126. van Wely M, Kwan I, Burt AL, et al. Recombinant versus urinary gonadotrophin for ovarian stimulation in assisted reproductive technology cycles. Cochrane Database Syst Rev 2011; CD005354.

127. Al-Inany H, Aboulghar M, Mansour R, Serour G. Meta-analysis of recombinant versus urinary-derived FSH: an update. Hum Reprod 2003; 18: 305–13.

128. European and Israeli Study Group on Highly Purified Menotropin versus Recombinant Follicle-Stimulating Hormone. Efficacy and safety of highly purified menotropin versus recombinant follicle-stimulating hormone in in vitro fertilization/intracytoplasmic sperm injection cycles: a randomized, comparative trial. Fertil Steril 2002; 78: 520–8.

129. Gordon UD, Harrison RF, Fawzy M, et al. A randomized prospective assessor-blind evaluation of luteinizing hormone dosage and in vitro fertilization outcome. Fertil Steril 2001; 75: 324–31.

130. Ng EH, Lau EY, Yeung WS, Ho PC. HMG is as good as recombinant human FSH in terms of oocyte and embryo quality: a prospective randomized trial. Hum Reprod 2001; 16: 319–25.

131. Westergaard LG, Erb K, Laursen SB, et al. Human menopausal gonadotropin versus recombinant follicle-stimulating hormone in normogonadotropic women down-regulated with a gonadotropin-releasing hormone agonist who were undergoing in vitro fertilization and intracytoplasmic sperm injection: a prospective randomized study. Fertil Steril 2001; 76: 543–9.

132. van Wely M, Westergaard LG, Bossuyt PMM, van der Veen F. Effectiveness of human menopausal gonadotropin versus recombinant follicle stimulating hormone for controlled ovarian hyperstimulation in assisted reproductive cycles. A meta-analysis. Fertil Steril 2003; 80:1086–93.

133. van Wely M, Westergaard LG, Bossuyt PM, van der Veen F. Human menopausal gonadotropin versus recombinant follicle stimulation hormone for ovarian stimulation in assisted reproductive cycles. Cochrane Database Syst Rev 2003; CD003973.

134. Al-Inany H, Aboulghar MA, Mansour RT, Serour GI. Ovulation induction in the new millennium: recombinant follicle-stimulating hormone versus human menopausal gonadotropin. Gynecol Endocrinol 2005; 20: 161–9.

135. Al-Inany HG, bou-Setta AM, Aboulghar MA, et al. Efficacy and safety of human menopausal gonadotrophins versus recombinant FSH: a meta-analysis. Reprod Biomed Online 2008; 16: 81–8.

136. Coomarasamy A, Afnan M, Cheema D, et al. Urinary hMG versus recombinant FSH for controlled ovarian hyperstimulation following an agonist long down-regulation protocol in IVF or ICSI treatment: a systematic review and meta-analysis. Hum Reprod 2008; 23: 310–15.

137. Lehert P, Schertz JC, Ezcurra D. Recombinant human follicle-stimulating hormone produces more oocytes with a lower total dose per cycle in assisted reproductive technologies compared with highly purified human menopausal gonadotrophin: a meta-analysis. Reprod Biol Endocrinol 2010; 8: 112.

138. Sunkara SK, Rittenberg V, Raine-Fenning N, et al. Association between the number of eggs and live birth in IVF treatment: an analysis of 400 135 treatment cycles. Hum Reprod 2011; 26: 1768–74.

139. Nardo LG, Fleming R, Howles CM, et al. Conventional ovarian stimulation no longer exists: welcome to the age of individualized ovarian stimulation. Reprod Biomed Online 2011; 23: 141–8.

140. Olivennes F, Howles CM, Borini A, et al. Individualizing FSH dose for assisted reproduction using a novel algorithm: the CONSORT study. Reprod Biomed Online 2009; 18: 195–204.

141. Howles CM, Saunders H, Alam V, Engrand P. Predictive factors and a corresponding treatment algorithm for controlled ovarian stimulation in patients treated with recombinant human follicle stimulating hormone (follitropin alfa) during assisted reproduction technology (ART) procedures. An analysis of 1378 patients. Curr Med Res Opin 2006; 22: 907–18.

142. Klinkert ER, Broekmans FJ, Looman CW, et al. The antral follicle count is a better marker than basal follicle-stimulating hormone for the selection of older patients with acceptable pregnancy prospects after in vitro fertilization. Fertil Steril 2005; 83: 811–14.

143. Popovic-Todorovic B, Loft A, Lindhard A, et al. A prospective study of predictive factors of ovarian response in 'standard' IVF/ICSI patients treated with recombinant FSH. A suggestion for a recombinant FSH dosage normogram. Hum Reprod 2003; 18: 781–7.

144. Broer SL, Mol B, Dolleman M, et al. The role of anti-Mullerian hormone assessment in assisted reproductive technology outcome. Curr Opin Obstet Gynecol 2010; 22: 193–201.

145. Broer SL, Dolleman M, Opmeer BC, et al. AMH and AFC as predictors of excessive response in controlled ovarian hyperstimulation: a meta-analysis. Hum Reprod Update 2011; 17: 46–54.

146. Nelson SM, Yates RW, Fleming R. Serum anti-Mullerian hormone and FSH: prediction of live birth and extremes of response in stimulated cycles–implications for individualization of therapy. Hum Reprod 2007; 22: 2414–21.

147. Nelson SM, Yates RW, Lyall H, et al. Anti-Mullerian hormone-based approach to controlled ovarian stimulation for assisted conception. Hum Reprod 2009; 24: 867–75.

148. Barad DH, Weghofer A, Gleicher N. Utility of age-specific serum anti-Mullerian hormone concentrations. Reprod Biomed Online 2011; 22: 284–91.

149. Nelson SM, Messow MC, Wallace AM, et al. Nomogram for the decline in serum antimullerian hormone: a population study of 9,601 infertility patients. Fertil Steril 2011; 95: 736–41.

150. Nelson SM, Messow MC, McConnachie A, et al. External validation of nomogram for the decline in serum anti-Mullerian hormone in women: a population study of 15,834 infertility patients. Reprod Biomed Online 2011; 23: 204–6.

151. Howles CM, Alam V, Tredway D, et al. Factors related to successful ovulation induction in patients with WHO group II anovulatory infertility. Reprod Biomed Online 2010; 20: 182–90.

152. Imani B, Eijkemans MJ, Faessen GH, et al. Prediction of the individual follicle-stimulating hormone threshold for gonadotropin induction of ovulation in normogonadotropic anovulatory infertility: an approach to increase safety and efficiency. Fertil Steril 2002; 77: 83–90.

153. van Wely M, Fauser BC, Laven JS, et al. Validation of a prediction model for the follicle-stimulating hormone response dose in women with polycystic ovary syndrome. Fertil Steril 2006; 86: 1710–15.

154. Mulders AG, Laven JS, Eijkemans MJ, et al. Patient predictors for outcome of gonadotrophin ovulation induction in women with normogonadotrophic anovulatory infertility: a meta-analysis. Hum Reprod Update 2003; 9: 429–49.

155. Kobayashi M, Nakano R, Ooshima A. Immunohistochemical localization of pituitary gonadotrophins and gonadal steroids confirms the 'two-cell, two-gonadotrophin' hypothesis of steroidogenesis in the human ovary. J Endocrinol 1990; 126: 483–8.

156. European Recombinant Human LH Study Group. Recombinant human luteinizing hormone (LH) to support recombinant human follicle-stimulating hormone (FSH)-induced follicular development in LH- and FSH-deficient anovulatory women: a dose-finding study. J Clin Endocrinol Metab 1998; 83: 1507–14.

157. Bosch E. Recombinant human FSH and recombinant human LH in a 2:1 ratio combination: a new tool for ovulation induction. Expert Rev Obstet Gynecol 2009; 4: 491–8.

158. Kolibianakis EM, Kalogeropoulou L, Griesinger G, et al. Among patients treated with FSH and GnRH analogues for in vitro fertilization, is the addition of recombinant LH associated with the probability of live birth? A systematic review and meta-analysis. Hum Reprod Update 2007; 13: 445–52.

159. Mochtar MH, van der Veen F, Ziech M, van Wely M. Recombinant luteinizing hormone (rLH) for controlled ovarian hyperstimulation in assisted reproductive cycles. Cochrane Database Syst Rev 2007; CD005070.

160. Howles CM. Luteininzing hormone supplementation in ART. In: Kovacs G, ed. How to Improve Your ART Success Rates. Gab Kovacs. Published by Cambridge University Press. UK © Cambridge University Press, 2011: 99–104.

161. Bosch E, Labarta E, Simón C, et al. The impact of luteinizing hormone supplementation in gonadotropin releasing hormone antagonist cycles. An age adjusted randomized trial. Fertil Steril 2008; 90: S41.

162. Humaidan P, Bungum M, Bungum L, Yding Andersen C. Effects of recombinant LH supplementation in women undergoing assisted reproduction with GnRH agonist down-regulation and stimulation with recombinant FSH: an opening study. Reprod Biomed Online 2004; 8: 635–43.

163. Marrs R, Meldrum D, Muasher S, et al. Randomized trial to compare the effect of recombinant human FSH (follitropin alfa) with or without recombinant human LH in women undergoing assisted reproduction treatment. Reprod Biomed Online 2004; 8: 175–82.

164. Matorras R, Prieto B, Exposito A, et al. Mid-follicular LH supplementation in women aged 35–39 years undergoing ICSI cycles: a randomized controlled study. Reprod Biomed Online 2009; 19: 879–87.

165. Fabregues F, Creus M, Penarrubia J, et al. Effects of recombinant human luteinizing hormone supplementation on ovarian stimulation and the implantation rate in down-regulated women of advanced reproductive age. Fertil Steril 2006; 85: 925–31.

166. Nilsson C, Pettersson K, Millar RP, et al. Worldwide frequency of a common genetic variant of luteinizing

hormone: an international collaborative research. International Collaborative Research Group. Fertil Steril 1997; 67: 998–1004.

167. de Castro F., Moron FJ, Montoro L, et al. Human controlled ovarian hyperstimulation outcome is a polygenic trait. Pharmacogenetics 2004; 14: 285–93.

168. Simoni M, Nieschlag E, Gromoll J. Isoforms and single nucleotide polymorphisms of the FSH receptor gene: implications for human reproduction. Hum Reprod Update 2002; 8: 413–21.

169. Lisi F, Rinaldi L, Fishel S, et al. Use of recombinant FSH and recombinant LH in multiple follicular stimulation for IVF: a preliminary study. Reprod Biomed Online 2001; 3: 190–4.

170. De Placido G, Alviggi C, Mollo A, et al. Effects of recombinant LH (rLH) supplementation during controlled ovarian hyperstimulation (COH) in normogonadotrophic women with an initial inadequate response to recombinant FSH (rFSH) after pituitary downregulation. Clin Endocrinol (Oxf) 2004; 60: 637–43.

171. De Placido G, Alviggi C, Mollo A, et al. Effects of recombinant LH (rLH) supplementation during controlled ovarian hyperstimulation (COH) in normogonadotrophic women with an initial inadequate response to recombinant FSH (rFSH) after pituitary downregulation. Clin Endocrinol (Oxf) 2004; 60: 637–43.

172. Ferraretti AP, Gianaroli L, Magli MC, et al. Exogenous luteinizing hormone in controlled ovarian hyperstimulation for assisted reproduction techniques. Fertil Steril 2004; 82: 1521–6.

173. Carmel PW, Araki S, Ferin M. Pituitary stalk portal blood collection in rhesus monkeys: evidence for pulsatile release of gonadotropin-releasing hormone (GnRH). Endocrinology 1976; 99: 243–8.

174. Schally AV, Arimura A, Kastin AJ, et al. Gonadotropin-releasing hormone: one polypeptide regulates secretion of luteinizing and folliclestimulating hormones. Science 1971; 173: 1036–8.

175. Amoss M, Burgus R, Blackwell R, et al. Purifi - cation, amino acid composition and N-terminus of the hypothalamic luteinizing hormone releasing factor (LRF) of ovine origin. Biochem Biophys Res Commun 1971; 44: 205–10.

176. Backstrom CT, McNeilly AS, Leask RM, Baird DT. Pulsatile secretion of LH, FSH, prolactin, oestradiol and progesterone during the human menstrual cycle. Clin Endocrinol (Oxf) 1982; 17: 29–42.

177. Reame N, Sauder SE, Kelch RP, Marshall JC. Pulsatile gonadotropin secretion during the human menstrual cycle: evidence for altered frequency of gonadotropin-releasing hormone secretion. J Clin Endocrinol Metab 1984; 59: 328–37.

178. Belchetz PE, Plant TM, Nakai Y, et al. Hypophysial responses to continuous and intermittent delivery of hypopthalamic gonadotropin-releasing hormone. Science 1978; 202: 631–3.

179. Suarez-Quian CA, Wynn PC, Catt KJ. Receptor mediated endocytosis of GnRH analogs: differential processing of gold-labeled agonist and antagonist derivatives. J Steroid Biochem 1986; 24: 183–92.

180. Schvartz I, Hazum E. Internalization and recycling of receptor-bound gonadotropin-releasing hormone agonist in pituitary gonadotropes. J Biol Chem 1987; 262: 17046–50.

181. Karten MJ, Rivier JE. Gonadotropin-releasing hormone analog design. Structure–function studies toward the development of agonists and antagonists: rationale and perspective. Endocr Rev 1986; 7: 44–66.

182. Coy DH, Labrie F, Savary M, et al. LH-releasing activity of potent LH-RH analogs in vitro. Biochem Biophys Res Commun 1975; 67: 576–82.

183. Lemay A, Metha AE, Tolis G, et al. Gonadotropins and estradiol responses to single intranasal or subcutaneous administration of a luteinizing hormone- releasing hormone agonist in the early follicular phase. Fertil Steril 1983; 39: 668–73.

184. Fogelman I. Gonadotropin-releasing hormone agonists and the skeleton. Fertil Steril 1992; 57: 715–24.

185. Sopelak VM, Hodgen GD. Infusion of gonadotropin releasing hormone agonist during pregnancy: maternal and fetal responses in primates. Am J Obstet Gynecol 1987; 156: 755–60.

186. Brogden RN, Buckley MM, Ward A. Buserelin. A review of its pharmacodynamic and pharmacokinetic properties, and clinical profile. Drugs 1990; 39: 399–437.

187. Golan A, Ron-El R, Herman A, et al. Fetal outcome following inadvertent administration of long-acting DTRP6 GnRH microcapsules during pregnancy: a case report. Hum Reprod 1990; 5: 123–4.

188. Dicker D, Goldman JA, Vagman I, et al. Pregnancy outcome following early exposure to maternal luteinizing-hormone-releasing hormone agonist (buserelin). Hum Reprod 1989; 4: 250–1.

189. Weissman A, Shoham Z. Favourable pregnancy outcome after administration of a long-acting gonadotrophin-releasing hormone agonist in the mid-luteal phase. Hum Reprod 1993; 8: 496–7.

190. Ron-El R, Golan A, Herman A, et al. Midluteal gonadotropin-releasing hormone analog administration in early pregnancy. Fertil Steril 1990; 53: 572–4.

191. Lahat E, Raziel A, Friedler S, et al. Long-term followup of children born after inadvertent administration of a gonadotrophin-releasing hormone agonist in early pregnancy. Hum Reprod 1999; 14: 2656–60.

192. Bajusz S, Kovacs M, Gazdag M, et al. Highly potent antagonists of luteinizing hormone-releasing hormone free of edematogenic effects. Proc Natl Acad Sci USA 1988; 85: 1637–41.

193. Ljungqvist A, Feng DM, Hook W, et al. Antide and related antagonists of luteinizing hormone release with long action and oral activity. Proc Natl Acad Sci USA 1988; 85: 8236–40.

194. Rivier J, Porter J, Hoeger C, et al. Gonadotropin-releasing hormone antagonists with N omega-triazolylornithine, -lysine, or -p-aminophenylalanine residues at positions 5 and 6. J Med Chem 1992; 35: 4270–8.

195. Nestor JJ Jr, Tahilramani R, Ho TL, et al. Potent gonadotropin releasing hormone antagonists with low histamine-releasing activity. J Med Chem 1992; 35: 3942–8.

196. Garnick MB, Campion M. Abarelix depot, a GnRH antagonist, v. LHRH superagonists in prostate cancer: differential effects on follicle-stimulating hormone. Abarelix Depot Study Group. Mol Urol 2000; 4: 275–7.

197. Cook T, Sheridan WP. Development of GnRH antagonists for prostate cancer: new approaches to treatment. Oncologist 2000; 5: 162–8.

198. Deghenghi R, Boutignon F, Wuthrich P, Lenaerts V. Antarelix (EP 24332) a novel water soluble LHRH antagonist. Biomed Pharmacother 1993; 47: 107–10.

199. Felberbaum R, Diedrich K. Ovarian stimulation for in vitro fertilization/intracytoplasmic sperm injection with gonadotrophins and gonadotrophinreleasing hormone analogues: agonists and antagonists. Hum Reprod 1999; 14(Suppl 1): 207–21.

200. Bajusz S, Csernus VJ, Janaky T, et al. New antagonists of LHRH. II. Inhibition and potentiation of LHRH by closely related analogues. Int J Pept Protein Res 1988; 32: 425–35.

201. Diedrich K, Diedrich C, Santos E, et al. Suppression of the endogenous luteinizing hormone surge by the gonadotrophin-releasing hormone antagonist cetrorelix during ovarian stimulation. Hum Reprod 1994; 9: 788–91.

202. Felberbaum RE, Albano C, Ludwig M, et al. Ovarian stimulation for assisted reproduction with hMG and concomitant midcycle administration of the GnRH antagonist cetrorelix according to the multiple dose protocol: a prospective uncontrolled phase III study. Hum Reprod 2000; 15: 1015–20.

203. Borm G, Mannaerts B. Treatment with the gonadotrophin-releasing hormone antagonist ganirelix in women undergoing ovarian stimulation with recombinant follicle stimulating hormone is effective, safe and convenient: results of a controlled, randomized, multicentre trial. The European Orgalutran Study Group. Hum Reprod 2000; 15: 1490–8.

204. The European Middle East Orgalutran Study Group. Comparable clinical outcome using the GnRH antagonist ganirelix or a long protocol of the GnRH agonist triptorelin for the prevention of premature LH surges in women undergoing ovarian stimulation. Hum Reprod 2001; 16: 644–51.

205. Fluker M, Grifo J, Leader A, et al. Efficacy and safety of ganirelix acetate versus leuprolide acetate in women undergoing controlled ovarian hyperstimulation. Fertil Steril 2001; 75: 38–45.

206. Mannaerts B, Gordon K. Embryo implantation and GnRH antagonists: GnRH antagonists do not activate the GnRH receptor. Hum Reprod 2000; 15: 1882–3.

207. Demirel LC, Weiss JM, Polack S, et al. Effect of the gonadotropin-releasing hormone antagonist ganirelix on cyclic adenosine monophosphate accumulation of human granulosa–lutein cells. Fertil Steril 2000; 74: 1001–7.

208. Ortmann O, Weiss JM, Diedrich K. Embryo implantation and GnRH antagonists: ovarian actions of GnRH antagonists. Hum Reprod 2001; 16: 608–11.

209. Raga F, Casan EM, Kruessel J, et al. The role of gonadotropin-releasing hormone in murine preimplantation embryonic development. Endocrinology 1999; 140: 3705–12.

210. The Ganirelix Dose-finding Study Group. A double-blind, randomized, dose-finding study to assess the efficacy of the gonadotrophin-releasing hormone antagonist ganirelix (Org 37462) to prevent premature luteinizing hormone surges in women undergoing ovarian stimulation with recombinant follicle stimulating hormone (Puregon). Hum Reprod 1998; 13: 3023–31.

211. Rackow BW, Kliman HJ, Taylor HS. GnRH antagonists may affect endometrial receptivity. Fertil Steril 2008; 89: 1234–9.

212. Prapas N, Prapas Y, Panagiotidis Y, et al. GnRH agonist versus GnRH antagonist in oocyte donation cycles: a prospective randomized study. Hum Reprod 2005; 20: 1516–20.

213. Saucedo de la Llata E, Moraga Sanchez MR, Batiza RV, et al. Comparison of GnRH agonists and antagonists in an ovular donation program. Ginecol Obstet Mex 2004; 72: 53–6.

214. Vlahos NF, Bankowski BJ, Zacur HA, et al. An oocyte donation protocol using the GnRH antagonist ganirelix acetate, does not compromise embryo quality and is associated with high pregnancy rates. Arch Gynecol Obstet 2005; 272: 1–6.

215. Devroey P, Aboulghar M, Garcia-Velasco J, et al. Improving the patient's experience of IVF/ICSI: a proposal for an ovarian stimulation protocol with GnRH antagonist co-treatment. Hum Reprod 2009; 24: 764–74.

216. Reissmann T, Felberbaum R, Diedrich K, et al. Development and applications of luteinizing hormone-releasing hormone antagonists in the treatment of infertility: an overview. Hum Reprod 1995; 10: 1974–81.

217. Tur-Kaspa I, Ezcurra D. GnRH antagonist, cetrorelix, for pituitary suppression in modern, patient-friendly assisted reproductive technology. Expert Opin Drug Metab Toxicol 2009; 5: 1323–36.

218. Al-Inany HG, Youssef MA, Aboulghar M, et al. Gonadotrophin-releasing hormone antagonists for assisted reproductive technology. Cochrane Database Syst Rev 2011; CD001750.

219. Youssef MA, Van d V, Al-Inany HG, et al. Gonadotropin-releasing hormone agonist versus HCG for oocyte triggering in antagonist assisted reproductive technology cycles. Cochrane Database Syst Rev 2011; CD008046.

220. Griesinger G, Schultz L, Bauer T, et al. Ovarian hyperstimulation syndrome prevention by gonadotropin-releasing hormone agonist triggering of final oocyte maturation in a gonadotropin-releasing hormone antagonist protocol in combination with a "freeze-all" strategy: a prospective multicentric study. Fertil Steril 2011; 95: 2029–33; 2033.

221. Weissman A, Lurie S, Zalel Y, et al. Human chorionic gonadotropin; Pharmacokinetics of subcutaneous administration. Gynecol Endocrinol 1996; 10: 273–6.

222. Trinchard-Lugan Khan A, Porchet HC, Muñato A. Pharmacokinetics and pharmacodynamics of recombinant human chorionic gonadotropin in healthy male and female volunteers. Reprod Biomed Online 2002; 4: 106–15.

38

The role of FSH and LH in ovulation induction: Current concepts

Juan Balasch

INTRODUCTION AND OVERVIEW

The ovary has two essential physiologic responsibilities: The periodic release of oocytes and the production of the steroid hormones, estradiol, and progesterone.

Both activities are integrated into the continuous repetitive process of follicle growth and maturation, ovulation, and corpus luteum formation and regression, which constitute the so-called ovarian cycle. The ovarian cycle is under pituitary gonadotropic control: Follicle-stimulating hormone (FSH) and luteinizing hormone (LH) are synthesized and secreted by the pituitary, and together they play a central part in regulating the menstrual cycle and ovulation. Therefore, a basic knowledge of gonadotropic control of ovarian function is an essential requirement for a proper understanding of ovulation-induction techniques using exogenously administered gonadotropins. Thus, this chapter begins with a review of the role of FSH and LH in the control of follicular growth and function. This is followed by a section addressing the development of pituitary gonadotropins, from urinary products to recombinant medications, and stressing the advantages of using the biotech drugs. The three gonadotropins involved in ovulation induction [FSH, LH, and human chorionic gonadotropin (hCG)] are now commercially available and produced in vitro by recombinant DNA technology (rhFSH, rhLH, rhCG). These highly specific monohormonal products have permitted important advances in our understanding of gonadotropin action at the cellular level, and also provide us with the perspective of preparing consistent-formulation regimens for ovulation induction or tailoring therapy with FSH and LH, individually or combined, according to the individual patient's needs (1–3). On the above evidence, the third section in this chapter is devoted to contemporary strategies for ovulation induction in the anovulatory patient. The object of ovulation induction is to restore the ovulatory state and restore fertility potential but producing ideally only one ovulatory follicle. Both the most appropriate gonadotropin to use and pros and cons of different regimens of gonadotropin administration are discussed separately for World Health Organization (WHO) group II and WHO group I anovulation. The chapter concludes by providing the reader with current therapeutic modalities for inducing multiple follicular developments (the so-called controlled ovarian hyperstimulation) in the already ovulating patient undergoing treatment with assisted reproductive techniques (ART). These different goals require different approaches to how the ovaries are stimulated.

GONADOTROPIC CONTROL OF FOLLICULAR GROWTH AND FUNCTION

Although the physiologic effects of FSH and LH are intimately connected, and both gonadotropins are necessary for normal gonadal function and gamete maturation, it has recently become possible to define better the specific spectrum of both FSH and LH actions. Although it is a continuum, the life cycle of a preovulatory follicle can be broken down into three successive phases:

1. Initiation, which occurs from birth to senescence independent of gonadotropic support.
2. FSH-dependent progression, requiring tonic stimulation by FSH.
3. LH-responsive maturation, when FSH-induced genes fall under LH control, leading to final follicular maturation and ovulation (4).

This subject has been reviewed elsewhere (2–8) and is summarized here.

Follicle-Stimulating Hormone

At birth, the human ovaries contain ~2,000,000 follicles arrested at the primordial stage of development. Throughout infancy, childhood, and adolescence, continuing throughout the reproductive years, this endowment is progressively depleted as individual follicles exit the primordial pool and folliculogenesis begins. However, ~99.9% of follicles will never complete their development; instead, they default to atresia, owing to inadequate stimulation by FSH. This means that only ~400 follicles sequentially mature and ovulate during an average woman's reproductive lifetime. Theoretically, every primordial follicle has the potential to mature, secrete estrogen, and ovulate. However, until puberty, blood concentrations of FSH and LH remain too low to stimulate full preovulatory follicular development.

The follicles start to grow more rapidly in the luteal phase of the cycle preceding ovulation, but pre-antral stages of follicular growth occur independently of gonadotropic stimulation. However, antrum formation requires tonic stimulation by FSH, beginning when follicles are ~0.25 mm in diameter (the so-called gonadotropin-regulated growth phase) (Fig. 38.1). The selective rise in serum FSH beyond a critical "threshold" level that occurs during the luteal–follicular transition is a potent stimulus for follicle recruitment (Fig. 38.2), and several early antral follicles begin to enlarge in this phase of the cycle because of the mitogenic action of FSH on granulosa cells. Only one of these follicles, however, is eventually "selected" to ovulate, while the others become atretic.

Selection of the dominant follicle can be explained by development-related changes in responsiveness to FSH and LH, which occur in granulosa and theca cells modulated by ovarian para(auto)crine mechanisms. The follicle whose granulosa cells are most responsive to FSH (lowest FSH "threshold") becomes first in the cohort to secrete estrogen, which feeds back through the hypothalamo–pituitary axis and begins to suppress pituitary FSH secretion. Blood FSH, therefore, declines to a concentration insufficient to sustain the development of other follicles that have higher FSH thresholds. These latter become non-ovulatory and undergo atresia, while the dominant follicle continues to mature and secrete estrogen. It is possible that the maturing follicle reduces its dependence on FSH by acquiring LH receptors, as discussed below (3,4,8).

Luteinizing Hormone

Traditionally, the roles of LH in folliculogenesis have been considered to be limited to stimulating theca cell androgen production, triggering ovulation, and supporting the corpus luteum. However, it is now accepted that in the late stages of follicle development, granulosa cells become receptive to LH stimulation and LH becomes capable of exerting its actions on both theca cells and granulosa cells (2,4,8).

At the mid-follicular phase, the dominant follicle reaches ≥10 mm in diameter, thus being recognizable as the largest healthy follicle in either ovary, and increasingly synthesizes estradiol. LH is capable of stimulating androgen-substrate production from theca cells, to be transformed into estrogen by FSH-stimulated aromatase activity in granulosa cells (the so-called two-cell, two-gonadotropin model). In addition, a major development-related response of granulosa cells to FSH is their increased expression of LH receptors, functionally coupled to steroid synthesis. LH receptors are constitutively present on theca cells, and appear on granulosa cells that have been adequately stimulated by FSH. This development enables mature granulosa cells in the preovulatory follicle (and subsequently in the corpus luteum) to respond directly to

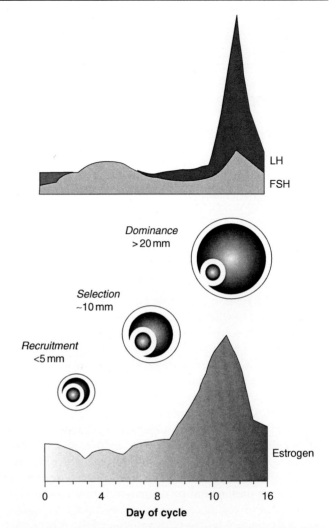

Figure 38.1   Gonadotropin-dependent stages in preovulatory follicular development. *Recruitment*: At the beginning of each menstrual cycle, plasma FSH concentrations increase sufficiently to stimulate the proliferation and functional maturation of granulosa cells in multiple immature follicles, including induction of LH receptors, aromatase activity, and inhibin biosynthesis. Tonic stimulation by LH maintains thecal androgen synthesis in these follicles. *Selection*: The next follicle that will ovulate emerges as the follicle that is most responsive to FSH (that is, has the lowest FSH "threshold"). *Dominance*: By the mid-follicular phase, the preovulatory follicle becomes recognizable as the largest healthy follicle in either ovary, containing granulosa cells that express LH receptors coupled to aromatase and inhibin synthesis. Since this follicle is uniquely responsive to both FSH and LH, it continues to grow and secrete estrogen despite decreasing plasma concentrations of FSH. Development-dependent paracrine signals (including inhibin) maintain the dominance of this follicle, amplifying its responsiveness to FSH and LH. *Abbreviations*: FSH, follicle-stimulating hormone; LH, luteinizing hormone. *Source*: From Ref. 3.

LH. Recent findings indicate that the process of preovulatory follicular development may be regulated by a single intracellular message (cyclic adenosine monophosphate, cAMP) which, in turn, is controlled in succession by two different messengers, FSH and LH (8). In fact, most of FSH's physiologic actions on granulosa cells, including stimulation of the aromatase system, can be exerted by LH once its receptors are expressed (2,4,8). As would be predicted by the common intracellular cAMP pathway,

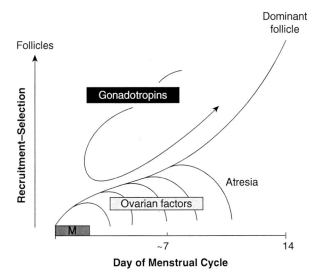

Figure38.2 Gonadotropin–ovarian interaction. Diagram of gonadotropin-mediated follicular recruitment, selection, and maturation of the dominant follicle by the rise in follicle-stimulating hormone (FSH) secretion at the beginning of the menstrual cycle. *Source*: From Ref. 9.

granulosa cells from FSH-stimulated follicles respond similarly to both FSH and LH, and, moreover, at nonsaturating levels of FSH and LH, the responses are additive (8). The overall significance of these findings is that while granulosa cells from early antral follicles are responsive only to FSH, granulosa cells from FSH-stimulated follicles are responsive to either FSH or LH (4,8). In fact, LH seems to be able to sustain preovulatory follicular endocrine activity previously induced by FSH (2,10,11), but definite in vivo evidence in the human is still lacking.

During the human menstrual cycle, LH released by the pituitary gland is also a major paracrine regulator (3,4). In fact, multiple growth/differentiation factors and sex steroids produced in response to ovarian stimulation with FSH and LH mediate short-loop feedback signaling between granulosa cells and theca during preovulatory follicular development. Ovarian paracrines include theca-derived androgens and granulosa-derived insulin-like growth factors (IGFs) and inhibins, which orchestrate preovulatory follicular estrogen secretion. Thus, there is experimental evidence that granulosa cells in immature follicles express androgen receptors, through which theca-derived androgens act to potentiate follicular responsiveness to FSH. Conversely, experimental studies have revealed that in the presence of minimal stimulation by LH, FSH is able to activate paracrine signaling (granulosa on theca signaling mediated by IGFs and inhibins), which sustains thecal androgen synthesis and thereby explains why treatment with FSH alone is capable of stimulating ovarian estrogen synthesis in many clinical situations (3,4). In spontaneous ovulatory cycles, the most responsive follicle to FSH at the beginning of the cycle is the first to produce estrogen and express granulosa-cell LH receptor. Paracrine signaling activated by FSH and LH sustains growth and estrogen secretion by the preovulatory follicle until ovulation.

In addition, both experimental and clinical evidence clearly indicates that while follicular growth may not require LH, LH plays a primary part in complete maturation of the follicle and oocyte competence (10,12–14). However, it is important to note that while LH, like FSH, is capable of dose-dependently stimulating steroid synthesis, with respect to granulosa cell proliferation, LH, unlike FSH, is inhibitory at high doses. This may provide a basis for interpreting some "antifolliculogenic" effects of inappropriately high concentrations of LH, which are discussed below.

Finally, when the mid-cycle LH surge occurs, LH follicle interactions disrupt granulosa cell contacts in the cumulus oophorus and induce oocyte maturation (meiosis), cause follicular rupture, and induce granulosa cell luteinization (7). Until now, no pharmaceutically pure human LH preparation has been commercially available; thus, hCG has been used for years in infertility treatment protocols as a surrogate for LH to stimulate ovulation. hCG acts on the ovary through a LH/CG receptor, exerting a luteinizing effect that is more prolonged than that of LH because of its longer half-life (15). This may have important implications with respect to the risk of developing ovarian hyperstimulation syndrome (OHSS), as discussed below.

The Window for LH: The "Threshold" Dose and "Ceiling" Value Concepts

There is basic, experimental, and clinical evidence unequivocally indicating that ovarian follicles have development-related requirements for stimulation by LH: That is, there is a "threshold" for LH requirements during folliculogenesis (2,4,16,17). The amount of LH activity actually necessary for normal follicle and oocyte development, however, is not known, but is likely to be very low, since less than 1% of follicular LH receptors need to be occupied to elicit a maximal steroidogenic response, and, accordingly, resting levels of LH (1–10 IU/l) should be sufficient to provide maximal stimulation to theca cells (18). Defining this threshold in clinical practice became possible when both rhFSH and rhLH were available as two separate preparations. Thus, two multicenter studies conducted in patients with hypogonadotropic hypogonadism (the ideal models for investigating gonadotropin actions on ovarian steroidogenesis and follicular development) confirmed the pivotal role of LH in normal follicular function, and established that a daily dose of 75 IU rhLH is sufficient for promoting optimal follicular development in most patients, as measured by estradiol secretion and the ability to luteinize when exposed to hCG (19,20). Remarkably, the dose-finding European multicenter study (19) showed that those patients who received the highest dose (225 IU/day) of rhLH developed a smaller number of growing follicles than those who received 75 IU rhLH/day, which may reflect an LH "ceiling" effect as discussed next.

Although LH is essential for estrogen synthesis and maintenance of follicular dominance, there is clinical evidence that excessive stimulation of the ovaries by LH adversely affects normal preovulatory development. Depending on the stage of development, follicles exposed to inappropriately high concentrations of LH enter atresia or become prematurely luteinized, and oocyte development may be compromised (2,18,21,22). Thus, developing follicles appear to have finite requirements for stimulation by LH, beyond which normal development ceases. Whereas each follicle has a threshold beyond which it must be stimulated by FSH to initiate preovulatory development, it may also have a "ceiling" within which it should be stimulated by LH, unless further normal development is terminated (Table 38.1) (2,23). The LH "ceiling" hypothesis is further supported by two well-known clinical conditions that may be associated with reproductive failure: Ovulation induction with clomiphene citrate in the anovulatory patient, and the use of the short protocol with gonadotropin-releasing hormone (GnRH) agonists in in vitro fertilization (IVF) (16). Clomiphene is used in WHO group II anovulatory patients [mainly polycystic ovary syndrome (PCOS)]. The main mode of action of clomiphene is to boost FSH in the early- to mid-follicular phase but, unfortunately, it also raises LH levels at this apparently critical stage and, mainly for those patients who already have a high baseline level, the additional discharge of LH may prejudice their chances to conceive. Both the lack of conception in the face of an apparent ovulatory pattern and an increased risk of miscarriage have been reported with clomiphene citrate. Inappropriate LH action interfering with follicular and oocyte maturation would explain these adverse reproductive effects (24). Similarly, exposure of the developing follicle to inappropriately high levels of LH with the flare-up protocol in assisted reproduction may adversely affect the reproductive process in the form of lower pregnancy rates and increased early pregnancy losses (25). Finally, it is noteworthy that a study in profoundly downregulated young oocyte donors showed that the inclusion of exogenous LH activity [in the form of 1 ampoule/day human menopausal gonadotropin (hMG) from stimulation day 5] in the ovarian stimulation protocol with rhFSH can have beneficial or detrimental effects on oocyte yield and quality, depending on the level of endogenous LH, thus supporting the concept of a "window" for LH requirement in ovarian stimulation (26).

In summary, current concepts of gonadotropic control of ovarian function and clinical evidence have established that both a "threshold" and a "ceiling" for LH levels (framing the so-called LH "window") exist during the follicular phase of menstrual and induced cycles. Therefore, levels of LH should be neither too high nor too low during ovulation induction (27). During the second half of the follicular phase, as plasma FSH concentrations decline, the LH-dependent phase of preovulatory follicular development proceeds normally only if LH is present at concentrations over the threshold level and beneath the ceiling value. When the ceiling is exceeded at the mid-cycle surge of LH, further division of granulosa cells ceases as luteinization proceeds (Fig. 38.3).

Clinical Implications

According to the above evidence, follicular responsiveness to FSH and LH is developmentally regulated. FSH plays a crucial part in recruitment, selection, and dominance, while LH contributes to dominance, final maturation, and ovulation. On the basis of physiology, now that pharmaceutically "pure" rhFSH and rhLH are available,

---

Table 38.1   The LH "Ceiling" Hypothesis (23)

- Ovarian follicles have development-related requirements for stimulation by LH.
- LH, beyond a certain "ceiling" level, suppresses granulosa proliferation, and initiates atresia (immature follicles) or premature luteinization (preovulatory follicles).
- Mature follicles are more resistant (higher "ceiling") to LH than immature ones.
- During ovulation induction, LH dose should not exceed the "ceiling" of the most mature follicles.

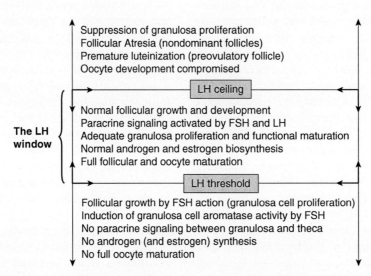

Figure 38.3   Diagram illustrating the "luteinizing hormone (LH) window" concept. *Abbreviation*: FSH, follicle-stimulating hormone. *Source*: Modified from Ref. 16.

it is possible to develop improved clinical strategies for stimulating ovarian function.

Those who stand to benefit are women receiving treatment for ovulatory dysfunction and those with normal ovarian function undergoing ART. The therapeutic aim in each group, however, is quite different. In the former, it is desirable to stimulate mono-ovulation with a view to conception occurring in vivo. In the latter, the aim is to stimulate multiple follicular development. The challenge is to tailor therapy with FSH and LH, alone or in combination, according to the outcome desired, based on the principles summarized here and the available gonadotropin preparations. This is discussed below.

DEVELOPMENTS IN GONADOTROPIN PREPARATIONS: FROM URINARY PRODUCTS TO RECOMBINANT GONADOTROPINS

Pharmaceutical preparations containing biologically active gonadotropins for ovulation induction have been in use for about 75 years. As previously reviewed (28), major advances in technology have brought the field of gonadotropin therapy a very long way since the era of animal-, human pituitary–, and urinary-derived hormones. For years, hMG has been the only urinary gonadotropin available for clinical use. The FSH and LH content of hMG is theoretically equal (75 IU of FSH and 75 IU of LH), albeit with different FSH/LH ratios. In addition, hMG has a low specific activity and is of <4% purity, as only ~3–4% of the protein content is gonadotropin. Over the past 20 years, urinary FSH-only preparations became new therapeutic options for ovulation induction. In the mid-1980s, urinary "purified" FSH (pFSH) (with <1% LH contamination but still having 95% protein impurity) was developed, which was followed by the availability of highly purified FSH (FSH-HP) in 1993. FSH-HP contained <0.1% LH contamination, and was the first highly pure biologic extract (~4% impurity), and, as a result of this, could be injected subcutaneously (SC), unlike the earlier preparations that had to be administered intramuscularly (IM). Biochemical analysis of a new formulation of hMG described as highly purified indicated that the hMG preparation contains a mixture of FSH, LH (0.85 IU/vial), and human chorionic gonadotropin (hCG; 11.3 IU/vial), together with other urinary proteins. Specific FSH activity was about 2000 IU/mg for the new hMG, compared with 8000 IU/mg of FSH-HP. The purity of the new hMG was estimated from high-performance liquid chromatography at 50–60% in terms of area percentage, compared with values of 99% for FSH-HP (29).

Recombinant human FSH (rhFSH), which is completely devoid of both LH activity and nonspecific urinary proteins, represents the final transition to a true drug, where the starting material and complete manufacture are under rigorous control (30). Two rhFSH preparations have been registered as follitropin α, which was marketed first in 1995 (Gonal-F; Merck-Serono International, Geneva, Switzerland), and follitropin β (Puregon; Merck Sharp & Dohme Corp., Whitehouse Station, New Jersey, USA). Both follitropins are structurally identical to native FSH, and each comprises the α and β subunits that compose this gonadotropin; the nomenclature for these recombinant products does not refer to those subunits, but is merely a means of distinguishing chronologically one from another (30). Recombinant DNA technologies have been used to develop longer-acting therapeutic proteins. One approach is to introduce sequences containing additional glycosylation sites. Using this technique, a new chimeric gene has been developed containing the coding sequences of the FSH β-subunit and the C-terminal peptide of the hCG β-subunit, which bears four O-linked oligosaccharide binding sites. Co-expression of the α-subunit and the chimeric FSH β-subunit produces a new recombinant molecule, named corifollitropin alfa (Elonva; Merck Sharp & Dohme Corp.) with a prolonged elimination half-life and enhanced in vivo bioactivity compared with wild-type FSH (31). Initial studies in pituitary suppressed female volunteers confirmed the extended half-life of the compound. Phase II studies have shown that corifollitropin alfa is able to induce and sustain multifollicular growth for an entire week in women undergoing ovarian stimulation using GnRH antagonist co-treatment for IVF. Corifollitropin alfa regimens have been developed with dosages of 100 mg and 150 mg, for patients with body weight ≤60 kg and >60 kg, respectively (31).

Like rhFSH, recombinant human LH (rhLH) (Luveris; Merck-Serono International) and recombinant hCG (rhCG) (Ovitrelle and Ovidrel; Merck-Serono International) are produced under the most stringent manufacturing conditions, and have been assessed successfully for clinical use (5,6,32–34). rhFSH and rhLH have been recently combined in a single product [Pergoveris (follitropin alfa/lutropin alfa 150 IU/75 IU); Merck-Serono International], thereby allowing administration of both gonadotropins in a convenient single injection at a 2:1 ratio. Follitropin alfa/lutropin alfa 150 IU/75 IU is indicated to induce ovulation in patients with hypogonadotropic hypogonadism. The fixed combination of follitropin alfa and lutropin alfa provides an equivalent activity to the same dose administered as a separate injection with the additional patient benefit of simplified treatment and a lower number of injections (35,36). Pergoveris may be also useful to induce multiple follicular development in IVF patients needing LH supplementation in rhFSH treated cycles (36).

The three gonadotropins now produced in vitro by recombinant DNA technology share several advantages over urinary products (28,30,33,37,38).

1. A fully controlled production process from bulk to finished product, a fact to be considered taking into account a recent report showing that there is transmission of prion infectivity from scrapie-infected mice with lymphocytic nephritis, and thus urine may provide a vector for prion transmission (39). Especially in the current era of "prion scare," this may be an important argument in favor of biotech substitutes (40).

2. Full traceability from the starting material (cell line) to the final product. "Traceability" means that for every manufactured batch of gonadotropin it is possible to identify the source. However, as far as urine collection goes, being able to record exactly which donor contributed to the pool of material used to produce the batch is impossible. This is noteworthy considering that there is a continuing and growing difficulty in maintaining control on the sourcing of large volumes of urine needed to supply commercial demands (28) and a consensus statement from an international panel of experts recommended that the urine should be sourced from donors not at risk from human transmissible spongiform encephalopathies (41). Along this line of action, national regulatory/health authorities from different countries encouraged the replacement of urinary-derived gonadotropins of human origin with recombinant products, advised that human plasma or urine used in the production of medicines should not be sourced from any country with one or more indigenous cases of human transmissible spongiform encephalopathies, outlined new labeling requirements for products derived from human urine (the labels are to state that risk of transmission of infective agents of known or unknown nature cannot be definitively excluded when administered products are derived from human urine), and required full traceability for urinary derived products. As an example, in 2002, an endogenous case of variant Creutzfeldt–Jakob disease was confirmed in Sicily (Italy), and as urine was sourced from this country for production of urinary FSH-HP, the product was withdrawn from the UK market as a precautionary measure (42).

3. High purity and specific activity, as reported above.

4. Unlimited supply with batch-to-batch consistency. This is important considering the current increasing demand for exogenous gonadotropins, which requires a big availability of raw material and the fact that an ampoule of urinary FSH labeled to contain 75 IU may range in true activity from 50 to 120 IU FSH (43). In addition, consistency in the biopotency of the preparation becomes important not to overstep the thin red line between mono- and multifollicular development, especially where small incremental dose rises are concerned (44) as discussed below.

5. Complete absence of contamination by the other gonadotropins (i.e., they are absolutely monohormonal products).

This leads to a circumvention of adverse immune reactions owing to contaminant urinary proteins, the possibility of s.c. self-administration with ready-to-use pen devices, ensuring patients an accurate and correct dose while facilitating treatment individualization, and prevention of variability in ovarian response to gonadotropin administration observed cycle-to-cycle in the same patient. Interestingly, a new filled-by-mass manufacturing process for follitropin α resulted in an even more consistent ovarian response, less need for dose adjustments, and fewer cancelled cycles (45–49).

At present, rhFSH, rhLH, and rhCG are commercially available and they offer risk reduction for patients as well as the assurance of superior quality control over the final product (28). In the clinical setting, these recombinant gonadotropins have proved to be, at least equal, or even more efficacious and/or efficient than their urinary counterparts, and thus they should be considered as the gold standard of today for ovarian stimulation (28,42). In fact, it has been claimed that unit for unit, rhFSH is more potent than urinary FSH (44). Remarkably, the first biotech drugs substitutes, which were introduced in the 1980s, namely recombinant insulin and recombinant growth hormone, have never really needed to show superiority compared with the previously used products they were replacing and the debate was not whether recombinant insulin was better than animal insulin, but whether it was not worse. Similarly, there has been a drive to use synthetic recombinant clotting factors in preference to plasma-derived products (40).

OVULATION INDUCTION IN THE ANOVULATORY PATIENT

Ovulatory disturbances are present in about 15–25% of couples presenting for an infertility evaluation (50–52). Most infertile anovulatory patients fall into the WHO group II (normogonadotropic anovulation) category, and the great majority of these women are diagnosed as having PCOS (51–53). These women are well estrogenized and have normal FSH levels, but LH may be elevated. In contrast, WHO group I anovulation or hypogonadotropic hypogonadism (HH) is a much less frequent condition, characterized by reduced hypothalamic or pituitary activity and resulting in abnormally low serum concentrations of FSH and LH and negligible estrogen activity. It can be caused by a number of abnormalities of endogenous hypothalamic GnRH secretion, all of which are incompatible with normal folliculogenesis and subsequent ovulation (52,54). Both groups of patients have different gonadotropin requirements for ovulation induction and are discussed separately.

The most important principle in ovulation induction is to provide as close as possible physiologic restoration of cyclic ovarian function. In particular, the aim should be to achieve the ovulation of a single follicle. Multiple follicular development is a complication which is characteristic of ovulation induction with exogenous gonadotropins, particularly in women having PCOS who are very sensitive to gonadotropin stimulation (55). Excessive follicular development (>35–40 follicles), usually associated with very high estradiol levels (>4000–5000 pg/ml), may lead to two important iatrogenic complications: OHSS and multifetal pregnancy. OHSS is a potentially lethal condition, the pathophysiologic hallmark of which is marked hemodynamic derangement caused by peripheral arterial vasodilatation and vascular leakage of fluid from the intravascular space into the peritoneum, causing ascites and hemoconcentration (56,57). Multifetal pregnancies are associated with considerable maternal–fetal morbidity and mortality, and, according to some studies, as many as 75% of iatrogenic multifetal pregnancies are due to ovulation induction in anovulatory women, whereas only the remaining 25% are the product of ART (58–62).

Induction of Ovulation in PCOS Patients (Who Group II Anovulation)

Which Gonadotropin to Use?

Elevated serum LH and disturbed intraovarian regulation of FSH action are endocrine features in PCOS (63,64) and early studies both in vitro (65) and in vivo (66) provided evidence that the self-perpetuating state of biochemical imbalance so characteristic of PCOS could be interrupted in a physiologic way when FSH is administered in a chronic low dose. Thus, although hMG and FSH preparations have both been used successfully for ovulation induction in PCOS (67), it is accepted that when endogenous LH is already elevated (for example in PCOS), FSH alone is conceptually better (2,5,64).

Elevated LH concentrations may directly or indirectly hasten late follicular phase meiotic maturation, and abnormal oocyte maturation may be responsible for the reduced fertility and increased miscarriage rates frequently encountered in women with PCOS (7,68,69). This notwithstanding, it has been questioned whether this can be applied to ovulation induction with gonadotropins on the basis that the administration of hMG to patients with PCOS who are not receiving GnRH agonist does not result in significant increases in serum LH concentrations (70–72). It is postulated that, during ovulation induction, gonadotropin-stimulated estrogens and inhibins feed back on the hypothalamic–pituitary axis and reduce endogenous gonadotropin secretion, and thus daily LH serum levels remain low (7). However, in those previous studies investigating LH levels during ovulation induction with hMG in PCOS patients, serum LH concentrations were judged by daily single blood samples. Owing to the pulsatile mode of LH secretion, no single blood sample can be used reliably to evaluate gonadotropin pathophysiology (73). This is because the 95% confidence limits of a single blood sample taken to measure LH range from 50% to 150% of the measured value (74). In addition, endogenous LH and exogenously administered LH (either urinary or recombinant) have a short terminal half-life of around 10–11 hours (75). Thus, it is not surprising that several studies have reported normal serum LH but abnormal urinary LH, and emphasized that early morning urinary measurements are more informative than those in serum because they reflect nocturnal LH secretion (76,77). Also, that fact may explain normal LH levels during exogenous LH administration, because blood sampling is performed after the hormone has been cleared from the serum. On the above evidence, we carried out a pharmacokinetic and endocrine comparison of rhFSH and hMG in PCOS patients, including LH measurements, in eight-hour urine samples reflecting overnight renal urine secretion (78). We found that a peak in LH serum levels was observed four hours after a single IM injection of 225 IU hMG, LH returning to basal values 10–11 hours later. Remarkably, in such patients receiving ovulation induction according to a low-dose step-up protocol with either rhFSH or hMG, we found that LH levels in urine were significantly higher in the hMG group (78).

Finally, two Cochrane reviews on clinical trials investigating gonadotropin therapy for ovulation induction in women with clomiphene-resistant PCOS concluded that no significant benefit could be demonstrated from urinary FSH versus hMG in terms of pregnancy rate, but a significant reduction in OHSS associated with FSH was observed (79,80). According to experimental data, this could be explained by the reciprocal paracrine signaling between LH-stimulated theca cells and FSH-stimulated granulosa cells, which could bring about follicular hypersensitivity to FSH (81).

As discussed above, hypersecretion of LH is one of the endocrine phenomena usually associated with PCOS. Thus, in principle, administration of exogenous LH for ovulation induction in these patients is not warranted. However, a new strategy for clinical research has been devised, which, on the basis of the "LH ceiling" hypothesis discussed above, explores the effect of exogenous administration of high doses of LH during ovarian stimulation in patients with PCOS having hypersensitive ovaries (17,82). The ultimate therapeutic goal in this line of research was to try and minimize the preovulatory follicles to reduce multiple pregnancy rates. A prospective, randomized, double-blind, multicenter, dose-finding study was carried out to evaluate the effects of four different doses of rhLH (6.8, 13.6, 30, or 60 µg daily for a maximum of seven days) administered in the late follicular phase in WHO group II anovulatory women overresponding to FSH treatment. It was concluded that doses of up to 30 µg rhLH/day appear to increase the proportion of patients developing a single dominant follicle, thus providing further support to the LH ceiling concept discussed above (83). Therefore, this study suggests the clinical efficacy of high-dose rhLH for inducing atresia of secondary follicles and promoting mono-ovulation in WHO group II anovulatory women.

Which Regimen of Gonadotropin Administration?

Gonadotropin induction of ovulation has been traditionally performed since the early 1970s by using hMG in the individualized conventional step-up dose regimen. This is characterized by initial daily doses of two ampoules of hMG (~150 IU of bioactive FSH), which is increased by ≥50% every 3–5 days until an ovarian response occurs. This treatment modality is effective, but the complication rate is relatively high (Table 38.2). On the other hand, the use of hMG containing fixed proportions of FSH and LH to stimulate ovarian function ignores the fact that follicular responsiveness to FSH and LH varies characteristically with preovulatory development, as discussed above (10,11). Thus, the need to reevaluate the use of gonadotropins became imperative once "LH-free" forms of urinary FSH became available, and led to the

Table 38.2   Results of Conventional Step-Up Protocol (Starting Dose Two Ampoules Human Menopausal Gonadotropin [hMG]/Day) for Gonadotropin Ovulation Induction in World Health Organization (WHO) Group II Infertile Patients

No of Patients	1047
No of cycles	>2500
Ovulatory cycles (%)	62–98
Conceptions (per ovulatory cycle) (%)	10–20
Multiple pregnancy rate (%)	15–36
Abortion rate (%)	24–42
Hyperstimulation rate (%)	1.1–14

Summary of six series.
Source: Adapted from Ref. 63.

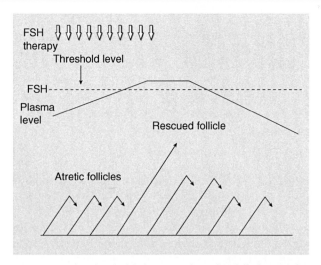

Figure 38.4   The threshold theory. When the follicle-stimulating hormone (FSH) level is above threshold, a follicle will be "rescued" (continue to growth).

implementation of low-dose treatment programs, which have been used in step-up, step-down, and sequential regimens (84).

Gonadotropins have a narrow therapeutic range: The difference between the dose that achieves adequate follicular growth and the dose that causes hyperstimulation is small, particularly in women with estrogenicity and anovulation (i.e., PCOS patients) (85). Thus, the three low-dose regimens proposed for treatment in WHO group II anovulation are focused to fulfill the two essential requirements for successful ovulation induction in PCOS patients: To allow FSH to rise slowly to just above the FSH threshold level (which is increased in PCOS patients – as evidenced by normal endogenous FSH concentrations – but has great inter-individual variability), while avoiding an "explosive" ovarian response because of the exquisite sensitivity of polycystic ovaries to exogenous gonadotropins (Fig. 38.4).

The chronic *low-dose step-up regimen* for gonadotropin induction of ovulation has been the preferred method of ovarian stimulation in PCOS patients since 1990 (55,63,67). This regimen is based on the threshold concept suggested by Brown et al. (86,87) and amplified by Zeleznik (88),which argues that the development of multiple follicles results from the failure to reproduce the precise dosage requirements that are normally maintained by feedback regulation. These authors established that initiation of follicular growth requires only a 10–30% increment in the dose of exogenous FSH, and thus advocated small, stepwise increments of FSH at five-day intervals. In practice, however, the results of this approach were complicated by an overstimulation rate of 3% and a 26% rate of multiple pregnancies (87). The failure to achieve a high proportion of uniovulatory cycles has been related to both too high a starting dose and too short a time before increasing the dose (89).

At present, this step-up approach is characterized by a low initial daily FSH dose, usually 75 IU, and the dose is increased gradually by small amounts (37.5 IU/day) until a dominant follicle emerges on ultrasound monitoring. According to the clinical features of the patient and history of multiple follicles developed within the first treatment week on 75 IU/day or OHSS in previous treatment

cycles, the starting dose may be lower (half to two-thirds ampoule per day). A feature of this regimen is that the first increase in the daily dose is performed only after 14 days of therapy if there is no evidence of an ovarian response on ultrasound (Fig. 38.5). Early large series of PCOS patients treated with this protocol have shown that this treatment modality is characterized by low complication rates while maintaining fair pregnancy rates (Table 38.3) (67,90–92). Also, two comparative prospective studies of the conventional regimen, with the chronic low-dose step-up protocol using urinary FSH (93) or rhFSH (94) for ovulation induction in PCOS patients, showed that the low-dose approach eliminated complications of OHSS and multiple pregnancies without jeopardizing the incidence of pregnancy. A review of results of published series of low (75 IU) starting-dose FSH therapy for women with PCOS, including 1391 cycles completed in 717 patients, indicates that mono-ovulatory cycles are observed consistently in approximately 70% of cases, pregnancy rates of 20% per cycle and 40% per woman are achieved, the incidence of OHSS is very low (0.14%), and the multiple pregnancy rate is only 6% (consisting of twins in 88% of cases) (95). The safety and effectiveness of chronic low-dose FSH administration for ovulation induction is further supported by a review of studies using this approach in intrauterine insemination (IUI) cycles and including 681 pregnancies among 6670 IUI cycles initiated and reporting a satisfactory pregnancy rate per initiated cycle (10%), with a mean rate of high-order multiple pregnancy of 0.3% (being 0% in most of the studies included) (96). Finally, a combined analysis of data from two clinical studies including 446 patients receiving rhFSH in a chronic low-dose (75 IU starting dose), step-up protocol, investigated factors related to successful ovulation induction in patients with WHO group II anovulatory infertility. It was concluded that low BMI, lower AFC, and higher (although still within the normal range) FSH concentration, at baseline, were associated with successful ovulation induction in normogonadotropic, oligo-, or anovulatory women undergoing a

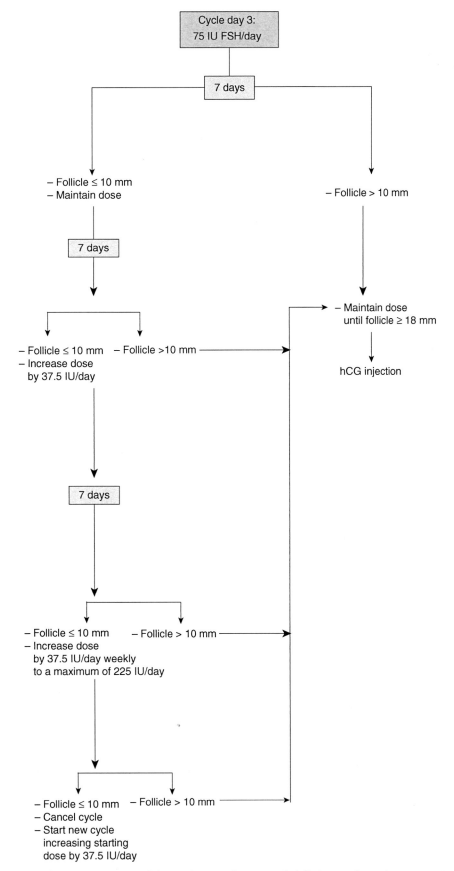

Figure 38.5   The chronic low-dose step-up protocol for ovulation induction with follicle-stimulating hormone (FSH) in polycystic ovarian syndrome (PCOS) patients. *Abbreviation*: HCG, human chorionic gonadotropin; IU, international unit.

Table 38.3 Results of Low-Dose Regimens for Gonadotropin Ovulation Induction in World Health Organization (WHO) Group II Infertile Women in Four Large Series

Parameter	Balen et al. (1994) (90)	White et al. (1996) (67)	Balasch et al. (1996) (91)	van Santbrink et al. (1995) (92)
Low-dose regimen	Step-up	Step-up	Step-up	Step-down
No of patients	103	225	234	82
No of cycles	603	934	534	234
Ovulatory cycles (%)	68	72	78	91
Cycle fecundity (per started cycle) (%)	14	11	17	16
Multiple pregnancy rate (%)	18	6	15	12
Abortion rate (%)	16	28	11	19
Severe OHSS	0.5	0	0	0

Abbreviation: OHSS, ovarian hyperstimulation syndrome.

chronic low-dose, step-up, follitropin alfa stimulation protocol (Howles et al., 2010) (97).

The *step-down protocol* applies decremental doses of gonadotropins once ovarian response is established, but the starting dose is higher than in the step-up approach (Fig. 38.6). The aim is to approximate physiologic circumstances mimicking the natural intercycle FSH elevation and the subsequent decreasing dependence of the dominant follicle with respect to FSH (63). According to this "threshold/window" concept, the duration, rather than the magnitude, of FSH increase affects follicle development (98). Monitoring of follicular growth is, however, more stringent than with the step-up approach. In addition, the long half-life of currently available FSH preparations makes it difficult to judge the correct reduction of dose to maintain follicle growth without risk of hyperstimulation (55). Notwithstanding the above, results from a pioneering team suggest that the step-down protocol is an effective approach for FSH administration in PCOS patients (92,99). However, difficult reproducibility of this approach in daily clinical practice may be a problem as suggested by a randomized multicenter study comparing the step-up versus step-down protocol in PCOS and concluding that the step-up protocol is more efficient in obtaining a monofollicular development and ovulation than the step-down protocol. In addition, it was found that although the duration of stimulation is longer, the rate of ovarian hyperstimulation is much lower using the step-up protocol (100).

An alternative method for ovulation induction with FSH in PCOS patients is the so-called sequential protocol, which combines an initial step-up gonadotropin administration followed by a step-down regimen after follicular selection (leading follicle ≥14 mm). In an early comparative study with a low-dose step-up regimen where the incremental dose increase was performed after seven days of treatment, both approaches were shown to be safe and effective (101). However, a large prospective multicenter study comparing the standard chronic low-dose step-up protocol versus the sequential approach showed that the chronic low-dose step-up regimen for rhFSH

administration is efficacious and safe for promoting monofollicular ovulation in women with WHO group II anovulation. In addition, this study confirmed that maintaining the same starting rhFSH dose (75 IU/day) for 14 days before increasing the dose in the step-up regimen is critical to adequately controlling the risk of over-response. During this interval, most women (>90%) will respond to a dose of 75 IU (102). Remarkably, rhFSH has proved to be effective and safe for ovulation induction in PCOS patients with a history of severe OHSS (103).

In summary, according to the current evidence, the strict adherence to the principle of the classic chronic low-dose step-up regimen, which is to employ a 75-IU FSH starting dose for 14 days and then use small incremental dose rises (37.5 IU) when necessary, at intervals of not less than seven days, until follicular development is initiated, should be the standard approach to be used for ovulation induction in patients with WHO group II anovulation.

Although rhFSH has been a major advance with respect to recombinant gonadotropins for the induction of ovulation in anovulatory infertility associated with PCOS, rhCG has also been successfully used in such a condition to trigger ovulation (when used instead of urinary hCG). The dose of 250 μg of rhCG provides the optimal dose for final follicular maturation in treatment cycles for timed intercourse or IUI, and this recombinant gonadotropin is better tolerated, as adverse reactions at the injection site are more likely to occur after treatment with the urinary hCG (104,105). hCG may also be used to support the luteal phase after ovulation induction. Although this is a controversial topic in PCOS patients (67,91,93),we are in favor of using repetitive hCG supplementation during the luteal phase (whenever no risk of OHSS exists), because it has been suggested that this may decrease pregnancy loss (106). In a large multicenter study (91), we found a 10% rate of spontaneous miscarriage, which contrasts sharply with spontaneous abortion rates >25–30% reported by others (67,93). New trends of ovulation induction include, according to some authors, more emphasis on maximizing efficacy of follicle maturing

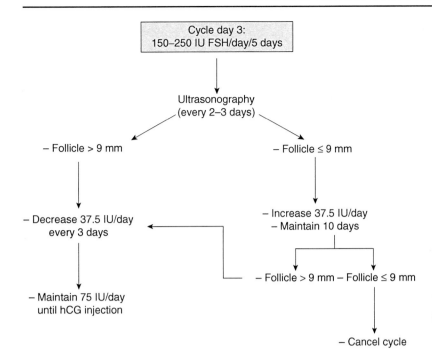

Figure 38.6 The step-down protocol for ovulation induction with follicle-stimulating hormone (FSH) in polycystic ovarian syndrome (PCOS) patients according to van Santbrink et al. (92). *Abbreviation*: hCG, human chorionic gonadotropin.

drugs, e.g., luteal phase support with progesterone, and carefully striving to find techniques to avoid over stimulation (107).

Ovulation Induction in Hypogonadotropic Hypogonadism (WHO Group I Anovulation)

In the HH woman having intact pituitary function, pulsatile GnRH therapy can be used to restore physiologically the periodic release of FSH and LH, resulting in ovulation and pregnancy rates of 75% and 18%, respectively (108). The alternative therapeutic option is gonadotropin treatment, and no definite consensus exists with respect to which of the two regimens is the more optimal, considering costs, drug availability, chances of ovulation and conception, risks and complications, patient's comfort, and physician's preferences (109–112).

Which Gonadotropin to Use?

The treatment of profoundly hypogonadotropic women with urinary FSH or rhFSH alone induces multiple follicle development but is associated with ovarian endocrine abnormalities and low oocyte fertilization rates (13,14,113–116). These findings, which are in agreement with the above-discussed current concepts on gonadotropic control of folliculogenesis, indicate that, in spite of apparently normal follicular development induced by FSH, some exogenous LH is required to optimize ovulation induction in terms of both drug requirements and clinical results. rhLH thus appears to be an ideal adjunct therapy to rhFSH in HH women. Until recently, hMG was the only source of exogenous LH for this group of anovulatory women. Over the past 10–15 years, however, a number of case reports and studies have suggested that

rhLH is effective and safe when administered in association with rhFSH in WHO group I anovulatory patients (13,19,20,117–119). The use of rhLH as a separate therapeutic agent allows the clinician to tailor the dose to stay below the "LH ceiling" discussed above (2,23,112).

Once the efficacy and safety of the combination of rhFSH and rhLH for ovulation induction in HH women were proved, the next step was to determine the minimal effective dose of rhLH for supporting rhFSH-induced follicular development in these LH- and FSH-deficient anovulatory patients. This was done in a multicenter dose-finding study, where patients were randomized to receive rhLH (0, 25, 75, or 225 IU/day) in addition to a fixed dose of rhFSH (150 IU/day) (19). The study concluded that rhLH was found to:

1. Promote dose-related increases in estradiol and androstenedione secretion by rhFSH-induced follicles.
2. Increase ovarian sensitivity to FSH, as demonstrated by the proportion of patients who developed follicles after the administration of a fixed dose of rhFSH.
3. Enhance the ability of these follicles to luteinize when exposed to hCG.

In the study (19) it was shown that a daily dose of 75 IU rhLH was effective in most women in promoting optimal follicular development, but a minority of patients may require up to 225 IU/day. Therefore, this pioneering study confirmed that there is individual variation in the dose of rhLH required to promote optimal follicular development. Furthermore, it was found that increasing exposure to LH during the follicular phase reduces the number of growing follicles, which might reflect an LH ceiling effect as discussed above (19).

Another multicenter study (20) confirmed that combined rhFSH and rhLH treatment induces follicular growth, ovulation, and pregnancy in a good proportion of hypogonadotropic anovulatory patients and is well tolerated. The doses of 150 IU rhFSH and 75 IU rhLH daily were found to be the most appropriate, but in some patients, doses >75 IU rhLH/day were necessary. Interestingly, this study clearly suggested that hypogonadotropic patients having very low levels of endogenous LH (<1 IU/l, i.e., below the threshold for normal estradiol biosynthesis and full follicular maturation) would need higher doses of gonadotropins, compared with women having basal LH levels of at least 1 IU/l, to reach the criteria necessary for hCG administration (20). In fact, there was individual variation in the dose of both LH and FSH necessary to induce ovulation depending on basal LH level (20), thus emphasizing the importance of administering FSH and LH separately, at least in some women.

Therefore, both studies (19,20) confirmed that there is individual variation in the dose of LH (and also FSH) required to promote optimal (mono)follicular development. The use of hMG containing fixed proportions of FSH and LH for ovulation induction in HH women has been linked to a high prevalence of multiple folliculogenesis, which is considered a major drawback to its use (108,110). Further refinement of the dosing schedule of both FSH and LH to minimize the likelihood of multiple ovulation occurring in these patients is now possible, with the availability of monotherapeutic recombinant gonadotropic agents (1,120). Thus, enhancing the LH environment would provide a means of inducing atresia in secondary follicles and promoting growth of a minimal number of preovulatory follicles ("LH ceiling concept"). In fact, a pilot study on the subject involved patients with HH who were treated with increasing doses (every seven days) of rhFSH (starting dose of 112.5 IU/day), according to patients' ovarian response, along with a fixed dose of 225 IU/day of rhLH. When at least one follicle reached a diameter of 10–13 mm, the patients were randomized to three different groups: The first group continued treatment with both drugs; the second group continued rhLH and received a placebo substitute for rhFSH; and the third group continued rhFSH and received a placebo substitute for rhLH. When one follicle reached 18 mm in mean diameter, ovulation was triggered by the administration of 10 000 IU of hCG. The results of this study clearly demonstrated that the number of follicles >11 mm in diameter on the day of hCG injection was significantly lower in the rhLH/placebo group in comparison with the rhFSH/placebo group (17,82). This study performed in HH patients, who are the best and only true models for investigating the physiology of gonadotropin actions on the ovary, emphasizes the delicate balance and need for both FSH and LH in normal follicular development. Thus, it is possible that a dual advantage of high-dose rhLH may exist in the form of promoting the terminal maturation of a single preovulatory follicle, and simultaneously arresting the development of multiple less mature follicles that would otherwise occur in response to treatment with FSH (27).

Apart from the above-discussed well-documented actions of LH on ovarian follicles, a recent study has investigated the effects of LH pretreatment on subsequent ovarian stimulation with FSH in longstanding HH women having negligible serum concentrations of FSH and LH (121). Pretreatment with rhLH (300 IU/d, SC, for seven days) immediately preceding the rhFSH treatment, significantly decreased the mean threshold (daily effective) FSH dose and tended to lower the total amount of FSH required to induce follicular maturation in association with appropriate serum estradiol levels and endometrial thickness. Unexpectedly, however, in HH women retaining functional pituitary tissue, pretreatment with rhLH evoked a consistent elevation of serum LH levels during FSH administration, an effect that was also induced, even at higher magnitude, by pretreatment with rhCG. Therefore, in addition to changes in FSH requirements for follicular maturation, pretreatment with rhLH/rhCG evoked unambiguous elevations in serum levels of endogenous LH during FSH treatment in HH patients with preserved pituitary function. This is suggestive of a novel regulatory loop of LH secretion involving gonadotropin-stimulated ovarian factors whose nature and physiological relevance are yet to be disclosed, ovarian-derived kisspeptins being appealing candidates (121).

Which Regimen of Gonadotropin Administration?

A chronic step-up regimen is the usual gonadotropin treatment approach (90,110,114). However, because these patients usually have long-standing HH associated with extremely low concentrations of FSH/LH and estradiol serum levels, the following facts should be considered when inducing ovulation:

1. Pretreatment with a sequential estrogen–progestin combination for one or two cycles "primes" the endometrium and cervical glands, and may result in a better response to gonadotropins.
2. Both the initial dose (traditionally 2 or 3 75-IU ampoules of hMG) and dose increments are usually higher than in low-dose protocols used in PCOS patients. In addition, the first dose adjustment is performed after seven rather than 14 days of therapy. This author prefers a combined step-down and step-up approach, where patients receive two to three ampoules daily of hMG [according to the patient's body mass index (BMI)] on stimulation days 1 and 2, and one ampoule on days 3–7. From day 8 onward, hMG is administered on an individual basis according to the ovarian response and the principles of the step-up regimen (Fig. 38.7). Now that rhLH is commercially available, it is possible to stimulate with 2 × 75 IU rhFSH coupled with 75 IU rhLH, or according to the individual needs of patients as discussed above. It has been proposed that in the first half of the stimulation cycle, the FSH dosage should exceed that of LH by 2:1, with an inverse ratio for the second half (112).

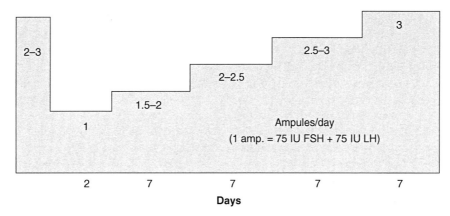

Figure 38.7   The combined (step-down and step-up) protocol for gonadotropin therapy in WHO group I anovulatory patients. *Abbreviations*: FSH, follicle-stimulating hormone; LH, luteinizing hormone; IU, international unit.

3. Because tonic ovarian stimulation by pituitary gonadotropin is absent in these patients, luteal phase support, preferentially with hCG, is indicated.

SUPEROVULATION OR STIMULATION OF MULTIPLE FOLLICULAR DEVELOPMENT

While the goal of induction of ovulation in anovulatory infertile women for conception in vivo is to approach the normal menstrual cycle as closely as possible, the aim of multiple follicular development (MFD) for ART is completely different: Here the objective is to interfere with the selection of a single dominant follicle to obtain multiple oocytes for IVF. In fact, exogenous gonadotropins are used to ensure the maintenance of a superthreshold level during the time of follicle recruitment, thus overriding ovarian mechanisms of follicle selection (Fig. 38.8). In addition, most ART patients are normally ovulating women. Therefore, as previously stressed (63) the use of the term "induction of ovulation" for ART is confusing and should be abandoned.

Which Gonadotropin to Use?

Although both urinary FSH (either in the form of hMG or pFSH/FSH-HP) and rhFSH alone can be successfully used for ovarian stimulation in non-downregulated cycles, (122,123) at present, most patients undergoing IVF or intracytoplasmic sperm injection (ICSI) also receive concomitant GnRH analogs to prevent spontaneous LH surges and improve follicular response. The low endogenous LH levels achieved with GnRH analogs in some cases may amplify the differences, if any, in treatment outcome seen with the use of hMG and FSH preparations. The recent availability of GnRH antagonists, which can cause more profound LH suppression than GnRH agonists, adds further interest to the subject.

Assisted Reproduction Treatment in General Population   Treatment with GnRH agonists does not usually result in total elimination of LH, and it is accepted that <1% of LH receptors needs to be occupied to elicit a maximal steroidogenic response (18). However, there seems to

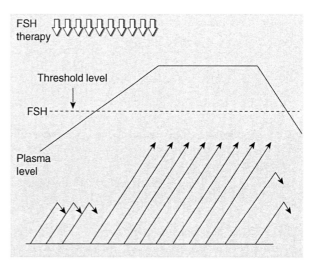

Figure 38.8   Stimulation of multiple follicular development for assisted reproductive techniques. Maintenance of a superthreshold follicle-stimulating hormone (FSH) level during the time of multiple follicular recruitment.

be a range of LH concentrations obtained in patients treated with GnRH agonists, and these can be maintained for a considerable duration; with FSH-only preparations containing negligible LH activity, it is possible that there may be a subgroup of patients with low LH concentrations in whom ovarian responses are influenced (81,124). This can become especially relevant considering the following:

1. Such women cannot be identified in advance by measuring LH levels after downregulation (125).
2. Oocyte maturity and fertilization rate in ART are influenced by the particular hormonal stimulation that preceded oocyte retrieval (126).
3. The availability of both rhFSH preparations, which are fully devoid of LH activity, and potent GnRH antagonists, suppressors of pituitary gonadotropin secretion.

Considerable debate exists as to whether the LH activity contained in hMG preparations could affect the outcome of ART in GnRH agonist–downregulated women. Some authors have postulated a negative impact of using "LH-free" gonadotropins for ovarian stimulation in ART. On the opposite side, the idea persists that elevated concentrations of LH (endogenous or superimposed through the use of hMG) during follicular development and in the periovulatory phase are unnecessary, and may not be desirable because of their potential detrimental effects on oocyte health and subsequent fertilization and implantation rates (18,127). Thus, while the relative importance of FSH and LH in the human process of follicular growth and maturation is still being investigated, considerable debate exists in the literature as to whether the LH component in hMG preparations could make a difference with regard to the outcome of ART treatment in GnRH agonist–downregulated women.

Several facts support the concept that LH administration is not needed in the vast majority of patients undergoing ART in cycles stimulated with rhFSH in downregulated women (long protocol of GnRH agonist) or in association with GnRH antagonist:

- The switch in stimulation regimens using downregulation with GnRH agonist to a more widespread use of FSH-only preparations, without LH supplementation, has been associated with an increased rate of overall program success (128–131).
- According to both case-control and cohort studies by us, LH serum measurements in the mid-follicular phase and even throughout the follicular phase during ovarian stimulation with rhFSH cannot predict ovarian response and ART outcome in downregulated women (132,133). Even in conditions of profound LH suppression, such as cycles treated with a depot GnRH and a fixed low gonadotropin dose (both of which are neither standard practices nor absolutely first choice in ART), we found that supplemental LH may be required in terms of treatment duration and gonadotropin consumption but, in spite of this, oocyte and embryo yield and quality were significantly higher with the use of rhFSH compared with hMG (134).
- rhLH supplementation to rhFSH does not improve ovarian stimulation and ART outcome in pituitary-suppressed women receiving the long protocol of GnRH agonist; even more, it may have a negative impact on oocyte maturation and/or implantation rates mainly in patients younger than 35 years (135,136).
- In the early clinical trials comparing GnRH agonist and GnRH antagonist for ART, pregnancy rates in the GnRH antagonist groups were similar irrespective of using rhFSH or hMG for ovarian stimulation (137). On the other hand, recent studies have shown that LH concentrations after GnRH antagonist administration do not influence pregnancy rates in IVF–embryo transfer, and even more, profound LH suppression after GnRH antagonist administration is associated with a significantly higher ongoing pregnancy rate after IVF (138,139). Finally, clinical trials

have demonstrated that rhLH supplementation to rhFSH during GnRH antagonist administration in ART cycles does not improve IVF outcome (140,141).
- A systematic review of the literature (142) concluded that the available evidence suggests that, among women with normal ovulation or WHO II oligo-anovulation, low endogenous LH levels during ovarian stimulation for IVF using GnRH analogs (agonist or antagonist) are not associated with a decreased probability of ongoing pregnancy beyond 12 weeks. On the contrary, this review concluded that there is evidence to suggest that the opposite may be true (142). In this respect, it is noteworthy that the inclusion of exogenous LH activity (in the form of hMG) to the ovarian stimulation protocol for downregulated young oocyte donors can have beneficial or detrimental effects on oocyte yield and quality depending on the level of endogenous LH (26).
- Another recent meta-analysis investigating the efficacy of rhLH supplementation to rhFSH for ovarian stimulation in GnRH antagonist protocol for IVF/ICSI cycles failed to show any statistically significant difference in implantation and pregnancy rates (143).

Therefore, according to the above evidence, it seems clear that there is no need to administer exogenous LH to a general ART population if daily doses of an appropriate GnRH agonist (in terms of the substance, formulation, and dosage) and the appropriate approach of rhFSH administration are used. Notwithstanding this, a need for some LH supplementation may be evidenced in some women, depending on the extent to which the endogenous serum LH is suppressed by concomitant GnRH agonist therapy, the direct effect of the latter on the ovary, and the protocol of gonadotropin administration used. Thus, randomized studies tested whether LH supplementation during controlled ovarian hyperstimulation, as opposed to increasing the daily rhFSH dose, can improve the outcome in downregulated normo-ovulatory normogonadotropic patients who show an initially hyporesponsiveness to rhFSH in the form of a steady response characterized by a normal follicular recruitment to age- and BMI appropriate rhFSH dosages on treatment days 5–7, but show a plateau on follicular growth (no increase in the estradiol level and in the follicular size) on days 8–10 of stimulation in spite of continuing the same rhFSH dosage (144–147). These women have to be distinguished from the typical poor responder in whom the detection of a few antral follicles during the early stages of stimulation is followed by later cancellation of the cycle due to insufficient follicular growth. From these studies (144–147), it was concluded that LH activity supplementation (in the form of hMG or rhLH) is more effective than increasing the dose of rhFSH in terms of ovarian outcome in patients showing a hyporesponsiveness to monotherapy with rhFSH in the mid-follicular phase of ART cycles. In addition, those studies demonstrated that the use of rhLH is more effective than hMG to rescue the ART cycles, and the daily dose of 150 IU rhLH seems to give better results than 75 IU in this regard (145,147). However, some of those studies employed a too-low daily starting dose (150 IU) of rhFSH, mainly considering that a depot GnRH agonist preparation (having a more profound suppressive effect on the pituitary and ovaries than daily doses) was used (145,146).

In fact, the agonist seems to be the major effect modifier (148), and it has been shown that the currently used dosages of GnRH agonists in ART are too high, resulting in unphysiologic low LH levels (149). Thus, using daily doses of an appropriate GnRH agonist (leuprolide or triptorelin having lower potency than buserelin) and a step-down regimen of rhFSH administration as described below, we found that the proportion of LH-suppressed women is lower than previously reported (132), and we need to add some LH during ovarian stimulation in no more than 1–2% of patients in our ART general program. These are patients usually having a low estradiol response and/or an apparent discrepancy between estradiol serum levels and developing follicles (16).

In conclusion, FSH-only products alone are useful tools for the vast majority of patients undergoing MFD under pituitary suppression for ART, provided that an appropriate GnRH agonist (substance, formulation, and dosage) is selected. The latter aspect is important considering that according to a recent IVF survey including as much as 151,000 cycles/yr performed in 273 centers worldwide, the use of GnRH-agonists was confirmed in 134,494 (89.1%) cycles (150).

Low Responders and Patients of Advanced Reproductive Age   The introduction of urinary purified FSH preparations first, and then rhFSH, was heralded as a stride forward for controlled ovarian hyperstimulation regimens. Thus, prospective studies in poor responders demonstrated significant benefits with rhFSH (151,152). Other investigators, however, have found that the association of LH activity in the form of hMG (153) or rhLH (154,155) to rhFSH during ovarian stimulation for ART improves success rates in previous poor responders or in patients with reduced ovarian reserve. Not infrequently, however, the use of hMG in previously poor responders to FSH-only preparations is associated with an increase in estradiol levels, but oocyte recovery and overall IVF results are still poor (16,156).

Age-related infertility is due to oocyte abnormalities and decreased ovarian reserve (157). Three recent reports (158–160) suggested that rhLH supplementation from the mid to late follicular phase in women undergoing assisted reproduction with GnRH agonist downregulation and stimulation with rhFSH may increase implantation rates in patients ≥35 years but not in younger women. One of these studies, (159) however, was based on a low number of patients aged ≥35 years, and, as stressed by the authors, their results required additional studies for confirmation. In the second study,(158) the clinical pregnancy rate was similar in women aged ≥35 years who received both rhFSH and rhLH and those stimulated with rhFSH alone, but the difference in clinical pregnancy rates was significantly higher in favor of the rhLH supplemented patients when

only the subgroup of women undergoing their first ART cycle were considered.

This subgroup of patients, however, also had significantly more embryos transferred in the rhFSH + rhLH group. Predicted clinical pregnancy rates from a regression logistic model adjusted for the number of embryos transferred indicated no significant difference between rhFSH + rhLH and rhFSH treatment groups, although the regression model also demonstrated that the higher number of embryos replaced in the LH-supplemented group did not explain the higher pregnancy rate (158). In the third study (160) including 131 patients treated with ICSI, no significant differences were observed in markers of either oocyte or embryo quality or quantity. However, higher rates of implantation and live birth per started cycle were observed with rhLH supplementation than with rhFSH alone.

In our prospective randomized clinical trial, comprising a total of 120 consecutive normogonadotropic infertile women aged ≥35 years undergoing their first cycle of ART, we concluded that rhLH supplementation does not increase ovarian response and implantation rates in patients of older reproductive age stimulated with rhFSH under pituitary suppression (161). Interestingly, a "ceiling effect" was evidenced in our study where rhLH-supplemented patients showed impaired follicular development and oocyte yield compared with patients receiving rhFSH alone (161). Considering some methodological differences between the three studies (148–150) mainly regarding the sample size, patients' selection criteria, the type of GnRH agonist used, the stimulation day when LH supplementation was started, and even the rhFSH/rhLH ratios used, further studies on the subject are warranted before a definite indication for routine rhLH supplementation in women of reproductive age undergoing ART is established. Thus, it has been reported that supplementation with rhLH 75 IU/day in ART patients over 38 years stimulated with rhFSH under pituitary downregulation may improve early follicular recruitment and the number of metaphase II oocytes obtained (162). However, no beneficial effect in the rhLH-treated group was observed in that study in terms of embryo yield and pregnancy rates. (162).In addition, we have recently presented the results of a prospective, randomized clinical trial to evaluate the effects of two daily doses of rhLH (37.5 IU or 75 IU) on ovarian stimulation and the implantation rate in downregulated women of advanced reproductive age undergoing follicular stimulation for IVF (163). As in our previous study (161) where the daily dose of rhLH used was 150 IU, we concluded on the lack of usefulness of LH supplementation in patients of older reproductive age in ovarian stimulation protocols where daily doses of an appropriate GnRH-a and a step-down regimen of rhFSH administration are used (163).

Interestingly, it has been reported that the effects of adding LH activity to GnRH analogue protocols in IVF cycles may differ according to age. Chung et al. (164) reported that with LH supplementation in the form of hMG in rhFSH and GnRH antagonist treated cycles, less oocytes were retrieved in women >40 years, which was not observed in those <40 years. Similarly, Kim et al. (165) recently reported that less oocytes were retrieved in women >35 years when supplemented with rhLH or hMG in GnRH antagonist/rhFSH protocols; however, this difference was not observed in women ≤35 years.

In fact, at present, the effects of adding LH activity in an IVF general population and more specifically in patients of advanced reproductive age are still unclear. It has been postulated that because of the greater stromal content in aging ovaries, older patients might be more sensitive to the potential adverse effects of LH (165). Others claim that excessive LH can induce postmaturity in already aged oocytes from women of advanced reproductive age, compromising further meiosis and mitosis process (147). Finally, others postulate that considering the fact that endogenous LH concentrations rise with age, older patients have probably LH concentrations high enough to ensure proper LH-mediated functions despite pituitary suppression. By further augmenting LH concentrations at larger follicular diameters via the use of FSH/LH protocol, patients may exceed desired ceiling levels for LH, resulting in negative outcome effects (166).

In conclusion, in spite of transient enthusiasm for specific stimulation protocols, no compelling advantage for one stimulation protocol over another has been established in poor responders and patients of advanced reproductive age. Currently, treatment of infertility when the cause is limited to decreased ovarian reserve is empiric, except for oocyte donation (157,167). However, at present, the possibility that androgen treatment directly (168–170) or indirectly through the use of an aromatase inhibitor (which induces a temporary accumulation of intraovarian androgens) (171,172), or rhLH (considering that androgens are a direct secretory product of LH action on thecal cells) (173), may amplify the FSH effects on the ovary, improving follicular recruitment, is a matter of great interest and research. As recently stressed by a group of experts, androgens and drugs that increase ovarian androgens, such as letrozole, may become important adjuncts for patients with low prognosis IVF (174).

Which Regimen of Gonadotropin Administration?

The daily dose of gonadotropin administered in ART cycles may be fixed, or progressively increased or tapered according to the given patient's response. We prefer a tapering (step-down) regimen after pituitary suppression, wherein the highest dose of FSH is given on stimulation days 1 and 2 (300–450 IU) and is then reduced to 150 IU/day once follicular recruitment has been achieved. This regimen has proved to be clinically efficacious (175,176) and is further supported by the following. First, it has been shown that for successful induction of multiple folliculogenesis in normally ovulating women, there is a critical period during the early follicular phase of the cycle when FSH values should remain above the physiologic level to stimulate follicle recruitment maximally

in the primary cohort (177,178). Second, follicles recruited by exogenous FSH require an FSH threshold concentration that is higher than that in the natural cycle (177). Third, marked inter-individual variation exists in FSH thresholds as well as in FSH metabolic clearance and ovarian sensitivity to FSH (179–181,181). Remarkably, in clinical studies, such a threshold level was reached with a single injection of six ampoules of FSH (75 IU/ampoule) on cycle day 2, and further growth of the follicles was obtained with extra FSH from cycle day 4 onward at the daily dose of two ampoules (177). Fourth, studies in primates have shown that the step-down regimen leads to greater synchronization of follicular maturation when compared with conventional step-up stimulation (182). Finally, it has been empirically observed that tapering of the FSH dose later in the course of ovarian stimulation for IVF reduces the risk of OHSS, despite a higher starting dose of stimulation. This would be explained by a reduction in circulating FSH levels during the days prior to the hCG injection (183).

The use of a step-down regimen of rhFSH administration may also be important with respect to ovarian paracrine signaling. If, as reported above, FSH activates a paracrine mechanism that up-regulates LH responsive androgen synthesis, and hence estradiol synthesis, it is tempting to postulate that higher doses of FSH used at a critical period of ovarian stimulation during the early follicular phase can overcome too low "residual" LH concentrations existing in some women once pituitary–ovarian suppression has been achieved. In vitro studies showing dose-dependent stimulation by FSH of paracrine regulators (inhibin and IGFs) production by granulosa cells from immature human ovarian follicles support that contention (3,4). This is important, taking into account that:

1. The LH isohormone profile may alter following GnRH agonist administration, resulting in differences in biopotency not reflected in immunoassays.
2. Measurements of serum LH either before or during ovarian stimulation are not useful to predict ovarian response.
3. Circulating LH measurements do not accurately reflect LH administration (19,20,144).

The above notwithstanding, defining the optimal starting dose of FSH for each patient is certainly one of the most important issues in the management of ART cycles. For a "standard" IVF patient, suggested optimal starting doses range from 100 to 350 IU of FSH per day, according to whether minimal or large numbers of oocytes are considered a success. An "appropriate" response has been arbitrarily defined as retrieval of 5–14 oocytes, but some European countries are now legally restricted in the number of oocytes that may be used in patients' treatment, and the ability to predict an appropriate response for each patient in this situation without wastage, both of oocytes and in cost of drugs, has become a crucial issue (184,185). Interestingly, in the largest data series so far analyzed to determine predictive factors of ovarian response, basal FSH, BMI, age, and the number of follicles <11 mm at screening were the most important variables in ART patients less than 35 years of age who were treated with rhFSH monotherapy. Using these four predictive factors, a follitropin α starting dose calculator was developed that can be used to select the FSH starting dose required for an optimal response. The relevance of this dose calculator is being evaluated in a prospective clinical trial where follitropin α filled by mass is used. As consistency in the biopotency of the preparation becomes important with respect to precise dose scheduling, the use of follitropin α filled by mass in that trial may enhance the modeling observed in the previous retrospective study (185). A recent meta-analysis including 10 studies (totaling 1952 IVF cycles) suggested that the optimal starting dose of rhFSH for IVF/ICSI is 150 IU daily in presumed normal responders younger than 39 years. This dose is associated with a more modest oocyte yield, but an equal pregnancy rate compared with higher doses (186).

Against the above evidence, it should be noted that a very recent study investigating the relationship between the number of eggs and live birth, across all female age groups, suggests that the number of eggs in IVF is a robust surrogate outcome for clinical success (187). The results in this study based on an analysis of more than 400, 000 IVF treatment cycles performed in the UK and compiled by the Human Fertilization and Embryology Authority, showed a strong relationship between the number of eggs and live birth rate following IVF treatment. The number of eggs to maximize the live birth rate is 15 (187). Remarkably, this is in agreement with early large studies showing that among women undergoing IVF, the chances of a live birth are related to the number of eggs fertilized, presumably because of the greater selection of embryos for transfer (188,189).

Irrespective of the regimen of FSH administration used, once MFD has been accomplished, hCG is used to induce final oocyte maturation in ART cycles. A Cochrane review concluded there is no evidence of a difference in clinical outcomes between urinary and recombinant gonadotropins used for induction of final follicular maturation in IVF/ICSI cycles, but rhCG showed better local tolerance (105).

Owing to marked differences in the manufacturing process, a potential additional advantage of rhCG over urinary hCG is in order to avoid the so-called empty follicle syndrome, a not frequent but frustrating condition causing expense and inconvenience that is considered to be a drug-related problem (190,191).

Apart from the potential usefulness of rhLH in inducing MFD in the ART general population receiving GnRH analogs (agonists or antagonists), low responders, and patients of advanced reproductive age, an important additional contribution of rhLH to ovulation induction in ART patients is related to the risk of developing OHSS. As manifestations of OHSS occur within a predictable time frame in the presence of hCG, this seems to indicate that the administration of hCG at culmination of the MFD cycle is the key event in the induction of OHSS. Clinical resolution of OHSS seems to parallel the decrease of residual exogenous hCG serum levels after induction of oocyte maturation in MFD cycles. Furthermore, pregnancy and its associated increase in endogenous hCG may prolong or worsen the course of an episode of OHSS or initiate a "late form" of OHSS. Finally, OHSS rarely occurs when hCG is withheld (192).

hCG is structurally related to the pituitary LH, and the actions of LH and hCG are mediated by the same receptor. Most important, both hormones have the same natural function: To cause luteinization and support lutein cells. The most relevant structural feature of hCG is its elevated content of sialic acid residues, which are responsible for its longer serum half-life and enhanced biologic activity. The potency of hCG appears to be approximately six- to sevenfold that of LH, although systematic information on this subject is limited (193). The longer serum half-life of hCG, with its prolonged effect on the follicle population (15), may be an undesirable characteristic in clinical practice. Thus, two studies have shown that rhLH is as effective (in terms of oocyte recovery) as, but safer (in terms of propagating OHSS) than, hCG when used in ART to induce final follicular maturation and luteinization (194,195). A single dose of rhLH, between 15,000 and 30,000 IU, gave the highest efficacy/safety ratio in IVF patients (194). It was comparable with 5000 IU urinary hCG in terms of efficacy, but resulted in a statistically significant reduction in moderate OHSS and mid-luteal serum progesterone levels. However, further studies are warranted to establish the protocol and dose for the optimal efficacy (number and competence of oocytes retrieved)/safety (incidence of OHSS) ratio when rhLH is given to induce final follicular maturation and luteinization in ART patients (196).

REFERENCES

1. Hillier SG. Ovarian manipulation with pure gonadotropins. J Endocrinol 1990; 127: 1–4.
2. Hillier SG. Current concepts of the roles of follicle stimulating hormone and luteinizing hormone in folliculogenesis. Hum Reprod 1994; 9: 188–91.
3. Hillier SG. Controlled ovarian stimulation in women. J Reprod Fertil 2000; 120: 201–10.
4. Hillier SG. Gonadotropic control of ovarian follicular growth and development. Mol Cell Endocrinol 2001; 179: 39–46.
5. Simoni M, Nieschlag E. FSH in therapy: Physiological basis, new preparations and clinical use. Reprod Med Rev 1995; 4: 163–77.
6. Zeleznik AJ, Hillier SG. The ovary: endocrine function. In: Hillier SG, Kitchener HC, Neilson JP, eds. Scientific Essentials of Reproductive Medicine. London: WB Saunders, 1996: 133–46.
7. Filicori M. The role of luteinizing hormone in folliculogenesis and ovulation induction. Fertil Steril 1999; 71: 405–14.
8. Zeleznik AJ. Follicle selection in primates: "Many are called but few are chosen." Biol Reprod 2001; 65: 655–9.
9. Yen SCC. The human menstrual cycle. In: Yen SCC, Jaffe RB, eds. Reproductive Endocrinology. 2nd edn. Philadelphia: WB, Saunders, 1986.

10. Sullivan MW, Stewart-Akers A, Krasnow JS, Berga SL, Zeleznik AJ. Ovarian responses in women to recombinant follicle-stimulating hormone and luteinizing hormone (LH): a role for LH in the final stages of follicular maturation. J Clin Endocrinol Metab 1999; 84: 228–32.

11. Balasch J, Fábregues F. Pregnancy after administration of high dose recombinant human LH alone to support final stages of follicular maturation in a woman with long-standing hypogonadotrophic hypogonadism. Reprod Biomed Online 2003; 6: 427–31.

12. Cortvrindt R, Hu Y, Smitz J. Recombinant luteinizing hormone as a survival and differentiation factor increases oocyte maturation in recombinant follicle stimulating hormone-supplemented mouse preantral follicle culture. Hum Reprod 1998; 13: 1292–302.

13. Balasch J, Miró F, Burzaco I, et al. The role of luteinizing hormone in human follicle development and oocyte fertility: evidence from in vitro fertilization in a woman with long-standing hypogonadotrophic hypogonadism and using recombinant human follicle stimulating hormone. Hum Reprod 1995; 10: 1678–83.

14. Fox R, Keroma A, Wardle P. Ovarian response to purified FSH in infertile women with longstanding hypogonadotropic hypogonadism. Aust NZ J Obstet Gynaecol 1997; 37: 92–4.

15. Peinado JA, Molina I, Pla M, et al. Recombinant human luteinizing hormone (rh-LH) as ovulatory stimulus in superovulated doses. J Assist Reprod Genet 1995; 12: 61–4.

16. Balasch J, Fábregues F. Is luteinizing hormone needed for optimal ovulation induction? Curr Opin Obstet Gynecol 2002; 14: 265–74.

17. Shoham Z. The clinical therapeutic window for luteinizing hormone in controlled ovarian stimulation. Fertil Steril 2002; 77: 1170–7.

18. Chappel SC, Howles C. Re-evaluation of the roles of luteinizing hormone and follicle-stimulating hormone in the ovulatory process. Hum Reprod 1991; 6: 1206–12.

19. The European Recombinant Human LH Study Group. Recombinant human luteinizing hormone (LH) to support recombinant human follicle-stimulating hormone (FSH)-induced follicular development in LH- and FSH-deficient anovulatory women: a dose-finding study. J Clin Endocrinol Metab 1998; 83: 1507–14.

20. Burgués S. The Spanish Collaborative Group on Female Hypogonadotrophic Hypogonadism. The effectiveness and safety of recombinant human LH to support follicular development induced by recombinant human FSH in WHO group I anovulation: evidence from a multicentre study in Spain. Hum Reprod 2001; 16: 2525–32.

21. Jacobs HS. The LH hypothesis. In: Shaw RW, ed. Polycystic Ovaries – A Disorder or a Symptom? Advances in Reproductive Endocrinology. Carnforth, UK: Parthenon Publishing, 1991: 3: 91–8.

22. Huirne JAF, van Loenen ACD, Schats R, et al. Dose-finding study of daily GnRH antagonists for prevention of premature LH surges in IVF/ICSI patients: optimal changes in LH and progesterone for clinical pregnancy. Hum Reprod 2005; 20: 359–67.

23. Hillier SG. Ovarian stimulation with recombinant gonadotrophins: LH as an adjunct to FSH. In: Jacobs HS, ed. The New Frontier in Ovulation Induction. UK: Carnforth Parthenon Publishing, 1993: 39–47.

24. Hughes E, Collins J, Vandekerckhove P. Gonadotrophin-releasing hormone analogue as an adjunct to gonadotrophin therapy for clomiphene resistant polycystic ovarian syndrome (Cochrane Review). In: The Cochrane Library. Oxford: Update Software, 2001.

25. Daya S. Gonadotrophin-releasing hormone agonist protocols for pituitary desensitization in in vitro fertilization and gamete intrafallopian transfer cycles (Cochrane Review). In: The Cochrane Library. Oxford: Update Software, 2001.

26. Tesarik J, Mendoza C. Effects of exogenous LH administration during ovarian stimulation of pituitary down-regulated young oocyte donors on oocyte yield and developmental competence. Hum Reprod 2002; 17: 3129–37.

27. Balasch J, Fábregues F. LH in the follicular phase: neither too high nor too low. Reprod Biomed Online 2006; 12: 406–15.

28. Lunenfeld B. Historical perspectives in gonadotrophin therapy. Hum Reprod Update 2004; 10: 453–67.

29. Giudice E, Crisci C, Altarocca V, O'Brien M. Characterisation of a partially purified human menopausal gonadotropin preparation. J Clin Res 2001; 4: 27–34.

30. Howles CM, Wikland M. The use of recombinant human FSH in in vitro fertilization. In: Shoham Z, Howles CM, Jacobs HS, eds. Female Infertility Therapy: Current Practice. London: Martin Dunitz, 1999: 103–14.

31. Fauser BCJM, Mannaerts BMJL, Devroey P, et al. Advances in recombinant DNA technology: corifollitropin alfa, a hybrid molecule with sustained follicle-stimulating activity and reduced injection frequency. Hum Reprod Update 2009; 15: 309–21.

32. Eshkol A. Recombinant gonadotrophins: an introduction. Hum Reprod 1996; 11(Suppl 1): 89–94.

33. Loumaye P, Martineau I, Piazzi A, et al. Clinical assessment of human gonadotrophins produced by recombinant technology. Hum Reprod 1996; 11(Suppl 1): 95–107.

34. Fonjallaz P, Loumaye E. Recombinant hCG (Ovidrel): Made by genetic engineering No. 13. J Biotechnol 2001; 87: 279–84.

35. Agostinetto R. Administration of follitropin alfa and lutropin alfa combined in a single injection: a feasibility assessment. Reprod Biol Endocrinol 2009; 7: 48.

36. Bosch E. Recombinant human follicular stimulating hormone and recombinant human luteinizing hormone in a 2:1 ratio combination. Pharmacological characteristics and clinical applications. Expert Opin Biol Ther 2010; 10: 1001–9.

37. Driebergen R, Baer G. Quantification of follicle stimulating hormone (follitropin alfa): Is in vivo bioassay still relevant in the recombinant age? Curr Med Res Opin 2003; 19: 41–6.

38. Bassett RM, Driebergen R. Continued improvements in the quality and consistency of follitropin alfa, recombinant human FSH. Reprod Biomed Online 2005; 10: 189–77.

39. Seeger H, Heikenwalder M, Zeller N, et al. Coincident scrapie infection and nephritis lead to prion excretion. Science 2005; 310: 324–6.

40. Zwart-van Rijkom JE, Broekmans FJ, Leufkens HG. From HMG through purified urinary FSH preparations

to recombinant FSH: a substitution study. Hum Reprod 2002; 17: 857–65.

41. Balen AH, Lumhotz IB. Consensus statement on the bio-safety of urinary-derived gonadotrophins with respect to Creutzfeldt–Jakob disease. Hum Reprod 2005; 20: 2994–9.

42. Howles CM. Recombinant gonadotrophins in reproductive medicine: the gold standard of today. Reprod Biomed Online 2006; 12: 11–13.

43. European Pharmacopoeia. 4th edn. Strasbourg: Council of Europe, 2002: 2101–3.

44. Homburg R. Gonadotropins. In: Homburg R, ed. Ovulation Induction and Controlled Ovarian Stimulation: A Practical Guide. London: Taylor & Francis, 2005: 53–8.

45. Hugues JN, Barlow DH, Rosenwaks Z, et al. Improvement in consistency of response to ovarian stimulation with recombinant human follicle stimulating hormone resulting from a new method for calibrating the therapeutic preparation. Reprod Biomed Online 2002; 6: 185–90.

46. Balasch J, Fábregues F, Peñarrubia J, et al. Outcome from consecutive assisted reproduction cycles in patients treated with recombinant follitropin alfa filled-by-bioassay and those treated with recombinant follitropin alfa filled-by-mass. Reprod Biomed Online 2004; 8: 408–13.

47. Lass A, McVeigh E; Gonal-f FbM PMS Group. Routine use of r-hFSH follitropin alfa filled-bymass for follicular development for IVF: a large multicentre observational study in the UK. Reprod Biomed Online 2004; 9: 604–10.

48. Wikland M, Hugues JN, Howles C. Improving the consistency of ovarian stimulation: follitropin alfa filled-by-mass. Reprod Biomed Online 2006; 12: 663–8.

49. Martinez G, Sanguineti F, Sepulveda J, et al. A comparison between follitropin α filled by mass and follitropin α filled by bioassay in the same egg donors. Reprod Biomed Online 2007; 14: 26–8.

50. Hull MGR. Epidemiology of infertility and polycystic ovarian disease: endocrinological and demographic studies. Gynecol Endocrinol 1987; 1: 235–45.

51. Speroff L, Glass RH, Kase NG. Clinical Endocrinology and Infertility. 5th edn. Baltimore: Williams and Wilkins, 1994.

52. American College of Obstetricians and Gynecologists. ACOG Practice Bulletin. Management of infertility caused by ovulatory dysfunction. Obstet Gynecol 2002; 99: 347–58.

53. Hill GA. The ovulatory factor and ovulation induction. In: Wentz AC, Herbert CM, Hill GA, eds. Gynecologic Endocrinology and Infertility. Baltimore: Williams, and, Wilkins, 1988: 147–60.

54. Santoro N, Filicori M, Crowley WF Jr. Hypogonadotropic disorders in men and women: diagnosis and therapy with pulsatile gonadotropinreleasing hormone. Endocrinol Rev 1986; 7: 11–23.

55. Franks S, Gilling-Smith C. Advances in induction of ovulation. Curr Opin Obstet Gynecol 1994; 6: 136–40.

56. Balasch J, Fábregues F, Arroyo V. Peripheral arterial vasodilation hypothesis: a new insight into the pathogenesis of ovarian hyperstimulation syndrome. Hum Reprod 1998; 13: 2718–30.

57. Elchalal U, Schenker JG. The pathophysiology of ovarian hyperstimulation syndrome – views and ideas. Hum Reprod 1997; 12: 1129–37.

58. Levene MI, Wild J, Steer P. Higher multiple births and the modern management of infertility in Britain. Br J Obstet Gynaecol 1992; 99: 607–13.

59. Hecht BR. Iatrogenic multifetal pregnancy. Assist Reprod Rev 1993; 3: 75–87.

60. Evans MI, Littmann L, Louis LS, et al. Evolving patterns of iatrogenic multifetal pregnancy generation: implications for aggressiveness of infertility treatments. Am J Obstet Gynecol 1995; 172: 1750–5.

61. Corchia C, Mastroiacovo P, Lanni R, et al. What proportion of multiple births are due to ovulation induction? A register-based study in Italy. Am J Public Health 1996; 86: 851–4.

62. Jones HW. Iatrogenic multiple births: a 2003 checkup. Fertil Steril 2007; 87: 453–5.

63. Fauser BC, Van Heusden AM. Manipulation of human ovarian function: physiological concepts and clinical consequences. Endocrinol Rev 1997; 18: 71–106.

64. Taymor ML. The regulation of follicle growth: some clinical implications in reproductive endocrinology. Fertil Steril 1996; 65: 235–47.

65. Erickson GF, Hsueh AJW, Quigley ME, Rebar RW, Yen SSC. Functional studies of aromatase activity in human granulosa cells from normal and polycystic ovaries. J Clin Endocrinol Metab 1979; 49: 514–19.

66. Seibel MM, Kamreva MM, MacArdle C, Taymor ML. Treatment of polycystic ovary disease with chronic low-dose follicle stimulating hormone: biochemical changes and ultrasound correlation. Int J Fertil 1984; 29: 39–43.

67. White DM, Polson DW, Kiddy D, et al. Induction of ovulation with low-dose gonadotropins in polycystic ovary syndrome: An analysis of 109 pregnancies in 225 women. J Clin Endocrinol Metab 1996; 81: 3821–4.

68. Shoham Z, Jacobs HS, Insler V. Luteinizing hormone: its role, mechanism of action, and detrimental effects when hypersecreted during the follicular phase. Fertil Steril 1993; 59: 1153–61.

69. Homburg R. Adverse effects of luteinizing hormone on fertility: fact or fantasy. Baillière's Clin Obstet Gynaecol 1998; 12: 555–63.

70. Anderson RE, Cragun JM, Chang RJ, et al. A pharmacodynamic comparison of human urinary follicle-stimulating hormone and humanmenopausal gonadotropin in normal women and polycystic ovary syndrome. Fertil Steril 1989; 52: 216–20.

71. Larsen T, Larsen JF, Schioler V, et al. Comparison of urinary human follicle-stimulating hormone and human menopausal gonadotropin for ovarian stimulation in polycystic ovarian syndrome. Fertil Steril 1990; 53: 426–31.

72. Sagle MA, Hamilton-Fairley D, Kiddy DS, Franks S. A comparative, randomized study of low-dose human menopausal gonadotropin and folliclestimulating hormone in women with polycystic ovarian syndrome. Fertil Steril 1991; 55: 56–60.

73. Li TC, Spuijbroek MDEH, Tuckerman E, et al. Endocrinological and endometrial factors in recurrent miscarriage. Br J Obstet Gynaecol 2000; 107: 1471–9.

74. Bergendahl M, Evans WS, Veldhuis JD. Current concepts on ultradian rhythms of luteinizing hormone secretion in the human. Hum Reprod Update 1996; 2: 507–18.

75. le Cotonnec JY, Porchet HC, Beltrami V, Munafo A. Clinical pharmacology of recombinant human

luteinizing hormone: Part I. Pharmacokinetics after intravenous administration to healthy female volunteers and comparison with urinary human luteinizing hormone. Fertil Steril 1998; 69: 189–94.

76. Clifford K, Rai R, Watson H, Regan L. An informative protocol for the investigation of recurrent miscarriage: preliminary experience of 500 consecutive cases. Hum Reprod 1994; 9: 1328–32.

77. Watson H, Kiddy DS, Hamilton-Fairley D, et al. Hypersecretion of luteinizing hormone and ovarian steroids in women with recurrent early miscarriage. Hum Reprod 1993; 8: 829–33.

78. Balasch J, Fábregues F, Casamitjana R, et al. A pharmacokinetic and endocrine comparison of recombinant follicle-stimulating hormone and human menopausal gonadotropin in polycystic ovary syndrome. Reprod Biomed Online 2003; 6: 296–301.

79. Hughes E, Collins J, Vandekerckhove P. Ovulation induction with urinary follicle stimulating hormone vs human menopausal gonadotropin for clomiphene-resistant polycystic ovary syndrome. Cochrane Database Syst Rev 2000:CD000087.

80. Nugent D, Vandekerckhove P, Hughes E, et al. Gonadotrophin therapy for ovulation induction in subfertility associated with polycystic ovary syndrome (Cochrane Review). In: The Cochrane Library. Oxford: Update Software, 2002.

81. Smyth CD, Miró F, Howles CM, Hillier SG. Effect of luteinizing hormone on follicle stimulating hormone-activated paracrine signalling in rat ovary. Hum Reprod 1995; 10: 33–9.

82. Loumaye E, Engrand P, Shoham Z, et al. Clinical evidence for an LH "ceiling" effect induced by administration of recombinant human LH during the late follicular phase of stimulated cycles in World Health Organization type I and type II anovulation. Hum Reprod 2003; 18: 314–22.

83. Hugues JN, Soussis J, Calderon I, et al. Recombinant LH Study Group. Does the addition of recombinant LH in WHO group II anovulatory women over-responding to FSH treatment reduce the number of developing follicles? A dose-finding study. Hum Reprod 2005; 20: 629–35.

84. Thessaloniki ESHRE/ASRM-Sponsored PCOS Consensus Workshop Group. Consensus on infertility treatment related to polycystic ovary syndrome. Hum Reprod 2008; 23: 462–77.

85. Wolf LJ. Ovulation induction. Clin Obstet Gynecol 2000; 43: 902–15.

86. Brown JB. Pituitary control of ovarian function – concepts derived from gonadotrophin therapy. Aust NZ J Obstet Gynaecol 1978; 18: 47–54.

87. Brown JB, Evans JH, Adey FD, et al. Factors involved in the induction of fertile ovulation with human gonadotrophins. J Obstet Gynaecol Br Commonw 1969; 76: 289–306.

88. Zeleznik AJ. Gonadotropic control of folliculogenesis: the threshold theory. In: Filicori M, Falmigni C, eds. Ovulation Induction: Basic Science and Clinical Advances. Amsterdam: Excerpta, Medica, 1994: 37–46.

89. Franks S, Hamilton-Fairley D. Ovulation induction: gonadotropins. In: Adashi EYRock JA, Rosenwaks Z, eds. Reproductive Endocrinology, Surgery, and Technology. Philadelphia: Lippincott- Raven, 1996: 1207–23.

90. Balen AH, Braat DD, West C, et al. Cumulative conception and live birth rates after the treatment of anovulatory infertility: safety and efficacy of ovulation induction in 200 patients. Hum Reprod 1994; 9: 1563–70.

91. Balasch J, Tur R, Peinado JA. The safety and effectiveness of stepwise and low-dose administration of follicle stimulating hormone in WHO group II anovulatory infertile women: evidence from a large multicenter study in Spain. J Assist Reprod Genet 1996; 13: 551–6.

92. van Santbrink EJ, Donderwinkel PF, van Dessel TJ, Fauser BC. Gonadotrophin induction of ovulation using a step-down dose regimen: single-centre clinical experience in 82 patients. Hum Reprod 1995; 10: 1048–53.

93. Homburg R, Levy T, Ben-Rafael Z. A comparative prospective study of conventional regimen with chronic low-dose administration of follicle-stimulating hormone for anovulation associated with polycystic ovary syndrome. Fertil Steril 1995; 63: 729–33.

94. Hedon B, Hugues JN, Emperaire JC, et al. A comparative prospective study of a chronic low dose versus a conventional ovulation stimulation regimen using recombinant follicle stimulating hormone in anovulatory infertile women. HumReprod 1998; 13: 2688–92.

95. Homburg R, Howles CM. Low-dose FSH therapy for anovulatory infertility associated with polycystic ovary syndrome: rationale, results, reflections and refinements. Hum Reprod Update 1999; 5: 493–9.

96. Ragni G, Caliari I, Nicolosi AE, et al. Preventing high order multiple pregnancies during controlled ovarian hyperstimulation and intrauterine insemination: 3 years' experience using low-dose recombinant follicle- stimulating hormone and gonadotropin-releasing hormone antagonists. Fertil Steril 2006; 85: 619–24.

97. Howles CM, Alam V, Tredway D, Homburg R, Warne DW. Factors related to successful ovulation induction in patients with WHO group II anovulatory infertility. Reprod BioMed Online 2010; 20: 182–90.

98. Schipper I, Hop WC, Fauser BC. The follicle-stimulating hormone (FSH) threshold/window concept examined by different interventions with exogenous FSH during the follicular phase of the normal menstrual cycle: duration, rather than magnitude, of FSH increase affects follicle development. J Clin Endocrinol Metab 1998; 83: 1292–8.

99. van Santbrink EJ, Fauser BC. Urinary follicle-stimulating hormone for normogonadotropic clomipheneresistant anovulatory infertility: prospective, randomized comparison between low dose step-up and step-down dose regimens. J Clin Endocrinol Metab 1997; 82: 3597–602.

100. Christin-Maitre S, Hugues JN. Recombinant FSH Study Group. A comparative randomized multicentric study comparing the step-up versus stepdown protocol in polycystic ovary syndrome. Hum Reprod 2003; 18: 1626–31.

101. Hugues JN, Cédrin-Durnerin I, Avril C, et al. Sequential step-up and step-down dose regimen: an alternative method for ovulation induction with follicle-stimulating hormone in polycystic ovarian syndrome. Hum Reprod 1996; 11: 2581–4.

102. Hugues JN, Cédrin-Durnerin I, Howles CM. Recombinant FSH OI Study Group. The use of a decremental

dose regimen in patients treated with a chronic low-dose step-up protocol for WHO Group II anovulation: a prospective randomized multicentre study. Hum Reprod 2006; 21: 2817–22.

103. Aboulghar MA, Mansour RT, Serour GI, et al. Recombinant follicle-stimulating hormone in the treatment of patients with history of severe ovarian hyperstimulation syndrome. Fertil Steril 1996; 66: 757–60.

104. The International Recombinant Human Chorionic Gonadotropin Study Group. Induction of ovulation in World Health Organization group II anovulatory women undergoing follicular stimulation with recombinant human follicle-stimulating hormone: A comparison of recombinant human chorionic gonadotropin (rhCG) and urinary hCG. Fertil Steril 2001; 75: 1111–18.

105. Al-Inany HG, Aboulghar M, Mansour R, Proctor M. Recombinant versus urinary human chorionic gonadotrophin for ovulation induction in assisted conception. Cochrane Database Syst Rev 2005:CD003719.

106. Blumenfeld Z, Nahhas F. Luteal dysfunction in ovulation induction: The role of repetitive human chorionic gonadotropin supplementation during the luteal phase. Fertil Steril 1988; 50: 403–7.

107. Check JH. The future trends of induction of ovulation. Minerva Endocrinol 2010; 35: 227–46.

108. Filicori M, Flamigni C, Dellai P, et al. Treatment of anovulation with pulsatile gonadotropin-releasing hormone: prognostic factors and clinical results in 600 cycles. J Clin Endocrinol Metab 1994; 79: 1215–20.

109. Filicori M, Flamigni C. Ovulation induction regimens: is a consensus possible? In: Filicori M, Flamigni C, eds. Ovulation Induction: Basic Science and Clinical Advances. Amsterdam: Elsevier Science, 1994: 371–87.

110. 110. Martin KA, Hall JE. Pulsatile GnRH in hypogonadotropic hypogonadism. In: Filicori M, Flamigni C, eds. Ovulation Induction. Update '98. New York: Parthenon Publishing, 1998: 47–54.

111. Messinis IE. Ovulation induction: A mini review. Hum Reprod 2005; 20: 2688–97.

112. Krause BT, Ohlinger R, Haase A. Lutropin alpha, recombinant human luteinizing hormone, for the stimulation of follicular development in profoundly LH-deficient hypogonadotropic hypogonadal women: A review. Bioloqics 2009; 3: 337–47.

113. Couzinet B, Lestrat N, Brailly S, et al. Stimulation of ovarian follicular maturation with pure folliclestimulating hormone in women with gonadotropin deficiency. J Clin Endocrinol Metab 1988; 66: 552–6.

114. Shoham Z, Balen A, Patel A, Jacobs HS. Results of ovulation induction using human menopausal gonadotropin or purified follicle-stimulating hormone in hypogonadotropic hypogonadism patients. Fertil Steril 1991; 56: 1048–53.

115. Schoot DC, Coelingh-Bennik HJ, Mannaerts BM, et al. Human recombinant follicle-stimulating hormone induces growth of preovulatory follicles without concomitant increase in androgen and estrogen biosynthesis in a woman with isolated gonadotropin deficiency. J Clin Endocrinol Metab 1992; 74: 1471–3.

116. Schoot DC, Harlin J, Shoham Z, et al. Recombinant human follicle-stimulating hormone and ovarian response in gonadotropin-deficient women. Hum Reprod 1994; 9: 1237–42.

117. Hull M, Corrigan E, Piazzi A, Loumaye E. Recombinant human luteinizing hormone: an effective new gonadotropin preparation. Lancet 1994; 344: 334–5.

118. Kousta E, White DM, Piazzi A, et al. Successful induction of ovulation and completed pregnancy using recombinant luteinizing hormone and follicle stimulating hormone in a woman with Kallmann's syndrome. Hum Reprod 1996; 11: 70–1.

119. Agrawal R, West C, Conway GS, et al. Pregnancy after treatment with three recombinant gonadotropins. Lancet 1997; 349: 29–30.

120. Hillier SG. Ovarian stimulation with recombinant gonadotropin: LH as an adjunct to FSH. In: Jacobs HS, ed. The New Frontier in Ovulation Induction. Carnforth, UK: Parthenon Publishing, 1993: 39–47.

121. Balasch J, Fábregues F, Carmona F, Casamitjana R, Tena-Sempere M. Ovarian luteinizing hormone priming preceding follicle-stimulating hormone stimulation: clinical and endocrine effects in women with long-term hypogonadotropic hypogonadism. J ClinEndocrinol Metab 2009; 94: 2367–73.

122. Jansen CA, Van Os MC. Puregon without analogs: an oxymoron. Gynecol Endocrinol 1996; 10(Suppl 1): 34.

123. Strowitzki T, Kentenich H, Kiesel L, et al. Ovarian stimulation in women undergoing in vitro fertilization and embryo transfer using recombinant human follicle stimulating hormone (Gonal-F) in non-downregulated cycles. Hum Reprod 1995; 10: 3097–101.

124. Fleming R, Chung CC, Yates RW, Coutts JR. Purified urinary follicle stimulating hormone induces different hormone profiles compared with menotrophins, dependent upon the route of administration and endogenous luteinizing hormone activity. Hum Reprod 1996; 11: 1854–8.

125. Loumaye E, Engrand P, Howles CM, O'Dea L. Assessment of the role of serum luteinizing hormone and estradiol response to follicle-stimulating hormone on in vitro fertilization outcome. Fertil Steril 1997; 67: 889–99.

126. Pieters MH, Dumoulin JC, Engelhart CM, et al. Immaturity and aneuploidy in human oocytes after different stimulation protocols. Fertil Steril 1991; 56: 306–10.

127. The Ganirelix Dose-Finding Study Group. A double-blind, randomised, dose-finding study to assess the efficacy of the GnRH antagonist Ganirelix (Org 37462) to prevent premature LH surges in women undergoing controlled ovarian hyperstimulation with recombinant FSH (Puregon). Hum Reprod 1998; 13: 3023–31.

128. FIVNAT. Dossier FIVNAT-99. Paris: Bilan de l'année 98, 1999.

129. FIVNAT. Dossier FIVNAT-2000. Paris: Bilan de l'année 99, 2000.

130. Wikland M. Progress of ART; the role of the clinician. Presented at the 11th World Congress on In Vitro Fertilization and Human Reproductive Genetics. Sydney, 1999.

131. Cramer DW, Liberman RF, Powers D, et al. Recent trends in assisted reproductive techniques and associated outcomes. Obstet Gynecol 2000; 95: 61–6.

132. Balasch J, Vidal E, Peñarrubia J, et al. Suppression of LH during ovarian stimulation: analysing threshold values and effects on ovarian response and the outcome of assisted reproduction in downregulated women stimulated with recombinant FSH. Hum Reprod 2001; 16: 1636–43.

133. Peñarrubia J, Fábregues F, Creus M, et al. LH serum levels during ovarian stimulation as predictors of ovarian response and assisted reproduction outcome in down-regulated women stimulated with recombinant FSH. Hum Reprod 2003; 18: 2689–97.
134. Balasch J, Peñarrubia J, Fábregues F, et al. Ovarian responses to recombinant FSH or HMG in normogonadotrophic women following pituitary desensitization by a depot GnRH agonist for assisted reproduction. Reprod Biomed Online 2003; 7: 35–42.
135. Balasch J, Creus M, Fábregues F, et al. The effect of exogenous luteinizing hormone (LH) on oocyte viability: evidence from a comparative study using recombinant human follicle-stimulating hormone (FSH) alone or in combination with recombinant LH for ovarian stimulation in pituitary-suppressed women undergoing assisted reproduction. J Assist Reprod Genet 2001; 18: 250–6.
136. Marrs R, Meldrum D, Muasher S, et al. Randomized trial to compare the effect of recombinant human FSH (follitropin alfa) with or without recombinant human LH in women undergoing assisted reproduction treatment. Reprod Biomed Online 2004; 8: 175–82.
137. Huirne JAF, Lambalk CB. Gonadotropin-releasinghormone-receptor antagonists. Lancet 2001; 358: 1793–803.
138. Kolibianakis EM, Zikopoulos K, Schiettecatte J, et al. Profound LH suppression after GnRH antagonist administration is associated with a significantly higher ongoing pregnancy rate in IVF. Hum Reprod 2004; 19: 2490–6.
139. Merviel P, Antoine JM, Mathieu E, et al. Luteinizing hormone concentrations after gonadotropinreleasing hormone antagonist administration do not influence pregnancy rates in in vitro fertilizationembryo transfer. Fertil Steril 2004; 82: 119–25.
140. Cédrin-Durnerin I, Grange-Dujardin D, Laffy A, et al. Recombinant human LH supplementation during GnRH antagonist administration in IVF/ICSI cycles: a prospective randomized study. Hum Reprod 2004; 19: 1979–84.
141. Griesinger G, Schultze-Mosgau A, Dafopoulos K, et al. Recombinant luteinizing hormone supplementation to recombinant follicle-stimulating hormone induced ovarian hyperstimulation in the GnRH-antagonist multiple-dose protocol. Hum Reprod 2005; 20: 1200–6.
142. Kolibianakis EM, Collins J, Tarlatzis B, et al. Are endogenous LH levels during ovarian stimulation for IVF using GnRH analogues associated with the probability of ongoing pregnancy? A systematic review. Hum Reprod Update 2006; 12: 3–12.
143. Baruffi RLR, Mauri AL, Petersen CG, et al. Recombinant LH supplementation to recombinant FSH during induced ovarian stimulation in the GnRH-antagonist protocol: A meta-analysis. Reprod Biomed Online 2007; 14: 14–25.
144. De Placido G, Mollo A, Alviggi C, et al. Rescue of IVF cycles by hMG in pituitary down-regulated normogonadotrophic young women characterized by a poor initial response to recombinant FSH. Hum Reprod 2001; 16: 1875–9.
145. De Placido G, Alviggi C, Mollo A, et al. Effects of recombinant LH (rLH) supplementation during controlled ovarian hyperstimulation (COH) in normogonadotrophic women with an initial inadequate response to recombinant FSH (rFSH) after pituitary downregulation. Clin Endocrinol 2004; 60: 637–43.
146. De Placido G, Alviggi C, Perino A, et al. Recombinant human LH supplementation versus recombinant human FSH (rFSH) step-up protocol during controlled ovarian stimulation in normogonadotrophic women with initial inadequate ovarian response to rFSH. A multicentre, prospective, randomized controlled trial. Hum Reprod 2005; 20: 390–6.
147. Ferraretti AP, Gianaroli L, Magli MC, et al. Exogenous luteinizing hormone in controlled ovarian hyperstimulation for assisted reproductive techniques. Fertil Steril 2004; 82: 1521–6.
148. Westergaard LG, Erb K, Laursen SB, et al. Human menopausal gonadotropin versus recombinant follicle stimulating hormone in normogonadotropic women down-regulated with a gonadotropin-releasing hormone agonist who were undergoing in vitro fertilization and intracytoplasmic sperm injection: a prospective study. Fertil Steril 2001; 76: 543–9.
149. Janssens RM, Lambalk CB, Vermeiden JP, et al. Dose-finding study of triptorelin acetate for prevention of a premature LH surge in IVF: a prospective, randomized, double-blind, placebo-controlled study. Hum Reprod 2000; 15: 2333–40.
150. Tur-Kaspa I, Fauser B. The use of GnRH agonist in IVF protocols, 2010. [Available from: www.IVF-Worldwide.com]
151. Raga F, Bonilla-Musoles F, Casañ EM, Bonilla F. Recombinant follicle stimulating hormone stimulation in poor responders with normal basal concentrations of follicle stimulating hormone and oestradiol: improved reproductive outcome. Hum Reprod 1999; 14: 1431–4.
152. De Placido G, Alviggi C, Mollo A, et al. Recombinant follicle stimulating hormone is effective in poor responders to highly purified follicle stimulating hormone. Hum Reprod 2000; 15: 17–20.
153. Meo F, Rainieri DM, Khadum I, Serhal P. Ovarian response and in vitro fertilization outcome in patients with reduced ovarian reserve who were stimulated with recombinant follicle-stimulating hormone or human menopausal gonadotropin. Fertil Steril 2002; 77: 630–2.
154. Laml T, Obruca A, Fischl F, Huber JC. Recombinant luteinizing hormone in ovarian hyperstimulation after stimulation failure in normogonadotropic women. Gynecol Endocrinol 1999; 13: 98–103.
155. Lisi F, Rinaldi L, Fishel S, et al. Use of recombinant FSH and recombinant LH in multiple follicular stimulation for IVF: A preliminary study. Reprod Biomed Online 2001; 3: 190–4.
156. Phelps JY, 0a L, Levine AS, et al. Exogenous luteinizing hormone (LH) increases estradiol response patterns in poor responders with low serum LH concentrations. J Assist Reprod Genet 1999; 16: 363–8.
157. Practice Committee of the American Society for Reproductive Medicine. Aging and infertility in women: A committee opinion. Fertil Steril 2006; 86(Suppl 4): S248–52.
158. Marrs R, Meldrum D, Muasher S, et al. Randomized trial to compare the effect of recombinant human FSH (follitropin alfa) with or without recombinant human LH in women undergoing assisted reproduction treatment. Reprod Biomed Online 2004; 8: 175–82.

159. Humaidan P, Bungum M, Bungum L, Yding Andersen C. Effects of recombinant LH supplementation in women undergoing assisted reproduction with GnRH agonist down-regulation and stimulation with recombinant FSH: an opening study. Reprod Biomed Online 2004; 8: 635–43.

160. Matorras R, Prieto B, Exposito A, et al. Mid-follicular LH supplementation in women aged 35–39 years undergoing ICSI cycles: A randomized controlled study. Reprod Biomed Online 2009; 19: 879–87.

161. Fábregues F, Creus M, Peñarrubia J, et al. Effects of recombinant human luteinizing hormone supplementation on ovarian stimulation and the implantation rate in down-regulated women of advanced reproductive age. Fertil Steril 2006; 85: 925–31.

162. Gómez-Palomares JL, Acevedo-Martin B, Andrés L, et al. LH improves early follicular recruitment in women over 38 years old. Reprod Biomed Online 2005; 11: 409–14.

163. Fábregues F, Iraola A, Casals G, et al. Evaluation of two doses of recombinant human luteinizing hormone supplementation in down-regulated women of advanced reproductive age undergoing follicular stimulation for IVF: a randomized clinical study. Eur J Obstet Gynecol Reprod Biol 2011; 158: 56–61.

164. Chung K, Krey L, Katz J, Noyes N. Evaluating the role of exogenous luteinizing hormone in poor responders undergoing in vitro fertilization with gonadotropin-releasing hormone antagonists. Fertil Steril 2005; 84: 313–18.

165. Kim YJ, Ku SY, Jee BC, et al. Effects of adding luteinizing hormone activity to gonadotropin releasing hormone antagonist protocols may differ according to age. Gynecol Endocrinol 2010; 26: 256–60.

166. Weghofer A, Munné S, Brannath W, et al. The impact of LH-containing gonadotropin stimulation on euploidy rates in preimplantation embryos: antagonist cycles. Fertil Steril 2009; 92: 937–42.

167. Mahuette NG, Arici A. Poor responders: Does the protocol make a difference? Curr Opin Obstet Gynecol 2002; 14: 275–81.

168. Balasch J, Fábregues F, Peñarrubia J, et al. Pretreatment with transdermal testosterone may improve ovarian response to gonadotrophins in poor-responder IVF patients with normal basal oncentrations of FSH. Hum Reprod 2006; 21: 1884–93.

169. Massin N, Cédrin-Durnerin I, Coussieu C, et al. Effects of transdermal testosterone application on the ovarian response to FSH in poor responders undergoing assisted reproductive technique – a prospective, randomized, double-blind study. Hum Reprod 2006; 21: 1204–11.

170. Fábregues F, Peñarrubia J, Creus M, et al. Transdermal testosterone may improve ovarian response to gonadotrophins in low-responder IVF patients: a randomized, clinical trial. Hum Reprod 2009; 24: 349–59.

171. García-Velasco JA, Moreno L, Pacheco A, et al. The aromatase inhibitor letrozole increases the concentration of intraovarian androgens and improves in vitro fertilization outcome in low responder patients: a pilot study. Fertil Steril 2005; 84: 82–7.

172. Lee VC, Ledger W. Aromatase inhibitors for ovulation induction and ovarian stimulation. Clin Endocrinol (Oxf) 2011; 74: 537–46.

173. Durnerin CI, Erb K, Fleming R, et al. Luveris Pretreatment Group. Effects of recombinant LH treatment on folliculogenesis and responsiveness to FSH stimulation. Hum Reprod 2008; 23: 421–6.

174. Meldrum DR, Chang RJ, de Ziegler D, et al. Adjuncts for ovarian stimulation: when do we adopt "orphan indications" for approved drugs? Fertil Steril 2009; 92: 13–18.

175. Balasch J, Fábregues F, Creus M, et al. Pure and highly purified follicle-stimulating hormone alone or in combination with human menopausal gonadotrophin for ovarian stimulation after pituitary suppression in in vitro fertilization. Hum Reprod 1996; 11: 2400–4.

176. Davis OK, Rosenwaks Z. In vitro fertilization. In: Adashi EY, Rock JA, Rosenwaks Z, eds. Reproductive Endocrinology, Surgery, and Technology. Philadelphia: Lippincott-Raven, 1996: 2: 2319–34.

177. Lolis DE, Tsolas O, Messinis IE. The follicle-stimulating hormone threshold level for folliclematuration in superovulated cycles. Fertil Steril 1995; 63: 1272–7.

178. Messinis IE, Templeton AA. The importance of follicle-stimulating hormone increase for folliculogenesis. Hum Reprod 1990; 5: 153–6.

179. Porchet HC, le Cotonnec JY, Loumaye E. Clinical pharmacology studies of recombinant human follicle-stimulating hormone. III. Pharmacokinetic–pharmacodynamic modeling after repeated subcutaneous administration. Fertil Steril 1994; 61: 687–95.

180. Ben-Rafael Z, Levy T, Schoemaker J. Pharmacokinetics of follicle stimulating hormone: clinical significance. Fertil Steril 1995; 63: 689–700.

181. van Santbrink EJ, Hop WC, van Dessel TJ, et al. Decremental follicle-stimulating hormone and dominant follicle development during the normal menstrual cycle. Fertil Steril 1995; 64: 37–43.

182. Abbasi R, Kenigsberg D, Danforth D, et al. Cumulative ovulation rate in human menopausal/human chorionic gonadotropin-treated monkeys: "step-up" versus "step-down" dose regimens. Fertil Steril 1987; 47: 1019–24.

183. Meldrum DR. Vascular endothelial growth factor, polycystic ovary syndrome, and ovarian hyperstimulation syndrome. Fertil Steril 2002; 78: 1170–1.

184. Popovic-Todorovis B, Loft A, Linhard A, et al. A prospective study of predictive factors of ovarian response in 'standard' IVF/ICSI patients treated with recombinant FSH. A suggestion for a recombinant FSH dosage normogram. Hum Reprod 2003; 18: 781–7.

185. Howles CM, Saunders H, Alam V, Engrand P. FSH Treatment Guidelines Clinical Panel. Predictive factors and a corresponding treatment algorithm for controlled ovarian stimulation in patients treated with recombinant human follicle stimulating hormone (follitropin alfa) during assisted reproductive technique (ART) procedures. An analysis of 1378 patients. Curr Med Res Opin. 2006; 22: 907–18.

186. Sterrenburg MD, Veltman-Verhulst SM, Eijkemans MJC, et al. Clinical outcomes in relation to the daily dose of recombinant follicle-stimulating hormone for ovarian stimulation in in vitro fertilization in presumed normal responders younger than 39 years: a meta-analysis. Hum Reprod Update 2011; 17: 184–96.

187. Sunkara SK, Rittenberg V, Raine-Fenning N, et al. Association between the number of eggs and live birth in IVF treatment: an analysis of 400 135 treatment cycles. Hum Reprod 2011; 26: 1768–74.

188. Templeton A, Morris JK. Reducing the risk of multiple births by transfer of two embryos after in vitro fertilization. N Engl J Med 1998; 339: 73–7.

189. Schieve LA, Peterson HB, Meikle SF, et al. Live-birth rates and multiple-birth risk using in vitro fertilization. JAMA 1999; 282: 1832–8.

190. Ndukwe G, Thornton S, Fishel. S, et al. "Curing" empty follicle syndrome. Hum Reprod 1997; 12: 21–3.

191. Peñarrubia J, Balasch J, Fábregues F, et al. Recurrent empty follicle syndrome successfully treated with recombinant human chorionic gonadotrophin. Hum Reprod 1999; 14: 1703–6.

192. Whelan JG III, Vlahos NF. The ovarian hyperstimulation syndrome. Fertil Steril 2000; 73: 883–96.

193. Stokman PG, de Leeuw R, van den Wijngaard HA, et al. Human chorionic gonadotropin in commercial human menopausal gonadotropin preparations. Fertil Steril 1993; 60: 175–8.

194. The European Recombinant LH Study Group. Recombinant human luteinizing hormone is as effective as, but safer than, urinary human chorionic gonadotropin in inducing final follicular maturation and ovulation in in vitro fertilization procedures: results of a multicenter double-blind study. J Clin Endocrinol Metab 2001; 86: 2607–18.

195. Manau D, Fábregues F, Arroyo V, et al. Hemodynamic changes induced by urinary human chorionic gonadotropin and recombinant luteinizing hormone used for inducing final follicular maturation and luteinization. Fertil Steril 2002; 78: 1261–7.

196. Engmann L, Benadiva C. Ovarian Hyperstimulation Syndrome Prevention Strategies: Luteal Support Strategies to Optimize Pregnancy Success in Cycles with Gonadotropin-Releasing Hormone Agonist Ovulatory Trigger. Sem Reprod Med 2010; 28: 506–12.

39

Endocrine characteristics of ART cycles

Jean-Noël Hugues and Isabelle Cédrin-Durnerin

INTRODUCTION

The hormonal control of ovarian function by gonadotropins plays a key role in the physiologic process of follicular growth and differentiation. Over the last two decades, the respective contributions of follicle-stimulating hormone (FSH) and luteinizing hormone (LH) to follicular development have been better defined mainly through clinical data obtained from assisted reproductive technique (ART) cycles performed with gonadotropin-releasing hormone (GnRH) agonist protocols. More recently, the introduction of GnRH antagonists to prevent the LH surge has provided a new model for assessing the respective role of FSH and LH. In each situation, measurements of plasma FSH and LH levels were used to evaluate the endocrine environment of the follicle. While it is clear that hormonal assays from blood sampling cannot adequately reflect the biological activity of gonadotropins, this approach has allowed an assessment of the required supply of exogenous FSH and LH in ART cycles.

Regarding the endocrine characteristics of stimulated cycles, plasma measurement of steroids is currently performed because it directly reflects the biological effect of gonadotropins on the ovary. Steroids are involved in the implantation process but may also play a paracrine or even an autocrine role on the cumulus–oocyte unit. Estradiol (E2) and progesterone measurements are currently done to adjust the daily dose of exogenous gonadotropins, whereas the determination of androgen production has been only performed in some clinical trials.

In this chapter, we will consider how therapeutic agents currently used in ART cycles (GnRH analogs, exogenous gonadotropins) specifically modify the endocrine environment and to what extent hormonal measurements can be helpful to better control ovarian stimulation and, eventually, to predict cycle outcome.

GONADOTROPIN PROFILES DURING OVARIAN STIMULATION FOR ART CYCLES

According to the two-cell-two-gonadotropin model (1), both FSH and LH are required for promoting follicular growth and differentiation. We will consider their respective contribution in stimulation regimens separately.

Follicle-Stimulating Hormone

It is well documented that FSH plays a crucial role in the recruitment, selection, and dominance processes during the whole follicular phase (2). On the one hand, FSH has a trophic effect on granulosa cells and is involved in the recruitment of the cohort at the early follicular phase. On the other hand, FSH stimulates transcription of several genes within the granulose cells, leading to the synthesis of proteins such as aromatase enzyme, inhibins, and LH receptor, which clearly reflect follicle differentiation.

From outstanding clinical studies performed by JB Brown in the late 1960s (3) it was demonstrated that a certain amount of FSH secretion, defined as the "FSH threshold," is required to induce follicular growth. Moreover, as the FSH threshold is not identical for the follicles of the same cohort, the FSH supply for inducing multifollicular development should overcome the threshold of the least FSH-sensitive follicles. This concept of FSH threshold led to the postulate that endogenous FSH supply in the early stage of the cycle is a key factor to induce follicular recruitment (Fig. 39.1).

Another aspect of the role of FSH in folliculogenesis is the concept of the "FSH window" described by Baird (4). It means that follicular growth is maintained as long as the FSH level is above the follicle's threshold. In a natural cycle, the progressive decrease in FSH secretion related to the feedback effect of ovarian factors at the pituitary level largely contributes to the dominance of the selected follicle over the others. In contrast, maintaining the FSH levels above the threshold of the dominant follicle opens the window until the final stages of follicular development and plays a key role to get a multifollicular recruitment.

These two concepts justify the assumption that FSH is the main therapeutic agent to control folliculogenesis in all situations except severe hypogonadotropic hypogonadism. Indeed, in this latter case, concomitant LH supply is absolutely required to ensure adequate steroid production according to the two-cell-two-gonadotropin model (5).

Both gonadotropin preparations and GnRH analogs are commonly used to achieve multifollicular development but the effects of each agent on FSH accumulation are quite different.

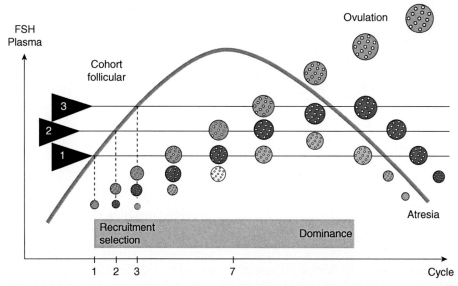

Figure 39.1   The FSH threshold and window concepts. This figure illustrates that follicular growth starts at the early follicular phase when plasma FSH concentration is above a threshold value. Differences in FSH threshold between each follicle of the same cohort account for the asynchrony of follicular development. Follicular growth will continue as long as the FSH window is opened, i.e., the plasma FSH value is above the threshold. Conversely, the reduction in plasma FSH induced by increased E2 secretion results in a progressive arrest of follicular growth. The follicle with the lowest threshold is only preserved because it becomes more sensitive to FSH and possesses LH receptor, which allows LH to contribute to ovarian steroidogenesis. *Abbreviation*: FSH, follicle-stimulating hormone.

As far as gonadotropin administration is concerned, it has been stated that, owing to the long elimination half-life (30–35 hours) of the FSH molecule, (6) a plateau of plasma FSH is obtained after five consecutive days of injection (7). Conversely, FSH accumulation, which seems to be a determinant factor for the size of final cohort of mature follicles, (8) is still observed during few days following the cessation of FSH administration (9). Furthermore, determination of plasma FSH levels following intramuscular or subcutaneous administration of FSH has shown that there is a modest and transient (4–8 hours) rise in plasma FSH values which cannot adequately reflect the actual bioactivity of the molecule. In another clinical study, (10) Schoemaker's group evaluated the role of plasma FSH measurements to determine the adequate threshold FSH dose. In this very sophisticated model, the dose of FSH administered in a pulsatile intravenous manner was adjusted daily according to the simultaneous evaluation of plasma FSH levels. This way, the authors were able to control the minimal supply of FSH required to select the most sensitive follicle of the cohort. However, the correlation between plasma FSH values and the FSH threshold dose was poor because of a large overlap of the plasma FSH values observed between patients who displayed follicular recruitment and those who did not (Fig. 39.2) Consequently, it appears that determination of plasma FSH levels is not a valuable tool to adjust exogenous FSH supply.

The effects of GnRH agonists (GnRH-a) on FSH secretion depend largely on the way these pharmaceutical agents are used. The initial flare-up effect of the agonist at the pituitary level is associated with a significant increase in plasma FSH levels that participates in the follicular recruitment when using the so-called short protocol. Several studies (11–13) have shown that the amplitude of the FSH response to GnRH-a is lower than that of LH. Furthermore, the dose dependence effect of the agonist on the gonadotroph response is far less evident for FSH than for LH, attesting to differences in the hypophyseal control of gonadotropin secretion. Since a lower dose of GnRH-a than that usually recommended may induce a larger increase in the FSH response, (14,15) there is a need to further evaluate the most appropriate dose of GnRH-a in this short-term protocol (16). Consistent with its lower dependence regarding GnRH control, the desensitizing effect of long-term GnRH-a administration upon FSH secretion is much less marked than for LH. Immunometric evaluation of plasma FSH has shown that the suppressive effect of the agonist is modest and may be dependent on the molecule used, buserelin being the most suppressive agent (17). Conversely, it has been also reported that FSH bioactivity may not actually decrease during GnRH-a administration (18,19). Thus, it is unlikely that determination of plasma FSH levels is relevant during the course of GnRH-a administration.

Later data concerning plasma FSH variations following administration of a GnRH antagonist provided similar conclusions. Indeed, the gonadotroph suppression was less marked for FSH than for LH, also attesting that FSH hypophyseal secretion is less dependent on GnRH control (20). Nevertheless, in clinical practice, the introduction of GnRH antagonists during ovarian stimulation can be associated with the need of higher dosage of gonadotropins to balance the suppressive effect of the antagonist on hypophyseal secretion.

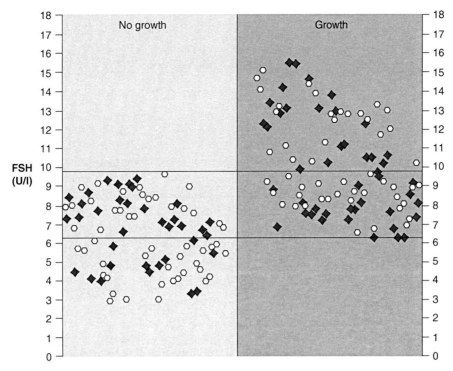

Figure 39.2 The FSH plasma threshold. FSH plasma "stable" concentrations according to follicular growth in anovulatory patients treated with hFSH (open symbols) or human menopausal gonadotropin (hMG; closed symbols). This figure shows the overlap of plasma FSH values between patients with (right panel) or without (left panel) follicular growth (10). *Abbreviation*: FSH, follicle-stimulating hormone.

To sum up these data on FSH variations during treatments for ART, it does appear that determination of plasma FSH is not contributive enough to tailor a gonadotropin regimen in a proper manner. Thus, it seems more appropriate to restrict this evaluation to clinical research studies.

Luteinizing Hormone

The role of LH on ovarian steroidogenesis depends on the stage of follicular development. On one hand, LH acts directly on theca cells where LH receptors are constitutively present and ensure a tonic production of androgens during the whole follicular phase. According to the two-cell-two-gonadotropin theory, androgens play a key role as substrates for aromatase activity and contribute to the production of E2 by granulosa cells. On the other hand, LH directly participates in the control of granulosa cell function through specific receptors that are gradually present as soon as cell differentiation is induced by FSH.

In vitro studies (21) clearly demonstrated that LH induces a dose-dependent protein synthesis (as aromatase activity) by granulosa cells. The pivotal role of LH on steroidogenesis has been also well documented in humans by studies performed in patients with hypogonadotropic hypogonadism. Indeed, in those patients deprived of hypophyseal gonadotroph production, substitution with recombinant FSH results in follicular growth but does not allow any concomitant steroid output. In contrast, addition of recombinant LH induces a dose-dependent increase in E2 production, a condition required to ensure endometrial preparation for embryo

implantation (5). This observation emphasizes that a minimal amount of LH, defined as the "LH threshold," is required for pregnancy. However, as discussed later on, determination of plasma LH concentrations by immunometric assays may not be helpful enough for an accurate assessment of the LH threshold. Alternatively, is there any evidence for an adverse effect of high endogenous LH environment? If we look at previous reports regarding the influence of the endogenous LH on the outcome of both natural and treated cycles, (22,23) presumably high endogenous LH levels are often associated with an increased incidence of infertility or miscarriages. Another study (24) performed in patients involved in an egg donation program suggests that this deleterious effect of high endogenous LH was related to a negative influence on the endometrium rather than on the oocyte/conceptus itself.

More recently, data reported in women suffering from hypogonadotropic hypogonadism demonstrated the synergistic effect of LH and FSH on folliculogenesis. In that study (25), LH administration (300 IU/day) was provided for seven days prior to FSH injection. Subsequent stimulation with FSH indicated that the daily effective dose of FSH was significantly reduced in women pre-treated with LH. These data eventually attest that LH acts in synergy with FSH to promote folliculogenesis.

However, using high doses of LH could negatively impact follicular development. This concept of the "LH ceiling" has been proposed by Hillier (26) on the basis of in vitro experiments showing an inhibitory effect of high LH doses on cell growth. Thus, LH, beyond a certain "ceiling" level, seems to suppress granulosa cell proliferation by inducing atresia of less mature follicles. Clinical data from patients with hypogonadotropic hypogonadism tend to support this concept: Indeed, substitution with recombinant LH alone in the late follicular phase induces a reduction in the size of the follicular cohort and in the number of large follicles (27). In addition, another study performed in patients with WHO II anovulation and treated with recombinant human FSH (rhFSH) also indicated that substitution by large doses of recombinant human LH (rhLH) (660 IU/day) when follicles reached 11–15 mm in diameter is able to reduce the number of developing follicles (28).

Altogether these data clearly demonstrated that LH plays, during the whole follicular phase, a critical role in synergy with FSH on both steroidogenesis and folliculogenesis.

Let us now consider plasma LH variations when using drugs for ART cycles. Urinary human menopausal gonadotropin (hMG) preparations have been commonly used with success over the last 30 years for ovulation induction. In regimens performed with gonadotropins alone, it has been demonstrated that LH is rapidly cleared from the circulation owing to its relatively short half-life (29). The pharmacokinetics of LH have been studied in detail

using rhLH and the terminal half-life was found to be approximately 12 hours, half that of FSH (30). Thus, in contrast to FSH, there is no evidence for plasma LH accumulation following a single injection of hMG (Fig. 39.3). However, in urine, LH concentrations in polycystic ovary (PCO) women treated according to a chronic low-dose step-up regimen are significantly elevated following hMG administration as compared to rhFSH (31). Furthermore, determination of plasma LH from a morning blood sample following a previous evening injection of gonadotropins is not very informative for evaluating the effects of LH content in hMG preparations. Thus, during gonadotropin therapy, plasma LH measurements are usually restricted to the detection of the endogenous LH surge, specially required for women undergoing intrauterine inseminations.

From 1982 until recently, GnRH agonists have been routinely adopted as adjunct therapy in controlled ovarian hyperstimulation. Taking advantage of the initial flare-up effect of GnRH-a injection, an ultrashort or a short-term administration of the analogs has been shown to promote follicular recruitment at the early follicular phase of the cycle. Indeed, within the 24 hours following

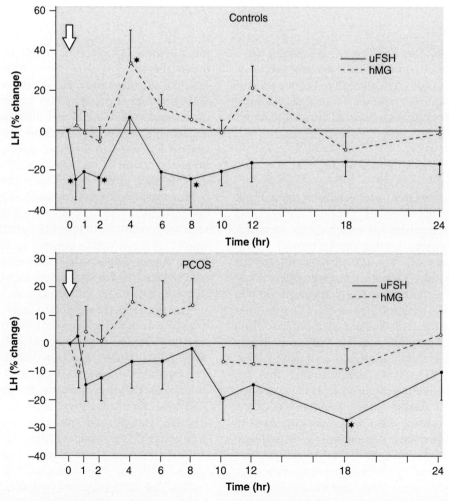

Figure 39.3 Pharmacodynamics of LH. Percent change in plasma LH after an intramuscular injection (arrow) of either hFSH or hMG (150 IU) in normal ovulatory controls (upper panel) and PCOS patients (lower panel). A significant increase in plasma LH levels is only minimal and transient (29). *Abbreviations*: hFSH, human follicle-stimulating hormone; LH, luteinizing hormone; hMG, human menopausal gonadotropin; PCOS, polycystic ovary syndrome.

the first GnRH-a administration, both endogenous FSH and LH are released from the hypophysis and, as mentioned earlier, the flare-up effect is more marked for LH than for FSH (11–13). Consequently, E2 secretion is stimulated and, as discussed below, the magnitude of E2 variation proves to be the best predictor of the ovarian sensitivity to gonadotropins. Thus, determination of plasma LH does not appear relevant during the flare-up period.

In contrast, measurements of plasma LH are routinely performed at the time of hypophyseal desensitization to make sure that gonadotropin secretion is adequately downregulated after a long-term administration of the GnRH-a. It is well documented that both the rapidity to achieve desensitization and the degree of LH suppression are critically dependent on numerous factors: The type of molecule, the time of its first administration in the cycle, the dose and duration of GnRH-a administration, and molecule formulation (32). As long as GnRH-a administration is maintained, the hypophysis is refractory to GnRH action, as attested by the disappearance of LH pulsatile secretion and a lack of response to exogenous GnRH or estradiol benzoate administration (33–35). It is also well documented that both intensity and duration of LH suppression are dose-dependent (36,37).

However, some questions remain unanswered regarding the state of hypophyseal desensitization. One of them is to elucidate the reasons why there is an inconstant need for higher amount of exogenous gonadotropins to obtain an adequate ovarian response. It is commonly stated that the more profound the hypophyseal desensitization, the worse the ovarian response to stimulation. This has led to the proposal of using a lower dose of GnRH-a specifically for patients with previous low response to gonadotropins. However, the effectiveness of this dose reduction is still a matter of debate.

In fact, the main issue to be addressed is the actual assessment of the residual bioactive LH secretion. Indeed, regular immunometric assays of LH cannot properly reflect the residual hormonal LH bioactivity. After a two-week GnRH administration, LH secretion seems to be completely suppressed but LH concentrations remain measurable by immunometric assays in relation to persistent secretion of presumed nonbiologically active hormones (α subunits and/or molecules with modified glycosylation) (38). It has also been shown that a daily GnRH-a administration leads to a partial release of measurable α subunit (34) and that stopping the daily agonist administration induces a sharp decrease in both plasma dimeric LH and α subunit concentrations (39,40) (Fig. 39.4). Thus, it is likely that the residual measurable LH secretion depends on both the type of GnRH-a formulation and the duration of administration.

This uncertainty in the evaluation of residual bioactive LH secretion is also reflected in the choice of gonadotropins. Indeed, with reference to the two-cell-two-gonadotropin theory, it could be predicted that administration of purified or recombinant FSH during the stimulation period would

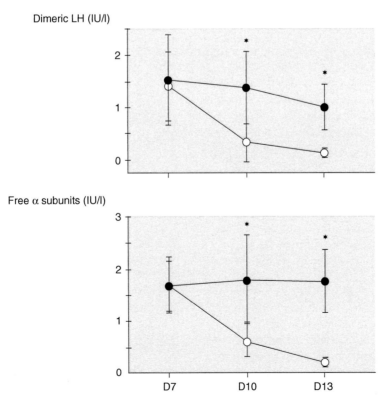

Figure 39.4 Effects of the duration of gonadotropin-releasing hormone (GnRH) agonist administration on plasma LH concentrations. Plasma dimeric LH and subunit concentrations in patients treated with GnRH agonist (decapeptyl 0.1 mg daily) for 7 (O) or 14 days (●) in short-term protocol. This figure illustrates that stopping GnRH-a administration at day 7 leads to a sharp and parallel decrease in both dimeric LH and subunit plasma concentrations. Thus, in contrast to GnRH antagonist, a daily agonist administration sustains a partial release of measurable subunit and LH from the hypophysis (39). *Abbreviation*: LH, luteinizing hormone.

not be effective in stimulating E2 production, but it is clear that it is not the case. Moreover, the largest studies previously published definitely showed that FSH administration alone is sufficient to yield an adequate number of good-quality oocytes and embryos and to obtain a high implantation rate (41,42). Other authors argued that, for some patients or in some situations with high LH suppression induced by some agonist formulations, the residual LH secretion may not be sufficient to ensure an appropriate E2 secretion. Westergaard et al. (43) as well as Fleming et al. (44) tried to identify this subgroup of patients by evaluating the outcome of ART cycles according to the plasma level of residual LH at the time of desensitization or during the mid-follicular phase. Selecting a subgroup of patients whose residual plasma levels were lower than 0.5 IU/l, they found a trend for a reduced plasma E2 concentration at the time of hCG administration and for a lower yield of oocytes and number of embryos. However, the rate of blastocyst development was unaffected. Thus, these data confirm the inability of plasma LH measurements to detect those patients who would need addition of LH to sustain ovarian stimulation. With another approach, Loumaye et al. (45) analyzed the E2/oocyte ratio, based on the previous observation in hypogonadotropic hypogonadal women, that the amplitude of E2 secretion per follicle is related directly to the dose of recombinant LH administered. In this model, it was shown that only a small population (less than 6% of patients) might benefit from exogenous LH administration and that measuring plasma LH levels after down-regulation is useless to identify this subgroup of patients. Collectively these data suggest that the LH threshold under which steroidogenesis and folliculogenesis may be impaired cannot be properly assessed by standard immunometric determination of plasma LH concentrations.

Finally, the introduction of GnRH antagonists in the field of ART therapy has provided another model for evaluating the need for LH in ART cycles. Acting as a competitor to endogenous GnRH at the receptor level, GnRH antagonists induce a rapid and reversible reduction in LH secretion without any interference with the hypophyseal machinery. In that respect, the hormonal situation induced by GnRH antagonist is easier to assess than that induced by GnRH agonist: A parallel decrease in plasma dimeric and α subunit LH concentrations is elicited by GnRH antagonist administration (46,47) and a rapid recovery of the pituitary–gonadal axis is predictable after discontinuation of treatment. A dose-finding study (48) showed that plasma LH concentrations decrease in a dose-dependent manner following the administration of Org 37462 (ganirelix), and no endogenous LH surge was observed whatever the dose used. This study also pointed out that the remaining endogenous LH concentrations during GnRH antagonist treatment may become critical when pituitary suppression is too profound. Consequently, assessment of residual LH concentrations could be helpful, specifically for patients who received a single (3 mg) GnRH antagonist dose.

To sum up these data on LH secretion during GnRH analog therapy (Fig. 39.5), we may consider that the

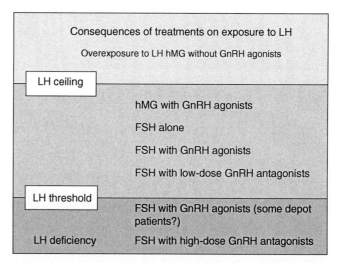

Figure 39.5 The LH threshold and ceiling concepts. This figure illustrates the interval defined by the respective values of LH threshold and LH ceiling. Within this interval, LH support is presumably sufficient to ensure steroidogenesis without negatively affecting follicular growth. Both gonadotropins and GnRH analogs jointly modify circulating LH levels in such a way that the residual plasma LH concentrations are most often included within these limits. *Abbreviation*: LH, luteinizing hormone.

limits of endogenous LH levels required for complete steroidogenesis and folliculogenesis are those defined by the LH ceiling and threshold values. Within this interval, residual endogenous LH secretion seems to be sufficient to provide adequate androgen synthesis to ensure E2 secretion and to participate in the control of follicular growth. This figure also emphasizes that the need for LH supplementation depends on the type and on the dose of GnRH analog prescribed.

STEROID PROFILES DURING OVARIAN STIMULATION FOR ART CYCLES

In contrast to gonadotropin hormones, the evaluation of steroid production is routinely performed during ART cycles. Indeed, plasma E2 measurement is a good indicator of granulosa cell differentiation and is helpful to evaluate follicular maturity before triggering ovulation. Plasma progesterone (P) determination has been also recommended to seek for any premature luteinization, which is uncommon since GnRH analogs are regularly prescribed in ART cycles. Finally, plasma androgen measurements are rarely performed except for clinical research.

Estradiol

E2 plays a critical role in the endocrine reproductive system, being involved in many tissues sensitive such as the uterus (cervical mucus production, endometrial proliferation), and the hypothalamic–pituitary network (mid-cycle LH surge). In contrast, the autocrine role of E2 in follicle development, firstly described in rats, has not been proven in humans, where E2 is not required for follicular growth. Thus, E2 synthesis is merely associated with dominant follicle development and plasma E2 concentration is a useful index for assessing follicular maturity.

During stimulation for ART cycles, plasma E2 measurements are routinely performed to adjust gonadotropin doses in conjunction with data obtained by ultrasound. Indeed, it is well admitted that E2 synthesis is directly related to follicular size and that the contribution of mature follicles to E2 output has been estimated at 200 pg/ml. Another aspect to be considered during ART cycles is the pattern of E2 secretion. In the early 1980s, at a time where GnRH analogs were not available for preventing any endogenous LH surge, particular attention has been paid to the pattern of plasma E2 levels. The Norfolk group described several E2 patterns well correlated to the outcome of the cycle (49).

When GnRH-a protocols became available, it was suggested that an increase in plasma E2 concentrations for six consecutive days could be optimal for the success of the cycle (50). Owing to the extreme diversity of protocols used in ART cycles, no optimal E2 pattern could be demonstrated. Nevertheless, some considerations seem to be valid whatever the protocol used. A plateau of plasma E2 values for more than three days is commonly associated with a poor outcome of the ART cycle. Conversely, measurements of plasma E2 are helpful to detect the risk of excessive ovarian response and to decide to proceed to coasting or cancellation of the cycle or of the embryo transfer. For these reasons, it seems that plasma E2 determination should be included in the monitoring of ART cycle treatment while some people claim that ultrasound assessment may be sufficient to make stimulation friendly.

Regarding hormonal determinations, plasma E2 variations can be used as a sensitive index of ovarian responsiveness to gonadotropins and, to some extent, as a predictor of the outcome of the ART cycle. For instance, following administration of a fixed dose of exogenous FSH (300 IU) at day 3 of the cycle, the relative increment of plasma E2 concentrations seems to be a better predictor of the ovarian response than the day 3 FSH value (51). Other authors (52) suggested that an early determination of plasma E2, after only few days of gonadotropin administration, may be useful to predict the subsequent ovarian response. Altogether, these data underline that an early determination of plasma E2 during ovarian stimulation may be a helpful predictor of a poor or high ovarian response.

A similar approach, based on the evaluation of E2 response to the endogenous gonadotropin flare-up induced by GnRH-a, was proposed by Padilla et al. (12). The test (Lupron screening test) aims at evaluating the increase in plasma E2 after a subcutaneous administration of leuprolide acetate (1 mg) on days 2–4 of the menstrual cycle. The authors found a good correlation between the E2 response and the ovarian response to controlled ovarian stimulation (COS) and described four patterns of E2 variations with different cycle outcomes. In contrast, Winslow et al., (53) using the same agonist, correlated the relative increment of plasma E2 from day 2 to day 3 (ΔE2) with the ovarian response to stimulation.

Table 39.1 Stimulation Tests Predictive of the Ovarian Response to Gonadotropins. Different Stimulation Tests Proposed to Evaluate Ovarian Sensitivity to Gonadotropins: HFSH (300 IU IM) (Efort Test) or Leuprolide Acetate (1 mg SC) or Triptorelin (0.1 mgSC after a Pretreatment by Norethisterone) (Gnrh-a Tests) are Administered at Day 2 of the Cycle. Plasma E2 Levels are Determined at Day 2 before Stimulation and 24 Hours Later at Day 3. ΔE2 Represents Differences between Plasma E2 Values. Figures Indicate the E2. Cut-Off Values Predictive of an Adequate Ovarian Response

Tests	ΔE2 (pg/ml)
Exogenous FSH (EFORT)	>30
Lupron screening test	>20
Triptorelin screening test	>5

Abbreviations: hFSH, human follicle-stimulating hormone; GnRH, gonadotropin-releasing hormone.

In a study using triptorelin as GnRH-a, we also demonstrated that the ΔE2 value is reduced by a pretreatment with progestogen in programmed cycles, but the relationship between the early events of the follicular phase and the subsequent pregnancy rate still exists (54). In clinical practice, determination of the E2 response to the flare-up effect of the agonist is relevant for an early detection of potential poor responders and for tailoring gonadotropin administration accordingly. To sum up these data, the predictive E2 values for each test are presented in Table 39.1.

When using long-term GnRH-a protocol, determination of plasma E2 is also recommended to assess if the hypophyseal desensitization is effective at the ovarian level. Indeed, as previously mentioned, plasma LH immunometric evaluation cannot adequately reflect the reality of pituitary desensitization. It is commonly stated that plasma E2 must be lower than 50 pg/ml to make sure that ovarian activity is actually suppressed, which usually occurs after two weeks of GnRH-a administration. Starting GnRH-a administration in the mid-luteal phase (55,56) or using a long-acting formulation of the agonist (57,58) may allow more rapid desensitization than when using short-acting formulations at the early follicular phase. However, it is still unclear whether there is any clinical advantage in achieving a prompt and profound desensitization. It was even suggested that a prompt desensitization would induce an ovarian refractoriness to exogenous gonadotropins (57). In every situation, it is recommended to start ovarian stimulation with FSH only when ovarian activity is suppressed, whatever the duration of GnRH-a administration needed to achieve it.

Finally, the recent availability of GnRH antagonist in ART cycles has challenged the interest of plasma E2 determination. Indeed, studies performed with GnRH antagonist protocol showed that the pattern of plasma E2 during the stimulation period actually differs from that observed with GnRH agonist protocol. Indeed, E2 plasma values are higher before the introduction of the GnRH antagonist. In contrast, when the antagonist is injected to control the LH surge, plasma E2 levels modestly increase, remain constant, or even decrease. However, there is no evidence that modest variations in plasma E2 have any negative impact on cycle outcome. Nevertheless, in clinical practice, physicians should be aware that adjustment of gonadotropin preparations used for GnRH agonist protocol cannot be strictly applied to regimens with GnRH antagonist.

Progesterone

Before the introduction of GnRH analogs in ART cycles, detection of premature endogenous LH surges was a constant concern because LH surges usually occurred when follicular development was still uncompleted with a high risk of oocyte retrieval or fertilization failure. At that time, determination of plasma progesterone (P) was considered as a complementary tool to detect partial luteinization of granulosa cells attributed to some small or short LH surges that could not have been detected even by daily LH measurement. The current use of both GnRH agonist and antagonist, highly effective to prevent LH surges, has limited the need for plasma P determination. However, measurement of this hormone is still recommended in different situations.

Plasma P concentration is commonly measured at the time of hypophyseal desensitization. Indeed, it seems worthwhile to make sure that the corpus luteum is not still active and has not been inadvertently rescued by the GnRH-a flare-up or by a spontaneous pregnancy. Moreover, at that time, if cyst formation is observed at ultrasound, any increase in plasma P concentrations could indicate the functional nature of the cyst and lead to perform ovarian puncture before FSH administration. Indeed, ovarian stimulation should not be started in a hormonal environment that may be deleterious for the oocyte or the endometrium. An increased steroid secretion at that time requires to extend the administration of GnRH agonist and to postpone ovarian stimulation. Similarly, it has been recommended to measure plasma P before starting ovarian stimulation in GnRH antagonist protocol and to postpone it if P values are >1.4 ng/ml (59).

With a similar concern regarding cycle outcome, special attention has been paid to other situations where an increase in plasma P is observed during the period of ovarian stimulation.

The first situation refers to the endocrine consequences of the flare-up effect induced by GnRH-a when a short-term protocol has been prescribed. As previously mentioned, the initial agonist administration induces a sharp increase in both gonadotropin and steroid secretion (60). Some reports (61–63) showed that increased plasma P levels during the early follicular phase may adversely affect follicular development, oocyte quality, and eventually the success rate of the cycle. However, these conclusions have been challenged by other studies.

For Sims et al., (64) it is only beyond a threshold of plasma P values that impairment of follicular development may be observed. Furthermore, a prospective randomized study demonstrated that cycle outcome was similar in two groups of patients pretreated or not by a progestogen that completely prevented any plasma P increase in the flare-up period (54). Thus, there is no evidence that any increase in plasma P is detrimental at the very early follicular phase of the cycle. It is no longer necessary to measure P levels during the flare-up of short-term GnRH a protocol.

During the late part of ovarian stimulation, plasma P determination should be performed. Indeed, despite an effective suppression of endogenous gonadotropins by GnRH analogs, increment in plasma P has been reported in a large range (5% to 35%) of stimulated cycles. Because this P increase usually occurs in absence of any LH surge, it cannot be considered as a premature luteinization. Several questions have been raised regarding this P elevation at the time of hCG administration.

First, the issue of the potential adverse effect of P increase on the cycle outcome has been addressed but is still a matter of debate: From the first reported studies, some authors (65–67) claimed a negative effect on the pregnancy rate through inadequate endometrial preparation, while others (68–71) could not find any significant relationship. A meta-analysis reported in 2007 (72) concluded for the lack of negative impact of elevated P values on pregnancy rate. However, this meta-analysis did not take into account the different threshold values used in these studies. Another study performed in patients treated with GnRH agonist and antagonist protocol eventually concluded for a negative impact of P elevation on cycle outcome above a threshold value of 1.5 ng/ml (73).

In addition, the mechanisms that account for this P plasma rise despite suppressed endogenous gonadotropins are not clearly understood. Surprisingly, a high ovarian response to FSH as well as an exposure to large doses of exogenous FSH for inadequate ovarian response can be associated with a risk of elevated plasma P. Therefore, the pathogenesis of P rise during the late phase of ovarian stimulation is still unclear (74). Indeed, P increases have been attributed to an over-response to normal doses of FSH with a high amount of granulosa cells or has been considered as the early expression of an occult ovarian failure (75). Furthermore, the contribution of the adrenal gland must be also considered because dexamethasone administration induces a partial reduction in plasma P levels (76).

Nevertheless, it is likely that the impact of exogenous gonadotropins on the ovary predominantly accounts for this process (77). FSH plays a major role by stimulating granulosa cell P production. The contribution of LH is more complex due to its dual effect on P synthesis by theca cells. In addition, LH may act on granulosa cells in the late part of the stimulation and participate in the P rise. Therefore, reducing the intensity of the ovarian response to FSH seems to be the best option to prevent any rise of P at the end of the stimulation.

ANDROGENS

Determination of plasma androgens, namely testosterone and Δ4 androstenedione, is not currently performed during monitoring of ART cycles. Indeed, while androgen production is strongly dependent on LH secretion, there is no evidence that assessment of androgen secretion is helpful in evaluating LH bioactivity. This is partly related to the fact that both ovary and adrenal gland contribute to androgen production in women with normal reproductive function. Conversely, excessive androgen production is commonly detected by plasma androgen measurement. With the exception of partial enzymatic adrenal defects where 17OH progesterone (17OHP) is helpful for diagnosis, most of hyperandrogenism situations are related to ovarian hyperandrogenism with or without LH hypersecretion.

During the last two decades, it became more evident that assessment of ovarian morphology by transvaginal probes allows a more accurate evaluation of polycystic ovary syndrome (PCOS) than plasma androgen measurement. However, some reports in monkeys (78) indicated that Testosterone (T) actually exerts a stimulatory effect on granulosa cell proliferation in human beings and may be involved in follicular recruitment. It is now believed that most of the effects of LH on folliculogenesis are actually mediated by androgens. In line with this concept, some studies reported a close relationship between baseline T values on day 3 and the ovarian response to FSH (79,80).

However, determination of plasma T is still highly dependent on the type of immunoassays used and a huge inter-assay variability has been reported (81). Testosterone measurement could not be the best parameter to assess theca cell function. Indeed, it has been recently shown that determining 17OHP concentrations following administration of GnRH agonist could be a better way to predict the ovarian response to FSH (82). Additionally, another study mentioned that the flare-up effect of GnRH-a induced by short-term protocol is associated with an increased androgen production. However, there is no significant evidence that oocyte quality may consequently be reduced (83). To sum up these data, it does seem that determination of plasma T should not be routinely included in the hormonal setting before ovarian stimulation, but further clinical research is required to assess its interest during last part of ovarian stimulation.

INHIBINS A AND B

Inhibins A and B are secreted from granulosa cells during the early follicular phase FSH secretion but additionally regulate FSH secretion throughout a negative pituitary feedback (84,85). These two heterodimers, composed of an α subunit and one of the two β subunits forming inhibin A (βA) and inhibin B (βB), also exhibit unique patterns of expression and secretion during the menstrual cycle. In vitro studies demonstrated that inhibin βB-subunit messenger ribonucleic acid (mRNA) is expressed predominantly in small antral follicles and βA mRNA is expressed in the preovulatory follicle in humans, whereas α-subunit mRNA expression is similar at both follicle stages (86). Therefore, small antral follicles have the potential to secrete inhibin B, whereas preovulatory follicles predominantly secrete inhibin A.

Many of the early observations concerning the physiology of inhibins were based on the relatively nonspecific Monash RIA, which detected both dimeric inhibins A and B as well as the inhibin α subunit. The availability of specific two-site assays for dimeric inhibin A and B measured by enzyme-linked immunosorbent (ELISA) (87) has led to reconsider the usefulness of their measurement in clinical practice. Serum inhibin B value in the early follicular phase of the menstrual cycle was shown to be a valuable tool to evaluate the size of the follicular cohort (88). Moreover, the FSH dependence of inhibin A and B secretion has been demonstrated in regularly menstruating women with normal ovaries as well as in women with PCOS (89,90).

Consequently, several studies have been performed to assess whether inhibin A and B measurements may be predictive of the ovarian response to gonadotropins, of the risk of hyperstimulation as well as of the pregnancy rate in controlled ovarian hyperstimulation. The results of the first study (91) indicated that inhibin A and pro αC are well correlated with E2 values and the number of follicles (>10 mm) during FSH stimulation, and may be useful markers for monitoring the effects of gonadotropin stimulation. However, a subsequent study (92) reported that neither inhibin A nor inhibin B measured at the time of human chorionic gonadotropin (hCG) administration provided additional information in predicting successful outcome over age and number of oocytes.

In clinical perspective, it is evident that the most useful markers are those that can be assessed in the early stage of ovarian stimulation. Therefore, other analyses were focused on the predictive value of inhibin B measurement as a marker of follicular recruitment. Indeed, it did appear that inhibin B measurement between days 4 and 6 of FSH stimulation provided an early indicator of the number of recruited follicles destined to form mature oocytes (93,94). Moreover, another study (95) showed that a similar relationship between inhibin B measured after two days of FSH stimulation and oocyte number may be applied in both normal and low responders. Therefore, inhibin B measurement in the early stage of ovarian stimulation may provide useful information to clinicians in making decision regarding cancellation of the cycle or modulation of the gonadotropin dose. Consequently, it has been stated that inhibin B determination on day 3 is likely to be a good predictor of the ovarian response to gonadotropins at least for patients treated with protocols that include hMG and GnRH antagonist (96). However, more reliable parameters of ovarian reserve have been described.

ANTI-MÜLLERIAN HORMONE

Anti-Müllerian hormone (AMH), a member of the transforming growth factor beta (TGF–β) family, is produced by granulosa cells (97). The highest level of AMH expression is present in granulosa cells of secondary, preantral, and small antral follicles up to 6 mm in diameter, (98) whereas, in follicles growing into dominance, this expression is progressively reduced (99,100). Consequently, AMH is barely detectable at birth, reaches the highest values after puberty, then decreases progressively with age and becomes undetectable at menopause (101,102). Serum AMH levels have been shown to strongly correlate with the number of antral follicles (103,104) and have the major advantage over other markers of ovarian reserve (FSH, E2, and inhibin B) of being cycle-independent. This allows blood sampling at any period of the cycle (105,106).

The main interest of measuring AMH prior to ART cycles is actually related to its ability to predict the ovarian responsiveness to FSH. It has been shown that as the number of antral follicles in the ovary is proportionally related to the size of primordial follicle stock from which they were recruited, (107) the antral follicular count (AFC) may be a useful predictor of poor response in the in vitro fertilization (IVF) program (108). Some studies have reported that AMH could also be one of the best predictors of the ovarian response to hyperstimulation (109,110) and even – albeit in only one study – predict the chance of becoming pregnant after IVF (111).

A systematic review has assessed the actual accuracy of AMH as a prognostic factor for the outcome of IVF/intracytoplasmic sperm injection (ICSI) treatment compared with AFC (112). Thirteen studies reporting on the capacity of AMH to predict ovarian response and/or non-pregnancy for IVF cycles, and considered suitable for data extraction and meta-analysis, were identified (104,113–124). Receiver Operating Characteristic (ROC) curves showed a high accuracy for AMH and AFC for the prediction of poor ovarian response, but limited accuracy for non-pregnancy prediction. Furthermore, these data did not suggest a better predictive ability for AMH than for AFC because the difference was not statistically significant ($p = 0.73$).

However, AMH determination has some advantages over AFC. Indeed, it does need to be carried out on a specific day of the cycle, because AMH levels fluctuate only marginally and prediction by samples of any cycle day will be equally accurate (105,120,125). Currently, the availability of the AMH assay may present some problems, but surely it will soon become part of one of the large automated platforms, with inherent validity checks and limited assay variation. In contrast, AFC necessitates skilled ultrasound operators who carefully identify, measure, and count ovarian follicles. Although observer bias may be limited technically, (126,127) a new source of bias may arise from the fact that the ultrasound operator is aware of the cut-off for test judgment and may become influenced by the consequences of the test for the treatment of the couple. Such test inflation has been suggested from a study in older IVF patients who were allowed or refused IVF treatment on the basis of this test (128). Also, AFC has to be carried out in the early follicular phase of the cycle, although variation of counts across the cycle may be very modest (129).

Finally, the performance for non-pregnancy prediction is clearly poor for both AMH and AFC. This observation makes sense because AMH, like AFC, is strongly thought to represent only the size of the cohort of FSH-sensitive follicles continuously present in the ovary while the relation between quantity and oocyte or embryo quality is much less clear.

Another issue to be addressed deals with the interest of measuring plasma AMH levels during ovarian stimulation. From experimental data mainly obtained in rodents, the potential functions of AMH are inhibition of the initial recruitment of primordial follicles (130), inhibition of aromatase activity in granulosa cells, (131,132) and decrease of FSH-stimulated follicle growth in the mouse, both in vitro and in vivo (133).

These data suggest that AMH is a negative regulator of follicle growth and reduces follicle sensitivity to FSH. Conversely, it has been suggested that AMH expression might be regulated by FSH itself. Indeed, in human follicular fluid, FSH exerts a negative influence on AMH secretion in small follicles (134). Furthermore, in vitro FSH treatment significantly reduced AMH expression in cultured granulosa cells retrieved from patients with PCOS (135). Additionally, in PCOS patients, during administration of low doses of recombinant hFSH according to a chronic low-dose step-up protocol to mimic the typical pattern of the FSH secretion of the early follicular phase of normal non-stimulated cycles, a significant AMH decrease was gradually observed up to the day of follicular dominance (136). Even if the precise mechanism is still not clearly understood, it is likely that the decrease in serum AMH observed prior to the establishment of dominance during FSH treatment in PCOS patients results from the shift of small antral follicles to larger ones expressing less AMH. Similarly, during COS for IVF in normo-ovulatory women, three studies have reported a marked serum AMH decline up to more than 50% in close relationship with the diminution of the small antral follicular number and the establishment of multifollicular dominance (99,137,138).

Therefore, in contrast to the physiological follicular phase where no significant change in plasma AMH levels is usually reported, (137,139) a decrease in AMH level can be mainly observed in situations such as ovarian stimulation in PCOS women or during COS in normal women undergoing IVF. Presumably, this decrease in plasma AMH levels might also result from the evolution of the unselected follicles to atresia (137). Accordingly, a contemporary decrease in the number of small follicles was observed at ultrasound in the IVF study (99). Overall, these data indicate that measurement of plasma AMH levels is not actually useful during ovarian stimulation, except in studies designed to investigate the regulation of follicular development and arrest.

CONCLUSIONS

It appears from this review that the endocrine characteristics of ART cycles depend largely on the drugs used to achieve COS. It is clear that, while FSH therapy is absolutely required in each stimulation, assessment of plasma FSH cannot predict the adequacy of FSH supply and should not be routinely determined. As far as plasma LH determinations are concerned, immunometric LH assays cannot properly reflect the bioactivity of the circulating residual LH following GnRH analog administration. Furthermore, there is no evidence that plasma LH measurement could be useful to detect patients who might benefit from LH supplementation during ART cycles. Consequently, plasma LH assessments can be restricted in order to ensure that there is not excessive pituitary desensitization.

Conversely, while minimizing the cost of ART cycle monitoring and paying more attention to ultrasound data during ovarian stimulation is proposed nowadays, a simultaneous assessment of E2 secretion should be recommended to assess the hormonal profile. Regarding plasma progesterone determination, it seems relevant in the final part of ovarian stimulation because values above a certain threshold (presumably 1.5 ng/ml) should lead the clinician to cryopreserve all the embryos. While baseline measurement of plasma androgen might partly predict the ovarian responsiveness to FSH, there is no evidence that androgen measurement is useful during ovarian stimulation. Finally, AMH determination is highly predictive of the potential responsiveness to FSH and should be used instead of inhibin B measurement to determine the starting dose of gonadotropins.

REFERENCES

1. Short R. Steroids in the follicular fluid and the corpus luteum of the mare: A "two-cell type" theory of ovarian steroid synthesis. J Endocrinol 1962; 24: 59–63.

2. Messinis IE, Templeton AA. The importance of follicle-stimulating hormone increase for folliculogenesis. Hum Reprod 1990; 5: 153–6.

3. Brown J. Pituitary control of ovarian function – concepts derived from gonadotrophin therapy. Aust NZ J Obstet Gynaecol 1978; 18: 47–54.

4. Baird DT. A model for follicular selection and ovulation: lessons from superovulation. J Steroid Biochem 1987; 27: 15–23.

5. The European Recombinant Human LH Study Group. Recombinant human luteinizing hormone (LH) to support recombinant human follicle-stimulating hormone (FSH)-induced follicular development in LH and FSH-deficient anovulatory women: a dosefinding study. J Clin Endocrinol Metab 1998; 83: 1507–14.

6. Le Cotonnec JY, Porchet HC, Beltrami V, et al. Clinical pharmacology of recombinant human follicle-stimulating hormone (FSH). I. Comparative pharmacokinetics with urinary human FSH. Fertil Steril 1994; 61: 669–78.

7. Diczfalusy E, Harlin J. Clinical pharmacological studies on human menopausal gonadotrophin. Hum Reprod 1988; 3: 21–7.

8. Ben-Rafael Z, Strauss JFD, Mastroianni L, Flickinger GL. Differences in ovarian stimulation in human menopausal gonadotropin treated women may be related to follicle-stimulating hormone accumulation. Fertil Steril 1986; 46: 586–92.

9. Mizunuma H, Takagi T, Yamada K, et al. Ovulation induction by step-down administration of purified urinary follicle-stimulating hormone in patients with polycystic ovarian syndrome. Fertil Steril 1991; 55: 1195–6.

10. Van Weissenbruch MM, Schoemaker HC, Drexhage HA. Pharmaco-dynamics of human menopausal gonadotrophin (HMG) and folliclestimulating hormone (FSH). The importance of the FSH concentration in initiating follicular growth in polycystic ovary-like disease. Hum Reprod 1993; 8: 813–21.

11. Lemay A, Metha AE, Tolis G, et al. Gonadotropins and estradiol responses to single intranasal or subcutaneous administration of a luteinizing hormone releasing hormone agonist in the early follicular phase. Fertil Steril 1983; 39: 668–73.

12. Padilla SL, Smith RD, Garcia JE. The Lupron screening test: tailoring the use of leuprolide acetate in ovarian stimulation for in vitro fertilization. published erratum appears in. Fertil Steril 1991; 56: 79–83.

13. Hugues JN, Attalah M, Herve F, et al. Effects of short-term GnRH agonist–human menopausal gonadotrophin stimulation in patients pre-treated with progestogen. Hum Reprod 1992; 7: 1079–84.

14. Deaton JL, Bauguess P, Huffman CS, Miller KA. Pituitary response to early follicular-phase minidose gonadotropin releasing hormone agonist (GnRH()) therapy: evidence for a second flare. J Assist Reprod Genet 1996; 13: 390–4.

15. Scott RT, Carey KD, Leland M, Navot D. Gonadotropin responsiveness to ultralow-dose leuprolide acetate administration in baboons. Fertil Steril 1993; 59: 1124–8.

16. Bständig B, Cédrin-Durnerin I, Hugues JN. Effectiveness of low dose of gonadotropin releasing hormone agonist on hormonal flare-up. J Assist Reprod Genet 2000; 17: 113–17.

17. Parinaud J, Oustry P, Perineau M, et al. Randomized trial of three luteinizing hormone-releasing hormone-analogues used for ovarian stimulation in an in vitro fertilization program. Fertil Steril 1992; 57: 1265–8.

18. Matikainen T, Ding YQ, Vergara M, et al. Differing responses of plasma bioactive and immunoreactive follicle-stimulating hormone and luteinizing hormone to gonadotropin-releasing hormone antagonist and agonist treatments in postmenopausal women. J Clin Endocrinol Metab 1992; 75: 820–5.

19. Huhtaniemi IT, Dahl KD, Rannikko S, Hsueh AJ. Serum bioactive and immunoreactive follicle-stimulating hormone in prostatic cancer patients during gonadotropin-releasing hormone agonist treatment and after orchidectomy. J Clin Endocrinol Metab 1988; 66: 308–13.

20. Gonzalez-Barcena D, Vadillo Buenfil M, Garcia Procel E, et al. Inhibition of luteinizing hormone, follicle-stimulating hormone and sex-steroid levels in men and women with a potent antagonist analog of luteinizing hormone-releasing hormone, Cetrorelix (SB-75). Eur J Endocrinol 1994; 131: 286–92.

21. Yong EL, Baird DT, Yates R, et al. Hormonal regulation of the growth and steroidogenic function of human granulosa cells. J Clin Endocrinol Metab 1992; 74: 842–9.

22. Stanger JD, Yovich JL. Reduced in vitro fertilization of human oocytes from patients with raised basal

luteinizing hormone levels during the follicular phase. Br J Obstet Gynaecol 1985; 92: 385–93.

23. Regan L, Owen EJ, Jacobs HS. Hypersecretion of luteinising hormone, infertility, and miscarriage. Lancet 1990; 336: 1141–4.

24. Ashkenazi J, Farhi J, Orvieto R, et al. Polycystic ovary syndrome patients as oocyte donors: the effect of ovarian stimulation protocol on the implantation rate of the recipient. Fertil Steril 1995; 64: 564–7.

25. Balasch J, Fabregues F, Carmona R, Casamitjana R, Tena-sempere M. Ovarian luteinizing hormone priming preceding Foolicle-Stimulating hormone stimulation: clinical and endocrine effects in women with long-term hypogonadotropic hypogonadism. J Clin Endocrinol Metab 2009; 94: 2367–73.

26. Hillier SG. Ovarian stimulation with recombinant gonadotropins: LH as an adjunct to FSH. In: Jacobs HS, ed. The new frontier in ovulation induction. Carnforth, UK: Parthenon Publishing, 1993: 39–47.

27. Loumaye E, Engrand P, Shoham Z, et al. Clinical evidence for an LH «ceiling» effect induced by administration of recombinant human LH during the late follicular phase of stimulated cycles in WHO type I and type II anovulation. Hum Reprod 2003; 18: 314–22.

28. Hugues JN, Soussis J, Calderon I, et al. On behalf of the recombinant LH Study Group. Does the addition of recombinant Luteinizing Hormone (r-hLH) in WHO Group II anovulatory women over-responding to FSH treatment reduce the number of developing follicles? A dose finding study. Hum Reprod 2005; 20: 629–35.

29. Anderson RE, Cragun JM, Chang RJ, et al. A pharmacodynamic comparison of human urinary follicle-stimulating hormone and human menopausal gonadotropin in normal women and polycystic ovary syndrome. Fertil Steril 1989; 52: 216–20.

30. Le Cotonnec JY, Porchet HC, Beltrami V, Munafo A. Clinical pharmacology of recombinant human luteinizing hormone: Part I. Pharmacokinetics after intravenous administration to healthy female volunteers and comparison with urinary human luteinizing hormone. Fertil Steril 1998; 69: 189–94.

31. Balasch J, Fábregues F, Casamitjana R, et al. A pharmacokinetic and endocrine comparison of recombinant follicle-stimulating hormone and human menopausal gonadotrophin in polycystic ovary syndrome. Reprod Biomed Online 2003; 6: 296–301.

32. Hugues JN, Cédrin-Durnerin I. Revisiting gonadotrophin-releasing hormone agonist protocols and management of poor ovarian responses to gonadotrophins. Hum Reprod Update 1998; 4: 83–101.

33. Fraser HM. Effect of oestrogen on gonadotrophin release in stumptailed monkeys (Macaca arctoides) treated chronically with an agonist analogue of luteinizing hormone releasing hormone. J Endocrinol 1981; 91: 525–30.

34. Broekmans FJ, Bernardus RE, Broeders A, et al. Pituitary responsiveness after administration of a GnRH agonist depot formulation: decapeptyl CR. Clin Endocrinol (Oxf) 1993; 38: 579–87.

35. Caraty A, Locatelli A, Delaleu B, et al. Gonadotropinreleasing hormone (GnRH) agonists and GnRH antagonists do not alter endogenous GnRH secretion in short-term castrated rams. Endocrinology 1990; 127: 2523–9.

36. Broekmans FJ, Hompes PG, Lambalk CB, et al. Short term pituitary desensitization: effects of different

doses of the gonadotrophin-releasing hormone agonist triptorelin. Hum Reprod 1996; 11: 55–60.

37. Oppenheim DS, Bikkal H, Crowley WFJ, Klibanski A. Effects of chronic GnRH analogue administration on gonadotrophin and alpha-subunit secretion in postmenopausal women. Clin Endocrinol (Oxf) 1992; 36: 559–64.

38. Meldrum DR, Tsao Z, Monroe SE, et al. Stimulation of LH fragments with reduced bioactivity following GnRH agonist administration in women. J Clin Endocrinol Metab 1984; 58: 755–7.

39. Cedrin-Durnerin I, Bidart JM, Robert P, et al. Consequences on gonadotropin secretion of an early discontinuation of gonadotrophin-releasing hormone agonist administration in short-term protocol for in vitro fertilization. Hum Reprod 2000; 15: 1009–14.

40. Sungurtekin U, Jansen RP. Profound luteinizing hormone suppression after stopping the gonadotropin releasing hormone-agonist leuprolide acetate. Fertil Steril 1995; 63: 663–5.

41. Hedon B, Out HJ, Hugues JN, et al. Efficacy and safety of recombinant follicle stimulating hormone (Puregon) in infertile women pituitary-suppressed with triptorelin undergoing in vitro fertilization: a prospective, randomized, assessor- blind, multicentre trial. Hum Reprod 1995; 10: 3102–6.

42. Bergh C, Howles CM, Borg K, et al. Recombinant human follicle stimulating hormone (r-hFSH; Gonal- F) versus highly purified urinary FSH (Metrodin HP): results of a randomized comparative study in women undergoing assisted reproductive techniques. Hum Reprod 1997; 12: 2133–9.

43. Westergaard LG, Erb K, Laursen S, et al. The effect of human menopausal gonadotrophin and highly purified, urine - derived follicle stimulating hormone on the outcome of in vitro fertilization in down-regulated normogonadotrophic women. Hum Reprod 1996; 11: 1209–13.

44. Fleming R, Lloyd F, Herbert M, et al. Effects of profound suppression of luteinizing hormone during ovarian stimulation on follicular activity, oocyte and embryo function in cycles stimulated with purified follicle stimulating hormone. Hum Reprod 1998; 13: 1788–92.

45. Loumaye E, Engrand P, Howles CM. Assessment of the role of serum luteinizing hormone and estradiol response to follicle-stimulating hormone on in vitro fertilization treatment outcome. Fertil Steril 1997; 67: 889–99.

46. Mortola JF, Sathanandan M, Pavlou S, et al. Suppression of bioactive and immunoreactive follicle-stimulating hormone and luteinizing hormone levels by a potent gonadotropin-releasing hormone antagonist: pharmacodynamic studies. Fertil Steril 1989; 51: 957–63.

47. Fluker MR, Monroe SE, Marshall LA, Jaffe RB. Contrasting effects of a gonadotropin - releasing hormone agonist and antagonist on the secretion of free alpha subunit. Fertil Steril 1994; 61: 573–5.

48. The Ganirelix Dose-finding Study Group. A double blind, randomized, dose-finding study to assess the efficacy of the gonadotrophin-releasing hormone antagonist ganirelix (Org 37462) to prevent premature luteinizing hormone surges in women undergoing ovarian stimulation with recombinant follicle

stimulating hormone (Puregon). Hum Reprod 1998; 13: 3023–31.

49. Jones HW, Acosta A, Andrews MC, et al. The importance of the follicular phase to success and failure in in vitro fertilization. Fertil Steril 1983; 40: 317–21.

50. Levran D, Lopata A, Nayudu PL, et al. Analysis of the outcome of in vitro fertilization in relation to the timing of human chorionic gonadotrophin administration by the duration of oestradiol rise in stimulated cycles. Fertil Steril 1995; 44: 335–41.

51. Fanchin R, de Ziegler D, Olivennes F, et al. Exogenous follicle stimulating hormone ovarian reserve test (EFORT): a simple and reliable screening test for detecting 'poor responders' in in vitro fertilization. Hum Reprod 1994; 9: 1607–1.

52. Phelps JY, Levine AS, Hickman TN, et al. Day 4 estradiol levels predict pregnancy success in women undergoing controlled ovarian hyperstimulation for IVF. Fertil Steril 1998; 69: 1015–19.

53. Winslow KL, Toner JP, Brzyski RG, et al. The gonadotrophin-releasing hormone agonist stimulation test - a sensitive predictor of performance in the flare-up in vitro fertilization cycle. Fertil Steril 1991; 56: 711–17.

54. Cédrin-Durnerin I, Herve F, Huet-Pecqueux L, et al. Progestogen pretreatment in the short-term protocol does not affect the prognostic value of the oestradiol flare-up in response to a GnRH agonist. Hum Reprod 1995; 10: 2904–8.

55. Urbancsek J, Witthaus E. Midluteal buserelin is superior to early follicular phase buserelin in combined gonadotrophin-releasing hormone analog and gonadotrophin stimulation in in vitro fertilization. Fertil Steril 1996; 65: 966–71.

56. Ron-El R, Raziel A, Herman A, et al. Ovarian response in repetitive cycles induced by menotrophin alone or combined with gonadotrophin releasing hormone analogue. Hum Reprod 1990; 5: 427–30.

57. Gonen Y, Dirnfeld M, Goldman S, et al. The use of long-acting gonadotropin-releasing hormone agonist (GnRH-a; decapeptyl) and gonadotropins versus short-acting GnRH-a (buserelin) and gonadotropins before and during ovarian stimulation for in vitro fertilization (IVF). J In Vitro Fert Embryo Transf 1991; 8: 254–9.

58. Vauthier D, Lefebvre G. The use of gonadotropin releasing hormone analogs for in vitro fertilization: comparison between the standard form and long-acting formulation of D-Trp-6-luteinizing hormone-releasing hormone. Fertil Steril 1989; 51: 100–4.

59. Kolibianakis EM, Zikopoulos K, Smitz J, et al. Elevated P at initiation of stimulation is associated with a lower ongoing pregnancy rate after IVF using GnRH antagonist. Hum Reprod 2004; 19: 1525–9.

60. Goswami SK, Chakravarty BN, Kabir SN. Significance of an abnormal response during pituitary desensitization in an in vitro fertilization and embryo transfer program. J Assist Reprod Genet 1996; 13: 374–80.

61. Loumaye E, Vankrieken L, Depreester S, et al. Hormonal changes induced by short-term administration of gonadotropin-releasing hormone agonist during ovarian hyperstimulation for in vitro fertilization and their consequences for embryo development. Fertil Steril 1989; 51: 105–11.

62. Brzyski RG, Muasher SJ, Droesch K, et al. Follicular atresia associated with concurrent initiation of

63. gonadotropin-releasing hormone agonist and follicle-stimulating hormone for oocyte recruitment. Fertil Steril 1988; 50: 917–21.

63. Antoine JM, Firmin C, Alvarez S. Hormonal levels in late follicular phase with long and short regimen of GnRH agonists. Contracept Fertil Sex 1988; 16: 630–1.

64. Sims JA, Seltman HJ, Muasher SJ. Early follicular rise of serum progesterone concentration in response to a flare-up effect of gonadotrophin-releasing hormone agonist impairs follicular recruitment for in vitro fertilization. Hum Reprod 1994; 9: 235–40.

65. Fanchin R, de Ziegler D, Taieb J, et al. Premature elevation of plasma progesterone alters pregnancy rates of in vitro fertilization and embryo transfer. Fertil Steril 1993; 59: 1090–4.

66. Schoolcraft W, Sinton E, Schlenker T, et al. Lower pregnancy rate with premature luteinization during pituitary suppression with leuprolide acetate. Fertil Steril 1991; 55: 563–6.

67. Shulman A, Ghetler Y, Beyth Y, Ben-Nun I. The significance of an early (premature) rise of plasma progesterone in in vitro fertilization cycles induced by a "long protocol" of gonadotropin releasing hormone analogue and human menopausal gonadotropins. J Assist Reprod Genet 1996; 13: 207–11.

68. Edelstein MC, Seltman HJ, Cox BJ, et al. Progesterone levels on the day of human chorionic gonadotropin administration in cycles with gonadotropin-releasing hormone agonist suppression are not predictive of pregnancy outcome [see comments]. Fertil Steril 1990; 54: 853–7.

69. Givens CR, Schriock ED, Dandekar PV, Martin MC. Elevated serum progesterone levels on the day of human chorionic gonadotropin administration do not predict outcome in assisted reproduction cycles. Fertil Steril 1994; 62: 1011–17.

70. Abuzeid MI, Sasy MA. Elevated progesterone levels in the late follicular phase do not predict success of in vitro fertilization–embryo transfer. Fertil Steril 1996; 65: 981–5.

71. Hofmann GE, Khoury J, Johnson CA, et al. Premature luteinization during controlled ovarian hyperstimulation for in vitro fertilization–embryo transfer has no impact on pregnancy outcome. Fertil Steril 1996; 66: 980–6.

72. Venetis CA, Kolibianakis EM, Papanikolaou E, et al. Is progesterone elevation on the day of human chorionic gonadotrophin administration associated with the probability of pregnancy in in vitro fertilization? A systematic review and meta-analysis. Hum Reprod 2007; 13: 343–55.

73. Bosch E., Labarta E, Crespo J, et al. Circulating progesterone levels and ongoing pregnancy rates in controlled ovarian stimulation cycles for in vitro fertilization-analysis of over 4000 cycles. Hum Reprod 2010; 25: 2092–100.

74. Fanchin R, de Ziegler D, Castracane VD, et al. Physiopathology of premature progesterone elevation. Fertil Steril 1995; 64: 796–801.

75. Younis JS, Haddad S, Matisky MBA. Premature luteinization: Could it be an early manifestation of low ovarian reserve? Fertil Steril 1998; 69: 461–5.

76. Eldar-Geva T, Margalioth EJ, Brooks B, et al. Elevated serum progesterone levels during pituitary suppression

may signify adrenal hyperandrogenism. Fertil Steril 1997; 67: 959–61.

77. Fanchin R, Righini C, Olivennes F, et al. Premature plasma progesterone and androgen elevation are not prevented by adrenal suppression in in vitro fertilization. Fertil Steril 1997; 67: 115–19.

78. Vendola KA, Zhou J, Adesanya OO, et al. Androgens stimulate early stages of follicular growth in the primate ovary. J Clin Invest 1998; 101: 2622–9.

79. Barbieri RL, Sluss PM, Powers RD, et al. Association of body mass index, age, and cigarette smoking with serum testosterone levels in cycling women undergoing in vitro fertilization. Fertil Steril 2005; 83: 302–8.

80. Frattarelli JL, Gerber MD. Basal and cycle androgen levels correlate with in vitro fertilization stimulation parameters but do not predict pregnancy outcome. Fertil Steril 2006; 86: 51–7.

81. Boots LR, Porter S, Potter HD, Azziz R. Measurement of total serum testosterone levels using commercially available kits. High degree of between kit variability. Fertil Steril 1998; 69: 286–92.

82. Hugues JN, Theron-Gerard L, Coussieu C, et al. Assessment of theca cell function prior to controlled ovarian stimulation: the predictive value of serum basal / stimulated steroid levels. Hum Reprod 2010; 25: 228–34.

83. San Roman GA, Surrey ES, Judd HL, Kerin JF. A prospective randomized comparison of luteal phase versus concurrent follicular phase initiation of gonadotropin - releasing hormone agonist for in vitro fertilization. Fertil Steril 1992; 58: 744–9.

84. Vale WW, Hunseult A, Rivier C, Yu J. The inhibin/ activin family of hormones and growth factors. In: Sporn MA, Roberts AB, eds. Peptide Growth Factors and their Receptors: Handbook of Experimental Physiology. Berlin: Springer-Verlag, 1990: 95: 211–48.

85. Baird DT, Smith KB. Inhibin and related-peptides in the regulation of reproduction. Oxf Rev Reprod Biol 1993; 15: 191–232.

86. Roberts VJ, Barth S, El-Roely A, Yen SSC. Expression of inhibin / activin subunits and follistatin messenger ribonucleic acids and proteins in ovarian follicles and the corpus luteum during the human menstrual cycle. J Clin Endocrinol Metab 1993; 77: 1402–10.

87. Groome NP, Illingworth PJ, O'Brien M, et al. Detection of dimeric inhibin throughout the human menstrual cycle by two-site enzyme enzyme immuno-assay. Clin Endocrinol (Oxf) 1994; 40: 717–23.

88. Seifer DB, Lambert Messerlian G, Hogan JW, et al. Day 3 serum inhibin-B is predictive of assisted reproductive techniques outcome. Fertil Steril 1997; 67: 110–14.

89. Burger HG, Groome NG, Robertson DM. Both inhibin A and B respond to exogenous follicle-stimulating hormone in the follicular phase of the human menstrual cycle. J Clin Endocrinol Metab 1998; 83: 4167–9.

90. Elting MW, Kwee J, Schats R, et al. The rise of estradiol and inhibin B after acute stimulation with follicle-stimulating hormone predict the follicular size in women with polycystic ovary syndrome, regularly menstruating women with polycystic ovaries and regularly menstruating women with normal ovaries. J Clin Endocrinol Metab 2001; 86: 1589–95.

91. Lockwood GM, Muttukrishna S, Groome NP, Keight PG, Ledger WL. Circulating inhibins and activin A during GnRH-analogue down regulation and ovarian hyperstimulation with recombinant FSH for in vitro fertilization–embryo transfer. Clin Endocrinol 1996; 45: 741–8.

92. Hall JE, Welt CK, Cramer DW. Inhibin A and inhibin B reflect ovarian function in assisted reproduction but are less useful at predicting outcome. Hum Reprod 1999; 14: 409–15.

93. Pennarubia J, Balasch J, Fábregues F, et al. Day 5 inhibin serum concentrations are predictors of assisted reproductive technique outcome in cycles stimulated with gonadotrophin-releasing hormone agonist–gonadotrophin treatment. Hum Reprod 2000; 15: 1499–504.

94. Eldar-Geva T, Robertson DM, Cahir N, et al. Relationship between serum inhibin A. and B and ovarian follicle development after a daily fixed dosed administration of recombinant follicle-stimulating hormone. J Clin Endocrinol Metab 2000; 65: 607–13.

95. Eldar-Geva T, Margalioth EJ, Ben-Chetrit A, et al. Serum inhibin B levels measured early during FSH administration for IVF may be of value in predicting the number of oocytes to be retrieved in normal and low responders. Hum Reprod 2002; 17: 2331–7.

96. Engel JB, Felberbaum RE, Reissmann T, et al. Inhibin A/B in HMG or recombinant FSH ovarian stimulation with cetrorelix medication. Reprod Biomed Online 2001; 3: 104–8.

97. Lee MM, Donahoe PK, Hasegawa T, et al. Müllerian inhibiting substance in humans: normal levels from infancy to adulthood. J Clin Endocrinol Metab 1996; 81: 571–6.

98. Weenen C, Laven JS, Von Bergh AR, et al. Anti-Müllerian hormone expression pattern in the human ovary: Potential implications for initial and cyclic follicle recruitment. Mol Hum Reprod 2004; 10: 77–83.

99. Fanchin R, Schonauer LM, Righini C, et al. Serum anti-Müllerian hormone dynamics during controlled ovarian hyper-stimulation. Hum Reprod 2003; 18: 328–32.

100. La Marca A, Malmusi S, Giulini S, et al. Anti-Müllerian hormone plasma levels in spontaneous menstrual cycle and during treatment with FSH to induce ovulation. Hum Reprod 2004; 19: 2738–41.

101. Hudson PL, Dougas I, Donahoe PK, et al. An immunoassay to detect human Müllerian inhibiting substance in males and females during normal development. J Clin Endocrinol Metab 1990; 70: 16–22.

102. de Vet A, Laven JS, de Jong FH, et al. Anti-Müllerian hormone serum levels: a putative marker for ovarian aging. Fertil Steril 2002; 77: 357–62.

103. Gruijters MJ, Visser JA, Durlinger AL, Themmen AP. Anti-Müllerian hormone and its role in ovarian function. Mol Cell Endocrinol 2003; 211: 85–90.

104. Van Rooij IA, Broekmans FJ, te Velde ER, et al. Serum anti-Müllerian hormone levels: a novel measure of ovarian reserve. Hum Reprod 2002; 17: 3065–71.

105. Hehenkamp WJ, Looman CW, Themmen AP, et al. Anti-Müllerian hormone levels in the spontaneous menstrual cycle do not show substantial fluctuation. J Clin Endocrinol Metab 2006; 91: 4057–63.

106. La Marca A, Stabile G, Artenisio AC, Volpe A. Serum anti-Müllerian hormone throughout the human menstrual cycle. Hum Reprod 2006; 21: 3103–7.

107. Gougeon A, Echochard R, Thalabard JC. Age-related changes of the population of human ovarian follicles: Increase in the disappearance rate of nongrowing and early-growing follicles in aging women. Biol Reprod 1994; 50: 653–63.

108. Hendriks DJ, Mol BW, Bancsi LF, et al. Antral follicle count in the prediction of poor ovarian response and pregnancy after in vitro fertilization: a meta-analysis and comparison with basal follicle-stimulating hormone level. Fertil Steril 2005; 83: 291–301.

109. Seifer DB, MacLaughlin DT, Christian BP, et al. Early follicular serum Müllerian-inhibiting substance levels are associated with ovarian response during assisted reproductive technique cycles. Fertil Steril 2002; 77: 468–71.

110. van Rooij IA, de Jong E, Broekmans FJ, et al. High follicle-stimulating hormone levels should not necessarily lead to the exclusion of subfertile patients from treatment. Fertil Steril 2004; 81: 1478–85.

111. Hazout A, Bouchard P, Seifer DB, et al. Serum anti-Müllerian hormone/Müllerian-inhibiting sub-stance appears to be a more discriminatory marker of assisted reproductive technique outcome than follicle-stimulating hormone, inhibin B, or estradiol. Fertil Steril 2004; 82: 1323–9.

112. Broer SL, Mol BWJ, Hendricks D, Broekmans FJM. The role of anti-Müllerian hormone in prediction of outcome after IVF: comparison with the antral follicle count. Fertil Steril 2009; 91: 705–14.

113. Muttukrishna S, McGarrigle H, Wakim R, et al. Antral follicle count, anti-Müllerian hormone and inhibin B: predictors of ovarian response in assisted reproductive technique? Br J Obstet Gynaecol 2005; 112: 1384–90.

114. Muttukrishna S, Suharjono H, McGarrigle H, Sathanandan M. Inhibin B and anti-Müllerian hormone: Markers of ovarian response in IVF/ICSI patients? Br J Obstet Gynaecol 2004; 111: 1248–53.

115. Penarrubia J, Fábregues F, Manau D, et al. Basal and stimulation day 5 anti-Müllerian hormone serum concentrations as predictors of ovarian response and pregnancy in assisted reproductive technique cycles stimulated with gonadotropin-releasing hormone agonist–gonadotropin treatment. Hum Reprod 2005; 20: 915–22.

116. Tremellen KP, Kolo M, Gilmore A, Lekamge DN. Anti-Müllerian hormone as a marker of ovarian reserve. Aust NZ J Obstet Gynaecol 2005; 45: 20–4.

117. Eldar-Geva T, Ben Chetrit A, Spitz IM, et al. Dynamic assays of inhibin B, anti-Müllerian hormone and estradiol following FSH stimulation and ovarian ultrasonography as predictors of IVF outcome. Hum Reprod 2005; 20: 3178–83.

118. McIlveen M, Skull JD, Ledger WL. Evaluation of the utility of multiple endocrine and ultrasound measures of ovarian reserve in the prediction of cycle cancellation in a high-risk IVF population. Hum Reprod 2007; 22: 778–85.

119. Ficicioglu C, Kutlu T, Baglam E, Bakacak Z. Early follicular anti-Müllerian hormone as an indicator of ovarian reserve. Fertil Steril 2006; 85: 592–6.

120. La Marca A, Giulini S, Tirelli A, et al. Anti-Müllerian hormone measurement on any day of the menstrual cycle strongly predicts ovarian response in assisted reproductive technique. Hum Reprod 2007; 22: 766–71.

121. Ebner T, Sommergruber M, Moser M, et al. Basal level of anti-Müllerian hormone is associated with oocyte quality in stimulated cycles. Hum Reprod 2006; 21: 2022–6.

122. Smeenk JM, Sweep FC, Zielhuis GA, et al. Anti-Müllerian hormone predicts ovarian responsiveness, but not embryo quality or pregnancy, after in vitro fertilization or intracytoplasmic sperm injection. Fertil Steril 2007; 87: 223–6.

123. Freour T, Mirallie S, Bach-Ngohou K, et al. Measurement of serum anti-Müllerian hormone by Beckman Coulter ELISA and DSL ELISA: comparison and relevance in assisted reproduction technique (ART). Clin Chim Acta 2007; 375: 162–4.

124. Kwee J, Schats R, McDonnell J, et al. Evaluation of anti-Müllerian hormone as test for the prediction of ovarian reserve. Fertil Steril 2008; 90: 737–43.

125. Cook CL, Siow Y, Taylor S, Fallat ME. Serum Müllerian-inhibiting substance levels during normal menstrual cycles. Fertil Steril 2000; 73: 859–61.

126. Hansen KR, Morris JL, Thyer AC, Soules MR. Reproductive aging and variability in the ovarian antral follicle count: application in the clinical setting. Fertil Steril 2003; 80: 577–83.

127. Scheffer GJ, Broekmans FJ, Bancsi LF, et al. Quantitative transvaginal two- and three-dimensional sonography of the ovaries: reproducibility of antral follicle counts. Ultrasound Obstet Gynecol 2002; 20: 270–5.

128. van Disseldorp J, Eijkemans MJ, Klinkert ER, et al. Cumulative live birth rates following IVF in 41- to 43-year-old women presenting with favourable ovarian reserve characteristics. Reprod Biomed Online 2007; 14: 455–63.

129. Pache TD, Wladimiroff JW, de Jong FH, et al. Growth patterns of non dominant ovarian follicles during the normal menstrual cycle. Fertil Steril 1990; 54: 638–42.

130. Durlinger AL, Visser JA, Themmen AP. Regulation of ovarian function: the role of anti-Müllerian hormone. Reproduction 2002; 124: 601–9.

131. Di Clemente N, Goxe B, Rémy JJ, et al. Inhibitory effect of AMH upon aromatase activity and LH receptors of granulosa cells of rat and porcine immature ovaries. Endocrine 1994; 2: 553–8.

132. Josso N, di Clemente N, Gouedard L. Anti-Müllerian hormone and its receptors. Mol Cell Endocrinol 2001; 179: 25–32.

133. Durlinger AL, Gruijters MJ, Kramer P, et al. Anti-Müllerian hormone attenuates the effects of FSH on follicle development in the mouse ovary. Endocrinology 2001; 142: 4891–9.

134. Andersen CY, Byskov AG. Estradiol and regulation of anti-Müllerian hormone, inhibin-A, and inhibin-B secretion: analysis of small antral and preovulatory human follicles' fluid. J Clin Endocrinol Metab 2006; 91: 4064–9.

135. Pellatt L, Hanna L, Brincat M, et al. Granulosa cell production of anti-Müllerian hormone is increased in polycystic ovaries. J Clin Endocrinol Metab 2007; 92: 240–5.

136. Catteau-Jonard S, Pigny P, Reyss AC, et al. Changes in serum anti-Müllerian hormone level during low dose

recombinant follicle-stimulating hormone therapy for anovulation in polycystic ovary syndrome. J Clin Endocrinol Metab 2007; 92: 4138–43.

137. La Marca A, Malmusi S, Giulini S, et al. Anti-Müllerian hormone plasma levels in spontaneous menstrual cycle and during treatment with FSH to induce ovulation. Hum Reprod 2004; 19: 2738–41.

138. Eldar-Geva T, Margalioth EJ, Gal M, et al. Serum anti-Müllerian hormone levels during controlled ovarian hyperstimulation in women with polycystic ovaries with and without hyperandrogenism. Hum Reprod 2005; 20: 1814–19.

139. Hehenkamp WJ, Looman CW, Themmen AP, et al. Anti-Müllerian hormone levels in the spontaneous menstrual cycle do not show substantial fluctuation. J Clin Endocrinol Metab 2006; 91: 4057–63.

40

The use of GnRH agonists

Roel Schats and Judith A. F. Huirne

INTRODUCTION

Gonadotropin-releasing hormone (GnRH) is the primary hypothalamic regulator of reproductive function. With the help of a very small amount (250 µg) of GnRH derived from 160,000 porcine hypothalami, a group of scientists at Andrew Schally's peptide laboratory in New Orleans was able to unravel the chemical structure of this compound in 1971 (1,2). Roger Guillemin was able to characterize and also synthesize independently this neuroendocrine hormone. They both received the Nobel Prize for their achievement. GnRH is a decapeptide that, like several other brain peptides, is synthesized as a part of a much larger precursor peptide, the GnRH-associated peptide (GAP). This peptide is made up of a sequence of 56 amino acids. The availability of the synthetic hormone for dynamic endocrine testing and receptor studies created new insights into the physiological role of GnRH in the hypothalamic–pituitary–gonadal axis (3).

GnRH is produced and released from a group of loosely connected neurons located in the medial basal hypothalamus, primarily within the arcuate nucleus, and in the preoptic area of the ventral hypothalamus. It is synthesized in the cell body, transported along the axons to the synapse, and released in a pulsatile fashion into the complex capillary net of the portal system of the pituitary gland (4). GnRH binds selectively to highly specific receptors of the anterior pituitary gonadotropic cells and activates intracellular signaling pathways via the coupled G proteins (Gαs), leading to the generation of several second messengers, among which are diacylglycerol and inositol-4,5-triphosphate. The former leads to activation of protein kinase C and the latter to the production of cyclic AMP and release of calcium ions from intracellular pools (5–7). Both events result in secretion and synthesis of luteinizing hormone (LH) and follicle-stimulating hormone (FSH). A pulsatile mode of GnRH release the hypothalamus to the pituitary is required to ensure gonadotropin secretion (8–10). In humans the pulsatile release frequencies range from the shortest interpulse frequency of about 71 minutes in the late follicular phase to an interval of 216 minutes in the late luteal phase (11–13). High frequent (>3 pulses/hour) and continuous exposure of the pituitary to GnRH failed to produce normal LH and FSH release patterns (14–16) owing to pituitary desensitization. This mechanism is still not clear except that postreceptor signaling is involved, true receptor loss (downregulation) having only an initial role (17). The pulsatile release by the GnRH neurons is hypothesized to be based on an ultrashort loop feedback by GnRH itself; this autocrine process could serve as a timing mechanism to control the frequency of pulsatile neurosecretion. Several mechanisms, based on calcium and cyclic AMP signaling, have been proposed to account for the pulse secretion. Another role of intracellular signaling in pulsatile generation has been suggested by the marked inhibition of Gi protein activation by LH, human chorionic gonadotropin (hCG), muscarine, estradiol (E2), and GnRH levels (7,18,19).

After the discovery of the chemical structure of native GnRH type I, which proved to be the classic reproductive neuroendocrine factor, many were synthetically produced. Most were able to elicit a huge FSH and LH release from the pituitary and were therefore called GnRH agonists. However, under continuous administration of a GnRH agonist the normal synthesis and subsequent release of LH, and to a lesser extent FSH, became blocked (Fig. 40.1). Other analogs caused an immediate fall in gonadotropin secretion from the pituitary by competitive receptor binding, and were designated GnRH antagonists. In contrast to the agonistic compounds, the introduction of the GnRH antagonists into clinical practice has been hampered for a long time by problems concerning solubility and direct allergy-like side effects due to histamine release (20,21). Recently, these problems have been resolved, leading to the third-generation GnRH antagonists: Two are on the market and many others are under investigation (22). Nowadays GnRH agonists have gained a wide field of clinical applications (23). Suppression of the pituitary ovarian (or testicular) axis for a limited or even an extended period is the main goal to be achieved in these treatments.

STRUCTURAL MODIFICATIONS

The elucidation of the structure, function, and metabolic pathways of native GnRH has prompted an intensive effort by research laboratories and the pharmaceutical industry

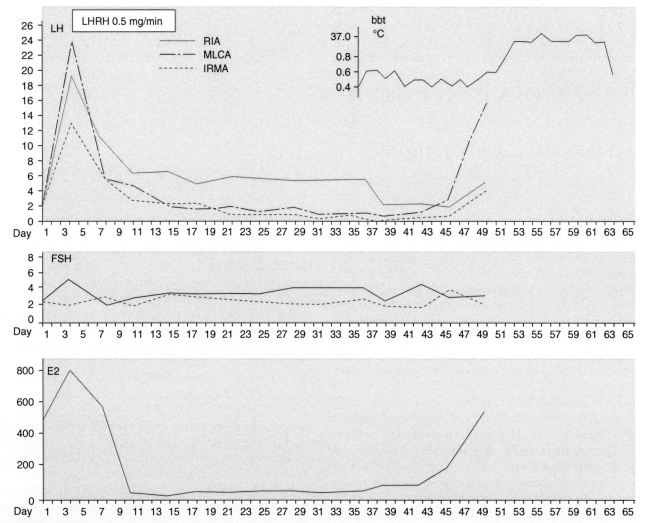

Figure 40.1 Hormone levels for FSH, LH, and E2 in a patient with continuous intravenous infusion of 0.5 mg/minute LHRH. LH was measured with three and FSH with two different assays. *Abbreviations*: RIA, radioimmunoassay; MLCA, Magic Lite chemoluminescence assay; IRMA, immunoradiometric assay; bbt, basal body temperature; LH, luteinizing hormone; FSH, follicle-stimulating hormone; E2, estradiol; LHRH, luteinizing hormone–releasing hormone. *Source*: Private collection Prof. J. Schoemaker.

to synthesize potent and longer-acting agonists and antagonists (24). Over the past three decades, thousands of analogs of GnRH have been synthesized. Only seven of the agonistic analogs of GnRH have been approved and have become clinically used drugs. The first major step in increasing the potency of GnRH was made with substitutions of glycine number 10 at the C terminus. Although 90% of the biologic activity is lost by the splicing of glycine number 10, most of it is restored with the attachment of NH2-ethylamide to the proline at position 9, leading to nonapeptides (25). The second major modification was the replacement of the glycine at position 6 by D-amino acids, which slows down enzymatic degradation. The combination of these two modifications was found to have synergistic biologic activity and proved to exhibit a higher receptor binding affinity. The affinity can be increased further by the introduction of larger, hydrophobic and more lipophilic D-amino acids at position number 6. The increased lipophilicity of the agonist is associated with a prolonged half-life, which may be attributed to reduced renal excretion through increased plasma protein binding,

or fat tissue storage of non-ionized fat-soluble compounds (25). For details about the structure see Table 40.1.

CLINICAL APPLICATIONS

The original goal for the development of agonistic analogs of GnRH was that they would eventually be used for the treatment of anovulation. However, soon after the elucidation of the structure of GnRH, the "paradoxical" ability of agonistic analogs to inhibit reproductive function in experimental animals was demonstrated (26). The most important clinical applications of the potent GnRH agonists were derived from their capacity to cause rapid desensitization of the pituitary gland as a result of prolonged non-pulsatile administration, leading to a decrease in serum gonadotropin levels and subsequently inhibition of ovarian steroidogenesis and follicular growth. The potential for reversibly inducing a state of hypogonadotropic hypogonadism, which was also termed "medical gonadectomy" or "medical hypophysectomy" allowed for the relatively rapid and extensive introduction of GnRH

Table 40.1 Amino Acid Sequence and Substitution of the GnRH Agonists

Compound						Position 6				Position 10
Amino acid no	1	2	3	4	5	6	7	8	9	10
Native GnRH	Glu	His	Trp	Ser	Tyr	Gly	Leu	Arg	Pro	GlyNH$_2$
Nonapeptides										
Leuprolide (Lupron, Lucrin)						Leu				N-Et-NH$_2$
Buserelin (Suprefact)						Ser(O'Bu)				N-Et-NH$_2$
Goserelin (Zoladex)						Ser(O'Bu)				AzaGlyNH$_2$
Histrelin (Supprelin)						D-His(Bzl)				AzaGlyNH$_2$
Deslorelin (Ovuplant)						D-Tr				N-Et-NH$_2$
Decapeptides										
Nafarelin (Synarel)						2Nal				GlyNH$_2$
Triptorelin (Decapeptyl)						Trp				GlyNH$_2$

agonists into clinical practice. For a variety of indications, complete abolition of gonadotropin secretion with subsequent suppression of gonadal steroids to the levels of castrated subjects was considered beneficial. This therapeutic approach has already had its efficacy and merits proved in the treatment of metastatic prostatic cancer, breast cancer, central precocious puberty, external endometriosis, uterine fibroids, hirsutism, and other conditions (27,28).

Since the first report on the use of the combination of the GnRH agonist buserelin and gonadotropins for ovarian stimulation for in vitro fertilization in 1984, (29) numerous studies have demonstrated the efficacy of this concept. Subsequently the use of GnRH agonists has gained widespread popularity, and the vast majority of assisted reproductive technique (ART) programs use this approach for controlled ovarian hyperstimulation (COH) in vitro fertilization (IVF). The major advantage initially offered by the agonists was the efficient abolition of the spontaneous LH surge (30). The incidence of premature LH surges and subsequent luteinization in cycles with exogenous gonadotropin stimulation, without the use of a GnRH agonist, was observed by several investigators to range between 20% and 50%, leading to an increased cancellation rate (31). Moreover, a deleterious effect on both fertilization and pregnancy rates was noted (30,32). A meta-analysis of randomized controlled trials has shown that the use of GnRH agonists has not only reduced cancellation rates but has also increased the number of oocytes and embryos, allowing better selection (33) so that, on average, the outcome in terms of pregnancy rates was improved (34).

A number of controversial issues remain concerning the use of GnRH agonists in assisted reproduction. The problems can be divided into the following four categories:

1. Which route of administration is the best?
2. Which agonist(s) should be used in ART?
3. What is the optimal dose?
4. What is the optimal scheme?

Which Route of Administration is the Best?

Administration routes of GnRH agonists are intramuscular or subcutaneous depot injection, intranasal, or subcutaneous

daily administration. Although there is an advantage for the patient in the usually single injection of the depot preparations, the duration of action is prolonged and rather unpredictable. The effect can last until the first weeks of pregnancy (35). Broekmans et al. showed that rapid induction of a hypogonadotropic and hypogonadal state is possible in regularly cycling women by administration of a single depot of triptorelin. However, suppression of pituitary and ovarian function appears to be continued until the eighth week after the injection (35). This is far longer than is actually needed. Devreker et al. found obvious negative effects of depot preparations: Longer stimulation phase, consequently more ampoules needed, but even more important: lower implantation and delivery rates (32.8 vs. 21.1%; 48.9 vs. 29.1%, respectively). Their conclusion was that since a long-acting GnRH agonist might interfere with the luteal phase and embryo development, short-acting GnRH agonists should be preferred in ART (36).

On the basis of a recent meta-analysis comparing depot versus daily administration, it can be concluded that no evident differences could be observed in terms of pregnancy rates. However, the use of depot GnRH analogs is associated with increased gonadotropin requirements and longer stimulation periods and should therefore not be advocated in terms of cost effectiveness (37). Moreover, on a theoretical basis it seems to be more elegant to avoid any possible direct effect on the embryo, although several authors claim a normal outcome of pregnancy following inadvertent administration of a GnRH agonist during early pregnancy (38–43). Lahat et al. reported a high incidence of attention deficit hyperactivity disorder (ADHD) in long-term follow-up of children inadvertently exposed to GnRH agonists early in pregnancy (44).

Thus, although depot preparations seem attractive because of their ease of administration for the patient, they cannot be advocated for routine use in IVF. One exception to this statement might be the prolonged use of GnRH analogs before IVF-ET in patients with severe endometriosis, which is associated with higher ongoing pregnancy rates (45).

With the intranasal route the absorption of the GnRH agonist fluctuates inter- and intra-individually, giving an unpredictable desensitization level, but most times this is sufficient to prevent premature LH surges. For research or study purposes the daily subcutaneous injections deserve preference, because of their more stable effect. The clinician has to make up the balance between comfort for the patient and a more stable effect in selecting the intranasal versus the subcutaneous route of administration.

Which Agonist(s) should be used in ART?

In Table 40.1 seven GnRH agonists are mentioned. In fact, only four are commonly used in IVF programs. An extensive search revealed only one article about the use of histrelin in IVF, (46) while deslorelin has never been applied in human IVF. Except for its combination with treatment of endometriosis, goserelin is not routinely used in ART, partly because it is only available as a depot preparation. Depot preparations also on the market for triptorelin and leuprolide are not to be used as first choice, as discussed earlier. Thirteen prospective randomized trials were traced in the literature comparing different agonists with each other (47–58). The problem with those studies is that the optimal dosage has not been determined for any of the applied individual agonists. Therefore, the value of these articles is limited with respect to elucidating the question as to which compound should be used. All the agonists seem effective and the differences in the studies can be explained by a dosage incompatibility. These studies make absolutely clear that proper dose-finding studies for the use of GnRH agonists in ART are still urgently needed. In fact, it is rather strange that they still have not been performed, more than 10 years after the introduction of the agonists in IVF. It is obvious that the dose required for the prevention of premature LH surges during controlled ovarian stimulation (COS) cycles in ART will be different from that to treat carcinoma of the prostate, which requires complete chemical castration (see below).

What is the Optimal Dose?

Finding the right dose in the treatment of infertility disorders has been notoriously difficult for obscure reasons. Proper dose-finding studies for the use of gonadotropins are lacking and it therefore took until the middle of the 1980s before an adequate treatment protocol, with a maximum of effect and a minimum of side effects, was introduced by Polson et al. (59). There is only one prospective, randomized, double-blind, placebo-controlled dose-finding study performed in IVF for the GnRH agonist triptorelin. This study demonstrated that the dosage needed for the suppression of the LH surge is much smaller, namely only 15–50% of the dosage needed for the treatment of a malignant disease (31). It is very likely that dose-finding studies for the other agonists will give similar results. As per the recent literature such studies are not performed.

What is the Optimal Scheme?

Many treatment schedules with the use of GnRH agonists in ART have been designed. The duration and initiation of agonist administration before the start of the actual ovarian stimulation varies widely. Initiation of the agonist treatment may be in either the early follicular or the mid-luteal phase of the preceding cycle. The cycle may be spontaneous or induced by progestogen and/or estrogen compounds. There is still much debate about the optimal GnRH agonist protocol. Tan published in 1994 a review article stating that the so-called long protocol was superior to the short and ultrashort protocols (60). Moreover, a major advantage of the long GnRH agonist protocol is its contribution to the planning of the ovum pick-up, since both the initiation of exogenous gonadotropins after pituitary desensitization and the administration of hCG can be delayed, without any detrimental effect on IVF outcome (61,62). A meta-analysis comparing ultrashort, short, and long IVF protocols showed a higher number of oocytes retrieved and higher pregnancy rates in the long protocol, although more ampoules of gonadotropins were needed (63). In terms of gonadotropin suppression and number of retrieved oocytes, the mid-luteal phase of the preceding cycle is the optimal moment for the initiation of the GnRH agonist, in comparison to the follicular, early, or late luteal phases (64–66).

However, a problem with (prospective randomized) clinical studies is that certain groups of patients, for example the poor responders (with or without elevated basal FSH) or patients with polycystic ovary syndrome (PCOS), are often excluded. There is a possibility that especially in the excluded groups other schemes are preferable. An unwanted side effect of starting the GnRH agonist in the luteal or follicular phase in the long protocol is the induction of the formation of functional cysts. Keltz et al. observed both a poor stimulation outcome and a reduction in pregnancy rates in a cycle with cyst formation (67). However, Feldberg et al. could not confirm this finding (68). Ovarian cyst formation was reduced when pretreatment with an oral contraceptive was applied (69). Damario et al. showed the beneficial effect of this strategy in high responder patients with respect to cancellation rates and pregnancy rates (70). A long GnRH agonist protocol in combination with an oral contraceptive seems to be advantageous, in prevention of functional ovarian cysts and especially for the larger IVF centers for programming of IVF cycles. Another practical advantage of including an oral contraceptive is the fact that the coincidence of GnRH agonist use and early pregnancy is prevented.

The mean desensitization phase with an agonist in the long protocols is about three weeks. Several investigators have tried to shorten this long duration of administration, leading to the so-called "early cessation protocol" (71–74). Increased hMG/FSH requirement and cancellation rates were reported after early cessation in 137 normal IVF patients, (74) but the opposite was found in a recent study that included 230 normo-ovulating IVF patients, (71) although pregnancy rates were the same in both studies (74). The paradoxical drop of serum LH following early cessation that leads to significantly lower estradiol levels on the day of hCG, may have a deleterious effect on IVF outcome (71,74). The early discontinuation protocol may improve ovarian response based on a hypothetical effect on the ovary, and was therefore additionally tested in poor responders. Although the number of retrieved oocytes was significantly higher and the amount of required gonadotropins was reduced after early cessation in comparison to the long protocol, this new approach reported no further advantages in these patients in terms of pregnancy and implantation rates (72,73). In conclusion, the currently available data do not favor an "early cessation" protocol, but this approach might have some beneficial effects in poor responders.

To prevent any detrimental effect of the profound suppression of circulating serum gonadotropins after cessation of GnRH agonist therapy, the opposite regimens have recently been developed in which the GnRH agonist administration is continued during the luteal phase, the so-called "continuous-long protocol". In a large prospective randomized study ($n = 319$) comparing this continued long protocol versus the standard long protocol, higher implantation and pregnancy rates were found in the continuous-long protocol (75).

Since the use of a long protocol in poor responders has been found to result in reduced ovarian responses to hormonal stimulation, the short GnRH agonist protocol has been proposed as providing better stimulation for these patients. In the "short or flare-up protocol," GnRH agonist therapy is started at cycle day 2 and gonadotropins treatment is started one day later. The immediate stimulatory action of the GnRH agonist serves as the initial stimulus for follicular recruitment (so-called flare-up). Adequate follicular maturation is on average reached in 12 days, which should allow enough time for sufficient pituitary desensitization to prevent any premature LH surges. The initial stimulatory effect of GnRH agonist on pituitary hormone levels may improve the ovarian response (76). On the other hand, this short protocol

might increase gonadotropins in the early phase, which induces enhanced ovarian androgen release. This is associated with declined oocyte quality and reduced ongoing pregnancy rates compared to the long protocol (77). Nevertheless, experience to date shows that the short protocol has an important role in the treatment of poor responders (78). Other investigators even promoted an "ultrashort protocol" in "poor responders," in which the agonist is given during a period of three days in the early follicular phase. At the second day of agonist administration, stimulation with gonadotropin administration (high dosages) is started (79–82).

In very high responders, in patients at risk of ovarian hyperstimulation syndrome (OHSS), the gonadotropin was discontinued whilst continuing the GnRH agonist; this so-called "coasting" might prevent the development of severe OHSS (83,84). This strategy allows a delay of a variable number of days in administering hCG injection until safe E2 levels are attained. However, sufficient randomized controlled trials comparing coasting with no coasting are lacking (85). Only one prospective comparative trial in 60 IVF patients showed a similar incidence of moderate and severe OHSS whether coasting was applied or not (86).

The most important advantages and disadvantages of the different GnRH agonist protocols are summarized in Table 40.2.

After the clinical availability of GnRH antagonists, an additional indication for the use of GnRH agonists became of interest. GnRH analogs may be used as an alternative way for hCG to trigger the endogenous LH and FSH surges and subsequent final maturation of the oocytes and ovulation (87,88). Since hCG is believed to contribute to the occurrence of OHSS owing to its prolonged circulating half-life time compared with native LH, this strategy seems to be an attractive alternative to prevent OHSS. In the early 1990s, it was already shown that single-dose

Table 40.2 Summary of Advantages and Disadvantages of the Different GnRH Agonist Protocols

GnRH agonist protocol	Route of administration	Administration days of cycle (CD)	Duration of administration	Advantages	Disadvantages
Ultrashort protocol	IN/SC	CD 2,3–4,5	3 days	Patient's comfort	Low PR
Short protocol	IN/SC	CD 2,3 until day of hCG	8–12 days	Patient's comfort	No programming
Long follicular	IN/SC	CD 2 until day of hCG	28–35 days	Programming, good PR	Long duration of administration
Long luteal	IN/SC	CD 21 until day of hCG	21–28 days	Programming, good PR	Long duration of administration
Menstrual early cessation	IN/SC	CD 21 until menses	7–12 days	Inconclusive	Low estradiol levels
Follicular early cessation	IN/SC	CD 21 until stim. day 6,7	13–20 days	Inconclusive	Low estradiol levels
Long follicular (depot)	Depot	CD 2	Once	Patient's comfort	(Too) long duration of action
Long luteal (depot)	Depot	CD 21	Once	Patient's comfort	(Too) long duration of action
Ultralong	IN/SC/depot	CD 2 or 21	8–12 weeks, depot 2 or 3 times	Only for special cases	Side effects due to estrogen deficiency

Abbreviations: PR, pregnancy rate.

GnRH agonists administrated in COH-IVF patients were able to induce an endogenous rise in both LH and FSH levels, leading to follicular maturation and pregnancy (89,90). Mean serum LH and FSH levels rose over 4–12 hours and were elevated for 24–34 hours after GnRH agonist, in comparison to approximately six days of elevated hCG levels after 5000 IU hCG administration. The capacity of a single administration of GnRH analog to trigger follicular rupture in anovulatory women or in preparation for IUI has been well established. This seems to induce lower OHSS rates with comparable or even improved results, despite short luteal phases, in comparison to hCG cycles (87,88,91). Interest in this approach was lost during the 1990s, because GnRH agonists were introduced in ovarian hyperstimulation protocols to prevent premature luteinization by pituitary desensitization, precluding stimulation of the endogenous LH surge. However, interest has returned following the introduction of GnRH antagonist protocols in which the pituitary responsiveness is preserved. This new concept of triggering final oocyte maturation after GnRH antagonist treatment by a single GnRH agonist injection was successfully tested in COH patients for IUI92 and in high responders for IVF (93). None of these patients developed OHSS. The efficacy and success of this new treatment regimen was established in a prospective multicenter trial, in which 47 patients were randomized to receive either 0.2 mg triptorelin, 0.5 mg leuprorelin, or 10,000 IU hCG (94). The LH surges peaked at four hours after agonist administration and returned to baseline after 24 hours; the luteal phase steroids levels were also closer to the physiologic range compared to the hCG groups. In terms of triggering the final stages of oocyte maturation similar outcomes were observed in all groups, as demonstrated by the similar fertilization rates and oocyte quality (94).

A prospective randomized study in 105 stimulated IUI cycles treated with a GnRH antagonist, in patients with clomiphene-resistant PCOS, showed significantly more clinical pregnancies statistically after ovulation triggering by a GnRH agonist in comparison to hCG (28.2% vs. 17% per completed cycle, respectively) (95). Thus, this new approach of ovulation triggering seems to be an attractive alternative for hCG in ART if administered in GnRH antagonist treated cycles, with lower OHSS and similar or improved IVF outcome.

CONCLUSIONS

GnRH agonists are widely used in IVF to control the endogenous LH surge and achieve augmentation of multifollicular development. Disadvantages, such as the necessity for luteal support, increased total gonadotropin dose per treatment cycle and consequently higher costs, appear to be outweighed by the observed increase in ability to control the cycle, higher yield of good quality oocytes and subsequently embryos, and consequent improvement of pregnancy rates. The introduction of GnRH agonists in IVF is not an example of excellent research, since proper dose-finding studies are still awaited. Further research in finding the right dose and

protocol can still improve the clinical benefits of the GnRH agonists. Initiatives to perform such studies are lacking. Daily administered short-acting preparations deserve preference to the depot formulations. Intranasal administration best fits a patient's comfort considerations, while the subcutaneous route may be advocated for research purposes. The long GnRH agonist protocols give the highest pregnancy rates in the normal responders. There is some evidence that the short flare-up protocol is the treatment of choice for patients with diminished ovarian reserve (poor responders). Dose reduction might be the key point in optimizing pregnancy rates. Finally, GnRH agonists can be used to induce final maturation and ovulation as an alternative to hCG in ART.

REFERENCES

1. Arimura A. The backstage story of the discovery of LHRH. Endocrinology 1991; 129: 1687–9.
2. Schally AV, Nair RM, Redding TW, et al. Isolation of the luteinizing hormone and follicle-stimulating hormone- releasing hormone from porcine hypothalami. J Biol Chem 1971; 246: 7230–6.
3. Clayton RN, Catt KJ. Gonadotropin-releasing hormone receptors: characterization, physiological regulation, and relationship to reproductive function. Endocrinol Rev 1981; 2: 186–209.
4. Carmel PW, Araki S, Ferin M. Pituitary stalk portal blood collection in rhesus monkeys: evidence for pulsatile release of gonadotropin-releasing hormone (GnRH). Endocrinology 1976; 99: 243–8.
5. Stojilkovic SS, Reinhart J, Catt KJ. Gonadotropin-releasing hormone receptors: structure and signal transduction pathways. Endocrinol Rev 1994; 15: 462–99.
6. Kaiser UB, Conn PM, Chin WW. Studies of gonadotropin-releasing hormone (GnRH) action using GnRH receptor-expressing pituitary cell lines. Endocrinol Rev 1997; 18: 46–70.
7. Catt KJ, Martinez-Fuentes AJ, Hu L, et al. Recent insights into the regulation of pulsatile GnRH secretion (abstract O–004). Gynecol Endocrinol 2003; 17: 2.
8. Neill JD, Patton JM, Dailey RA, et al. Luteinizing hormone releasing hormone (LHRH) in pituitary stalk blood of rhesus monkeys: Relationship to level of LH release. Endocrinology 1977; 101: 430–4.
9. Levine JE, Pau KY, Ramirez VD, et al. Simultaneous measurement of luteinizing hormone-releasing hormone and luteinizing hormone release in unanesthetized, ovariectomized sheep. Endocrinology 1982; 111: 1449–55.
10. Levine JE, Norman RL, Gliessman PM, et al. In vivo gonadotropin-releasing hormone release and serum luteinizing hormone measurements in ovariectomized, estrogen-treated rhesus macaques. Endocrinology 1985; 117: 711–21.
11. Backstrom CT, McNeilly AS, Leask RM, et al. Pulsatile secretion of LH, FSH, prolactin, oestradiol and progesterone during the human menstrual cycle. Clin Endocrinol (Oxf) 1982; 17: 29–42.
12. Reame N, Sauder SE, Kelch RP, et al. Pulsatile gonadotropin secretion during the human menstrual cycle: evidence for altered frequency of gonadotropin-releasing hormone secretion. J Clin Endocrinol Metab 1984; 59: 328–37.

13. Crowley WF Jr, Filicori M, Spratt DI, et al. The physiology of gonadotropin-releasing hormone (GnRH) secretion in men and women. Recent Prog Horm Res 1985; 41: 473–531.

14. Belchetz PE, Plant TM, Nakai Y, et al. Hypophysial responses to continuous and intermittent delivery of hypothalamic gonadotropin-releasing hormone. Science 1978; 202: 631–3.

15. Gharib SD, Wierman ME, Shupnik MA, et al. Molecular biology of the pituitary gonadotropins. Endocrinol Rev 1990; 11: 177–99.

16. Nillius SJ, Wide L. Variation in LH and FSH response to LH-releasing hormone during the menstrual cycle. J Obstet Gynaecol Br Common 1972; 79: 865–73.

17. Conn PM, Crowley WF Jr. Gonadotropin-releasing hormone and its analogs. Annu Rev Med 1994; 45: 391–405.

18. Krsmanovic LZ, Martinez-Fuentes AJ, Arora KK, et al. Local regulation of gonadotroph function by pituitary gonadotropin-releasing hormone. Endocrinology 2000; 141: 1187–95.

19. Merchenthaler I. Identification of estrogen receptor-B in the GnRH neurons of the rodent hypothalamus (abstract O–024). Gynecol endocrinol 2003; 17: 12.

20. Reissmann T, Diedrich K, Comaru-Schally AM, et al. Introduction of LHRH-antagonists into the treat- ment of gynaecological disorders. Hum Reprod 1994; 9: 769.

21. Gordon K, Hodgen GD. Will GnRH antagonists be worth the wait? Reprod Med Rev 1992; 1: 189–94.

22. Huirne JA, Lambalk CB. Gonadotropin-releasing-hormone-receptor antagonists. Lancet 2001; 358: 1793–803.

23. Andreyko JL, Marshall LA, Dumesic DA, et al. Therapeutic uses of gonadotropin-releasing hormone analogs. Obstet Gynecol Surv 1987; 42: 1–21.

24. Nestor JJ Jr. Developments of agonistic LHRH analogs. In: Vickery BH, Nestor JJ Jr, Hafez ESE, eds. LHRH and its Analogs. Lancaster: MTP Press, 1984: 3–15.

25. Karten MJ, Rivier JE. Gonadotropin-releasing hormone analog design. Structure–function studies toward the development of agonists and antagonists: rationale and perspective. Endocrinol Rev 1986; 7: 44–66.

26. Corbin A, Beattie CW. Post-coital contraceptive and uterotrophic effects of luteinizing hormone releasing hormone. Endocrinol Res Commun 1975; 2: 445–58.

27. Conn PM, Crowley WF Jr. Gonadotropin-releasing hormone and its analogs. N Engl J Med 1991; 324: 93–103.

28. Klijn JGM. LHRH-agonist therapy in breast cancer (abstract O–016). Gynecol endocrinol 2003; 17: 8.

29. Porter RN, Smith W, Craft IL, et al. Induction of ovulation for in vitro fertilisation using buserelin and gonadotropins. Lancet 1984; 2: 1284–5.

30. Fleming R, Coutts JR. Induction of multiple follicular growth in normally menstruating women with endogenous gonadotropin suppression. Fertil Steril 1986; 45: 226–30.

31. Janssens RM, Lambalk CB, Vermeiden JP, et al. Dose-finding study of triptorelin acetate for prevention of a premature LH surge in IVF: a prospective, randomized, double-blind, placebo-controlled study. Hum Reprod 2000; 15: 2333–40.

32. Loumaye E. The control of endogenous secretion of LH by gonadotrophin-releasing hormone agonists during ovarian hyperstimulation for in vitro fertilization and embryo transfer. Hum Reprod 1990; 5: 357–76.

33. Templeton A, Morris JK. Reducing the risk of multiple births by transfer of two embryos after in vitro fertilization. N Engl J Med 1998; 339: 573–7.

34. Hughes EG, Fedorkow DM, Daya S, et al. The routine use of gonadotropin-releasing hormone agonists prior to in vitro fertilization and gamete intrafallopian transfer: a meta-analysis of randomized controlled trials. Fertil Steril 1992; 58: 888–96.

35. Broekmans FJ, Bernardus RE, Berkhout G, et al. Pituitary and ovarian suppression after early follicular and mid-luteal administration of a LHRH agonist in a depot formulation: decapeptyl CR. Gynecol Endocrinol 1992; 6: 153–61.

36. Devreker F, Govaerts I, Bertrand E, et al. The long-acting gonadotropin-releasing hormone analogues impaired the implantation rate. Fertil Steril 1996; 65: 122–6.

37. Albuquerque LE, Saconato H, Maciel MC. Depot versus daily administration of gonadotrophin releasing hormone agonist protocols for pituitary desensitization in assisted reproduction cycles. The Cochrane Library 2003. Oxford: Update Software, 2003; Issue 1.

38. Weissman A, Shoham Z. Favourable pregnancy outcome after administration of a long-acting gonadotrophin-releasing hormone agonist in the mid-luteal phase. Hum Reprod 1993; 8: 496–7.

39. Balasch J, Martinez F, Jove I, et al. Inadvertent gonadotrophin-releasing hormone agonist (GnRHa) administration in the luteal phase may improve fecundity in in vitro fertilization patients. Hum Reprod 1993; 8: 1148–51.

40. Ron-El R, Lahat E, Golan A, et al. Development of children born after ovarian superovulation induced by long-acting gonadotropin-releasing hormone agonist and menotropins, and by in vitro fertilization. J Pediatr 1994; 125: 734–7.

41. Cahill DJ, Fountain SA, Fox R, et al. Outcome of inadvertent administration of a gonadotrophin-releasing hormone agonist (buserelin) in early pregnancy. Hum Reprod 1994; 9: 1243–6.

42. Gartner B, Moreno C, Marinaro A, et al. Accidental exposure to daily long-acting gonadotrophin-releasing hormone analogue administration and pregnancy in an in vitro fertilization cycle. Hum Reprod 1997; 12: 2557–9.

43. Taskin O, Gokdeniz R, Atmaca R, et al. Normal pregnancy outcome after inadvertent exposure to long-acting gonadotrophin-releasing hormone agonist in early pregnancy. Hum Reprod 1999; 14: 1368–71.

44. Lahat E, Raziel A, Friedler S, et al. Long-term follow-up of children born after inadvertent administration of a gonadotrophin-releasing hormone agonist in early pregnancy. Hum Reprod 1999; 14: 2656–60.

45. Surrey ES, Silverberg KM, Surrey MW, et al. Effect of prolonged gonadotropin-releasing hormone agonist therapy on the outcome of in vitro fertilization-embryo transfer in patients with endometriosis. Fertil Steril 2002; 78: 699–704.

46. de Ziegler D, Cedars MI, Randle D, et al. Suppression of the ovary using a gonadotropin releasing-hormone agonist prior to stimulation for oocyte retrieval. Fertil Steril 1987; 48: 807–10.

47. Balasch J, Jove IC, Moreno V, et al. The comparison of two gonadotropin-releasing hormone agonists in an in vitro fertilization program. Fertil Steril 1992; 58: 991–4.

48. Parinaud J, Oustry P, Perineau M, et al. Randomized trial of three luteinizing hormone-releasing hormone analogues used for ovarian stimulation in an in vitro fertilization program. Fertil Steril 1992; 57: 1265–8.

49. Penzias AS, Shamma FN, Gutmann JN, et al. Nafarelin versus leuprolide in ovulation induction for in vitro fertilization: a randomized clinical trial. Obstet Gynecol 1992; 79: 739–42.

50. Tapanainen J, Hovatta O, Juntunen K, et al. Subcutaneous goserelin versus intranasal buserelin for pituitary down-regulation in patients undergoing IVF: a randomized comparative study. Hum Reprod 1993; 8: 2052–5.

51. Dantas ZN, Vicino M, Balmaceda JP, et al. Comparison between nafarelin and leuprolide acetate for in vitro fertilization: preliminary clinical study. Fertil Steril 1994; 61: 705–8.

52. Goldman JA, Dicker D, Feldberg D, et al. A prospective randomized comparison of two gonadotrophin- releasing hormone agonists, nafarelin acetate and buserelin acetate, in in vitro fertilization-embryo transfer. Hum Reprod 1994; 9: 226–8.

53. Tarlatzis BC, Grimbizis G, Pournaropoulos F, et al. Evaluation of two gonadotropin-releasing hormone (GnRH) analogues (leuprolide and buserelin) in short and long protocols for assisted reproductive techniques. J Assist Reprod Genet 1994; 11: 85–91.

54. Lockwood GM, Pinkerton SM, Barlow DH. A prospective randomized single-blind comparative trial of nafarelin acetate with buserelin in long-protocol gonadotrophin-releasing hormone analogue controlled in vitro fertilization cycles. Hum Reprod 1995; 10: 293–8.

55. Tanos V, Friedler S, Shushan A, et al. Comparison between nafarelin acetate and D-Trp6–LHRH for temporary pituitary suppression in in vitro fertilization (IVF) patients: A prospective crossover study. J Assist Reprod Genet 1995; 12: 715–19.

56. Oyesanya OA, Teo SK, Quah E, et al. Pituitary down-regulation prior to in vitro fertilization and embryo transfer: a comparison between a single dose of Zoladex depot and multiple daily doses of Suprefact. Hum Reprod 1995; 10: 1042–4.

57. Avrech OM, Goldman GA, Pinkas H, et al. Intranasal nafarelin versus buserelin (short protocol) for controlled ovarian hyperstimulation before in vitro fertilization: a prospective clinical trial. Gynecol Endocrinol 1996; 10: 165–70.

58. Corson SL, Gutmann JN, Batzer FR, et al. A double-blind comparison of nafarelin and leuprolide acetate for down-regulation in IVF cycles. Int J Fertil Menopausal Stud 1996; 41: 446–9.

59. Polson DW, Mason HD, Saldahna MB, et al. Ovulation of a single dominant follicle during treatment with low-dose pulsatile follicle stimulating hormone in women with polycystic ovary syndrome. Clin Endocrinol (Oxf) 1987; 26: 205–12.

60. Tan SL. Luteinizing hormone-releasing hormone agonists for ovarian stimulation in assisted reproduction. Curr Opin Obstet Gynecol 1994; 6: 166–72.

61. Chang SY, Lee CL, Wang ML, et al. No detrimental effects in delaying initiation of gonadotropin administration after pituitary desensitization with gonadotropin-releasing hormone agonist. Fertil Steril 1993; 59: 183–6.

62. Dimitry ES, Oskarsson T, Conaghan J, et al. Beneficial effects of a 24 h delay in human chorionic gonadotrophin administration during in vitro fertilization treatment cycles. Hum Reprod 1991; 6: 944–6.

63. Daya S. Gonadotrophin-releasing hormone agonist protocols for pituitary desensitization in in vitro fertilization and gamete intrafallopian transfer cycles. The Cochrane Library 2001. Oxford: Update Software, 2001; Issue 1.

64. Pellicer A, Simon C, Miro F, et al. Ovarian response and outcome of in vitro fertilization in patients treated with gonadotrophin-releasing hormone analogues in different phases of the menstrual cycle. Hum Reprod 1989; 4: 285–9.

65. Kondaveeti-Gordon U, Harrison RF, Barry-Kinsella C, et al. A randomized prospective study of early follicular or midluteal initiation of long protocol gonadotropin-releasing hormone in an in vitro fertilization program. Fertil Steril 1996; 66: 582–6.

66. San Roman GA, Surrey ES, Judd HL, et al. A prospective randomized comparison of luteal phase versus concurrent follicular phase initiation of gonadotropin-releasing hormone agonist for in vitro fertilization. Fertil Steril 1992; 58: 744–9.

67. Keltz MD, Jones EE, Duleba AJ, et al. Baseline cyst formation after luteal phase gonadotropin-releasing hormone agonist administration is linked to poor in vitro fertilization outcome. Fertil Steril 1995; 64: 568–72.

68. Feldberg D, Ashkenazi J, Dicker D, et al. Ovarian cyst formation: a complication of gonadotropin-releasing hormone agonist therapy. Fertil Steril 1989; 51: 42–5.

69. Biljan MM, Mahutte NG, Dean N, et al. Pretreatment with an oral contraceptive is effective in reducing the incidence of functional ovarian cyst formation during pituitary suppression by gonadotropin-releasing hormone analogues. J Assist Reprod Genet 1998; 15: 599–604.

70. Damario MA, Barmat L, Liu HC, et al. Dual suppression with oral contraceptives and gonadotrophin releasing-hormone agonists improves in vitro fertilization outcome in high responder patients. Hum Reprod 1997; 12: 2359–65.

71. Cedrin-Durnerin I, Bidart JM, Robert P, et al. Consequences on gonadotrophin secretion of an early discontinuation of gonadotropin-releasing hormone agonist administration in short-term protocol for in vitro fertilization. Hum Reprod 2000; 15: 1009–14.

72. Dirnfeld M, Fruchter O, Yshai D, et al. Cessation of gonadotropin-releasing hormone analogue (GnRH-a) upon down-regulation versus conventional long GnRH-a protocol in poor responders undergoing in vitro fertilization. Fertil Steril 1999; 72: 406–11.

73. Garcia-Velasco JA, Isaza V, Requena A, et al. High doses of gonadotrophins combined with stop versus non-stop protocol of GnRH analogue administration in low responder IVF patients: a prospective, randomized, controlled trial. Hum Reprod 2000; 15: 2292–6.

74. Fujii S, Sagara M, Kudo H, et al. A prospective randomized comparison between long and discontinuous-long protocols of gonadotropin-releasing hormone agonist for in vitro fertilization. Fertil Steril 1997; 67: 1166–8.

75. Fujii S, Sato S, Fukui A, et al. Continuous administration of gonadotrophin-releasing hormone agonist during the luteal phase in IVF. Hum Reprod 2001; 16: 1671–5.

76. Padilla SL, Dugan K, Maruschak V, et al. Use of the flare-up protocol with high dose human follicle stimulating

hormone and human menopausal gonadotropins for in vitro fertilization in poor responders. Fertil Steril 1996; 65: 796–9.

77. Loumaye E, Coen G, Pampfer S, et al. Use of a gonadotropin-releasing hormone agonist during ovarian stimulation leads to significant concentrations of peptide in follicular fluids. Fertil Steril 1989; 52: 256–63.

78. Fasouliotis SJ, Simon A, Laufer N. Evaluation and treatment of low responders in assisted reproductive technique: A challenge to meet. J Assist Reprod Genet 2000; 17: 357–73.

79. Acharya U, Irvine S, Hamilton M, et al. Prospective study of short and ultrashort regimens of gonadotropin-releasing hormone agonist in an in vitro fertilization program. Fertil Steril 1992; 58: 1169–73.

80. Scott RT, Navot D. Enhancement of ovarian responsiveness with microdoses of gonadotropin-releasing hormone agonist during ovulation induction for in vitro fertilization. Fertil Steril 1994; 61: 880–5.

81. Feldberg D, Farhi J, Ashkenazi J, et al. Minidose gonadotropin-releasing hormone agonist is the treatment of choice in poor responders with high follicle-stimulating hormone levels. Fertil Steril 1994; 62: 343–6.

82. Surrey ES, Bower J, Hill DM, et al. Clinical and endocrine effects of a microdose GnRH agonist flare regimen administered to poor responders who are undergoing in vitro fertilization. Fertil Steril 1998; 69: 419–24.

83. Sher G, Zouves C, Feinman M, et al. 'Prolonged coasting': an effective method for preventing severe ovarian hyperstimulation syndrome in patients undergoing in vitro fertilization. Hum Reprod 1995; 10: 3107–9.

84. Fluker MR, Hooper WM, Yuzpe AA. Withholding gonadotropins ("coasting") to minimize the risk of ovarian hyperstimulation during superovulation and in vitro fertilization-embryo transfer cycles. Fertil Steril 1999; 71: 294–301.

85. D'Angelo A, Amso N. "Coasting" (withholding gonadotrophins) for preventing ovarian hyperstimulation syndrome. Cochrane Database Syst Rev 2002; CD002811.

86. Egbase PE, Sharhan MA, Grudzinskas JG. Early unilateral follicular aspiration compared with coasting for the prevention of severe ovarian hyperstimulation syndrome: a prospective randomized study. Hum Reprod 1999; 14: 1421–5.

87. Emperaire JC, Ruffie A. Triggering ovulation with endogenous luteinizing hormone may prevent the ovarian hyperstimulation syndrome. Hum Reprod 1991; 6: 506–10.

88. Lanzone A, Fulghesu AM, Villa P, et al. Gonadotropin-releasing hormone agonist versus human chorionic gonadotropin as a trigger of ovulation in polycystic ovarian disease gonadotropin hyperstimulated cycles. Fertil Steril 1994; 62: 35–41.

89. Gonen Y, Balakier H, Powell W, et al. Use of gonadotropin-releasing hormone agonist to trigger follicular maturation for in vitro fertilization. J Clin Endocrinol Metab 1990; 71: 918–22.

90. Itskovitz J, Boldes R, Levron J, et al. Induction of preovulatory luteinizing hormone surge and prevention of ovarian hyperstimulation syndrome by gonadotropin-releasing hormone agonist. Fertil Steril 1991; 56: 213–20.

91. Romeu A, Monzo A, Peiro T, et al. Endogenous LH surge versus hCG as ovulation trigger after low-dose highly purified FSH in IUI: a comparison of 761 cycles. J Assist Reprod Genet 1997; 14: 518–24.

92. Olivennes F, Fanchin R, Bouchard P, et al. Triggering of ovulation by a gonadotropin-releasing hormone (GnRH) agonist in patients pretreated with a GnRH antagonist. Fertil Steril 1996; 66: 151–3.

93. Itskovitz-Eldor J, Kol S, Mannaerts B. Use of a single bolus of GnRH agonist triptorelin to trigger ovulation after GnRH antagonist ganirelix treatment in women undergoing ovarian stimulation for assisted reproduction, with special reference to the prevention of ovarian hyperstimulation syndrome: preliminary report: short communication. Hum Reprod 2000; 15: 1965–8.

94. Fauser BC, de Jong D, Olivennes F, et al. Endocrine profiles after triggering of final oocyte maturation with GnRH agonist after cotreatment with the GnRH antagonist ganirelix during ovarian hyperstimulation for in vitro fertilization. J Clin Endocrinol Metab 2002; 87: 709–15.

95. Egbase PE, Grudzinskas JG, Al Sharhan M, Ashkenazi L. HCG or GnRH agonist to trigger ovulation in GnRH antagonist-treated intrauterine insemination cycles: a prospective randomized study. Hum Reprod 2002; 17: 2–O–006.

41

GnRH-antagonists in ovarian stimulation for IVF

Efstratios M. Kolibianakis, Georg Griesinger, and Basil C. Tarlatzis

INTRODUCTION

Although the first successful in vitro fertilization (IVF) was a procedure that did not involve ovarian stimulation (1), it was soon accepted that the role of IVF as an efficient therapeutic modality for subfertile couples could only be served through multifollicular development, achieved with the use of gonadotropins (2).

Gonadotropin use, however, was frequently associated with premature luteinizing hormone (LH) surge prior to oocyte retrieval, which led to cycle cancellation (3). The estimated proportion of patients who will exhibit a premature LH surge under gonadotropin stimulation only is 23% (95% CI: 14 to 35) (4).

Thanks to the pioneering work of Schally in 1971 (5), the problem of premature LH surge was managed by the introduction of gonadotropin-releasing hormone (GnRH)–agonists in ovarian stimulation (6). Although antagonistic analogues were also available, they were not used for this purpose due to the associated allergic reactions provoked by their administration (7). It was the GnRH-agonists that changed the way ovarian stimulation was performed in the early 1980s.

Following pituitary downregulation by GnRH-agonists, the unhindered use of gonadotropins, devoid from the problem of premature LH surge, allowed for flexibility in ovarian stimulation, collection of more oocytes, and an increase in the number of good quality embryos available for transfer (8). This led to an increase in pregnancy rates, compared to cycles where no suppression of premature LH surge was performed, as was shown by one of the first meta-analyses in reproductive medicine (9).

The use of GnRH-agonists became universal through the 1980s, 1990s, and until the early 2000s, since they were the only clinically available GnRH-analogue for suppressing premature LH surge. IVF throughout this period, from an ovarian stimulation point of view, can be identified as the GnRH-agonist era (10).

Despite this, there is probably no much doubt that if GnRH-antagonist usage was not associated with allergic reactions, the analogue of choice for suppressing premature LH rise back in the early 1980s should have been GnRH antagonist instead of GnRH agonist. This is mainly due to the fact that GnRH-antagonist action starts immediately after their administration as opposed to the lengthy downregulation period, which characterizes GnRH-agonists use. Thus GnRH-antagonists are available for immediate action when needed.

Moreover, although GnRH-agonists solved the problem of premature LH surge, their use resulted in new problems, such as the presence of estrogen deprivation symptoms during the downregulation period, the occurrence of cyst formation at initiation of stimulation and of ovarian hyperstimulation syndrome (OHSS) after the administration of human chorionic gonadotropin (hCG).

For the above reasons, the introduction of the third generation of GnRH-antagonists, lacking histamine release problems and thus, allergic reactions in the early 2000s (11,12), was perceived by the scientific community as a great opportunity to simplify and optimize ovarian stimulation.

GNRH-AGONISTS VS. GNRH-ANTAGONISTS

GnRH-antagonists were initially introduced by five large, comparative trials with GnRH-agonists, which were sponsored by the pharmaceutical industry. Following the completion of these trials a meta-analysis by the Cochrane library suggested that the use of GnRH-antagonists was associated with a significantly lower chance of clinical pregnancy compared to GnRH-agonists (13). The difference was of marginal clinical significance (5%) and no clear explanation was available to justify its presence. Nevertheless, it created a lot of anxiety amongst clinicians willing to adopt GnRH-antagonists for ovarian stimulation, limiting their popularity. According to the German registry, GnRH-antagonists as compared to GnRH-agonists were used in patients with a worse prognosis for becoming pregnant, such as those with a higher number of previously failed cycles and those who were older (14). GnRH-antagonist usage by the end of the last decade remained at approximately 30% of the IVF cycles preformed worldwide (15).

The initial meta-analysis of the Cochrane library that generated a lot of skepticism regarding the efficacy of GnRH-antagonists was updated twice, in 2006 and in 2011 (16,17). Interestingly, the reanalysis of the five initial studies that generated a significant concern in the scientific community, using the figures published in 2011 by the Cochrane group, shows that a significant difference in clinical pregnancy rate was not present back in 2001 (Fig. 41.1) and thus the concern generated, which led to a bad reputation of GnRH-antagonists was not justified.

This had already been suggested in an earlier meta-analysis (18) comparing GnRH-agonists with GnRH-antagonists. In that meta-analysis, it was pointed out that a significant difference in live birth rate, which is the outcome measure that should be used to evaluate treatments that aim to alleviate subfertility (19), was not present in 2001, after the initial studies were performed, as well as in 2006 with the addition of more comparative RCTs (18).

The most important evolution in the debate regarding the comparison between GnRH-agonists and GnRH-antagonists was the recent meta-analysis of the Cochrane group comparing GnRH-agonists with GnRH-antagonists (17). This suggested that a move away from the standard GnRH-agonist long protocol to a GnRH antagonist protocol is justified, given the significantly increased safety of

GnRH-antagonists compared with GnRH-agonists, combined with their equal effectiveness regarding live birth rate.

Unfortunately, this occurred 11 years after the introduction of GnRH-antagonists, although a difference in live birth rate per woman randomized was never present. During this period, from the multiple comparisons between the two analogues, certain quantitative advantages of GnRH-antagonists emerged, such as a shorter duration of stimulation and a decreased occurrence of OHSS by more than 50% (risk ratio 0.45 95% CI:0.34 to 0.59) (18). The latter represents one of the most important GnRH-antagonist advantages.

Apparently, complicated and sometimes difficult to follow meta-analyses comparing GnRH-agonists versus GnRH-antagonists are not necessary to understand that GnRH-antagonist use makes ovarian stimulation more patient friendly and, from a physician's point of view, a rational procedure. It is difficult to defend GnRH agonist use as a rational way to inhibit premature LH rise in

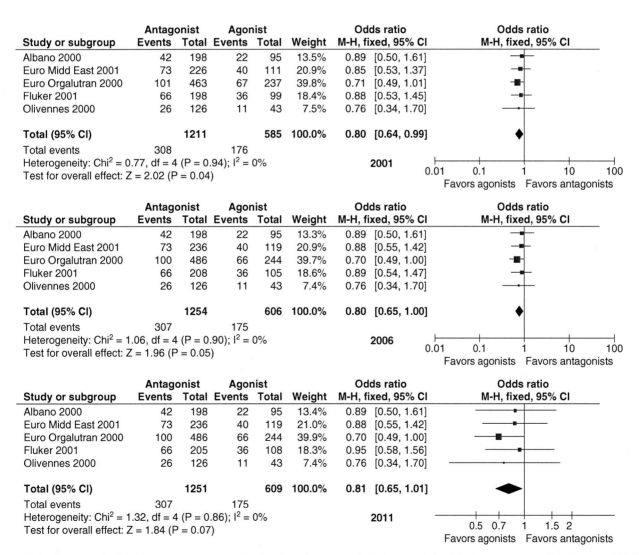

Figure 41.1   Analysis of clinical pregnancy rates in the five introductory trials that generated a lot of concern regarding the use of GnRH-antagonists, according to the figures published by the Cochrane group in the initial (13) and the updated meta-analyses (16,17). The figures published regarding clinical pregnancies differ in each update and there is no difference in clinical pregnancy rates according to the figures published in 2011 (17).

2011, when GnRH-agonist is administered approximately three weeks before such an event is possible.

Following the publication of the updated Cochrane meta-analysis (17) it is clear that the long-standing debate regarding the efficacy of GnRH-antagonists compared to GnRH-agonists has come to an end, probably heralding the end of the GnRH-agonist era as well.

DOSE, SCHEME, AND TIMING OF GNRH-ANTAGONIST ADMINISTRATION

GnRH-antagonists can be administered according to a daily- (20) or a single-dose scheme (21), the latter inhibiting premature LH rise for four days. The single-dose scheme can be combined with daily GnRH-antagonist administration if necessary. Two types of third generation GnRH-antagonists have been developed: Ganirelix (Organon, Oss, Netherlands) (22) and Cetrorelix (ASTA-Medica, Frankfurt/M, Germany) (23). On the basis of dose-finding studies, the optimal dose for the daily-dose scheme is 0.25 mg for both Cetrorelix and Ganirelix (24,25) and 3 mg for the single-dose scheme (Cetrorelix) (26).

The majority of GnRH-antagonist cycles performed today follow the daily-dose scheme (20), although a stratified analysis of two relevant comparative trials between the single- and the daily-dose scheme (27,28) did not show a difference in the probability of clinical pregnancy [Rate Difference (RD): −2% in favor of the daily dose protocol; 95% CI: −16 to + 11].

GnRH-antagonist initiation can be performed either in a fixed or in a flexible way. The fixed mode of GnRH-antagonist administration assumes that after a fixed number of stimulation days, LH rise or LH surge becomes imminent in the majority of patients and thus routine GnRH-antagonist administration is justified. In the early introductory antagonist studies this was thought to be the case on day 6 of stimulation (29), while in the more recent studies (24) GnRH-antagonist initiation in a fixed mode has been moved forward to day 5 of stimulation (30).

In a flexible GnRH-antagonist administration scheme, GnRH-antagonist is administered only after certain endocrine and/or sonographic criteria, which are thought to indicate a risk for LH rise/surge, are present. These criteria have differed between studies (31).

Apparently, fixed GnRH-antagonist initiation is a simpler protocol that requires less monitoring compared to the flexible one. However, flexible GnRH-antagonist administration might avoid unnecessary GnRH-antagonist administration, in a proportion of patients in whom an LH surge is unlikely to occur on day 5 of stimulation due to absence of follicular development.

Four RCTs have been published comparing fixed versus flexible GnRH-antagonist administration in patients undergoing IVF (31–34). A stratified analysis of these RCTs suggests that no significant difference appears to exist in clinical pregnancy rates (odds ratio 0.79, 95% CI: 0.53 to 1.16) (Fig. 41.2). This is in line with the results of an earlier meta-analysis (35).

PROGRAMMING THE INITIATION OF A GNRH-ANTAGONIST CYCLE

One of the basic differences between a GnRH-agonist and a GnRH-antagonist cycle is that in the latter, initiation of stimulation is dependent on the occurrence of menstruation. In a long luteal GnRH-agonist protocol, gonadotropin stimulation starts after downregulation is confirmed, which might be soon after menstruation but can also be postponed, if deemed necessary.

There are two basic reasons for programming the initiation of an IVF cycle: First, the prevention of oocyte retrievals on Sundays or on weekends, and second, the avoidance of concomitant initiation of too many cycles in very busy centers that can increase the center's workload beyond what is considered as manageable.

Regarding the second case, knowing the type and length of patients' cycles makes it feasible to avoid too many cycles starting on the same days by simply planning cycle initiation. Avoiding oocyte retrievals on Sundays for centers working six days per week or weekend for centers working five days per week is more difficult, both for GnRH-agonists and for GnRH-antagonists cycles. It would be ideal if gonadotropin stimulation lasted a fixed period of days. If this was the case, then by scheduling initiation of stimulation on a certain day, inevitably oocyte retrieval would occur on a specific, known day, and the problem would be solved, at least in GnRH-agonist cycles. However, both in GnRH-agonist and in GnRH-antagonist cycles, duration of

Study or subgroup	Flexible Events	Total	Fixed Events	Total	Weight	Odds ratio M-H, fixed, 95% CI	Year	Odds ratio M-H, fixed, 95% CI
Ludwig	20	50	26	59	24.9%	0.85 [0.39, 1.82]	2002	
Escudero	7	40	4	20	7.6%	0.85 [0.22, 3.33]	2004	
Mochtar	23	101	34	103	45.2%	0.60 [0.32, 1.11]	2004	
Kolibianakis	18	73	17	73	22.3%	1.08 [0.50, 2.31]	2011	
Total (95% CI)		264		255	100.0%	0.79 [0.53, 1.16]		
Total events	68		81					

Heterogeneity: Chi^2 = 1.45, df = 3 (P = 0.69); I^2 = 0%
Test for overall effect: Z = 1.22 (P = 0.22)

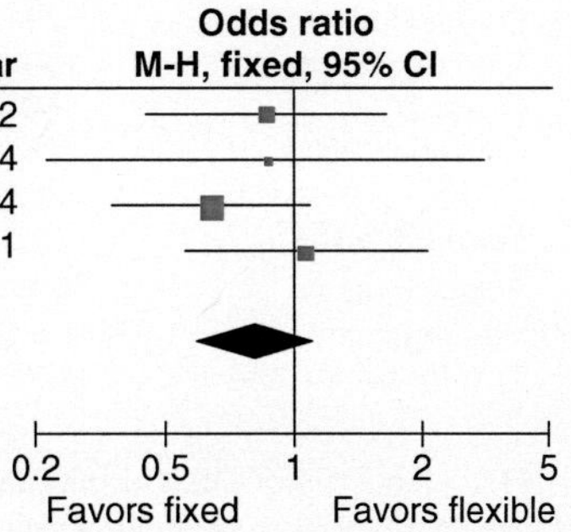

0.2   0.5   1   2   5
Favors fixed   Favors flexible

Figure 41.2 Stratified analysis of clinical pregnancy rates in four RCTs comparing fixed versus flexible antagonist administration in patients undergoing IVF.

stimulation is characterized by a significant inter- and even intra-individual variation, which makes this a challenging task. Nevertheless, in GnRH-antagonist cycles it is also possible to manage this problem effectively by altering the day of starting gonadotropin stimulation from day 2 to day 3 of the cycle and/or by delaying hCG administration by one day, if necessary (36). It should be noted, however, that delaying hCG administration for ≥ two days after ≥ three follicles of ≥17 mm are present at ultrasound is associated with a significantly decreased probability of pregnancy in GnRH-antagonist cycles (37).

Use of the oral contraceptive pills (OCP) as a pretreatment, to program the initiation of an antagonist IVF cycle should probably be avoided, as, according to recent meta-analysis, it is associated with a decreased probability of ongoing pregnancy (relative risk: 0.80, 95% CI: 0.66 to 0.97; p = 0.02; rate difference: −5%, 95% CI: −10% to −1%; p = 0.02). OCP pretreatment in GnRH-antagonist cycles is also associated with an increased duration of stimulation [weighted mean difference (WMD): +1.35 days, 95% CI: +0.62 to +2.07; p < 0.01] and gonadotropin consumption (WMD: +360 IUs, 95% CI: +158 to +563; p < 0.01) (38).

GONADOTROPHIN STIMULATION IN A GNRH-ANTAGONIST CYCLE

Determining the starting dose of gonadotropins is performed subjectively in IVF, although efforts to develop an objective procedure have also been made (39,40). A starting dose of 150 IU is generally considered appropriate for a typical patient. Two studies have been performed in GnRH-antagonist cycles to determine whether a higher (200 IU or 225 IU) than the "standard" (150 IU) dose would increase the probability of pregnancy (41,42). Although a limited number of patients were analyzed in these studies, it does not appear that pregnancy rates are increased by using a higher than the "standard" dose of FSH (odds ratio for clinical pregnancy 0.81, 95% CI: 0.51 to 1.28).

In GnRH-antagonist cycles FSH stimulation can start either on day 2 or day 3 of the cycle (43,44). Data from reanalysis of the recently published ENGAGE trial (30,36) suggest that such an intervention (starting on day 2 or 3 of menses) does not alter the probability of pregnancy. A later initiation of FSH stimulation, on day 5, is also possible in the so-called "mild stimulation protocols" (45), the target of which is increased safety and decreased drug consumption (46,47).

Increase of FSH dose at GnRH-antagonist initiation versus no increase has been evaluated in two trials by Aboulghar et al. (2004) and by Propst et al. (2006), which did not show a significant increase in the probability of clinical pregnancy (17.2% vs. 19.1% and 60% vs.70%, respectively) (48,49).

LH addition has so far been tested in a limited number of studies, which have been summarized in three meta-analyses. These suggest that LH addition does not appear to be necessary in GnRH-antagonist cycles (50–52).

ENDOCRINE ASSOCIATIONS IN A GNRH-ANTAGONIST CYCLE

Elevated progesterone at initiation of stimulation in a spontaneous cycle with natural luteal phase is a rather infrequent event in antagonist cycles (~5% of patients). If, in those patients, initiation of stimulation is postponed for one or two days, progesterone levels will normalize in the majority of cases (80%). However, pregnancy rates in this group are expected to be significantly lower compared with patients with normal progesterone levels at initiation of stimulation (53). Thus, postponing IVF attempt until the next menstruation is worth considering. The same is true, if elevated estradiol (E2) levels are present on day 2 of the cycle, which might be indicative of an ovarian cyst.

Elevated progesterone levels on the day of triggering final oocyte maturation have been associated with a significantly decreased probability of pregnancy (risk ratio: 0.76; 95% CI: 0.60 to 0.97) (54). If progesterone elevation occurs, it is worth considering freezing all embryos and performing the transfer in a subsequent cycle.

According to a systematic review, low LH levels during ovarian stimulation with GnRH-antagonists are not a concern and cannot serve as a rationale for LH addition to FSH (55).

TRIGGERING OF FINAL OOCYTE MATURATION IN A GNRH-ANTAGONIST CYCLE

Although the incidence of OHSS is significantly decreased in GnRH-antagonists as compared to GnRH-agonist cycles (17), it can still occur, depending on the type of patient stimulated and the intensity of gonadotropin stimulation.

OHSS is invariably associated with administration of hCG for triggering final oocyte maturation. Thus, the unique to GnRH-antagonists option of triggering final oocyte maturation with GnRH-agonists, represents one of the most important aspects of the antagonistic protocol. This is due to the fact that the incidence of OHSS after agonist triggering is practically zero (56). Thus, by performing GnRH-antagonist stimulation, not only is the incidence of OHSS reduced by half compared to a GnRH-agonist cycle, but in case of an excessive ovarian response in high risk for OHSS patients, GnRH agonist can replace hCG, saving patients from lengthy hospitalizations, increased costs, and potentially serious risks for their health.

GnRH-agonist triggering is currently associated with a significantly decreased probability of pregnancy (57), if embryo transfer is performed in the same cycle and thus when administered to replace hCG in high risk for OHSS patients, all embryos should be frozen and transferred safely in a subsequent frozen-thawed cycle (58). This also ensures that patients will not develop late pregnancy-associated OHSS.

For the above reasons GnRH-antagonists/FSH stimulation combined with GnRH-agonist triggering is the standard mode of stimulation for oocyte donors (59).

LUTEAL SUPPORT IN GNRH-ANTAGONIST CYCLES

The major reason for supporting the luteal phase in IVF is the presence of endometrium abnormalities and very low LH levels following oocyte retrieval. Both these problems are associated with gonadotropin stimulation and are independent of the type of analogue used to inhibit premature LH surge (60). Micronized progesterone is frequently used for luteal phase support while the addition of E2 appears not to be beneficial for pregnancy rates (61).

NEW CONCEPTS IN OVARIAN STIMULATION USING GNRH-ANTAGONISTS

GnRH-antagonists have rendered IVF a patient-friendly and safe procedure of high efficacy. Concomitantly they have stimulated scientific thinking in developing new concepts in ovarian stimulation. These include the modified natural cycle, mild IVF (62), agonist triggering and cryopreservation of all 2PN oocytes (58), reinitiation of antagonist in case of severe established OHSS (63–65) and many more which are currently under investigation.

The recent introduction of long acting FSH (30), which is used only in GnRH-antagonist cycles, is a step further in simplifying ovarian stimulation and making it as patient friendly as possible, while retaining its efficacy regarding the achievement of live birth.

REFERENCES

1. Steptoe PC, Edwards RG. Birth after the reimplantation of a human embryo. Lancet 1978; 2: 366.
2. Trounson AO, Leeton JF, Wood C, Webb J, Wood J. Pregnancies in humans by fertilization in vitro and embryo transfer in the controlled ovulatory cycle. Science 1981; 212: 681–2.
3. Loumaye E. The control of endogenous secretion of LH by gonadotrophin-releasing hormone agonists during ovarian hyperstimulation for in-vitro fertilization and embryo transfer. Hum Reprod 1990; 5: 357–76.
4. Janssens RM, Lambalk CB, Vermeiden JP, et al. Dose-finding study of triptorelin acetate for prevention of a premature LH surge in IVF: a prospective, randomized, double-blind, placebo-controlled study. Hum Reprod 2000; 15: 2333–40.
5. Schally AV, Arimura A, Baba Y, et al. Isolation and properties of the FSH and LH-releasing hormone. Biochem Biophys Res Commun 1971; 43: 393–9.
6. Porter RN, Smith W, Craft IL, Abdulwahid NA, Jacobs HS. Induction of ovulation for in-vitro fertilisation using buserelin and gonadotropins. Lancet 1984; 2: 1284–5.
7. Hahn DW, McGuire JL, Vale WW, Rivier J. Reproductive/endocrine and anaphylactoid properties of an LHRH-antagonist, ORF 18260 [Ac-DNAL1(2), 4FDPhe2,D-Trp3, D-Arg6]-GnRH. Life Sci 1985; 37: 505–14.
8. Meldrum DR. Ovulation induction protocols. Arch Pathol Lab Med 1992; 116: 406–9.
9. Hughes EG, Fedorkow DM, Daya S, et al. The routine use of gonadotropin-releasing hormone agonists prior to in vitro fertilization and gamete intrafallopian transfer: a meta-analysis of randomized controlled trials. Fertil Steril 1992; 58: 888–96.
10. Marcus SF, Ledger WL. Efficacy and safety of long-acting GnRH agonists in in vitro fertilization and embryo transfer. Hum Fertil (Camb) 2001; 4: 85–93.
11. Duijkers IJ, Klipping C, Willemsen WN, et al. Single and multiple dose pharmacokinetics and pharmacodynamics of the gonadotrophin-releasing hormone antagonist Cetrorelix in healthy female volunteers. Hum Reprod 1998; 13: 2392–8.
12. Mannaerts B, Gordon K. Embryo implantation and GnRH antagonists: GnRH antagonists do not activate the GnRH receptor. Hum Reprod 2000; 15: 1882–3.
13. Al-Inany H, Aboulghar M. Gonadotrophin-releasing hormone antagonists for assisted conception. Cochrane Database Syst Rev 2001: CD001750.
14. Griesinger G, Felberbaum R, Diedrich K. GnRH antagonists in ovarian stimulation: a treatment regimen of clinicians' second choice? Data from the German national IVF registry. Hum Reprod 2005; 20: 2373–5.
15. D.I.R. Jahrbuch 2008.
16. Al-Inany HG, Abou-Setta AM, Aboulghar M. Gonadotrophin-releasing hormone antagonists for assisted conception. Cochrane Database Syst Rev 2006; 3: CD001750.
17. Al-Inany HG, Youssef MA, Aboulghar M, et al. Gonadotrophin-releasing hormone antagonists for assisted reproductive technology. Cochrane Database Syst Rev 2011; 5: CD001750.
18. Kolibianakis EM, Collins J, Tarlatzis BC, et al. Among patients treated for IVF with gonadotrophins and GnRH analogues, is the probability of live birth dependent on the type of analogue used? A systematic review and meta-analysis. Hum Reprod Update 2006; 12: 651–71.
19. Land JA, Evers JL. Risks and complications in assisted reproductive techniques: Report of an ESHRE consensus meeting. Hum Reprod 2003; 18: 455–7.
20. Diedrich K, Diedrich C, Santos E, et al. Suppression of the endogenous luteinizing hormone surge by the gonadotrophin-releasing hormone antagonist Cetrorelix during ovarian stimulation. Hum Reprod 1994; 9: 788–91.
21. Olivennes F, Fanchin R, Bouchard P, et al. The single or dual administration of the gonadotropin-releasing hormone antagonist Cetrorelix in an in vitro fertilization-embryo transfer program. Fertil Steril 1994; 62: 468–76.
22. Rabinovici J, Rothman P, Monroe SE, Nerenberg C, Jaffe RB. Endocrine effects and pharmacokinetic characteristics of a potent new gonadotropin-releasing hormone antagonist (Ganirelix) with minimal histamine-releasing properties: studies in postmenopausal women. J Clin Endocrinol Metab 1992; 75: 1220–5.
23. Klingmuller D, Schepke M, Enzweiler C, Bidlingmaier F. Hormonal responses to the new potent GnRH antagonist Cetrorelix. Acta Endocrinol (Copenh) 1993; 128: 15–18.
24. Group Tgd-fs. A double-blind, randomized, dose-finding study to assess the efficacy of the gonadotrophin-releasing hormone antagonist ganirelix (Org 37462) to prevent premature luteinizing hormone surges in women undergoing ovarian stimulation with recombinant follicle stimulating hormone (Puregon). Hum Reprod 1998; 13: 3023–31.
25. Albano C, Smitz J, Camus M, et al. Comparison of different doses of gonadotropin-releasing hormone antagonist

Cetrorelix during controlled ovarian hyperstimulation. Fertil Steril 1997; 67: 917–22.

26. Olivennes F, Alvarez S, Bouchard P, et al. The use of a GnRH antagonist (Cetrorelix) in a single dose protocol in IVF-embryo transfer: a dose finding study of 3 versus 2 mg. Hum Reprod 1998; 13: 2411–14.

27. Lee TH, Wu MY, Chen HF, et al. Ovarian response and follicular development for single-dose and multiple-dose protocols for gonadotropin-releasing hormone antagonist administration. Fertil Steril 2005; 83: 1700–7.

28. Wilcox J, Potter D, Moore M, Ferrande L, Kelly E. Prospective, randomized trial comparing cetrorelix acetate and ganirelix acetate in a programmed, flexible protocol for premature luteinizing hormone surge prevention in assisted reproductive techniques. Fertil Steril 2005; 84: 108–17.

29. Borm G, Mannaerts B. Treatment with the gonadotrophin-releasing hormone antagonist ganirelix in women undergoing ovarian stimulation with recombinant follicle stimulating hormone is effective, safe and convenient: results of a controlled, randomized, multicentre trial. The European Orgalutran Study Group. Hum Reprod 2000; 15: 1490–8.

30. Devroey P, Boostanfar R, Koper NP, et al. A double-blind, non-inferiority RCT comparing corifollitropin alfa and recombinant FSH during the first seven days of ovarian stimulation using a GnRH antagonist protocol. Hum Reprod 2009; 24: 3063–72.

31. Kolibianakis EM, Venetis CA, Kalogeropoulou L, Papanikolaou E, Tarlatzis BC. Fixed versus flexible gonadotropin-releasing hormone antagonist administration in in vitro fertilization: a randomized controlled trial. Fertil Steril 2011; 95: 558–62.

32. Escudero E, Bosch E, Crespo J, et al. Comparison of two different starting multiple dose gonadotropin-releasing hormone antagonist protocols in a selected group of in vitro fertilization-embryo transfer patients. Fertil Steril 2004; 81: 562–6.

33. Mochtar MH. The effect of an individualized GnRH antagonist protocol on folliculogenesis in IVF/ICSI. Hum Reprod 2004; 19: 1713–18.

34. Ludwig M, Katalinic A, Banz C, et al. Tailoring the GnRH antagonist cetrorelix acetate to individual patients' needs in ovarian stimulation for IVF: results of a prospective, randomized study. Hum Reprod 2002; 17: 2842–5.

35. Al-Inany H, Aboulghar MA, Mansour RT, Serour GI. Optimizing GnRH antagonist administration: meta-analysis of fixed versus flexible protocol. Reprod Biomed Online 2005; 10: 567–70.

36. Gordon K, Levy MJ, Ledger W, Kolibianakis EM, IJzerman-Boon PC. Reducing the incidence of weekend oocyte retrievals in a rFSH/GnRH -antagonist protocol by optimizing the start day of rFSH and delaying human chorionic gonadotropin (hCG) by 1 Day. Fertil Steril 2011; 95: s16.

37. Kolibianakis EM, Albano C, Camus M, et al. Prolongation of the follicular phase in in vitro fertilization results in a lower ongoing pregnancy rate in cycles stimulated with recombinant follicle-stimulating hormone and gonadotropin-releasing hormone antagonists. Fertil Steril 2004; 82: 102–7.

38. Griesinger G, Kolibianakis EM, Venetis C, Diedrich K, Tarlatzis B. Oral contraceptive pretreatment significantly reduces ongoing pregnancy likelihood in gonadotropin-releasing hormone antagonist cycles: an updated meta-analysis. Fertil Steril 2010; 94: 2382–4.

39. Popovic-Todorovic B, Loft A, Lindhard A, et al. A prospective study of predictive factors of ovarian response in 'standard' IVF/ICSI patients treated with recombinant FSH. A suggestion for a recombinant FSH dosage normogram. Hum Reprod 2003; 18: 781–7.

40. Olivennes F, Howles CM, Borini A, et al. Individualizing FSH dose for assisted reproduction using a novel algorithm: the CONSORT study. Reprod Biomed Online 2009; 18: 195–204.

41. Wikland M, Bergh C, Borg K, et al. A prospective, randomized comparison of two starting doses of recombinant FSH in combination with cetrorelix in women undergoing ovarian stimulation for IVF/ICSI. Hum Reprod 2001; 16: 1676–81.

42. Out HJ, David I, Ron-El R, et al. A randomized, double-blind clinical trial using fixed daily doses of 100 or 200 IU of recombinant FSH in ICSI cycles. Hum Reprod 2001; 16: 1104–9.

43. Albano C, Felberbaum RE, Smitz J, et al. Ovarian stimulation with HMG: results of a prospective randomized phase III European study comparing the luteinizing hormone-releasing hormone (LHRH)-antagonist cetrorelix and the LHRH-agonist buserelin. European Cetrorelix Study Group. Hum Reprod 2000; 15: 526–31.

44. Group EaMEOS. Comparable clinical outcome using the GnRH antagonist ganirelix or a long protocol of the GnRH agonist triptorelin for the prevention of premature LH surges in women undergoing ovarian stimulation. Hum Reprod 2001; 16: 644–51.

45. 45. Hohmann FP, Macklon NS, Fauser BC. A randomized comparison of two ovarian stimulation protocols with gonadotropin-releasing hormone (GnRH) antagonist cotreatment for in vitro fertilization commencing recombinant follicle-stimulating hormone on cycle day 2 or 5 with the standard long GnRH agonist protocol. J Clin Endocrinol Metab 2003; 88: 166–73.

46. Verberg MF, Macklon NS, Nargund G, et al. Mild ovarian stimulation for IVF. Hum Reprod Update 2009; 15: 13–29.

47. Verberg MF, Eijkemans MJ, Macklon NS, et al. The clinical significance of the retrieval of a low number of oocytes following mild ovarian stimulation for IVF: a meta-analysis. Hum Reprod Update 2009; 15: 5–12.

48. Propst AM, Bates GW, Robinson RD, et al. A randomized controlled trial of increasing recombinant follicle-stimulating hormone after initiating a gonadotropin-releasing hormone antagonist for in vitro fertilization-embryo transfer. Fertil Steril 2006; 86: 58–63.

49. Aboulghar MA, Mansour RT, Serour GI, et al. Increasing the dose of human menopausal gonadotrophins on day of GnRH antagonist administration: randomized controlled trial. Reprod Biomed Online 2004; 8: 524–7.

50. Baruffi RL, Mauri AL, Petersen CG, et al. Recombinant LH supplementation to recombinant FSH during induced ovarian stimulation in the GnRH-antagonist protocol: a meta-analysis. Reprod Biomed Online 2007; 14: 14–25.

51. Kolibianakis EM, Kalogeropoulou L, Griesinger G, et al. Among patients treated with FSH and GnRH analogues for in vitro fertilization, is the addition of recombinant LH associated with the probability of live

birth? A systematic review and meta-analysis. Hum Reprod Update 2007; 13: 445–52.

52. Mochtar MH, Van der V, Ziech M, van Wely M. Recombinant Luteinizing Hormone (rLH) for controlled ovarian hyperstimulation in assisted reproductive cycles. Cochrane Database Syst Rev 2007: CD005070.

53. Kolibianakis EM, Zikopoulos K, Smitz J, et al. Elevated progesterone at initiation of stimulation is associated with a lower ongoing pregnancy rate after IVF using GnRH antagonists. Hum Reprod 2004; 19: 1525–9.

54. Kolibianakis EM, Venetis CA, Bontis J, Tarlatzis BC. Significantly Lower Pregnancy Rates in the Presence of Progesterone Elevation in Patients Treated with GnRH Antagonists and Gonadotrophins: A Systematic Review and Meta-Analysis. Curr Pharm Biotechnol 2012; 13: 464–70.

55. Kolibianakis EM, Collins J, Tarlatzis B, Papanikolaou E, Devroey P. Are endogenous LH levels during ovarian stimulation for IVF using GnRH analogues associated with the probability of ongoing pregnancy? A systematic review. Hum Reprod Update 2006; 12: 3–12.

56. Griesinger G, Diedrich K, Tarlatzis BC, Kolibianakis EM. GnRH-antagonists in ovarian stimulation for IVF in patients with poor response to gonadotrophins, polycystic ovary syndrome, and risk of ovarian hyperstimulation: a meta-analysis. Reprod Biomed Online 2006; 13: 628–38.

57. Griesinger G, Diedrich K, Devroey P, Kolibianakis EM. GnRH agonist for triggering final oocyte maturation in the GnRH antagonist ovarian hyperstimulation protocol: a systematic review and meta-analysis. Hum Reprod Update 2006; 12: 159–68.

58. Griesinger G, Berndt H, Schultz L, Depenbusch M, Schultze-Mosgau A. Cumulative live birth rates after GnRH-agonist triggering of final oocyte maturation in patients at risk of OHSS: a prospective, clinical cohort study. Eur J Obstet Gynecol Reprod Biol 2010; 149: 190–4.

59. Bodri D, Sunkara SK, Coomarasamy A. Gonadotropin-releasing hormone agonists versus antagonists for controlled ovarian hyperstimulation in oocyte donors: a systematic review and meta-analysis. Fertil Steril 2011; 95: 164–9.

60. Beckers NG, Macklon NS, Eijkemans MJ, et al. Nonsupplemented luteal phase characteristics after the administration of recombinant human chorionic gonadotropin, recombinant luteinizing hormone, or gonadotropin-releasing hormone (GnRH) agonist to induce final oocyte maturation in in vitro fertilization patients after ovarian stimulation with recombinant follicle-stimulating hormone and GnRH antagonist cotreatment. J Clin Endocrinol Metab 2003; 88: 4186–92.

61. Kolibianakis EM, Venetis CA, Papanikolaou EG, et al. Estrogen addition to progesterone for luteal phase support in cycles stimulated with GnRH analogues and gonadotrophins for IVF: a systematic review and meta-analysis. Hum Reprod 2008; 23: 1346–54.

62. Pelinck MJ, Knol HM, Vogel NE, et al. Cumulative pregnancy rates after sequential treatment with modified natural cycle IVF followed by IVF with controlled ovarian stimulation. Hum Reprod 2008; 23: 1808–14.

63. Lainas TG, Sfontouris IA, Zorzovilis IZ, et al. Live births after management of severe OHSS by GnRH antagonist administration in the luteal phase. Reprod Biomed Online 2009; 19: 789–95.

64. Lainas TG, Sfontouris IA, Zorzovilis IZ, et al. Management of severe OHSS using GnRH antagonist and blastocyst cryopreservation in PCOS patients treated with long protocol. Reprod Biomed Online 2009; 18: 15–20.

65. Lainas TG, Sfontouris IA, Zorzovilis IZ, et al. Management of severe early ovarian hyperstimulation syndrome by re-initiation of GnRH antagonist. Reprod Biomed Online 2007; 15: 408–12.

42

The use of AMH to tailor ovarian stimulation for IVF

Scott M. Nelson

INTRODUCTION

Anti-Müllerian hormone (AMH) is a novel biomarker that has a critical role in follicular and testicular development. In males, AMH is secreted by Sertoli cells and its biological function in the fetus is to induce regression of the Müllerian ducts during fetal life, whilst in postnatal males it has a regulatory function in the gonad impacting on reproductive fertility. In women, AMH is secreted by granulosa cells to inhibit the early stages of follicular development (1).

AMH displays several unique characteristics that have led to its widespread adoption in the field of reproductive endocrinology and assisted conception. First, AMH appears to be solely derived from the ovary, since bilateral oophorectomy in premenopausal women and menopause are associated with undetectable AMH levels (2). Second, in the ovary it is the only hormone produced by a single-type cell, namely granulosa cells (3–5), permitting its use as a biochemical marker of granulosa cell function. Moreover, it is synthesized and secreted only by granulosa cells from primary to small antral follicles ($\leq$4–6 mm) (5,6). Despite this, serum AMH concentrations also correlate with primordial follicle number in humans (7) as in rodents (8). Other characteristics such as being independent of circulating FSH (9) and being relatively stable across the menstrual cycle (10) and between cycles (11), combined with its ability to be measured by a commercially available Enzyme-linked immunosorbent assay (ELISA), have all contributed to its overall appeal.

In this chapter we will detail recent developments in the AMH assay, the relationship of AMH with ovarian reserve, the interpretation of AMH in an age-specific manner, the association of circulating AMH to oocyte yield and consequently live birth, and ultimately the use of this information to counsel patients and individualize treatment strategies.

CLINICAL MEASUREMENT OF AMH

In the last 20 years there has been a constant evolution of the assay from single laboratory versions through to the more recent Diagnostic Systems Lab Inc (DSL) and Immunotech (IOT) [also branded as the Immunotech Beckman Coulter (IBC)] assays. Consequently at present half of the published articles have used the DSL assay and the other half the IOT assay. However, these current assays utilize two different primary antibodies against AMH and different standards, and consequently, the crude values reported by authors and between papers can differ substantially, with the IOT assay giving values for AMH that are higher than those obtained with the DSL assay. A new assay, the AMH Generation II assay (AMH Gen II assay), which is a hybrid of the previous two assays combining the DSL antibodies and thereby cross species reactivity, but calibrated to the IOT standards, has now been developed and is in the process of replacing the DSL and the IOT assays (12). Although potentially confusing, clinicians historically accustomed to interpreting the IOT assay should not be troubled since the new AMH Gen II assay has been calibrated identically to the old IOT assay and will therefore give the same values. Whereas those using the DSL assay should be prepared that the new AMH Gen II assay will give values for AMH that are approximately 40% higher than they are accustomed to. In the foreseeable future, assay automation and alternative suppliers will be additional issues to contend with, however, it is hoped that any future assays will have similar calibration to that of the current AMH Gen II assay from Beckman Coulter.

STABILITY OF AMH ACROSS THE MENSTRUAL CYCLE

Nonsignificant variation of AMH throughout the menstrual cycle has been reported by several groups (10,13–15). Although others have reported significant cyclical fluctuations in AMH levels with a rapid decrease in the early luteal phase, (14,16) the excursions from mean levels are relatively small (+3% to –19%). These variations are similar to reported inter-cycle variability for AMH (17). Consequently, in the clinical setting, the inter- and intra-cycle variability in serum AMH levels may be considered to be low enough to permit random timing of AMH measurement during the menstrual cycle.

AGE-SPECIFIC INTERPRETATION OF AMH

Given the recognition that AMH declines prior to the menopause and is associated with the date of the final menstrual period (18–22), there has been considerable interest in being able to place any given individuals AMH in context and predict for an individual woman her reproductive life span. Thus, many clinicians and patients are keen to know not only what their actual AMH is but how this relates to woman of a similar age, i.e., an age-specific AMH centile. To date, nomograms have primarily focused on adult populations attending infertility clinics, with the largest externally validated nomogram being developed for the DSL assay (n = 25,341; Fig. 42.1) (23,24). More recently, we have utilized a data aggregation approach for healthy populations from birth through to the menopause, and have calibrated this to the AMH Gen II assay values (Fig. 42.2), thereby allowing interpretation of AMH from conception to menopausal ages (25).

RELATIONSHIP OF AMH TO OVARIAN RESERVE

As outlined in other chapters, the human ovary establishes its complete complement of primordial follicles during fetal life. Recruitment and thereby depletion of this dormant primordial follicle pool is required for normal fertility but ultimately leads to reproductive senescence. AMH is the principal regulator of early follicular recruitment from the primordial pool, with AMH null mice demonstrating accelerated depletion of primordial follicle number and an almost threefold increase in smaller growing follicles (26). This increase in number of growing follicles occurs despite lower serum follicle-stimulating hormone (FSH) concentrations (27), suggesting that in the absence of AMH, follicles are more sensitive to FSH and progress through the early stages of follicular development.

The prepubertal endocrine environment is markedly different from the adult with low and non-cyclical gonadotropins: The relevance of this to AMH secretion is incompletely understood although follicle growth through the pre-antral stages and occasionally to early antral stages (i.e., across the full range of stages that secrete AMH) is observed in childhood. A recent study has reported an increase in initial primordial follicular recruitment rates up to the age of puberty, and then a progressive decline to the menopause (28). This suggests that AMH concentrations at any given age in both childhood and adulthood may mirror primordial follicular recruitment rates, rather than simply primordial follicle number. Consequently, across the female life span, circulating AMH will potentially exhibit an initial increase followed by a nonlinear decline as is well established for the primordial follicle pool (28–31).

In adult women, serum AMH concentrations correlate with the size of the stereologically determined primordial follicle pool (7), despite AMH production being restricted to later stages of follicular development. Analyses of the relationships between circulating AMH and the primordial follicle population have recently been undertaken (Fig. 42.3) (25). This demonstrated that from birth to peak AMH, the primordial follicle population is

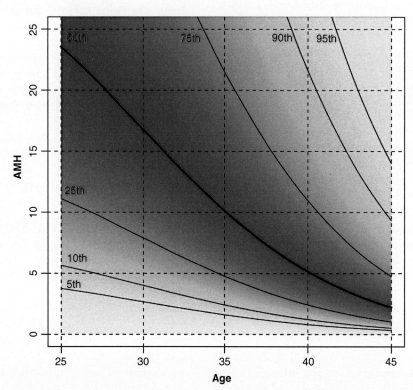

Figure 42.1 Age-related nomogram for AMH (pmol/l) determined using the DSL assay. Model derived and validated in 9178 European women, then externally validated in 15,834 U.S. women. Produced by the author and a version originally presented in Ref. 23. *Abbreviation:* AMH, anti-Müllerian hormone.

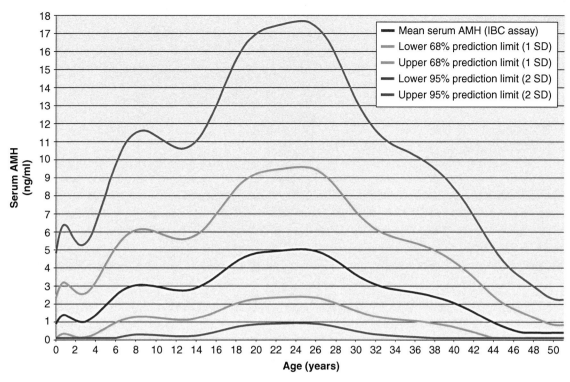

Figure 42.2   A validated model of serum anti-Müllerian hormone (AMH) from conception to menopause. The red line is the log-unadjusted validated AMH model using Immunotech (IOT) assay values. The blue and green lines are the 68% and 95% prediction limits for the model (+ and − 1 and 2 standard deviations respectively). The dataset was derived from over 3500 subjects with ages ranging from −0.3 years to 68 years. Produced by the author with a version originally presented in Ref. 25. *Abbreviations*: AMH, anti-Müllerian hormone; IBC assay, Immunotech Beckman Coulter assay.

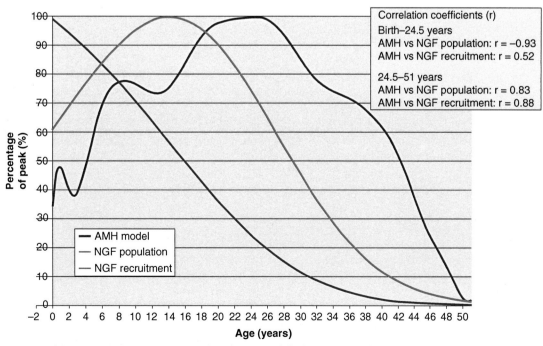

Figure 42.3   Comparison of serum AMH concentrations with nongrowing follicle (NGF) population and with NGF recruitment. The red line is the log-unadjusted validated AMH model (Kelsey et al. 2011), peaking at 24.5 years. The blue line denotes the decline in NGF population (Wallace & Kelsey, 2010), with peak population at 18–22 weeks gestation. The green line denotes the numbers of NGFs recruited toward maturation population (Wallace & Kelsey, 2010), with peak numbers lost at age 14.2 years on average. Each quantity has been normalized so that the peak occurs at 100%. Correlation coefficients (r) are given for AMH concentrations against the other two curves for birth to 24.5 years and for 24.5 to 51 years. Produced by the author with a version originally presented in Ref. 52. *Abbreviations*: AMH, anti-Müllerian hormone, NGF, nongrowing follicle.

strongly negatively correlated with AMH (r = −0.93), since nongrowing follicle (NGF) populations are falling while AMH concentrations are rising in general (Fig. 42.3). Over the same age range, AMH is positively but less closely correlated with rate of NGF recruitment (r = 0.52). The finding that during childhood AMH tends to rise with time/age while NGF number falls does not imply that individuals with highest AMH will have the lowest NGF number, although you may anticipate them to have the lowest NGF recruitment based on the known biology of AMH. The relationship between AMH and NGF appeared to change in early adulthood, probably reflecting the absence of larger AMH-producing follicles in childhood that will change postpuberty, thus causing a rise in AMH independent of NGF number.

Close relationships were also demonstrated between AMH concentrations and NGF populations from peak AMH until the menopause. From 24.5 years to 51 years both NGF population and NGF recruitment correlate well and positively with AMH (r = 0.83 and r = 0.88 respectively). Consequently, circulating AMH concentrations in adult women fall in line with the rate of loss of nongrowing follicles. AMH concentrations also broadly rise in line with this rate in children and young adults, but with a delay of about 10 years between the two peaks. The relationship of AMH to the total number of primordial follicles remaining in the pool for future recruitment therefore has two distinct phases, with the direction of association changing in early adulthood. This reflects the change with puberty in the stages at which follicles atrese.

Given these strong relationships between AMH and NGF recruitment rates, one would anticipate that AMH would be strongly associated with oocyte yield, particularly if stimulation strategies like the long course agonist approach that are designed to maximize oocyte yield are used.

AMH AND OOCYTE YIELD

Several studies have now consistently demonstrated a strong positive association between basal serum AMH levels and the number of oocytes retrieved in women undergoing ovarian stimulation (Fig. 42.4) (32). Recent analysis of all retrospective and prospective studies have found that this correlation with oocyte yield is substantially better than the associations observed for the age of the patient, day 3 FSH, estradiol, or inhibin B (33). With respect to ultrasound markers, AMH appears to have equivalent performance to that of antral follicle count (AFC) in prediction of oocyte yield, with a comparative meta-analysis analyzing 17 AFC and 13 AFC studies, indicating no significant differences between the performance of AMH and AFC in predicting oocyte yield (34). Our desire to exploit this strong association with oocyte yield underlies our approach to use AMH to stratify both prognosis and individualized treatment.

PREDICTION OF A POOR OVARIAN RESPONSE

A proportion (2–30%) of women undergoing controlled ovarian stimulation will experience a poor ovarian response. Although there has been a multitude of studies assessing its pathogenesis, clinical characterization, and possible treatment, a major limitation has been the lack of an internationally accepted definition. A recent European Society of Human Reproduction and Embryology (ESHRE) consensus proposed the following criteria to define a poor response (35), with at least two of the following three features required to be present:

1. Advanced maternal age (≥40 years) or any other risk factor for poor ovarian response.
2. A previous poor ovarian response (≤3 oocytes with a conventional stimulation protocol).
3. An abnormal ovarian reserve test (i.e., AFC <5–7 follicles or AMH <0.5–1.1 ng/ml).

Alternatively, two episodes of poor ovarian response after maximal stimulation are sufficient to define a patient as a poor responder in the absence of advanced maternal age or abnormal ovarian reserve test.

By definition, the term poor ovarian response requires at least one stimulated cycle to be diagnosed. The consensus

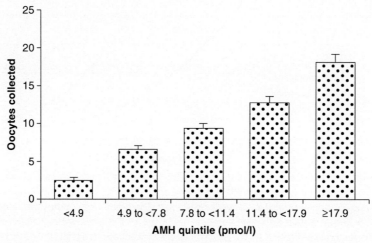

Figure 42.4   Mean oocyte yield per AMH quintile. Values are mean ± standard error of the mean (SEM). Produced by the author with a version originally presented in Ref. 32. *Abbreviation*: AMH, anti-Müllerian hormone.

statement suggested that for patients over 40 years of age with an abnormal ovarian reserve test may be classified as expected poor responders since both advanced age and an abnormal ovarian reserve test may indicate a reduced ovarian reserve.

The inclusion of AMH and AFC within the definition reflects the strengths of their associations with oocyte yield. Several meta-analyses have demonstrated that AMH and AFC had the best sensitivity and specificity for predicting ovarian response. However, both of these markers at even their best cutoff values are associated with a false–positive rate of 10–20% (Fig. 42.5) (36). Although the use of multiple tests would intuitively improve diagnostic accuracy, this was not demonstrated in a meta-analysis of cohort studies. This finding was subsequently confirmed in an individualized patient data meta-analysis, with no significant improvement in classification of a poor response, above a basal AMH when age, FSH, or AFC were also taken into account. In reality many will assess AFC as part of a baseline transvaginal scan performed during the infertility work up, this will therefore allow confirmation of a low ovarian reserve in a woman with an unexpected low AMH, or direct reassessment of the ovarian reserve if AMH was assessed previously.

The AMH cutoff values for prediction of a poor response in clinical practice, range from 0.5 – 1.1 ng/ml (≤3.6 to 7.8 pmol/l), whereas for AFC the values range from less than five to seven (Fig. 42.5). These values have been set at an extreme value since they are demonstrated

a high specificity (low false–positive rate) accepting that sensitivity will be compromised. It is important to note that even with these low levels, women identified as potential poor responders still have the capacity to become pregnant and have live births. In particular, young poor responders have a better prognosis from older women. The greatest utility of the early identification of a poor responder may therefore be managing their expectations of treatment, ensuring maximal therapy in the first cycle and in the research environment where accurate classification of patients will allow comparability of patients across clinical trials. Although it is tempting to exclude poor prognosis patients from clinical programmes, at present there has been limited economic, ethical, or psychological evaluation of such an approach.

PREDICTION OF AN EXCESSIVE RESPONSE TO OVARIAN STIMULATION

At the other extreme of ovarian response, an excessive response to gonadotropin stimulation is associated with abdominal discomfort, painful oocyte retrieval, cycle cancellation, and a reduced chance of pregnancy. It is also a major risk factor for ovarian hyperstimulation syndrome (OHSS), a potentially life-threatening condition. Accurate identification of patients at risk of an excessive response therefore allows primary prevention strategies to be undertaken with concomitant improvements in the overall safety of ovarian stimulation.

Unfortunately there is no consensus definition for excessive response and consequently different definitions ranging from ≥14 up to ≥21 oocytes, or development of OHSS has been used when assessing the performance of predictive factors. Despite these methodological differences, a meta-analysis of 11 studies assessing AMH and AFC clearly demonstrated their predictive power for an excessive response. The plot of sensitivity–specificity combinations in an Receiver operating characteristic (ROC) space is shown in Figure 42.6 (37). For AMH the sensitivity varied between 40% and 95% and the specificity between 31% and 96%. Using bivariate modeling that can account for the heterogeneity of the studies, and gives greater weight to the larger studies, the summary of estimates for sensitivity were 82% (95% CI 52–95%) and 76% (95% CI 43–93%) for specificity. For AFC the sensitivity varied between 20% and 94% and specificity varied between 33% and 98%. The summary estimates for AFC were 82% (95% CI 30–98%) for sensitivity and 80% (95% CI 31–97%) for specificity.

This meta-analysis was, however, limited in the derivation of values for predicting an excessive response, due to the different AMH assays that were historically used and that for AFC different studies included follicles of sizes 2–5 or 2–10 mm. Four prospective studies using the DSL assay have however, reported relevant values for AMH in the prediction of an excessive response and OHSS (33). Three of these independently calculated a similar performance of AMH for the prediction of an excessive response when a cutoff value of 3.5 ng/ml (25 pmol/l) (DSL assay) was used.

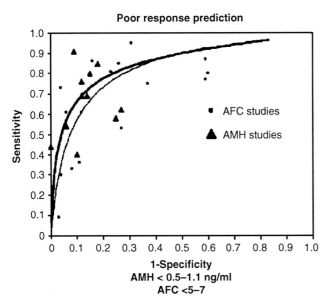

Figure 42.5 Estimated ROC curve and sensitivity–specificity points for studies reporting on the performance of basal anti-Müllerian hormone (AMH) and antral follicle count (AFC) in the prediction of a poor response. The accuracy of AMH and AFC for predicting a poor response in regularly cycling women is considered adequate and these two markers are considered superior to inhibin B, FSH, ovarian volume, and age of women in the prediction of ovarian response to stimulation. Most frequently used cutoff values for follicle-stimulating hormone (FSH), AMH, and AFC are reported. *Source*: Reproduced from Ref. 36.

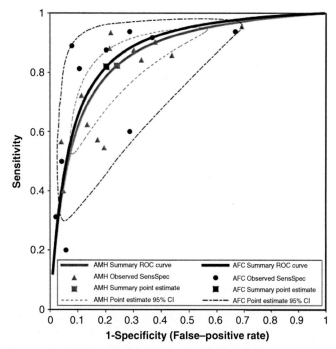

Figure 42.6 Anti-Müllerian hormone (AMH) and antral follicle count (AFC) in the prediction of an excessive response. Regardless of the number of cutoffs mentioned per study, only one cut-off was taken into analysis. For the observed values of sensitivity–specificity points, all cut-offs are displayed. *Source*: Reproduced from Ref. 37.

UTILIZING AMH TO PERSONALIZE REPRODUCTIVE HEALTH CARE

The philosophy underlying the ethos of personalized medicine is to tailor medical treatment to the individual characteristics of each patient. Potentially more important is the ability to predict the risk of disease or its presence before clinical signs and symptoms appear. This information underlies a health care strategy focused on prevention and early intervention, rather than a reaction to advanced disease. An important step in achieving these goals is the accurate stratification into biological subgroups. Recognition of the strong association of AMH with oocyte yield, the reproductive life span, and its ability to predict poor, normal, and excessive response to ovarian stimulation is an important first step in attaining this goal for fertility and assisted conception.

PREDICTING REPRODUCTIVE LIFE SPAN

The clear associations of AMH with the reproductive life span and its ability to predict the menopause, presents exciting opportunities in the field of preventative medicine. For example women who have undergone chemotherapy during childhood, may postpuberty have regular periods and therefore a false reassurance regarding their reproductive potential. However, the true extent to which their ovarian reserve has been impaired and when they will undergo the menopause has to date been largely unknown. Measuring AMH as part of the routine follow-up of these women will allow accurate identification of those women at risk of premature ovarian insufficiency

and also inform them of their potential reproductive life span. Fertility preservation measures including oocyte freezing can then be undertaken early to ensure that these young women have an opportunity to potentially avoid oocyte donation in the future. It is tempting to apply a similar approach to generic health screening for young women, regarding their potential reproductive life span. However, as age of the menopause demonstrates strong heritability, AMH would need to do substantially better than just asking when their mother went through the menopause and extrapolating back.

PREDICTING LIVE BIRTH AFTER ASSISTED CONCEPTION

A variety of prognostic models have described the probability of an ongoing pregnancy or a live birth following assisted conception (38). To date these models have predominantly been established using patient baseline characteristics and although they have been heterogeneous in their performance they consistently demonstrated that certain patient characteristics such as female age, duration of infertility, pregnancy history, diagnostic category, and BMI are associated with IVF/ICSI success (39). Alternative models have incorporated the characteristics of the intermediate results of the first treatment cycle thereby improving the accuracy of probability estimates for future cycles (40). The variables used in these models include the number of retrieved oocytes, the fertilization rate, and the embryo number and quality. Moreover, it has been clearly demonstrated that in models predicting pregnancy based on intermediate results (at embryo transfer), the number of retrieved and fertilized oocytes have the highest prognostic value (35). This suggests that any marker that can predict the number of retrieved oocytes prior to ovarian stimulation may be of value in initial baseline prognostic models.

Although there has been much written about the inability of AMH to predict pregnancy, there are now several studies all showing that AMH is associated with live birth but that this is independent of age (32,41–43). Collectively, this suggests that while age is the principal determinant of oocyte quality, for any given age, women with a higher AMH will do better in IVF due to the higher number of oocytes retrieved. This is in line with a recent analysis of 400,135 IVF cycles demonstrating that live birth rates steadily increased up to 15 eggs (44). Although the studies assessing AMH have been performed on small cohorts and their clinical utility is therefore limited due to the wide confidence intervals, it does suggest that the next step would be to examine whether AMH can improve classification of more complex well-calibrated models for prediction of live birth.

AMH STRATIFICATION FOR ALTERING TREATMENT STRATEGIES

The ability to identify the likely response to ovarian stimulation by a pretreatment AMH can ensure that patients are treated optimally in their very first treatment

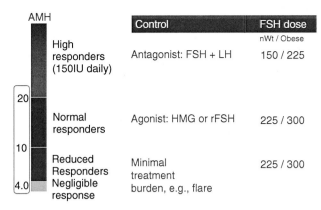

AMH		Control	FSH dose
			nWt / Obese
High responders (150IU daily)		Antagonist: FSH + LH	150 / 225
Normal responders		Agonist: HMG or rFSH	225 / 300
Reduced Responders Negligible response		Minimal treatment burden, e.g., flare	225 / 300

Figure 42.7 Current approach for anti-Müllerian hormone (AMH)– stratified ovarian stimulation. AMH values in pmol/l as measured by the AMH generation II assay (Beckman Coulter). nWT - BMI <30 kg/m², obese - BMI ≥30 kg/m². *Abbreviations*: FSH, follicle-stimulating hormone; rFSH, recombinant follicle-stimulating hormone; LH, luteinizing hormone; HMG, human menopausal gonadotrophin.

cycle. We previously proposed, then adopted, and subsequently validated an AMH-stratified approach to controlled ovarian stimulation (32,45,46). This is summarized in Figure 42.7. For women with a very low or poor ovarian reserve (AMH <1.0 pmol/l), although pregnancy is feasible, the likelihood of success is limited. Withholding treatment and pursuing alternatives like oocyte donation have been suggested as a cost-effective approach, but for many moving on to donor gametes without first pursuing attempts at IVF and the inherently low success rates is not an option. Instead, accurate counseling to ensure that their expectations regarding risk of cycle cancellation, reduced oocyte yield, low embryo number, and a reduced chance of success are set appropriately, will potentially minimize the associated disappointment of a negative outcome. Although it may be feasible to identify these extremely poor responders in advance of stimulation, at present none of the adjuvant therapies including dehydroepiandrosterone (DHEA) or growth hormone supplementation, have consistently demonstrated substantial efficacy (47). Novel strategies including changing the focus from an individual stimulation cycle and its outcome to considering multiple oocyte vitrification cycles, and then a single defrost, to allow ICSI and optimal embryo selection have been proposed. The rationale being that the psychological stress associated with multiple cycles where the oocytes are just banked is less than repeated failures and drop out rates substantially reduced, with an overall increase in cumulative live birth rate across the stimulation cycles. Whether this approach is more widely adopted remains to be seen.

To date the optimal treatment strategy for the expected poor responder has yet to be achieved. In line with others experiences, our recent prospective exploration of five different and novel strategies trying to ensure synchronized follicular recruitment, avoiding premature luteinization, and minimizing the treatment burden failed to improve clinical pregnancy or live birth rates. Given the preselection based on an AMH <5 pmol/l (DSL assay), as expected, cycle outcomes were solely determined by maternal age. Given the overall poor rates of success per cycle in women with a low AMH, minimization of treatment burden and promotion of maximal follicular recruitment continue to be the priorities. In the future, combining depot GnRH agonists as a flare, with long-acting gonadotropin preparations and then human chorionic gonadotropin (hCG) for oocyte maturation and for luteal support, may allow the development of a truly minimally invasive approach, with only four needle sticks. The inherent low risk of ovarian hyperstimulation in women with a low AMH would allow both the long-acting gonadotropin preparations and hCG to be used safely.

For women with a normal ovarian reserve as indicated by an AMH of 7–20 pmol/l, an agonist-based approach is feasible, accepting a small risk of OHSS, which is principally restricted to those women at the top end of this spectrum. Whether recombinant or urinary products are used, it will influence this risk given the greater biological potency of the recombinant products. Although GnRH antagonist–based strategies are now increasingly suggested as an optimal treatment for all patients, there remain potentially significant issues that may compromise the overall effectiveness in this normal ovarian reserve group where the OHSS risk is still low. These weaknesses have recently been recognized by the original proponents of mild ovarian stimulation (48). They include lower pregnancy rates and live birth rates per cycle, a reduced margin for suboptimal laboratory performance, fewer embryos being available for cryopreservation, difficulties with programming of the cycle and scheduling of workload, a lack of individualized FSH-dosing algorithms, and an overall relative lack of robustness with a reduced window for scheduling hCG. We would therefore suggest that an agonist-based approach can still be safely used within this group provided accurate monitoring and hCG is timed relative to the lead follicle development.

Despite these difficulties with antagonist strategies, for women with a high ovarian reserve (AMH >20 pmol/l) and a substantial risk of OHSS, failure to use GnRH antagonist–based approach may be potentially regarded as clinically negligible. This is particularly the case given the overwhelming evidence from (29) randomized controlled trials that antagonists significantly reduce the OHSS risk (OR 0.43, 95% CI 0.33 to 0.57) (49). In contrast to using it for all women, in patients with a high AMH the use of GnRH antagonist–based stimulation strategies significantly improves fresh clinical pregnancy rates while not compromising the number of embryos cryopreserved. As one would anticipate, it also substantially reduces the risk of an excessive response, OHSS, and hospitalization. It is this ability to identify patients at risk of OHSS, alter their treatment, and improve the overall safety of IVF that is potentially the greatest tangible benefit of AMH, and would in itself justify its widespread adoption.

Altruistic oocyte donors can be optimally selected based on their AMH to have a high oocyte yield. To facilitate repeat donations, the treatment burden should, however, be minimal and safe. In these women, antagonist strategies have the additional benefit of being able to use a GnRH agonist trigger, thereby negating the risk of OHSS. At present this approach is not been recommended for all, as a meta-analysis of eight studies suggesting that in fresh autologous cycles use of a GnRH trigger was associated with a markedly reduced live birth rate as compared to hCG (OR 0.45, 95% CI 0.31 to 0.65) (50). Although some units combine this with a low dose of hCG (1500 IU) to avoid any risk of failure to mature oocytes complications, it is still unclear whether this is associated with an improvement in live birth rates.

Others have now externally validated our AMH-stratified approach, and have confirmed the initial findings of higher pregnancy and live birth rates and reduced incidence of OHSS and failed fertilization (51). This clinical success was also accompanied by a reduction in cost. Further developments and refinements of our stimulation approaches are inevitable and welcomed.

CONCLUSIONS

Stratification of reproductive health care based on phenotypic and biomarker characteristics is now feasible. AMH is the latest of these biomarkers, and its inclusion in the diagnostic armamentarium will allow patients to be accurately counseled, treatment to be individualized, and clinical outcomes improved.

REFERENCES

1. Durlinger ALL, Gruijters MJG, Kramer P, et al. Anti-Mullerian Hormone Inhibits Initiation of Primordial Follicle Growth in the Mouse Ovary. Endocrinology 2002; 143: 1076–84.
2. La Marca A, Pati M, Orvieto R, et al. Serum anti-mullerian hormone levels in women with secondary amenorrhea. Fertil Steril 2006; 85: 1547–9.
3. Baarends WM, Uilenbroek JT, Kramer P, et al. Anti-mullerian hormone and anti-mullerian hormone type II receptor messenger ribonucleic acid expression in rat ovaries during postnatal development, the estrous cycle, and gonadotropin-induced follicle growth. Endocrinology 1995; 136: 4951–62.
4. Bezard J, Vigier B, Tran D, Mauleon P, Josso N. Immunocytochemical study of anti-Mullerian hormone in sheep ovarian follicles during fetal and post-natal development. J Reprod Fertil 1987; 80: 509–16.
5. Weenen C, Laven JSE, von Bergh ARM, et al. Anti-Mullerian hormone expression pattern in the human ovary: potential implications for initial and cyclic follicle recruitment. Mol Hum Reprod 2004; 10: 77–83.
6. Visser JA, Themmen AP. Anti-Mullerian hormone and folliculogenesis. Mol Cell Endocrinol 2005; 234:81–6.
7. Hansen KR, Hodnett GM, Knowlton N, Craig LB. Correlation of ovarian reserve tests with histologically determined primordial follicle number. Fertil Steril 2011; 95: 170–5.
8. Kevenaar ME, Meerasahib MF, Kramer P, et al. Serum Anti-Mullerian Hormone Levels Reflect the Size of the Primordial Follicle Pool in Mice. Endocrinology 2006; 147: 3228–34.
9. Fanchin R, Schonäuer LM, Righini C, et al. Serum anti-Müllerian hormone dynamics during controlled ovarian hyperstimulation. Hum Reprod 2003; 18: 328–32.
10. La Marca A, Stabile G, Artenisio AC, Volpe A. Serum anti-Mullerian hormone throughout the human menstrual cycle. Hum Reprod 2006; 21: 3103–7.
11. van Disseldorp J, Lambalk CB, Kwee J, et al. Comparison of inter- and intra-cycle variability of anti-Mullerian hormone and antral follicle counts. Hum Reprod 2010; 25: 221–7.
12. Nelson SM, La Marca A. The journey from the old to the new AMH assay: How to avoid getting lost in the values. Reprod Biomed Online 2011.
13. Hehenkamp WJ, Looman CW, Themmen AP, et al. Anti-Mullerian hormone levels in the spontaneous menstrual cycle do not show substantial fluctuation. J Clin Endocrinol Metab 2006; 91: 4057–63.
14. Streuli I, Fraisse T, Chapron C, et al. Clinical uses of anti-Mullerian hormone assays: Pitfalls and promises. Fertil Steril 2009; 91: 226–30.
15. Tsepelidis S, Devreker F, Demeestere I, et al. Stable serum levels of anti-Mullerian hormone during the menstrual cycle: A prospective study in normo-ovulatory women. Hum Reprod 2007; 22: 1837–40.
16. Wunder DM, Bersinger NA, Yared M, Kretschmer R, Birkhauser MH. Statistically significant changes of antimullerian hormone and inhibin levels during the physiologic menstrual cycle in reproductive age women. Fertil Steril 2008; 89: 927–33.
17. Fanchin R, Taieb J, Lozano DHM, et al. High reproducibility of serum anti-Müllerian hormone measurements suggests a multi-staged follicular secretion and strengthens its role in the assessment of ovarian follicular status. Hum Reprod 2005; 20: 923–7.
18. van Rooij IA, Tonkelaar I, Broekmans FJ, et al. Anti-mullerian hormone is a promising predictor for the occurrence of the menopausal transition. Menopause 2004; 11(6 Pt 1): 601–6.
19. La Marca A, De Leo V, Giulini S, et al. Anti-Mullerian hormone in premenopausal women and after spontaneous or surgically induced menopause. J Soc Gynecol Investig 2005; 12: 545–8.
20. Sowers MR, Eyvazzadeh AD, McConnell D, et al. Anti-mullerian hormone and inhibin B in the definition of ovarian aging and the menopause transition. J Clin Endocrinol Metab 2008; 93: 3478–83.
21. Soto N, Iniguez G, Lopez P, et al. Anti-Mullerian hormone and inhibin B levels as markers of premature ovarian aging and transition to menopause in type 1 diabetes mellitus. Hum Reprod 2009; 24: 2838–44.
22. Broer SL, Eijkemans MJ, Scheffer GJ, et al. Anti-mullerian hormone predicts menopause: A long-term follow-up study in normoovulatory women. J Clin Endocrinol Metab 2011; 96: 2532–9.
23. Nelson SM, Messow MC, Wallace AM, Fleming R, McConnachie A. Nomogram for the decline in serum antimullerian hormone: A population study of 9,601 infertility patients. Fertil Steril 2011; 95: 736–41.
24. Nelson SM, Messow MC, McConnachie A, et al. External validation of nomogram for the decline in serum anti-Mullerian hormone in women: A population study

of 15,834 infertility patients. Reprod Biomed Online 2011; 23: 204–6.

25. Kelsey TW, Wright P, Nelson SM, Anderson RA, Wallace WH. A validated model of serum anti-mullerian hormone from conception to menopause. PLoS One 2011; 6: e22024.

26. Durlinger ALL, Kramer P, Karels B, et al. Control of Primordial Follicle Recruitment by Anti-Mullerian Hormone in the Mouse Ovary. Endocrinology 1999; 140: 5789–96.

27. Durlinger ALL, Gruijters MJG, Kramer P, et al. Anti-Mullerian Hormone Attenuates the Effects of FSH on Follicle Development in the Mouse Ovary. Endocrinology 2001; 142: 4891–9.

28. Wallace WH, Kelsey TW. Human ovarian reserve from conception to the menopause. PLoS One 2010; 5: e8772.

29. Faddy MJ. Follicle dynamics during ovarian ageing. Molecular and Cellular Endocrinology 2000; 163: 43–8.

30. Faddy MJ, Gosden RG. Ovary and ovulation: A model conforming the decline in follicle numbers to the age of menopause in women. Hum Reprod 1996; 11: 1484–6.

31. Faddy MJ, Gosden RG, Gougeon A, Richardson SJ, Nelson JF. Accelerated disappearance of ovarian follicles in mid-life: Implications for forecasting menopause. Hum Reprod 1992; 7: 1342–6.

32. Nelson SM, Yates RW, Fleming R. Serum anti-Mullerian hormone and FSH: Prediction of live birth and extremes of response in stimulated cycles implications for individualization of therapy. Hum Reprod 2007; 22: 2414–21.

33. La Marca A, Sighinolfi G, Radi D, et al. Anti-Mullerian hormone (AMH) as a predictive marker in assisted reproductive technique (ART). Hum Reprod Update 2010; 16: 113–30.

34. Broer SL, Mol BW, Hendriks D, Broekmans FJ. The role of antimullerian hormone in prediction of outcome after IVF: comparison with the antral follicle count. Fertil Steril 2009; 91: 705–14.

35. Ferraretti AP, La Marca A, Fauser BC, et al. ESHRE consensus on the definition of 'poor response' to ovarian stimulation for in vitro fertilization: The Bologna criteria. Hum Reprod 2011; 26: 1616–24.

36. Broer SL, Mol BWJ, Hendriks D, Broekmans FJM. The role of antimullerian hormone in prediction of outcome after IVF: Comparison with the antral follicle count. Fertil Steril 2009; 91: 705–14.

37. Broer SL, Dólleman M, Opmeer BC, et al. AMH and AFC as predictors of excessive response in controlled ovarian hyperstimulation: A meta-analysis. Hum Reprod Update 2011; 17: 46–54.

38. Leushuis E, van der Steeg JW, Steures P, et al. Prediction models in reproductive medicine: A critical appraisal. Hum Reprod Update 2009; 15: 537–52.

39. Nelson SM, Lawlor DA. Predicting live birth, preterm delivery, and low birth weight in infants born from in vitro fertilisation: A prospective study of 144,018 treatment cycles. PLoS Med 2011; 8: e1000386.

40. Banerjee P, Choi B, Shahine LK, et al. Deep phenotyping to predict live birth outcomes in in vitro fertilization. Proc Natl Acad Sci USA 2010; 107: 13570–5.

41. Lee TH, Liu CH, Huang CC, et al. Impact of female age and male infertility on ovarian reserve markers to predict outcome of assisted reproductive technique cycles. Reprod Biol Endocrinol 2009; 7: 100.

42. La Marca A, Nelson SM, Sighinolfi G, et al. Anti-Mullerian Hormone (AMH) based prediction model for the live birth in assisted reproductive technique (ART). RBM online 2010: in press.

43. Gleicher N, Weghofer A, Barad DH. Anti-Mullerian hormone (AMH) defines, independent of age, low versus good live-birth chances in women with severely diminished ovarian reserve. Fertil Steril 2010; 94: 2824–7.

44. Sunkara SK, Rittenberg V, Raine-Fenning N, et al. Association between the number of eggs and live birth in IVF treatment: An analysis of 400 135 treatment cycles. Hum Reprod 2011; 26: 1768–74.

45. Nelson SM, Yates RW, Lyall H, et al. Anti-Mullerian hormone-based approach to controlled ovarian stimulation for assisted conception. Hum Reprod 2009; 24: 867–75.

46. Nelson SM, Fleming R. Low AMH and GnRH-antagonist strategies. Fertil Steril 2009; 92: e40; author reply e1.

47. Yakin K, Urman B. DHEA as a miracle drug in the treatment of poor responders; hype or hope? Hum Reprod 2011; 26: 1941–4.

48. Fauser BCJM, Nargund G, Andersen AN, et al. Mild ovarian stimulation for IVF: 10 years later. Hum Reprod 2010; 25: 2678–84.

49. Al-Inany HG, Youssef MA, Aboulghar M, et al. Gonadotrophin-releasing hormone antagonists for assisted reproductive technique. Cochrane Database Syst Rev 2011: CD001750.

50. Youssef MA, Van der Veen F, Al-Inany HG, et al. Gonadotropin-releasing hormone agonist versus HCG for oocyte triggering in antagonist assisted reproductive technique cycles. Cochrane Database Syst Rev 2010: CD008046.

51. Yates AP, Rustamov O, Roberts SA, et al. Anti-Müllerian hormone-tailored stimulation protocols improve outcomes whilst reducing adverse effects and costs of IVF. Hum Reprod 2011; 26: 2353–62.

52. Kelsey TW, Anderson RA, Wright P, Nelson SM, Wallace WH. Data-driven assessment of the human ovarian reserve. Mol Hum Reprod 2012; 18: 79–87.

43

Monitoring ovarian response in IVF cycles

Matts Wikland and Torbjörn Hillensjö

INTRODUCTION

Historically, monitoring of ovarian response, by means of measuring ovarian hormones, came into the use for ovulation induction due to the complications of gonadotropin therapy. In ovulation induction cycles with gonadotropins, Klopper and coworkers showed that success complication rates were not dependant on monitoring as such, but on the treatment protocol used (1). If more gonadotropins are given, successes increase, as do complications such as ovarian hyperstimulation syndrome (OHSS) and multiple births.

Monitoring merely gives us the possibility to decide how far we want to go (1). This may be true for ovulation induction cycles but not for IVF cycles, where the number of transferred embryos can be restricted and thereby at least the risk for multiple births can be minimized and probably also the severity of OHSS if no embryos are transferred. Due to the dramatic increase in the number of IVF cycles worldwide, and the various ovarian stimulation protocols used, different ways of monitoring have been tested. Of all the methods described for monitoring IVF cycles, ultrasound imagining of the utero-ovarian response to gonadotropins has become clinically most useful. This method was first evaluated in the natural cycle, but it was soon realised that it was in stimulated cycles where it really could be useful (2,3). One problem though, was that the size (mean diameter as well as the volume) of the mature follicle seems to vary greatly (4,5). To overcome this problem, several studies have been performed to determine the value of combining serum estradiol (E2) measurements and ultrasound monitoring of follicular maturation in stimulated cycles (6–9). This combination of ultrasound and hormonal monitoring seemed to be important in protocols with clomiphene citrate and gonadotropins alone where the endogenous luteinizing hormone (LH) peek could not be controlled. With the introduction of gonadotropin-releasing hormone (GnRH) analogues combined with gonadotropins, the risk for high tonic levels of LH or premature LH peaks has disappeared (10). Thus, with the use of GnRH agonists or lately GnRH antagonists, there seems to be less need for extensive hormonal monitoring of IVF cycles (11). Ultrasound alone or in certain cases combined with one or two serum E2 measurements seems to be sufficient in the majority of women entering an IVF cycle (12). Thus, nowadays in most IVF units ultrasound imaging has become the method of choice for monitoring ovarian stimulation during an IVF cycle.

WHY MONITOR THE CYCLE?

Ovarian stimulation with gonadotropins in IVF cycles is performed merely for one reason and that is to achieve as many mature healthy oocytes as possible. The more mature oocytes that can be retrieved in one cycle the better is the chance of having several good embryos of which one can be transferred and the others frozen for future use, one at a time. With such a philosophy the number of started stimulated cycles could be reduced probably to a minimum before a full-term pregnancy is achieved. Up to date available data from large database analysis clearly indicate that the more high quality embryos in one stimulated cycle the better chance to achieve a pregnancy (13). With the protocols used today for controlled ovarian hyperstimulation (COH), to our opinion, there are five reasons for monitoring the cycle.

1. Beforehand predict the ovarian response to gonadotropins
2. Monitoring the effect of pituitary downregulation
3. During the stimulation evaluate if the dose of gonadotropin is adequate
4. To avoid OHSS
5. Find the optimal time for human chorionic gonadotropin (hCG) administration.

Monitoring before starting COH may identify poor responders as well as women at risk for ovarian OHSS (14–16). Furthermore, if a protocol with a GnRH agonist has been used, pituitary downregulation has to be verified before starting with gonadotropins. Since multiple follicular development plays a major role in the success of IVF, ovarian stimulation with FSH or FSH plus LH is nowadays routine for COH. However, identifying adequate follicular development during stimulation and finally optimizing the time of hCG administration also requires monitoring, preferably by a simple method, since it sometimes has to be repeated over a short period of time. Ideally, the method should be noninvasive and tell us when the oocytes are mature. Unfortunately, there is no such method. All methods are indirect with regard to assessment of oocyte maturity. The fact that there is no method by which oocyte maturation can be directly monitored in vivo and the huge number of IVF cycles performed today, monitoring has to be simple but still tell us enough about oocyte maturity. In this respect, ultrasound imagining of follicular development during COH has proved to be the most practical way of monitoring IVF cycles.

PREDICTION OF OVARIAN RESPONSE TO GONADOTROPINS

Prediction of ovarian response prior to stimulation is important since it helps us to choose an optimal starting dose of gonadotropins. Traditionally, the ovarian reserves have been evaluated by means of basal day 3 FSH measurement or a clomiphene citrate challenge test (17). However, measuring the number of small antral follicles in both ovaries by vaginal ultrasound has proved to be a reliable predictor of the ovarian reserve (18) as well as anti-Müllerian Hormone (AMH) in serum. In a study by Ng and coworkers they were able to show that the number of antral follicles as measured by vaginal ultrasound was even superior to basal day 3 FSH as well as BMI for predicting the number of oocytes retrieved for IVF (18). They demonstrated that in women with fewer antral follicles, a longer duration and higher dose of gonadotropin were required but still significantly less oocytes were retrieved. They could also show that if there were less than six antral follicles found in a cycle prior to the start of stimulation, there is an increased risk that cycles were cancelled before egg collection. Furthermore, those women at risk for OHSS can be identified. Women with typical polycystic ovary (PCO) appearance as well as those with multifollicular ovaries (MFO) can easily be identified. It seems as if women with more than 10 antral follicles have an increased risk for OHSS. In our program we nowadays routinely perform a vaginal scan in the early follicular phase in the cycle prior to the IVF cycle. The purpose is to identify those who could be poor as well as high responders. By doing so, it seems easier to identify an optimal starting dose of FSH and in certain cases also decide upon the type of protocol to be used particularly in poor responders where sometimes a GnRH antagonist protocol can be beneficial.

MONITORING PITUITARY DOWNREGULATION

As mentioned above, an often-used protocol for IVF cycles is the long GnRH agonist protocol with pituitary downregulation. When using such a protocol, one has to verify the downregulation before starting with gonadotropins. If the GnRH agonist is started in the late luteal phase a menstrual bleeding normally indicates that the estrogen is low and stimulation with gonadotropins can start. However, measuring suppression of ovarian/pituitary hormones in blood will clearly confirm pituitary downregulation. This can also be performed by ultrasound by checking that the endometrium is thin (<4 mm) and that there are no large cystic structures in the ovaries. In GnRH agonist cycles, hormone analyses are believed to be mandatory for confirming pituitary supression. However, even in this group it has been demonstrated that ultrasound imaging seems to be enough to verify downregulation (19). It has also been shown that color flow Doppler velocimetry of the utero-ovarian arteries can be used for verifying pituitary desensitization in those women. Dada and coworkers did show that that the ovarian artery resistance index was the best Doppler predictor of pituitary suppression and a mean discriminatory cutoff value of 0.9 was found to have the highest specificity and positive predictive value (20) in women that had started the GnRH in the early follicular phase.

MONITORING FOLLICULAR MATURATION

There are five methods that clinically can be used for monitoring follicular maturation in IVF cycles.

1. Serum E2
2. Ultrasound measurements of follicular growth and endometrial thickness
3. Ultrasound and serum E2 combined
4. Perifollicular blood flow by means of power Doppler imaging
5. Three-dimensional ultrasound of follicles

There is extensive literature regarding the use of all the above methods for monitoring the ovarian response in assisted reproductive technique (ART). There are enough data today showing that ultrasound imagining (UI) of the follicular and endometrial growth is sufficient for monitoring response to COH in IVF cycles in the majority of cases (21,22). It has been said that ultrasound should be used for timing hCG administration and the E2 to avoid complications (23). Which of the two methods is more reliable for the clinician's decision to increase, decrease, or stop the gonadotropin administration seems to be very much dependent on experience and/or routines used at the clinic. Furthermore, there is no consensus about how often the monitoring has to be done during ovarian stimulation. The frequency of monitoring seems to be arbitrarily chosen and thus varies considerably between different clinics. Thus, there are simple as well as complicated methods on how to monitor IVF cycles by means of serum E2 and/or ultrasound. However, irrespective of the method chosen, there seems to be no difference in the outcome of the IVF cycle as measured by live birth rate.

MONITORING WITH SERUM E2 ALONE

Serum E2, the only method for monitoring ART cycles stimulated with gonadotropins, was mainly used in the early days of IVF. The method for monitoring was based on the experience from monitoring of ovulation induction cycles. Some groups have tried to identify a certain serum E2 level that should be reached before hCG is given (24). Others have claimed that the number of days E2 increased was important and thus administered hCG accordingly (25). Even though some groups still continue to use E2 measurements as the sole monitoring modality, the majority of groups using serum E2 for monitoring of ovarian stimulation in IVF cycles also use ultrasound.

MONITORING WITH ULTRASOUND

Ultrasound monitoring of follicular diameter and endometrial thickness is a noninvasive method. It can be performed by the clinician and gives an actual status of the number and size of growing follicles. Endometrial thickness as measured by ultrasound can be used as a bioassay of the total follicular estrogen production. Vaginal ultrasound scanning of the utero-ovarian response to gonadotropin stimulation is a simple and reliable method that is the most practical way of monitoring IVF cycles.

Since the end of 1991 our group has utilized a monitoring system where ultrasound alone has been used in the majority of IVF cycles. In women not at risk for OHSS or poor responders (normally identified before the treatment cycle) only one ultrasound scan was performed on stimulation day 9 or 10. If the patient at that day had three follicles of 18 mm (mean of two diameters), less than 15 follicles, and an endometrial thickness of 7 mm or more, hCG was given and oocyte pickup performed 36–38 hours later. If the follicles did not fulfill this criteria at the day for the scan, a follicular growth of 2 mm/24 hours was predicted and hCG given according to that. The 18 mm diameter as well as the figure of 15 follicles has been arbitrarily chosen.

Retrospectively comparing 361 ART cycles performed during the year 1989 when several ultrasound and serum E2 measurements were used for monitoring each cycle, with 500 cycles performed during 1991 with the above simplified method, the take home baby rates were 17% and 26%, respectively (26). Another retrospective analysis of our data with the same simplified method of monitoring follicular maturation by ultrasound only once during COH showed a take home baby rate per started cycle of 31% and 1.8% of OHSS (11). During 1991–2002 this simplified monitoring system was utilized in our IVF program for 7325 cycles. During that period the take home baby rate per started cycle was 25% and mild to moderate OHSS occurred in 2.7% of the cycles. These figures show that it is possible to use simple monitoring by ultrasound only and still achieve a good pregnancy rate. Our experience has been confirmed by others (14). Later, Lass and coworkers showed in a multicenter prospective randomized study that ultrasound for monitoring of IVF in normal responders was enough for timing hCG administration without lowering the pregnancy rate or increasing the risk of OHSS (21).

In GnRH antagonist protocols, it has been recommended to start ultrasound monitoring on stimulation day 6 since that has been the day for starting with the GnRH antagonist in the majority of patients (27). However, in our IVF program, nowadays the antagonist is started when the largest follicle is ≥12 mm in diameter,

irrespective of the day in the cycle. In normal responders it means that the first scan can be performed on stimulation day 7–8.

The most important advantage of monitoring the IVF cycle only once or occasionally twice by ultrasound, is that the woman has to spend less time in the clinic. The simplified monitoring will thus bring down the costs for the treatment.

The disadvantage of using a simple monitoring system as described above is that there is no possibility of increasing the dose of gonadotropins early in the cycle. However, whether such an early increase of gonadotropin dose may affect the outcome of the IVF cycle has up to date not been proven.

MONITORING BY SERUM E2 AND ULTRASOUND

To date randomized trials do not support the notion that cycle monitoring by ultrasound plus serum E2 is more efficacious than cycle monitoring by ultrasound only in terms of live birth and pregnancy rates (22). However, combining ultrasound and serum E2 in women at risk for OHSS should be retained as a precautionary good practice point until adequately powered randomized trials, assessing the effects of different monitoring protocols on OHSS rate have been performed (28).

MONITORING BY COLOUR DOPPLER AND THREE-DIMENSIONAL ULTRASOUND

Doppler duplex system combining pulsed Doppler and grayscale ultrasound made it possible to noninvasively study ovarian blood flow and use that as a measurement of ovarian angiogenesis. From animal studies it is well known that there is a correlation between follicular vascularity and oocyte maturation. In a classic clinical study by Nargund and coworkers they could show a significant increased oocyte recovery from follicles with a high peak systolic velocity as measured by pulsed Doppler and grayscale ultrasound (29). Furthermore, they found that oocytes from poorly vascularized follicles produced morphologically poor embryos as compared to oocytes from highly vascularized follicles. Later, in a very elegant study, Van Blerkom and coworkers have shown by means of color Doppler imaging (CDI) that follicles with normal perifollicular blood flow contained oocytes free of cytoplasmic or chromosomal/spindle defects (30). However, CDI is time consuming and cannot be used in daily clinical setting. In 1994 a new color Doppler technique called power Doppler imaging (PDI) was described (31). The PDI technique has many advantages as compared to CDI, as it is more sensitive, enables flow with lower volumes and velocity to be displayed, and can thus display areas where the mean velocity is zero. Thus, PDI has proved to be a technique that can be used for measuring perifollicular blood flow and is simple enough to be used in the daily clinical setting.

Chui and coworkers adopted the PDI technique in their IVF program and showed that high-grade follicular vascularity resulted in oocytes/embryos that had an increased potential for becoming a full-term pregnancy (32). Further studies using PDI for monitoring perifollicular blood flow have shown that the technique can be used clinically for identifying follicles with oocytes that seem to have a better chance of resulting in good quality embryos (33).

Combining power Doppler angiography (PDA) and three-dimensional ultrasonography (3D-US) has been used for prediction and monitoring ovarian response in IVF-ET (embryo transfer) cycles (34,35). However, whether this technique really improves the outcome of the cycle is still unclear. Another interesting technique used for monitoring ovarian response in IVF cycles is the Sonography-based Automated Volume Count (SonoAVC), which is a relatively new three-dimensional (3D) US technology, that automatically generates a set of measurements including the mean follicular diameter (MFD) and a volume-based diameter [d(V)] for each follicle in the ovaries (36). Ata and coworkers recently published data indicating that this automatic follicle monitoring technique as compared to conventional two-dimensional ultrasound measurements is equally accurate but less time-consuming (37).

CONCLUSION

Ultrasound scanning of follicular size is the method of choice for monitoring ovarian response in stimulated IVF cycles irrespective of protocol used. It is to date the most practical, reliable, and cost-effective method for monitoring ovarian stimulation.

REFERENCES

1. Klopper A, Aiman J, Besser M. Ovarian steroidogenesis resulting from treatment with menopausal gonadotropin. Eur J ObstetGynecol Reprod Biol 1974; 4: 25–30.
2. Hackeloer BJ, Nitsche S, Daume E, Sturm G, Bucholz R. Ultraschaldarstellung von ovarveranderungen bei gonadotropinstimulierung. Geburtsh Fruenheilk 1977; 37: 185–9.
3. Ylöstalo P, Lindgren P, Nillius SJ. Ultrasonic measurment of ovarian follicles, ovarian and uterine size during induction of ovulation with human gonadotrophins. Acta Endocrinol 1981; 98: 592–8.
4. Vargyas JM, Marrs R, Kletzky OA, Mishell DR. Correlation of ultrasonic measurment of ovarian follicle size and serum estradiol levels in ovulatorypatients following clomiphene citrate for in vitro fertilization. Am J Obstet Gynecol 1982; 144: 569–73.
5. Wittmaack FM, Kreger DO, Blasco L, et al. Effect of follicular size on oocyte retrieval, fertilization, cleavage, and embryo quality in in vitro fertilization cycles: a 6-year data collection. Fertil Steril 1994; 62: 1205–10.
6. Cabau A, Bessis R. Monotoring of ovulation induction with human menopausal gonadotropin and human chorionic gonadotropin by ultrasound. Fertil Steril 1981; 36: 178–82.
7. McArdle C, Seibel M, Hann LE, Weinstein F, Taymor M. The diagnosis of ovarian hyperstimulation(OHS): the impact of ultrasound. Fertil Steril 1983; 39: 464–7.
8. Salam MN, Marinho AO, Collins WP, Rodeck CH, Campbell S. Monitoring gonadotrophin therapy by real-time ultrasonic scanning of ovarian follicles. Br J Obstet Gynaecol 1982; 89: 155–9.
9. Venturoli S, Fabbri R, Paradisi R, et al. Induction of ovulation with human urinary follicle stimulating hormone: endocrine pattern and ultrasound monitoring. Eur J Obstet Gynecol Reprod Biol 1983; 16: 135–45.
10. Messinis IE, Tempelton AA, Baird DT. Endogenous luteinizing hormone surge during superovulation induction with sequential use of clomiphene citrate and pulsatile human menopausal gonadortophin. J Clin Endocrin Metab 1985; 61: 1076–81.
11. Wikland M, Borg J, Hamberger L, Svalander P. Simplification of IVF. Minimal monitoring and the use of subcutaneous highly purified FSH administration for ovulation induction. Hum Reprod 1994; 9: 1430–6.
12. Bergh C, Howles C, Borg K, et al. Recombinant human follicle stimulating hormone(r-hFSH; Gonal-F) versus highly purified urinary FSH (Metrodin HP): results of a randomized comparative study in women undergoing assisted. Hum Reprod 1997; 12: 2133–9.
13. Templeton A, Morris JK. Reducing the risk of multiple births by transfer of two embryos after in vitro fertilization. N Engl J Med 1998; 27: 573–7.
14. Forman R, Robinson J, Egan J, et al. Follicular monitoring and outcome of in vitro fertilization in gonadotrophin-releasing hormone agonist-treated cycles. Fertil Steril 1991; 55: 567–73.
15. Shoham Z, Di Carlo C, Patel A, Conway G, Jacobs H. Is it possible to run a successful ovulation program based solely on ultrasound monitoring? The importance of endometrial measurements. Fertil Steril 1991; 56: 836–41.
16. Tomas C, Nuojua-Huttunen S, Martikainen H. Pretreatment transvaginal ultrasound examination predicts ovarian responsiveness to gonadotrophjins in in-vitro fertilization. Hum Reprod 1997; 12: 220–3.
17. Scott RT, Hofmann GE. Prognostic assessment of ovarian reserve. Fertil Steril 1995; 63: 1–11.
18. Ng EH, Tang OS, Ho PC. The significance of the number of antral follicles prior to stimulation in predicting ovarian responses in an IVF programme. Hum Reprod 2000; 15: 1937–42.
19. Barash A, Weissman A, Manor M, et al. Prospective evaluation of endometrial thickness as a predictor of pituitary down-regulation after gonadotropin-releasing hormone analogue administration in an in vitro fertilization program. Fertil Steril 1998; 69: 496–9.
20. Dada T, Salaha O, Allgar V, Sharma V. Utero-ovarian blood flow characteristics of pituitary desensitisation. Hum Reprod 2002; 16: 1663–70.
21. Lass A. UK Timing of hCG Group. Monitoring of in vitro fertilization-embryo transfer cycles by ultrasound versus ultrasound and hormonal levels: a prospective, multicenter, randomised study. Fertil Steril 2003; 80: 80–5.
22. Kwan I, Bhattacharya S, McNeil A, van Rumste MM. Monitoring of stimulated cycles in assisted reproduction (IVF and ICSI). Cochrane Database Syst Rev 2008; 6: CD005289.
23. Schoemaker J, Meer M, Weissenbruch M. Re-evaluation of the role of estrogens as a marker for ovulation induction. In: Linenfelt B, ed. FSH alone in ovulation induction. New York: The Parthenon Publishing Group, 1993: 23–7.
24. Wramsby H, Sundstrom P, Liedholm P. Pregnancy rate in relation to number of cleaved eggs replaced after in-vitro

fertilization in stimulated cycles monitored by serum levels of oestradiol and progesterone as sole index. Hum Reprod 1987; 2: 325–8.

25. Levran D, Lopata A, Nayudu PL, et al. Analysis of the outcome of in vitro fertilization in relation to the timing of human chorionic gonadotropin administration by the duration of estradiol rise in stimulated cycles. Fertil Steril 1985; 44: 335–41.

26. Wikland M. Vaginal ultrasound in sssisted reproduction. In: Hamberger H, Wikland M, eds. Asisted Reproduction (Elsevier's, Bailliere's Clinical obstetrics and Gynaecology). 1992: 2: 283–96.

27. Ganarelix dose-finding study group. A double-blind, randomized, dose-finding study to assess the efficacy of the GnRH-antagonist ganarelix(Org 37462) to prevent premature luteinizing hormone surges in women undergoing controlled ovarian hyperstimulation with recombinant follicle stimulating hormone. Hum Reprod 1998; 13: 3023–31.

28. Forman R, Frydman R, Egan D. Severe ovarian hyperstimulation syndrome using agonists of gonadotropin-releasing hormone for in vitro fertilization: a European series and a proposal for prevention. Fertil Steril 1990; 55: 502.

29. Nargund G, Bourne T, Doyle P, et al. Associations between ultrasound indices of follicular blood flow and oocyte recovery and preimplantation embryo quality. Hum Reprod 1996; 11: 109–13.

30. Van Blerkom J, Antczak M, Schrader R. The developmental potential of human oocytes is related to the dissolved oxygen content of follicular fluid: association with vascular endothelial growth factor levels and perifollicular blood flow characteristics. Hum Reprod 1997; 12: 1047–55.

31. Rubin JM, Bude RO Carson PL, Bree RL, Adler RS. Power Doppler US: potential useful alternative to mean frequency-based color Doppler US. Radiology 1994; 190: 853–6.

32. Chui DK, Pugh ND, Walker SM, Gregory M, Shaw RW. Follicular vascularity-the predictive value of transvaginal ultrasonography in an in vitro-fertilization program: a preliminary study. Hum Reprod 1997; 12: 191–6.

33. Bhal PS, Pugh ND, Gregory L, O'Brien S, Shaw RW. Perifollicular vascularity as a potential variable affecting outcome in stimulated intrauterine insemination treatment cycles: a study using transvaginal power Doppler. Hum Reprod 2001; 16: 1682–9.

34. Vlaisavljevic V, Reljic M, Gavric Lovrec V, Zazula D, Sergent N. Measurment of perifollicular blood flow of the dominant follicle using three-dimensional power Doppler. Ultrasound Obstet Gynecol 2003; 22: 520–6.

35. Mercé LT, Barco MJ, Bau S, Troyano JM. Prediction of ovarian response and IVF/ICSI outcome by three-dimensional ultrasonography and power Doppler angiography. Eue J Obstet Gynecol Reprod Biol 2007; 132: 93–100.

36. Raine-Fenning N, Jayaprakasan K, Clewes J, et al. Sono-AVC: a novel method of automatic volume calculation. Ultrasound Obstet Gynecol 2008; 31: 691–6.

37. Ata B, Seyhan A, Reinblatt SL, et al. Comparison of automated and manual follicle monitoring in an unrestricted population of 100 women undergoing controlled ovarian stimulation for IVF. Hum Reprod 2011; 26: 127–33.

44

Oocyte collection

Gab Kovacs

HISTORY

The very first human pregnancy using in vitro fertilization (IVF) was achieved using laparotomy for obtaining the oocyte by de Kretzer et al. in 1973 (1). Meanwhile, Morgenstern and Soupart in 1972 (2) had described an experimental procedure for both abdominal and vaginal approaches to oocyte recovery, in conjunction with gynecological surgery, using a special oocyte recovery unit (ORU). As laparoscopy was just being applied to gynecology, the laparoscopic approach became routine by the late 1970s (3,4).

It was the expertise with laparoscopy of Patrick Steptoe, and his successful partnership with Bob Edwards that resulted in the birth of Louise Brown in 1978 (5). However, it was the laparoscopic approach with modification of the collection needle (6) and lining it with Teflon to give a continuous column without obstacles and turbulence that was used in the stimulated/controlled cycles, which resulted in the next eight births from the Monash team during 1981, which converted IVF from a research tool to clinical treatment. The laparoscopic approach was also used by the Jones' team when they applied the use of human menopausal gonadotropin to achieve the first pregnancies in the United States (7).

During the early 1980s, IVF became practiced worldwide, using laparoscopic oocyte collection. It was the pioneering work of Susan Lenz in Copenhagen (8) and Wilfred Feichtinger in Vienna (9) that changed oocyte collection to a transvaginal ultrasound-guided technique. With its efficacy being proven to be as good as laparoscopy, (10) most of the world's IVF units abandoned laparoscopy for the transvaginal ultrasound-guided route.

ANESTHESIA/ANALGESIA

The use of anesthesia and sedation for oocyte collection are discussed in detail in chapter 53, so only a brief summary will be given here. With the change to transvaginal ultrasound-guided oocyte collection, relaxant anesthesia was no longer required. Currently there is great variation in the type of analgesia used for oocyte collection. In many centers, oocyte collection is undertaken without any analgesia, whereas in other places some intravenous sedation or even general anesthesia is administered. This depends on several factors including cultural expectations, the facility used for the oocyte collection, and the medical financial rebate system. A balance has to be reached with minimal risk and cost, but without causing the women unacceptable discomfort. A survey of anesthetic practice employed for oocyte collection in the United Kingdom (11) found that intravenous sedation was the preferred method of sedation, being used in 62.4% of units. General anesthesia was the primary method in 24.6% of units. Sedation was administered by non-anesthetic doctors in 46% and by nurses in 8%. A review of anesthetic practices used in the United States and Europe undertaken by Vlahos and colleagues (12) found that conscious sedation was the most popular method of anesthesia used in IVF, with a combination of propofol, fentanyl, and midazolam used frequently. They also found a relatively low incidence of adverse effects especially on oocyte and embryo quality.

A study comparing women who underwent monitored anesthesia care (MAC) technique with a remifentanil infusion versus general anesthesia consisting of alfentanil, propofol, and nitrous oxide, which was maintained with isoflurane or propofol infusion, was undertaken in Germany by Wilhelm and colleagues (13). They found that pregnancy rates in women were significantly higher with a remifentanil-based MAC technique than with a general anesthetic technique. In contrast, a meta-analysis by Kim and colleagues (14) found that cleavage and pregnancy rates were not significantly different in between the general anesthesia and locoregional anesthesia groups.

CLEANSING/STERILIZING THE VAGINA

There is little data on the need or effectiveness of vaginal cleansing prior to vaginal oocyte collection. As early as 1992 van Os and colleagues (15) showed in a prospective randomized study that there was no difference in outcome whether povidon iodine 1% was used to cleanse the vagina or normal saline, when assessing fertilization, cleavage, and pregnancy rates. However, the clinical pregnancy rate per embryo transfer was significantly higher in the normal saline group (17.2% vs. 30.3%). As no increase in infections occurred in the saline group, it can be included that there was no indication to used iodine. When studying a group of patients with increased risk of infection (16), those with endometriomas, pre-retrieval vaginal douching with aqueous povidone iodine followed by normal saline irrigation immediately before oocyte retrieval, was effective in preventing the pelvic infection without compromising the outcome of IVF treatment. There was no difference in the fertilization rate (81.2% vs. 79.8%, P > 0.05), implantation rate (19.2% vs. 23.3%, P > 0.05), clinical pregnancy rate (39.3% vs. 46.2%, P > 0.05), but whereas there was no infection in patients treated with povidone iodine, there were two women in the control group who developed pelvic abscess and needed surgical intervention. So whilst povidone douche may decrease the incidence of infection in "high risk" patients, with van Os et al. (15) data suggesting a harmful effect on clinical pregnancy rates, the use of antiseptic douching is not indicated.

THE EQUIPMENT

The Suction Source

In the early days, manual suction with a needle, plastic tubing, and syringe were used (2) and Berger and colleagues in 1975 (3) devised a special aspiration unit, with a 20-gauge -inch needle connected by polyethylene tube to a 10 cc Vacutainer, which then connected to a vacuum bottle with an adjustable pressure gauge. The suction was turned on or off by a thumb valve. The technique then was modified with the use of suction pump operated by a foot pump (6). Today, sophisticated suction pumps with adjustable aspiration pressure are widely available commercially.

The Suction

There has been surprisingly little study undertaken on the physical aspects of oocyte recovery. We published the findings of experiments on bovine eggs carried out in the laboratories of Cook Medical Technology in Brisbane (17). Some of the observations of these studies are outlined below. In this study, we measured the velocity and flow rates of oocytes through the collection system, and observed the damaging effect of non-laminar flow on the oocyte.

Application of Vacuum to the Follicle

Vacuum Applied after the Needle Entry into the Follicle After application of the vacuum, the pressure within the system equilibrates, resulting in a steady flow rate until the fluid volume decreases and follicle collapses, so that the follicular wall blocks the lumen of the needle. The time for the system to equilibrate depends on the vacuum pressure, the diameter of the needle, and the volume of the follicle. Maximum flow is achieved when the pressure is at a steady state. Should air be sucked into the system, by entering around where the needle pierced the follicle wall, frothing with non-laminar flow results, which I call the "cappuccino effect." This has deleterious effect on the oocyte, as it is thrown around the collection system.

Vacuum Deactivated before the Needle was Withdrawn from the Follicle If the pressure is deactivated whilst the needle is still in the follicle (and there are no leaks), the pressure within the needle and collecting tube drops, and there is often back flow toward the follicle. This can result in the oocyte being sucked back and possibly lost. The amount of backflow depends on how much air enters the system and how much higher the collection tube is above the patients pelvis.

The Vacuum Profiles within the Aspiration System It was estimated that using the system at 150 kPa, it took 5 seconds for the system to stabilize. The pressure within the follicle before penetration varies depending on the size (maturity), shape, and position of the follicle. The internal pressure increases correlating with size. However, due to the pressure caused by the needle deforming the surface of the follicle at the time of puncture, the pressure within the follicle may be much higher (up to 60 mmHg). The more blunt the needle, the higher the resultant pressure. This may result in follicular fluid being lost as it spurts out during the process. If the pressure is already applied, some/most of this fluid will be aspirated as it escapes along the outer wall of the follicle.

There is a pressure gradient down the collection system, so that the pressure at the tip of the needle is only 5% of the pressure at the pump. The oocyte is therefore exposed to ever-increasing pressures as it travels along the needle, the collection tube, and the collecting test tube. Excessive pressure can cause the ovum to swell and the zona to crack.

Follicle and Needle Volumes Table 44.1 lists the respective volumes contained in follicles between 6 and 20 mm in diameter. A 6-mm follicle only contains 0.1 ml, so that 10 to 12 follicles need to be emptied before the

Table 44.1 The Diameter to Volume Ratio of Typical Follicles

Follicle diameter (mm)	Follicle volume (ml)
6	0.1
7	0.2
8	0.3
9	0.4
10	0.5
11	0.7
12	0.9
13	1.1
14	1.4
15	1.8
16	2.1
17	2.6
18	3.0
19	3.6
20	4.2

The typical dead space of needle and collecting tubule are 1.0 to 1.2 ml.

dead space of 1.0 to 1.2 ml in a standard needle and collecting tube is filled, and fluid reaches the collection test tube. This is relevant in the technique of collecting oocytes from unstimulated ovaries for in vitro maturation (IVM) (18).

Application of the Vacuum Following the penetration of the follicle by the needle and the application of suction, the pressure within the follicle, the needle, and the collecting tube equilibrates. If there is a tight seal around the needle (that is the needle was sharp and was introduced precisely through the follicular wall and the hand is kept still so that tearing does not result), when the suction pressure is reduced, there will be backflow of fluid into the follicle. This can result in the oocyte being lost. On the other hand, if the needle is withdrawn whilst the suction is still applied, there is sudden change of pressure at the needle tip from the high vacuum of the follicle to atmospheric pressure, with a rapid surge of fluid toward the collection tube. If the oocyte is contained in the terminal portion of the fluid, it is subjected to increased speeds of travel as well as turbulence, resulting in loss of the cumulus mass and even fracture of the zona pellucida.

Damage within the Follicle During aspiration, the oocyte has to accelerate from a resting state to the velocity of fluid within the needle. If this is too rapid, the cumulus may be stripped off. The higher the aspiration pressure the greater the risk, and the smaller the follicle the higher the pressure that is needed. This may also be very relevant in the collection of immature oocytes for IVM.

Damage to Oocytes It was noted that high velocities may strip the cumulus from the oocyte. Even with laminar flow there are significant differences in velocity of the follicular fluid within the center of the needle compared to the periphery. This can result in "drag" on the outer layers of cumulus, resulting in potential damage. The longer the needle the smaller its internal diameter, the greater the pressure required to maintain the same velocity. It was found that when a 17-gauge collection needle was used, all oocytes lost their cumulus mass when the aspiration pressure reached 20 kPa (150 mmHg). It is therefore recommended that pressures be kept below 120 mmHg.

Apart from the speed of travel, turbulent non-laminar flow can also damage the oocyte, either stripping its cumulus mass or fracturing the zona. It is believed that an intact cumulus may be important in preventing damage to oocytes.

The Needle

Initially only a single lumen needle was used, and it was disconnected at a hub that was inserted through the cork of the suction test tube to allow flushing. This meant that with a dead space of 1.0 to 1.2 ml, the oocyte was often flushed up and down in the collection system, only being recovered in the final aspiration which we called "the needle wash." To allow more efficient flushing, double lumen needles were introduced. Scott and colleagues (19) compared a single-lumen needle (SLN; N = 22) or a double-lumen needle (DLN; N = 22) to compare recovery rates and the technical aspects of their use. Two hundred and ten and 202 follicles were aspirated with each needle, respectively. One or more washes were performed when using the DLN and the SLN was withdrawn each time to recover the fluid in the dead space of the needle. The distribution of follicular sizes was the same for both needles. Oocyte recovery rates (SLN = 65.7%; DLN = 63.9%) and the incidence of fractured zonae (SLN = 9.1%; DLN = 6.4%) was the same for both needles (alpha > 0.50; beta < 0.01). Although there were no differences between the two needles in the number of oocytes provided for IVF, there were technical differences. The DLN needle was more flexible and frequently deviated from the projected path as observed by ultrasound. The SLN may be preferable because it is technically easier to use; however, there may remain specific indications for the use of the DLN. It is now our policy to utilize a single-lumen needle without flushing unless there are four or less follicles present for aspiration.

TECHNIQUE

Flushing or Rapid Oocyte Collection

When transvaginal oocyte collection was first undertaken, the technique of laparoscopic harvesting was transferred to the transvaginal approach. Follicles were initially aspirated, and then repeatedly flushed to try and recover as many oocytes as possible. This required the use of a double-lumen needle. This, however, is time consuming and also uses large quantities of culture medium. It was soon recognized that most oocytes can be recovered by just aspirating, and that the follicular fluid from the next follicle will often flush the oocyte into the collection tube. This technique was called the rapid oocyte recovery (ROC).

Scott and colleagues from Norfolk Virginia (19) reported no advantage from using a flushing technique with DLN.

More recently, Haydardedeoglu and colleagues (20) compared the retrieval efficiency of single- (only follicular aspiration) and double-lumen needle (aspiration with follicular flushing) procedures in normal-responder IVF cycles in a prospective randomized study. They did not demonstrate a beneficial effect of double-lumen needle retrieval compared with single-lumen needle retrieval in terms of retrieved oocytes, clinical pregnancy rates, and live birth rates.

Wongtra-Ngan and colleagues from Thailand (21) undertook a Cochrane Systematic Review to determine whether flushing yields a larger number of oocytes and a higher potential for pregnancy than aspiration only. They reviewed randomized controlled trials that compared follicular aspiration and flushing with aspiration alone.

Trials were excluded if the flushing method comparison was confounded by comparisons of other methods. They found that no studies reported on the primary outcome of live birth. There was no evidence (three studies, 164 patients) to suggest an association between follicular aspiration and flushing and ongoing or clinical pregnancy per woman randomized (OR 1.17, 95% CI 0.57 to 2.38). There was no evidence of a difference in adverse events reported between follicular aspiration and flushing, and aspiration only. There was no evidence of significant differences in increased oocyte yield per woman randomized (one study, 44 patients). Without flushing, the operative time was significantly shorter, by three to 15 minutes (three studies, $P < 0.001$) and the dose of pethidine required was significantly less (50 mg vs. 100 mg, $P < 0.00001$). They concluded that there is no evidence that follicular aspiration and flushing is associated with improved clinical outcome.

Whilst the evidence for flushing in conventional IVF is not convincing, with minimal stimulation IVF the topic has been revisited. Mendez-Lozano and colleagues in 2007 (22) showed that flushing improved pregnancy rates when the number of follicles were limited.

Peter Steiner has developed a new type of needle to make flushing more efficient (23). He devised a quasi double-lumen needle where the needle's diameter increases approximately 7 cm from its tip, where holes communicating with a plastic tube make it possible to flush the tube from the outside. This allows efficient flushing of follicles via a single-lumen needle with minimal time added to the procedure.

This topic was recently reviewed by Hill and Levens (24). They concluded that "Randomized controlled trials consistently demonstrate no benefit and increased procedural time with follicular flushing in both normal and poor-responding ART patients. Nonrandomized data suggest a possible role for follicular flushing in natural cycle or minimal stimulation ART and in those undergoing IVM cycles."

It is the clinical protocol at Monash IVF that if four or fewer follicles are present, a double-lumen needle should be used and follicles flushed. If more than four follicles are present then a single-lumen needle is used and follicles are sequentially aspirated. Flushing of follicles requires the use of a double-lumen needle, as with a single-lumen needle with a dead space of 1.0 to 1.2 ml, the oocyte is likely to be flushed up and down within the system.

Curetting the Follicle

Dahl and colleagues (25) made a point that the follicles should be curetted at the completion of aspiration to increase oocyte yield. With curetting, 13.9 ± 0.6 oocytes collected compared to 11.4 ± 0.6 oocytes without curetting ($P = 0.003$).

Avoiding Turbulent Flow

When aspirating follicles, it is important to recognise that to fill the "dead space" between the needle tip and the aspiration tube, somewhere between 1 and 2 ml of follicular fluid is needed.

As described above, it is desirable to avoid damage to the cumulus-oocyte mass during aspiration. The aim is to avoid non-laminar flow within the collection tube, which is likely to damage the oocyte. Attention should be paid to filling the tubing with fluid prior to aspiration, gentle changes in aspiration pressure, limiting the suction pressure, and stopping aspiration whilst withdrawing the needle to avoid the aspiration of air causing turbulence ("The Cappuccino effect").

Temperature Control

Another important point is to deliver oocytes to the laboratory in the best condition including being aware of the effect of cooling. Redding and colleagues from New Zealand (26) investigated the effects of IVF aspiration on the temperature, pH, and dissolved oxygen of bovine follicular fluid. They found that the temperature of follicular fluid dropped by $7.7 \pm 1.3\,°C$ upon aspiration. Dissolved oxygen levels rose by 5 ± 2 vol.%. The pH increased by 0.04 ± 0.01, and they concluded that these changes could be detrimental to oocyte health and efforts should be made to minimize these changes. The collection tubes are therefore kept in a test-tube warmer whilst they are waiting to be connected to the collection system.

THE APPROACH

Any ultrasound machine with the capacity to use a transvaginal probe with a needle guide can be used. The ovaries are visualized and ovarian follicles are then aspirated in a systematic fashion. It is my habit to always commence with the right ovary, and then to aspirate follicles sequentially. It is best to keep the needle within the ovary if possible, to minimize the amount of trauma to the ovarian capsule. When all follicles within the right ovary are aspirated, the needle is withdrawn from the vagina and the needle is flushed with the medium to clear any blood. The pressure is retested, and the left ovary is then aspirated.

A Checklist of Oocyte Collection

A technique that I learnt from Aircraft Pilots' procedures is that there should be a checklist used in association with each oocyte collection procedure, which the diligent clinician should physically or at least mentally – less reliable method –tick off (Table 44.2).

COMPLICATIONS

Whilst these are discussed in detail in chapter 62, a brief synopsis is provided here.

Transvaginal oocyte collection has become the method of choice during the last two decades. However, although complications are rare, several possible complications of transvaginal oocyte collection have been reported.

Table 44.2   Oocyte Collection Checklist

Check patient's ID details against history. Obtain/confirm "informed consent"

Review previous oocyte collections/outcomes

Review most recent ultrasound

Check ultrasound machine is working, orientation, needle guide line(s)

Check suction pump is functioning, pressure calibrated appropriately – not excessive

Check connection of tubing

Select needle (single or double lumen)

Test aspiration system

Check/confirm that collection tubes are correctly labeled with patient details

Proceed with aspiration

Clean out blood from the vagina (if there is subsequent blood loss its new bleed)

Complete operative notes

Leave message for patient about number of eggs

Contact partner to reassure/inform regarding egg numbers

The commonest operative complications are:

- Hemorrhage
- Trauma to pelvic structures
- Pelvic infection, tubo-ovarian, or pelvic abscess

Rarely reported complications include:

- Ovarian torsion
- Rupture of ovarian endometriosis
- Appendicitis
- Ureteral obstruction (27)
- Uretero vaginal fistula (28)
- Vertebral osteomyelitis (29)
- Anesthetic complications

The incidence of postoperative acute abdomen was reported by Dicker and colleagues in 1994 from Israel (30). They reported 14 cases, out of 3656 patients undergoing the procedure, presenting with a clinical picture of acute abdomen. In nine patients tubo-ovarian and pelvic abscess were diagnosed. In three cases severe intra-abdominal bleeding occurred with one requiring laparotomy and hemostasis. Ruptured endometriotic cysts caused acute abdomen in two patients.

Tureck from Philadelphia (31) published a retrospective analysis of 674 patients who underwent transvaginal retrieval of oocytes during a three-year period. Ten (1.5%) required hospital admission because of perioperative complications. Nine of these patients needed intravenous antibiotics and one required admission and observation for an expanding broad-ligament hematoma.

Hemorrhage can result in vaginal bleeding at and after the oocyte collection, (overt bleeding) or intra-abdominal bleeding (covert bleeding). Bennet and colleagues (32) from a four-year prospective study carried out at King's College London of 2670 consecutive procedures reported that vaginal hemorrhage occurred in 229 (8.6%) of the cases, with a significant loss (classified as more than 100 ml) in 22 (0.8%). Hemorrhage from the ovary with hemoperitoneum formation was seen on two occasions and necessitated emergency laparotomy in one instance. A single case of pelvic hematoma formation from a punctured iliac vessel was also recorded; this settled without intervention.

Aragona and colleagues (33) have recently reported on the complications observed after transvaginal oocyte retrievals in 7098 IVF cycles. They found that frequency of severe complications was 0.08%, of which four cases were of intraperitoneal bleeding (0.06%) and two were cases of ovarian abscess (0.03%).

As bleeding appears to be the commonest complication, it has been suggested that maybe patients should undergo routine screening for coagulation abnormalities before oocyte retrieval. Revel and colleagues (34) in Jerusalem, Israel carried out a cross-sectional retrospective study to assess the value of coagulation screening to prevent procedure-related bleeding. Among 1032 patients evaluated, they found that 534 coagulation tests were needed to prevent one case of bleeding associated with an abnormal coagulation test result, thus making the procedure not cost effective.

Risquez and Confino (35) using color Doppler ultrasound to assess hemorrhagic complications found that 56/898 patients had significant peritoneal bleeding after Vaginal pick up (VPU).

Jayakrishnan and colleagues (36) reported a pseudoaneurysm after oocyte retrieval resulting in massive hematuria causing hemodynamic instability.

As early as the 1990s it was recognized that preexisting endometrioma was a risk factor for pelvic infection after oocyte collection with Younis and colleagues from Israel (37) reporting on three infertile women with ovarian endometriomata, who presented with late manifestation of severe pelvic abscess 40, 24, and 22 days after oocyte collection respectively. It is now accepted that ovarian endometriomata seems to be a significant risk factor for pelvic abscess development. Late manifestation of pelvic abscess supports the notion that the presence of old blood in an endometrioma provides a culture medium for bacteria to grow slowly after transvaginal inoculation. Moini and colleagues (38), working in Tehran, reported that during a six-year period, when 5958 transvaginal ultrasound-guided oocyte retrievals were carried out, 10 cases of acute pelvic inflammatory disease (0.12%) were observed. Eight of the 10 patients were diagnosed infertile because of endometriosis. They concluded that this supports the previous reports that endometriosis can raise the risk of pelvic inflammatory disease after oocyte retrieval. More vigorous antibiotic prophylaxis and better vaginal preparation was recommended when oocyte pickup is performed in patients with endometriosis.

Overall the risk of significant pelvic infection is between 1:200 and 1:500. Consequently, prophylactic antibiotics are not indicated, unless an endometrioma is entered, or there is a past history of pelvic infection, and then it is our policy to administer a single dose of intravenous antibiotic, e.g., Gentamicin.

Very Uncommon Complications

Ureteric Obstruction

There is a case report from Greenville, South Carolina, U.S.A., of a case of acute ureteral obstruction following seemingly uncomplicated oocyte retrieval. Prompt diagnosis and ureteral stenting led to rapid patient recovery with no long-term urinary tract sequelae (27).

Severe Hematuria Cystic Pseudoaneurysm

Jayakrishnan and colleagues (36) reported a pseudoaneurysm after oocyte retrieval resulting in massive hematuria causing hemodynamic instability.

Uretero-Vaginal Fistula

Von Eyre and colleagues (28) reported a case of ureterovaginal fistula secondary to transvaginal oocyte retrieval. The woman presented with immediate right lower abdominal pain with radiation to the suprapubic area and associated with vaginal discharge. Vaginal examination and excretory urography confirmed the diagnosis. Treatment was the insertion of a double-J catheter under general anesthesia. Vaginal leakage ceased a few hours after catheter insertion. The double-J catheter was removed 21 days after its placement. Imaging studies done six weeks later demonstrated a normal urinary tract morphology.

Vertebral Osteomyelitis

The most bizarre complication reported after oocyte collection is vertebral osteomyelitis reported from Tel Aviv by Almog and colleagues (29). They described a case of vertebral osteomyelitis as a complication of transvaginal oocyte retrieval in a 41-year-old woman. After she returned with severe low back pain, vertebral osteomyelitis was diagnosed and treated with antibiotics.

Cullen's Sign (Periumbilical Hematoma)

Bentov and colleagues (39) described two cases of periumbilical hematoma (Cullen's sign) following ultrasound-guided transvaginal oocyte retrieval. Spontaneous resolution of the symptoms occurred within two weeks. They concluded that the appearance of a periumbilical hematoma (Cullen's sign) following ultrasound-guided transvaginal oocyte retrieval reflects a retroperitoneal hematoma.

TROUBLESHOOTING

It is important that before commencing oocyte collection, the system is tested by aspirating some culture medium. This also provides a column of fluid into which to collect the follicular fluid, thus encouraging laminar flow.

Should suction then subsequently decrease or stop, the following steps should be undertaken:

1. Ensure that suction pump is turned on and that the suction pedal is functioning (many aspiration pumps have a light that goes on, and some have audible signals when pump is activated)
2. Check that all connections of tubing between the aspiration tube and the pump are tightly connected
3. Exclude any cracks in the aspiration test tube
4. Ensure that the collection tubing is not kinked or damaged
5. Rotate the needle within the follicle to ensure that it is not blocked by follicular wall tissue
6. If still no suction, remove the needle and perform a "retrograde flush" to clear any blockage
7. Before re-inserting the needle, recheck by aspirating some culture medium.

Failure to get Oocytes – Empty Follicle Syndrome

Sometimes several follicles are aspirated, and no oocytes are recovered. If the fluid collected is very clear and devoid of cells (granulosa and cumulus), suspicion may be raised that the patient has not had her trigger human chorionic gonadotropin (hCG). It is suggested that before follicles from the second ovary are aspirated, some of the follicular fluid is tested with a urinary pregnancy test strip. As these turn blue (react positive) when the concentration exceeds 25 mIU/ml, if the hCG was administered, there should be sufficient hCG in the follicle to give a positive result. If the test is negative, it is possible to abandon the collection, administer hCG, and defer the collection from the other ovary till about 36 hours later.

Although the number of oocytes collected will be limited to one ovary, it is still possible to salvage the cycle.

Pretreatment of Pathology

It has long been suggested that tubal disease, and particularly hydrosalpinx, has a detrimental effect on the outcome of IVF. To determine whether surgical removal of hydrosalpinges improved outcome, Johnson and colleagues (40) undertook a Cochrane analysis of all trials comparing a surgical treatment for tubal disease with a control group generated by randomization. The studied outcomes were live birth (and ongoing pregnancy), pregnancy, ectopic pregnancy, miscarriage, multiple pregnancy, and complications. Three randomized controlled trials involving 295 couples were included in this review. The odds of ongoing pregnancy and live birth were increased with laparoscopic salpingectomy for hydrosalpinges prior to IVF. The odds of pregnancy were also increased but there was no significant difference in the odds of ectopic pregnancy. They recommended that laparoscopic salpingectomy should be considered for all women with hydrosalpinges prior to IVF treatment. They also concluded that the role of surgery for tubal disease in the absence of a hydrosalpinx is unclear and merits further evaluation. The role of surgery for hydrosalpinges was recently reviewed in detail by van Voorst and Johnson (41).

Endometriosis

Al-Fadhli and colleagues (42) reported a study to evaluate the effects of different stages of endometriosis on the outcome of treatment in an IVF program. They found that the presence of endometriosis, including stages III and IV, does not affect IVF outcome. However, women with endometriosis required more gonadotropins than those with no endometriosis. Women with an obliterated cul-de-sac have fewer oocytes retrieved. The effect of endometriosis in IVF treatment was recently reviewed by Adamson and Abusief (43).

Assessing Clinical Competence

It is recommended that prior to undertaking oocyte collections, a structured training program for clinicians is carried out. One approach is that the instructor aspirates one side, and having collected some eggs, the trainee should do the other side. The number of supervised collections probably varies between 20 and 40 before the trainees are credentialed to perform collections on their own. Indeed, Goldman et al. (44) conducted a retrospective study to determine a minimum number of procedures required for proficiency in oocyte retrieval and to characterize skill acquisition. The majority of individual fellows in training demonstrate proficiency in follicular aspirations within 20 procedures; however, a minority may require 50 procedures to achieve the proficiency of an attending physician.

Ongoing assessment of clinical competence should then be regularly reassessed. Our clinical indicator is the oocyte collection rate; the number of oocytes aspirated per follicle (>13 mm) on the pre-hCG scan. The collection rates are then compared between clinicians working within the unit. Other indicators that could be recorded are the time taken for the oocyte collection, the complication rate, although the incidence of bleeding and infection is so low that it is probably meaningless unless there are a large number of cases that can be studied.

REFERENCES

1. De Kretzer D, Dennis P, Hudson B, et al. Transfer of a human zygote. Lancet 1973; 2: 728–9.
2. Morgenstern LL, Soupart P. Oocyte recovery from the human ovary. Fertil Steril 1972; 23: 751–8.
3. Berger MJ, Smith DM, Taymor ML, Thompson RS. Laparoscopic recovery of mature human oocytes. Fertil Steril 1975; 26: 513–22.
4. Steptoe PC, Edwards RG. Laparoscopic recovery of pre-ovulatory human oocytes after priming of ovaries with gonadotrophins. Lancet 1970; 1: 683–9.
5. Steptoe PC, Edwards RG. Birth after the reimplantation of a human embryo. Lancet 1978; 2: 366.
6. Renou P, Trounson AO, Wood C, Leeton JF. The collection of human oocytes for in vitro fertilization. I. An instrument for maximizing oocyte recovery rate. Fertil Steril 1981; 35: 409–12.
7. Jones HW Jr, Acosta AA, Garcia J. A technique for the aspiration of oocytes from human ovarian follicles. Fertil Steril 1982; 37: 26–9.
8. Lenz S. Ultrasonic-guided follicle puncture under local anesthesia. J In Vitro Fert Embryo Transf 1984; 1: 239–43.
9. Feichtinger W, Kemeter P. Laparoscopic or ultrasonically guided follicle aspiration for in vitro fertilization? J In Vitro Fert Embryo Transf 1984; 1: 244–9.
10. Kovacs GT, King C, Cameron I, et al. A comparison of vaginal ultrasonic-guided and laparoscopic retrieval of oocytes for in vitro fertilization. Asia Oceania J Obstet Gynaecol 1990; 16: 39–43.
11. Yasmin E, Dresner M, Balen A. Sedation and anaesthesia for transvaginal oocyte collection: an evaluation of practice in the UK. Hum Reprod 2004; 19: 2942–5.
12. Vlahos NF, Giannakikou I, Vlachos A, Vitoratos N. Analgesia and anesthesia for assisted reproductive techniques. Int J Gynaecol Obstet 2009; 105: 201–5.
13. Wilhelm W, Hammadeh ME, White PF, et al. General anesthesia versus monitored anesthesia care with remifentanil for assisted reproductive techniques: effect on pregnancy rate. J Clin Anesth 2002; 14: 1–5.
14. Kim WO, Kil HK, Koh SO, Kim JI. Effects of general and locoregional anesthesia on reproductive outcome for in vitro fertilization: a meta-analysis. J Korean Med Sci 2000; 15: 68–72.
15. van Os HC, Roozenburg BJ, Janssen-Caspers HA, et al. Vaginal disinfection with povidon iodine and the outcome of in-vitro fertilization. Hum Reprod 1992; 7: 349–50.
16. Tsai YC, Lin MY, Chen SH, et al. Vaginal disinfection with povidone iodine immediately before oocyte retrieval is effective in preventing pelvic abscess formation without compromising the outcome of IVF-ET. J Assist Reprod Genet 2005; 22: 173–5.
17. Horne R, Bishop CJ, Reeves G, Wood C, Kovacs GT. Aspiration of oocytes for in-vitro fertilization. Hum Reprod Update 1996; 2: 77–85.
18. Barnes FL, Kausche A, Tiglias J, et al. Production of embryos from in vitro-matured primary human oocytes. Fertil Steril 1996; 65: 1151–6.
19. Scott RT, Hofmann GE, Muasher SJ, et al. A prospective randomized comparison of single- and double-lumen needles for transvaginal follicular aspiration. J In Vitro Fert Embryo Transf 1989; 6: 98–100.
20. Haydardedeoglu B, Cok T, Kilicdag EB, et al. In vitro fertilization-intracytoplasmic sperm injection outcomes in single- versus double-lumen oocyte retrieval needles in normally responding patients: a randomized trial. Fertil Steril 2011; 95: 812–14.
21. Wongtra-Ngan S, Vutyavanich T, Brown J. Follicular flushing during oocyte retrieval in assisted reproductive techniques. Cochrane Database Syst Rev 2010: CD004634.
22. Mendez Lozano DH, Fanchin R, Chevalier N, et al. The follicular flushing duplicate the pregnancy rate on semi natural cycle IVF. J Gynecol Obstet Biol Reprod (Paris) 2007; 36: 36–41.
23. Steiner HP. Optimising technique in follicular aspiration and flushing. In: Chavez-badiola A, Allahbadia GN, eds. Technique of Minimal Stimulation in IVF-Milder, Mildest or Back to Nature. New Delhi, India: Jaypee Brothers Medical Publishers, 2011: 98–102.
24. Hill MJ, Levens ED. Is there a benefit in follicular flushing in assisted reproductive technique? Curr Opin Obstet Gynecol 2010; 22: 208–12.

25. Dahl SK, Cannon S, Aubuchon M, et al. Follicle curetting at the time of oocyte retrieval increases the oocyte yield. J Assist Reprod Genet 2009; 26: 335–9.

26. Redding GP, Bronlund JE, Hart AL. The effects of IVF aspiration on the temperature, dissolved oxygen levels, and pH of follicular fluid. J Assist Reprod Genet 2006; 23: 37–40.

27. Miller PB, Price T, Nichols JE Jr, Hill L. Acute ureteral obstruction following transvaginal oocyte retrieval for IVF. Hum Reprod 2002; 17: 137–8.

28. von Eye Corleta H, Moretto M, D'Avila AM, Berger M. Immediate ureterovaginal fistula secondary to oocyte retrieval—a case report. Fertil Steril 2008; 90: 2006. e1–3.

29. Almog B, Rimon E, Yovel I, et al. Vertebral osteomyelitis: a rare complication of transvaginal ultrasound-guided oocyte retrieval. Fertil Steril 2000; 73: 1250–2.

30. Dicker D, Ashkenazi J, Feldberg D, et al. Severe abdominal complications after transvaginal ultrasonographically guided retrieval of oocytes for in vitro fertilization and embryo transfer. Fertil Steril 1993; 59: 1313–15.

31. Tureck RW, Garcia CR, Blasco L, Mastroianni L. Jr., Perioperative complications arising after transvaginal oocyte retrieval. Obstet Gynecol 1993; 81: 590–3.

32. Bennett SJ, Waterstone JJ, Cheng WC, Parsons J. Complications of transvaginal ultrasound-directed follicle aspiration: a review of 2670 consecutive procedures. J Assist Reprod Genet 1993; 10: 72–7.

33. Aragona C, Mohamed MA, Espinola MS, et al. Clinical complications after transvaginal oocyte retrieval in 7,098 IVF cycles. Fertil Steril 2011; 95: 293–4.

34. Revel A, Schejter-Dinur Y, Yahalomi SZ, Simon A, Zelig O Revel-Vilk S. Is routine screening needed for coagulation abnormalities before oocyte retrieval? Fertil Steril 2011; 95: 1182–4.

35. Risquez F, Confino E. Can Doppler ultrasound-guided oocyte retrieval improve IVF safety? Reprod Biomed Online 2010; 21: 444–5.

36. Jayakrishnan K, Raman VK, Vijayalakshmi VK, Baheti S, Nambiar D. Massive hematuria with hemodynamic instability–complication of oocyte retrieval. Fertil Steril 2011; 96: e22–4.

37. Younis JS, Ezra Y, Laufer N, Ohel G. Late manifestation of pelvic abscess following oocyte retrieval, for in vitro fertilization, in patients with severe endometriosis and ovarian endometriomata. J Assist Reprod Genet 1997; 14: 343–6.

38. Moini A, Riazi K, Amid V, et al. Endometriosis may contribute to oocyte retrieval-induced pelvic inflammatory disease: report of eight cases. J Assist Reprod Genet 2005; 22: 307–9.

39. Bentov Y, Levitas E, Silberstein T, Potashnik G. Cullen's sign following ultrasound-guided transvaginal oocyte retrieval. Fertil Steril 2006; 85: 227.

40. Johnson NP, Mak W, Sowter MC. Surgical treatment for tubal disease in women due to undergo in vitro fertilisation. Cochrane Database Syst Rev 2004: CD002125.

41. van Voorst SF, Johnson NP. Management of hydrosalpinges. In: Kovacs G, ed. How to Improve your ART Success Rates? An Evidence-Based Review of Adjuncts to IVF. UK: Cambridge University Press Cambridge, 2011: 57–62.

42. Al-Fadhli R, Kelly SM, Tulandi T, Tanr SL. Effects of different stages of endometriosis on the outcome of in vitro fertilization. J Obstet Gynaecol Can 2006; 28: 888–91.

43. Adamson GD, Abusief M. How to improve your IVF pregnancy rate: An evidence-based medicine review of adjunctive treatments to IVF. In: Kovacs G, ed. How to Improve your ART Success Rates? An Evidence-Based Review of Adjuncts to IVF. UK: Cambridge University Press Cambridge, 2011: 51–6.

44. Goldman KN, Moon KS, Yauger BJ, et al. Proficiency in oocyte retrieval: how many procedures are necessary for training? Fertil Steril 2011; 95: 2279–82.

45

Luteal support in ART

Dominique de Ziegler, Isabelle Streuli, Vanessa Gayet, Usama Bajouh, Juliane Berdah, and Charles Chapron

INTRODUCTION

From inception, assisted reproduction technique (ART) – initially called in vitro fertilization (IVF) – endorsed the principle that inducing multiple ovulation would improve reliability and outcome (1). This approach – now referred to as controlled ovarian stimulation (COS) – has been intimately associated with the practice of ART (2–4). Introducing COS is recognized as the single most effective measure ever taken for improving ART outcome. This explains that over the years, the results of COS – the number of oocytes collected – have too often served as surrogate marker for ART outcome, often erroneously so (5). In spite of being a quarter century old, pundits of COS still fiercely argue over the best products to use and objectives to set – the number of collected oocytes (3). It is indeed easy to err on the side of either too many, or too few. Moreover, while COS helps boosting ART's results, all concur to recognize today that the luteal phase is altered in COS. Experience indicates however that this can be mended by human chorionic gonadotropin (hCG) or progesterone supplementation, a concept referred to as luteal phase support (LPS) (6). We will review here the evidence for the needs of providing progesterone supplements in ART as part of LPS and discuss the various modalities to choose from. Once pregnancy is established, hCG, not LH, drives the corpus luteum. As will be discussed, this fact bears relevance on the proposed duration for LPS.

In certain circumstances the efficacy of LPS confronts conditions that are characterized by progesterone resistance. This is notably the case in endometriosis (7,8) and certain forms of polycystic ovary syndrome (PCOS) associated with androgen elevation (9). In case of progesterone resistance, the primary measure will be to restore progesterone responsiveness prior to initiating ART (10). Only then will classical LPS be efficient in these disorders, as in regular ART patients.

We will also discuss the possible needs for adjunct therapy to be prescribed in addition to progesterone, a generally controversial topic because of the lack of hard evidence. The most debated of these adjunct therapies are (i) estradiol (E2) and (ii) gonadotropin-releasing

hormone (GnRH) agonist (GnRH-a). Finally, we will address the much talked about and still unresolved issue of endometrial receptivity when ovulation is triggered with GnRH-a in antagonist COS cycles.

THE PATHOPHYSIOLOGY OF THE LUTEAL PHASE IN ART

Several pathophysiological mechanisms have been put forth over the years for explaining that COS alters the luteal production of progesterone. In the heydays of ART, concerns were raised about the possibility that follicular fluid aspiration when retrieving oocytes might disrupt and/or diminish the number of granulosa cells undergoing luteinization (11,12). This ultimately could diminish the progesterone-producing capacity of the corpus luteum (CL) and thus, reduce progesterone levels (12). Numerous studies have rapidly disclaimed these early fears about the progesterone-producing capacity of CL in ART (13).

The elevation of serum E2 to supra-physiological levels as a result of COS was seen as prone to alter endometrial receptivity by causing an imbalance of the E2/progesterone ratio (14). We later demonstrated that even an extreme alteration of the E2 to progesterone ratio did not impact on endometrial morphology (15), a finding subsequently confirmed by others (16). In spite of this, endometrial alterations encountered in strong COS responders were attributed to the high E2 levels that characterize these cycles (17). We have now found converging evidence indicating that these endometrial alterations actually result from ovarian factors other than E2 (18). But as discussed below, the high levels of E2 in COS may be the play of feedback mechanisms reducing the progesterone production, if not affecting its action on the endometrium.

Today there is mounting evidence that the primary cause maiming progesterone production in the luteal phase of COS is the suppression of pulsatile LH production. LH suppression results from: (i) the use of GnRH analogues (19,20); (ii) the high levels of E2 (21) and; (iii) triggering ovulation with hCG instead of LH (22,23). As discussed later, identifying that impaired progesterone production stems from LH dysfunction in the luteal phase implies a return to physiology at the beginning of pregnancy, with the CL then being driven by hCG.

DONOR EGG ART (DE-ART), THE REFERENCE FOR PROGESTERONE EFFICACY

In DE-ART, oocytes recipients have absent, inactive, or suppressed ovaries. Endometrial receptivity to embryo implantation is therefore fostered with the sole help of exogenous hormones, E2, and progesterone. Quite unexpectedly at the outset, implantation and pregnancy rates achieved in DE-ART were found to be astonishingly good, surpassing in general the results of the corresponding regular ART programs (24). Logically therefore, E2 and progesterone cycles designed for DE-ART have served as a reference for studying the hormonal control of endometrial receptivity (25,26). The primary lessons thought by DE-ART are three: (i) the optimal timing for embryo transfers depends on the duration of exposure to progesterone, not the circulating levels (18). In regular ART, the endometrium may therefore become asynchronous with embryo development in case of premature – preovulatory – progesterone elevation (27,28); (ii) optimal receptivity for cleavage-stage and blastocyst embryos is on day 3–4 and 5 of progesterone exposure, respectively (24); (iii) contrary to prevailing self-proclaimed dogmas of yesteryears, the E2 to progesterone ratio does not influence the course of secretory changes induced by progesterone in the endometrium.

Moreover, the E2 and progesterone cycles designed for DE-ART have served as test bench for new candidate products for luteal support in ART (29,30). This strategy was rooted in the postulate that any progesterone preparation capable of decidualizing the endometrium in the absence of endogenous progesterone will necessarily work in the presence of endogenous progesterone (30). The principle that equipments resisting an exposure to acid will resist anything else led to coining of the expression of "acid test." Hence, the DE-ART regimen was seen as an "acid test" for checking the efficacy of any new progesterone preparation. For example, a new aqueous progesterone preparation (31) for subcutaneous administration was recently submitted to and passed the acid test, as did before the vaginal progesterone gel Crinone® (30,32). Certain progestins failed the acid test, however, being incapable of pre-decidualizing the endometrium in total absence of endogenous progesterone. This is notably the case of oral progesterone (33,34) and the synthetic progesterone analogue, dydrogesterone (35). In the latter case, dydrogesterone failed to foster pre-decidual transformation in absence of endogenous progesterone in spite of reports suggesting efficacy for LPS in regular ART (36). In our eyes this discrepancy is troublesome. Indeed, it indicates that the marginally effective product – here dydrogesterone – appears effective in a tested environment – a typical normal ART population.

But because of the failed acid test, uncertainties remain as to whether the preparation – dydrogesterone – will be actually effective in all ART patients, possibly different from the tested population. For this reason we do not recommend using dydrogesterone for luteal support in ART until more is known, as we abstain ourselves.

THE EXISTING EVIDENCE SUPPORTING THE NEED FOR LUTEAL SUPPORT IN ART

Any progesterone – vaginal or IM – when compared to placebo was associated with higher clinical and ongoing pregnancy rates (37). Likewise, hCG resulted in higher ART outcome. In this early meta-analysis, higher pregnancy rates were associated with IM as compared to vaginal progesterone (37). The latter findings probably stemmed from the weight given to one of the studies that suffered methodological errors with notably a larger fraction of older patients in the vaginal progesterone arm (38).

A more recent meta-analysis identified 12 randomized controlled trials (RCTs) comparing hCG with progesterone, seven with IM and four with vaginal (6). Ultimately, no significant differences were found with a seemingly random distribution of upward and downward trends. In the latter meta-analysis, 32 RCTs involving 9839 women looked at possible differences in ART outcomes between the different progesterone preparations and the routes of administration used (6). Generally, these comparisons showed no differences thus leading to the conclusion that IM and vaginal progesterone are equally effective at providing LPS. There were also no differences between the different COS regimens used. Concern once existed regarding the efficacy of the vaginal progesterone gel delivering 90 mg/day, as compared to the higher doses provided by all the other vaginal progesterone preparations. Nine RCTs reported on such a comparison. For both agonist and antagonist protocols all vaginal progesterone preparations were found equivalent. This probably put to rest the early fears regarding the efficacy of the vaginal progesterone gel in ART. The latter primarily stemmed from one poorly conducted trial that showed poorer outcome with the vaginal progesterone gel, but in a population richer in older patients, as compared to controls.

BEYOND PROGESTERONE, DEAL WITH RESISTANCE TO PROGESTERONE

There is now ample evidence for the existence of endometrial alterations – in the eutopic endometrium – in case of endometriosis (39–41). In endometriosis, these alterations are associated with resistance to progesterone (42,7), a phenomenon involving the progesterone receptor (PR) co-activator Hic-5 (43). In case of endometriosis, ART outcome was improved by three to six months of ovarian suppression by GnRH-a (44–46). More recently, we reported that shorter ovarian suppression – six to eight weeks – with oral contraceptive (OC) normalized implantation and pregnancy rates in women suffering from endometriosis (10).

While in the case of endometriosis, pre-ART ovarian suppression using GnRH-a for three to six months or OC for six to eight weeks improves outcome (10,44), it is unknown whether similar treatment might benefit PCOS. There is indeed a consensus convening that endometrial receptivity is altered in hyper-androgenic PCOS and that ovarian suppression can lower the circulating levels of androgens (47,48). It is also unsure whether higher progesterone levels can overcome the state of resistance to progesterone that is encountered in endometriosis and PCOS.

PRACTICAL OPTIONS FOR LUTEAL SUPPORT

Different options for administering progesterone exist, whereas certain possibilities used in other facets of gynecology are non-options as far LPS in ART is concerned. These are illustrated in Figure 45.1. When in micronized form, progesterone is absorbed orally but highly metabolized during the first liver pass (49,50). This explains that oral administration of progesterone fails to induce the pre-decidual transformation of E2-primed endometrium (51) and was demonstrated ineffective at providing LPS in ART (6). The transdermal route – amply developed for delivering E2 – is not an option for progesterone administration. This is due to: (i) the doses needed – 25 mg/24 hours – for duplicating daily production in the luteal phase being >100 times superior to the E2 doses commonly administered transdermally; (ii) poor skin permeability and; (iii) metabolic inactivation of absorbed progesterone by 5α-reductase contained in the skin.

Progesterone in oil has been available for IM injections with daily administration leading to sustained levels (52)

years before ART ever existed. These IM preparations were indicated for managing luteal phase defect and miscarriages threats (53). In ART, the commonly prescribed dose is 50 mg/day, but reports on using 25 mg/day uniformly showed similar efficacy. The side effects of IM progesterone are pain and local irritation at the site of injection. The latter may occasionally evolve to the stage of full-blown sterile abscess.

Considering the hindrance at administering progesterone orally (ineffective) or transdermally (impossible), investigators have looked at the vaginal route as only remaining alternative to injections. Experience existed with vaginal progesterone for the treatment of luteal phase defect (54). In the heydays of DE-ART, it rapidly became evident that the endometrial effects induced by vaginal progesterone were highly effective and predictable (55) in spite of subnormal progesterone levels. The discrepancy between low circulating levels and endometrial efficacy was substantiated by Miles et al. who documented unexpectedly high tissue concentrations with vaginal progesterone (56). These latter findings having been challenged at medical meetings as possibly resulting from contamination of the endometrial sampling by progesterone present in the vagina led us to reproduce the experiment. In the new study paradigm the possibility of vaginal contamination of the endometrial sampler was excluded by collecting the endometrial tissue at the time of hysterectomy (57). These observations led us to postulate the existence of a direct vagina-to-uterus transport or first uterine pass effect (FUPE) (18). We subsequently provided evidence in support of the concept that FUPE results from countercurrent exchanges (58) that affects the upper one-third of the vagina (59). The principle of countercurrent exchange with vein-to-artery transport is illustrated in Figure 45.2.

Progesterone preparations available

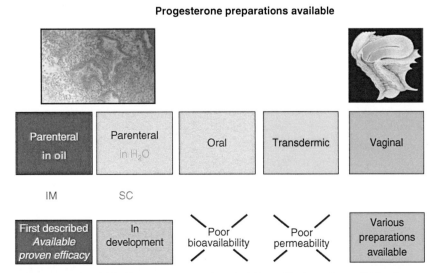

Figure 45.1   Progesterone preparations available. Progesterone can be administered by injections – IM in oil preparations or soon in aqueous solution subcutaneously – or vaginally. Preferential direct transport to the uterus exists in this latter case. Progesterone cannot be administered orally in ART because of poor bioavailability due to high level of metabolism during the first liver pass. Progesterone cannot be administered transdermally because of the doses needed (>40× higher than E2), poor bioavailability, and skin inactivation by 5-α reductase.

The various progesterone preparations available with their routes and commonly used doses are summarized in Table 45.1. Practically speaking, progesterone is administered in ART by injections (25–50 mg/day) or vaginally (90 mg/day–200 mg TID), starting on the day of oocytes retrieval.

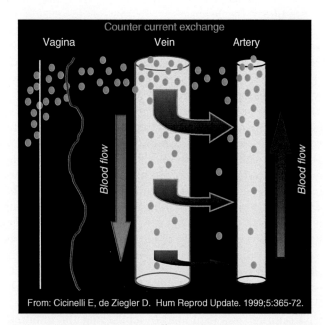

Figure 45.2 First uterine pass effect. Direct vagina to uterus transport or first uterine pass effect (FUPE), a functional portal system, connects the upper one-third of the vagina to the uterus. FUPE function by countercurrent transport with vein-to-artery exchange. The existence of an FUPE accounts for the exceptionally high uterine tissue concentration of progesterone encountered following vaginal administration of progesterone. *Source*: From Ref. 58.

DURATION OF LUTEAL SUPPORT

Onset of Luteal Support

The onset of luteal support in ART has been debated with seemingly now a generally recognized consensus (6,60). Starting progesterone on the day of oocyte retrieval was documented to decrease uterine contractility on the day of embryo transfer as compared to starting two days later (61). In this trial the earlier start protocol for luteal support was associated with a trend for higher pregnancy rates (61). These findings are in keeping with the prior observation of an inverse correlation between uterine contractility on the day of transfer and ART outcome in the absence of exogenous progesterone (62). In a prospective trial, we demonstrated that uterine contractility was higher four days after hCG administration in ART, as compared four days after LH surge in the preceding menstrual cycle (63). Uterine contractility being similar in this trial on the day of LH surge and hCG administration, one concludes that the higher E2 levels encountered in ART do further enhance uterine contractility, as compared to the menstrual cycle (63). The slower decrease in uterine contractility in ART as compared to the menstrual cycle is taken as evidence for uterine resistance to the utero-relaxing properties of progesterone, probably caused by E2 (63).

The above reported data amounts to quelling some earlier concerns about the risk that starting progesterone support as early as on the day of oocyte retrieval might unduly advance the endometrium (64). This latter concern had momentarily motivated using antiprogestin early in the luteal phase (65), a practice not retained today. These concerns for endometrial advancement were revived with the documentation that vaginal administration of progesterone

Table 45.1 Types of Progesterone Preparations Available

Product	Onset of treatment	End of treatment	Route	Doses	Side effects, comments
Progesterone	In principle, on the day of oocyte retrieval. Reduces uterine contractions on the day of transfer. Earlier onset may unduly advance endometrium	At time of luteo-placental shift (8–10 weeks after embryo transfer).	Oral Transdermic IM (peanut/sesame oil preparation) Subcutaneous (aqueous preparation) Vaginal	NA: not inducing pre-decidualized endom. NA: poorly absorbed and metabolized in skin 25–50 mg/day 25 mg/day 300–600–800 mg/day (bio-adhesive gel 90 mg/day	Not reliable Not recommended; drowsiness NA Pain at injection site, sterile abcesses Local irritation Vaginal discharge, gel accumulation, not desired by certain patients
Synthetic progestin dydrogester-one	Same as progesterone	Same as progesterone	Oral	10 mg BID Not recommended in DE-ART, no pre-deci-dualization of endometrium	Not known.
hCG	In principle, 3 days after triggering of ovulation. Repeated every 3 days, 2–3 times.	On luteal day 6 or 9	IM or SC Purified from urine or recombinant source	1,500–2,000 IU	Undue increase in risk of OHSS (>10x). Not recommended

results in elective tissue concentration in the uterus (56) through direct transport (18). The concerns for possible harm in starting of luteal support on the day of oocyte retrieval were definitively silenced by recent meta-analysis of the clinical evidence (6).

Discontinuation of Luteal Support

The timing for discontinuation of luteal support in case of pregnancy occurring in ART remains a matter for debate. On the one side, there is a consensus for convening that there is no need for pursuing luteal support beyond the first trimester. In humans, contrary to most mammalian species, hormone production in pregnancy shifts from corpus luteum (CL) to placenta, which ultimately takes over entirely. From the seminal work of Csapo et al. we know that continuation of pregnancy is independent from corpus luteum (CL) function as early as by 8–10 weeks of pregnancy (66). At that time ovariectomy can be performed harmlessly for the developing pregnancy, as hormone production is entirely taken over by placental function. The CL is not inactive in late pregnancy, as it produces peptides such as relaxin, the function of which remains obscure in humans (67,68).

On the other side, diverting views and clinical practices exist regarding early stopping. Certain studies, including RCT by Schmidt et al. (69), have indicated that there are no benefits in pursuing luteal support beyond the positive pregnancy test. Specifically, these authors discontinued progesterone supplementation on the day of positive pregnancy test (βhCG >250 mIU/mL), two weeks after embryo transfer (69). There were no differences in ongoing pregnancy rates in women who stopped progesterone support at the positive pregnancy test or three to four weeks later, at 88.7% and 90.8%, respectively. Likewise, miscarriages rates were similar. Others have provided evidence that there is no harm in stopping at the time of the first ultrasound, four to six weeks after embryo transfer (70). In their RCT, Aboulghar et al. randomly assigned 257 women who were pregnant after Intra Cytoplasmic Sperm Injection (ICSI) to either discontinue luteal support on the day of the first ultrasound or continue for three more weeks. Beyond the first ultrasound showing fetal heart rate activity, miscarriage rate was 4.6% (6/132) and 4.8% (6/125) in women who continued or stopped luteal support at the first ultrasound. Likewise, bleeding was not different between the two treatment groups.

In spite of this accumulating data supporting early stop of luteal support, the larger share of ART programs – it includes ours at Cochin Hospital in Paris – continue luteal support for 8–10 weeks after embryo transfer. Admittedly, the primary reason sustaining this latter practice is lack of courage, as well as the perception of lack of risk in unnecessarily pursuing until the end of the first trimester of pregnancy.

THE GNRH-A ENIGMA

In a seminal publication, Gonen et al. reported the possibility of triggering ovulation with a single injection of leuprolide acetate (LA) instead of hCG (71). A group of 14 patients receiving similar no-GnRH analog COS protocols were randomized to receive a single injection of either GnRH-a (LA 0.5 mg) or hCG (5,000 IU). Plasma luteinizing hormone (LH) and follicle-stimulating hormone (FSH) were elevated for 34 hours after GnRH-a, but not in the hCG group. Plasma E2 concentrations were lower in the GnRH-a group as compared to hCG group (P < 0.02). A similar number of oocytes and embryos were retrieved in both groups and embryo quality was also similar. In the GnRH-a group, three out of seven patients became pregnant but none in the hCG group without worthy conclusions possible, considering the small number of patients included.

Using GnRH-a for triggering ovulation was ignored during the years of routine and exclusive use of GnRH-a in ART, because the lasting gonadotropin suppression precluded it. The GnRH-a for-triggering-ovulation option was revived with the advent of GnRH antagonists. Indeed, a pilot report on five patients showed that GnRH-a could displace the competitive pituitary blockage exerted by antagonists and manage to trigger a functional LH surge in spite of the antagonist (72).

Later a meta-analysis reported on testing the GnRH-a options in poor responders (eight trials) or PCOS (four trials) (73). This report's sobering conclusion was that triggering of ovulation with GnRH-a led to decreased outcome. This indeed blew the whistle about possible adverse effects of this procedure. Surprisingly, this contradicted prior results of an RCT emanating from the same group of authors (74). Evidence from oocyte donation later indicated that the lower results when using GnRH-a for-triggering-ovulation resulted from an endometrial effect. In a large trial on oocyte donors, the triggering of ovulation with GnRH-a did not reduce pregnancy chances but totally prevented the risk of OHSS (75). This approach was later satisfactorily adopted by numerous oocyte donation programs, including our own, thus confirming that oocytes quality is unharmed.

In a subsequent publication Humaidan et al. reported that pregnancy rates could be preserved when GnRH-a was used for triggering ovulation if complement hCG (1500 IU) was administered on the oocyte retrieval day (76). In our hands, this approach used in PCOS patients at risk of OHSS remained associated with a seemingly unacceptable incidence of severe OHSS, and was thus abandoned. Until more is known, we use GnRH-a (triptorelin 0.3 mg) for triggering ovulation routinely in DE-ART. In regular ART, we use GnRH-a for triggering in antagonist cycles in case of OHSS threat, but with systematic cryopreservation of oocytes (vitrification) or 2PN-stage embryos (slow freezing).

ADJUNCT PRODUCTS OFFERED IN THE LUTEAL PHASE

E2

The addition of E2 in the luteal phase of ART was motivated by the gruesome finding that E2 levels sometimes drop in mid-luteal phase in ART. In prior studies, we (15) and later others (16) showed that discontinuation of E2, in E2 and progesterone cycles, was without consequences on endometrial morphology. Through years of ART practice, the fear from the drop in E2 levels prevailed over the clinical science indicating that luteal E2 probably does not affect implantation (15). In total, 11 trials challenged the value of adding E2 together with progesterone for luteal phase support in ART. In a prospective randomized trial, Lukaszuk et al. found that in long-GnRH-a protocols, addition of E2 to progesterone induced a dose-dependent increase in ART outcome (77). In their meta-analysis, Fatemi et al. found no differences between the groups supplemented by E2 and progesterone as compared to progesterone alone (78). The latter authors, however, did not include two of the RCTs (77) that reported positive results when adding E2 to LPS.

GnRH-a

Despite the lack of putative mechanisms, there have been attempts of administrating GnRH-a – triptorelin 0.1 mg – three days after embryo transfer for improving implantation (79). Following this preliminary report, there have been five RCTs looking at the effects of GnRH-a on implantation in both agonist and antagonist COS cycles (80–84). No statistically significant benefit was seen in the three studies in agonist protocols (n = 983). Conversely, pregnancy rates were statistically improved by 46% (RR = 1.46, 95%; CI: 1.04, 2.06; p = 0.03), in the pooled data from three studies in antagonist protocols (n = 459). Likewise, there was a statistically significant increase in live birth rates in the pooled data from the two studies reporting on this (RR = 3.29, 95%; CI: 1.15, 9.47; p = 0.03).

CONCLUSION

Overwhelming evidence supports the need for providing LPS in ART. This stems from the documented dysfunction of LH support to CL function during the luteal phase of ART cycles. Partaking in this are the use of GnRH analogues (agonists or antagonists), triggering of ovulation by hCG instead of LH, and harboring abnormally high levels of E2 induced by COS that exert anti-gonadotropin effects.

Luteal support is best initiated on the day of oocyte retrieval or alternatively on the morning after. For LPS, progesterone – in injectable or vaginal preparations – was found as effective as repeated hCG injections. The latter is best avoided, however, in light of the marked increase in OHSS risk. Issues regarding the timing for discontinuing progesterone administration, needs for E2 support, and/or other adjunct products such as uterorelaxing substances and possibly GnRH-a remain debated. The optimal luteal support following triggering of ovulation by GnRH-a in GnRH antagonist cycles remain an enigma as of today. This leads us and others to recommend cryopreservation when ovulation is triggered by an agonist.

In conclusion, LPS is mandatory in ART for optimizing outcome. One of several options, using injectable or vaginal progesterone preparation, should be offered to all ART patients, starting on the day of oocyte retrieval until anywhere from two to eight weeks after embryo transfer.

REFERENCES

1. Edwards RG, Fishel SB, Cohen J, et al. Factors influencing the success of in vitro fertilization for alleviating human infertility. J In Vitro Fert Embryo Transf 1984; 1: 3–23.
2. Simonetti S, Veeck LL, Jones HW Jr. Correlation of follicular fluid volume with oocyte morphology from follicles stimulated by human menopausal gonadotropin. Fertil Steril 1985; 44: 177–80.
3. Macklon NS, Stouffer RL, Giudice LC, Fauser BC. The science behind 25 years of ovarian stimulation for in vitro fertilization. Endocr Rev 2006; 27: 170–207.
4. Baart EB, Macklon NS, Fauser BJ. Ovarian stimulation and embryo quality. Reprod Biomed Online 2009; 18(Suppl 2): 45–50.
5. De Ziegler D, Streuli MI, Borghese B, et al. Infertility and endometriosis: a need for global management that optimizes the indications for surgery and ART. Minerva Ginecol 2011; 63: 365–73.
6. van der Linden M, Buckingham K, Farquhar C, Kremer JA, Metwally M. Luteal phase support for assisted reproduction cycles. Cochrane Database Syst Rev 2011: CD009154.
7. Aghajanova L, Velarde MC, Giudice LC. Altered gene expression profiling in endometrium: evidence for progesterone resistance. Semin Reprod Med 2010; 28: 51–8.
8. Cakmak H, Taylor HS. Molecular mechanisms of treatment resistance in endometriosis: the role of progesterone-hox gene interactions. Semin Reprod Med 2010; 28: 69–74.
9. Cermik D, Selam B, Taylor HS. Regulation of HOXA-10 expression by testosterone in vitro and in the endometrium of patients with polycystic ovary syndrome. J Clin Endocrinol Metab 2003; 88: 238–43.
10. de Ziegler D, Gayet V, Aubriot FX, et al. Use of oral contraceptives in women with endometriosis before assisted reproduction treatment improves outcomes. Fertil Steril 2010; 94: 2796–9.
11. Frydman R, Testart J, Giacomini P, et al. Hormonal and histological study of the luteal phase in women following aspiration of the preovulatory follicle. Fertil Steril 1982; 38: 312–17.
12. Garcia J, Jones GS, Acosta AA, Wright GL Jr. Corpus luteum function after follicle aspiration for oocyte retrieval. Fertil Steril 1981; 36: 565–72.
13. de Ziegler D, Fanchin R, de Moustier B, Bulletti C. The hormonal control of endometrial receptivity: estrogen (E2) and progesterone. J Reprod Immunol 1998; 39: 149–66.
14. Forman R, Fries N, Testart J, et al. Evidence for an adverse effect of elevated serum estradiol concentrations on embryo implantation. Fertil Steril 1988; 49: 118–22.
15. de Ziegler D, Bergeron C, Cornel C, et al. Effects of luteal estradiol on the secretory transformation of human endometrium and plasma gonadotropins. J Clin Endocrinol Metab 1992; 74: 322–31.

16. Younis JS, Ezra Y, Sherman Y, et al. The effect of estradiol depletion during the luteal phase on endometrial development. Fertil Steril 1994; 62: 103–7.

17. Basir GS, WS O, EH Ng, PC Ho. Morphometric analysis of peri-implantation endometrium in patients having excessively high oestradiol concentrations after ovarian stimulation. Hum Reprod 2001; 16: 435–40.

18. de Ziegler D. Hormonal control of endometrial receptivity. Hum Reprod 1995; 10: 4–7.

19. Broekmans FJ, Bernardus RE, Berkhout G, Schoemaker J. Pituitary and ovarian suppression after early follicular and mid-luteal administration of a LHRH agonist in a depot formulation: decapeptyl CR. Gynecol Endocrinol 1992; 6: 153–61.

20. Smitz J, Erard P, Camus M, et al. Pituitary gonadotrophin secretory capacity during the luteal phase in superovulation using GnRH-agonists and HMG in a desensitization or flare-up protocol. Hum Reprod 1992; 7: 1225–9.

21. Macklon NS, Fauser BC. Impact of ovarian hyperstimulation on the luteal phase. J Reprod Fertil Suppl 2000; 55: 101–8.

22. Van Steirteghem AC, Smitz J, Camus M, et al. The luteal phase after in-vitro fertilization and related procedures. Hum Reprod 1988; 3: 161–4.

23. Smitz J, Devroey P, Camus M, et al. The luteal phase and early pregnancy after combined GnRH-agonist/HMG treatment for superovulation in IVF or GIFT. Hum Reprod 1988; 3: 585–90.

24. Rosenwaks Z, Navot D, Veeck L, et al. Oocyte donation. The Norfolk Program. Ann N Y Acad Sci 1988; 541: 728–41.

25. Navot D, Anderson TL, Droesch K, et al. Hormonal manipulation of endometrial maturation. J Clin Endocrinol Metab 1989; 68: 801–7.

26. Navot D, Bergh PA, Williams M, et al. An insight into early reproductive processes through the in vivo model of ovum donation. J Clin Endocrinol Metab 1991; 72: 408–14.

27. Fanchin R, Righini C, Olivennes F, et al. Premature progesterone elevation does not alter oocyte quality in in vitro fertilization. Fertil Steril 1996; 65: 1178–83.

28. Fanchin R, Righini C, Olivennes F, et al. Consequences of premature progesterone elevation on the outcome of in vitro fertilization: insights into a controversy. Fertil Steril 1997; 68: 799–805.

29. Fanchin R, De Ziegler D, Bergeron C, et al. Transvaginal administration of progesterone. Obstet Gynecol 1997; 90: 396–401.

30. Gibbons WE, Toner JP, Hamacher P, Kolm P. Experience with a novel vaginal progesterone preparation in a donor oocyte program. Fertil Steril 1998; 69: 96–101.

31. Hamoudi M, Fattal E, Gueutin C, Nicolas V, Bochot A. Beads made of cyclodextrin and oil for the oral delivery of lipophilic drugs: in vitro studies in simulated gastrointestinal fluids. Int J Pharm 2011; 416: 507–14.

32. Toner JP. Vaginal delivery of progesterone in donor oocyte therapy. Hum Reprod 2000; 15(Suppl 1): 166–71.

33. Bourgain C, Devroey P, Van Waesberghe L, Smitz J, Van Steirteghem AC. Effects of natural progesterone on the morphology of the endometrium in patients with primary ovarian failure. Hum Reprod 1990; 5: 537–43.

34. Tavaniotou A, Smitz J, Bourgain C, Devroey P. Comparison between different routes of progesterone administration as luteal phase support in infertility treatments. Hum Reprod Update 2000; 6: 139–48.

35. Fatemi HM, Bourgain C, Donoso P, et al. Effect of oral administration of dydrogestrone versus vaginal administration of natural micronized progesterone on the secretory transformation of endometrium and luteal endocrine profile in patients with premature ovarian failure: a proof of concept. Hum Reprod 2007; 22: 1260–3.

36. Chakravarty BN, Shirazee HH, Dam P, et al. Oral dydrogesterone versus intravaginal micronised progesterone as luteal phase support in assisted reproductive technology (ART) cycles: results of a randomised study. J Steroid Biochem Mol Biol 2005; 97: 416–20.

37. Daya S, Gunby J. Luteal phase support in assisted reproduction cycles. Cochrane Database Syst Rev 2004; 3: CD004830.

38. Propst AM, Hill JA, Ginsburg ES, et al. A randomized study comparing Crinone 8% and intramuscular progesterone supplementation in in vitro fertilization-embryo transfer cycles. Fertil Steril 2001; 76: 1144–9.

39. Engemise SL, Willets JM, Taylor AH, Emembolu JO, Konje JC. Changes in glandular and stromal estrogen and progesterone receptor isoform expression in eutopic and ectopic endometrium following treatment with the levonorgestrel-releasing intrauterine system. Eur J Obstet Gynecol Reprod Biol 2011; 157: 101–6.

40. Anaf V, Simon P, El Nakadi I, et al. Hyperalgesia, nerve infiltration and nerve growth factor expression in deep adenomyotic nodules, peritoneal and ovarian endometriosis. Hum Reprod 2002; 17: 1895–900.

41. Tokushige N, Markham R, Russell P, Fraser IS. Different types of small nerve fibers in eutopic endometrium and myometrium in women with endometriosis. Fertil Steril 2007; 88: 795–803.

42. Aghajanova L, Hamilton A, Kwintkiewicz J, Vo KC, Giudice LC. Steroidogenic enzyme and key decidualization marker dysregulation in endometrial stromal cells from women with versus without endometriosis. Biol Reprod 2009; 80: 105–14.

43. Aghajanova L, Velarde MC, Giudice LC. The progesterone receptor coactivator Hic-5 is involved in the pathophysiology of endometriosis. Endocrinology 2009; 150: 3863–70.

44. Surrey ES, Silverberg KM, Surrey MW, Schoolcraft WB. Effect of prolonged gonadotropin-releasing hormone agonist therapy on the outcome of in vitro fertilization-embryo transfer in patients with endometriosis. Fertil Steril 2002; 78: 699–704.

45. Rickes D, Nickel I, Kropf S, Kleinstein J. Increased pregnancy rates after ultralong postoperative therapy with gonadotropin-releasing hormone analogs in patients with endometriosis. Fertil Steril 2002; 78: 757–62.

46. Sallam HN, Garcia-Velasco JA, Dias S, Arici A. Long-term pituitary down-regulation before in vitro fertilization (IVF) for women with endometriosis. Cochrane Database Syst Rev 2006: CD004635.

47. Daftary GS, Taylor HS. Endocrine regulation of HOX genes. Endocr Rev 2006; 27: 331–55.

48. Martin R, Taylor MB, Krikun G, et al. Differential cell-specific modulation of HOXA10 by estrogen and specificity protein 1 response elements. J Clin Endocrinol Metab 2007; 92: 1920–6.

49. Nahoul K, Dehennin L, Jondet M, Roger M. Profiles of plasma estrogens, progesterone and their metabolites

after oral or vaginal administration of estradiol or progesterone. Maturitas 1993; 16: 185–202.

50. Nahoul K, de Ziegler D. "Validity" of serum progesterone levels after oral progesterone. Fertil Steril 1994; 61: 790–2.

51. Devroey P, Palermo G, Bourgain C, et al. Progesterone administration in patients with absent ovaries. Int J Fertil 1989; 34: 188–93.

52. Fatemi HM, Popovic-Todorovic B, Papanikolaou E, Donoso P, Devroey P. An update of luteal phase support in stimulated IVF cycles. Hum Reprod Update 2007; 13: 581–90.

53. Huang KE, Muechler EK, Schwarz KR, Goggin M, Graham MC. Serum progesterone levels in women treated with human menopausal gonadotropin and human chorionic gonadotropin for in vitro fertilization. Fertil Steril 1986; 46: 903–6.

54. Rosenberg SM, Luciano AA, Riddick DH. The luteal phase defect: the relative frequency of, and encouraging response to, treatment with vaginal progesterone. Fertil Steril 1980; 34: 17–20.

55. Schmidt CL, de Ziegler D, Gagliardi CL, et al. Transfer of cryopreserved-thawed embryos: the natural cycle versus controlled preparation of the endometrium with gonadotropin-releasing hormone agonist and exogenous estradiol and progesterone (GEEP). Fertil Steril 1989; 52: 609–16.

56. Miles RA, Paulson RJ, Lobo RA, et al. Pharmacokinetics and endometrial tissue levels of progesterone after administration by intramuscular and vaginal routes: a comparative study. Fertil Steril 1994; 62: 485–90.

57. Cicinelli E, de Ziegler D, Bulletti C, et al. Direct transport of progesterone from vagina to uterus. Obstet Gynecol 2000; 95: 403–6.

58. Cicinelli E, de Ziegler D. Transvaginal progesterone: evidence for a new functional 'portal system' flowing from the vagina to the uterus. Hum Reprod Update 1999; 5: 365–72.

59. Cicinelli E, De Ziegler D, Morgese S, Bulletti C, Luisi D. Schonauer LM. "First uterine pass effect" is observed when estradiol is placed in the upper but not lower third of the vagina. Fertil Steril 2004; 81: 1414–16.

60. de Ziegler D, Fanchin R. Progesterone and progestins: applications in gynecology. Steroids 2000; 65: 671–9.

61. Fanchin R, Righini C, de Ziegler D, et al. Effects of vaginal progesterone administration on uterine contractility at the time of embryo transfer. Fertil Steril 2001; 75: 1136–40.

62. Fanchin R, Righini C, Olivennes F, et al. Uterine contractions at the time of embryo transfer alter pregnancy rates after in-vitro fertilization. Hum Reprod 1998; 13: 1968–74.

63. Ayoubi JM, Epiney M, Brioschi PA, et al. Comparison of changes in uterine contraction frequency after ovulation in the menstrual cycle and in in vitro fertilization cycles. Fertil Steril 2003; 79: 1101–5.

64. Kolb BA, Paulson RJ. The luteal phase of cycles utilizing controlled ovarian hyperstimulation and the possible impact of this hyperstimulation on embryo implantation. Am J Obstet Gynecol 1997; 176: 1262–7; discussion 1267–1269.

65. Paulson RJ, Sauer MV, Lobo RA. Potential enhancement of endometrial receptivity in cycles using controlled ovarian hyperstimulation with antiprogestins: a hypothesis. Fertil Steril 1997; 67: 321–5.

66. Csapo AI, Pulkkinen MO, Wiest WG. Effects of luteectomy and progesterone replacement therapy in early pregnant patients. Am J Obstet Gynecol 1973; 115: 759–65.

67. Weiss G, O'Byrne EM, Steinetz BG. Relaxin: a product of the human corpus luteum of pregnancy. Science 1976; 194: 948–9.

68. Quagliarello J, Szlachter N, Steinetz BG, Goldsmith LT, Weiss G. Serial relaxin concentrations in human pregnancy. Am J Obstet Gynecol 1979; 135: 43–4.

69. Schmidt KL, Ziebe S, Popovic B, et al. Progesterone supplementation during early gestation after in vitro fertilization has no effect on the delivery rate. Fertil Steril 2001; 75: 337–41.

70. Aboulghar MA, Amin YM, Al-Inany HG, et al. Prospective randomized study comparing luteal phase support for ICSI patients up to the first ultrasound compared with an additional three weeks. Hum Reprod 2008; 23: 857–62.

71. Gonen Y, Balakier H, Powell W, Casper RF. Use of gonadotropin-releasing hormone agonist to trigger follicular maturation for in vitro fertilization. J Clin Endocrinol Metab 1990; 71: 918–22.

72. Olivennes F, Fanchin R, Bouchard P, Taieb J, Frydman R. Triggering of ovulation by a gonadotropin-releasing hormone (GnRH) agonist in patients pretreated with a GnRH antagonist. Fertil Steril 1996; 66: 151–3.

73. Griesinger G, Diedrich K, Tarlatzis BC, Kolibianakis EM. GnRH-antagonists in ovarian stimulation for IVF in patients with poor response to gonadotrophins, polycystic ovary syndrome, and risk of ovarian hyperstimulation: a meta-analysis. Reprod Biomed Online 2006; 13: 628–38.

74. Lainas TG, Sfontouris IA, Papanikolaou EG, et al. Flexible GnRH antagonist versus flare-up GnRH agonist protocol in poor responders treated by IVF: a randomized controlled trial. Hum Reprod 2008; 23: 1355–8.

75. Bodri D, Guillen JJ, Trullenque M, et al. Early ovarian hyperstimulation syndrome is completely prevented by gonadotropin releasing-hormone agonist triggering in high-risk oocyte donor cycles: a prospective, luteal-phase follow-up study. Fertil Steril 2010; 93: 2418–20.

76. Humaidan P, Ejdrup Bredkjaer H, Westergaard LG, Yding Andersen C. 1,500 IU human chorionic gonadotropin administered at oocyte retrieval rescues the luteal phase when gonadotropin-releasing hormone agonist is used for ovulation induction: a prospective, randomized, controlled study. Fertil Steril 2010; 93: 847–54.

77. Lukaszuk K, Liss J, Lukaszuk M, Maj B. Optimization of estradiol supplementation during the luteal phase improves the pregnancy rate in women undergoing in vitro fertilization-embryo transfer cycles. Fertil Steril 2005; 83: 1372–6.

78. Fatemi HM, Kolibianakis EM, Camus M, et al. Addition of estradiol to progesterone for luteal supplementation in patients stimulated with GnRH antagonist/rFSH for IVF: a randomized controlled trial. Hum Reprod 2006; 21: 2628–32.

79. Tesarik J, Hazout A, Mendoza C. Enhancement of embryo developmental potential by a single administration of GnRH agonist at the time of implantation. Hum Reprod 2004; 19: 1176–80.

80. Ata B, Yakin K, Balaban B, Urman B. GnRH agonist protocol administration in the luteal phase in ICSI-ET cycles stimulated with the long GnRH agonist protocol: a

randomized, controlled double blind study. Hum Reprod 2008; 23: 668–73.

81. Isik AZ, Caglar GS, Sozen E, et al. Single-dose GnRH agonist administration in the luteal phase of GnRH antagonist cycles: a prospective randomized study. Reprod Biomed Online 2009; 19: 472–7.

82. Pirard C, Donnez J, Loumaye E. GnRH agonist as novel luteal support: results of a randomized, parallel group, feasibility study using intranasal administration of buserelin. Hum Reprod 2005; 20: 1798–804.

83. Qublan H, Amarin Z, Al-Qudah M, et al. Luteal phase support with GnRH-a improves implantation and pregnancy rates in IVF cycles with endometrium of <or = 7 mm on day of egg retrieval. Hum Fertil (Camb) 2008; 11: 43–7.

84. Tesarik J, Hazout A, Mendoza-Tesarik R, Mendoza N, Mendoza C. Beneficial effect of luteal-phase GnRH agonist administration on embryo implantation after ICSI in both GnRH agonist- and antagonist-treated ovarian stimulation cycles. Hum Reprod 2006; 21: 2572–9.

46

Treatment strategies in assisted reproduction for the poor responder patient

Ariel Weissman and Colin M. Howles

OVERVIEW

In a spontaneous menstrual cycle, only one follicle out of a cohort of 10–20 usually completes maturation and ovulates to release a mature oocyte. The aim of controlled ovarian stimulation (COS) in assisted reproductive technique (ART) protocols is to overcome the selection of a dominant follicle and to allow the growth of a cohort of follicles. This strategy leads to an increase in the number of oocytes and hence embryos available for transfer, thereby increasing the chance of transferring viable embryos. However, the chance of pregnancy and also live birth begins to dramatically decline after the age of 35 years, and successful treatment for these patients continues to be a major challenge in ART programs. Preimplantation genetic screening (PGS) studies over the last decade have identified a dramatic increase in the rate of aneuploidy as a major contributor to the reduction in embryo viability in older patients. It has also been demonstrated that women of advanced maternal age (AMA) may have oocytes that are compromised by a significant reduction in the amount of mitochondrial DNA in their cytoplasm.

In this chapter we describe the current strategies aimed at augmenting follicular recruitment and improving cytoplasmic integrity either in patients who are about to start COS and were estimated to have low ovarian reserve, or have been found to be poor responders in previous COS attempts. By standard and modified COS protocols as well as by various methods of manipulating endocrinology, the prognosis for these women is expected to be improved.

INTRODUCTION

The decline in female fecundity associated with increasing age is well documented: The decrease occurs slowly through the 30s, and then accelerates to reach nearly zero between the ages of 45 and 50 years (1). This decline can be based on a variety of age-related conditions, including an increase in gynecological disorders such as endometriosis or fibroids, an increase in ovulatory disorders due to effects on the hypothalamic–pituitary–ovarian axis, or a compromised uterine vascular supply that may impede implantation (2). Spontaneous conception is rare in women >45 years: A study carried out in orthodox Jewish sects that are proscribed from using contraceptives showed that natural pregnancies and deliveries after the age of 45 years constitute only 0.2% of total deliveries, and >80% of these are in grand multiparas (3). Similar findings have been described in Bedouin women as well (4). In infertile couples, in vitro fertilization (IVF) may be a reasonable option for such women of AMA (>40 years), but at the age of 45 years and more deliveries are a rare event (5).

The peak number of oocytes present in the human ovary occurs during fetal gestation, and follicles are continually lost thereafter through the mechanism of apoptosis, a process known as atresia (6). A cohort of growing follicles is recruited each month, and the cohort enters the final stages of follicle maturation during the first half of the menstrual cycle. This maturation phase is gonadotropin dependent. Painstaking histological and in vitro studies carried out by Gougeon suggest that follicles require a period of approximately 70 days from the time they enter the preantral stage (0.15 mm) to reach a size of 2 mm. These 2-mm follicles have very low steroidogenic activity, and they are impervious to cyclic follicle-stimulating hormone (FSH) and luteinizing hormone (LH) changes in terms of granulosa cell (GC) proliferation. Over a four- to five-day period during the late luteal phase, follicles that are 2–5 mm in diameter enter a recruitment stage, and cyclic changes in FSH drive the development of the follicle and proliferation of GC; GC aromatase activity is not affected during this stage. Thus, as the follicle develops, it becomes increasingly responsive to gonadotropins.

In the perspective of treatment management, this means that to influence the size of the recruitable pool of follicles, it would be necessary to "boost" continued healthy follicle development over a protracted period of time (≥70 days). However, gonadotropins play a role only during the phases of recruitment and final follicular maturation, which occur over the last 20 days or so of this 70-day period. Therefore, extrapolating from knowledge about basic physiology, different agents would be required at different times to successfully reverse the age-related decline in follicle numbers.

It has also been suggested that the rate of ovarian oocyte depletion further accelerates after the age of 37 years (7), so that older women have a decreased reserve of healthy oocytes in their ovarian pool. Women who postpone childbearing until their late 30s or early 40s are therefore frequently faced with the distressing realization that their chance of achieving a pregnancy is significantly reduced, and that they may require the help of ART, with further complex difficulties that can jeopardize their quest for successful conception.

In Europe for the year 2004, women undergoing IVF or intracytoplasmic sperm injection (ICSI) procedures in the age group >40 years represented approximately 15% and 12.5%, respectively, of those attending IVF clinics (8). A number of different variables can affect success rates in ART, and the negative impact of increasing age is one feature that is well recognized. Not only does the response to stimulation steadily deteriorate, requiring larger amounts of gonadotropins, but also the cancellation rate is higher, and there is a significant increase in the rate of miscarriages.

Data from the United States (Center for Disease Control 2008 report on ART success rates) (9) clearly shows that the potential for embryo implantation and successful delivery of a live birth decreases rapidly in women >35 years (Fig. 46.1). This same report also documents the increased incidence of pregnancy loss that is related to increased maternal age, going from less than 12% in women <35 years, then increasing from the mid 30s to reach 29.8% at 40 years and 57% in women >44 years. These data suggest that the lower age limit to define women of AMA should be considered as ≥35 years.

The most effective treatment option for infertile women of AMA is oocyte donation from young donors, but this is not an option in some parts of the world. Dal Prato et al. (10) reported a single case of a woman who successfully delivered a child after IVF treatment at the age of 46 years, but emphasized that this is an extraordinary event, and is not a cost-effective option compared with oocyte donation.

Although chronological age is the most important predictor of ovarian response to stimulation, the rate of reproductive aging and ovarian sensitivity to gonadotropins varies considerably among individuals (11). Biological and chronological age are not always equivalent, and biological age is more important in predicting the outcome of ART (11). Biological aging often renders the ovaries increasingly resistant to gonadotropin stimulation, with the result that the number of oocytes harvested may be very low.

Any strategy that might enhance the efficacy of treatment for these women would be of great benefit, and different areas of research have recently been explored, such as the use of pharmacogenomics to assess response to gonadotropin stimulation, manipulating the endocrinology of the treatment cycle, and screening of embryos for aneuploidy.

DEFINITIONS AND TERMINOLOGY

Over the years, a plethora of papers on different aspects of pathogenesis and management of poor ovarian response (POR) have been published. One of the major problems in comparing these studies was the lack of a uniform definition of a poor response. The considerable heterogeneities in the definition of POR (inclusion criteria, outcome measures, etc.) made it almost impossible to develop or asses any protocol to improve the outcome.

Very recently, a working group from the European Society of Human Reproduction and Embryology (ESHRE) attempted to standardize the definition of POR to stimulation in a simple and reproducible manner (The Bologna consensus) (12). POR to ovarian stimulation usually indicates a reduction in follicular response, resulting in a reduced number of retrieved oocytes. The group recommended that two of the following three features should be present for a diagnosis of POR: (i) advanced maternal age (≥40 years) or other risk factor for POR (ii) a previous POR (≤3 oocytes with a conventional stimulation protocol) (iii) an abnormal ovarian reserve test (ORT) [i.e., antral follicles count (AFC) <5–7 follicles or anti-Müllerian hormone (AMH) <0.5–1.1 ng/mL (3.57–7.85 pmol/l)]. Two episodes of POR after maximal stimulation were considered sufficient to define a patient as a poor responder in the absence of AMA or abnormal ORT. Patients of AMA with an abnormal ORT may be more properly defined as "expected poor responders." The development of this definition is an important "stake in the ground" and is already the subject of some examination (13). One thing is clear that we have not heard the end of this debate!

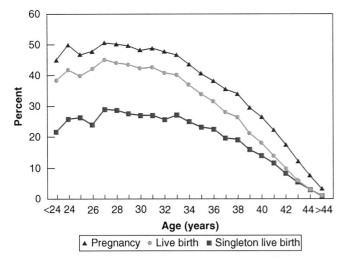

Figure 46.1 ART success rates in the United States, 2008: CDC report (9). Over the age of 35 years there is a further acceleration in the decline in pregnancy rates following ART procedures.

ASSESSMENT AND PREDICTION OF OVARIAN RESPONSE TO STIMULATION

The ability to accurately assess and predict ovarian response would reduce the burdens imposed by failure because of inadequate response to stimulation. Unfortunately, the response to stimulation cannot be reliably predicted, even for young patients with no evidence of endocrine disorders. Parameters that have been identified as exerting an influence include age (14–17), cause of infertility (9), body weight (16,18), and body mass index (BMI) (19). Ovarian characteristics have also been assessed by ultrasound, such as the number and size of antral follicles, ovarian volume, and ovarian vascular resistance measured by Doppler ultrasound.

There is a clear correlation between the number of antral follicles (defined as ≥2mm to ≥10mm) seen at the beginning of the follicular phase during a natural cycle and subsequent ovarian response to stimulation. However, there is as yet no consensus of agreement regarding the minimum number of antral follicles below which an influence can be seen (20–24); a minimum of less than five follicles of 2–5mm diameter has been suggested as a predictive parameter (25). One of the major reasons for this was a lack of standardized definition for assessment of the AFC, whose accuracy of measurement is highly operator dependent (26). Small ovaries and high resistance to vascular flow have also been shown to correlate with POR to gonadotropins (22,25,27,28). Klinkert et al. (25) suggest that patients with an AFC of <5 follicles of 2–5mm diameter are expected to have a poor response, and in a randomized controlled trial (RCT) they recently demonstrated that doubling the starting doses of gonadotropins does not lead to an improvement in response for these patients during IVF treatment. In this study of 52 patients, more than half were aged >40 years, and 13 had basal FSH levels >15 IU/l. A meta-analysis (29) showed that the predictive performance of ovarian volume for poor response is clearly inferior compared with that of AFC.

Basal hormone assessment at the start of the follicular phase has been used to predict ovarian response, including FSH (4,14,30–36), estradiol (E2), (36,37) and inhibin-B (36–41). Anti-Müllerian hormone (AMH) is an accurate marker of oocyte yield and live birth (42–47). Circulating levels of AMH decline with increasing biological ovarian age but remain relatively stable throughout each menstrual cycle (48,49), leading to it being measureable at any time during the cycle. A comparison of AMH and FSH as predictors of retrieved oocyte numbers and clinical pregnancy rates showed that AMH was clearly superior in predicting IVF outcomes (50). Moreover, a meta-analysis comparing AMH and AFC showed that AMH had at least the same level of accuracy and clinical value as AFC for the prediction of poor response in IVF (51). A prospective cohort study of 538 patients undergoing their first ART cycle with differential COS strategies based on an AMH measurement showed that AMH was associated with oocyte yield and that a low AMH (1 to <5 pmol/l) was associated with a reduced clinical pregnancy rate (52). Similarly, other investigators showed that AMH-based prediction of ovarian response was independent of age and polycystic ovary syndrome (PCOS) in 165 patients undergoing a first COS cycle for ART (53). AMH was a significantly better predictor of poor response compared with FSH but not AFC. Various AMH cutoff values to predict a poor response have been

explored (51). It has been suggested that an AMH cutoff level of <1.0 ng/ml (7.14 pmol/l) may have modest sensitivity and specificity in predicting a poor response to COS (53) (see Figure 42.5).

Individualized, AMH-guided treatment protocols significantly improved pregnancy rate per treated cycle and live birth rate compared with conventional treatment in a retrospective study of 796 women (54). The incidence of ovarian hyperstimulation syndrome (OHSS) was also significantly lower with AMH-tailored versus conventional treatment. An age-related AMH nomogram is available for pretreatment patient counseling (48).

There have been attempts to develop models for ovarian response based upon algorithms made up of multiple predictive factors. For instance, Popovic-Todorovic and colleagues developed a scoring system for calculating the FSH starting dose, based on four predictors: the total number of antral follicles, total Doppler score, serum testosterone levels, and smoking habit (22). This model was tested prospectively in a two-site clinical study, in which an ongoing pregnancy rate of 36.6% was reported using the algorithm to assign starting FSH doses between 100 and 250 IU, compared with an ongoing pregnancy rate of 24.4% with a standard protocol using 150 IU FSH (55). Another predictive algorithm to predict the recombinant human FSH (r-hFSH) (follitropin alfa) starting dose has been described but is only applicable to young (<35 years), normogonadotropic women (56). The four factors identified as significantly predictive of ovarian response were baseline serum FSH levels, BMI, age, and AFC. The basal and dynamic tests for prediction of ovarian reserve and response to stimulation are described in further detail in chapter 54.

From a practical perspective, it is interesting to note that a comprehensive systematic review of tests predicting ovarian reserve and IVF outcome (57) concluded that entry into the first IVF cycle without prior testing currently seems to be the best strategy, as a POR to treatment per se provides information on ovarian reserve status (especially if the stimulation is maximal); however, with the increased availability and use of AMH this may be revised as a first step.

This chapter will focus on classic and specialized protocols designed for poor responder patients, as well as on hormonal and pharmacologic manipulations that are expected to improve ovarian response. A large variety of strategies have been developed to improve outcome in patients with diminished ovarian reserve. There is no established intervention or treatment protocol for poor responders (58,59). Indeed, all of the currently available COS protocols have been used, with or without modifications, for the treatment of poor responders. Unfortunately, each of these approaches has achieved only limited success (58–63).

HIGH-DOSE GONADOTROPINS

It is generally believed that the dose of gonadotropins should be adjusted upward in an attempt to overcome the age-related decline in ovarian response to FSH stimulation. Patients who responded poorly to conventional doses (150–225 IU of FSH) may produce more follicles when given 300–450 IU or even 600 IU per day. It is expected that an enhanced response would lead to an increased number of oocytes retrieved, number of available embryos, and, ultimately, higher pregnancy and live birth rates (64–68). These expectations, however, are not always met, and this strategy is often of limited effectiveness.

Although higher circulating levels may be achieved by increasing the quantity of gonadotropins being administered, at some point saturation kinetics are attained (64,69) and the ovarian response is determined more by the number of follicles available for recruitment than by circulating gonadotropin levels. This is of particular importance, since poor responders generally have markedly diminished numbers of follicles available for recruitment, as reflected in low AFC. Furthermore, Ben-Rafael and colleagues (65) reported poorer oocyte quality with the use of incrementally higher gonadotropin doses in their normally responding patients. It is not clear, however, whether poor oocyte quality results from exposure to high-dose gonadotropins or, more likely, is another reflection of poor ovarian reserve. However, in a recent study (70) of young normogonadotropic ART patients there was no indication of an adverse effect on pregnancy outcomes of higher daily doses, if FSH was given according to an algorithm based on the four patient characteristics described by Howles et al. (56).

Very few studies have been conducted on the effects of increasing the dose of gonadotropins in poor responders, the vast majority of the studies being small and retrospective. The studies available suffer from heterogeneity with regard to the definition of poor responders, treatment protocols [use or nonuse of gonadotropin-releasing hormone (GnRH) agonists], and main outcome measures.

An interesting question is whether it is possible to rescue a cycle with initial poor response by doubling the gonadotropin dose after stimulation has already started. An RCT (71) evaluated the effect of doubling the human menopausal gonadotropin (hMG) dose in the current cycle in which the ovarian response after five days of ovarian stimulation with 225 IU/day was considered "low." No effect of doubling the hMG dose was noted with regards to the length of ovarian stimulation, peak E2 values, number of follicles >11mm and >14mm in diameter on the day of human chorionic gonadotropin (hCG) administration, number of cancelled cycles, number of oocytes retrieved, and the number of patients with ≤3 oocytes retrieved. It was concluded that doubling the hMG dose in the course of an IVF cycle is not effective in enhancing ovarian response. This is in accordance with current understanding of follicular growth dynamics, which states that follicular recruitment occurs only in the late luteal and early follicular phase of the previous menstrual cycle.

Another relevant issue is whether high-dose stimulation should be continued throughout the stimulation phase, or the gonadotropin dose can be reduced (step down) without compromising ovarian response. In an RCT (72), a high fixed versus a step-down dose of gonadotropins on a flare-up GnRH agonist (GnRH-a) regimen were compared. Patients were pretreated for 14 days with progestin, followed by 100 mcg triptorelin from day 1, reduced to 25 mcg/day from day 3 of the cycle. Purified FSH at a dose of 450 IU/day was administered on days 3–5 and on cycle day 6 patients were randomized to receive either a fixed dose of 450 IU/day or decreased to 300 IU/day, and finally to 150 IU/day. Cancellation rates, serum E2, oocyte yield, fertilization, and pregnancy rates were similar for both groups. The duration of stimulation and gonadotropin requirements were both significantly reduced with the step-down regimen. It was concluded that in poor responders undergoing COS on a short protocol with high-dose gonadotropins, the dose of gonadotropins can be safely reduced during the second part of the follicular phase, when follicles have attained high sensitivity to gonadotropins, without compromising cycle outcome. Thus, the step-down regimen offers a substantial economic benefit and some centers routinely use this approach to ensure that the available follicle cohort is exposed as early as possible to elevated FSH concentrations so as to reduce the possibility of late cycle cancellation (73).

In summary, increasing the starting dose of gonadotropins in poor responders is a rational approach that is widely practiced. A common starting dose would be at least 300 IU/day. Nevertheless, further dose increments are of limited effectiveness, and clinically meaningful improvements are only rarely obtained with doses >450 IU/day.

GNRH AGONISTS IN THE TREATMENT OF POOR RESPONDERS

Long GnRH-a Protocols

The use of GnRH-a has gained widespread popularity and most ART programs use this approach as the predominant method of ovarian stimulation. A meta-analysis of randomized and quasi-RCTs showed that use of GnRH-a reduced cancellation rates, increased the number of oocytes retrieved, and improved clinical pregnancy rates per cycle commenced and per embryo transfer (ET), compared with conventional stimulation regimens without the use of GnRH analogs (74). The aim of the long protocol is to achieve pituitary downregulation with suppression of endogenous gonadotropin secretion before stimulation with exogenous gonadotropins. Once pituitary downregulation and ovarian suppression are achieved, ovarian stimulation with exogenous gonadotropins is commenced while GnRH-a administration is continued concomitantly until the day of hCG administration. In the general IVF population, the long protocol has been found to be superior in terms of efficacy compared with the short protocol (75) and is therefore used most frequently. However, the matter of which GnRH-a protocol is preferable in poor responders remains controversial.

Because of its substantial medical and practical advantages, the use of the long GnRH-a protocol was extended also to the treatment of poor responder patients undergoing IVF. Although early studies were optimistic and suggested that long GnRH-a protocols could be beneficial for poor responders (76–80), subsequent clinical experience has yielded disappointing results. Downregulation of the hypothalamic–pituitary–ovarian axis prior to gonadotropin therapy is often associated with prolongation of the follicular phase and a significant increase in the number of gonadotropin ampoules required for achieving adequate follicular development. The extent of this increase is far greater than what could be attributed to simply delaying hCG administration to the point where larger cohorts of homogeneously well-synchronized large follicles are present. Moreover, in some relatively young patients with normal ovarian reserve, it was difficult to induce any ovarian response in the presence of pituitary downregulation, even with very large doses of exogenous gonadotropins (81–85). Normal ovarian function was restored in these patients after withdrawal of the GnRH-a, with subsequent normal response to hMG (83,84). These early observations indicated that GnRH-a may induce a state of ovarian hyporesponsiveness, the mechanism of which has never been clearly clarified.

Several theories have been suggested in an attempt to explain the dramatic (often a twofold) increase in exogenous gonadotropin requirements during pituitary downregulation:

1. Diminished circulating endogenous gonadotropin levels (81,82).
2. Altered biologic activity of endogenous gonadotropins (86–88).
3. Interference with follicular recruitment (89).
4. Direct ovarian inhibition effects by GnRH-a (90–92).

Thus, in many poor responder patients, ovarian suppression with GnRH-a resulted in excessive dampening of the ovarian response to COS and complete refractoriness to gonadotropin stimulation (93). Consequently, cancellation rates due to lack of ovarian response were unacceptably high, and hormonal stimulation was excessively prolonged, with increased cost and duration of treatment and only a marginal benefit in the mean E2 maximum response and the yield of mature oocytes (94–96).

It has been well established that there is a dose-dependent duration of ovarian suppression after single implant injections of GnRH-a, and that in a suppressed pituitary gland the dose needed to maintain suppression gradually decreases with the length of treatment (97). This supports the concept of step-down GnRH-a protocols, where the dose of the agonist is decreased once the criteria for ovarian suppression have been achieved. Furthermore, the minimal effective dose for sufficient pituitary suppression with GnRH-a has not been thoroughly studied before their actual introduction to clinical practice. Regarding triptorelin, for example, Janssens et al., (98) in a prospective, placebo-controlled, double-blind study, demonstrated that daily administration of 15 mcg of triptorelin is sufficient to prevent a premature LH surge, and that 50 mcg is equivalent to 100 mcg in terms of IVF results.

In an attempt to maximize ovarian response without losing the benefits of GnRH-a downregulation, Feldberg et al. (99) introduced the use of the mini-dose GnRH-a protocol in poor responders. They found that patients with elevated basal FSH levels who received daily triptorelin, 100 mcg SC from the mid-luteal phase until menstruation and 50 mcg thereafter, had higher peak E2 levels, more oocytes recovered, and more embryos transferred. They also noted a trend toward improved pregnancy and implantation rates and a lower spontaneous abortion rate.

Olivennes et al. (100) studied 98 IVF patients with a high basal FSH concentration who were previously treated by the long protocol with a GnRH-a in a depot formulation. The same patients received SC leuprolide acetate (LA) 0.1 mg/day from cycle day 21, reducing it to 0.05 mg/day upon downregulation. The comparison was made using the previous IVF cycle of the same patient as a control. The use of a low-dose agonist protocol resulted in significantly reduced gonadotropin requirements, a shorter duration of stimulation, a higher E2 concentration on stimulation day 8, a higher number of mature oocytes, and a higher number of good-quality embryos. The cancellation rate was lower (11% vs. 24%). Kowalik et al. (90) have demonstrated that lowering the dose of LA resulted in a faster E2 rise and higher mean peak E2 level. The higher E2 levels were obtained with a lower total gonadotropin dose. The oocyte yield was not affected. It was concluded that lowering the dosage of LA allows higher E2 response, which suggests an inhibitory in vivo effect of LA on ovarian steroidogenesis. Davis and Rosenwaks (85) reported similar results using a low-dose LA protocol.

Weissman et al. (101) prospectively compared two stimulation protocols specifically designed for poor responder patients. Sixty poor responders who were recruited on the basis of response in previous cycles received either a modified flare-up protocol in which a high dose of triptorelin (500 mcg) was administered for the first four days, followed by a standard dose (100 mcg), or a mini-dose long protocol in which 100 mcg triptorelin was used until pituitary downregulation, after which the triptorelin dose was halved during stimulation. Twenty-nine cycles were performed with the modified flare-up protocol and 31 were performed with the mini-dose long protocol. Significantly more oocytes were obtained with the modified long protocol than the modified flare protocol. The number and quality of embryos available for transfer were similar in both groups. One clinical pregnancy (3.4%) was achieved with the modified flare protocol, and seven pregnancies (22.5%) were achieved using the mini-dose long protocol.

Ovarian cyst formation is a common complication of the long GnRH-a protocol. It has been suggested as being typical for poor responders and as being a reliable predictor of poor stimulation and low pregnancy rates in a given cycle (102,103). Although the pathophysiology of

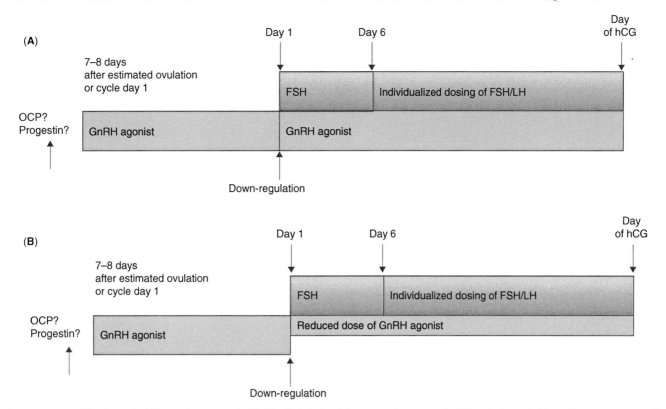

Figure 46.2 (**A**) The long GnRH agonist protocol. (**B**) The "mini-dose" long agonist protocol. *Abbreviations*: OCP, oral contraceptive pills; GnRH, gonadotropin-releasing hormone; FSH, follicle-stimulating hormone; LH, luteinizing hormone; hCG, human chorionic gonadotropin.

ovarian cyst formation following GnRH-a administration has not been completely elucidated, the higher the serum progesterone level at the time of commencing GnRH-a administration, the lower the incidence of cyst formation (104). Progestogen pretreatment directly inhibits endogenous gonadotropin secretion and influences the pattern of gonadotropin and hypothalamic GnRH secretion. Three RCTs have demonstrated the successful use of progestins to prevent ovarian cyst formation during pituitary suppression in IVF cycles (105–107). We have also successfully included progestogen pretreatment in the long mini-dose protocol (101).

Summarizing the above studies and observations, it appears that if the long GnRH-a protocol is to be used in poor responders, then a reduced agonist dose ("mini-dose") is superior to a standard agonist dose in terms of oocyte yield and cycle outcome, and this approach should be preferably employed (Fig. 46.2).

GnRH-a "Stop" Protocols

Pituitary recovery and resumption of gonadotropin secretion following GnRH-a treatment may take up to several weeks, depending on the dose and route of administration of the agonist. For example, with intranasal buserelin acetate (BA), suppression of endogenous gonadotropin secretion seems to continue for at least 12 days after the discontinuation of the agonist (108), as was also reported for SC BA (109). Interestingly, using the "ultrashort protocol," suppression of endogenous LH secretion was more profound when LA administration was stopped

after five days of administration, compared with continuous LA administration, and no premature LH peak was recorded (110). This forms the basis for a variety of discontinuous or "stop" GnRH-a protocols.

The above observations prompted several studies in which GnRH-a were administered in the long protocol, but agonist administration was withheld once gonadotropin stimulation had started (111–115). The majority of studies have shown favorable results in terms of both clinical outcome and cost-effectiveness, but studies showing discouraging results were also reported (115). Corson et al. (111) prospectively evaluated the effect of stopping GnRH-a (SC LA) therapy upon initiation of ovarian stimulation versus simultaneous GnRH-a and gonadotropin therapy. Both groups were found comparable in terms of the duration of stimulation and amount of exogenous gonadotropins required, as well as for any other stimulation or outcome parameter studied. Stopping LA upon initiation of ovarian stimulation did not reduce its efficacy in suppressing LH secretion, as in neither group was a premature LH surge detected.

Similar results were obtained in a prospective study that compared two protocols with variable duration of BA administration in an IVF/gamete intrafallopian transfer program (112). No spontaneous premature LH surges were recorded in any of the groups, and all parameters of ovarian response to stimulation were found comparable for both groups. A trend toward a higher pregnancy rate per ET was noted in the discontinuous BA arm. Simons et al. (113) compared the efficacy of two early cessation protocols of triptorelin treatment with the conventional long protocol in IVF. In a multicenter RCT, 178 women were randomized to one of three treatment groups at the start of stimulation. SC triptorelin was started at the mid-luteal phase of the previous cycle and continued until the first day of gonadotropin treatment, or up to and including the fourth day of gonadotropin treatment or the day of hCG injection. One premature LH surge was observed in the second group. Both early cessation protocols were at least as effective as the standard long protocol with regard to the number of oocytes, number of embryos, and ongoing pregnancy rate. It was concluded that early cessation of triptorelin on day 1 of gonadotropin treatment is as effective as the traditional long protocol in preventing a premature LH surge and results in similar reproductive outcome.

In contrast, Fujii et al. (115) reported on an RCT, where 900 mcg/day of intranasal BA were administered from the mid-luteal phase of the previous cycle until cycle day 7, when normal responding patients were randomized to receive either gonadotropin stimulation alone or combined BA and gonadotropin therapy. The duration and total dose of gonadotropins administered were significantly increased in the early GnRH-a cessation group, compared with the conventional long protocol. The number of fertilized oocytes and embryos transferred were significantly lower and the cancellation rate and rate of failed oocyte retrieval were significantly higher in the discontinuous long protocol. Although premature LH surges were not recorded in either group, serum progesterone and LH concentrations were significantly increased on the day of hCG administration with the discontinuous long protocol. Clinical pregnancy rates per transfer were similar for both protocols. It was concluded that early discontinuation of the GnRH-a is not beneficial and not cost-effective because of its adverse effects on follicular development and increased exogenous gonadotropin requirements, respectively. A reason for this could be because stopping daily agonist administration combined with ovarian stimulation leads to a further reduction in circulating LH concentrations (116), which supports the concept that there is still a small release of LH following daily agonist administration.

Discontinuous protocols were considered to be potentially beneficial for poor responder patients undergoing IVF–ET (117). Several trials with contradictory results have been reported. Faber et al. (118) conducted a single group uncontrolled study, in which poor responder patients were treated with LA, 0.5 mg/day, starting at the mid-luteal phase of the previous cycle. With the onset of menses, LA was discontinued and high-dose gonadotropin therapy was initiated. The cancellation rate was 12.5% (28/224 cycles), and only one case of premature LH surge was observed. Despite the uncontrolled nature of the study, a clinical pregnancy rate per transfer of 32% and ongoing pregnancy rate per transfer of 23%, which seemed highly favorable for the specific subgroup of poor responder patients, were achieved.

Subsequently, Wang et al. (119) conducted a prospective non-randomized study to determine the efficacy of a "stop" protocol in previously poor responders to a standard long protocol. Fifty patients were scheduled for 52 cycles of the modified "stop" agonist protocol. All patients received GnRH-a from the mid-luteal phase of the previous cycle to the onset of menstruation, followed by high-dose gonadotropin stimulation. Six of the 52 cycles (11.8%) were canceled because of POR. One premature ovulation was noted, and in the other 45 cycles, an average of 6.3 mature oocytes was retrieved. A favorable embryo implantation rate (11.5%) and clinical pregnancy rate (20.5%) were noted.

In a prospective study with historical controls involving 36 poor responders, the use of intranasal nafarelin (600 mcg/day), commenced in the mid-luteal phase and discontinued on day 5 of ovarian stimulation, was evaluated (120). The cancellation rate was 8.3%, and there was a trend toward increased peak E2 levels and an increase in the number of oocytes retrieved. The ongoing pregnancy rate per ET was 15%. A significant improvement in both the number and the quality of cleaving embryos was observed, and it was suggested therefore that discontinuation of the GnRH-a leads to improved oocyte quality.

In another prospective study with historical controls (121), 39 "stop" nafarelin cycles in 30 previously poor responder patients were compared to 60 past cycles in the same individuals. A significantly higher number of oocytes were retrieved and a higher number of embryos were available for transfer. No cases of premature LH surge were recorded. Pregnancy rates per ET and per cycle were 10.4% and 7.7%, respectively.

In contrast, Dirnfeld et al. (122) reported on an RCT involving 78 cycles, in which a "stop agonist" regimen was compared with a standard long luteal protocol. Intranasal BA (1 mg/day) or SC triptorelin (100 mcg/day) was initiated on day 21 of the previous cycle and ceased once pituitary suppression was confirmed. Ovarian stimulation was induced with the use of 225–375 IU/day hMG or purified FSH, commencing on the day of down-regulation. A significantly higher cancellation rate was noted with the stop regimen compared with the controls (22.5% vs. 5%, respectively). The stop and long regimens resulted in similar stimulation characteristics and clinical pregnancy rates (11% vs. 10.3%, respectively). Only in patients with a basal FSH level that was not persistently high did the stop regimen result in a significantly higher number of retrieved oocytes compared with the standard long protocol (7.6 vs. 4.0, respectively). It was concluded that, for most poor responders, the stop regimen offers no further advantage over the standard long protocol.

Garcia-Velasco et al. (123) designed an RCT to evaluate whether early cessation of the GnRH-a (LA) is more beneficial than just increasing the doses of gonadotropins in poor responder patients. Seventy poor responder patients with normal basal FSH concentrations and a previous canceled IVF cycle were randomly allocated to either a standard long protocol or a stop protocol. A significantly higher number of mature oocytes were obtained with the stop protocol compared with the standard long protocol (8.7 vs. 6.2). The stop protocol significantly reduced the gonadotropin requirements. Both protocols resulted in a similar cancellation rate (2.7% vs. 5.8%), pregnancy rate

(14.3% vs. 18.7%), and implantation rate (12.1% vs. 8.8%). It was concluded that the stop protocol combined with high doses of gonadotropins permitted the retrieval of a significantly higher number of oocytes, but did not influence the reproductive outcome.

Short GnRH-a Regimen

In patients who fail to obtain adequate multifollicular growth with the long GnRH-a protocol, one of the options is to decrease the length of suppression by decreasing the duration of GnRH-a use (short and ultrashort regimens). The short protocol consists of early follicular phase initiation of GnRH-a, with minimal delay before commencing gonadotropin ovarian stimulation. It takes advantage of the initial agonistic stimulatory effect of GnRH-a on endogenous FSH and LH secretion, also known as the flare-up effect. In theory, it eliminates excessive ovarian suppression associated with prolonged agonist use. The duration of the endogenous gonadotropin flare has not been completely characterized, but pituitary desensitization is generally achieved within five days of initiating treatment (124), and therefore, patients are protected from premature LH surges by the end of the stimulation phase. The short protocol has been proposed by many authors as a better stimulation protocol for poor responders (125–127).

Although widely used in poor responders, no RCTs comparing the efficacy of the short protocol with standard long protocols have been published. In an early prospective study with historical controls and using an ultrashort protocol, Howles et al. (127) treated seven patients who had previously responded poorly to stimulation with clomiphene citrate (CC) and hMG with 0.5 mg/day BA during only the first three days of the cycle (ultrashort protocol). All seven patients had oocytes recovered, and embryos replaced, and three out of these seven conceived (42.9%). Similarly, Katayama et al. (128) reported improved cycle outcomes in seven prior poor responder patients with the short regimen. Garcia et al. (126) conducted a non-randomized prospective trial comparing long luteal and short flare-up agonist initiation in 189 cycles. They noted a significant decrease in exogenous gonadotropin requirements, higher pregnancy rates, and decreased miscarriage rates in patients receiving the flare-up regimen. In a retrospective comparison, Toth et al. (129) also reported that pregnancy and implantation rates were significantly higher and cancellation rates lower in patients with basal serum FSH levels ≥15 mIU/ml undergoing a flare-up regimen versus a long luteal agonist regimen. In a prospective uncontrolled study, Padilla et al. (125) administered a flare-up protocol with high-dose gonadotropins to 53 patients who were thought to be at risk for poor response after a "leuprolide acetate screening test." The cancellation rate was higher in poor flare-up LA test responders (11.3%) compared with good flare-up LA responders (1.1%) and luteal phase long protocols cycles (1.8%). Despite a low number of oocytes retrieved, the ongoing pregnancy rate was 29% per retrieval and was considered favorable for this group of potentially poor responder patients.

Despite these encouraging findings, other authors failed to confirm any substantial benefit of using a classic flare-up protocol. In a prospective study with historical controls (130), 80 poor responders were treated using a classic flare-up regimen with LA 0.5 mg/day from cycle day 2, and high-dose hMG from cycle day 3. While the number of retrieved oocytes was increased (10 ± 6.6), the cancellation rate was high (23.4%), and the ongoing pregnancy rate of 6.5% per retrieval and 7.6% per transfer were disappointing. Brzyski et al. (131) reported that not only did concomitant initiation of GnRH-a with purified urinary FSH result in poorer cycle outcome, but also an increased number of atretic oocytes were retrieved. A significant increase in LH and progesterone levels during the follicular phase was noted. Other groups using this approach also reported failure to improve ovarian response or cycle outcome in generally similar patient populations (132–134).

In an RCT, San Roman et al. (135) have shown that a combination of early follicular phase LA administration and hMG stimulation was associated with a significant increase in serum LH levels, beginning with the first follicular phase agonist dose, and with significant increases in serum progesterone and testosterone levels during the follicular phase, compared with mid-luteal GnRH-a administration. The live birth rate/retrieval for the long protocol was 25% compared with 3.8% in the flare-up group. All these adverse effects may result through the initial flare-up effect of GnRH-a on LH secretion, with a subsequent increase in intrafollicular androgen levels. The androgen-rich environment may interfere with the process of folliculogenesis by untimely inhibition of meiosis-inhibiting factors, leading to over aging of oocytes, with a significant reduction in their fertilization and implantation capacity (136–138). Evidence of an adverse effect of high endogenous LH level during the follicular phase has led to the establishment of the ceiling theory (139). According to this theory, beyond a certain ceiling level, LH suppresses GC proliferation and initiates atresia of less mature follicles.

Further support for this view comes from a study of Gelety et al. (140), who performed a prospective randomized crossover study of five regularly cycling women to determine the short-term pituitary and ovarian effects of GnRH-a administered during differing phases of the menstrual cycle in the absence of gonadotropin stimulation. Each patient was administered LA 1 mg/day SC for five days beginning on cycle day 3, eight days post-LH surge, and 13 days post-LH surge with an intervening "washout" month. Significant increases in serum LH, E2, estrone, androgens, and progesterone levels were noted in the early follicular phase group, compared with the mid-luteal group. Early follicular initiation of the agonist resulted in a more pronounced suppression of FSH. It was suggested that relative FSH suppression and marked androgen elevations could have potential detrimental effects on oocytes of the developing cohort that are often observed with flare-up regimens.

Can the adverse effects of the gonadotropin flare be prevented without losing the potential benefits of the short protocol? Two possible solutions have been suggested: The first is pretreatment with an oral contraceptive pill (OCP) or a progestin. Cédrin-Durnerin et al. (141) noted that pretreatment with a 12–20 day course of the progestin norethisterone before initiation of a flare-up regimen effectively lowered LH and progesterone levels during the early stages of gonadotropin stimulation. Many clinicians thus regard pretreatment with an OCP or a progestin as integral in flare-up regimens, although this issue also became a matter of controversy (142). The second solution is dose reduction of the GnRH-a causing the flare, which forms the basis for the "microdose flare" regimen (Fig. 46.3).

Microdose Flare GnRH-a Regimen

In theory, micro-flare regimens decrease the enhanced LH, progesterone, and androgen secretion associated with standard flare-up regimens, as described above. Bstandig et al. (143) studied the hormonal profiles during the flare-up period using 25 mcg and 100 mcg of triptorelin in the short protocol. No significant difference in the magnitude of FSH and E2 release was observed between the two groups, but the maximal plasma LH level was significantly reduced after injection of 25 mcg of triptorelin. It was suggested that in the flare protocol, a lower dose of GnRH-a induces a hormonal flare-up that is more conducive for optimal follicular recruitment. Deaton et al. (144) have demonstrated that an extremely low dose of LA (25 or 50 mcg) is needed to cause a pituitary flare of gonadotropins. Following a

flare from 25 mcg of LA on cycle day 2, the pituitary is able to recover and respond with a repeat flare on cycle day 5. These observations support the rationale behind the so-called microdose flare protocols.

Navot et al. (145) studied the effect of very low doses of GnRH-a in cynomolgus monkeys and humans and established that 10 mg of historelin in four divided doses (microdoses) could induce ovarian hyperstimulation in humans. Scott et al. (146) reported that an increase in gonadotropin levels could be induced in baboons with LA doses as low as 0.017 mg/kg. Although the minimal and optimal effective dose of GnRH-a that can be successfully used to induce a gonadotropin flare in humans has not been thoroughly evaluated, several investigators have reported an improved outcome with doses as low as 20–40 mcg of LA twice daily in poor responders.

In a prospective study with historical controls, Scott and Navot (146) treated 34 poor responder patients with an OCP followed by 20 mcg LA twice daily, beginning on cycle day 3 and supplemented with exogenous gonadotropins, beginning on cycle day 5. Ovarian responsiveness was enhanced with the microdose GnRH-a stimulation cycle when compared with previous stimulation cycles. Specifically, the patients had a more rapid rise in E2 levels, much higher peak E2 levels, the development of more mature follicles, and the recovery of larger numbers of mature oocytes. None of the patients had a premature LH surge.

Impressive results using the microdose flare protocol were also reported in a prospective study with historical

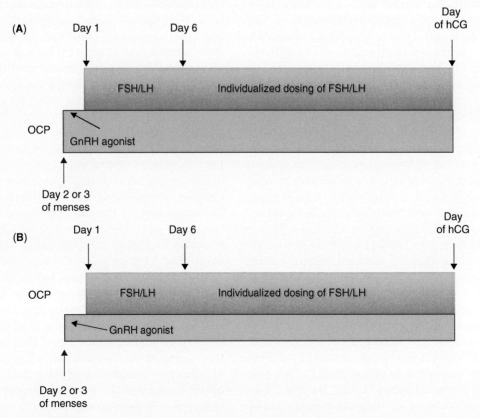

Figure 46.3 (**A**) The short GnRH agonist protocol. (**B**) The "microdose" flare GnRH agonist protocol. *Abbreviations*: OCP, oral contraceptive pills; GnRH, gonadotropin-releasing hormone; FSH, follicle-stimulating hormone; LH, luteinizing hormone; hCG, human chorionic gonadotropin.

controls by Schoolcraft et al. (147). Thirty-two patients, whose prior long luteal agonist cycles had been canceled because of poor response, were now pretreated with an OCP followed by follicular phase administration of 40 mcg LA twice daily beginning on cycle day 3 and high-dose FSH supplemented with human growth hormone (hGH) beginning on cycle day 5. Compared with the prior long luteal GnRH-a cycle, there was a higher E2 response, more oocytes retrieved (10.9 per patient), fewer cycle cancellations (12.5%), and no premature LH surge or luteinization. For patients who were not canceled, a favorable ongoing pregnancy rate of 50% was achieved.

In a prospective non-randomized trial with historical controls, Surrey et al. (148) treated 34 patients with a prior poor response to a standard mid-luteal long protocol with an OCP followed by LA 40 mcg twice daily and high-dose gonadotropins. Cycle cancellation rates were dramatically reduced, and the mean maximal serum E2 levels obtained were significantly higher. The ongoing pregnancy rates per ET were 33% in patients ≤39 years and 18.2% in patients >39 years. Significant increases in circulating FSH levels occurred after five days of gonadotropin stimulation. No abnormal rises in LH, progesterone, or testosterone during the follicular phase were noted. This could result from either the lower GnRH-a dose, the OCP pretreatment, or a combination of the two.

Detti et al. reported on a retrospective cohort study that assessed the efficacy of three different GnRH-a stimulation regimens to improve ovarian response in poor responders (117). Women diagnosed as poor responders underwent three different stimulation regimens during IVF cycles:

1. Stop protocol: LA 500 mcg/day administered from the mid-luteal phase to the start of menses, then gonadotropins from day 2 of cycle.
2. Microdose flare: LA 20 mcg administered twice daily with gonadotropins from day 2 to the day of hCG administration.
3. Regular dose flare: Gonadotropins beginning with LA on day 2 at 1 mcg/day for three days, followed by 250 LA mcg/day until the day of hCG administration.

Since only 61 cycles were included in the analysis, none of the comparisons reached statistical significance; however, the microdose flare group demonstrated a trend toward a higher delivery rate.

It is noteworthy that, in a general IVF population (excluding poor responders), retrospective analysis failed to find the microdose flare protocol superior over the long mid-luteal agonist regimen (149). Significantly higher cancellation rates (22.5% vs. 8.2%), lower clinical pregnancy rates (47.3% vs. 60%, NS; Not Significant), and a decreased number of oocytes retrieved per cycle (13.3 vs. 16.5, NS) were noted with the microdose flare-up regimen.

Overall, all studies evaluating the microdose flare protocols were retrospective in nature. Obviously, large prospective RCTs are needed to validate the true efficacy of the microdose flare-up GnRH-a regimens in poor responder patients.

GNRH ANTAGONISTS IN THE TREATMENT OF POOR RESPONDERS

GnRH antagonists competitively block the GnRH receptor in the pituitary gland, producing an immediate dose-related suppression of gonadotropin release. Within six hours of GnRH antagonist (GnRH-ant) administration, LH levels are significantly reduced. On the principle of maximizing potential endogenous pituitary stimulation, a GnRH-ant can be administered later in the follicular phase to suppress the LH surge (150,151), thus avoiding suppression during the phase of early follicular recruitment. In the general IVF population, the GnRH-ants offer comparable therapeutic efficacy to agonists and have a number of potential advantages over agonists for use in ovarian stimulation protocols, such as avoiding the initial "flare-up" of LH, shortening the overall treatment period, reducing the risk of OHSS, and menopausal side effects (150,151).

The GnRH-ants are administered in the late follicular phase, either according to the fixed or the flexible protocol (see chap. 41). Thus, at the beginning of COS, the pituitary is fully susceptible to GnRH pulses. This may allow us to obtain a more natural follicular recruitment without any inhibitory effect possibly induced by the GnRH-a. It has been therefore suggested as a suitable protocol for poor responders. GnRH-ants also permit the revival of stimulation protocols of the pre-agonist era using, for example, CC (152). The combination of CC treatment in the early follicular phase and subsequent, overlapping, gonadotropin stimulation has been a standard therapy in the past (152,153). Owing to the synergistic effect of these compounds, the amount of gonadotropins required is lower and so are the costs (154,155). In addition, the gonadotropins counteract the detrimental effects of CC on the endometrium (154). As a result of the high rate of premature LH surges, and therefore the high cancellation rate, this stimulation regimen was abandoned when GnRH-a were introduced in IVF (Fig. 46.4).

Craft et al. (156) were first to suggest the use of GnRH-ants for COS in poor responders. In a small retrospective series, 18 previously poor responders were stimulated with a combination of gonadotropins and CC, and started on a GnRH-ant according to the flexible protocol. Compared to their poor response in a previous GnRH-a cycle, modest improvements in cycle cancellation rates (29% vs. 57%),

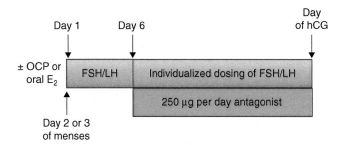

Figure 46.4 GnRH antagonist protocol. *Abbreviations*: OCP, oral contraceptive pills; E2, estradiol; FSH, follicle-stimulating hormone; LH, luteinizing hormone; hCG, human chorionic gonadotropin.

oocyte yield (6.4 vs. 4.7), and gonadotropin requirements (4506 IU vs. 5468 IU) were noted with the GnRH-ant. Two live births resulted (11.8%). Several studies were subsequently undertaken to examine the efficacy of GnRH-ants in COS regimens designed for poor responders. The majority of these studies were of small scale and retrospective. Retrospective studies will be presented first, followed by more recently reported RCTs.

Retrospective Studies

Nikolettos et al. (157) compared 21 poor responders who underwent IVF–ICSI and were treated with a GnRH-ant protocol with 21 matched poor responders treated according to the long GnRH-a protocol. Fifteen patients of the GnRH-ant group were treated with the combination of CC plus gonadotropins, while six patients were treated with gonadotropins alone. The use of the GnRH-ant protocol resulted in a significantly shorter treatment duration and lower gonadotropin consumption as compared with the use of the long GnRH-a protocol. Three pregnancies (14.3%) were achieved with the antagonist and two (9.5%) with the long agonist protocol (NS).

Several retrospective studies have compared the GnRH-ant protocol with GnRH-agonist flare-up and microdose flare regimens. In a retrospective cohort study, Posada et al. (158) compared the clinical outcome of COS in unselected patients undergoing IVF with a GnRH-ant (133 cycles) versus a four-day ultrashort GnRH-a regimen (236 cycles). The GnRH-ant protocol was shown to reduce treatment duration and amount of gonadotropin used. In younger women, the antagonist protocol was associated with significantly better pregnancy and implantation rates, but no difference was observed in pregnancy rates in patients >38 years.

Mohamed et al. (159) retrospectively compared the agonist flare-up and antagonist protocols in the management of poor responders to the standard long protocol. One hundred and thirty-four patients undergoing IVF–ICSI treatment, who responded poorly to the standard long protocol in their first treatment cycle, were studied. In the second cycle, 77 patients received a short GnRH-a flare-up regimen and 57 patients received an antagonist protocol, based solely on physician preference. There were no cycle cancellations in the flare-up protocol and a 7% cancellation rate in the antagonist protocol due to lack of response. A significantly higher number of patients had ET in the flare-up protocol. Similar numbers of oocytes (5.4 vs. 5.2) and similar implantation and pregnancy rates per cycle (12.8% and 17.5% vs. 12.8% and 24.7%) were reported in the antagonist and flare-up groups, respectively. It was concluded that both the flare-up and the antagonist protocols significantly improved the ovarian response of previously poor responders. However, a significantly higher cycle cancellation rate and less patients having ET in the antagonist group suggested a higher efficacy for the flare-up regimen.

Conflicting results were reported by Fasouliotis et al. (160) who also conducted a retrospective analysis between the flare-up and antagonist regimens in poor responders. Of 56 poor responders treated with flare-up protocol, 53 who failed to conceive were subsequently treated in the next cycle with a GnRH-ant regimen. While ovarian response did not differ between the two protocols, the number of embryos transferred was significantly higher in the GnRH-ant group (2.5 ± 1.6 vs. 2.0 ± 1.4). The clinical pregnancy and implantation rates per transfer in the GnRH-ant group tended to be higher than in the flare-up group, but did not reach significance (26.1% and 10.7% compared with 12.2% and 5.9%, respectively). However, the ongoing pregnancy rate per transfer was significantly higher in the GnRH-ant than in the GnRH-a flare-up group (23.9% vs. 7.3%, respectively).

Copperman (161) conducted a retrospective analysis with historic controls comparing cycle outcomes in poor responders who had stimulation protocols that included an antagonist with those with the microdose flare protocol. Patients were placed in the antagonist or microdose flare treatment group usually after failing in an LA downregulation cycle, and often according to physician preference. The results of this retrospective analysis indicated that, for poor responders, the inclusion of a GnRH antagonist in the treatment regimen significantly increased clinical pregnancy rates and significantly lowered cancellation rates compared with patients treated with the microdose flare protocol.

The use of OCP pretreatment in antagonist cycles for poor responder patients is also of clinical relevance, as their ovarian reserve may be especially sensitive to suppression of endogenous gonadotropins by the pill. Copperman (161) reported a retrospective study of 1343 patients, where poor responders were given a starting dose of 450 IU of gonadotropin. In the OCP pretreatment group, patients were administered OCP for 18–24 days, beginning on cycle day 3. Patients were first administered a combination of r-hFSH and hMG on cycle day 3, and were administered GnRH-ant when their lead follicle reached 14 mm. An additional 75 IU of hMG was administered beginning the first day of antagonist. Patients whose antagonist stimulation cycle included OCP pretreatment had a significantly higher pregnancy rate and a significantly lower cancellation rate. In addition, a higher proportion of patients obtained more than eight oocytes following OCP pretreatment. In contrast, Shapiro et al. (162) reported significantly increased cancellation rates (23%) in a group of poor responder patients pretreated with an OCP compared with patients not receiving OCP pretreatment (9%). The two studies, however, differed both in inclusion criteria and in the use of LH in the stimulation protocol.

Prospective Studies

Akaman et al. (163) compared a GnRH-ant protocol to a protocol using gonadotropins alone in poor responders. In total, 20 women were randomized to each group. Women assigned to the antagonist arm received 0.25 mg of cetrorelix according to the flexible protocol, and all women were initially stimulated with 600 IU of urinary-derived gonadotropin. There was no statistically significant difference between the groups for cancellation rates, gonadotropin requirements, number of mature oocytes retrieved, E2 concentrations on the day of hCG administration, fertilization rates, and number of embryos transferred. The clinical pregnancy and implantation rates in the antagonist group appeared higher, but were not significantly different (20% and 13.33% compared with 6.25% and 3.44%, respectively) because of the small numbers involved.

There are several RCTs that compare the agonist flare-up with the antagonist protocols. Akman et al. (164) compared clinical outcomes of 48 poor responder patients who were treated with either a microdose flare (LA, 40 mcg SC per day) protocol or the antagonist (cetrorelix 0.25 mg daily) protocol. All patients received 300 IU of highly purified FSH and 300 IU of hMG for four days, followed by individual adjustments in the dose of highly purified FSH. Patients in the microdose flare group also received OCP pretreatment. There was no difference in the median total treatment doses of gonadotropins between the two groups. Serum E2 levels on the day of hCG administration and the number of oocytes retrieved were significantly lower in the antagonist group. No differences were observed between the two groups for fertilization rates, number of embryos transferred, and most importantly, implantation rates and ongoing pregnancy rates per transfer. It was concluded that the efficacy of these stimulation protocols in poor responder patients was comparable, but larger studies were needed.

De Placido et al. (165) randomized 133 women "at risk for poor ovarian response" to undergo COS by either a modified GnRH-ant protocol or a short flare-up regimen. Patients in the antagonist arm were treated by the flexible regimen with 300 IU of r-hFSH given from cycle day 2. When the lead follicle reached a diameter of 14 mm, cetrurelix 0.125 was given daily for two days, followed by 0.25 cetrurelix daily until the day of hCG administration. Beginning on the same day of GnRH-ant administration, a daily dose of 150 IU of r-hLH (Luveris) was also added until the day of hCG. Patients in the flare-up arm received daily a dose of triptorelin (0.1 mg) SC, beginning on the same day of the first r-hFSH administration. In addition, in this group, a dose of 150 IU/day of r-hLH was added when at least one follicle reached 14 mm. The mean number of Metaphase II (M II) oocytes (primary end point) was significantly higher in the antagonist group (5.73 ± 3.57 vs. 4.64 ± 2.23, respectively; p < 0.05). Cancellation rates, gonadotropin requirements, implantation, and clinical and ongoing pregnancy rates were all comparable for the two groups.

Demirol and Gurgan (166) conducted an RCT comparing the short micro-flare and the flexible GnRH-ant protocol in 90 poor responder patients. In the micro-flare group, 45 patients received an OCP and on the third day of menstruation, 40 mcg SC twice daily of LA followed by 450 IU/day hMG. In the antagonist group, 45 patients received 450 IU/day hMG starting on day 3 and 0.25 mg cetrorelix administered daily when more

than two follicles reached 13–14 mm in diameter. The total gonadotropin dose used was significantly higher in the antagonist group, while the number of oocytes retrieved was significantly greater in the micro-flare group (4.3 ± 2.13 vs. 3.1 ± 1.09; p = 0.001). Implantation rate was significantly higher in the micro-flare group than in the antagonist group (22% vs. 11%; p = 0.017). It was concluded that the short micro-flare protocol seems to have a better outcome in poor-responder patients, with a significantly higher mean number of mature oocytes retrieved and higher implantation rate.

Kahraman et al. (167) conducted another RCT comparing the micro-flare and the antagonist protocols in patients who previously had a low response to the long GnRH-a protocol. Twenty-one patients received LA (50 mcg twice daily) starting on the second day of post OCP bleeding. The other 21 patients received 0.25 mg of cetrorelix daily when the leading follicle reached 14 mm in diameter. Stimulation in both groups consisted of 300–450 daily doses of r-hFSH. The mean serum E2 concentration on the day of hCG administration was significantly higher in the micro-flare group than in the antagonist group (1904 vs. 1362 pg/mL; p = 0.042) but all other outcome variables studied were found comparable for the two groups. It was concluded that the micro-flare agonist and multiple dose GnRH-ant protocol seem to have similar efficacy in improving treatment outcomes of poor responder patients. Very similar findings were recently reported by Devasa et al. (168) who compared the micro-flare agonist and multiple dose antagonist protocols in 221 poor prognosis patients based on previous cycles or clinical criteria. Except for significantly higher serum E2 levels on hCG day in the micro-flare group, all other outcome variables were found to be comparable for the two groups.

Schmidt et al. (169) randomized 48 previously poor responder patients to either a GnRH-ant protocol (ganirelix 0.25 mg daily in a flexible manner) or a micro-dose flare regimen (LA, 40 mcg b.i.d, after OCP pretreatment). Ovarian stimulation consisted of 300 IU of r-hFSH every morning and 150 IU of hMG every evening. Cancellation rates due to an inadequate response were equally high, close to 50% in both groups. While only 13 women in the antagonist group and 11 women who received a microdose flare completed their cycle, no significant differences in oocyte yield (8.9 vs. 9), fertilization rate (69.1% vs. 63.5%), or clinical pregnancy rate (38.5% vs. 36.4%) were detected. It was concluded that the antagonist protocol appears to be as effective as the microdose flare protocol for COS in poor responders, but could be a superior choice in terms of cost and convenience for the patient.

Malmusi et al. (170) compared the efficacy of the flare-up GnRHa protocol to the flexible GnRH-ant in poor responders. Fifty-five poor responder patients undergoing IVF–ICSI were randomized to receive either triptorelin (100 mcg daily) from the first day of menstruation, followed by exogenous gonadotropins from the second day of menstruation (30 cycles), or exogenous gonadotropins from the first day of menstrual cycle, and later ganirelix (0.25 mg daily) once the leading follicle reached

14 mm in diameter (25 cycles). Gonadotropin requirements were significantly reduced with the flare-up protocol. The number of mature oocytes retrieved, fertilization rate, and top-quality embryos transferred were significantly increased in the flare-up compared to the GnRH-ant group. The implantation and pregnancy rates were similar in both groups.

Very few RCTs comparing the long GnRH-a and the GnRH-ant for COS in poor responders have been published (171–174) (Table 46.1). Studies vary and suffer from considerable heterogeneities in terms of almost all possible aspects such as inclusion criteria, agonist and antagonist administration regimens, and outcome variables reported. For example, in two studies (171,173) a depot preparation of a GnRH agonist was used, which is not a recommended administration route for low responders. In contrast, in the study by Tazegul et al. (172) a mini-dose agonist protocol was used, a certainly more appropriate administration route for low responders. Since these studies are not readily comparable, only general conclusions can be made. It appears that the GnRH-ant protocol is as effective as the long agonist protocol in poor responders. Gonadotropin consumption and stimulation duration both appear to be reduced with the antagonist protocol, a considerable practical advantage for patients. Clinical pregnancy and live birth rates appear to be similar. A recent meta-analysis compared the different COS regimens used for low responders (59). Very few studies were available for analysis in each category. It was therefore concluded that "there is insufficient evidence to support the routine use of any particular intervention either for pituitary downregulation, ovarian stimulation, or adjuvant therapy in the management of poor responders to controlled ovarian stimulation in IVF. More robust data from good quality RCTs with relevant outcomes are needed."

Representing a novel approach, a prospective cohort study of 538 patients undergoing their first IVF cycle was conducted to compare outcomes of GnRH-a versus GnRH-ant protocols in an attempt to individualize treatment using baseline AMH (52). Predetermined AMH values were used to dictate either FSH dose in a GnRH-a controlled program or a program of modified GnRH analog strategy. GnRH-ant (vs. agonist) co-treatment resulted in a reduced cycle cancellation rate and treatment burden for poor responders [AMH <0.16 to 0.7 ng/ml (1 to <5 pmol/l)]. A higher fresh clinical pregnancy rate per oocyte retrieval (p < 0.001) was achieved by a profound reduction in excessive response to COS and an increased proportion of fresh ET (vs. agonist co-treatment).

Alternative Approaches and Treatment Protocols using GnRH Antagonists

GnRH antagonists are recently gaining much popularity in COS protocols for normal, high, and poor responder patients. Much work, however, remains to be done in optimizing the antagonist protocols and individualizing them to different patient and cycle characteristics. Several of such recent attempts in poor responder patients are outlined below.

The baseline FSH level is commonly used as an indicator of ovarian reserve and predictor of IVF performance. It is well known that wide inter-cycle fluctuation of baseline hormones occurs in poor responder patients. Because GnRH-ant protocols do not require pituitary desensitization, an unaltered, up-to-date baseline hormonal assessment of ovarian reserve may be obtained during the actual cycle of stimulation. It has been suggested that it is better to start a treatment cycle when baseline FSH levels are low, representing a presumably healthier and large cohort of recruitable follicles during that cycle. A retrospective analysis by Jurema et al. (175) suggests that restricting the initiation of COS with GnRH-ant in poor prognosis patients to cycles in which the day 3 FSH was <8 IU/l would have halved the cycle cancellation rate, and almost tripled the clinical pregnancy rate in this patient population.

One of the problems often seen in poor responding patients is a shortened follicular phase, which limits the ability to recruit a sizable cohort of follicles. Frankfurter et al. (176) described a novel use of a GnRH-ant before ovarian stimulation in an attempt to lengthen the follicular phase, aiming to lengthen the recruitment phase of the cycle to allow for the rescue of more follicles once gonadotropin stimulation was initiated. Twelve patients who previously exhibited a poor response to a standard (long, short, or antagonist) protocol were included. According to the new regimen, patients received two doses of 3 mg of cetrorelix, the first on cycle days 5–8, and the second four days later. With cetrorelix start, medroxyprogesterone acetate (MPA, 10 mg daily) was given and was continued until ovarian suppression was confirmed. Then, a combination of r-hFSH (225 IU SC, twice a day) and recombinant hCG (2.5 mg SC, four times a day) was initiated, and MPA was discontinued to allow for vaginal bleeding. When a lead follicle size of 13 mm was observed, daily cetrorelix (0.25 mg SC) was started and continued until hCG triggering. By using a GnRH-ant in the follicular phase before ovarian stimulation, a significant improvement in oocyte, zygote, and embryo yield was achieved. A trend toward improved implantation (21%), clinical pregnancy (41.7%), and ongoing pregnancy (25%) rates in the follicular GnRH-ant cycle was also noted. More prospective studies are needed to examine the efficacy of this novel therapeutic approach.

Orvieto et al. (177) described the combination of the micro-flare GnRH-a protocol and a GnRH-ant protocol in poor responders. This protocol combines the benefits of the stimulatory effect of the micro-flare on endogenous FSH release with the immediate LH suppression induced by the GnRH-ant, and was therefore suggested as a valuable new tool for treating poor responders (177,178). The stimulation characteristics of 21 consecutive ultrashort GnRH-a/GnRH-ant cycles in 21 patients were compared with their previous failed cycles (177). Triptorelin (100 mcg SC) was started on the first day of menses and continued for three consecutive days, followed by high-dose gonadotropins, which were initiated two days later. Once the lead follicle reached a size of 14 mm or/and E2 levels exceeded 400 pg/ml, cetrorelix (0.25 mg/day) was

Table 46.1 Cycle Characteristics of RCTs Comparing the Long GnRH Agonist and the GnRH Antagonist Protocols in Poor Responder Patients Undergoing IVF

Authors	Inclusion criteria	Number of patients agonist	Number of patients antagonist	Long protocol	Antagonist protocol	Gonadotropin type and dose	Cancellation rate (%)	Stimulation duration (days)	Gonadotropin consumption ampoules or FSH units	No. of oocytes retrieved	Implantation rate (%)	Clinical pregnancy rate started cycle(%)	Ongoing/live birth rate (%)
D'Amato et al. (171)	<3 oocytes retrieved in >2 long agonist cycles or cancelled cycles	60	85	Depot leuprolide, dose not given	Multidose Cetrurelix, flexible	Agonist: rec-FSH, individualized dose; Antagonist: Clomiphene 100mg days 2–6 plus rec-FSH 300 IU	34 GnRH-a 4.8 GnRH-ant		50.05 ± 5.11 GnRH-a 83.48 ± 7.05 GnRH-ant	3.36 ± 1.3 agonist 5.56 ± 1.13 antagonist	7.6 agonist 13.5 antagonist	15.3 agonist 22.2 antagonist	NA
Cheung et al. (174)	<3 mature follicles on previous long protocol or basal FSH >10 IU/L	31	32	Luteal, nasal buserelin 60 mcg daily following OCP	Cetrurelix multiple dose, fixed (S6)	Rec-FSH 300 IU	34.4 GnRH-a 38.7 GnRH-ant	11.5 ± 2.4 GnRH-a 10.5 ± 2.7 GnRH-ant	3445 ± 730 GnRH-a 3150 ± 813 GnRH-ant	5.62 ± 4.17 GnRH-a 5.89 ± 3.02 GnRH-ant	13.3 GnRH-a 13.6 GnRH-ant	9.4 GnRH-a 16.1 GnRH-ant	NA
Marci et al. (173)	<3 oocytes retrieved and E2 max<600 pg/mL on a previous standard long protocol	30	30	Luteal, depot leuprolide 3.75 mg	Cetrurelix, multiple dose, flexible	Rec-FSH 375 IU	13.3 GnRH-a 3.3 GnRH-ant	14.6 ± 1.2 GnRH-a 9.8 ± 0.8 GnRH-ant	72.6 ± 6.8 GnRH-a 49.3 ± 4.3 GnRH-ant	4.3 ± 2.2 GnRH-a 5.6 ± 1.6 GnRH-ant	NA	6.6 GnRH-a 16.6 GnRH-ant	0 GnRH-a 13.3 GnRH-ant
Tazegul et al. (172)	FSH< 13 mIU/mL, E2 max< 500 pg/mL on hCG day, <3 mature follicles, <4 oocytes retrieved	45	44	Luteal leuprolide 1 mg, decreased to 0.5 mg upon downregulation	Cetrurelix/Ganirelix, multiple dose, flexible	Rec-FSH 300 IU and 300 IU hMG	6.8 GnRH-a 9.0 GnRH-ant	12.03 ± 2.86 GnRH-a 10.6 ± 1.63 GnRH-ant	3872.7 ± 1257.1 GnRH-a 2467.7 ± 342.4 GnRH-ant	5.47 ± 2.45 GnRH-a 5.44 ±1.29 GnRH-ant	NA	24.4 GnRH-a 22.7 GnRH-ant	22.2 GnRH-a 18.1 GnRH-ant

Abbreviations: OCP, oral contraceptive pill; hCG, human chorionic gonadotropin; hMG, human menopausal gonadotropin.

introduced and continued up to and including the day of hCG administration. The number of follicles >14mm on the day of hCG administration, number of oocytes retrieved, and number of embryos transferred were all significantly higher in the study protocol as compared with the historic control cycles. A reasonable clinical pregnancy rate (14.3%) was achieved.

Another innovative protocol using GnRH-a/antagonist conversion with estrogen priming (AACEP) in poor responders has been reported by Fisch et al. (179) and is described later in this chapter (section on luteal phase manipulations).

NATURAL AND MODIFIED NATURAL CYCLE

The yield of lengthy high dose and cost stimulation regimens used in poor responders to increase the number of oocytes retrieved is often disappointing. It was therefore suggested to perform natural cycle IVF in such cases, an approach which is less invasive and less costly for the patient.

Terminology

Recently, the International Society for Mild Approaches in Assisted Reproduction (ISMAAR) has recommended revised definitions and terminology for natural cycle IVF and different protocols used in ovarian stimulation for IVF (180). This was the result of the broad inconsistencies existing in the terminology used for definitions and protocols for ovarian stimulation in IVF cycles, as will be later seen in this text. The term natural cycle (NC) IVF should be used when IVF is carried out with oocytes collected from a woman's ovary or ovaries in a spontaneous menstrual cycle without administration of any medication at any time during the cycle. The aim of this cycle is to collect a naturally selected single oocyte at the lowest possible cost. The term modified natural cycle (MNC) should be applied when exogenous hormones or any drugs are used when IVF is being performed during a spontaneous cycle with the aim of collecting a naturally selected single oocyte but with a reduction in chance of cycle cancellation. This could include the following scenarios: (i) The use of hCG to induce final oocyte maturation. Luteal support may/may not be administered. (ii) The administration of GnRH-ant to block the spontaneous LH surge with or without FSH or hMG as add-back therapy. An hCG injection and luteal support are administered.

The above-mentioned terminology has not yet been well incorporated into clinical practice. In all of the following studies presented on NC-IVF, hCG was used for ovulation triggering, and the term MNC is used when a combination of GnRH-ant and gonadotropins is given. In a prospective study with historical controls, Bassil et al. (181) analyzed 11 patients who underwent 16 natural cycles (with hCG administration) for IVF. These were compared with 25 previous failed cycles with poor response in the same patients. The cancellation rate in natural cycles was 18.8% compared with

48% in stimulated cycles. Three ongoing pregnancies were obtained in natural cycles (18.8% per started cycle) compared with none in stimulated cycles. In another prospective study with historical controls, Feldman et al. (182) compared 44 unstimulated IVF cycles in 22 poor responder patients with those of 55 stimulated cycles of the same patients during the 12 months prior to the study. Eighteen (82%) patients had at least one oocyte retrieved, while nine (41%) had at least one cycle with ET. Two (9%) patients each gave birth to a healthy term baby. These results were comparable with those of the stimulated cycles. In a small retrospective study (183), 30 patients who had previously been cancelled because of POR underwent 35 natural cycles, achieving an ongoing pregnancy rate of 16.6% per oocyte retrieval and an implantation rate of 33%. All patients, however, were <40 years of age and had a mean day 3 FSH of 11.1 IU/l.

Similar results were found in an observational study with no controls, in which patients aged 44–47 years were included (184). These patients were recruited based on age only, without prior demonstration of poor response. Out of 48 treatment cycles conducted in 20 women, oocyte retrieval was successful in 22 cycles (46%). Fertilization and cleavage rates of 48% and 100%, respectively, were obtained. One biochemical and one ongoing pregnancy were achieved. Thus, the ongoing pregnancy rate was 5% per patient and 2.08% per cycle.

In addition, Check et al. (185) reported on 259 retrieval cycles and 72 transfers in poor responders using minimal or no gonadotropin stimulation and without GnRH-a or antagonists. These patients were divided into four age groups (<35, 36–39, 40–42, and >43 years) and their mean serum day-3 FSH levels were 19.7, 20.6, 18.8, and 21.9 mIU/ml, respectively. In total, 12 deliveries were achieved after 259 IVF cycles (4.6%). Eliminating the oldest age group, the delivery rate for 47 embryo transfers in women ≤42 years of age was 25.5%. Approximately 50% of retrievals resulted in an embryo (about half were transferred fresh and half frozen). The median number of embryos transferred was one. The implantation rate was 21.6% for the three groups and was 33.3% for patients aged <35 years and 28.6% for women aged 36–39 years. It was concluded that the pregnancies and live births can be achieved in poor prognosis/poor responder patients with elevated basal FSH levels, and age was found to be a more adverse infertility factor than elevated serum FSH.

The only RCT on this topic (186) compared the efficacy of NC IVF with the microdose GnRH-a flare protocol in poor responders. A total of 129 patients who were poor responders in a previous IVF cycle were included: 59 women underwent 114 attempts of NC IVF and 70 women underwent 101 attempts of IVF with COS by microdose agonist flare. In the NC patients, the oocyte retrieval procedure was performed in 114 cycles, and oocytes were found in 88 of these (77.2%). The poor responders treated with NC IVF and those treated with microdose GnRH-a flare showed similar pregnancy rates per cycle and per transfer (6.1% and 14.9% vs. 6.9% and

10.1%, respectively). The women treated with NC IVF showed a statistically significant higher implantation rate (14.9%) compared with controls (5.5%). When subdivided into three groups according to age (≤ 35 years, 36–39 years, and >40 years), younger patients had a better pregnancy rate than the other two groups. It was concluded that in poor responders, NC IVF is at least as effective as COS, especially in younger patients, with a higher implantation rate.

Finally, Papaleo et al. (187) reported on a series of poor psrognosis patients, all of them with AMA, elevated serum FSH, and reduced AFC, who underwent NC IVF. A total of 26 natural cycles in 18 patients were analyzed. Pregnancy was achieved in three patients, of which two patients were ongoing (11.5% per cycle, 20.0% per ET). It was suggested that since the overall pregnancy rates achieved were comparable with those of conventional IVF–ET in poor responders, considering the lower costs and risks and the patient-friendly nature of such protocols, NC IVF can provide an acceptable alternative option for persistent poor responders.

Modified Natural Cycle

The efficacy of natural cycle IVF is hampered by high cancellation rates because of premature LH rise and premature ovulations (188). The possibility of enhancing the efficacy of unstimulated IVF cycles by the concomitant addition of a GnRH-ant and exogenous gonadotropins in the late follicular phase was introduced by Paulson et al. as early as 1994 (189). This protocol, later known as the "modified natural cycle" (MNC), is expected to reduce the rate of premature ovulation and to improve control of gonadotropin delivery to the developing follicle.

In a preliminary report on 44 cycles in 33 young normal responder patients (190), the cancellation rate was 9%, and in 25% of retrievals no oocyte was obtained. ET was performed in 50% of the started cycles, leading to a clinical pregnancy rate of 32.0% per transfer and 17.5% per retrieval, of which five (22.7% per transfer) were ongoing. It was suggested that the MNC could represent a first-choice IVF treatment with none of the complications and risks of current COS protocols, a considerably lower cost, and an acceptable success rate.

Considerable experience with the MNC protocol in the general IVF population has been accumulated by the Dutch group in Groningen (191–193). In a preliminary report, the cumulative ongoing pregnancy rate after three cycles with this protocol was 34% and the live birth rate per patient was 32% (192). Summarizing a much larger experience, the same group (193) later reported on a total of 336 patients who completed 844 cycles (2.5 per patient). The overall ongoing pregnancy rate per started cycle was 8.3% and the cumulative ongoing pregnancy rate after up to three cycles was 20.8% per patient. In a recent report of further follow-up of up to nine cycles (191), a total of 256 patients completed 1048 cycles (4.1 per patient). The ET rate was 36.5% per started cycle. The ongoing pregnancy rate was 7.9% per started cycle and 20.7% per ET. Including treatment-independent

pregnancies, the observed clinical pregnancy rate after up to nine cycles was 44.4% [95% confidence interval (CI) 38.3–50.5] per patient. Pregnancy rates per started cycle did not decline in higher cycle numbers (overall 9.9%), but dropout rates were high (overall 47.8%).

Several studies have been reported on the use of the MNC protocol in poor responders. Kolibianakis et al. (194) evaluated the use of the MNC for IVF in poor responders with an extremely poor prognosis, as a last resort prior to oocyte donation. Thirty-two patients with regular menstrual cycles, basal FSH levels >12 IU/l, and one or more failed IVF cycles with ≤5 oocytes retrieved were included. Recombinant hFSH 100 IU and ganirelix 0.25 mg/day were started concomitantly when a follicle with a mean diameter of 14 mm was identified. hCG was administered as soon as the mean follicular diameter was ≥16 mm. Twenty-five out of 78 cycles performed (32.1%) did not result in oocyte retrieval. In nine out of 53 cycles (16.9%), in which oocyte retrieval was performed, no oocytes were retrieved. ET was performed in 19 out of 44 cycles in which oocytes were retrieved (43.2%), but no ongoing pregnancy was achieved in 78 MNC cycles. It was concluded that the MNC does not offer a realistic chance of live birth in poor prognosis/poor responder patients, when offered as a last resort prior to oocyte donation.

Studies with somewhat more encouraging outcome were also reported. Elizur et al. (195) retrospectively evaluated 540 cycles in 433 poor responders who were divided by treatment protocol into MNC, GnRH-ant, and long agonist groups: There were 52 MNC cycles, 200 GnRH-ant cycles, and 288 long GnRH-a cycles. In the MNC protocol, a GnRH-ant 0.25 mg/day and 2–3 ampoules of hMG were administered daily once the lead follicle reached a diameter of 13 mm. The mean number of oocytes retrieved in the MNC group was significantly lower than in the stimulated antagonist and long agonist groups (1.4 ± 0.5 vs. 2.3 ± 1.1 and 2.5 ± 1.1, respectively, p < 0.05). The respective implantation and pregnancy rates were comparable, 10% and 14.3%, 6.75% and 10.2%, and 7.4% and 10.6%. The number of canceled cycles was significantly higher in the MNC group. Cancellations due to premature luteinization or failure to respond to stimulation were significantly more common in patients aged >40 years. As pregnancy rates were comparable for all groups, it was concluded that the MNC is a reasonable alternative to COS in poor responders.

The only RCT on this issue was performed to investigate the value of MNC–IVF compared with the conventional GnRH-ant cycle in low responders (196). The study population consisted of 90 patients with low response in previous cycles who had undergone 90 IVF cycles. Forty-five patients were randomly allocated into the MNC–IVF protocol and 45 into the GnRH-ant protocol. In the MNC arm, SC injections of 0.25 mg cetrorelix and 150 IU r-hFSH were started concomitantly when the lead follicle reached 13–14 mm in diameter and were continued daily until the day of hCG administration. In the antagonist group patients received a conventional, multiple dose, flexible GnRH-ant protocol with 225 IU of r-hFSH administered daily from cycle day 3. In the MNC group, eight out of 45 cycles initiated (17.8%) had to be cancelled before ET because no oocytes were available. Four out of 45 cycles initiated (8.9%) did not result in oocyte retrieval owing to no follicular development or premature ovulation and no oocytes were found in four out of 41 cycles (9.8%) in which oocyte retrieval was performed. In the antagonist group, 3/45 cycles initiated (6.7%) were cancelled before ET. Despite the difference in cancellation rate between the two groups it was not statistically significant. The numbers of oocytes, mature oocytes, fertilized oocytes, grade 1 or 2 embryos, and embryos transferred were all significantly lower in the MNC group. Gonadotropin requirements and number of days of r-hFSH required for COS were significantly fewer in the MNC group than in the antagonist group. Finally, clinical pregnancy rates per cycle initiated and per ET of the MNC group were similar to those of the antagonist group (13.3% and 17.8%; 16.2% and 19% respectively). Live-birth rates per ET and implantation rates were also comparable between the two groups (13.5% and 16.7%; 12.5% and 9.8%, respectively). It was concluded that the MNC provides comparable pregnancy rates to GnRH antagonist-based COS with lower doses and shorter duration of FSH administration and thus can be a patient-friendly and cost-effective alternative in low responders.

In summary, the option of NC or MNC IVF is a safe, patient friendly treatment with low cost of medication, especially in those who are refractory to COS and decline the option of oocyte donation. Despite the advantages of this approach, its low efficiency has restricted its widespread use. Patients should be fully informed of the advantages and disadvantages of NC or MNC IVF protocols. From the above studies it is evident that the likelihood of retrieving an oocyte is between 45–80%, likelihood of reaching embryo transfer is around 50%, and the likelihood of pregnancy and live birth is between 0–20% (generally around 5%), depending largely on age and ovarian reserve. Younger patients with diminished ovarian reserve (DOR) have a much better prognosis (197). The use of Indomethacin during the late follicular phase has been suggested to decrease the spontaneous ovulation rate and hence provide a higher oocyte retrieval success rate in MNC IVF (197,198).

In addition, it should be also mentioned that in patients undergoing COS, failure to respond to a long or short GnRH-a regimen does not necessarily mean cycle cancellation. Agonist administration can be withdrawn, but gonadotropin stimulation continued. The cycle can be converted either to an antagonist or an MNC regimen, once ovarian response is observed.

The exact role of NC and MNC protocols in patients with DOR has yet to be determined, as are also several key issues that have not yet been subjected to testing such as:

1. Is the MNC protocol superior to the simple NC protocol? No study so far has evaluated these two regimens.
2. What is the best timing for hCG administration and what is the ideal time interval between hCG administration and egg retrieval? Different authors have used different criteria for triggering ovulation. While many authors regard follicle size ≥16 mm as threshold (186,194,199,200) others prefer to administer hCG at 17–18 mm (196), or even ≥18 mm (181,183,195). Segawa et al. (201) prefer the use of GnRH-a for ovulation triggering rather than hCG. While no consensus exists, the best estimate is that early ovulation triggering (i.e., ≥16 mm) is beneficial (202).
3. Are oocyte and embryo quality improved in natural cycles? While there is a common belief that "natural" is better, this assumption has never been directly tested.
4. How many attempts should be made? Schimberni et al. report fairly constant implantation and pregnancy rates through five NC cycles (199). Castelo-Branco et al. (200) have reported a cumulative pregnancy rate of 35.2% after three MNC cycles. The best estimate is that three to five cycles should be offered.
5. What is the role of follicle flushing? While in the general IVF population the use of follicular flushing was abandoned, there are studies suggesting that flushing may improve oocyte yield in poor responders (203–205). Others (206), however, failed to show any beneficial effect.
6. Should cleavage- or blastocyst-stage transfers be performed?
7. Which dose of gonadotropins should be administered in the MNC protocol? Different authors have used doses ranging from 100 IU r-hFSH (194) or 150 IU (200) and up to 225 IU (195). The optimal dose needed to support a single follicle in conjunction with GnRH antagonist administration has not been determined.
8. Should LH be included in the gonadotropin regimen? In patients with POR the addition of LH to the stimulation regimen might be beneficial (207), as will be later discussed.

More research is needed before these questions can be effectively answered.

MANIPULATING ENDOCRINOLOGY

The Role of FSH

Inherent biological mechanisms such as follicle sensitivity to FSH and pharmacodynamics of drug metabolism or receptor interaction (208) may affect the individual ovarian response to stimulation. Recent genetic and pharmacogenomic research has revealed other factors that may facilitate improved cycle management.

FSH secreted from the pituitary is a heterodimer glycoprotein hormone with two covalently linked subunits, alfa and beta. The molecule is glycosylated by posttranslational modification, and the presence and composition of the carbohydrate glycan moieties determine its in vivo biological activity (Fig. 46.5) (209,210). In vivo, the native FSH hormone consists of a family of at least 20 different isohormones that differ in their pattern of glycosylation.

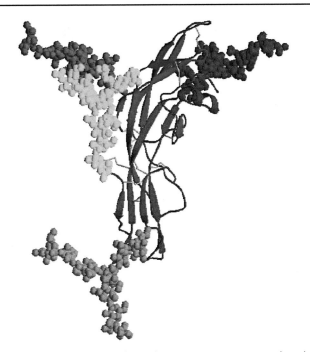

Figure 46.5 Follicle-stimulating hormone (FHS) is a complex gly-coprotein with two noncovalently associated alfa and beta protein subunits. Two oligosaccharides are linked to each protein subunit. (Molecular model created by Merck Serono Reproductive Biology Unit, USA.)

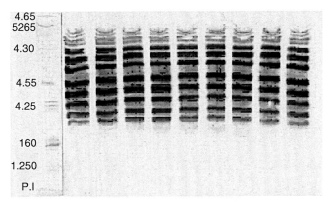

Figure 46.6 Isoelectric focusing (IEF) gel showing the follicle-stimulating hormone (FSH) isoform pattern of nine batches of follitropin-alfa filled by mass (GONAL-f). First lane pI markers, lanes 2–10, nine batches of follitropin-alfa. *Source*: Reproduced from Ref. 211 with permission.

For follitropin-alfa, isoelectric focusing has identified seven major bands of FSH isoforms between pI 4.2 and 5.05, five minor bands between pI 5.25 and 6.30, and one minor band at pI 4.20. These have been demonstrated to be consistent between different manufactured batches (Fig. 46.6) (211). The ovarian response to stimulation by FSH relies on an interaction of the hormone with membrane receptors (FSHR) on GCs, and a normal response is dependent on correct molecular structure of the hormone, the receptor, and factors associated with their interaction. Any defect in the genes encoding FSH or its receptor may result in ovarian resistance, and therefore genotype may play a fundamental role in determining the physiological response to FSH stimulation.

The FSHR is a member of the family of G-protein receptors linked to adenyl cyclase signaling, with extensive extracellular ligand-binding domains. The gene encoding the FSHR is located on the short arm of chromosome 2, and is made up of 2085 nucleotides that translate into a polypeptide with 695 amino acids. This molecule has four potential N-linked glycosylation sites located at amino acids 191, 199, 293, and 318. Mutations in the receptor gene can result in amino acid changes that affect function, and mutations that result in complete FSH resistance (212) as well as partial loss of FSHR function have been identified (213). Screening different populations for mutations of the FSHR gene have shown that single nucleotide polymorphisms can be identified, and two discrete polymorphisms have been studied: (1) position 307 (Ala or Thr) in the extracellular domain, and (2) position 680 (Asn or Ser) in the intracellular domain. Both polymorphic sites give rise to two discrete allelic variants of the FSHR, i.e., Thre307/Asn680 and

Ala307/Ser680. There is an association between these polymorphisms and ovarian response in patients undergoing ART (214,215), and their frequency may vary among different ethnic groups. Women with the Ser/Ser polymorphism at position 680 have an increased total menstrual cycle length and time from luteolysis to ovulation compared with Asn/Asn controls (216). This Ser/Ser genotype occurs less frequently in Asian women than in Caucasians (Table 46.2).

In a Korean IVF patient population, Jun et al. (215) grouped 263 young patients according to their FSHR genotype, and found that basal FSH levels differed between the groups. The Ser/Ser (p.N680S) homozygous group required higher total doses of gonadotropins to achieve multiple follicular development compared with the other two groups (Asn/Asn and Asn/Ser at position 680). Additionally, significantly fewer oocytes were recovered in patients with the Ser/Ser FSHR genotype.

Perez Mayorga et al. (214) also suggest that the FSHR genotype plays a fundamental role in determining the physiological response to FSH stimulation, and that subtle differences in FSHR might fine-tune the action of FSH in the ovary. In a study conducted in 161 ovulatory young (<40 years) women who underwent IVF treatment, a wide variation in the number of ampoules of FSH required to achieve an adequate response was observed. They confirmed that this observation could be correlated with the patient's FSHR genotype, i.e., type of polymorphism.

Behre et al. (217) also carried out an RCT to further investigate this observation, and found that the Ser/Ser (p.N680S) homozygous group results in lower E2 levels following FSH stimulation. This lower FSHR sensitivity could be overcome by higher FSH doses in the trial patients.

Achrekar et al. have shown that the AA genotype at the −29 position in the 5′-untranslated region of the FSHR gene may be associated with the poor ovarian response to COS (218). Women with the AA genotype required a large total dose of exogenous FSH and only low numbers of preovulatory follicles were produced and oocytes retrieved. In addition, E2 levels on the day of hCG administration were significantly lower in women with the AA versus GA genotypes.

Table 46.2 The Frequency of the FSH Receptor Polymorphism at p.N680S in Published Reports

Author	Ethnic origin	Patient number (diagnosis)	SNP680		
			Asn/Asn (%)	Asn/Ser (%)	Ser/Ser (%)
Perez Mayorga et al. (214)	Caucasian	161 (male/tubal)	29%	45%	26%
Sudo et al. (375)	Japanese	522 (mixed)	41%	46.9%	12.1%
Laven et al. (376)	Caucasian	148(anovulatory)	16%	44%	40%
Laven et al. (376)	Caucasian	30 (ovulatory)	23%	61%	16%
De Castro et al. (377)	Caucasian	102(male/tubal/both)	31.4%	50%	18.6%
Daelemans et al. (378)	Caucasian	99 (non-IVF control)	38%	45%	17%
Daelemans et al. (378)	Caucasian	130 (mixed?)	24%	51%	25%
Daelemans et al. (378)	Caucasian	37 (mixed–OHSS)	16%	54%	32%
Choi et al. (379)	Korean	172 (mixed, non-PCOS)	41.9%	47.7%	10.5%
Schweickhardt 2004–unpublished thesis	Not stated (USA)	663 (mixed)	30.6%	48.7%	20.7%

The Ser/Ser (p.N680S) homozygous group is generally lower in Asian populations than in Caucasian populations.
Abbreviation: OHSS, ovarian hyperstimulation syndrome; PCOS, polycystic ovarian syndrome.

In recent years, there has been a paradigm shift in the use of gonadotropins. The outdated "one size fits all" approach to fertility treatment has been superseded by individualized COS (219,220). Individualized COS is designed to maximize the efficacy and safety for each patient, and is discussed more fully in Chapters 35 and 40.

Accordingly, an analysis was undertaken to assess whether specific factors could optimally predict a response to stimulation in ART, and then to develop a corresponding treatment algorithm that could be used to calculate the optimal starting dose of r-hFSH (follitropin-alfa) for selected patients (56). Backward stepwise regression modeling indicated that in ART patients <35 years ($N = 1378$) who were treated with r-hFSH monotherapy, predictive factors for ovarian response included basal FSH, BMI, age, and number of follicles <11mm at baseline screening. The concordance probability index was 59.5% for this model. Using these four predictive factors, a follitropin-alfa starting dose calculator was developed that could be used to select the FSH starting dose required for an optimal response. A prospective cohort study has been completed using this r-hFSH starting dose calculator and demonstrated a similar number of oocytes and pregnancy rates across the doses used (221).

Taken together, these studies suggest that, in the future, it might be possible to tailor FSH therapy to the patient's genetic background, and thereby adjust the doses and the timing of stimulation. This would be of particular benefit in the treatment of older women, who cannot afford any delay in their race against the biological clock.

The Role of LH

Ovulation induction studies in hypogonadotropic women using r-hFSH have demonstrated that FSH can induce follicular growth to the preovulatory stage, but E2 and androstenedione concentrations remain extremely low (222,223). This suggests that follicular maturation depends on the action of LH to stimulate androstenedione

biosynthesis as a substrate for aromatase activity. Below a minimal level of LH, follicular development will plateau – this has been observed in patients with profound pituitary downregulation after GnRH-a depot (224,225). In women with hypogonadotropic hypogonadism, E2 concentrations may be inadequate for cytoplasmic maturation of the follicle, endometrial proliferation, and corpus luteum function (222,223).

Adequate folliculogenesis and steroidogenesis required for successful fertilization and implantation therefore depend upon a certain threshold level of LH. Although the amount of LH necessary for normal follicle and oocyte development is not known, it is likely to be very low, since a maximal steroidogenic response can be elicited when <1% of follicular LH receptors are occupied (226). On this basis, resting levels of LH (1–10 IU/l) should be sufficient to provide maximal stimulation of thecal cells (227). There is also evidence that excessive levels of LH can have an adverse effect on follicular development (228), associated with impaired fertilization and pregnancy rates, as well as higher miscarriage rates, the so-called "ceiling" effect (Fig. 46.7). LH levels must be below this ceiling for the LH-dependent phase of development to proceed normally. It seems that there is a clinical therapeutic window (229,230): "Low-dose" treatment with LH generally enhances steroidogenesis, but "high-dose" treatment can enhance progesterone synthesis, suppress aromatase activity, and inhibit cell growth.

Huirne et al. (231) administered different GnRH-ant doses to five groups of patients and measured the subsequent change in LH levels between the groups. The aim of this study was to deliberately induce different LH levels, and assess the effect of an LH range on IVF outcome to estimate what the optimal level might be. No pregnancies were observed in relation to either very high or very low LH, suggesting an optimal window. However, their data led them to conclude that not the absolute levels, but instead excessive changes in LH – either increases or

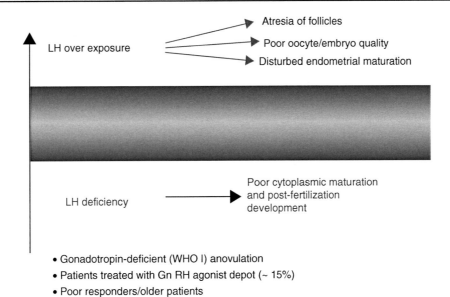

Figure 46.7   The LH therapeutic window concept. *Abbreviations*: LH, luteinizing hormone; GnRH, gonadotropin-releasing hormone.

decreases – were the more significant parameter. They suggest that the correct sequence of stages in oocyte maturation, together with synchrony between nuclear and cytoplasmic maturation, is dependent upon an appropriate endocrine milieu. Excessive fluctuations in LH levels might disrupt this balance, as well as affect maturation of the endometrium – i.e., stable and appropriate LH levels are needed during IVF cycles. It is possible that specific patient groups, such as those with PCOS or DOR may be prone to larger changes in LH levels and sensitive to high fluctuations. In addition, serum LH levels assayed by immunoassay do not necessarily reflect circulating LH bioactivity, particularly in these specific patient groups.

A common variant of the LH gene is recognized (Trp8Arg and Ile15Thr of the beta subunit) that encodes a protein with altered in vitro and in vivo activity (232). It has been suggested that this variant may be less effective at supporting FSH-stimulated multifollicular growth, resulting in suboptimal ovarian response to standard COS regimens and higher drug consumption (233). An increased prevalence of this gene has been reported in Japanese patients with infertility (234) and premature ovarian failure (235), and it has been postulated that women with this gene variant could benefit from exogenous LH supplementation during COS (11).

The initial availability of a pure recombinant human LH (r-hLH) (Luveris®, Merck Serono International, Geneva, Switzerland) preparation has provided a new tool that allows the endocrinology of ovarian stimulation to be examined more accurately. This has been followed by the recent commercial availability of a combination r-hFSH/r-hLH (2:1 ratio) preparation (Pergoveris®, Merck Serono International, Geneva, Switzerland) indicated for use in women with severe gonadotropin deficiency. The use of r-hLH in COS protocols has been recently reviewed (236). A clear relationship between the dose of r-hLH and serum E2 has been found in hypogonadotropic patients

(237). The optimal LH levels required to provide the best results in IVF are still a matter of debate, and a number of studies have tried to assess the role of LH supplementation in GnRH-a and GnRH antagonist cycles.

LH supplementation may have an effect via intraovarian mechanisms that affect steroid biosynthesis, and therefore oocyte maturation. Foong et al. (238) recently conducted a study that included patients who showed an inadequate response to r-hFSH-only stimulation, and reported that although peak E2 levels were similar to those found in normal responders, intrafollicular E2 levels were significantly lower, and progesterone was significantly higher in poor responders to FSH. E2 plays an important role in human oocyte cytoplasmic maturation in vitro (239), as manifested by improved fertilization and cleavage rates. hGH has also been shown to stimulate E2 production by follicular cells (240,241). High intrafollicular E2 concentrations in the preovulatory follicle predict an increased chance of pregnancy (242). On the other hand, androstenedione can irreversibly block the effect of E2 (243), and it is clear that maintaining an appropriate steroid balance within the follicle is very important. In the ovine, E2 is associated with an upregulation of oocyte DNA repair enzymes (244). In the rhesus monkey, adding an aromatase inhibitor during the late stages of follicular development, just prior to the period of ovulation, resulted in a reduced capacity of the oocyte to mature, and a reduced rate of fertilization in vitro (245). Overall, it seems that LH may have a beneficial effect through a mechanism that improves oocyte cytoplasmic maturation (increasing mitochondrial function and/or upregulating DNA repair enzymes), either through E2 or some other intraovarian factor. However, an additional effect on the endometrium itself cannot be excluded.

A number of further studies have examined the effect of LH supplementation in poor responders (246) or patients who respond inadequately to FSH stimulation

(224,225,247). Following stratification of the data, a subset of patients aged ≥35 years has been identified, who seem to benefit from LH supplementation in terms of an increased number of mature oocytes retrieved and improved implantation and pregnancy rates. This benefit was maintained even when LH supplementation was initiated from stimulation day 6 or 8. This seems logical in terms of physiology, as the GCs, through FSH stimulation, acquire LH receptors only after the follicle reaches a diameter of at least 11 mm (248). In hyporesponsive women, the need for higher FSH doses might be an individual biological index of LH deficiency, with an effect on oocyte competence.

A requirement for LH supplementation to achieve good ovarian response and follicular maturation in patients of AMA could be based on a number of theoretical explanations. With age and the onset of the menopause, endogenous LH as well as FSH levels increase and testosterone levels decrease (249,250). The number of functional LH receptors also decreases with age (251). Kim et al. (252) found that the best predictor of ovarian reserve (reproductive age) in normally cycling women was the combination of the FSH and LH levels on menstrual cycle day 1. There is also evidence that endogenous LH may be less biologically active or potent than it should be, or the immunologic LH many not be comparable to the biologically active LH (253,254). Overall, this could result in an increasing ovarian resistance to LH-mediated events.

It has been suggested that follicular recruitment in women >38 years can be improved by supplementing r-hFSH stimulation with LH-containing preparations (255,256). Since hMG contains hCG and a number of unknown contaminating proteins in addition to FSH and LH, Gomez-Palomares et al. (257) conducted a prospective randomized cohort study comparing the effects of hMG with r-hLH supplementation in a group of women 38–40 years to determine whether LH is the hMG component that favors early follicular recruitment. The patients were randomly assigned to one of two groups: 58 patients received r-hFSH 225 plus hMG (one ampoule), and 36 were treated with r-hFSH 225 plus r-hLH 75 until day 6. Follicular recruitment was evaluated on day 6, and stimulation was continued with r-hFSH alone, without further hMG or r-hLH. Both groups recruited a similar number of follicles after five days of stimulation, but the r-hLH group showed a significant increase in the number of metaphase II oocytes retrieved, and higher clinical pregnancy rate (47% vs. 26%; NS).

In a group of patients representing about 10–15% of young women, ovarian response to COS using r-hFSH in GnRH-a protocols is suboptimal (rather than poor), despite the presence of normal circulating FSH and/or LH levels (258). Such patients have normal follicular development up to cycle days 5–7, but this response plateaus on days 8–10. As described previously, suboptimal ovarian response to FSH may be due to an LH-beta variant polymorphism (259), or due to polymorphic variants of the FSH receptor (208,260). Early evidence suggests that LH supplementation may improve outcomes in patients with suboptimal response to FSH stimulation

(224,246,247). Lisi et al. showed a significant improvement in fertilization and clinical pregnancy rates with the addition of r-hLH to r-hFSH in women who required high doses of r-hFSH in previous cycles (246). Ferraretti et al. demonstrated that supplementation from the mid-to-late stimulation phase with r-hLH but not hMG was associated with significantly improved implantation and clinical pregnancy rates in patients who responded inadequately to FSH-only stimulation (247). This is an interesting category of ART patients and it seems that such a response may be more common in a GnRH-a depot regimen (224,225). de Placido and colleagues also described the beneficial use of r-hLH supplementation administered following the occurrence of a plateau in E2 secretion and a lack of continued follicle growth around day 7 of FSH stimulation (224,225).

Several studies have also supported the need for additional LH in poor responders when short and long protocols of GnRH agonists are used (261–263). From such studies, it has been theorized that ovarian stimulation in patients with diminished ovarian reserve may be enhanced by the LH-induced production of E2 precursors such as androstenedione.

Because of the sudden and often dramatic inhibition of LH secretion associated with the use of GnRH-ant, there has been interest in the potential need for exogenous LH supplementation. A recent meta-analysis of data on 1764 women (aged 18–39 years) from six RCTs showed that the amount of endogenous LH during GnRH-ant protocols was sufficient to support r-hFSH in COS prior to IVF or ICSI (264). No association between endogenous LH level and pregnancy rate in normogonadotropic women was found (264).

There is, however, a paucity of data on the potential use of LH supplementation in poor responders or patients with AMA undergoing COS using a GnRH-ant protocol. In a retrospective cohort study (265), 240 GnRH-ant cycles in poor responders were evaluated. Of 153 that reached the stage of oocyte retrieval, 75 patients received r-hFSH for ovarian stimulation, and 66 received hMG in combination with r-hFSH. In patients aged <40 years, there were no significant differences between treatment groups in the amount and duration of treatment, number of oocytes retrieved, and number of embryos. In patients aged ≥40 years, significantly fewer oocytes were retrieved in patients who received exogenous LH in their stimulation, resulting in significantly fewer fertilized embryos. Implantation and clinical pregnancy rates did not differ by treatment group. It was concluded that outcomes in poor responders undergoing IVF with GnRH-ants are comparable whether COS is performed with or without supplementary LH.

Similar results from an RCT using a GnRH-a flare-up protocol were reported by Barrenetxea et al. (266) Patients (n = 84) who had a basal FSH level of >10 mIU/ml, were aged >40 years, and undergoing their first IVF cycle, were randomly allocated into two study groups: Group A, in which ovarian stimulation included GnRH-a flare-up and r-hFSH and r-hLH; and group B, in which patients received no LH. The overall pregnancy rate was 22.6%. The pregnancy wastage rate was 30.0% in group A and 22.2% in group B. There were no differences in the ongoing pregnancy rate per retrieval and implantation rate per ET. The duration of stimulation, E2 level on hCG administration day, number of developed follicles, number of retrieved oocytes, number of normally fertilized zygotes, cumulative embryo score, and number of transferred embryos were all comparable for the two groups. It was concluded that the addition of r-hLH at a given time of follicular development produces no further benefit in poor responder patients stimulated with the short protocol, and a reduced ovarian response cannot be overcome by changes in the COS protocol.

Very recently, Hill et al. (207) conducted a systematic review and meta-analysis in order to evaluate the effect of r-hLH in ART cycles in patients of AMA. All published RCTs comparing r-hLH plus r-hFSH versus r-hFSH only in patients 35 years and older undergoing assisted reproduction were evaluated. Seven trials were identified that met inclusion criteria and comprised 902 cycles. In a fixed effect model, implantation rate was higher in the r-hLH-supplemented group (odds ratio 1.36, 95% confidence interval 1.05–1.78). Similarly, clinical pregnancy was increased in the r-hLH-supplemented group (odds ratio 1.37, 95% confidence interval 1.03–1.83) (Fig. 46.8). It was concluded that the addition of r-hLH to ART cycles may improve implantation and clinical pregnancy in patients of AMA.

In summary, the addition of LH to the COS regimen of poor responders remains controversial. This is probably because of the heterogeneity of the patient population so far studied. Future large-scale studies with a prospective randomized design in well-defined patient subgroups are needed to define the circumstances under which LH supplementation could be beneficial.

The Role of Androgens

The human follicle has internal (granulosa) and external (theca) cell layers, and folliculogenesis is regulated by endocrine and paracrine factors that interact within a microenvironment; steroidogenesis is coordinated by the two different cell types (Fig. 46.9). Pituitary LH acts on theca cells through surface receptors to promote androgen synthesis in the early follicular phase, and FSH acts through membrane-associated GC receptors to promote their proliferation and differentiation. GCs then express an aromatase enzyme system that catalyzes the conversion of androgens to estrogen (267). For normal folliculogenesis to continue, adequate levels of bioavailable estrogen are needed, and paracrine signaling activated by FSH and LH (steroids, cytokines, and other growth factors) sustains growth and estrogen secretion as the follicle develops. Theca cell enzyme activity is increased to enhance androgen production, thus contributing further to estrogen synthesis within the follicle. FSH also stimulates GC LH receptor expression in the late follicular phase, so that they become receptive to LH stimulation. Larger follicles with GC LH receptors continue to grow, and LH can then also stimulate the GC aromatase system. FSH and LH together stimulate GCs to produce inhibin, which has a synergistic effect on theca cells to further promote androgen synthesis.

Androgens are synthesized in thecal cells through cell-specific expression of P450C17alpha (CYP17), which is under LH control, and GCs express androgen receptors (AR) throughout antral development. During the late stages of follicle development prior to ovulation, transcription of the granulosa AR gene and AR protein levels decline, so that GC responsiveness to gonadotropins is diminished. This mechanism could delay terminal differentiation until the LH surge signals the onset of ovulation, when the cells begin to switch their steroid synthesis to progesterone for the luteal phase.

The rate-limiting step in androgen synthesis, conversion of cholesterol to pregnenolone, occurs within theca cells, and close cooperation between the two types of somatic cells ensures that sufficient E2 is produced during oocyte maturation (238). In the primate ovary, androgens stimulate early stages of follicular growth (268), and primate experiments indicate that androgens may influence the responsiveness of ovaries to gonadotropins. In rhesus monkeys, treatment with dihydrotestosterone or testosterone (T) augments follicular FSHR

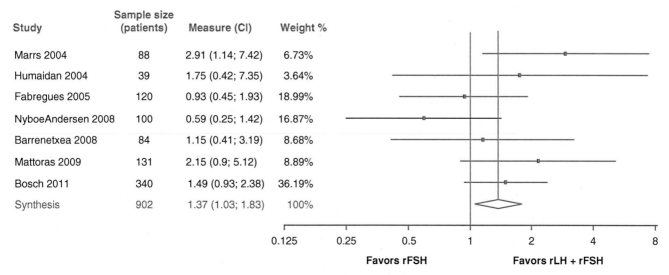

Study	Sample size (patients)	Measure (CI)	Weight %
Marrs 2004	88	2.91 (1.14; 7.42)	6.73%
Humaidan 2004	39	1.75 (0.42; 7.35)	3.64%
Fabregues 2005	120	0.93 (0.45; 1.93)	18.99%
NyboeAndersen 2008	100	0.59 (0.25; 1.42)	16.87%
Barrenetxea 2008	84	1.15 (0.41; 3.19)	8.68%
Mattoras 2009	131	2.15 (0.9; 5.12)	8.89%
Bosch 2011	340	1.49 (0.93; 2.38)	36.19%
Synthesis	902	1.37 (1.03; 1.83)	100%

Figure 46.8 Comparison of clinical pregnancy rate in patients of AMA undergoing COS using r-hFSH plus r-hLH and r-hFSH alone (207).

expression in GCs, promotes initiation of primordial follicle growth, and increases the number of growing preantral and small antral follicles. These studies strongly suggest that androgen treatment may amplify the effects of FSH on the ovary. Hillier and Tetsuka (136) confirmed that T enhances FSH-induced GC gene expression, and that androgens also exert a paracrine effect in the early follicular phase (269).

Hugues and Cédrin-Durnerin (270) have recently reviewed the role of androgens in fertility treatment. They suggest that androgen status should be more carefully

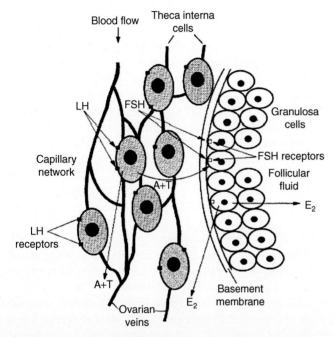

Figure 46.9 Schematic diagram of the "two cells–two gonadotropins theory," which interacts to produce estradiol (E2). Luteinizing hormone (LH) acts on the theca cells, which produce androgens. Through follicle-stimulating hormone (FSH) stimulation, granulosa cell aromatase converts androgens into E2. *Abbreviations*: A, Androstenedione; T, Testosterone.

assessed prior to treatment. Thus, androgens might have two separate roles:

1. During early follicle growth before the follicle becomes sensitive to gonadotropins (reducing apoptosis?)
2. Enhancing FSH action during the early gonadotropin-sensitive phase of follicular growth.

In premenopausal cycling women, circulating T is derived from direct secretion by the ovary and adrenal, and from conversion of precursors such as androstenedione (Fig. 46.10). Testosterone circulates in three forms: free, bound to albumin, and bound to sex hormone-binding globulin (SHBG). The free and albumin-bound fractions are believed to be bioavailable, and the fraction bound to SHBG is thought to be unavailable for action in the periphery. With increasing age, androgen levels in women decline significantly (271,272).

Frattarelli et al. (273) evaluated androgen levels in 43 normo-ovulatory women before IVF treatment, and observed that patients who had a low level of T after downregulation (<20 ng/dl) required a higher FSH dose, a longer duration of stimulation, and were less likely to achieve a pregnancy than patients with higher baseline T levels.

Barbieri et al. (274) investigated the association of BMI, age, and cigarette smoking with serum T levels in women undergoing IVF. They observed that T levels decreased significantly with advancing age, and suggest that this may be because LH stimulation of ovarian androgen secretion begins to decline during the decade of the 30s. This effect occurs before a decline in ovarian estrogen secretion, possibly due to the fact that a compensatory increase in FSH with ovarian aging at 35–45 years maintains ovarian estrogen secretion but does not maintain ovarian androgen secretion. They also found a positive correlation between serum T and the number of oocytes retrieved; advancing age and

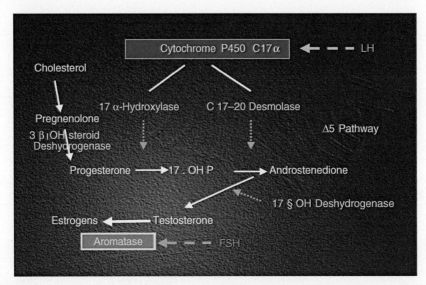

Figure 46.10 Steroid biosynthesis in the human ovary; the Δ5 pathway predominates in the follicle for estrogen synthesis. *Abbreviation*: FSH, follicle-stimulating hormone.

years of cigarette smoking were associated with a decreased number of oocytes.

GnRH-a administration during ART treatment cycles reduces the level of circulating LH, and therefore the amount or bioactivity of aromatizable androgen substrate available for FSH-induced E2 synthesis is reduced. It is therefore suggested that in women with diminished ovarian reserve who undergo ART treatment, boosting intraovarian androgens might increase the number of follicles available to enter the recruitment stage, as well as the process of follicle recruitment itself. Three different strategies have been proposed:

1. Stimulating theca cells with r-hLH prior to r-hFSH stimulation in the long agonist protocol.
2. Testosterone or dehydroepiandrosterone (DHEA) supplementation prior to gonadotropin stimulation.
3. Blocking intraovarian androgen conversion with the use of an aromatase enzyme inhibitor.

Pretreatment with r-hLH

Normogonadotropic women ($n = 146$) were treated in a long depot GnRH-a protocol and were randomized to receive r-hLH (Luveris, 300 IU/day) for a fixed seven days, or no r-hLH treatment. This was followed by a standard r-hFSH stimulation regimen (GONAL-f®, Merck Serono SA, Geneva, Switzerland, 150 IU/day). Pretreatment with r-hLH was associated with an increase in small antral follicles prior to FSH stimulation ($p = 0.007$), and an increased yield of normally fertilized (2 PN) embryos ($p = 0.03$) (275).

Androgen Supplementation

Androgens might have two separate roles in enhancing follicular recruitment and function: 1. During early follicle growth, before the follicles reach gonadotropin sensitivity. Clinical applications of androgens targeted at these stages would require a protracted course. One example is supplementation with DHEA. 2. Enhancing FSH action during the early gonadotropin-sensitive phase of follicular growth. This would require a relatively short treatment approach, and would lead to improved function rather than increased follicular numbers, as the number of antral follicles present has been determined by other, preceding, factors. Examples for short course treatment include supplementation with T and blocking androgen conversion to estrogen with aromatase inhibitors.

Testosterone   Massin et al. (276) treated poor responders with transdermal T application for 15 days prior to FSH stimulation. Testosterone gel application resulted in a significant increase in plasma T levels but did not significantly improve the AFC. Furthermore, after gel application, the main parameters of ovarian response (numbers of preovulatory follicles, total and mature oocytes, and embryos) did not sig-

nificantly differ between T and placebo-treated patients. It was concluded that no significant beneficial effects of androgen administration on ovarian response to FSH can be demonstrated.

Balasch et al. (73) investigated the usefulness of T pretreatment in poor responders. In a prospective, therapeutic, self-controlled clinical trial, 25 consecutive infertile patients who had a background of the first and second IVF treatment cycle cancellations due to poor follicular response, in spite of vigorous gonadotropin ovarian stimulation and having normal basal FSH levels, were included. In their third IVF attempt, all patients received transdermal T treatment (20 mcg/kg per day) during the five days preceding gonadotropin treatment. Twenty patients (80%) showed an increase of over fivefold in the number of recruited follicles, produced 5.8 oocytes, received two or three embryos, and achieved a clinical pregnancy rate of 30% per oocyte retrieval. There were 20% cancelled cycles. It was concluded that pretreatment with transdermal T may be a useful approach for women known to be poor responders but having normal basal FSH concentrations.

Further evidence of a potentially beneficial effect of T was recently provided by Kim et al. in an RCT of 110 poor responders to COS (277). Poor responders were defined as patients who failed to produce three follicles with a mean diameter of ≥16 mm, leading to the retrieval of ≤3 oocytes, despite the use of a high gonadotropin dose (>2,500 IU) in a previous failed IVF/ICSI cycle. Transdermal T gel, 12.5 mg, was applied daily for 21 days in the cycle preceding COS. Testosterone pretreatment significantly increased the numbers of oocytes retrieved, mature oocytes, fertilized oocytes, and good-quality embryos versus the control group. Embryo implantation rate and clinical pregnancy rate per started cycle were also significantly higher in the women pretreated with T gel.

DHEA   Casson et al. (278) postulated that DHEA administration to poor responders might augment the effect of gonadotropin stimulation, via a paracrine effect mediated by insulin-like growth factor I (IGF-I). In a preliminary small series of five patients (<41 years) with documented poor response to high doses of gonadotropins, DHEA was administered orally (80 mg/day) for two months, and continued during ovarian stimulation prior to intrauterine insemination (IUI). After two months of treatment, all patients showed increased serum androgen and E2 levels during the stimulation cycle, and all had an improved response to stimulation by approximately twofold, even after controlling for gonadotropin dose. One of the patients delivered twins after IUI.

This preliminary report was extended by several publications reported primarily by Gleicher, Barad, and their colleagues (279–285). The initiative for the use of DHEA was an unusual case report (281) on a 42.7-year-old woman with presumed severe DOR who requested embryo banking. This patient underwent serial COS cycles with concomitant use of DHEA dietary supplementation as well as acupuncture. In her first treatment cycle, peak E2 was 1211 pmol/mL. After seven months of DHEA supplementation, her peak E2 in cycle 8 was >18,000 pmol/mL. Because of fear of hyperstimulation her gonadotropin dose was reduced by 25%. The patient had undergone nine treatment cycles while continuously and dramatically improving her ovarian response and banking of 66 embryos overall. Subsequently, the effect of DHEA supplementation on fertility outcomes among women with DOR was evaluated in a case–control study (280). Twenty-five women with significant DOR had one IVF cycle before and after DHEA treatment, with otherwise identical hormonal stimulation. Women received 75 mg of DHEA daily for an average of 17.6 ± 2.1 weeks. Paired analysis of IVF cycle outcomes before and after DHEA supplementation, demonstrated significant increases in fertilized oocytes, normal day-3 embryos, embryos transferred, and average embryo scores per oocyte after DHEA treatment. This study supported the previously reported beneficial effects of DHEA supplementation on ovarian function in women with diminished ovarian reserve.

Another case–control study from the same group (279) included 190 women with DOR. The study group included 89 patients who used supplementation with 75 mg/day of oral, micronized DHEA for up to four months prior to entry into IVF. The definition of DOR was based on age-specific FSH concentrations. The control group comprised 101 couples who received infertility treatment but did not use DHEA. Cumulative clinical pregnancy rates were significantly higher in the study group (28.4% vs. 11.9%; $p < 0.05$).

Data from the same group also suggest improvement in ovarian function and oocyte and embryo quality following DHEA supplementation. This is reflected by: (i) An increase in AMH levels in patients with DOR in parallel with the duration of DHEA use (285), (ii) Significantly lower miscarriage rates in women who had used DHEA compared with those rates reported in the National US IVF database (283), (iii) A lower rate of embryonic aneuploidy as detected by preimplantation genetic screening (284). A recent review by Gleicher and Barad summarizes the experience with DHEA supplementation suggesting that DHEA improves ovarian function, increases pregnancy chances, and by reducing aneuploidy, lowers miscarriage rates (282). The authors further comment that DHEA may represent a first agent beneficially affecting aging ovarian environments.

In another self-controlled study from Turkey, Sonmezer et al. (286) compared the IVF performance of 19 women with POR before and after DHEA supplementation. The definition of POR was a history of cycle cancellation due to low E2 levels (<130 pg/ml) on the sixth day of cycle or on the hCG day (<450 pg/ml) or <4 retrieved oocytes. After 90–180 days of DHEA supplementation, these patients had an increased number of follicles (3 ± 0.7 vs. 1.9 ± 1.3, $p < 0.05$) and metaphase II oocytes (4 ± 1.8 vs. 2.1 ± 1.8, $p < 0.05$), an increased number of day 3 high quality embryos (1.9 ± 0.8 vs.0.7 ± 0.6, $p < 0.05$) as well as higher pregnancy rates (47.4% vs. 10.5%, $p < 0.01$).

Wiser et al. (287) reported the results of the only RCT published so far on the use of DHEA in patients with POR. A total of 33 women received either DHEA 75 mg/day before and during IVF (n = 17), or no supplementation (n = 16). The long GnRH-a protocol was used for COS, and up to two cycles per patient (total 51 cycles) were carried out. The DHEA group demonstrated a nonsignificant improvement in E2 levels on day of hCG (p = 0.09) and improved embryo quality during treatment (p = 0.04) between first and second cycles. Patients in the DHEA group also had a significantly higher live birth rate compared with controls (23.1% vs. 4.0%; p = 0.05), respectively. It was concluded that DHEA supplementation can have a beneficial effect on ovarian reserve for poor responder patients undergoing IVF.

It should be mentioned, however, that despite of all the encouraging data presented above, the current level of evidence on the effectiveness of DHEA is rather low and insufficient, and DHEA supplementation is therefore under an intense ongoing debate. There is a lack of well powered and designed RCTs, and there are many methodological problems associated with most of the studies that have been published so far (288,289). In addition, in many countries DHEA is sold as a food supplement without prescription, and even in countries where a prescription is necessary, DHEA is produced in a variety of formulations by many manufacturers without clear data or control on its biologic activity (290). Therefore, currently, the efficacy of DHEA supplementation in patients with POR awaits confirmation by more data and high quality evidence.

Blocking Intraovarian Androgen Conversion

Aromatase inhibitors were initially approved to suppress estrogen levels in postmenopausal women with breast cancer. They inhibit the enzyme by competitive binding to the heme of the cytochrome P450 subunit, blocking androgen conversion into estrogens so that there is a temporary accumulation of intraovarian androgens. Mitwally and Casper (291) were first to show that aromatase inhibition improves ovarian response to FSH in poor responder patients undergoing COS and IUI. Garcia-Velasco et al. (292) assessed whether aromatase inhibitors improve ovarian response and IVF outcomes in patients with POR, using an OCP/GnRH-ant protocol. Patients with at least one previously cancelled IVF attempt with ≤4 16-mm follicles received a high-dose gonadotropin regimen supplemented with 2.5 mg letrozole for the first five days of COS (n = 71), or the high-dose gonadotropin regimen alone (n = 76). In this study, letrozole-treated patients showed significantly higher levels of follicular fluid T and androstenedione, and had more oocytes retrieved (6.1 vs. 4.3) and a higher implantation rate (25% vs. 9.4%), despite similar doses of gonadotropins.

In a recent RCT, Ozmen et al. (293) randomized 70 poor-responder patients into two groups. In the study group, letrozole (5 mg/day) was administered along with a fixed dosage (450 IU/day) of r-hFSH, whereas controls were treated with the same r-hFSH dosage alone. A flexible regimen of GnRH-ant was used in both groups. The mean total dose of r-hFSH and serum concentrations of E2 on the day of hCG administration were significantly lower in the letrozole group compared with controls, respectively. The rate of cycle cancellation due to poor ovarian response was lower in the study group (8.6%) than in controls (28.6%), (p < 0.05). The costs of achieving a clinical pregnancy were significantly reduced in the letrozole group, and the clinical pregnancy rates per ET were comparable (25.8% and 20%, in the letrozole group and controls, respectively). It was concluded that adjunctive letrozole administration is beneficial since it reduces both cycle cancellation rate and cycle cost without an adverse effect on outcome.

Lee et al. (294) compared the sequential use of letrozole and hMG with hMG only in poor responders undergoing IVF. Patients (n = 53) with less than four oocytes retrieved in previous IVF cycles or less than five antral follicles were randomized to either letrozole for five days followed by hMG or hMG alone. The letrozole group required a lower dosage of hMG (p < 0.001), had a shorter duration of hMG treatment (p < 0.001) but fewer oocytes retrieved (p = 0.001) when compared with controls. Live-birth rate was comparable with a lower miscarriage rate in the letrozole group (p = 0.038). Serum E2 concentrations were lower in the letrozole group from day 4 until the hCG day (all p < 0.001). Follicular fluid concentrations of testosterone, androstenedione, FSH, and AMH were all significantly increased in the letrozole group.

Studies with less favorable outcome with letrozole use were also reported. In a prospective controlled trial, Schoolcraft et al. (295) compared the efficacy of a microdose GnRH-a flare with a GnRH-ant/letrozole protocol in poor responders. Five hundred thirty-four infertile women classified as past or potential poor responders based on clinic-specific criteria were prospectively assigned to a microdose flare or antagonist/letrozole protocol in a 2:1 ratio, respectively. There were no significant differences in mean age, number of oocytes, fertilization rates, number of embryos transferred, or embryo score. Peak E2 levels were significantly lower in the antagonist/letrozole group. Ongoing pregnancy rates were significantly higher in the microdose flare group (52% vs. 37%). Trends toward increased implantation and lower cancellation rates were also noted, but did not reach statistical significance. In another study involving 94 patients, the administration of letrozole with FSH/hMG in a GnRH-ant protocol resulted in significantly lower implantation and fertilization rates, and significantly lower metaphase II oocytes and top-quality embryos compared with a microdose GnRH-a flare protocol with FSH or hMG (296).

Finally, a meta-analysis of controlled trials of androgen adjuvants, such as T and DHEA, and androgen-modulating agents, such as letrozole, showed no significant difference in the number of oocytes retrieved or pregnancy/live birth rates with androgen supplementation or modulation compared with controls (297). The authors concluded that there was insufficient evidence from the few RCTs performed (n = 9) to support the use of androgen supplementation or modulation to improve live birth outcome in poor responders undergoing IVF or ICSI treatment (297).

A recent review of the current clinical approaches aiming at increasing androgen availability in the ovary has highlighted the conflicting nature of results (298). Therefore, additional studies using proper strategies to achieving higher intraovarian androgen concentrations for longer intervals are required to define the clinical efficiency of androgens in poor responders.

The Role of hGH

The use of hGH in the management of female and male subfertility was reported in the early 1990s (299,300) and there has been a great deal of controversy about its use in patient management since that time. There are substantial data that demonstrate the critical importance of the IGF–IGFBP family (the growth factors IGF-I, IGF-II, and their binding proteins) to follicular development. In particular, IGF-I is GH-dependent and is involved in potentiating the effect of FSH (301,302).

Abir et al. (303) have demonstrated the expression of hGH receptor in human ovaries from fetuses as well as women/girls and of GH in human fetal ovaries. The hGH receptor mRNA is also expressed in human oocytes and throughout preimplantation embryonic development. Mendoza et al. (304) reported that the low hGH concentrations in follicular fluid were associated with cleavage failure and poor embryo morphology, whereas the addition of hGH to culture medium improves in vitro maturation of immature human oocytes. Izadyar et al. (305) suggested that hGH stimulates cytoplasmic maturation and may have a positive role in increasing total cell number in the embryo and in decreasing apoptosis, as described in the bovine species (306). It may also stimulate the mechanisms of DNA repair, as described in the liver (307). Further studies are eagerly awaited to elucidate the mechanisms through which hGH may exert a positive effect on embryonic development (Fig. 46.11).

Early trials were promising, showing improvements in follicular responsiveness and pregnancy rates (308–310). Similarly, in a cohort of poor responders, Kim et al. (311) found that co-treatment with pyridostigmine, an hGH releasing agent, enhanced the ovarian response to stimulation and resulted in a non-statistically significant higher clinical pregnancy rate. Subsequent studies using hGH or GH-releasing factor in IVF poor responders demonstrated no improvement in stimulation characteristics, clinical pregnancy, or live birth rates, and the interest and use of adjuvant hGH has subsided (312–317). This was further confirmed by a Cochrane Review published in the year 2000, which reported a meta-analysis of the trials assessing the effectiveness of adjuvant hGH therapy in women undergoing COS (318). In previous poor responders treated with hGH, the common OR for pregnancy per cycle instituted was 2.55 (95% CI 0.64–10.12). No significant difference was noted in either the number

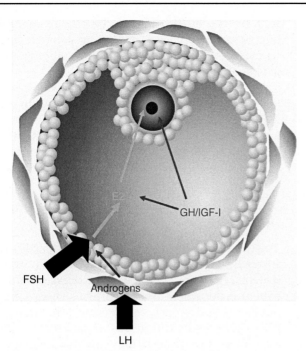

- In vitro GH stimulates E_2 production 240,241
- Oocytes from follicles with high antral fluid GH levels have better developmental potential than oocytes from low GH follicles 304
- GH receptor mRNA in human oocyte and preimplantation embryos (Menezo et al. 304a)
- Nuclear and cytoplasmic maturation enhanced by GH (bovine – Izadyar et al. 305)
- Role for GH in stimulation of DNA repair (as in liver, Thompson et al. 307)
- Improvement in normal fertilization and embryo development

Figure 46.11   E2 and GH/IGF-I may enhance oocyte quality by enhancing and coordinating cytoplasmic and nuclear maturation. *Abbreviations*: GH, growth hormone; IGF-1, insulin-like growth factor I; FSH, follicle-stimulating hormone; LH, luteinizing hormone.

of follicles and oocytes, or gonadotropin usage. It was concluded that a trend toward improved outcome with hGH treatment deserved further study.

Several recent studies have re-raised the interest in the use of hGH for COS in poor responders. In a randomized, placebo-controlled study, Tesarik et al. reported the use of hGH in women >40 years undergoing ART (319). They used a high-dose FSH stimulation regimen (600 IU FSH) supplemented with 8 IU/day hGH from FSH stimulation day 7 until day +1 hCG. Although no improvement in the number of oocytes retrieved was observed, significantly higher plasma and intrafollicular E2 levels were found in the hGH group, and the clinical pregnancy and live birth rates were also significantly higher in the hGH-treated group. They concluded that hGH may improve the potential for oocyte development. The action of GH in vitro in stimulating E2 production by follicular cells has been previously reported (240,241).

In a more recent RCT, Kucuk et al. (320) assessed the efficacy of hGH co-stimulation in a long luteal GnRH-a regimen in poor responders. The study involved 61 patients who previously responded poorly to high dose gonadotropin treatment. The study group (n = 31) received prolonged hGH co-treatment, daily SC injection of 4 mg (equivalent to 12 IUI) from day 21 of preceding cycle along with GnRH-a, until the day of hCG. A control group (n = 30) received the same treatment protocol except for the hGH co-treatment. Although the gonadotropins requirements were significantly reduced, the average cost of the cycle was more than double with hGH co-treatment. Significantly more mature oocytes, zygotes, and embryos available for transfer were achieved following hGH administration. This, however, did not translate into improved cycle outcome, as implantation rate was significantly higher in the control group as compared to the hGH-treated group (31.5% vs. 11.7%, respectively; p < 0.05). Pregnancy rates were comparable for both groups.

In a sequential crossover study (321), hGH supplementation was assessed in poor-prognosis patients, categorized on the basis of past failure to conceive (mean 3.05 cycles) due to low response to high-dose stimulation (<3 metaphase II oocytes) or poor-quality embryos. Pregnancy rates in both fresh and frozen transfer cycles and the total productivity rates (fresh and frozen pregnancies per egg collection) were compared. In all, 159 patients had 488 treatment cycles: 221 with hGH and 241 without hGH. These cycles were also compared with 1572 uncategorized cycles from the same period. hGH co-treatment significantly improved the clinical pregnancy rate per fresh transfer (p < 0.001) as well as per frozen-thawed embryo derived from hGH cycles (p < 0.05) creating a highly significant productivity rate (p < 0.001). The effect was significant across all age groups, especially in younger patients, and was independent of stimulation modality or number of transfers. hGH cycles resulted in significantly more babies delivered per transfer than non-hGH cycles (20% vs. 7%; p < 0.001), although less than the uncategorized cycles (53%). The data uniquely show that the effect of hGH is directed at oocyte and subsequent embryo quality.

Meta-analyses regarding hGH have been recently updated. A meta-analysis of 22 RCTs that evaluated 15 interventions to increase pregnancy rates in poor responders to IVF found that the addition of hGH to ovarian stimulation was one of only two interventions that increased the probability of pregnancy (322). Interestingly, the other beneficial intervention was ET on day 2 rather than day 3 (322). Similarly, an updated meta-analysis (323) focusing on the use of hGH co-treatment in poor responders has shown that hGH addition increases the probability of clinical pregnancy and live birth. It was, however, mentioned that the total number of patients analyzed was small and thus further RCTs are warranted to prove or disprove this finding.

In summary, considering the extra cost and limited data available, there is currently no well-established clinical role for adjuvant hGH in the treatment of poor responders. Further studies should be directed at defining the dose of hGH, and determining if select populations may benefit from hGH co-treatment (324).

OCP Pretreatment

It has been suggested that the use of an OCP in the previous cycle may increase pregnancy rates in IVF (325). Because OCPs have a putative role in enhancement of estrogen receptor sensitization due to their estrogen content, in addition to exerting pituitary suppression, they have been used in combination with GnRH-a. Biljan et al. (326) reported that pituitary suppression with OC and a GnRH-a was superior to GnRH-a alone regarding the time required to achieve pituitary suppression, as well as pregnancy and implantation rates.

Because of these promising effects, OCPs have also been used in poor responders. However, there are only very few retrospective studies evaluating the actual contribution of OCPs in this group of patients. Lindheim et al. (327) found higher pregnancy rates with OCP alone compared with GnRH-a–treated cycles (both long and short protocols). They concluded that the good outcome associated with OCP pretreatment might reflect production or alterations of local ovarian growth factors and/or changes at the endometrial level. In contrast with the above observations, Kovacs et al. (328) also compared retrospectively the use of OCPs with GnRH-a for hypothalamic–pituitary suppression in poor responder IVF patients. Hypothalamic–pituitary suppression was performed with either an OCP or a GnRH-a followed by stimulation with gonadotropins. Cycle outcomes, including cancellation rates, gonadotropin requirements, number of oocytes retrieved, number of embryos transferred, and embryo quality, were similar. Patients in the OCP group required fewer days of stimulation to reach oocyte retrieval. Pregnancy rates were similar in the two groups. Overall, there was no improvement in IVF cycle outcome in poor responders who received OCPs to achieve pituitary suppression instead of a GnRH-a.

In summary, although there is a general feeling that OCP pretreatment might be of assistance in the ovarian response of poor responders, especially in flare-up regimens, only a minimal amount of published data exist to support this approach.

Luteal Phase Manipulations

During the early follicular phase of the menstrual cycle, antral follicle sizes are often markedly heterogeneous. These follicle size discrepancies may, at least in part, result from the early exposure of FSH-sensitive follicles to gradient FSH concentrations during the preceding luteal phase. This phenomenon, which often occurs in women with poor ovarian reserve, and in particular those with short cycles, may potentially affect the results of ovarian stimulation. Preexisting follicle size discrepancies may encumber coordinated follicular growth during ovarian stimulation, thereby reducing the number of follicles that reach maturation at once. Interventions aimed at coordinating follicular growth by manipulations at the mid-luteal phase of the preceding cycle are largely based on the innovative work of Fanchin et al. (329).

To investigate this issue, three clinical studies were conducted to test the hypothesis that luteal FSH suppression could coordinate subsequent follicular growth. First, luteal FSH concentrations were artificially lowered by administering physiological E2 doses and follicular characteristics were measured on the subsequent day 3 in healthy volunteers (330). In this study, luteal E2 administration was found to reduce the size and to improve the homogeneity of early antral follicles on day 3.

Second, it was verified whether luteal E2 administration could promote the coordination of follicular growth during ovarian stimulation and improve its results (331). Ninety IVF patients were randomly pretreated with 17 beta-estradiol (4 mg/day) from cycle day 20 until next cycle day 2 ($n = 47$) or controls ($n = 43$). On cycle day 3, all women started r-hFSH treatment followed by a GnRH-ant in the flexible protocol. The authors focused on the dynamics of follicular development, including magnitude of size discrepancy of growing follicles on day 8 of r-hFSH treatment and number of follicles >16 mm in diameter on the day of hCG administration. On day 8, follicles were significantly smaller (9.9 ± 2.5 vs. 10.9 ± 3.4 mm) and their size discrepancies attenuated in the treatment group compared with controls. This was associated with more >16 mm follicles, and more mature oocytes and embryos in the E2-treated group. It was concluded that luteal E2 administration reduces the pace of growth, improves size homogeneity of antral follicles on day 8 of r-hFSH treatment, and increases the number of follicles reaching maturation at once.

Third, the effects of premenstrual GnRH-ant administration on follicular characteristics were assessed during the early follicular phase (332). Twenty-five women underwent measurements of early antral follicles by ultrasound and serum FSH and ovarian hormones on cycle day 2 (control/day 2). On day 25, they received a single dose of 3 mg cetrorelix acetate. On the subsequent day 2 (premenstrual GnRH-ant/day 2), participants were re-evaluated as on control/day 2. The main outcome measure was the magnitude of follicular size discrepancies. Follicular diameters (4.1 ± 0.9 vs. 5.5 ± 1.0 mm) and follicle-to-follicle size differences decreased on premenstrual GnRH-ant/day 2 compared with control/day 2. Consistently, FSH (4.5 ± 1.9 vs. 6.7 ± 2.4 mIU/ml), E2 (23 ± 13 vs. 46 ± 26 pg/ml), and inhibin B (52 ± 30 vs. 76 ± 33 pg/ml) were lower on GnRH-ant/day 2 than on control/day 2. It was concluded that premenstrual GnRH-ant administration reduces diameters and size disparities of early antral follicles, probably through the prevention of luteal FSH elevation and early follicular development.

Taken together, the results of the above studies suggest that luteal FSH suppression by either E2 or GnRH-ant administration improves the size homogeneity of early antral follicles during the early follicular phase, an effect that persists during ovarian stimulation. Coordination of follicular development has the potential to optimize ovarian response to COS protocols, and constitutes an attractive approach for improving their outcome.

An opposite approach of enhancing follicular recruitment by initiating FSH therapy during the late luteal as opposed to the early follicular phase has been attempted in prior poor responders but without success. In an RCT, Rombauts et al. (333) failed to demonstrate any benefit of this regimen, with the exception that follicular maturation was achieved sooner after the onset of menses.

Several studies evaluated the effects of combining pretreatment with E2 and/or GnRH-ant during the luteal phase of the preceding cycle on the outcome of COS in poor responders. Dragisic et al. (334) reported lower cancellation rates and improved IVF outcome via a combination of estrogen patch therapy and GnRH-ant started in the mid-luteal phase of the preceding menstrual cycle. Frattarelli et al. (335) reported a retrospective paired cohort analysis where they compared embryo and oocyte data between a standard protocol and a luteal phase E2 protocol. The results of 60 poor responder patients who underwent IVF with a luteal phase oral E2 protocol were compared to 60 cycles in the same patients without E2 pretreatment. The luteal phase E2 protocol showed significant increases in the number of embryos with >7 cells, number of oocytes retrieved, number of mature oocytes, and number of embryos generated than did the standard protocol. There was no difference between the two protocols with respect to basal AFC, days of stimulation, number of follicles >14 mm on day of hCG administration, or endometrial thickness. A trend toward improved pregnancy outcomes was found with the luteal E2 protocol.

Several studies compared the luteal phase E2 with subsequent GnRH-ant protocol with the short micro-flare agonist protocol. DiLuigi et al. (336) performed an RCT to compare IVF outcomes in 54 poor responder patients undergoing a microdose LA flare protocol or a GnRH-ant protocol incorporating both a luteal phase E2 patch and GnRH-ant in the preceding menstrual cycle. Cancellation rates (32.1% vs. 23.1%), number of oocytes retrieved (5.4 ± 4.7 vs. 5.2 ± 4), clinical pregnancy rates (28.6% vs. 34.6%), and ongoing pregnancy rates (25% vs. 23.1%) were similar for the micro-flare and luteal E2/GnRH-ant, respectively. Similarly, Weitzman et al. (337) retrospectively compared IVF outcomes in poor-responder patients undergoing COS after luteal phase E2 patch and subsequent GnRH-ant protocol (n = 45) versus microdose GnRH-a flare protocol (n = 76). The cancellation rate (28.9% vs. 30.3%), mean number of oocytes (9.1 ± 4.1 vs. 8.9 ± 4.3), fertilization rates (70.0% ± 24.2% vs. 69.9% ± 21.5%), the number of embryos transferred (2.5 ± 1.1 vs. 2.7 ± 1.3), implantation rates (15.0% vs. 12.5%), clinical

pregnancy rates (43.3% vs. 45.1%), and ongoing pregnancy rate per transfer (33.3% vs. 26.0%) were all comparable for both groups. Focusing on young poor responders (age <35 years), Shastri et al. (338) retrospectively compared COS with a luteal E2 and subsequent GnRH-ant protocol versus an OCP microdose LA flare protocol. Patients in the luteal E2/GnRH-ant group had increased gonadotropin requirements (71.9 ± 22.2 vs. 57.6 ± 25.7 ampoules) and lower E2 level (1178.6 ± 668 vs. 1627 ± 889 pg/mL), yet achieved similar numbers of oocytes retrieved and fertilized, and a greater number of embryos transferred (2.3 ± 0.9 vs. 2.0 ± 1.1) with a better mean grade (2.14 ± .06 vs. 2.7 ± 1.8) compared with the micro-flare group. The luteal E2/GnRH-ant group exhibited a trend toward improved implantation rates (30.5% vs. 21.1%) and ongoing pregnancy rates per started cycle (37% vs. 25%). From the above studies (336–338) it can be concluded that both protocols remain viable options for poor responders undergoing IVF, and that adequately powered, randomized clinical comparison appears justified.

When luteal E2 and antagonist (n = 256) was compared with luteal E2 only (n = 57) before GnRH-ant protocol in low responders (339), the addition of GnRH-ant to luteal E2 for luteal suppression did not improve IVF outcome.

Elassar et al. (340) recently compared IVF outcomes after COS using letrozole/antagonist (LA) versus luteal-phase E2/GnRH-ant in poor responders. In a retrospective study, 99 women with ≥2 prior failed cycles with poor response were included. In the luteal intervention group (n = 52), both transdermal E2 and GnRH-ant were administered in the preceding luteal phase, with gonadotropins started on the second day of menstruation. In the LA group (n = 47), letrozole 5 mg/day was initiated on the second day of spontaneous menstruation for five days and then gonadotropins were added on day 5; for both groups a flexible antagonist protocol was used. The total dose of gonadotropins administered and E2 levels on day of hCG administration were significantly lower with the LA protocol. Cancellation rates (55.3% vs. 36.5%), the number of oocytes retrieved (6.1 ± 3.0 vs. 7.9 ± 4.8), number of transferred embryos (2.2 ± 1.0 vs. 2.4 ± 1.4), ongoing pregnancy rates per transfer (40% vs. 21.2%) and per initiated cycle (19.1% vs. 13.5%) were similar in the LA and luteal intervention groups, respectively. It was concluded that both aromatase inhibitor regimens and luteal intervention regimens can be feasible alternatives in recurrent POR.

Using a slightly different approach, Fisch et al. (179) described their experience with a protocol using GnRH-a/ antagonist conversion with estrogen priming (AACEP) in poor responders with prior IVF failures. The AACEP protocol focuses on promoting estrogenic dominance in the stimulated ovary, and opposing the potential ill effects of the LH flare and overproduction of androgens, which are commonly seen in GnRH-a flare, and in antagonist protocols. Patients received an OCP and a GnRH-a overlapping the last five to seven days of the pill until the onset of menses. From cycle day 2, low-dose GnRH-ant (0.125 mg/day), and estradiol valerate (2 mg) was given intramuscularly every three days for two doses, followed by estrogen suppositories until a dominant follicle was detected. Ovarian stimulation consisted of high-dose FSH/hMG. Although women aged <38 years and those on 600 IU/day produced more mature eggs and fertilized embryos than women aged 38–42 years, there were no differences in peak serum E2, endometrial thickness, or embryos transferred. Outcomes were similar for all patients, regardless of age or FSH dosage. Ongoing pregnancy rates were 27% for all patients, 25% for patients aged <38 years, and 28% for patients aged 38–42 years. It was concluded that the AACEP protocol may improve the prognosis and outcome for poor responders with prior IVF failures.

In summary, manipulating the luteal phase preceding the IVF treatment cycle may improve the coordination of follicular development and increase the number and quality of embryos achieved in poor responder patients. Ultimately, this may translate into improved cycle and pregnancy outcomes in these patients. It remains to be seen whether this approach is superior to pretreatment with an OCP, which is commonly practiced in various protocols designed for poor responders. Properly designed RCTs are needed to test this innovative therapeutic approach.

ADDITIONAL INTERVENTIONS

Low-Dose Aspirin

Low-dose aspirin therapy has been demonstrated to enhance blood perfusion in multiple different organ systems. This may be accomplished by proportionally greater inhibition of vasoconstricting prostaglandins (thromboxane A2) than the vasodilating prostaglandins (prostacyclin).

Early reports on the use of aspirin in ART were encouraging. Rubinstein et al. (341) reported an RCT of the impact of daily 100 mg aspirin on multiple outcome parameters, including ovarian responsiveness, oocyte number, implantation rates, and pregnancy rates in a general IVF population. Dramatic improvements in gonadotropin responsiveness, pregnancy rates, and implantation rates were reported. Low-dose aspirin therapy was also found to improve implantation rates in oocyte donation recipients with a thin endometrium (342), as well as in IUI cycles (343). Following these early encouraging reports, multiple studies were conducted on general IVF populations, yielding conflicting results. Finally, two meta-analyses published in 2007 have reached a similar conclusion that currently available evidence does not support the use of aspirin in IVF or ICSI treatment (344,345). Interestingly, Ruopp et al. (346) reanalyzed the effects of low-dose aspirin in IVF and raised methodological questions regarding the analysis by Gelbaya et al. (344). They concluded that aspirin may increase clinical pregnancy rates and that more data are needed to resolve the issue. In their opinion there is no reason to change clinical management and discontinue the use of aspirin, reflecting the ongoing controversy regarding the use of low-dose aspirin in IVF.

The use of low-dose aspirin was specifically studied in poor responder patients as well. Lok et al. (347) conducted an RCT evaluating the effect of adjuvant low-dose aspirin on utero-ovarian blood flow and ovarian responsiveness in poor responders undergoing IVF. Sixty patients received 80 mg aspirin daily or placebo during long downregulation protocol. Doppler measurements of intraovarian and uterine pulsatility index were performed before (baseline) and after ovarian stimulation. Duration of use and dose of gonadotropins, cycle cancellation rate, number of mature follicles recruited, and oocytes retrieved were also compared. High cancellation rates were found in both groups (33.3% vs. 26.7%, placebo vs. treatment). There were no significant differences in gonadotropin requirements, median number of mature follicles recruited (3.5 vs. 3.0), or median number of oocytes retrieved (4 vs. 3). No significant differences were found in either intraovarian or uterine artery pulsatility index measured at baseline or on the day of hCG administration. It was concluded that supplementation with low-dose aspirin failed to improve either ovarian and uterine blood flow or ovarian responsiveness in poor responders undergoing IVF.

Scoccia et al. (348) reported a retrospective cohort study, where 133 poor responder cycles were reviewed. There were 108 patients who received 81 mg aspirin daily during ovarian stimulation and 25 who did not. There was no improvement with aspirin use in pregnancy or live birth rates. However, there was a trend (p = 0.05) toward an improved implantation rate in cycles without aspirin. Recently, another retrospective cohort analysis was reported by Frattarelli et al. (349). A total of 1250 poor responder patients undergoing IVF were studied, of which 417 patients used 81 mg of aspirin before and during the IVF cycle, and 833 did not. Patients taking 81 mg of aspirin had significantly higher basal AFCs, required more days of stimulation, needed more ampoules of gonadotropins, achieved higher peak E2 levels, and had more follicles that were ≥14 mm in diameter on the day of hCG administration. There was a decrease in the overall fertilization rate for the patients taking aspirin. There was no difference in IVF outcome (implantation, pregnancy, loss, or live birth). Overall, no improvement in IVF outcome secondary to 81-mg aspirin intake was found.

Currently available evidence does not support the use of aspirin in poor responder patients undergoing IVF. However, the paucity of RCTs highlights the need for additional trials.

Aneuploidy Screening

Oocytes produced in women of AMA may have inadequate reserves of energy, due to age-related accumulated effects on their mitochondrial DNA (350). Energy produced by mitochondria is necessary for correct function throughout the processes of oocyte maturation and the final stages of meiosis, and mitochondrial dysfunction can lead to an increase in the frequency of nondysjunction, abnormalities in chromatid separation, and increased rates of apoptosis. As a result, the oocytes retrieved during ART procedures may be biochemically or chromosomally defective. Tzeng et al. (351) transferred a homologous mitochondrial enriched fraction of cytoplasm obtained from cumulus granulosa cells (CGs) to compromised oocytes, and reported an increase in fertilization, embryo development, and pregnancies.

It has long been known that women over the age of 35 years are at increased risk of having a fetus with a chromosome abnormality, and this is probably due to an age-related increase in oocyte aneuploidy. Chromosome abnormalities are the primary cause of embryo wastage in patients aged >35 years and up to 80% of embryos in women over 40 years may be aneuploid (Table 46.3). Therefore, screening oocytes or embryos for aneuploidy so that only chromosomally normal embryos are transferred should increase implantation rates, reduce spontaneous abortion, and increase live-birth rates. Munné et al. (355) conducted a controlled clinical study to assess the incidence of chromosomal aneuploidy in women with a history of recurrent miscarriage presenting for assisted reproduction treatment. This group was compared with a group undergoing PGS because of AMA. Each embryo was biopsied on day 3, and blastomeres were analyzed using fluorescent probes for chromosomes X, Y, 13, 15, 16, 17, 18, 21, and 22. Their findings confirmed that for women aged ≥35 years, PGS significantly reduced pregnancy losses and increased the number of viable pregnancies.

Taranissi et al. (356) also assessed the influence of maternal age on the outcome of PGS in IVF cycles carried out in patients with recurrent implantation failure. Their prospective study included 160 couples with a history of three or more failed fresh IVF attempts; the study population was divided into two groups: 78 patients aged ≤40 years, and 38 patients aged ≥41 years. Their results also confirmed the detrimental effects of increasing age: Younger patients have a significantly higher proportion of euploid oocytes/embryos, cycles reaching ET, clinical pregnancy (36.1% vs. 16.6%), and ongoing delivery (32% vs. 12.5%) per ET.

Similarly, Rubio et al. (357) performed 341 PGS cycles in women ≥38 years (mean age = 40.5 years), and compared the results with a control group of women aged <37 years. Their study confirmed a significant increase in the percentage of abnormal embryos in women of AMA (70.3% vs. 33.1% in the control group; $p < 0.05$). They were able to achieve acceptable ongoing pregnancy rates with PGS until the age of 42 years (28.8%), but women >42 years had a poorer prognosis.

Conflicting results, however, were recently reported by Mastenbroek et al. (358), who conducted a multicenter, randomized, double-blind, controlled trial comparing three cycles of IVF with and without PGS in women aged 35–41 years: 408 women (206 assigned to PGS and 202 assigned to the control group) underwent 836 cycles of IVF (434 cycles with and 402 cycles without PGS). The ongoing pregnancy rate was significantly lower in the women assigned to PGS (25%) than in those not assigned to PGS (37%; rate ratio = 0.69; 95% CI 0.51–0.93). The women assigned to PGS also had significantly lower live birth rate (24%) versus (35%; (rate ratio = 0.68; 95% CI 0.50–0.92). It was concluded that PGS did not increase but instead significantly reduced the rates of ongoing pregnancies and live births after IVF in women of AMA. There were, however, problems with the study design and implementation that may have led to the damage of biopsied embryos leading to lower viability. This issue has been examined and confirmed in a recent study by Treff et al. (359) in a paired analysis of co-transferred biopsied and non-biopsied sibling embryos.

New test methodologies for aneuploidy employing microarray comparative genomic hybridization analysis are now yielding extremely reliable data which has the potential to provide help to poor prognosis patients (360).

The identification of high-quality embryos in all women undergoing IVF, including poor responders, remains a high priority. In the future, accurate noninvasive methods for assessing oocyte and embryo quality may also become available, such as gene expression profiling of cumulus cells surrounding the oocyte, and metabolomics and proteomics. Cumulus cells are typically discarded during classical IVF and ICSI, are easily accessible and plentiful. Gene expression signatures have been identified using transcriptomic data of cumulus cells (361,362). This noninvasive approach is based on the level of expression of potential biomarkers in cumulus cells to assess the potential and quality of the

Table 46.3   The Majority of Embryos are Chromosomally Abnormal in Older Patients

Abnormality	Age (years)		
	20–34	35–39	40–47
Aneuploidy (9 chromosomes)[a]	24%	27%	39% (p < 0.001)
Other aneuploidy (by CGH)	5%	6%	8%
Postmeiotic abnormalities[b]	35%	36%	35% (NS)
Total abnormal	64%	69%	82% (p < 0.001)

[a]Aneuploidy for chromosomes X, Y, 13, 15, 16, 17, 18, 21, and 22.
[b]Mosaics, polyploid, ha.
Abbreviation: CGH, comparative genomic hybridization.
Source: From Refs. (352–354).

embryo. Additionally, analysis of the proteins contained in the surrounding embryo culture medium may provide a noninvasive method of using proteomic techniques to identify novel biomarkers of embryo viability (363). Metabolomic technology is being used in the development of a new method for aneuploidy detection. This approach is based on the assumption that an embryo with a missing or extra chromosome may have modified metabolism. By correlating metabolomic profiles with the results of subsequently performed PGS, it has been possible to differentiate between embryos with normal and abnormal chromosome numbers, and even classify embryos according to their chromosomal anomaly (364).

Assisted Hatching

Assisted hatching (AH) involves the artificial thinning or breaching of the zona pellucida (ZP) and has been proposed as one technique to improve implantation and pregnancy rates following IVF. The AH procedure is generally performed on day 3 after fertilization using various methods. These include the creation of an opening in the zona either by drilling with acidified Tyrode's solution, partial zona drilling (PZD) with a glass microneedle, laser photoablation, or use of a piezo-micromanipulator. The ZP can be artificially thinned without breaching its integrity with proteolytic enzymes, acidified Tyrode's solution, or laser. For a comprehensive review on AH the reader is referred to Chapter 14.

An RCT on AH suggested an improvement in implantation rates when the procedure was selectively applied to embryos with a poor prognosis (based on zona thickness, blastomere number, fragmentation rates, maternal age, etc) (365). Since its introduction, many ART programs have incorporated the use of AH in efforts to improve clinical outcomes. Success rates following the use of AH have varied considerably. However, differences in patient populations, operator experience, hatching technique, and study design make it difficult to compare directly reports from different centers.

Assisted hatching has been suggested for increasing the chance for implantation and pregnancy in poor prognosis women, such as those with multiple IVF failures or those >38 years (365,366). The role of AH in the treatment of poor responders has never been directly assessed, but poor responders have been often included as poor prognosis patients either because of AMA or because of multiple previous failed IVF attempts. Schoolcraft et al. (367) compared prospectively 33 poor prognosis IVF patients (elevated day 3 FSH level, age ≥39 years, and multiple prior IVF failures) who were treated with AH, with 43 control subjects without AH. The implantation and ongoing pregnancy rate in the AH group were 33% and 64%, compared with 6.5% and 19% in the control group, respectively. It was concluded that AH, when applied to poor prognosis patients, improves embryonic implantation and pregnancy rates.

Similarly, Stein et al. (366) have demonstrated that, in a selected group of patients (aged >38 years, who have failed to conceive in >3 previous IVF attempts), AH significantly increases the clinical pregnancy rate (23.9% in the study group compared with only 7% of the controls). Focusing on maternal age, Meldrum et al. (368) demonstrated that following AH, the implantation rate was increased in women aged 35–39 years and markedly increased in women aged 40–42 years, but not in women over 43 years.

Magli et al. (369) conducted an RCT on the efficacy of AH in poor prognosis patients with: (i) maternal age ≥38 years (45 cycles); (ii) ≥3 failed IVF attempts (70 cycles), and (iii) patients possessing both inclusion criteria (20 cycles). The control groups included patients with similar characteristics who did not undergo AH. The clinical pregnancy rate per cycle following AH was significantly higher than in controls for the first (31% vs. 10%) and second groups (36% vs. 17%), but not for the third group. Similarly, higher implantation rates were obtained (11.5%, 15%, and 11%) compared with the respective controls (4%, 6.3%, and 1.5%).

Finally, in an RCT, Mansour et al. (370) demonstrated that transfer of zona-free embryos significantly increased pregnancy rates in poor prognosis patients (age ≥40 years, and/or ≥2 previous failed IVF–ICSI attempts) compared with controls (23% vs. 7.3%), but not in good prognosis patients (age <40 years undergoing the first ICSI attempt).

Other RCTs have failed to find a benefit for AH in women with AMA. Bider et al. (371) focused on patients >38 years undergoing IVF. A total of 839 embryos from 211 patients underwent AH during 312 cycles of therapy and compared to 540 non-hatched embryos transferred to 174 patients during 274 cycles of therapy. The pregnancy rate was not statistically different between the groups (8.9% in the AH group vs. 5.1% in the controls) as were implantation rates (3.75% and 3.55%, respectively), and delivery rates (3.8% and 3.4%, respectively). It was concluded that AH in patients aged >38 years does not increase the take-home baby rate after IVF. Lanzendorf et al. (372) reached similar conclusions in an RCT in which patients ≥36 years were treated with ($n = 41$) or without ($n = 48$) AH. No significant differences were observed in the rates of implantation (11.1% vs. 11.3%), clinical pregnancy (39.0% vs. 41.7%), and ongoing pregnancy (29.3% vs. 35.4%) between the hatched and control groups, respectively. These results suggest that AH may have no significant impact on IVF success rates in the patient population studied.

A recent comprehensive review and meta-analysis (373) identified 28 RCTs involving 3646 women undergoing AH during ART. Only seven of the studies included in the analysis reported on live birth rates. There was no significant difference in the odds of live births in the AH compared with control groups (OR 1.13, 95% CI 0.83–1.55). Women undergoing AH were significantly more likely to achieve clinical pregnancy (28 RCTs, OR 1.29, 95% CI 1.12–1.49). Miscarriage rates per women were similar in both groups (14 RCTs; OR 1.13, 95% CI 0.74 to 1.73). Multiple pregnancy rates per woman were significantly increased in women who were randomized to AH compared with women in control groups (12 RCTs; OR 1.67, 95% CI 1.24 to 2.26). The authors commented that the improvement in clinical pregnancy rate means that a clinic with a success rate of 25% could anticipate improving the clinical pregnancy rate to between 29% and 49%. However, despite significantly improved odds of clinical pregnancy, but due to lack of power, it is not possible to make conclusions on its effect to improve live birth rate.

The most recent meta-analysis on the role of AH in ART (374) has reached somewhat conflicting results. There were 28 studies with 5507 participants included. Additional analysis was performed in these subgroups: (i) Fresh embryos transferred to unselected or non-poor prognosis women; (ii) Fresh embryos transferred to women with previous repeated failure; (iii) Fresh embryos transferred to women of advanced age; (iv) Frozen-thawed embryos transferred to unselected or non-poor prognosis women. AH was related to a trend toward increased clinical pregnancy for all participants (RR = 1.11, 95% CI = 1.00–1.24), with a significant increase in subgroups 2 (RR = 1.73; 95% CI = 1.37–2.17) and 4 (RR = 1.36; 95% CI = 1.08–1.72, p < 0.01), but not for subgroups 1 and 3. For multiple pregnancy, a significant increase was observed for all participants (RR = 1.45; 95% CI = 1.11–1.90) and for subgroups 2 (RR = 2.53; 95% CI = 1.23–5.21) and 4 (RR = 3.40; 95% CI = 1.93–6.01). AH was related to increased clinical pregnancy and multiple pregnancy rates in women with previous repeated failure or frozen-thawed embryos. However, they reported that AH is unlikely to increase clinical pregnancy rates when performed in fresh embryos transferred to unselected or non-poor prognosis women or to women of AMA. Due to the small sample evaluated by the pool of included studies, no proper conclusions could be drawn regarding miscarriage or live birth.

Currently, there is insufficient evidence to recommend AH to patients with AMA or POR. Large RCTs involving documented poor responders should be conducted to assess the efficacy of this intervention in this subgroup of patients.

SUMMARY: PRACTICAL CONSIDERATIONS

There are several key issues that make the challenge of developing treatment strategies for poor responder patients difficult and frustrating:

1. Historically, there was no universally accepted definition of poor responders. While many papers are referenced in this text, all use a large variety of inclusion criteria and are therefore not readily comparable. It is hoped that the recently published ESHRE definition of POR (12) may assist future comparisons of published data on poor responders.
2. The lack of large-scale, prospective, RCTs of the different management strategies prevents any definitive conclusion to be drawn.

The following practical considerations represent a combination of the evidence presented above with long-standing clinical experience.

High-Dose Gonadotropins

Patients with either diminished ovarian reserve (by testing prior to treatment) or POR in previous cycles may benefit from high-dose gonadotropin therapy (300–450 IU of FSH daily) to maximize oocyte yield.

Long GnRH-a Protocol

The long GnRH-a protocol might be the protocol of choice if ovarian reserve is estimated to be poor but not critically diminished. If the long protocol is to be used, progestagen pretreatment may reduce the incidence of cyst formation. Reducing the dose of the GnRH-a once pituitary downregulation has been achieved (mini-dose agonist), might help to augment ovarian response. Depot GnRH-a preparations should not be used.

Short or Microdose Flare GnRH-a Protocol

Oral contraceptive pretreatment is extremely important in short GnRH-a regimens, as it may prevent the adverse effects of elevated LH and androgen secretion caused by the endogenous gonadotropin flare.

Failure to Respond to a GnRH-a Regimen

Failure to respond to a long or short GnRH-a regimen does not necessarily mean cycle cancellation. Agonist administration can be withdrawn, but gonadotropin stimulation can be continued. The cycle can be converted either to an antagonist or a modified natural cycle regimen, once ovarian response is observed.

Addition of LH activity

Since there is evidence suggesting that patients with AMA and/or poor responders may benefit from the addition of LH activity to the stimulation regimen, and it is not currently possible to identify those patients who are LH deficient following GnRH-a or antagonist administration, it is recommended to add LH (a minimum of 150 IU daily) during the final stages of follicle and oocyte maturation (from stimulation day 6 onward).

CONCLUSIONS

Women who have entered the declining years of fecundity and then require assisted reproduction have always been a major challenge in ART treatment. The poor response that is commonly observed in women of AMA is directly related to diminished ovarian reserve. The associated reduction in oocyte quality as manifested by the increase in aneuploidy embryos is most likely due to suboptimal cytoplasmic maturation (including reduced capacity of oocyte mitochondria to generate sufficient quantities of energy required for fertilization and cell division). In addition to the obstacles of diminished ovarian reserve, resistance to ovarian stimulation, and higher frequency of potential gynecological disorders, they are also at higher risk of producing aneuploid oocytes and embryos. Uterine factors, as well as the possibility of aneuploid embryos, result in an increased miscarriage rate. Their situation is further compounded by the psychological stress of knowing that the "biological clock" is ticking, and that time is against them.

Although the use of donor oocytes has proved to be a very successful alternative treatment, this is not an option in many parts of the world, and efforts must be made to maximize each patient's potential to use her own oocytes. If a sufficient number of oocytes and embryos can be obtained, aneuploidy screening by PGS may allow abnormal embryos to be eliminated, thus increasing the chance of implantation and reducing miscarriage rates. In the future, accurate noninvasive methods for assessing oocyte and embryo quality may also become available, such as gene expression profiling of cumulus cells surrounding the oocyte, and metabolomics and proteomics. These strategies, utilizing pharmacogenomics and manipulating endocrinology, may provide a means of augmenting follicular recruitment and cytoplasmic integrity, and thus improve the prognosis for these women.

Currently, there is insufficient evidence of benefit of any particular intervention for pituitary downregulation, COS, or adjuvant therapy in the management of poor responders (59). Recent studies indicate that androgen supplementation may be one area to explore further. The availability of r-hLH has made it possible to investigate the role of LH in the endocrinology of follicular recruitment: It appears that a defect in the balance of LH/FSH might be involved in the subtle age-related decline in follicular recruitment, and patients of older reproductive age undergoing ART might benefit from the addition of LH and/or hGH. Further data from good-quality RCTs with relevant outcomes are required to investigate the physiological mechanisms behind this observation, and to assess the possible effect of r-hLH and/or hGH supplementation on the age-related decline in pregnancy rate.

REFERENCES

1. Menken J, Trussell J, Larsen U. Age and infertility. Science 1986; 233: 1389–94.
2. Borini A, Bafaro G, Violini F, et al. Pregnancies in postmenopausal women over 50 years old in an oocyte donation program. Fertil Steril 1995; 63: 258–61.
3. Laufer N, Simon A, Samueloff A, et al. Successful spontaneous pregnancies in women older than 45 years. Fertil Steril 2004; 81: 1328–32.
4. Gielchinsky Y, Mazor M, Simon A, Mor-Yossef S, Laufer N. Natural conception after age 45 in Bedouin women, a uniquely fertile population. J Assist Reprod Genet 2006; 23: 305–9.
5. Spandorfer SD, Bendikson K, Dragisic K, et al. Outcome of in vitro fertilization in women 45 years and older who use autologous oocytes. Fertil Steril 2007; 87: 74–6.
6. Baker TG. Radiosensitivity of mammalian oocytes with particular reference to the human female. Am J Obstet Gynecol 1971; 110: 746–61.
7. Faddy MJ, Gosden RG, Gougeon A, Richardson SJ, Nelson JF. Accelerated disappearance of ovarian follicles in mid-life: implications for forecasting menopause. Hum Reprod 1992; 7: 1342–6.
8. Andersen AN, Goossens V, Ferraretti AP, et al. Assisted reproductive technology in Europe, 2004. results generated from European registers by ESHRE. Hum Reprod 2008; 23: 756–71.
9. http://www.cdc.gov/art/ART2008/sect2_fig6–15. htm#15
10. Dal Prato L, Borini A, Cattoli M, et al. Live birth after IVF in a 46-year-old woman. Reprod Biomed Online 2005; 11: 452–4.
11. Alviggi C, Humaidan P, Howles CM, Tredway D, Hillier SG. Biological versus chronological ovarian age: implications for assisted reproductive technology. Reprod Biol Endocrinol 2009; 7: 101.
12. Ferraretti AP, La Marca A, Fauser BC, et al. ESHRE consensus on the definition of 'poor response' to ovarian stimulation for in vitro fertilization: the Bologna criteria. Hum Reprod 2011; 26: 1616–24.
13. Polyzos NP, Devroey P. A systematic review of randomized trials for the treatment of poor ovarian responders: is there any light at the end of the tunnel? Fertil Steril 2011; 96: 1058–61; e7.
14. Chuang CC, Chen CD, Chao KH, et al. Age is a better predictor of pregnancy potential than basal follicle-stimulating hormone levels in women undergoing in vitro fertilization. Fertil Steril 2003; 79: 63–8.
15. Marrs R, Meldrum D, Muasher S, et al. Randomized trial to compare the effect of recombinant human FSH (follitropin alfa) with or without recombinant human LH in women undergoing assisted reproduction treatment. Reprod Biomed Online 2004; 8: 175–82.
16. McClure N, McQuinn B, McDonald J, et al. Body weight, body mass index, and age: predictors of menotropin dose and cycle outcome in polycystic ovarian syndrome? Fertil Steril 1992; 58: 622–4.
17. Templeton A, Morris JK. Reducing the risk of multiple births by transfer of two embryos after in vitro fertilization. N Engl J Med 1998; 339: 573–7.
18. Imani B, Eijkemans MJ, Faessen GH, et al. Prediction of the individual follicle-stimulating hormone threshold for gonadotropin induction of ovulation in normogonadotropic anovulatory infertility: an approach to increase safety, efficiency. Fertil Steril 2002; 77: 83–90.
19. Hohmann FP, Laven JS, de Jong FH, Eijkemans MJ, Fauser BC. Low-dose exogenous FSH initiated during the early, mid or late follicular phase can induce multiple dominant follicle development. Hum Reprod 2001; 16: 846–54.
20. Nahum R, Shifren JL, Chang Y, et al. Antral follicle assessment as a tool for predicting outcome in IVF–is it a better predictor than age and FSH? J Assist Reprod Genet 2001; 18: 151–5.
21. Pohl M, Hohlagschwandtner M, Obruca A, et al. Number and size of antral follicles as predictive factors in vitro fertilization and embryo transfer. J Assist Reprod Genet 2000; 17: 315–18.
22. Popovic-Todorovic B, Loft A, Lindhard A, et al. A prospective study of predictive factors of ovarian response in 'standard' IVF/ICSI patients treated with recombinant FSH. A suggestion for a recombinant FSH dosage normogram. Hum Reprod 2003; 18: 781–7.

23. Scheffer GJ, Broekmans FJ, Looman CW, et al. The number of antral follicles in normal women with proven fertility is the best reflection of reproductive age. Hum Reprod 2003; 18: 700–6.

24. Kupesic S, Kurjak A. Predictors of IVF outcome by three-dimensional ultrasound. Hum Reprod 2002; 17: 950–5.

25. Klinkert ER, Broekmans FJ, Looman CW, Habbema JD, te Velde ER. The antral follicle count is a better marker than basal follicle-stimulating hormone for the selection of older patients with acceptable pregnancy prospects after in vitro fertilization. Fertil Steril 2005; 83: 811–14.

26. Broekmans FJ, de Ziegler D, Howles CM, et al. The antral follicle count: practical recommendations for better standardization. Fertil Steril 2010; 94: 1044–51.

27. Bassil S, Wyns C, Toussaint-Demylle D, et al. The relationship between ovarian vascularity and the duration of stimulation in in-vitro fertilization. Hum Reprod 1997; 12: 1240–5.

28. Lass A, Skull J, McVeigh E, Margara R, Winston RM. Measurement of ovarian volume by transvaginal sonography before ovulation induction with human menopausal gonadotrophin for in-vitro fertilization can predict poor response. Hum Reprod 1997; 12: 294–7.

29. Hendriks DJ, Kwee J, Mol BW, te Velde ER, Broekmans FJ. Ultrasonography as a tool for the prediction of outcome in IVF patients: a comparative meta-analysis of ovarian volume and antral follicle count. Fertil Steril 2007; 87: 764–75.

30. Toner JP, Philput CB, Jones GS, Muasher SJ. Basal follicle-stimulating hormone level is a better predictor of in vitro fertilization performance than age. Fertil Steril 1991; 55: 784–91.

31. Abdalla H, Thum MY. An elevated basal FSH reflects a quantitative rather than qualitative decline of the ovarian reserve. Hum Reprod 2004; 19: 893–8.

32. Bancsi LF, Broekmans FJ, Mol BW, Habbema JD, te Velde ER. Performance of basal follicle-stimulating hormone in the prediction of poor ovarian response and failure to become pregnant after in vitro fertilization: a meta-analysis. Fertil Steril 2003; 79: 1091–100.

33. Fenichel P, Grimaldi M, Olivero JF, et al. Predictive value of hormonal profiles before stimulation for in vitro fertilization. Fertil Steril 1989; 51: 845–9.

34. Gurgan T, Urman B, Yarali H, Duran HE. Follicle-stimulating hormone levels on cycle day 3 to predict ovarian response in women undergoing controlled ovarian hyperstimulation for in vitro fertilization using a flare-up protocol. Fertil Steril 1997; 68: 483–7.

35. Scott RT, Toner JP, Muasher SJ, et al. Follicle-stimulating hormone levels on cycle day 3 are predictive of in vitro fertilization outcome. Fertil Steril 1989; 51: 651–4.

36. Tinkanen H, Blauer M, Laippala P, Tuohimaa P, Kujansuu E. Prognostic factors in controlled ovarian hyperstimulation. Fertil Steril 1999; 72: 932–6.

37. Fawzy M, Lambert A, Harrison RF, et al. Day 5 inhibin B levels in a treatment cycle are predictive of IVF outcome. Hum Reprod 2002; 17: 1535–43.

38. Bancsi LF, Broekmans FJ, Eijkemans MJ, et al. Predictors of poor ovarian response in in vitro fertilization: a prospective study comparing basal markers of ovarian reserve. Fertil Steril 2002; 77: 328–36.

39. Eldar-Geva T, Margalioth EJ, Ben-Chetrit A, et al. Serum inhibin B levels measured early during FSH administration for IVF may be of value in predicting the number of oocytes to be retrieved in normal and low responders. Hum Reprod 2002; 17: 2331–7.

40. Ficicioglu C, Kutlu T, Demirbasoglu S, Mulayim B. The role of inhibin B as a basal determinant of ovarian reserve. Gynecol Endocrinol 2003; 17: 287–93.

41. Seifer DB, Lambert-Messerlian G, Hogan JW, et al. Day 3 serum inhibin-B is predictive of assisted reproductive technologies outcome. Fertil Steril 1997; 67: 110–14.

42. Nelson SM, Yates RW, Fleming R. Serum anti-Mullerian hormone and FSH: prediction of live birth and extremes of response in stimulated cycles–implications for individualization of therapy. Hum Reprod 2007; 22: 2414–21.

43. Lekamge DN, Barry M, Kolo M, et al. Anti-Mullerian hormone as a predictor of IVF outcome. Reprod Biomed Online 2007; 14: 602–10.

44. Kwee J, Schats R, McDonnell J, et al. Evaluation of anti-Mullerian hormone as a test for the prediction of ovarian reserve. Fertil Steril 2008; 90: 737–43.

45. Wunder DM, Guibourdenche J, Birkhauser MH, Bersinger NA. Anti-Mullerian hormone and inhibin B as predictors of pregnancy after treatment by in vitro fertilization/intracytoplasmic sperm injection. Fertil Steril 2008; 90: 2203–10.

46. Feyereisen E, Mendez Lozano DH, Taieb J, et al. Anti-Mullerian hormone: clinical insights into a promising biomarker of ovarian follicular status. Reprod Biomed Online 2006; 12: 695–703.

47. Wunder DM, Guibourdenche J, Birkhauser MH, Bersinger NA. Anti-Mullerian hormone and inhibin B as predictors of pregnancy after treatment by in vitro fertilization/intracytoplasmic sperm injection. Fertil Steril 2008; 90: 2203–10.

48. Nelson SM, Messow MC, Wallace AM, Fleming R, McConnachie A. Nomogram for the decline in serum antimullerian hormone: a population study of 9,601 infertility patients. Fertil Steril 2011; 95: 736–41; e1–3.

49. van Disseldorp J, Lambalk CB, Kwee J, et al. Comparison of inter- and intra-cycle variability of anti-Mullerian hormone and antral follicle counts. Hum Reprod 2010; 25: 221–7.

50. Barad DH, Weghofer A, Gleicher N. Comparing anti-Mullerian hormone (AMH) and follicle-stimulating hormone (FSH) as predictors of ovarian function. Fertil Steril 2009; 91: 1553–5.

51. Broer SL, Mol BW, Hendriks D, Broekmans FJ. The role of antimullerian hormone in prediction of outcome after IVF: comparison with the antral follicle count. Fertil Steril 2009; 91: 705–14.

52. Nelson SM, Yates RW, Lyall H, et al. Anti-Mullerian hormone-based approach to controlled ovarian stimulation for assisted conception. Hum Reprod 2009; 24: 867–75.

53. Nardo LG, Gelbaya TA, Wilkinson H, et al. Circulating basal anti-Mullerian hormone levels as predictor of ovarian response in women undergoing ovarian stimulation for in vitro fertilization. Fertil Steril 2009; 92: 1586–93.

54. Yates AP, Rustamov O, Roberts SA, et al. Anti-Mullerian hormone-tailored stimulation protocols

improve outcomes whilst reducing adverse effects and costs of IVF. Hum Reprod 2011; 26: 2353–62.

55. Popovic-Todorovic B, Loft A, Bredkjaeer HE, et al. A prospective randomized clinical trial comparing an individual dose of recombinant FSH based on predictive factors versus a 'standard' dose of 150 IU/day in 'standard' patients undergoing IVF/ICSI treatment. Hum Reprod 2003; 18: 2275–82.

56. Howles CM, Saunders H, Alam V, Engrand P. Predictive factors and a corresponding treatment algorithm for controlled ovarian stimulation in patients treated with recombinant human follicle stimulating hormone (follitropin alfa) during assisted reproduction technology (ART) procedures. An analysis of 1378 patients. Curr Med Res Opin 2006; 22: 907–18.

57. Broekmans FJ, Kwee J, Hendriks DJ, Mol BW, Lambalk CB. A systematic review of tests predicting ovarian reserve and IVF outcome. Hum Reprod Update 2006; 12: 685–718.

58. Ubaldi FM, Rienzi L, Ferrero S, et al. Management of poor responders in IVF. Reprod Biomed Online 2005; 10: 235–46.

59. Pandian Z, McTavish AR, Aucott L, Hamilton MP, Bhattacharya S. Interventions for 'poor responders' to controlled ovarian hyper stimulation (COH) in in-vitro fertilisation (IVF). Cochrane Database Syst Rev 2010; CD004379.

60. Keay SD, Liversedge NH, Mathur RS, Jenkins JM. Assisted conception following poor ovarian response to gonadotrophin stimulation. Br J Obstet Gynaecol 1997; 104: 521–7.

61. Karande V, Gleicher N. A rational approach to the management of low responders in in-vitro fertilization. Hum Reprod 1999; 14: 1744–8.

62. Fasouliotis SJ, Simon A, Laufer N. Evaluation and treatment of low responders in assisted reproductive technology: a challenge to meet. J Assist Reprod Genet 2000; 17: 357–73.

63. Tarlatzis BC, Zepiridis L, Grimbizis G, Bontis J. Clinical management of low ovarian response to stimulation for IVF: a systematic review. Hum Reprod Update 2003; 9: 61–76.

64. Ben-Rafael Z, Strauss JF 3rd, Mastroianni L Jr, Flickinger GL. Differences in ovarian stimulation in human menopausal gonadotropin treated woman may be related to follicle-stimulating hormone accumulation. Fertil Steril 1986; 46: 586–92.

65. Ben-Rafael Z, Benadiva CA, Ausmanas M, et al. Dose of human menopausal gonadotropin influences the outcome of an in vitro fertilization program. Fertil Steril 1987; 48: 964–8.

66. Hofmann GE, Toner JP, Muasher SJ, Jones GS. High-dose follicle-stimulating hormone (FSH) ovarian stimulation in low-responder patients for in vitro fertilization. J In Vitro Fert Embryo Transf 1989; 6: 285–9.

67. Karande VC, Jones GS, Veeck LL, Muasher SJ. High-dose follicle-stimulating hormone stimulation at the onset of the menstrual cycle does not improve the in vitro fertilization outcome in low-responder patients. Fertil Steril 1990; 53: 486–9.

68. Crosignani PG, Ragni G, Lombroso GC, et al. IVF: induction of ovulation in poor responders. J Steroid Biochem 1989; 32: 171–3.

69. Ben-Rafael Z, Levy T, Schoemaker J. Pharmacokinetics of follicle-stimulating hormone: clinical significance. Fertil Steril 1995; 63: 689–700.

70. Olivennes F, Howles CM, Borini A, et al. Individualizing FSH dose for assisted reproduction using a novel algorithm: the CONSORT study. Reprod Biomed Online 2009; 18: 195–204.

71. van Hooff MH, Alberda AT, Huisman GJ, Zeilmaker GH, Leerentveld RA. Doubling the human menopausal gonadotrophin dose in the course of an in-vitro fertilization treatment cycle in low responders: a randomized study. Hum Reprod 1993; 8: 369–73.

72. Cedrin-Durnerin I, Bstandig B, Herve F, et al. A comparative study of high fixed-dose and decremental-dose regimens of gonadotropins in a minidose gonadotropin-releasing hormone agonist flare protocol for poor responders. Fertil Steril 2000; 73: 1055–6.

73. Balasch J, Fabregues F, Penarrubia J, et al. Pretreatment with transdermal testosterone may improve ovarian response to gonadotrophins in poor-responder IVF patients with normal basal concentrations of FSH. Hum Reprod 2006; 21: 1884–93.

74. Hughes EG, Fedorkow DM, Daya S, et al. The routine use of gonadotropin-releasing hormone agonists prior to in vitro fertilization and gamete intrafallopian transfer: a meta-analysis of randomized controlled trials. Fertil Steril 1992; 58: 888–96.

75. Daya S. Optimal protocol for gonadotropin-releasing hormone agonist use in ovarian stimulation. In: Gomel V, Cheung PCK, eds. In Vitro Fertilization and Assisted Reproduction. Italy, Bologna: Monduzzi Editore, 1997: 405–15.

76. Belaisch-Allart J, Testart J, Frydman R. Utilization of GnRH agonists for poor responders in an IVF programme. Hum Reprod 1989; 4: 33–4.

77. Cummins JM, Yovich JM, Edirisinghe WR, Yovich JL. Pituitary down-regulation using leuprolide for the intensive ovulation management of poor prognosis patients having in vitro fertilization (IVF)-related treatments. J In Vitro Fert Embryo Transf 1989; 6: 345–52.

78. Neveu S, Hedon B, Bringer J, et al. Ovarian stimulation by a combination of a gonadotropin-releasing hormone agonist and gonadotropins for in vitro fertilization. Fertil Steril 1987; 47: 639–43.

79. Serafini P, Stone B, Kerin J, et al. An alternate approach to controlled ovarian hyperstimulation in "poor responders": pretreatment with a gonadotropin-releasing hormone analog. Fertil Steril 1988; 49: 90–5.

80. Sharma V, Williams J, Collins W, et al. The sequential use of a luteinizing hormone-releasing hormone (LH-RH) agonist and human menopausal gonadotropins to stimulate folliculogenesis in patients with resistant ovaries. J In Vitro Fert Embryo Transf 1988; 5: 38–42.

81. Ben-Rafael Z, Bider D, Dan U, et al. Combined gonadotropin releasing hormone agonist/human menopausal gonadotropin therapy (GnRH-a/hMG) in normal, high, and poor responders to hMG. J In Vitro Fert Embryo Transf 1991; 8: 33–6.

82. Chetkowski RJ, Rode RA, Burruel V, Nass TE. The effect of pituitary suppression and the women's age on embryo viability and uterine receptivity. Fertil Steril 1991; 56: 1095–103.

83. Lessing JB, Cohen JR, Yovel I, et al. Atypical response to luteinizing hormone-releasing hormone (LH-RH) agonist (suprefact nasal) in induction of ovulation in in vitro fertilization (IVF). J In Vitro Fert Embryo Transf 1991; 8: 314–16.

84. Ben-Nun I, Jaffe R, Goldberger S, et al. Complete ovarian unresponsiveness to hMG stimulation after prolonged GnRH analogue administration. Gynecol Endocrinol 1990; 4: 151–5.

85. Davis OK, Rosenwaks Z. The ovarian factor in assisted reproductive technology. In: Adashi EY, Leung P, ed. The Ovary. New York: Raven Press, 1993: 545–60.

86. Meldrum DR, Tsao Z, Monroe SE, et al. Stimulation of LH fragments with reduced bioactivity following GnRH agonist administration in women. J Clin Endocrinol Metab 1984; 58: 755–7.

87. Cedars MI, Surey E, Hamilton F, Lapolt P, Meldrum DR. Leuprolide acetate lowers circulating bioactive luteinizing hormone and testosterone concentrations during ovarian stimulation for oocyte retrieval. Fertil Steril 1990; 53: 627–31.

88. Dahl KD, Pavlou SN, Kovacs WJ, Hsueh AJ. The changing ratio of serum bioactive to immunoreactive follicle-stimulating hormone in normal men following treatment with a potent gonadotropin releasing hormone antagonist. J Clin Endocrinol Metab 1986; 63: 792–4.

89. Scott RT, Neal GS, Illions EH, Hayslip CA, Hofmann GE. The duration of leuprolide acetate administration prior to ovulation induction does not impact ovarian responsiveness to exogenous gonadotropins. Fertil Steril 1993; 60: 247–53.

90. Kowalik A, Barmat L, Damario M, et al. Ovarian estradiol production in vivo. Inhibitory effect of leuprolide acetate. J Reprod Med 1998; 43: 413–17.

91. Latouche J, Crumeyrolle-Arias M, Jordan D, et al. GnRH receptors in human granulosa cells: anatomical localization and characterization by autoradiographic study. Endocrinology 1989; 125: 1739–41.

92. Yoshimura Y, Nakamura Y, Ando M, et al. Direct effect of gonadotropin-releasing hormone agonists on the rabbit ovarian follicle. Fertil Steril 1992; 57: 1091–7.

93. Muasher SJ. Treatment of low responders. J Assist Reprod Genet 1993; 10: 112–14.

94. Brzyski RG, Jones GS, Oehninger S, et al. Impact of leuprolide acetate on the response to follicular stimulation for in vitro fertilization in patients with normal basal gonadotropin levels. J In Vitro Fert Embryo Transf 1989; 6: 290–3.

95. Droesch K, Muasher SJ, Brzyski RG, et al. Value of suppression with a gonadotropin-releasing hormone agonist prior to gonadotropin stimulation for in vitro fertilization. Fertil Steril 1989; 51: 292–7.

96. Sathanandan M, Warnes GM, Kirby CA, Petrucco OM, Matthews CD. Adjuvant leuprolide in normal, abnormal, and poor responders to controlled ovarian hyperstimulation for in vitro fertilization/gamete intrafallopian transfer. Fertil Steril 1989; 51: 998–1006.

97. Sandow J, Stoeckemann K, Jerabek-Sandow G. Pharmacokinetics, endocrine effects of slow release formulations of LHRH analogues. J Steroid Biochem Mol Biol 1990; 37: 925–31.

98. Janssens RM, Lambalk CB, Vermeiden JP, et al. Dose-finding study of triptorelin acetate for prevention of a premature LH surge in IVF: a prospective, randomized, double-blind, placebo-controlled study. Hum Reprod 2000; 15: 2333–40.

99. Feldberg D, Farhi J, Ashkenazi J, et al. Minidose gonadotropin-releasing hormone agonist is the treatment of choice in poor responders with high follicle-stimulating hormone levels. Fertil Steril 1994; 62: 343–6.

100. Olivennes F, Righini C, Fanchin R, et al. A protocol using a low dose of gonadotrophin-releasing hormone agonist might be the best protocol for patients with high follicle-stimulating hormone concentrations on day 3. Hum Reprod 1996; 11: 1169–72.

101. Weissman A, Farhi J, Royburt M, et al. Prospective evaluation of two stimulation protocols for low responders who were undergoing in vitro fertilization-embryo transfer. Fertil Steril 2003; 79: 886–92.

102. Keltz MD, Jones EE, Duleba AJ, et al. Baseline cyst formation after luteal phase gonadotropin-releasing hormone agonist administration is linked to poor in vitro fertilization outcome. Fertil Steril 1995; 64: 568–72.

103. Session DR, Saad AH, Salmansohn DD, Kelly AC. Ovarian activity during follicular-phase down regulation in in vitro fertilization is associated with advanced maternal age and a high recurrence rate in subsequent cycles. J Assist Reprod Genet 1995; 12: 301–4.

104. Margalioth EJ, Kafka I, Friedler S, et al. The incidence of ovarian cysts formation following GnRH analog treatment in IVF cycles is related to serum progesterone on the day of analog treatment initiation. In: 7th Anuual Meeting of the ESHRE. Paris, France, 1991. 15.

105. Aston K, Arthur I, Masson GM, Jenkins JM. Progestogen therapy and prevention of functional ovarian cysts during pituitary desensitisation with GnRH agonists. Br J Obstet Gynaecol 1995; 102: 835–7.

106. Ditkoff EC, Sauer MV. A combination of norethindrone acetate and leuprolide acetate blocks the gonadotrophin-releasing hormone agonistic response and minimizes cyst formation during ovarian stimulation. Hum Reprod 1996; 11: 1035–7.

107. Engmann L, Maconochie N, Bekir J, Tan SL. Progestogen therapy during pituitary desensitization with gonadotropin-releasing hormone agonist prevents functional ovarian cyst formation: a prospective, randomized study. Am J Obstet Gynecol 1999; 181: 576–82.

108. Smitz J, Devroey P, Camus M, et al. Inhibition of gonadotropic and ovarian function by intranasal administration of D-Ser (TBU)6-EA10-LHRH in normo-ovulatory women and patients with polycystic ovary disease. J Endocrinol Invest 1988; 11: 647–52.

109. Calogero AE, Macchi M, Montanini V, et al. Dynamics of plasma gonadotropin and sex steroid release in polycystic ovarian disease after pituitary-ovarian inhibition with an analog of gonadotropin-releasing hormone. J Clin Endocrinol Metab 1987; 64: 980–5.

110. Sungurtekin U, Jansen RP. Profound luteinizing hormone suppression after stopping the gonadotropin-releasing hormone-agonist leuprolide acetate. Fertil Steril 1995; 63: 663–5.

111. Corson SL, Batzer FR, Gocial B, et al. Leuprolide acetate-prepared in vitro fertilization-gamete intrafallopian transfer cycles: efficacy versus controls and cost analysis. Fertil Steril 1992; 57: 601–5.

112. Pantos K, Meimeth-Damianaki T, Vaxevanoglou T, Kapetanakis E. Prospective study of a modified gonadotropin-releasing hormone agonist long protocol in an in vitro fertilization program. Fertil Steril 1994; 61: 709–13.

113. Simons AH, Roelofs HJ, Schmoutziguer AP, et al. Early cessation of triptorelin in in vitro fertilization: a double-blind, randomized study. Fertil Steril 2005; 83: 889–96.

114. Beckers NG, Laven JS, Eijkemans MJ, Fauser BC. Follicular and luteal phase characteristics following early cessation of gonadotrophin-releasing hormone agonist during ovarian stimulation for in-vitro fertilization. Hum Reprod 2000; 15: 43–9.

115. Fujii S, Sagara M, Kudo H, et al. A prospective randomized comparison between long and discontinuous-long protocols of gonadotropin-releasing hormone agonist for in vitro fertilization. Fertil Steril 1997; 67: 1166–8.

116. Cedrin-Durnerin I, Bidart JM, Robert P, et al. Consequences on gonadotrophin secretion of an early discontinuation of gonadotrophin-releasing hormone agonist administration in short-term protocol for in-vitro fertilization. Hum Reprod 2000; 15: 1009–14.

117. Detti L, Williams DB, Robins JC, Maxwell RA, Thomas MA. A comparison of three downregulation approaches for poor responders undergoing in vitro fertilization. Fertil Steril 2005; 84: 1401–5.

118. Faber BM, Mayer J, Cox B, et al. Cessation of gonadotropin-releasing hormone agonist therapy combined with high-dose gonadotropin stimulation yields favorable pregnancy results in low responders. Fertil Steril 1998; 69: 826–30.

119. Wang PT, Lee RK, Su JT, et al. Cessation of low-dose gonadotropin releasing hormone agonist therapy followed by high-dose gonadotropin stimulation yields a favorable ovarian response in poor responders. J Assist Reprod Genet 2002; 19: 1–6.

120. Schachter M, Friedler S, Raziel A, et al. Improvement of IVF outcome in poor responders by discontinuation of GnRH analogue during the gonadotropin stimulation phase–a function of improved embryo quality. J Assist Reprod Genet 2001; 18: 197–204.

121. Pinkas H, Orvieto R, Avrech OM, et al. Gonadotropin stimulation following GnRH-a priming for poor responders in in vitro fertilization-embryo transfer programs. Gynecol Endocrinol 2000; 14: 11–14.

122. Dirnfeld M, Fruchter O, Yshai D, et al. Cessation of gonadotropin-releasing hormone analogue (GnRH-a) upon down-regulation versus conventional long GnRH-a protocol in poor responders undergoing in vitro fertilization. Fertil Steril 1999; 72: 406–11.

123. Garcia-Velasco JA, Isaza V, Requena A, et al. High doses of gonadotrophins combined with stop versus non-stop protocol of GnRH analogue administration in low responder IVF patients: a prospective, randomized, controlled trial. Hum Reprod 2000; 15: 2292–6.

124. Bider D, Ben-Rafael Z, Shalev J, et al. Pituitary, ovarian suppression rate after high dosage of gonadotropin-releasing hormone agonist. Fertil Steril 1989; 51: 578–81.

125. Padilla SL, Dugan K, Maruschak V, Shalika S, Smith RD. Use of the flare-up protocol with high dose human follicle stimulating hormone and human menopausal gonadotropins for in vitro fertilization in poor responders. Fertil Steril 1996; 65: 796–9.

126. Garcia JE, Padilla SL, Bayati J, Baramki TA. Follicular phase gonadotropin-releasing hormone agonist and human gonadotropins: a better alternative for ovulation induction in in vitro fertilization. Fertil Steril 1990; 53: 302–5.

127. Howles CM, Macnamee MC, Edwards RG. Short term use of an LHRH agonist to treat poor responders entering an in-vitro fertilization programme. Hum Reprod 1987; 2: 655–6.

128. Katayama KP, Roesler M, Gunnarson C, Stehlik E, Jagusch S. Short-term use of gonadotropin-releasing hormone agonist (leuprolide) for in vitro fertilization. J In Vitro Fert Embryo Transf 1988; 5: 332–4.

129. Toth TL, Awwad JT, Veeck LL, Jones HW Jr. Muasher SJ. Suppression and flare regimens of gonadotropin-releasing hormone agonist. Use in women with different basal gonadotropin values in an in vitro fertilization program. J Reprod Med 1996; 41: 321–6.

130. Karande V, Morris R, Rinehart J, et al. Limited success using the "flare" protocol in poor responders in cycles with low basal follicle-stimulating hormone levels during in vitro fertilization. Fertil Steril 1997; 67: 900–3.

131. Brzyski RG, Muasher SJ, Droesch K, et al. Follicular atresia associated with concurrent initiation of gonadotropin-releasing hormone agonist and follicle-stimulating hormone for oocyte recruitment. Fertil Steril 1988; 50: 917–21.

132. Gindoff PR, Hall JL, Stillman RJ. Ovarian suppression with leuprolide acetate: comparison of luteal, follicular, and flare-up administration in controlled ovarian hyperstimulation for oocyte retrieval. J In Vitro Fert Embryo Transf 1990; 7: 94–7.

133. Anserini P, Magnasco A, Remorgida V, et al. Comparison of a blocking vs. a flare-up protocol in poor responders with a normal and abnormal clomiphene citrate challenge test. Gynecol Endocrinol 1997; 11: 321–6.

134. Karacan M, Erkan H, Karabulut O, et al. Clinical pregnancy rates in an IVF program. Use of the flare-up protocol after failure with long regimens of GnRH-a. J Reprod Med 2001; 46: 485–9.

135. San Roman GA, Surrey ES, Judd HL, Kerin JF. A prospective randomized comparison of luteal phase versus concurrent follicular phase initiation of gonadotropin-releasing hormone agonist for in vitro fertilization. Fertil Steril 1992; 58: 744–9.

136. Hillier SG, Tetsuka M. Role of androgens in follicle maturation and atresia. Baillieres Clin Obstet Gynaecol 1997; 11: 249–60.

137. Erickson GF, Magoffin DA, Dyer CA, Hofeditz C. The ovarian androgen producing cells: a review of structure/function relationships. Endocr Rev 1985; 6: 371–99.

138. McNatty KP, Smith DM, Makris A, Osathanondh R, Ryan KJ. The microenvironment of the human antral follicle: interrelationships among the steroid levels in antral fluid, the population of granulosa cells, and the status of the oocyte in vivo and in vitro. J Clin Endocrinol Metab 1979; 49: 851–60.

139. Hillier SG. Roles of follicle stimulating hormone and luteinizing hormone in controlled ovarian hyperstimulation. Hum Reprod 1996; 11(Suppl 3): 113–21.

140. Gelety TJ, Pearlstone AC, Surrey ES. Short-term endocrine response to gonadotropin-releasing hormone agonist initiated in the early follicular, midluteal, or late luteal phase in normally cycling women. Fertil Steril 1995; 64: 1074–80.

141. Cedrin-Durnerin I, Bulwa S, Herve F, et al. The hormonal flare-up following gonadotrophin-releasing hormone agonist administration is influenced by a progestogen pretreatment. Hum Reprod 1996; 11: 1859–63.

142. al-Mizyen E, Sabatini L, Lower AM, et al. Does pretreatment with progestogen or oral contraceptive pills in low responders followed by the GnRHa flare protocol improve the outcome of IVF-ET? J Assist Reprod Genet 2000; 17: 140–6.

143. Bstandig B, Cedrin-Durnerin I, Hugues JN. Effectiveness of low dose of gonadotropin releasing hormone agonist on hormonal flare-up. J Assist Reprod Genet 2000; 17: 113–17.

144. Deaton JL, Bauguess P, Huffman CS, Miller KA. Pituitary response to early follicular-phase minidose gonadotropin releasing hormone agonist (GnRHa) therapy: evidence for a second flare. J Assist Reprod Genet 1996; 13: 390–4.

145. Navot D, Rosenwaks Z, Anderson F, Hodgen GD. Gonadotropin-releasing hormone agonist-induced ovarian hyperstimulation: low-dose side effects in women and monkeys. Fertil Steril 1991; 55: 1069–75.

146. Scott RT, Carey KD, Leland M, Navot D. Gonadotropin responsiveness to ultralow-dose leuprolide acetate administration in baboons. Fertil Steril 1993; 59: 1124–8.

147. Schoolcraft W, Schlenker T, Gee M, Stevens J, Wagley L. Improved controlled ovarian hyperstimulation in poor responder in vitro fertilization patients with a microdose follicle-stimulating hormone flare, growth hormone protocol. Fertil Steril 1997; 67: 93–7.

148. Surrey ES, Bower J, Hill DM, Ramsey J, Surrey MW. Clinical and endocrine effects of a microdose GnRH agonist flare regimen administered to poor responders who are undergoing in vitro fertilization. Fertil Steril 1998; 69: 419–24.

149. Leondires MP, Escalpes M, Segars JH, Scott RT Jr. Miller BT. Microdose follicular phase gonadotropin-releasing hormone agonist (GnRH-a) compared with luteal phase GnRH-a for ovarian stimulation at in vitro fertilization. Fertil Steril 1999; 72: 1018–23.

150. Albano C, Felberbaum RE, Smitz J, et al. Ovarian stimulation with HMG: results of a prospective randomized phase III European study comparing the luteinizing hormone-releasing hormone (LHRH)-antagonist cetrorelix and the LHRH-agonist buserelin. European Cetrorelix Study Group. Hum Reprod 2000; 15: 526–31.

151. Howles CM. The place of gonadotrophin-releasing hormone antagonists in reproductive medicine. Reprod Biomed Online 2002; 4(Suppl 3): 64–71.

152. Quigley MM. The use of ovulation-inducing agents in in-vitro fertilization. Clin Obstet Gynecol 1984; 27: 983–92.

153. Lehmann F, Baban N, Webber B. Ovarian stimulation for in-vitro fertilization: clomiphene and HMG. Hum Reprod 1988; 3(Suppl 2): 11–21.

154. Ronen J, Bosschieter J, Wiswedel K, Hendriks S, Levin M. Ovulation induction for in vitro fertilisation using clomiphene citrate and low-dose human menopausal gonadotrophin. Int J Fertil 1988; 33: 120–2.

155. Tummon IS, Daniel SA, Kaplan BR, Nisker JA, Yuzpe AA. Randomized, prospective comparison of luteal leuprolide acetate and gonadotropins versus clomiphene citrate and gonadotropins in 408 first cycles of in vitro fertilization. Fertil Steril 1992; 58: 563–8.

156. Craft I, Gorgy A, Hill J, Menon D, Podsiadly B. Will GnRH antagonists provide new hope for patients considered 'difficult responders' to GnRH agonist protocols? Hum Reprod 1999; 14: 2959–62.

157. Nikolettos N, Al-Hasani S, Felberbaum R, et al. Gonadotropin-releasing hormone antagonist protocol: a novel method of ovarian stimulation in poor responders. Eur J Obstet Gynecol Reprod Biol 2001; 97: 202–7.

158. Posada MN, Vlahos NP, Jurema MW, et al. Clinical outcome of using ganirelix acetate versus a 4-day follicular phase leuprolide acetate protocol in unselected women undergoing in vitro fertilization. Fertil Steril 2003; 80: 103–10.

159. Mohamed KA, Davies WA, Allsopp J, Lashen H. Agonist "flare-up" versus antagonist in the management of poor responders undergoing in vitro fertilization treatment. Fertil Steril 2005; 83: 331–5.

160. Fasouliotis SJ, Laufer N, Sabbagh-Ehrlich S, et al. Gonadotropin-releasing hormone (GnRH)-antagonist versus GnRH-agonist in ovarian stimulation of poor responders undergoing IVF. J Assist Reprod Genet 2003; 20: 455–60.

161. Copperman AB. Antagonists in poor-responder patients. Fertil Steril 2003; 80(Suppl 1): S16–24.

162. Shapiro D, Carter M, Mitchell-Leef D, Wininger D. Plateau or drop in estradiol (E2) on the day after initiation of the GnRH antagonist antagon™ in in-vitro fertilization (IVF) treatment cycles does not affect pregnancy outcome. Fertil Steril 2002; 78: S22–3.

163. Akman MA, Erden HF, Tosun SB, et al. Addition of GnRH antagonist in cycles of poor responders undergoing IVF. Hum Reprod 2000; 15: 2145–7.

164. Akman MA, Erden HF, Tosun SB, et al. Comparison of agonistic flare-up-protocol and antagonistic multiple dose protocol in ovarian stimulation of poor responders: results of a prospective randomized trial. Hum Reprod 2001; 16: 868–70.

165. De Placido G, Mollo A, Clarizia R, et al. Gonadotropin-releasing hormone (GnRH) antagonist plus recombinant luteinizing hormone vs. a standard GnRH agonist short protocol in patients at risk for poor ovarian response. Fertil Steril 2006; 85: 247–50.

166. Demirol A, Gurgan T. Comparison of microdose flare-up and antagonist multiple-dose protocols for poor-responder patients: a randomized study. Fertil Steril 2009; 92: 481–5.

167. Kahraman K, Berker B, Atabekoglu CS, et al. Microdose gonadotropin-releasing hormone agonist flare-up protocol versus multiple dose gonadotropin-releasing hormone antagonist protocol in poor responders undergoing intracytoplasmic sperm injection-embryo transfer cycle. Fertil Steril 2009; 91: 2437–44.

168. Devesa M, Martinez F, Coroleu B, et al. Poor prognosis for ovarian response to stimulation: results of a randomised trial comparing the flare-up GnRH agonist

protocol vs. the antagonist protocol. Gynecol Endocrinol 2010; 26: 509–15.

169. Schmidt DW, Bremner T, Orris JJ, et al. A randomized prospective study of microdose leuprolide versus ganirelix in in vitro fertilization cycles for poor responders. Fertil Steril 2005; 83: 1568–71.

170. Malmusi S, La Marca A, Giulini S, et al. Comparison of a gonadotropin-releasing hormone (GnRH) antagonist and GnRH agonist flare-up regimen in poor responders undergoing ovarian stimulation. Fertil Steril 2005; 84: 402–6.

171. D'Amato G, Caroppo E, Pasquadibisceglie A, et al. A novel protocol of ovulation induction with delayed gonadotropin-releasing hormone antagonist administration combined with high-dose recombinant follicle-stimulating hormone and clomiphene citrate for poor responders and women over 35 years. Fertil Steril 2004; 81: 1572–7.

172. Tazegul A, Gorkemli H, Ozdemir S, Aktan TM. Comparison of multiple dose GnRH antagonist and mini-dose long agonist protocols in poor responders undergoing in vitro fertilization: a randomized controlled trial. Arch Gynecol Obstet 2008; 278: 467–72.

173. Marci R, Caserta D, Dolo V, et al. GnRH antagonist in IVF poor-responder patients: results of a randomized trial. Reprod Biomed Online 2005; 11: 189–93.

174. Cheung LP, Lam PM, Lok IH, et al. GnRH antagonist versus long GnRH agonist protocol in poor responders undergoing IVF: a randomized controlled trial. Hum Reprod 2005; 20: 616–21.

175. Jurema MW, Bracero NJ, Garcia JE. Fine tuning cycle day 3 hormonal assessment of ovarian reserve improves in vitro fertilization outcome in gonadotropin-releasing hormone antagonist cycles. Fertil Steril 2003; 80: 1156–61.

176. Frankfurter D, Dayal M, Dubey A, Peak D, Gindoff P. Novel follicular-phase gonadotropin-releasing hormone antagonist stimulation protocol for in vitro fertilization in the poor responder. Fertil Steril 2007; 88: 1442–5.

177. Orvieto R, Kruchkovich J, Rabinson J, et al. Ultrashort gonadotropin-releasing hormone agonist combined with flexible multidose gonadotropin-releasing hormone antagonist for poor responders in in vitro fertilization/embryo transfer programs. Fertil Steril 2008; 90: 228–30.

178. Berger BM, Ezcurra D, Alper MM. The agonist-antagonist protocol: a novel protocol for treating the poor responder [abstract]. Fertil Steril 2004; 82: S126.

179. Fisch JD, Keskintepe L, Sher G. Gonadotropin-releasing hormone agonist/antagonist conversion with estrogen priming in low responders with prior in vitro fertilization failure. Fertil Steril 2008; 89: 342–7.

180. Nargund G, Fauser BC, Macklon NS, et al. The ISMAAR proposal on terminology for ovarian stimulation for IVF. Hum Reprod 2007; 22: 2801–4.

181. Bassil S, Godin PA, Donnez J. Outcome of in-vitro fertilization through natural cycles in poor responders. Hum Reprod 1999; 14: 1262–5.

182. Feldman B, Seidman DS, Levron J, et al. In vitro fertilization following natural cycles in poor responders. Gynecol Endocrinol 2001; 15: 328–34.

183. Lindheim SR, Vidali A, Ditkoff E, Sauer MV, Zinger M. Poor responders to ovarian hyperstimulation may benefit from an attempt at natural-cycle oocyte retrieval. J Assist Reprod Genet 1997; 14: 174–6.

184. Bar-Hava I, Ferber A, Ashkenazi J, et al. Natural-cycle in vitro fertilization in women aged over 44 years. Gynecol Endocrinol 2000; 14: 248–52.

185. Check ML, Check JH, Wilson C, Choe JK, Krotec J. Outcome of in vitro fertilization-embryo transfer according to age in poor responders with elevated baseline serum follicle stimulation hormone using minimal or no gonadotropin stimulation. Clin Exp Obstet Gynecol 2004; 31: 183–4.

186. Morgia F, Sbracia M, Schimberni M, et al. A controlled trial of natural cycle versus microdose gonadotropin-releasing hormone analog flare cycles in poor responders undergoing in vitro fertilization. Fertil Steril 2004; 81: 1542–7.

187. Papaleo E, De Santis L, Fusi F, et al. Natural cycle as first approach in aged patients with elevated follicle-stimulating hormone undergoing intracytoplasmic sperm injection: a pilot study. Gynecol Endocrinol 2006; 22: 351–4.

188. Pelinck MJ, Hoek A, Simons AH, Heineman MJ. Efficacy of natural cycle IVF: a review of the literature. Hum Reprod Update 2002; 8: 129–39.

189. Paulson RJ, Sauer MV, Lobo RA. Addition of a gonadotropin releasing hormone (GnRH) antagonist and exogenous gonadotropins to unstimulated in vitro fertilization (IVF) cycles: physiologic observations and preliminary experience. J Assist Reprod Genet 1994; 11: 28–32.

190. Rongieres-Bertrand C, Olivennes F, Righini C, et al. Revival of the natural cycles in in-vitro fertilization with the use of a new gonadotrophin-releasing hormone antagonist (Cetrorelix): A pilot study with minimal stimulation. Hum Reprod 1999; 14: 683–8.

191. Pelinck MJ, Vogel NE, Arts EG, et al. Cumulative pregnancy rates after a maximum of nine cycles of modified natural cycle IVF and analysis of patient drop-out: A cohort study. Hum Reprod 2007; 22: 2463–70.

192. Pelinck MJ, Vogel NE, Hoek A, et al. Minimal stimulation IVF with late follicular phase administration of the GnRH antagonist cetrorelix and concomitant substitution with recombinant FSH: A pilot study. Hum Reprod 2005; 20: 642–8.

193. Pelinck MJ, Vogel NE, Hoek A, et al. Cumulative pregnancy rates after three cycles of minimal stimulation IVF and results according to subfertility diagnosis: a multicentre cohort study. Hum Reprod 2006; 21: 2375–83.

194. Kolibianakis E, Zikopoulos K, Camus M, et al. Modified natural cycle for IVF does not offer a realistic chance of parenthood in poor responders with high day 3 FSH levels, as a last resort prior to oocyte donation. Hum Reprod 2004; 19: 2545–9.

195. Elizur SE, Aslan D, Shulman A, et al. Modified natural cycle using GnRH antagonist can be an optional treatment in poor responders undergoing IVF. J Assist Reprod Genet 2005; 22: 75–9.

196. Kim CH, Kim SR, Cheon YP, et al. Minimal stimulation using gonadotropin-releasing hormone (GnRH) antagonist and recombinant human follicle-stimulating hormone versus GnRH antagonist multiple-dose protocol in low responders undergoing in vitro fertilization/intracytoplasmic sperm injection. Fertil Steril 2009; 92: 2082–4.

197. Kadoch IJ, Phillips SJ, Bissonnette F. Modified natural-cycle in vitro fertilization should be considered as the first approach in young poor responders. Fertil Steril 96: 1066–8.

198. Kadoch IJ, Al-Khaduri M, Phillips SJ, et al. Spontaneous ovulation rate before oocyte retrieval in modified natural cycle IVF with and without indomethacin. Reprod Biomed Online 2008; 16: 245–9.

199. Schimberni M, Morgia F, Colabianchi J, et al. Natural-cycle in vitro fertilization in poor responder patients: a survey of 500 consecutive cycles. Fertil Steril 2009; 92: 1297–301.

200. Castelo Branco A, Achour-Frydman N, Kadoch J, et al. In vitro fertilization and embryo transfer in seminatural cycles for patients with ovarian aging. Fertil Steril 2005; 84: 875–80.

201. Segawa T, Yelian Y, Kato K, et al. Natural cycle IVF is an excellent treatment option for women with advanced age. Fertil Steril 2009; 92: S54.

202. Ellenbogen A, Gidoni Y, Atamna R, et al. Last chance before egg donation: modified natural cycle in vitro fertilization in poor responder patients; the role of follicle diameter on the day of hCG administration in order to improve results. Fertil Steril 2009; 92: S162.

203. Ellenbogen A, Michaeli M, Ballas S. Egg collection with a double lumen needle in poor responder patients undergoing in vitro fertilization treatment. Fertil Steril 2003; 80: 127.

204. Méndez Lozano DH, Brum Scheffer J, Frydman N, et al. Optimal reproductive competence of oocytes retrieved through follicular flushing in minimal stimulation IVF. Reprod Biomed Online 2008; 16: 119–23.

205. Mendez Lozano DH, Fanchin R, Chevalier N, et al. The follicular flushing duplicate the pregnancy rate on semi natural cycle IVF. J Gynecol Obstet Biol Reprod (Paris) 2007; 36: 36–41.

206. Levens ED, Whitcomb BW, Payson MD, Larsen FW. Ovarian follicular flushing among low-responding patients undergoing assisted reproductive technology. Fertil Steril 2009; 91: 1381–4.

207. Hill MJ, Levens ED, Levy G, et al. The use of recombinant luteinizing hormone in patients undergoing assisted reproductive techniques with advanced reproductive age: a systematic review and meta-analysis. Fertility and sterility 2012; 97: 1108–14 e1.

208. Simoni M, Nieschlag E, Gromoll J. Isoforms and single nucleotide polymorphisms of the FSH receptor gene: implications for human reproduction. Hum Reprod Update 2002; 8: 413–21.

209. Flack MR, Froehlich J, Bennet AP, Anasti J, Nisula BC. Site-directed mutagenesis defines the individual roles of the glycosylation sites on follicle-stimulating hormone. J Biol Chem 1994; 269: 14015–20.

210. Howles CM. Genetic engineering of human FSH (Gonal-F). Hum Reprod Update 1996; 2: 172–91.

211. Bassett RM, Driebergen R. Continued improvements in the quality and consistency of follitropin alfa, recombinant human FSH. Reprod Biomed Online 2005; 10: 169–77.

212. Aittomaki K, Herva R, Stenman UH, et al. Clinical features of primary ovarian failure caused by a point mutation in the follicle-stimulating hormone receptor gene. J Clin Endocrinol Metab 1996; 81: 3722–6.

213. Touraine P, Beau I, Gougeon A, et al. New natural inactivating mutations of the follicle-stimulating hormone receptor: correlations between receptor function, phenotype. Mol Endocrinol 1999; 13: 1844–54.

214. Perez Mayorga M, Gromoll J, Behre HM, et al. Ovarian response to follicle-stimulating hormone (FSH) stimulation depends on the FSH receptor genotype. J Clin Endocrinol Metab 2000; 85: 3365–9.

215. Jun JK, Yoon JS, Ku SY, et al. Follicle-stimulating hormone receptor gene polymorphism and ovarian responses to controlled ovarian hyperstimulation for IVF-ET. J Hum Genet 2006; 51: 665–70.

216. Greb RR, Grieshaber K, Gromoll J, et al. A common single nucleotide polymorphism in exon 10 of the human follicle stimulating hormone receptor is a major determinant of length and hormonal dynamics of the menstrual cycle. J Clin Endocrinol Metab 2005; 90: 4866–72.

217. Behre HM, Greb RR, Mempel A, et al. Significance of a common single nucleotide polymorphism in exon 10 of the follicle-stimulating hormone (FSH) receptor gene for the ovarian response to FSH: a pharmacogenetic approach to controlled ovarian hyperstimulation. Pharmacogenet Genomics 2005; 15: 451–6.

218. Achrekar SK, Modi DN, Desai SK, et al. Poor ovarian response to gonadotrophin stimulation is associated with FSH receptor polymorphism. Reprod Biomed Online 2009; 18: 509–15.

219. Bosch E, Ezcurra D. Individualised controlled ovarian stimulation (iCOS): maximising success rates for assisted reproductive technology patients. Reprod Biol Endocrinol 2011; 9: 82.

220. Nardo LG, Fleming R, Howles CM, et al. Conventional ovarian stimulation no longer exists: welcome to the age of individualized ovarian stimulation. Reprod Biomed Online 2011; 23: 141–8.

221. Olivennes F, Howles CM, Borini A, et al.; CONSORT study group. Individualizing FSH dose for assisted reproduction using a novel algorithm: the CONSORT study. Reprod Biomed Online. 2009; 18: 195–204. PubMed PMID: 19192339.

222. Balasch J, Miro F, Burzaco I, et al. The role of luteinizing hormone in human follicle development and oocyte fertility: evidence from in-vitro fertilization in a woman with long-standing hypogonadotrophic hypogonadism and using recombinant human follicle stimulating hormone. Hum Reprod 1995; 10: 1678–83.

223. Hull M, Corrigan E, Piazzi A, Loumaye E. Recombinant human luteinising hormone: an effective new gonadotropin preparation. Lancet 1994; 344: 334–5.

224. De Placido G, Alviggi C, Mollo A, et al. Effects of recombinant LH (rLH) supplementation during controlled ovarian hyperstimulation (COH) in normogonadotrophic women with an initial inadequate response to recombinant FSH (rFSH) after pituitary downregulation. Clin Endocrinol (Oxf) 2004; 60: 637–43.

225. De Placido G, Alviggi C, Perino A, et al. Recombinant human LH supplementation versus recombinant human FSH (rFSH) step-up protocol during controlled ovarian stimulation in normogonadotrophic women with initial inadequate ovarian response to rFSH. A multicentre, prospective, randomized controlled trial. Hum Reprod 2005; 20: 390–6.

226. Howles CM. Role of LH, FSH in ovarian function. Mol Cell Endocrinol 2000; 161: 25–30.

227. Chappel SC, Howles C. Reevaluation of the roles of luteinizing hormone and follicle-stimulating hormone in the ovulatory process. Hum Reprod 1991; 6: 1206–12.

228. Hillier SG. Current concepts of the roles of follicle stimulating hormone and luteinizing hormone in folliculogenesis. Hum Reprod 1994; 9: 188–91.

229. Balasch J, Fabregues F. Is luteinizing hormone needed for optimal ovulation induction? Curr Opin Obstet Gynecol 2002; 14: 265–74.

230. Shoham Z. Treatment of female infertility with recombinant human luteinising hormone: is there a benefit over other available drugs? Expert Opin Pharmacother 2003; 4: 1985–94.

231. Huirne JA, van Loenen AC, Schats R, et al. Dose-finding study of daily GnRH antagonist for the prevention of premature LH surges in IVF/ICSI patients: optimal changes in LH and progesterone for clinical pregnancy. Hum Reprod 2005; 20: 359–67.

232. Haavisto AM, Pettersson K, Bergendahl M, Virkamaki A, Huhtaniemi I. Occurrence and biological properties of a common genetic variant of luteinizing hormone. J Clin Endocrinol Metab 1995; 80: 1257–63.

233. Alviggi C, Clarizia R, Pettersson K, et al. Suboptimal response to GnRHa long protocol is associated with a common LH polymorphism. Reprod Biomed Online 2009; 18: 9–14.

234. Takahashi K, Kurioka H, Ozaki T, et al. Increased prevalence of luteinizing hormone beta-subunit variant in Japanese infertility patients. Hum Reprod 1998; 13: 3338–44.

235. Takahashi K, Ozaki T, Okada M, et al. Increased prevalence of luteinizing hormone beta-subunit variant in patients with premature ovarian failure. Fertil Steril 1999; 71: 96–101.

236. Caglar GS, Asimakopoulos B, Nikolettos N, Diedrich K, Al-Hasani S. Recombinant LH in ovarian stimulation. Reprod Biomed Online 2005; 10: 774–85.

237. The European Recombinant Human LH Study Group. Recombinant human luteinizing hormone (LH) to support recombinant human follicle-stimulating hormone (FSH)-induced follicular development in LH- and FSH-deficient anovulatory women: a dose-finding study. J Clin Endocrinol Metab 1998; 83: 1507–14.

238. Foong SC, Abbott DH, Lesnick TG, et al. Diminished intrafollicular estradiol levels in in vitro fertilization cycles from women with reduced ovarian response to recombinant human follicle-stimulating hormone. Fertil Steril 2005; 83: 1377–83.

239. Tesarik J, Mendoza C. Nongenomic effects of 17 beta-estradiol on maturing human oocytes: relationship to oocyte developmental potential. J Clin Endocrinol Metab 1995; 80: 1438–43.

240. Mason HD, Martikainen H, Beard RW, Anyaoku V, Franks S. Direct gonadotrophic effect of growth hormone on oestradiol production by human granulosa cells in vitro. J Endocrinol 1990; 126: R1–4.

241. Lanzone A, Fortini A, Fulghesu AM, et al. Growth hormone enhances estradiol production follicle-stimulating hormone-induced in the early stage of the follicle maturation. Fertil Steril 1996; 66: 948–53.

242. Mendoza C, Ruiz-Requena E, Ortega E, et al. Follicular fluid markers of oocyte developmental potential. Hum Reprod 2002; 17: 1017–22.

243. Tesarik J, Mendoza C. Direct non-genomic effects of follicular steroids on maturing human oocytes: oestrogen versus androgen antagonism. Hum Reprod Update 1997; 3: 95–100.

244. Murdoch WJ, Van Kirk EA. Estrogenic upregulation of DNA polymerase beta in oocytes of preovulatory ovine follicles. Mol Reprod Dev 2001; 58: 417–23.

245. Zelinski-Wooten MB, Hess DL, Baughman WL, et al. Administration of an aromatase inhibitor during the late follicular phase of gonadotropin-treated cycles in rhesus monkeys: effects on follicle development, oocyte maturation, and subsequent luteal function. J Clin Endocrinol Metab 1993; 76: 988–95.

246. Lisi F, Rinaldi L, Fishel S, et al. Use of recombinant FSH and recombinant LH in multiple follicular stimulation for IVF: a preliminary study. Reprod Biomed Online 2001; 3: 190–4.

247. Ferraretti AP, Gianaroli L, Magli MC, et al. Exogenous luteinizing hormone in controlled ovarian hyperstimulation for assisted reproduction techniques. Fertil Steril 2004; 82: 1521–6.

248. Richards JS, Jahnsen T, Hedin L, et al. Ovarian follicular development: from physiology to molecular biology. Recent Prog Horm Res 1987; 43: 231–76.

249. Robertson DM, Burger HG. Reproductive hormones: ageing and the perimenopause. Acta Obstet Gynecol Scand 2002; 81: 612–16.

250. Piltonen T, Koivunen R, Ruokonen A, Tapanainen JS. Ovarian age-related responsiveness to human chorionic gonadotropin. J Clin Endocrinol Metab 2003; 88: 3327–32.

251. Vihko KK, Kujansuu E, Morsky P, Huhtaniemi I, Punnonen R. Gonadotropins and gonadotropin receptors during the perimenopause. Eur J Endocrinol 1996; 134: 357–61.

252. Kim YK, Wasser SK, Fujimoto VY, et al. Utility of follicle stimulating hormone (FSH), luteinizing hormone (LH), oestradiol and FSH:LH ratio in predicting reproductive age in normal women. Hum Reprod 1997; 12: 1152–5.

253. Mitchell R, Hollis S, Rothwell C, Robertson WR. Age related changes in the pituitary-testicular axis in normal men; lower serum testosterone results from decreased bioactive LH drive. Clin Endocrinol (Oxf) 1995; 42: 501–7.

254. Huhtaniemi IT, Pettersson KS. Alterations in gonadal steroidogenesis in individuals expressing a common genetic variant of luteinizing hormone. J Steroid Biochem Mol Biol 1999; 69: 281–5.

255. De Placido G, Mollo A, Alviggi C, et al. Rescue of IVF cycles by HMG in pituitary down-regulated normogonadotrophic young women characterized by a poor initial response to recombinant FSH. Hum Reprod 2001; 16: 1875–9.

256. Loutradis D, Drakakis P, Milingos S, Stefanidis K, Michalas S. Alternative approaches in the management of poor response in controlled ovarian hyperstimulation (COH). Ann N Y Acad Sci 2003; 997: 112–19.

257. Gomez-Palomares JL, Acevedo-Martin B, Andres L, Ricciarelli E, Hernandez ER. LH improves early follicular recruitment in women over 38 years old. Reprod Biomed Online 2005; 11: 409–14.

258. Alviggi C, Mollo A, Clarizia R, De Placido G. Exploiting LH in ovarian stimulation. Reprod Biomed Online 2006; 12: 221–33.

259. Nilsson C, Pettersson K, Millar RP, et al. Worldwide frequency of a common genetic variant of luteinizing hormone: an international collaborative research. International Collaborative Research Group. Fertil Steril 1997; 67: 998–1004.

260. de Castro F, Moron FJ, Montoro L, et al. Human controlled ovarian hyperstimulation outcome is a polygenic trait. Pharmacogenetics 2004; 14: 285–93.

261. Loutradis D, Elsheikh A, Kallianidis K, et al. Results of controlled ovarian stimulation for ART in poor responders according to the short protocol using different gonadotrophins combinations. Arch Gynecol Obstet 2004; 270: 223–6.

262. Laml T, Obruca A, Fischl F, Huber JC. Recombinant luteinizing hormone in ovarian hyperstimulation after stimulation failure in normogonadotropic women. Gynecol Endocrinol 1999; 13: 98–103.

263. Ferrari B, Barusi L, Coppola F. Clinical and endocrine effects of ovulation induction with FSH and hCG supplementation in low responders in the midfollicular phase. A pilot study. J Reprod Med 2002; 47: 137–43.

264. Griesinger G, Shapiro DB, Kolibianakis EM, Witjes H, Mannaerts BM. No association between endogenous LH and pregnancy in a GnRH antagonist protocol: part II, recombinant FSH. Reprod Biomed Online 2011; 23: 457–65.

265. Chung K, Krey L, Katz J, Noyes N. Evaluating the role of exogenous luteinizing hormone in poor responders undergoing in vitro fertilization with gonadotropin-releasing hormone antagonists. Fertil Steril 2005; 84: 313–18.

266. Barrenetxea G, Agirregoikoa JA, Jimenez MR, et al. Ovarian response and pregnancy outcome in poor-responder women: a randomized controlled trial on the effect of luteinizing hormone supplementation on in vitro fertilization cycles. Fertil Steril 2008; 89: 546–53.

267. Adashi EY. The ovarian follicular apparatus. In: Adashi EY, Rock J, Rosenwaks Z, eds. Reproductive Endocrinology, Surgery and Technology. Philadelphia: Lippincott-Raven, 1996: 7–40.

268. Weil SJ, Vendola K, Zhou J, et al. Androgen receptor gene expression in the primate ovary: cellular localization, regulation, and functional correlations. J Clin Endocrinol Metab 1998; 83: 2479–85.

269. Hillier SG. Gonadotropic control of ovarian follicular growth and development. Mol Cell Endocrinol 2001; 179: 39–46.

270. Hugues JN, Durnerin IC. Impact of androgens on fertility – physiological, clinical and therapeutic aspects. Reprod Biomed Online 2005; 11: 570–80.

271. Piltonen T, Koivunen R, Perheentupa A, et al. Ovarian age-related responsiveness to human chorionic gonadotropin in women with polycystic ovary syndrome. J Clin Endocrinol Metab 2004; 89: 3769–75.

272. Guay A, Munarriz R, Jacobson J, et al. Serum androgen levels in healthy premenopausal women with and without sexual dysfunction: part A. Serum androgen levels in women aged 20–49 years with no complaints of sexual dysfunction. Int J Impot Res 2004; 16: 112–20.

273. Frattarelli JL, Peterson EH. Effect of androgen levels on in vitro fertilization cycles. Fertil Steril 2004; 81: 1713–14.

274. Barbieri RL, Sluss PM, Powers RD, et al. Association of body mass index, age, and cigarette smoking with serum testosterone levels in cycling women undergoing in vitro fertilization. Fertil Steril 2005; 83: 302–8.

275. Durnerin CI, Erb K, Fleming R, et al. Effects of recombinant LH treatment on folliculogenesis and responsiveness to FSH stimulation. Hum Reprod 2008; 23: 421–6.

276. Massin N, Cedrin-Durnerin I, Coussieu C, et al. Effects of transdermal testosterone application on the ovarian response to FSH in poor responders undergoing assisted reproduction technique–a prospective, randomized, double-blind study. Hum Reprod 2006; 21: 1204–11.

277. Kim CH, Howles CM, Lee HA. The effect of transdermal testosterone gel pretreatment on controlled ovarian stimulation and IVF outcome in low responders. Fertil Steril 2011; 95: 679–83.

278. Casson PR, Lindsay MS, Pisarska MD, Carson SA, Buster JE. Dehydroepiandrosterone supplementation augments ovarian stimulation in poor responders: a case series. Hum Reprod 2000; 15: 2129–32.

279. Barad D, Brill H, Gleicher N. Update on the use of dehydroepiandrosterone supplementation among women with diminished ovarian function. J Assist Reprod Genet 2007; 24: 629–34.

280. Barad D, Gleicher N. Effect of dehydroepiandrosterone on oocyte and embryo yields, embryo grade and cell number in IVF. Hum Reprod 2006; 21: 2845–9.

281. Barad DH, Gleicher N. Increased oocyte production after treatment with dehydroepiandrosterone. Fertil Steril 2005; 84: 756.

282. Gleicher N, Barad DH. Dehydroepiandrosterone (DHEA) supplementation in diminished ovarian reserve (DOR). Reprod Biol Endocrinol 2011; 9: 67.

283. Gleicher N, Ryan E, Weghofer A, Blanco-Mejia S, Barad DH. Miscarriage rates after dehydroepiandrosterone (DHEA) supplementation in women with diminished ovarian reserve: a case control study. Reprod Biol Endocrinol 2009; 7: 108.

284. Gleicher N, Weghofer A, Barad DH. Dehydroepiandrosterone (DHEA) reduces embryo aneuploidy: direct evidence from preimplantation genetic screening (PGS). Reprod Biol Endocrinol 2010; 8: 140–4.

285. Gleicher N, Weghofer A, Barad DH. Improvement in diminished ovarian reserve after dehydroepiandrosterone supplementation. Reprod Biomed Online 2010; 21: 360–5.

286. Sonmezer M, Ozmen B, Cil AP, et al. Dehydroepiandrosterone supplementation improves ovarian response and cycle outcome in poor responders. Reprod Biomed Online 2009; 19: 508–13.

287. Wiser A, Gonen O, Ghetler Y, et al. Addition of dehydroepiandrosterone (DHEA) for poor-responder patients before and during IVF treatment improves the pregnancy rate: a randomized prospective study. Hum Reprod 2010; 25: 2496–500.

288. Kolibianakis EM, Venetis CA, Tarlatzis BC. DHEA administration in poor responders. Hum Reprod 2011; 26: 730–1; author reply 731.

289. Yakin K, Urman B. DHEA as a miracle drug in the treatment of poor responders; hype or hope? Hum Reprod 2011; 26: 1941–4.

290. Thompson RD, Carlson M, Thompson RD, Carlson M. Liquid chromatographic determination of dehydroepiandrosterone (DHEA) in dietary supplement products. J AOAC Int 2000; 83: 847–57.

291. Mitwally MF, Casper RF. Aromatase inhibition improves ovarian response to follicle-stimulating hormone in poor responders. Fertil Steril 2002; 77: 776–80.

292. Garcia-Velasco JA, Moreno L, Pacheco A, et al. The aromatase inhibitor letrozole increases the concentration of intraovarian androgens and improves in vitro fertilization outcome in low responder patients: a pilot study. Fertil Steril 2005; 84: 82–7.

293. Ozmen B, Sonmezer M, Atabekoglu CS, Olmus H. Use of aromatase inhibitors in poor-responder patients receiving GnRH antagonist protocols. Reprod Biomed Online 2009; 19: 478–85.

294. Lee VC, Chan CC, Ng EH, Yeung WS, Ho PC. Sequential use of letrozole and gonadotrophin in women with poor ovarian reserve: a randomized controlled trial. Reprod Biomed Online 2011; 23: 380–8.

295. Schoolcraft WB, Surrey ES, Minjarez DA, Stevens JM, Gardner DK. Management of poor responders: can outcomes be improved with a novel gonadotropin-releasing hormone antagonist/letrozole protocol? Fertil Steril 2008; 89: 151–6.

296. Davar R, Oskouian H, Ahmadi S, Firouzabadi RD. GnRH antagonist/letrozole versus microdose GnRH agonist flare protocol in poor responders undergoing in vitro fertilization. Taiwan J Obstet Gynecol 2010; 49: 297–301.

297. Sunkara SK, Pundir J, Khalaf Y. Effect of androgen supplementation or modulation on ovarian stimulation outcome in poor responders: a meta-analysis. Reprod Biomed Online 2011; 22: 545–55.

298. Fanchin R, Frydman N, Even M, et al. Androgens and poor responders: are we ready to take the plunge into clinical therapy? Fertil Steril 2011; 96: 1062–5.

299. Shoham Z, Homburg R, Owen EJ, et al. The role of treatment with growth hormone in infertile patients. Baillieres Clin Obstet Gynaecol 1992; 6: 267–81.

300. Owen EJ, Shoham Z, Mason BA, Ostergaard H, Jacobs HS. Cotreatment with growth hormone, after pituitary suppression, for ovarian stimulation in in vitro fertilization: a randomized, double-blind, placebo-control trial. Fertil Steril 1991; 56: 1104–10.

301. Adashi EY, Resnick CE, Hurwitz A, et al. Insulin-like growth factors: the ovarian connection. Hum Reprod 1991; 6: 1213–19.

302. Adashi EY, Resnick CE, Hernandez ER, et al. Insulin-like growth factor I as an intraovarian regulator: basic and clinical implications. Ann NY Acad Sci 1991; 626: 161–8.

303. Abir R, Garor R, Felz C, et al. Growth hormone and its receptor in human ovaries from fetuses and adults. Fertil Steril 2008; 90: 1333–9.

304. Mendoza C, Cremades N, Ruiz-Requena E, et al. Relationship between fertilization results after intracytoplasmic sperm injection, and intrafollicular steroid, pituitary hormone and cytokine concentrations. Hum Reprod 1999; 14: 628–35.

304a. Menezo YJ, el Mouatassim S, Chavrier M, et al. Human oocytes and preimplantation embryos express mRNA for growth hormone receptor. Zygote 2003; 11: 293–7.

305. Izadyar F, Van Tol HT, Hage WG, Bevers MM. Preimplantation bovine embryos express mRNA of growth hormone receptor and respond to growth hormone addition during in vitro development. Mol Reprod Dev 2000; 57: 247–55.

306. Kolle S, Stojkovic M, Boie G, Wolf E Sinowatz F. Growth hormone inhibits apoptosis in in vitro produced bovine embryos. Mol Reprod Dev 2002; 61: 180–6.

307. Thompson BJ, Shang CA, Waters MJ. Identification of genes induced by growth hormone in rat liver using cDNA arrays. Endocrinology 2000; 141: 4321–4.

308. Ibrahim ZH, Matson PL, Buck P, Lieberman BA. The use of biosynthetic human growth hormone to augment ovulation induction with buserelin acetate/human menopausal gonadotropin in women with a poor ovarian response. Fertil Steril 1991; 55: 202–4.

309. Wu MY, Chen HF, Ho HN, et al. The value of human growth hormone as an adjuvant for ovarian stimulation in a human in vitro fertilization program. J Obstet Gynaecol Res 1996; 22: 443–50.

310. Busacca M, Fusi FM, Brigante C, et al. Use of growth hormone-releasing factor in ovulation induction in poor responders. J Reprod Med 1996; 41: 699–703.

311. Kim CH, Chae HD, Chang YS. Pyridostigmine cotreatment for controlled ovarian hyperstimulation in low responders undergoing in vitro fertilization-embryo transfer. Fertil Steril 1999; 71: 652–7.

312. Howles CM, Loumaye E, Germond M, et al. Does growth hormone-releasing factor assist follicular development in poor responder patients undergoing ovarian stimulation for in-vitro fertilization? Hum Reprod 1999; 14: 1939–43.

313. Suikkari A, MacLachlan V, Koistinen R, Seppala M, Healy D. Double-blind placebo controlled study: human biosynthetic growth hormone for assisted reproductive technology. Fertil Steril 1996; 65: 800–5.

314. Shaker AG, Fleming R, Jamieson ME, Yates RW, Coutts JR. Absence of effect of adjuvant growth hormone therapy on follicular responses to exogenous gonadotropins in women: normal and poor responders. Fertil Steril 1992; 58: 919–23.

315. Hughes SM, Huang ZH, Morris ID, et al. A double-blind cross-over controlled study to evaluate the effect of human biosynthetic growth hormone on ovarian stimulation in previous poor responders to in-vitro fertilization. Hum Reprod 1994; 9: 13–18.

316. Dor J, Seidman DS, Amudai E, et al. Adjuvant growth hormone therapy in poor responders to in-vitro fertilization: a prospective randomized placebo-controlled double-blind study. Hum Reprod 1995; 10: 40–3.

317. Younis JS, Simon A, Koren R, et al. The effect of growth hormone supplementation on in vitro fertilization outcome: a prospective randomized placebo-controlled double-blind study. Fertil Steril 1992; 58: 575–80.

318. Kotarba D, Kotarba J, Hughes E. Growth hormone for in vitro fertilization. Cochrane Database Syst Rev 2000; CD000099.

319. Tesarik J, Hazout A, Mendoza C. Improvement of delivery and live birth rates after ICSI in women aged >40 years by ovarian co-stimulation with growth hormone. Hum Reprod 2005; 20: 2536–41.

320. Kucuk T, Kozinoglu H, Kaba A. Growth hormone cotreatment within a GnRH agonist long protocol in patients with poor ovarian response: a prospective,

randomized, clinical trial. J Assist Reprod Genet 2008; 25: 123–7.

321. Yovich JL, Stanger JD. Growth hormone supplementation improves implantation and pregnancy productivity rates for poor-prognosis patients undertaking IVF. Reprod Biomed Online 2010; 21: 37–49.

322. Kyrou D, Kolibianakis EM, Venetis CA, et al. How to improve the probability of pregnancy in poor responders undergoing in vitro fertilization: a systematic review and meta-analysis. Fertil Steril 2009; 91: 749–66.

323. Kolibianakis EM, Venetis CA, Diedrich K, Tarlatzis BC, Griesinger G. Addition of growth hormone to gonadotrophins in ovarian stimulation of poor responders treated by in-vitro fertilization: a systematic review and meta-analysis. Hum Reprod Update 2009; 15: 613–22.

324. de Ziegler D, Streuli I, Meldrum DR, Chapron C. The value of growth hormone supplements in ART for poor ovarian responders. Fertil Steril 2011; 96: 1069–76.

325. Gonen Y, Jacobson W, Casper RF. Gonadotropin suppression with oral contraceptives before in vitro fertilization. Fertil Steril 1990; 53: 282–7.

326. Biljan MM, Mahutte NG, Dean N, et al. Effects of pretreatment with an oral contraceptive on the time required to achieve pituitary suppression with gonadotropin-releasing hormone analogues and on subsequent implantation and pregnancy rates. Fertil Steril 1998; 70: 1063–9.

327. Lindheim SR, Barad DH, Witt B, Ditkoff E, Sauer MV. Short-term gonadotropin suppression with oral contraceptives benefits poor responders prior to controlled ovarian hyperstimulation. J Assist Reprod Genet 1996; 13: 745–7.

328. Kovacs P, Barg PE, Witt BR. Hypothalamic-pituitary suppression with oral contraceptive pills does not improve outcome in poor responder patients undergoing in vitro fertilization-embryo transfer cycles. J Assist Reprod Genet 2001; 18: 391–4.

329. Fanchin R, Mendez Lozano DH, Schonauer LM, Cunha-Filho JS, Frydman R. Hormonal manipulations in the luteal phase to coordinate subsequent antral follicle growth during ovarian stimulation. Reprod Biomed Online 2005; 10: 721–8.

330. Fanchin R, Salomon L, Castelo-Branco A, et al. Luteal estradiol pre-treatment coordinates follicular growth during controlled ovarian hyperstimulation with GnRH antagonists. Hum Reprod 2003; 18: 2698–703.

331. Fanchin R, Cunha-Filho JS, Schonauer LM, et al. Coordination of early antral follicles by luteal estradiol administration provides a basis for alternative controlled ovarian hyperstimulation regimens. Fertil Steril 2003; 79: 316–21.

332. Fanchin R, Castelo Branco A, Kadoch IJ, et al. Premenstrual administration of gonadotropin-releasing hormone antagonist coordinates early antral follicle sizes and sets up the basis for an innovative concept of controlled ovarian hyperstimulation. Fertil Steril 2004; 81: 1554–9.

333. Rombauts L, Suikkari AM, MacLachlan V, Trounson AO, Healy DL. Recruitment of follicles by recombinant human follicle-stimulating hormone commencing in the luteal phase of the ovarian cycle. Fertil Steril 1998; 69: 665–9.

334. Dragisic KG, Davis OK, Fasouliotis SJ, Rosenwaks Z. Use of a luteal estradiol patch and a gonadotropin-releasing hormone antagonist suppression protocol before gonadotropin stimulation for in vitro fertilization in poor responders. Fertil Steril 2005; 84: 1023–6.

335. Frattarelli JL, Hill MJ, McWilliams GD, et al. A luteal estradiol protocol for expected poor-responders improves embryo number and quality. Fertil Steril 2008; 89: 1118–22.

336. DiLuigi AJ, Engmann L, Schmidt DW, Benadiva CA, Nulsen JC. A randomized trial of microdose leuprolide acetate protocol versus luteal phase ganirelix protocol in predicted poor responders. Fertil Steril 2011; 95: 2531–3.

337. Weitzman. VN, EngmannL, DiLuigi A, Maier D, Nulsen J, Benadiva C. Comparison of luteal estradiol patch and gonadotropin-releasing hormone antagonist suppression protocol before gonadotropin stimulation versus microdose gonadotropin-releasing hormone agonist protocol for patients with a history of poor in vitro fertilization outcomes. Fertil Steril 2009; 92: 226–30.

338. Shastri SM, Barbieri E, Kligman I, et al. Stimulation of the young poor responder: comparison of the luteal estradiol/gonadotropin-releasing hormone antagonist priming protocol versus oral contraceptive microdose leuprolide. Fertil Steril 2011; 95: 592–5.

339. Elassar A, Mann JS, Engmann L, Nulsen Benadiva C. Luteal phase estradiol versus luteal phase estradiol and antagonist protocol for controlled ovarian stimulation before in vitro fertilization in poor responders. Fertil Steril 2011; 95: 324–6.

340. Elassar A, Engmann L, Nulsen J,Benadiva C. Letrozole and gonadotropins versus luteal estradiol and gonadotropin-releasing hormone antagonist protocol in women with a prior low response to ovarian stimulation. Fertil Steril 2011; 95: 2330–4.

341. Rubinstein M, Marazzi A, Polak de Fried E. Low-dose aspirin treatment improves ovarian responsiveness, uterine and ovarian blood flow velocity, implantation, and pregnancy rates in patients undergoing in vitro fertilization: a prospective, randomized, double-blind placebo-controlled assay. Fertil Steril 1999; 71: 825–9.

342. Weckstein LN, Jacobson A, Galen D, Hampton K, Hammel J. Low-dose aspirin for oocyte donation recipients with a thin endometrium: prospective, randomized study. Fertil Steril 1997; 68: 927–30.

343. Hsieh YY, Tsai HD, Chang CC, Lo HY, Chen CL. Low-dose aspirin for infertile women with thin endometrium receiving intrauterine insemination: a prospective, randomized study. J Assist Reprod Genet 2000; 17: 174–7.

344. Gelbaya TA, Kyrgiou M, Li TC, Stern C, Nardo LG. Low-dose aspirin for in vitro fertilization: a systematic review and meta-analysis. Hum Reprod Update 2007; 13: 357–64.

345. Khairy M, Banerjee K, El-Toukhy T, Coomarasamy A, Khalaf Y. Aspirin in women undergoing in vitro fertilization treatment: a systematic review and meta-analysis. Fertil Steril 2007; 88: 822–31.

346. Ruopp MD, Collins TC, Whitcomb BW, Schisterman EF. Evidence of absence or absence of evidence? A reanalysis of the effects of low-dose aspirin in in vitro fertilization. Fertil Steril 2008; 90: 71–6.

347. Lok IH, Yip SK, Cheung LP, Yin Leung PH, Haines CJ. Adjuvant low-dose aspirin therapy in poor responders undergoing in vitro fertilization: a prospective, randomized, double-blind, placebo-controlled trial. Fertil Steril 2004; 81: 556–61.

348. Scoccia H, Puccini M, Horlick N, Winston N. Advancing Maternal Age and Low-Dose Aspirin Effect in Poor Responders Undergoing In Vitro Fertilization. Fertil Steril 2005; 84: S248.

349. Frattarelli JL, McWilliams GD, Hill MJ, Miller KA, Scott RT Jr. Low-dose aspirin use does not improve in vitro fertilization outcomes in poor responders. Fertil Steril 2008; 89: 1113–17.

350. May-Panloup P, Chretien MF, Jacques C, et al. Low oocyte mitochondrial DNA content in ovarian insufficiency. Hum Reprod 2005; 20: 593–7.

351. Tzeng CR, Hsieh RH, Au HK, et al. Mitochondria transfer (MIT) into oocyte from autologous cumulus granulosa cells (cGCs). Fertil Steril 2004; 82: S53.

352. Munne S, Alikani M, Tomkin G, Grifo J, Cohen J. Embryo morphology, developmental rates, and maternal age are correlated with chromosome abnormalities. Fertility and sterility 1995; 64: 382–91.

353. Marquez C, Sandalinas M, Bahce M, Alikani M, Munne S. Chromosome abnormalities in 1255 cleavage-stage human embryos. Reproductive biomedicine online 2000; 1: 17–26.

354. Gutierrez-Mateo C, Wells D, Benet J, et al. Reliability of comparative genomic hybridization to detect chromosome abnormalities in first polar bodies and metaphase II oocytes. Hum Reprod 2004; 19: 2118–25.

355. Munne S, Chen S, Fischer J, et al. Preimplantation genetic diagnosis reduces pregnancy loss in women aged 35 years and older with a history of recurrent miscarriages. Fertil Steril 2005; 84: 331–5.

356. Taranissi M, El-Toukhy T, Gorgy A, Verlinsky Y. Influence of maternal age on the outcome of PGD for aneuploidy screening in patients with recurrent implantation failure. Reprod Biomed Online 2005; 10: 628–32.

357. Rubio C, Rodrigo L, Perez-Cano I, et al. FISH screening of aneuploidies in preimplantation embryos to improve IVF outcome. Reprod Biomed Online 2005; 11: 497–506.

358. Mastenbroek S, Twisk M, van Echten-Arends J, et al. In vitro fertilization with preimplantation genetic screening. N Engl J Med 2007; 357: 9–17.

359. Treff NR, Ferry KM, Zhao T, et al. Cleavage stage embryo biopsy significantly impairs embryonic reproductive potential while blastocyst biopsy does not: a novel paired analysis of cotransferred biopsied and non-biopsied sibling embryos. Fertil Steril 2011; 96: S2.

360. Forman EJ, Treff NR, Tao X, et al. Comprehensive chromosome screening (CCS) results in significantly higher pregnancy rates and lower loss rates from single embryo transfer (SET) in a poor prognosis population. Fertil Steril 2011; 96: S17.

361. Assou S, Haouzi D, De Vos J, Hamamah S. Human cumulus cells as biomarkers for embryo and pregnancy outcomes. Mol Hum Reprod 2010; 16: 531–8.

362. Assou S, Haouzi D, Mahmoud K, et al. A non-invasive test for assessing embryo potential by gene expression profiles of human cumulus cells: a proof of concept study. Mol Hum Reprod 2008; 14: 711–19.

363. Dominguez F, Gadea B, Esteban FJ, et al. Comparative protein-profile analysis of implanted versus non-implanted human blastocysts. Hum Reprod 2008; 23: 1993–2000.

364. Sanchez-Ribas I, Dominguez F, Barr J, et al. Metabolomic profile as a novel non-invasive tool for human embryo aneuploidy assessment. Fertil Steril 2008; 90: S100.

365. Cohen J, Alikani M, Trowbridge J, Rosenwaks Z. Implantation enhancement by selective assisted hatching using zona drilling of human embryos with poor prognosis. Hum Reprod 1992; 7: 685–91.

366. Stein A, Rufas O, Amit S, et al. Assisted hatching by partial zona dissection of human pre-embryos in patients with recurrent implantation failure after in vitro fertilization. Fertil Steril 1995; 63: 838–41.

367. Schoolcraft WB, Schlenker T, Gee M, Jones GS, Jones HW Jr. Assisted hatching in the treatment of poor prognosis in vitro fertilization candidates. Fertil Steril 1994; 62: 551–4.

368. Meldrum DR, Wisot A, Yee B, et al. Assisted hatching reduces the age-related decline in IVF outcome in women younger than age 43 without increasing miscarriage or monozygotic twinning. J Assist Reprod Genet 1998; 15: 418–21.

369. Magli MC, Gianaroli L, Ferraretti AP, et al. Rescue of implantation potential in embryos with poor prognosis by assisted zona hatching. Hum Reprod 1998; 13: 1331–5.

370. Mansour RT, Rhodes CA, Aboulghar MA, Serour GI, Kamal A. Transfer of zona-free embryos improves outcome in poor prognosis patients: a prospective randomized controlled study. Hum Reprod 2000; 15: 1061–4.

371. Bider D, Livshits A, Yonish M, Yemini Z, Mashiach Dor J. Assisted hatching by zona drilling of human embryos in women of advanced age. Hum Reprod 1997; 12: 317–20.

372. Lanzendorf SE, Nehchiri F, Mayer JF, Oehninger Muasher SJ. A prospective, randomized, double-blind study for the evaluation of assisted hatching in patients with advanced maternal age. Hum Reprod 1998; 13: 409–13.

373. Das S, Blake D, Farquhar C, Seif MM. Assisted hatching on assisted conception (IVF and ICSI). Cochrane Database Syst Rev 2009; CD001894.

374. Martins WP, Rocha IA, Ferriani RA, Nastri CO. Assisted hatching of human embryos: a systematic review and meta-analysis of randomized controlled trials. Hum Reprod Update 2011; 17: 438–53.

375. Sudo S, Kudo M, Wada S, et al. Genetic and functional analyses of polymorphisms in the human FSH receptor gene. Mol Hum Reprod 2002; 8: 89–90.

376. Laven JS, Mulders AG, Suryandari DA, et al. Follicle-stimulating hormone receptor polymorphisms in women with normogonadotropic anovulatory infertility. Fertil Steril 2003; 80: 986–92.

377. de Castro F, Moron FJ, Montoro L, et al. Pharmacogenetics of controlled ovarian hyperstimulation. Pharmacogenomics 2005; 6: 629–37.

378. Daelemans C, Smits G, de Maertelaer V, et al. Prediction of severity of symptoms in iatrogenic ovarian hyperstimulation syndrome by follicle-stimulating hormone receptor Ser680Asn polymorphism. J Clin Endocrinol Metab 2004 89: 6310–15.

379. Choi D, Lee EY, Yoon S, et al. Clinical correlation of cycline D2 mRNA expression in human luteinized granulosa cells. J Assist Reprod Genet 2000; 17: 574–9.

47

Repeated implantation failure

Mark A. Damario and Zev Rosenwaks

OVERVIEW

The treatment of human infertility through the assisted reproductive techniques (ART) continues to be comparatively inefficient. Despite the common practice of multiple embryo transfers, all in vitro fertilization–embryo transfer (IVF–ET) procedures performed in the United States in 2006 resulted in a mean 35.4% delivery rate per embryo transfer (1). Although this IVF–ET delivery rate is actually an improvement over the preceding years, it is obvious that the majority of IVF–ET cycles still fail. While a clearly attributed cause for cycle failure may occasionally be present, in most circumstances there is no apparent explanation other than failure of the implantation process. Although both subclinical and clinical pregnancy losses occur, the largest percentage of failed IVF–ET cycles simply exhibit lack of implantation. In some patients, implantation failure occurs repeatedly. These latter patients continue to present unique challenges for the infertility specialist.

Age is perhaps the most important single variable influencing outcome in assisted reproduction. The effect of advancing female age on clinical IVF–ET is manifested not only in the pattern of ovarian response to gonadotropin stimulation but also in reduced implantation efficiency and in an increased spontaneous abortion rate (2). Determination of diminished ovarian reserve by timed hormonal evaluation provides useful prognostic information regarding assisted reproductive treatment (3,4). Ovarian reserve testing, however, still does not provide 100% sensitivity in the detection of women with reduced IVF–ET treatment potential.

Embryonic loss, which occurs repeatedly after assisted reproduction, may be attributable to many factors. These include embryonic genetic abnormalities, a lack of endometrial receptivity, and suboptimal laboratory culture conditions. Genetic abnormalities may perhaps account for at least as many as 30–40% of implantation failures (5). It is likely that, even in the best of circumstances, some embryonic loss occurs due to the artificial laboratory environment. This is supported by the differences in morphology and cleavage rates of in vivo human embryos and human embryos that have been supported in vitro (6).

This chapter summarizes several of the contemporary strategies used to enhance IVF–ET outcome in cases of repeated implantation failure.

METHODS

Prophylactic Salpingectomy

It has become apparent that patients with severe tubal damage have a poor prognosis with IVF–ET. In many retrospective reports, patients with hydrosalpinges have been identified as having lower implantation and pregnancy rates than patients suffering other types of tubal damage (7–9). Similar adverse effects on embryonic implantation specifically attributable to hydrosalpinges were noted in two meta-analyses of published comparative studies (10,11).

Different theories have evolved to explain the mechanism behind the association of hydrosalpinges with poorer pregnancy outcome. Reflux of hydrosalpinx fluid into the uterine cavity may simply result in mechanical factors diminishing embryonic endometrial apposition (12). Hydrosalpinx fluid is commonly slightly alkaline and may also contain cytokines, prostaglandins, or other inflammatory compounds (13). These inflammatory mediators may result in either direct embryotoxicity or adverse effects on the endometrium (14,15). One group has demonstrated an association of hydrosalpinges with altered endometrial histology and a lack of expression of endometrial adhesion molecules (integrins), which may play important roles in the implantation process (16).

Clinical evidence has shown that improved clinical outcomes are seen after prophylactic bilateral salpingectomy. Several retrospective studies have demonstrated that bilateral salpingectomy results in improved implantation as well as pregnancy rates compared with controls who harbor hydrosalpinges (17,18).

Assisted Hatching

It has been found that only a relatively small percentage of human embryos cleave beyond the eight-cell stage in vitro to form expanded blastocysts. In addition, fewer than 25% of such expanded blastocysts have been shown to hatch in vitro, presumably secondary to abnormal zona hardening (19). It was also noted that cleavage-stage embryos with a reduced zona thickness seemed to have a good prognosis for implantation (20). Furthermore, microsurgically fertilized embryos with artificial gaps in their zonae (from partial zona dissection) seemed to have higher rates of implantation (21).

From these observations, techniques were developed to promote improved embryo implantation efficiency. Assisted hatching was first tested experimentally by introducing small incisions in the zonae of four-cell embryos by a mechanical method (22). However, the observation of embryonic entrapment in the narrow zona openings during hatching (23) and the potential for embryo damage due to micromanipulation prior to the formation of blastomere structural junctions led to the development of an alternative zona drilling procedure that is performed with acidified Tyrodes solution on three-day-old embryos (24). Assisted hatching has also been accomplished utilizing a piezo-micromanipulator (25) and a laser (26).

Early randomized, prospective trials examining the efficacy of assisted hatching were undertaken at the Center for Reproductive Medicine and Infertility at the Weill Cornell Medical College and New York-Presbyterian Hospital (27). The initial trials included patients with normal basal follicle-stimulating hormone (FSH) concentrations. Assisted hatching appeared to benefit patients with thick zonae (>15 μm). Further trials employed zona biometric criteria as the indication for zona drilling. These latter selective assisted hatching trials indicated that women aged >38 years appeared to derive the most benefit from the procedure.

Preimplantation Genetic Diagnosis (Aneuploidy Screening)

There is significant evidence that implantation failure in women of advanced maternal age is closely linked to embryonic aneuploidy. This is based on data from spontaneous abortions (28) as well as data on oocytes and embryos (29,30). Utilizing blastomere biopsy and fluorescent in situ hybridization (FISH) to diagnose X, Y, 18, 13, and 21 aneuploidy, Munné et al. noted that even in embryos judged to be of good quality, aneuploidy rates were 4.0%, 9.4%, and 37.2%, in women aged 20–34, 35–39, and 40–47 years, respectively (30). A relationship between maternal age and aneuploidy for chromosome 16 was also identified (31). Therefore, considering only these data, rates of aneuploidy in women aged 40 years would be expected to exceed 40%. There remains a possibility that the rate of embryonic aneuploidy may be even higher in these women when further assessment of additional chromosomes is included.

Methods have been developed for the detection of aneuploidy in older women undergoing IVF–ET. These methods were developed to improve the implantation efficiency, reduce the spontaneous abortion rate, as well as decrease the incidence of chromosomal abnormalities at term. The first method involves embryo biopsy on day 3, in which one to two blastomeres are removed from an eight- to 10-cell embryo. Early work suggested that removing single blastomeres from eight-cell embryos did not affect their viability or ability to progress to the blastocyst stage (32). While analyses of two blastomeres may be preferable to reduce misdiagnoses, there is presently less clinical experience with two-blastomere biopsies. Following blastomere biopsy, the cells are fixed on a slide and analyzed by FISH. Most studies to date have been carried out with a multiple probe technique in a time frame compatible with clinical IVF (embryo transfer on day 4 or 5) (33). Up to five chromosomes can be detected by FISH at the single-cell level. Further investigations suggest that even more chromosomes may be investigated incorporating techniques of FISH–FISH cell recycling in which two or more rounds of hybridization are employed (34).

Recent work has included the use of comparative genomic hybridization (CGH) on single blastomeres for the purpose of aneuploidy screening. CGH is a molecular cytogenetic technique that allows for the simultaneous assessment of every chromosome in single interphase cells (35). Investigators have applied CGH to single human blastomeres from disaggregated human embryos (36). The clinical application of CGH for preimplantation detection of embryonic aneuploidy has also been reported (37,38). Chief limitations of single-cell CGH are that it is complex and requires three to four days to complete, thereby requiring initial freezing of biopsied embryos and later thawing prior to transfer.

The use of first polar body analysis for aneuploidy detection has also been proposed as an alternative to blastomere analysis since most aneuploidies originate from maternal meiosis I nondisjunction (39,40). To further uncover aneuploidies deriving from errors in the second meiotic division, the sequential analysis of the first and second polar bodies using multiprobe FISH has also been reported (41). Polar body analyses, however, are hampered by the inability to diagnose paternally derived chromosome abnormalities as well as those resulting from postfertilization events.

To overcome some of the known limitations of polar body and cleavage-stage aneuploidy screening, there has been recent focus on the use of trophectoderm biopsy for the cytogenetic analysis of human blastocysts. Utilizing a single nucleotide polymorphism (SNP) microarray-based 24-chromosome aneuploidy screening technology, Northrop et al. demonstrated euploid results in a significant proportion of embryos previously determined to be aneuploid by cleavage-stage FISH (42). Explanations for this phenomenon include that findings of cleavage-stage mosaicism may be significantly overrepresented by FISH-based analyses and that embryo self-correction capabilities may also occur (43). Further studies suggest that either CGH or microarray-CGH are accurate methodologies for blastocyst-stage aneuploidy screening (44). Clinical application of aneuploidy screening utilizing trophectoderm biopsy, blastocyst vitrification, comprehensive chromosomal screening utilizing CGH, and subsequent frozen embryo transfer has also had encouraging preliminary results (45).

Blastocyst Culture and Transfer

In attempts to improve the overall efficiency of human IVF–ET, investigators have strived to identify embryos with higher implantation potential. One method that has been repeatedly explored is the culture of human embryos to the blastocyst stage (day 5 of culture). In the human embryo, activation of the embryonic genome occurs at the eight- to 10-cell stage (day 3 of culture). Embryos that cleave after day 3 in culture therefore are no longer dependent on maternal RNA transcripts and have made the successful transition from maternal to embryonic genomic control. Embryos that progress to the blastocyst stage may thereby represent embryos with higher implantation potential. Blastocyst culture and transfer approaches may potentially provide certain patients with a history of repeated implantation failures an improved chance for pregnancy.

Early attempts to culture human embryos to the blastocyst stage, however, were discouraging as it was clear that the culture medium in use was primitive and would not support long-term growth of human embryos. In 1992, significant improvements were obtained when human embryos were cocultured in vitro along with Vero cell monolayers (46). The availability of sequential culture media furthered interest in the culture of human embryos to the blastocyst stage (47). Sequential culture media have been designed specifically for the first two days after fertilization (early cleavage) and the third to fifth days of embryo growth (morula and blastocyst). These new sequential culture media systems clearly have resulted in improved blastocyst culture and transfer results over those seen with conventional culture media (48).

A few investigators have suggested that blastocyst culture and transfer may potentially improve clinical outcome in women with repeated implantation failure (49,50). Since cleaving embryos do not normally reside in the uterine cavity, it is felt that there is a possibility that some embryos may experience nutritional or homeostatic stress when introduced during day 2–3 transfers.

Of perhaps more significance is the fact that blastocyst culture and transfer may allow for better embryo selection. A higher incidence of aneuploidy has been detected in embryos that fail to progress to the blastocyst stage in vitro (51). On the other hand, progression to blastocyst stage certainly would not be expected to guarantee chromosomal normality. Blastocyst culture and transfer, however, may be used as an additional tool in older women with a history of repeated implantation failure. Owing to the current limited efficiency of blastocyst culture and transfer techniques, this would be expected to work favorably only if satisfactory ovarian responses can be achieved.

Coculture Methods

The quality of in vitro culture conditions is one of the most crucial aspects of successful IVF–ET. Studies in many lower mammalian species have suggested that growth, biochemical synthetic activity, and survival after transfer are inferior in in vitro derived embryos when compared with in vivo derived embryos (52–54). Embryonic developmental blocks are frequently encountered during the transition from maternal to embryonic genomic activation.

Various attempts at improving in vitro culture conditions by modifying the medium electrolyte and energy sources have met with limited success (55). An alternative approach has been the development of coculture systems in which a variety of "helper cells" have provided a more efficient means to maintain human embryos in vitro. Various cell types have been used, including tubal or endometrial epithelium (from humans or animals), autologous cumulus or granulosa cells, or an established cell line [monkey kidney epithelial cells (Vero cells)] (56–60). Use of coculture methods has produced somewhat variable results, although most investigators have noted at least improvements in embryonic developmental rates (58,59). The variability in success rates associated with coculture systems probably is attributable to differences in cell lines, maintenance of the cells, and various environmental factors within each laboratory.

Although the beneficial effects of coculture systems have been demonstrated by a number of researchers, the mechanism of action of these helper cells remains uncertain. Coculture cells have been demonstrated to both produce embryotrophic factors (61) as well as serve to detoxify the culture medium (62). There is a fair consensus that coculture improves embryo morphology, blastocyst development, and hatching (63). In addition, a better synchrony between embryo development and the uterine environment may occur.

At the Center for Reproductive Medicine and Infertility at the Weill Cornell Medical College and New York-Presbyterian Hospital, we have developed a unique coculture system that uses the patient's own endometrial cells and successfully applied this system to our clinical IVF–ET program (64,65). In this system, patients undergo an endometrial biopsy performed in the mid to late luteal phase of a cycle preceding their actual IVF–ET treatment cycle. Endometrial glandular epithelial and stromal cells are then separated by differential sedimentation and plated until monolayers are obtained. The cells are then cryopreserved and later thawed at a precise time in synchrony with the patient's treatment. An equal mixture of glandular epithelial and stromal cells is seeded into a four-well tissue plate containing Ham's F-10 medium supplemented with 15% patient's serum. In general, approximately 75% confluence is achieved by the time embryos are placed into the system (Fig. 47.1). Embryos are introduced into the coculture system after fertilization checks (Fig. 47.2) and maintained with the autologous endometrial cells until day 3 (Fig. 47.3) when embryo transfer is performed.

RESULTS

Prophylactic Salpingectomy

In women with tubal factor infertility, the presence of hydrosalpinges has been related to poorer IVF outcomes in comparison to women without hydrosalpinges in

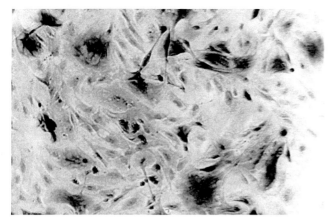

Figure 47.1 Autologous endometrial cell cultures at confluence consisting of a mixture of glandular epithelial cells and stromal cells.

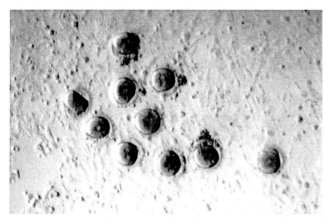

Figure 47.2 Pronuclear oocytes placed on autologous endometrial coculture.

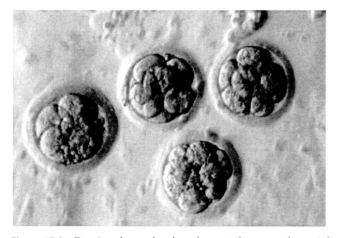

Figure 47.3 Day 3 embryos developed on autologous endometrial coculture.

numerous retrospective studies (7–9). It seems that there may be a relation between the size of the hydrosalpinx and reduced implantation, as one group of investigators has noted that only when hydrosalpinges were large enough to be visualized by ultrasonography were clinical outcomes diminished (66). Two meta-analyses estimated that hydrosalpinges diminished implantation rates by 35–50% (10,11). In addition, both meta-analyses also

reported an increased risk of early pregnancy loss in patients with hydrosalpinges.

Two prospective randomized trials involving prophylactic salpingectomy in patients with severe tubal factor infertility and hydrosalpinges have explored whether implantation rates and clinical outcomes can be improved in these patients (67,68). In the first monocentric study, Dechaud et al. (67) reported an improved implantation rate (10.4%) in the group with salpingectomy in comparison to the group without salpingectomy (4.6%) during the first IVF attempt. For all IVF–ET attempts, the respective implantation rates in the two groups were 13.4% and 8.6%, respectively. In addition, the ongoing pregnancy rate per transfer was 34.2% in the group with salpingectomy compared with 18.7% in the group without salpingectomy. A prospective randomized multicenter trial of salpingectomy prior to IVF was conducted in Scandinavia (68). Inclusion criteria included the presence of unilateral or bilateral hydrosalpinges as determined by either hysterosalpingography or laparoscopy and age <39 years. A total of 204 patients were available for an intention to treat analysis and 192 actually started IVF. Clinical pregnancy rates per included patient were 36.6% in the salpingectomy group and 23.9% in the nonintervention group (not significant, $p = 0.067$). Subgroup analyses, however, revealed significant differences in favor of salpingectomy in patients with bilateral hydrosalpinges (implantation rates of 25.6% vs. 12.3%, $p = 0.038$) and in patients with ultrasound visible hydrosalpinges (clinical pregnancy rates of 45.7% vs. 22.5%, $p = 0.029$; delivery rates of 40.0% vs. 17.5%, $p = 0.038$). In addition, the delivery rate was increased 3.5-fold in patients who had exhibited bilateral hydrosalpinges on ultrasound ($p = 0.019$).

Further studies have only strengthened the evidence that IVF clinical outcomes in women with severe tubal disease are improved following bilateral salpingectomy. Strandell et al. (69) reported on the effect of cumulative cycles after reviewing further data from the Scandinavian randomized, prospective trial. After taking into account the number of cycles per patient and the presence of salpingectomy after a previous transfer, salpingectomy resulted in a significant increase in birth rate [hazard ratio = 2.1, 95% confidence interval (CI) 1.6–3.6, $p = 0.014$]. Similar findings were included in a Cochrane review (70). In this meta-analysis of published randomized, controlled trials, the odds ratios (ORs) for both pregnancy and live birth were statistically increased with laparoscopic salpingectomy prior to IVF. One retrospective study has reported improved pregnancy rates in patients with severe tubal factor infertility who underwent laparoscopic salpingectomy after experiencing repeated implantation failure (71).

One can therefore conclude that patients with severe tubal factor infertility have improved clinical outcomes following prophylactic salpingectomy, particularly if they have either bilateral hydrosalpinges or hydrosalpinges large enough to be visualized by ultrasound. Laparoscopic salpingectomy appears to improve clinical outcomes in patients who have hydrosalpinges and repeated implantation failures. On the other hand, the clinical efficacy of prophylactic salpingectomy in the presence of either unilateral hydrosalpinges or hydrosalpinges that are not visible on ultrasound requires further study.

Assisted Hatching

The clinical results after assisted hatching in poor prognosis patients undergoing IVF–ET have been mixed. In the initial randomized clinical trials from our institution, it appeared that breaches in the zona pellucida impaired the clinical pregnancy rate after transfers of drilled embryos with a thin zona pellucida (<13 µm), while facilitating the implantation of embryos in the setting of a thick zona pellucida (>15 µm), compared to controls (27). In a later trial, selective assisted hatching was performed only on those embryos with a thick zona pellucida or poor morphology (<5 cells or >20% fragmentation on day 3). The overall implantation rates per transferred embryos were improved in the selectively zona drilled group (25%) when compared with controls (18%) (p <0.05). Selective assisted hatching, however, seemed to have the largest impact in improving the implantation rate of women >38 years (16% vs. 3%, p < 0.05).Women with elevated basal FSH concentrations greater than 15 mIU/ml also seemed to particularly benefit, although this has not been subsequently corroborated.

In non-randomized studies using historical controls, several investigators reported improved implantation efficiency following assisted hatching in poor prognosis patients (>40 years or several IVF–ET failures) (72–74). Most of these centers attempted to use assisted hatching globally rather than selectively according to zona characteristics. One investigator challenged the zona thickness theory by reporting no differences in mean zona thickness in subsequently pregnant (18.5 µm) as opposed to nonpregnant (18.7 µm) patients (75). Other investigators also failed to demonstrate clinical benefits from assisted hatching in patients selected for advanced age, zona thickness, or previous failed attempts (76).

There have been relatively few prospective, randomized controlled trials examining the efficacy of assisted hatching in poor prognosis patients. Magli et al. (77) reported the clinical efficacy of assisted hatching in 135 cycles with a poor prognosis for pregnancy: (i) Maternal age ≥38 years (45 cycles); (ii) Three or more previous failed IVF–ET attempts (70 cycles); and (iii) Patients possessing both criteria (20 cycles). The control group (113 cycles) included patients possessing the same characteristics (42, 53, and 18 cycles, respectively) who did not undergo the assisted hatching procedure. The percentage of clinical pregnancies per cycle was significantly higher for the first (31% vs. 10%, p < 0.05) and second groups (36% vs. 17%, p < 0.05). No significant difference in pregnancy rates was noted in the third group, although the numbers were limited. Chao et al. (78) also reported a prospective randomized study of assisted hatching exclusively in patients with a history of repeatedly failed IVF–ET and noted significantly improved pregnancy and

implantation rates in the assisted hatching group following transcervical, but not transtubal, embryo transfers. Lanzendorf et al., (79) however, were unable to ascertain any statistically significant benefits of assisted hatching in a prospective randomized study that comprised unselected patients >36 years. In addition, a recent Cochrane systematic review of randomized trials reported that, despite the significantly improved odds of clinical pregnancy, there was insufficient evidence to demonstrate an improvement in live birth rates with assisted hatching in unselected patients (80). An additional systematic review of randomized controlled trials performed additional analyses regarding subgroups of patients and identified increased clinical pregnancy and multiple pregnancy rates in women with repeated implantation failure or frozen-thawed embryos (81).

To account for some of the variable clinical results seen with assisted hatching, investigators have examined some of the different available techniques of assisted hatching. Hsieh et al. (26) reported that the 1.48 µm noncontact diode laser was more effective for assisted hatching than the chemical method in older patients. In a multicenter prospective randomized trial, Primi et al. (82) showed that following recurrent implantation failure, implantation and pregnancy rates trended higher with assisted hatching with the diode laser. In contrast, Balaban et al. (83) did not find any appreciable differences when selective assisted hatching was performed by either the partial zona dissection, acid Tyrodes, diode laser, or pronase thinning methods. Other researchers have reported on a modification of the laser-assisted hatching technique in which the zona is partially thinned without a total breach (84). In fact, Mantoudis et al. (85) reported that the highest pregnancy rates occurred in patients treated with laser partial thinning extended to a quarter segment of the zona. A further prospective randomized study by Petersen et al. (86) demonstrated significantly higher implantation rates (p = 0.02) in patients with recurrent implantation failure who received quarter-laser zona thinning.

Meldrum et al. (74) have suggested that results of chemical-assisted hatching are highly technique dependent. They noted a time-dependent improvement in clinical results associated with the technique which they attributed to increasing technical experience. With experience, embryologists can perform the procedure rapidly, thus limiting temperature and pH changes around the embryo. In addition, the size and shape of the gap in the zona may be fashioned in a more consistent manner. Although hard to assess, perhaps operator-related variables have contributed to some of the inconsistent reported clinical results seen with assisted hatching.

Preimplantation Genetic Diagnosis (Aneuploidy Screening)

The extensive use of polar body testing for aneuploidy to improve IVF–ET outcome has been reported by Verlinsky et al. (87). These investigators reported the application of first and second polar body testing with multi-probe FISH in 659 cycles of women of advanced maternal age (>35 years). Specific probes for chromosomes 13, 18, and 21 were used. FISH results were available for 3217 (81.6%) of 3943 oocytes studied, of which 1388 (43.1%) had aneuploidies; 35.7% of aneuploidies were of first meiotic division origin, and 26.1% of second meiotic division origin. The transfer of embryos derived from 1558 aneuploidy-free oocytes in 614 treatment cycles resulted in 131 clinical pregnancies (21.3%) and 88 healthy children born (with an additional 18 pregnancies ongoing). As this was a non-randomized study, the precise impact of the preselection of aneuploidy-free oocytes on the overall IVF–ET efficiency is hard to determine.

A larger body of literature is available on the use of blastomere biopsy approaches in the screening for aneuploidy in patients with a poor prognosis (older women and those with repeated IVF–ET failure) (88–91). In an initial non-randomized trial, Gianaroli et al. (88) reported on preimplantation genetic diagnosis (PGD) for aneuploidy of chromosomes X, Y, 13, 18, and 21 on 196 embryos from 36 infertile patients classified with a poor prognosis due to: (i) Maternal age ≥ 38 years ($n = 11$); (ii) Repeated IVF failure ($n = 22$); and (iii) Altered karyotype (46XX/45XO mosaics) ($n = 3$). The percentage of abnormal embryos was comparable in the three groups: maternal age (63%), repeated IVF failure (57%), and mosaic karyotype (62%). They noted an increase in the percentage of chromosomally abnormal embryos that was directly proportional to the number of IVF failures. This led these investigators to propose that the high rate of chromosomally abnormal embryos may have been the cause of implantation failure. Subsequently, these investigators performed a prospective randomized controlled trial using a similar PGD scheme in women with either maternal age ≥38 years or ≥3 previous IVF failures (89). Assisted hatching was performed on day 3 embryos in the control group. In the study group, a total of 61 embryos were analyzed, with 55% detected to be chromosomally abnormal. Embryo transfer with at least one normal embryo was carried out in 10 cycles, resulting in four clinical pregnancies and a 28.0% implantation rate. In the control group, 41 embryos were transferred in 17 cycles, resulting in four clinical pregnancies and a statistically lower implantation rate (11.9%).

A later multicenter PGD for aneuploidy study was performed in women aged ≥35 years (90). Initially, this study was intended to be randomized. Owing to lack of available data at the time supporting a beneficial clinical effect of aneuploidy screening, however, few patients agreed to the study, and those who committed to it rejected randomization. Therefore, PGD cases were matched retrospectively with controls based on maternal age, number of previous IVF cycles, duration of stimulation, estradiol concentration, and number of mature follicles. One or two cells per embryo were biopsied on day 3 and analyzed by FISH. In most cases, embryos classified as normal after PGD were transferred on the same day of analysis. During the beginning of the trial, probes for the simultaneous detection of chromosomes X, Y, 18, and the shared alpha satellite region of chromosomes

13 and 21 were used ($n = 14$). Later, specific probes for X, Y, 13, 18, and 21 ($n = 22$) were used. Even later, a probe for chromosome 16 was added to the previous mixture and used in an additional proportion of cases ($n = 50$). Finally, a small fraction of cases ($n = 31$) benefited from having the biopsied cells analyzed with the X, Y, 13, 16, 18, and 21-probe mixture and then reanalyzed with a second probe mixture specific for chromosomes 14, 15, and 22. Only embryos classified as normal were transferred after PGD. The rates of fetal heartbeat (FHB)/embryo transferred were similar between the test and control groups. However, spontaneous abortions, measured as FHB aborted/FHB detected, decreased after PGD (24.2% vs. 9.6%, $p <0.05$) and ongoing fetuses or delivered babies per embryo transferred increased after PGD (15.9% vs. 10.6%, $p <0.05$). From this trial, the authors concluded that while increased implantation efficiency was not proven, PGD for aneuploidy reduced the rate of embryo loss after implantation.

Later trials have further expanded the testing capabilities of FISH on biopsied blastomeres (33,91,92). In one trial, Gianaroli et al. (91) reported on the outcomes of patients of maternal age ≥36 years, ≥3 previous IVF failures, or abnormal karyotypes who underwent PGD testing, including two rounds of FISH (initial analysis of chromosomes X, Y, 13, 16, 18, and 21 followed by reanalysis for chromosomes 14, 15, and 22). In many of these cases, embryo transfer was carried out on day 4 to allow time for the two rounds of FISH analysis. The investigators reported in a randomized controlled trial that an increase in the ongoing implantation rate (22.5% vs. 10.2%, $p <0.001$) was achieved in the PGD patients compared with controls. The clinical benefits of PGD were most notable in women ≥38 years and in carriers of an altered karyotype. In a further large randomized controlled aneuploidy screening (AS) trial, Staessen et al. (92) compared blastocyst transfer combined with PGD–AS using FISH for chromosomes X, Y, 13, 16, 18, 21, and 22, with a control group without PGD–AS, in couples with advanced maternal age (mean = 39 years in control and 40 years in study groups, respectively). The implantation rates were similar (17.1% and 11.5%, respectively), but a significantly higher number of embryos were replaced in the control group. In PGD–AS cycles with genetically normal embryos, no morula or blastocyst formation occurred in 11 of 148 cycles. The authors reported that in patients from which an expanded blastocyst on day 5 results, the chance of selecting a genetically normal embryo is 65% versus 41.3% if an eight-cell stage embryo is selected on day 3.

Mastenbroek et al. (93) reported on a multicenter randomized controlled trial comparing three cycles of IVF with and without preimplantation genetic screening (PGS) in women 35–41 years old. The PGS method used in this trial included analysis for chromosomes 1, 16, and 17, followed by analysis for chromosomes 13, 18, 21, X, and Y. In this report, 206 women were assigned to PGS and 202 women were assigned to the control group. Ultimately, 434 cycles with PGS and 402 cycles without were performed. Interestingly, in this report of consecutive PGS cycles, the ongoing pregnancy rate was actually significantly lower in the women assigned to PGS (25%) than in those not assigned to PGS (37%). The women receiving PGS also demonstrated a lower live birth rate (24% vs. 35%; rate ratio = 0.68; 95% CI 0.50–0.92). A recent systematic review and meta-analysis of randomized, controlled trials also reported no beneficial effect for PGS after IVF (94). On the contrary, for women of advanced age, PGS appears to significantly lower live birth rates.

Further trials have looked specifically at the outcomes of PGD for aneuploidy screening in recurrent implantation failure patients (95–98). Pehlivan et al. (95) reported using FISH on one or two blastomeres from 49 implantation failure patients (defined as three or more failed IVF attempts) and compared them with nine fertile controls. In each case, three rounds of FISH were utilized (assessing chromosomes 13, 16, 18, 21, 22, X, and Y) and transfer was undertaken on day 5. There was a significantly higher rate of chromosomal abnormalities in the implantation failure patients (67.4%) than in controls (36.3%). Following PGD–AS, the implantation failure patients demonstrated a pregnancy rate of 34.0% and implantation rate of 19.8%, which was comparable to controls (33.1% and 24.1%, respectively). On the other hand, Munné et al. (96) reported that the major clinical effect seen with PGD–AS was in women of advanced maternal age with eight or more 2-pronuclear zygotes. In this report, an increase in implantation rate was not observed in patients with two or more previous IVF attempts or in patients with fewer than eight zygotes. Taranissi et al. (96) reported on the use of FISH of the first and second polar bodies using probes specific for chromosomes 13, 16, 18, 21, and 22 in couples with recurrent implantation failure. Subsequent diploid oocytes that cleaved were further tested using the same probes on a single blastomere from day 3 embryos and subsequent chromosomally normal embryos were replaced on day 5. In this study, patients aged <40 years had a significantly higher proportion of euploid oocytes and embryos, cycles reaching embryo transfer, and ongoing delivery rates per transfer (32% vs. 12.5%) than patients aged ≥41 years. Finally, Blockeel et al. (97) reported a randomized, controlled trial of PGD–AS in patients with recurrent implantation failure and observed no clinically significant differences in either implantation or clinical pregnancy rates between the study and control groups.

Voullaire et al. (38) reported on the use of CGH in single blastomeres from 20 women with repeated implantation failure. Biopsied embryos were initially cryopreserved. Individual blastomeres underwent alkaline lysis followed by whole genome amplification and CGH. Abnormalities detected include aneuploidy for one or two chromosomes (25%) and complex chromosomal abnormalities (29%). Approximately 40% of the embryos were considered suitable for transfer, although the investigators did not report on clinical outcomes. In comparison to CGH, multicolor FISH utilizing a five-probe set would have detected 77% of the abnormalities and incorrectly diagnosed 38% of abnormal embryos. In comparison to CGH, repetitive rounds of FISH utilizing a nine-probe set would have detected 85% of the abnormalities but still incorrectly diagnosed 25% of abnormal embryos as normal.

Further studies utilizing SNP microarray-based chromosome aneuploidy screening have demonstrated that cleavage-stage FISH remains poorly predictive in determining aneuploidy in embryos that progressed to the blastocyst stage (42). Northrop et al. (42) reported that of all blastocysts evaluated following trophectoderm biopsy, 58% were euploid in all sections despite an aneuploid FISH result. Treff et al. (43) reported that embryonic mosaicism was significantly less commonly observed by microarray than FISH. The limitations associated with cleavage-stage FISH, including mosaicism, self-correction of aneuploidy within the embryo, evaluation of only a limited number of chromosomes, and the potential for an adverse impact of embryo biopsy, have resulted in professional society statements that reiterate the lack of clinical benefit of this technique for patients of advanced maternal age. The European Society of Human Reproduction and Embryology recently suggested that future randomized controlled trials be performed examining alternative biopsy timing (polar body and/or trophectoderm biopsy) and technologies that allow for more comprehensive testing of all chromosomes (microarray-based testing) to determine whether PGS shows clinical benefit (99).

Blastocyst Culture and Transfer

As stated earlier, it has been hypothesized that in some patients cleavage-stage embryos prematurely transferred into the uterine environment may undergo nutritive and homeostatic stress (100). On the other hand, uterine hostility to cleavage-stage embryos seems doubtful in lieu of the excellent clinical results achieved in some clinics. In addition, perhaps blastocyst culture and transfer may serve as an indirect method of screening out aneuploidic embryos as it is known that the rate of aneuploidy is increased in embryos which arrest in culture (51).

Since the proportion of aneuploidic embryos appears to increase directly with the number of failed previous IVF–ET cycles, (88) blastocyst culture and transfer may be of clinical benefit in patients with a history of repeated implantation failure. Cruz et al. (101) reported the use of blastocyst culture and transfer in patients who had previously failed three or more IVF cycles and who had at least three eight- to 12-cell embryos on day 3. In this non-randomized small trial using a selected "poor prognosis" patient group, a statistically significant increase in clinical pregnancy and implantation rates was seen in the blastocyst group compared with controls. Guerif et al. (102) similarly reported the use of blastocyst transfer in a non-randomized analysis in patients who previously failed at least two cleavage-stage embryo transfers with at least two good-quality embryos. These investigators reported that live birth rate and implantation rates were subsequently higher when day 5 or day 6 transfers were used. Barrenetxea et al. (103) performed a retrospective analysis of day 5 and day 6 transfers in patients with repeated implantation failure. In this analysis, day 5 transfers had nearly fivefold the implantation rate as day 6 transfers (23% vs. 5%, respectively). Finally, Levitas et al. (104) performed a prospective randomized study utilizing patients with recurrent cleavage-stage implantation failure. In this trial, the clinical pregnancy rates per oocyte retrieval were 21.7% and 12.9% per blastocyst and day 2–3 embryo transfers, respectively.

The main disadvantage of blastocyst culture and transfer is that the rate of blastocyst development is still limited. Even with newer sequential culture media, blastocyst formation occurs in only <55% of embryos. While a higher proportion of embryos that fail to develop to the blastocyst stage in culture are apparently chromosomally abnormal, it is still uncertain whether some embryos may fail to progress simply because of suboptimal culture conditions. In addition, it remains difficult to fully evaluate the clinical benefits of blastocyst culture and transfer since many trials have used selected patient groups. Patients who are high responders to gonadotropin stimulation seem to be excellent candidates for blastocyst culture since they are not only likely to have many embryos available for transfer but also the ability to select among available blastocysts in many instances probably also enhances the implantation rate (105). The clinical efficacy of blastocyst culture and transfer in unselected patient groups is less certain. In particular, patients with multiple failed previous IVF–ET cycles will frequently exhibit poor responses to gonadotropin therapy and have few embryos available. Therefore, blastocyst culture and transfer may not be the best approach for all patients with repeated implantation failure.

Coculture Methods

Favorable clinical results have been achieved utilizing various cellular preparations (both human and animal) in coculture systems. Vero cells (monkey kidney epithelial cells) have been documented to be beneficial in long-term cocultures of embryos, resulting in an increase in the total number and quality of blastocysts when compared to embryos that were not cultured in the presence of Vero cells (106). Use of bovine oviductal epithelial cells in combination with the use of assisted hatching and day 3 embryo replacements were noted to yield relatively high pregnancy rates in poor prognosis patients (107,108). Coculture of human embryos with buffalo rat liver cells seemed to exhibit a favorable trend toward improving pregnancy rates in patients with previous in vitro fertilization failure (34% coculture vs. 28% control) (109).

Because of the potential infectious risks associated with the use of animal cells, investigators have focused on utilizing human cells (both autologous and homologous) in coculture systems. To mimic the in vivo environment of the fallopian tube, tubal cells from the ampullary portion of the fallopian tube have been used (110,111). In these reports, the cells were harvested during postpartum tubal ligations or hysterectomies and

passaged several times to achieve adequate numbers of cells for multiple patients. Embryonic viability, morphological appearance, and the number of blastocysts were reported to be enhanced with the tubal epithelial coculture system (110). Further clinical benefits of tubal epithelial coculture have included a higher pregnancy rate, a higher implantation rate, lower spontaneous abortion rate, and an increased number of spare embryos available for cryopreservation (111).

Autologous systems for coculture have also been developed. One of the simplest involves the use of granulosa or cumulus cells derived from the cells collected during the patient's retrieval. The use of autologous cells in coculture is relatively safe and ethical for the patient, although it can be time consuming as each coculture is individualized. Furthermore, since the granulosa or cumulus cells are plated after retrieval, any coculture benefit provided to either the gametes or early embryo is probably limited. Nevertheless, Plachot et al. (112) noted convincing evidence of the benefits of granulosa cell coculture. Using each patient as her own control, half of the zygotes were cultured using either standard methods or autologous granulosa cell coculture. Eighty-three percent of granulosa cell coculture embryos were available for transfer compared with only 3% of controls. Other investigators have also noted beneficial morphological effects with cumulus cells utilized in the coculture of supernumerary embryos (113,114). Carrell et al. (115) reported that the use of autologous cumulus coculture improved embryo morphology, implantation rates, and clinical pregnancy rates following IVF.

At The Center for Reproductive Medicine and Infertility at the Weill Medical College and New York-Presbyterian Hospital, we have developed a unique coculture system using autologous cryopreserved endometrial cells. Advantages of this system include use of a readily available source of autologous cells, avoidance of the infectious and ethical risks when using either animal or homologous cell lines, and use of cells in which preimplantation embryo development is known to take place. In addition, there is rather convincing evidence of a chemical dialogue between the developing embryo and the maternal endometrium (116,117). Coculture with human endometrial epithelial cells has been noted to be beneficial to blastocyst development, presumably owing to the induction of embryonic paracrine secretion (118). Furthermore, endometrial cells may be cryopreserved so that a proper cellular confluence can be timed to allow a beneficial effect for the early developing embryo.

Coculture of embryos on autologous endometrial cells prior to transfer in patients with repeated failures of implantation was first reported by Jayot et al. (119). With this approach, these investigators reported a pregnancy rate of 21% versus 8% in patients' previous cycles. These investigators used a mixture of stromal and epithelial cells following one month of subculture and multiple tissue flask passages. Nieto et al. (120) used cryopreserved autologous endometrial (predominantly epithelial) cells and reported a positive effect on the proportion of embryos with minimal or no fragmentation. Simon et al.

(121) further developed a coculture system using autologous endometrial epithelial cells that were previously cryopreserved. In 168 cycles in patients with a history of implantation failure (>3 previous failed cycles), a 49.2% blastocyst formation, 11.8% implantation rate, and a 20.2% pregnancy rate were achieved using a day 6 transfer approach. Eyeheremendy et al. (122) also demonstrated a beneficial effect utilizing autologous endometrial cell coculture and day 3 transfer in patients with repeated implantation failure.

We have used an autologous endometrial coculture system incorporating both stromal and epithelial cells in equal proportions. It is highly likely that endometrial stromal cells also play a significant role in implantation. Our system isolates endometrial stromal and epithelial cells through differential sedimentation, obtaining cell lines of >90% purity. Cells are then cryopreserved and subsequently thawed in synchrony with the patient's IVF cycle so that a developing monolayer of both epithelial and stromal cells is available by the time the fertilized oocytes have reached the pronuclear stage. Zygotes are then placed on coculture and incubated until day 3, when transfer is undertaken.

The initial trial using our autologous endometrial coculture system was undertaken in women who had a history of at least one previously failed IVF–ET attempt with poor embryo quality (defined as <6 cells or <grade 2 morphology on day 3) (64). In this trial, half of available embryos were allocated to coculture and the other half allocated to conventional medium. The morphologically best embryos were transferred back to the patient irrespective of the culture system. From this study, although it was found that an approximately equal number of embryos were transferred from either group, embryos derived from autologous endometrial coculture had a statistically lower percentage of fragmentation and higher mean number of blastomeres at the time of transfer (Table 47.1).

A second trial utilized autologous endometrial coculture in patients with a history of at least one previously failed IVF–ET attempt with poor embryo quality (65). In this trial, all available embryos were allocated to coculture. Again, it was noted that coculture resulted in a significant improvement in the mean number of blastomeres compared to that in the patient's previous non-coculture cycle. The implantation and clinical pregnancy rates in these coculture cycles were 15% and 29%, respectively.

In subsequent trials, we have noted that enhancement of cleavage rates and the lowering of the degree of fragmentation associated with autologous endometrial coculture appears to be related to the timing of the initial endometrial biopsy (Tables 47.2, 47.3) (123). In particular, better results were obtained when the endometrial biopsy was obtained in the mid to late luteal phase as opposed to the early luteal phase of the menstrual cycle. With this in mind, we have further optimized our coculture system.

Table 47.1 Characteristics of Human Embryos Developed on Autologous Endometrial Coculture and Conventional Medium

Embryo characteristics	Coculture	Conventional medium	Wilcoxon matched-pairs test
No. of embryos	203	186	
Mean (± SD) no. of blastomeres (day 3)	5.9 ± 1.5	5.5 ± 1.4	0.19
Mean (± SD) % of fragmentation	21 ± 13	24 ± 11	0.045
No. of embryos transferred	90	83	
Mean (± SD) no. of blastomeres (transfer)	7.4 ± 1.3	6.7 ± 1.9	0.032

Table 47.2 Cleavage Characteristics of Human Embryos Developed on Autologous Endometrial Coculture (AECC) and Conventional Medium (CM) According to Timing of the Endometrial Biopsy

	No. of blastomeres AECC	No. of blastomeres CM	p value
All patients (n = 79)	6.2 ± 1.4	5.5 ± 1.3	0.0015
Early luteal (n = 33)	6.0 ± 1.6	5.6 ± 1.4	0.19
Mid/late luteal (n = 46)	6.3 ± 1.2	5.5 ± 1.2	0.0024

Table 47.3 Degree of Fragmentation of Human Embryos Developed on Autologous Endometrial Coculture (AECC) and Conventional Medium (CM) According to Timing of the Endometrial Biopsy

	% Fragmentation AECC	% Fragmentation CM	p value
All patients (n = 79)	17.7 ± 12.3	21.6 ± 11	0.04
Early luteal (n = 33)	19.4 ± 13	20 ± 11	0.87
Mid/late luteal (n = 46)	16.5 ± 12	22.8 ± 11	0.012

With the availability of sequential media, the role for coculture has been somewhat questioned (124). Some investigators utilizing refined coculture systems, however, have reported potential unique advantages and clinical superiority of coculture in comparison to sequential media. Dominquez et al. (125) reported experience with endometrial epithelial cell (EEC) system and sequential media on the embryologic outcome and secretome profile of implanted blastocysts of patients undergoing IVF with either own or donor oocytes. Pregnancy rates (39.1% vs. 27.5%) and implantation rates (33.3% vs. 20.9%) were statistically higher in EEC culture versus sequential media. Furthermore, interleukin-6 (IL-6) was the most secreted protein in EEC culture, as opposed to sequential media for which IL-6 levels were noted to be diminished. A meta-analysis regarding the role of coculture in IVF was also reported (126). Analysis of 17 prospective, randomized trials revealed that although the data was heterogeneous, cocultured embryos had greater numbers of blastomeres. Coculture also demonstrated a statistically significant improvement in implantation as well as clinical and ongoing pregnancy rates.

COMPLICATIONS

Prophylactic Salpingectomy

Some investigators have expressed concern that salpingectomy prior to IVF may impair ovarian response. The mechanism in which salpingectomy might cause reduced ovarian response is not clear, but unilateral or bilateral removal of the fallopian tubes may have a detrimental effect on the ovarian arterial blood supply. Lass et al. (127) have demonstrated that there were fewer follicles and, consequently, fewer oocytes retrieved from the ipsilateral ovary in women who had previously undergone a unilateral salpingectomy. Other investigators have not demonstrated diminished ovarian responses in women who had undergone bilateral salpingectomy as compared to a tubal factor control group (128). For women with already suspected diminished ovarian reserve, however, the potential detrimental effect of unilateral or bilateral salpingectomy on ovarian response must be considered. In these cases, either interruption of tubal uterine patency or ultrasound-guided drainage of hydrosalpinges might also be considered (129,130).

Moreover, salpingectomy is not a procedure without the recognized complications of operative laparoscopy and/or laparotomy in addition to the rare complications of subsequent interstitial (131) or abdominal pregnancies (132).

Assisted Hatching

The risk of injury to the embryo during the performance of assisted hatching techniques should be minimal in experienced hands. Because the breach in the zona pellucida may reduce some of the embryo's natural defenses to bacteriologic and other pathogenic organisms, many investigators have advocated the concurrent use of corticosteroids and antibiotics in this setting. In a short series, Cohen et al. reported that the implantation rate of partial

zona dissected embryos reached 28% (11 out of 39) in patients who received immunosuppressive treatment, whereas implantation rates were only 7% in patients who did not (2 out of 31) (133). Nevertheless, there are roughly an equal number of reports describing a positive action of corticosteroids as there are those that do not in the literature (134,135).

Another concern regarding zona manipulation procedures is a possible increased rate of monozygotic twins (136,137). This risk has been attributed to the use of small openings in the zona, which may be prone to bisecting the embryo during the hatching process. While some reports have suggested that the increased risk of monozygotic twinning seen after assisted hatching reflects just the overall increased monozygotic twinning seen with assisted reproduction techniques, (138) other reports have suggested otherwise (139).

Lastly, because assisted hatching increases the implantation rate of embryos that otherwise may be of poor prognosis and unable to escape from the zona pellucida, it was feared that the technique could result in the implantation of poor-quality embryos destined to abort. Fortunately, an increase in spontaneous abortions has not been seen in contemporary large trials using the technique (72–77).

Preimplantation Genetic Diagnosis (Aneuploidy Screening)

Potential adverse effects of PGD for aneuploidy focus mostly on the likelihood of misdiagnosis. A drawback of blastomere analysis at the cleavage stage is that the result may not be representative of the whole embryo, due to the high frequency of chromosomal mosaicism (140,141). Thus, haploid or aneuploid mosaicism could lead to genetic misdiagnosis and transfer of chromosomally abnormal embryos. An analysis of two blastomeres could theoretically decrease the likelihood of misdiagnosis and improve the detection rate of mosaic embryos. There remains less clinical experience with two blastomere biopsies, however, at the present time. In addition, the actual biologic significance of early cleavage-stage embryonic mosaicism remains unclear. Some investigators have suggested that abnormal cells may be subsequently eliminated or diverted to the trophectoderm (142). Therefore, detecting and discarding mosaic embryos, which is the current preferred approach, might lead to the loss of potentially normal embryos.

Although FISH is relatively efficient, FISH failure or misinterpretation can also occur. Harper et al. (143) reported that a clear FISH signal is obtained in 97% of fixed blastomere nuclei. Interpretation of FISH signals can also be complicated by overlapping probe signals. In an early trial, Munné et al. (30) reported that PGD using FISH for the common aneuploidies was associated with an error rate of 5.4%. Lastly, it is still under debate which chromosomes need to be tested for aneuploidy (34).

The question of whether embryo biopsy might adversely affect implantation and live birth rates as well as its possible impact on birth defects or more subtle developmental problems in the children must be further investigated. Polar biopsy diagnosis is less invasive, although is hampered by the inability to detect paternally derived chromosomal abnormalities as well as abnormalities derived from postfertilization events. Trophectoderm biopsy is less invasive and potentially more accurate when utilizing microarray technology, although further research is needed to determine its clinical utility.

Blastocyst Culture and Transfer

One of the intriguing questions regarding the use of blastocyst culture and transfer is whether some of the remaining arrested embryos would have otherwise implanted had they been transferred earlier. Blastocyst development still does not exceed 55%, even with the new sequential culture media. While it seems that a higher proportion of embryos that fail to develop to the blastocyst stage in culture are chromosomally abnormal, it is possible that some may still not progress because of suboptimal laboratory conditions.

In addition, limited information is available on the use of blastocyst culture and transfer either in unselected patient groups or in patients who are not high responders to gonadotropin therapy where small numbers of blastocysts may preclude selection of the "best embryos" and offer no significant advantage. In addition, there is also the risk that a particular patient may have no blastocysts available for transfer. These latter risks may also be potentially increased in patients with a history of repeated implantation failure, many of whom may also be marginal responders to gonadotropin therapy.

Coculture Methods

Although the use of well-characterized animal cells such as Vero cells in human IVF–ET has been documented to be safe, it presents certain medical and ethical challenges. One potential risk is the transmission of infectious agents, including possibly those that may not ordinarily infect humans. The risk of transmission of infectious agents with the use of accessory homologous cells in human IVF–ET also exists. Regulatory agencies have recommended screening and testing for human immunodeficiency virus (HIV), hepatitis B, and hepatitis C for all donors of reproductive cells and tissue. In addition, the risks of syphilis as well as transmissible spongiform encephalopathies, including Creutzfeldt–Jakob disease (CJD), must also be considered.

Use of autologous cells averts these infectious risks. Since various cellular preparations and protocols exist, however, laboratories employing coculture technologies are obligated to assess whether their particular method is embryotrophic and enhances clinical outcomes. A coculture system may occasionally result in poor cellular proliferation and an increased fraction of nonviable cells. Clinical judgment is required in these instances to ensure that the best environment for human embryos is being provided.

FUTURE DIRECTIONS AND CONTROVERSIES

Technologies for PGS for aneuploidies in women with diminished IVF–ET prognoses are evolving, although their clinical utility has not been fully defined. In addition, methods to culture embryos to the blastocyst stage using sequential culture media are continuing to evolve. In particular, little is known regarding whether the latter technique may help women with repeated implantation failure. Results with assisted hatching and coculture methodologies are variable, although on the whole seem to result in improved clinical outcomes in women with repeated implantation failure.

An additional significant amount of focus has been placed on potential immunological causes of repeated implantation failure. Much work has been performed attempting to associate antiphospholipid antibodies and in vitro fertilization failure. The proposed mechanism of such failure includes abnormal implantation, abnormal placentation, and early embryonic compromise. Intravenous immunoglobulin and anti-thrombogenic therapy, including aspirin and heparin, have been proposed as treatments (144,145). Although an association between antiphospholipid abnormalities and IVF failure has been shown in some retrospective studies, (146,147) prospective studies have failed to reveal an association (148). Additional work has focused on the relationship between acquired and inherited thrombophilias and recurrent implantation failure, which similarly has been shown to have an association in some retrospective studies, (149) but not others (150).

Certain micromanipulation techniques have recently been described that attempt to "rescue" poor-quality embryos. These include microsurgical embryonic fragment removal and cytoplasmic transfer (151,152). Results of these techniques, however, are very preliminary and have not been studied systematically in a controlled fashion. In addition, techniques such as cytoplasmic transfer present certain theoretical risks (transfer of third-party mitochondrial DNA) that need to be carefully considered. The interpretation that cytoplasmic transfer is a form of gene therapy has currently resulted in the technique receiving a heightened level of regulatory scrutiny in the United States. Finally, there is a recent renewed interest in the techniques of embryo transfer and variables that may affect success (153). Significantly different outcomes with varying embryo transfer catheters, embryo transfer methods, and physician experience have all highlighted the importance of optimal embryo transfer techniques. The use of ultrasound-guided embryo transfer rather than blind catheter insertion is currently attracting increased interest. In fact, one report suggests that transvaginal ultrasound-guided embryo transfer improves outcomes in patients with repeated implantation failure (154). A recent controlled study at our institute, however, did not reveal an advantage of this technique by experienced operators.

CONCLUSIONS

Although treatment of patients with a history of repeated implantation failure has been historically discouraging, new techniques and methodologies are being developed that provide this difficult group of patients with a better prognosis. If severe tubal factor and bilateral hydrosalpinges are visible by ultrasonography, patients seem to clearly benefit from prophylactic salpingectomy. Most studies have found that assisted hatching, whether globally or selectively used, provides clinical benefits. PGD techniques for the detection of aneuploidic embryos have considerable promise, although their precise clinical roles need to be further defined. Blastocyst culture and transfer may offer some theoretic advantages in patients with previous IVF failures, particularly in patients who are good responders to gonadotropin therapy. Lastly, coculture methods have also shown promise in improving both embryo quality and clinical outcomes in patients with previous IVF failures. In particular, we have found that the use of autologous cryopreserved endometrial cells offers significant advantages as a coculture method.

APPENDIX: AUTOLOGOUS ENDOMETRIAL COCULTURE TECHNIQUE

Endometrial tissue is obtained during a luteal phase endometrial biopsy performed in a cycle before the patient's IVF procedure with the use of a Pipelle Endometrial Suction Curette (Unimar, Wilton, CT, USA). The sample is transferred to the laboratory in a sterile container filled with normal saline solution. A small portion of each endometrial biopsy is also placed in 10% neutral buffered formalin solution for histological assessment. All tissue samples have revealed secretory morphologic changes ranging from cycle day 16 to cycle day 25. The remaining tissue is then minced into small pieces ($1–2\,mm^2$) and washed with Hank's balanced salt solution (HBSS) (Gibco, Grand Island, NY, USA) supplemented with $5000\,\mu g$ per $100\,ml$ of penicillin–streptomycin (Gibco) to remove excess red blood cells and mucus.

The tissue is then enzymatically digested using four steps into separate glandular epithelial and stromal cells. The method involves a slight modification to previously published differential sedimentation techniques developed in our laboratory (155). Initially, we incubate the tissue pieces for five minutes at 37°C in a shaking water bath in $10\,ml$ of HBSS containing 0.2% collagenase type 2 (Sigma, St. Louis, MO, USA) and $5000\,\mu g$ per $100\,ml$ of penicillin–streptomycin. Cell clumps are then dispersed by brisk aspiration through a sterile transfer pipette. The digested tissue pieces are then allowed to settle by differential sedimentation at unit gravity for five minutes. After sedimentation, the supernatant (containing a mixture of single stromal cells and small intact glands) is transferred into a separate $15\,ml$ polyethylene test tube and centrifuged at $400 \times g$ for 5 minutes. The pellet is then resuspended in RPMI medium 1640 (Gibco) supplemented with 10% patient's serum (RPMI-10% serum) and $5000\,\mu g$ per $100\,ml$ of penicillin–streptomycin.

The above steps are repeated four times, resulting in a combined $4\,ml$ of single stromal cells mixed with small glands. This stroma and small gland sample undergoes another differential sedimentation at unit gravity for 45 minutes to separate most small glands from the stromal cells. The supernatant (containing the stroma-enriched fraction) is centrifuged at $400 \times g$ for five minutes and the cell pellet resuspended in RPMI-10% serum. A small aliquot of the final sample is diluted 1:1 with 0.4% trypan blue stain (Gibco) with cell yield and viability determined quantitatively on a hemocytometer. Tissue culture flasks ($25\,cm^2$) are then seeded with approximately 5×10^5 cells.

The pellet which remains after four digestions contains predominately intact glands mixed with undigested connective tissue and stromal clumps. The glandular epithelial cells are purified by further resuspending this pellet in $10\,ml$ of HBSS. After approximately 30 seconds, the largest fragments (stromal clumps and undigested tissue) settle on the bottom of the $15\,ml$ test tube while the top $8\,ml$ contains glands and single stromal cells. The top $8\,ml$ (which has a typical snowflake appearance) is then transferred to another $15\,ml$ test tube and allowed to settle for 30 minutes at unit gravity. This sedimentation allows most of the glands to form a pellet at the bottom of the test tube while leaving the remaining single stromal cells in the supernatant that is removed and discarded. This glandular-enriched pellet is then resuspended in RPMI-10% serum and plated into one to three 25-cm^2 tissue culture flasks, depending on a gross estimate of the yield.

The seeded tissue flasks are maintained at 37°C in 5% $CO2$ air atmosphere, with the culture medium changed every two to three days. After about one week, the cells generally reach confluence. Although not representing entirely purified cellular populations, immunostaining studies using monoclonal antipancytokeratin and desmin antibodies have revealed >90% endometrial epithelial and stromal cells, respectively, in the respective cell cultures at time of confluence. After confluence is achieved, the cells are then released with trypsin-ethylenediamine tetra-acetic acid (EDTA) (Gibco). The cells are cryopreserved in a 15% glycerol solution at −70°C overnight and then transferred to liquid nitrogen storage.

Approximately equal mixtures of glandular and stromal cells are thawed on the estimated day prior to administration of human chorionic gonadotropin (hCG) during the patient's subsequent IVF--ET treatment cycle. Cell count and viability are determined, and approximately 3×10^5 cells (both glandular and stromal) are seeded into a four-well tissue culture plate containing $1\,ml$ of Ham's F-10 medium (Gibco) supplemented with 15% patient's serum. Approximately 75% confluence is achieved at the time embryos are placed into the coculture system.

Following identification of fertilization, zygotes are removed from the insemination droplet and allocated to growth in conventional medium (human tubal fluid + 15% maternal serum) or autologous endometrial coculture incorporating Ham's F-10 medium supplemented with 15% maternal serum. In studies where embryos were allocated to either conventional media or coculture, the morphologically best embryos were transferred back to the patient 72 hours after retrieval, irrespective of the culture system.

After embryo transfer, the coculture cells are fixed in 4% paraformaldehyde. Immunostaining of these coculture cells using a monoclonal antipancytokeratin antibody (Sigma, St. Louis, MO) have typically shown 25–50% glandular epithelial cells per coculture well.

REFERENCES

1. Sunderam S, Chang J, Flowers L, et al. Centers for disease control and Prevention (CDC). Assisted reproductive technology surveillance-United States, 2006. MMWR Surveill Summ 2009; 58: 1–25.
2. Rosenwaks Z, Davis OK, Damario MA. The role of maternal age in assisted reproduction. Hum Reprod 1995; 10(Suppl 1): 165–73.
3. Scott RT, Toner JP, Muasher SJ, et al. Follicle-stimulating hormone levels on cycle day 3 are predictive of in vitro fertilization outcome. Fertil Steril 1989; 51: 651–4.
4. Licciardi FL, Liu H-C, Rosenwaks Z. Day 3 estradiol serum concentrations as prognosticators of stimulation response and pregnancy outcome in patients undergoing in vitro fertilization. Fertil Steril 1995; 64: 991–4.
5. Plachot M. Chromosome analysis of oocytes and embryos. In: Verlinsky Y, Kuriev A, eds. Preimplantation Genetics. New York: Plenum Press, 1991: 103–12.
6. Edwards RG, Fishel S, Cohen J, et al. Factors influencing the success of IVF for alleviation of human infertility. J In Vitro Fertil Embryo Transf 1984; 1: 3–23.
7. Strandell A, Waldenstrom U, Nilsson L, Hamberger L. Hydrosalpinx reduces in vitro fertilization/embryo transfer pregnancy rates. Hum Reprod 1994; 9: 861–3.
8. Vandromme J, Chasse E, Jejeune B, et al. Hydrosalpinges in in vitro fertilization: an unfavorable prognostic feature. Hum Reprod 1995; 10: 576–9.
9. Fleming C, Hull MG. Impaired implantation after in vitro fertilization treatment associated with hydrosalpinx. Br J Obstet Gynaecol 1996; 103: 268–72.
10. Zeyneloglu HB, Arici A, Olive DL. Adverse effects of hydrosalpinx on pregnancy rates after in vitro fertilization-embryo transfer. Fertil Steril 1998; 70: 492–9.
11. Camus E, Poncelet C, Goffinet F, et al. Pregnancy rates after in vitro fertilization in cases of tubal infertility with and without hydrosalpinx: a metaanalysis of published comparative studies. Hum Reprod 1999; 14: 1243–9.
12. Sharara FI. The role of hydrosalpinx in IVF: simply mechanical? Hum Reprod 1999; 14: 557–78.
13. David A, Garcia CR, Czernobilsky B. Human hydrosalpinx: histologic study and chemical composition of fluid. Am J Obstet Gynecol 1969; 105: 400–11.
14. Mukherjee T, Copperman AB, McCaffrey C, et al. Hydrosalpinx fluid has embryotoxic effects on murine embryogenesis: a case for prophylactic salpingectomy. Fertil Steril 1996; 66: 851–3.
15. Ben-Rafael Z, Orvieto R. Cytokines – involvement in reproduction. Fertil Steril 1992; 58: 1093–9.
16. Meyer WR, Castelbaum AJ, Somkuti S, et al. Hydrosalpinges adversely affect markers of endometrial receptivity. Hum Reprod 1997; 12: 1393–8.
17. Murray DL, Sagostin AW, Widra EA, Levy MJ. The adverse effect of hydrosalpinges on in vitro fertilization pregnancy rates and the benefit of surgical correction. Fertil Steril 1998; 69: 41–5.
18. Bredkjaer H, Ziebe S, Hamid B, et al. Delivery rates after in vitro fertilization following bilateral salpingectomy due to hydrosalpinges: a case control study. Hum Reprod 1999; 14: 101–5.
19. Fehilly CB, Cohen J, Simons RF, et al. Cryopreservation of cleaving embryos and expanded blastocysts in the human: a comparative study. Fertil Steril 1985; 44: 638–44.
20. Cohen J, Inge KL, Suzman M, et al. Videocinematography of fresh and cryopreserved embryos: a retrospective analysis of embryonic morphology and implantation. Fertil Steril 1989; 51: 820–7.
21. Cohen J. Assisted hatching of human embryos. J In Vitro Fertil Embryo Transf 1991; 8: 179–80.
22. Cohen J, Elsner C, Kort H, et al. Impairment of the hatching process following in vitro fertilization in the human and improvement of implantation by assisting hatching using micromanipulation. Hum Reprod 1990; 5: 7–13.
23. Malter HE, Cohen J. Blastocyst formation and hatching in vitro following zona drilling of mouse and human embryos. Gamete Res 1989; 24: 67–80.
24. Gordon JW, Talansky BE. Assisted fertilization by zona drilling: a mouse model for correction of oligospermia. J Exp Zool 1986; 239: 347–54.
25. Nakayama T, Fujiwara H, Tatsumi K, et al. A new assisted hatching technique using a piezomicromanipulator. Fertil Steril 1998; 69: 784–8.
26. Hsieh YY, Huang CC, Cheng TC, et al. Laser assisted hatching of embryos is better than the chemical method for enhancing the pregnancy rate in women with advanced age. Fertil Steril 2002; 78: 179–82.
27. Cohen J, Alikani M, Trowbridge J, Rosenwaks Z. Implantation enhancement by selective assisted hatching using zona drilling of human embryos with poor prognosis. Hum Reprod 1992; 7: 685–91.
28. Hassold T, Chiu D. Maternal age-specific rates of numerical chromosome abnormalities with special reference to trisomy. Hum Genet 1985; 70: 11–17.
29. Dailey T, Dale B, Cohen J, Munné S. Association between non-disjunction and maternal age in meiosis-II human oocytes detected by FISH analysis. Am J Hum Genet 1996; 59: 176–84.
30. Munné S, Alikani M, Tomkin G, Grifo J, Cohen J. Embryo morphology, developmental rates and maternal age are correlated with chromosome abnormalities. Fertil Steril 1995; 64: 382–91.
31. Benadiva CA, Kligman I, Munné S. Aneuploidy 16 in human embryos increases significantly with maternal age. Fertil Steril 1996; 66: 248–55.
32. Hardy K, Martin KL, Leese HJ, Winston RML, Handyside AH. Human preimplantation development in vitro is not adversely affected by biopsy at the 8-cell stage. Hum Reprod 1990; 5: 708–14.
33. Gianaroli L, Magli MC, Munné S, Fortini D, Ferraretti AP. Advantages of day 4 embryo transfer in patients undergoing preimplantation genetic diagnosis of aneuploidy. J Assist Reprod Genet 1999; 16: 170–5.

34. Bahce M, Cohen J, Munné S. Preimplantation genetic diagnosis of aneuploidy: were we looking at the wrong chromosomes? J Assist Reprod Genet 1999; 16: 176–81.

35. Wells D, Sherlock JK, Handyside AH, Delhanty JDA. Detailed chromosomal and molecular genetic analysis of single cells by whole genome amplification and comparative genomic hybridization. Nucleic Acids Res 1999; 27: 1214–18.

36. Voullaire L, Slater H, Williamson R, Wilton L. Chromosome analysis of blastomeres from human embryos by using comparative genomic hybridization. Hum Genet 2000; 106: 210–17.

37. Wilton L, Williamson R, McBain J, et al. Birth of a healthy infant after preimplantation confirmation of euploidy by comparative genomic hybridization. N Engl J Med 2001; 345: 1537–41.

38. Voullaire L, Wilton L, McBain J, et al. Chromosome abnormalities identified by comparative genomic hybridization in embryos from women with repeated implantation failure. Mol Hum Reprod 2002; 8: 1035–41.

39. Munné S, Dailey T, Sultan KM, et al. The use of first polar bodies for preimplantation diagnosis of aneuploidy. Hum Reprod (Mol Hum Reprod vol. 1) 1995; 10: 1014–20.

40. Verlinsky Y, Cieslak J, Friedine M, et al. Pregnancies following pre-conception diagnosis of common aneuploidies by fluorescent in situ hybridization. Hum Reprod (Mol Hum Reprod vol. 1) 1995; 10: 1923–7.

41. Verlinsky Y, Cieslak J, Ivakhnenko V, et al. Preimplantation diagnosis of common aneuploidies by first- and second-polar body FISH analysis. J Assist Reprod Genet 1998; 15: 285–9.

42. Northrop LE, Treff NR, Levy B, Scott RT Jr. SNP microarray-based 24 chromosome aneuploidy screening demonstrates that cleavage-stage FISH poorly predicts aneuploidy in embryos that develop to morphologically normal blastocysts. Mol Hum Reprod 2010; 16: 590–600.

43. Treff NR, Levy B, Su J, et al. SNP microarray based 24 chromosome aneuploidy screening is significantly more consistent than FISH. Mol Hum Reprod 2010; 16: 583–9.

44. Fragouli E, Alfarawati S, Daphnis DD, et al. Cytogenetic analysis of human blastocysts with the use of FISH, CGH and aCGH: scientific data and technical evaluation. Hum Reprod 2011; 26: 480–90.

45. Schoolcraft WB, Fragouli E, Stevens J, et al. Clinical application of comprehensive chromosomal screening at the blastocyst stage. Fertil Steril 2010; 94: 1700–6.

46. Menezo Y, Hazout A, Dumont M, Herbaut N, Nicollet B. Co-culture of embryos on Vero cells and transfer of blastocysts in the human. Hum Reprod 1992; 7(Suppl 1): 101–6.

47. Gardner DK, Vella P, Lane M, et al. Culture and transfer of human blastocysts increases implantation rates and reduces the need for multiple embryo transfers. Fertil Steril 1998; 69: 84–8.

48. Gardner DK, Schoolcraft WB, Wagley L, et al. A prospective randomized trial of blastocyst culture and transfer in in vitro fertilization. Hum Reprod 1998; 13: 3434–40.

49. Jones GM, Trounson AO, Lolatgis N, Wood C. Factors affecting the success of human blastocyst development and pregnancy following in vitro fertilization and embryo transfer. Fertil Steril 1998; 70: 1022–9.

50. Meldrum DR. Blastocyst transfer – a natural evolution. Fertil Steril 1999; 72: 216–17.

51. Magli MC, Jones GM, Gras L, et al. Chromosome mosaicism in day 3 aneuploid embryos that develop to morphologically normal blastocysts in vitro. Hum Reprod 2000; 15: 1781–6.

52. Harlow GM, Quinn P. Development of mouse preimplantation embryos in vivo and in vitro. Aust J Biol Sci 1982; 35: 187–93.

53. Jung T, Fischer B. Correlation between diameter and DNA or protein synthetic activity in rabbit blastocysts. Biol Reprod 1988; 39: 1111–16.

54. Carney EW, Foote RH. Effect of superovulation, embryo recovery, culture system and embryo transfer on development of rabbit embryos in vivo and in vitro. J Reprod Fertil 1990; 89: 543–51.

55. Quinn P, Kerin JF, Warnes GM. Improved pregnancy rate in human in vitro fertilization with the use of a medium based on the composition of human tubal fluid. Fertil Steril 1985; 44: 493–8.

56. Yeung WSB, Lau EYL, Chan STH, Ho PC. Coculture with homologous oviductal cells improved the implantation of human embryos – a prospective randomized clinical trial. J Assist Reprod Genet 1996; 13: 762–7.

57. Nieto FS, Watkins WB, Lopata A, Baker HW, Edgar DH. The effects of coculture with autologous cryopreserved endometrial cells on human in vitro fertilization and early embryo morphology: a randomized study. J Assist Reprod Genet 1996; 13: 386–9.

58. Plachot M, Antoine JM, Alvarez S, et al. Granulosa cells improve human embryo development in vitro. Hum Reprod 1993; 8: 2133–40.

59. Quinn P, Margalit R. Beneficial effects of coculture with cumulus cells on blastocyst formation in a prospective trial with supernumerary human embryos. J Assist Reprod Genet 1996; 13: 9–14.

60. Sakkas D, Jaquenoud N, Leppens G, Campana A. Comparison of results after in vitro fertilized human embryos are cultured in routine medium and in coculture on Vero cells: a randomized study. Fertil Steril 1994; 61: 521–5.

61. Barmat LI, Worrilow KC, Payton BV. Growth factor expression by human oviduct and buffalo rat liver coculture cells. Fertil Steril 1997; 67: 775–9.

62. Fukui Y, McGowan LT, James RW, et al. Factors affecting the in vitro development of blastocysts of bovine oocytes matured and fertilized in vitro. J Reprod Fertil 1991; 92: 125–31.

63. Menezo Y, Guerin JF, Czyba JC. Improvement of human early embryo development in vitro by coculture on monolayers of Vero cells. Biol Reprod 1990; 42: 301–6.

64. Barmat LI, Liu HC, Spandorfer SD, et al. Human pre-embryo development on autologous endometrial coculture versus conventional medium. Fertil Steril 1998; 70: 1109–13.

65. Barmat LI, Liu H-C, Spandorfer SD, et al. Autologous endometrial co-culture in patients with repeated failures of implantation after in vitro fertilization-embryo transfer. J Assist Reprod Genet 1999; 16: 121–7.

66. de Wit W, Gowrising CJ, Kuik DJ, et al. Only hydrosalpinges visible on ultrasound are associated with

reduced implantation and pregnancy rates after in vitro fertilization. Hum Reprod 1998; 13: 1696–701.

67. Dechaud H, Daures JP, Arnal F, et al. Does previous salpingectomy improve implantation and pregnancy rates in patients with severe tubal factor infertility who are undergoing in vitro fertilization? A pilot prospective randomized study. Fertil Steril 1998; 69: 1020–5.

68. Strandell A, Lindhard A, Waldenstrom U, et al. Hydrosalpinx and IVF outcome: a prospective, randomized multicentre trial in Scandinavia on salpingectomy prior to IVF. Hum Reprod 1999; 14: 2762–9.

69. Strandell A, Lindhard A, Waldenstrom U, Thornburn J. Hydrosalpinx and IVF outcome: cumulative results after salpingectomy in a randomized controlled trial. Hum Reprod 2001; 16: 2403–10.

70. Johnson NP, Mak W, Sowter MC. Laparoscopic salpingectomy for women with hydrosalpinges enhances the success of IVF: a Cochrane review. Hum Reprod 2002; 17: 543–8.

71. Dechaud H, Anahory T, Aligier N, et al. Salpingectomy for repeated embryo nonimplantation after in vitro fertilization in patients with severe tubal factor infertility. J Assist Reprod Genet 2000; 17: 200–6.

72. Schoolcraft WB, Schlenker T, Gee M, et al. Assisted hatching in the treatment of poor prognosis in vitro fertilization candidates. Fertil Steril 1994; 62: 551–4.

73. Stein A, Rufas O, Amit S, et al. Assisted hatching by partial zona dissection of human pre-embryos in patients with recurrent implantation failure after in vitro fertilization. Fertil Steril 1995; 63: 838–41.

74. Meldrum DR, Wisot A, Yee B, et al. Assisted hatching reduces the age-related decline in IVF outcome in women younger than age 43 without increasing miscarriage or monozygotic twinning. J Assist Reprod Genet 1998; 15: 418–21.

75. Janssens R, Carle M, De Clerk E, et al. Can zona pellucida thickness predict the implantation rate (abstr)? Hum Reprod 1994; 9(Suppl 4): 78.

76. Edirisinghe WR, Ahnonkitpanit V, Promviengchai S, et al. A study failing to determine significant benefits from assisted hatching: patients selected for advanced age, zonal thickness of embryos, and previous failed attempts. J Assist Reprod Genet 1999; 16: 294–301.

77. Magli MC, Gianaroli L, Ferraretti AP, et al. Rescue of implantation potential in embryos with poor prognosis by assisted zona hatching. Hum Reprod 1998; 13: 1331–5.

78. Chao KH, Chen SU, Chen HF, et al. Assisted hatching increases the implantation and pregnancy rate of in vitro fertilization (IVF)-embryo transfer (ET), but not that of IVF-tubal ET in patients with repeated IVF failures. Fertil Steril 1997; 67: 904–8.

79. Lanzendorf SE, Nehchiri F, Mayer JF, et al. A prospective, randomized, double-blind evaluation of assisted hatching in patients of advanced maternal age. Hum Reprod 1998; 13: 409–13.

80. Das S, Blake D, Farquhar C, Seif MM. Assisted hatching on assisted conception (IVF & ICSI). Cochrane Database Syst Rev 2009; (2): CD001894.

81. Martins WP, Rocha IA, Ferriani R, Nastri CO. Assisted hatching of human embryos: a systematic review and meta-analysis of randomized controlled trails. Hum Reprod Update 2011; 17: 438–53.

82. Primi M-P, Senn A, Montag M, et al. A European multicentre prospective randomized study to assess the use of assisted hatching with a diode laser and the benefit of an immunosuppressive/antibiotic treatment in different patient populations. Hum Reprod 2004; 19: 2325–33.

83. Balaban B, Urman B, Alatas C, et al. A comparison of four different techniques of assisted hatching. Hum Reprod 2002; 17: 1239–43.

84. Blake DA, Forsberg AS, Johansson BR, Wikland M. Laser zona pellucida thinning – an alternative approach to assisted hatching. Hum Reprod 2001; 16: 1959–64.

85. Mantoudis E, Podsiadly BT, Gorgy A, et al. A comparison between quarter, partial and total laser assisted hatching in selected infertility patients. Hum Reprod 2001; 16: 2182–6.

86. Petersen CG, Mauri AL, Baruffi RL, et al. Implantation failures: success of assisted hatching with quarter-laser zona thinning. Reprod Biomed Online 2004; 10: 224–9.

87. Verlinsky Y, Cieslak J, Ivakhnenko V, et al. Prevention of age-related aneuploidies by polar body testing of oocytes. J Assist Reprod Genet 1999; 16: 165–9.

88. Gianaroli L, Magli MC, Munné S, et al. Will preimplantation genetic diagnosis assist patients with a poor prognosis to achieve pregnancy? Hum Reprod 1997; 12: 1762–7.

89. Gianaroli L, Magli MC, Ferraretti AP, et al. Preimplantation genetic diagnosis increases the implantation rate in human in vitro fertilization by avoiding the transfer of chromosomally abnormal embryos. Fertil Steril 1997; 68: 1128–31.

90. Munné S, Magli C, Cohen J, et al. Positive outcome after preimplantation diagnosis of aneuploidy in human embryos. Hum Reprod 1999; 14: 2191–9.

91. Gianaroli L, Magli MC, Ferraretti AP, Munné S. Preimplantation diagnosis for aneuploidies in patients undergoing in vitro fertilization with a poor prognosis: identification of the categories for which it should be proposed. Fertil Steril 1999; 72: 837–44.

92. Staessen C, Platteau P, Van Assche E, et al. Comparison of blastocyst transfer with or without preimplantation genetic diagnosis for aneuploidy screening in couples with advanced maternal age: a prospective randomized controlled trial. Hum Reprod 2004; 19: 2849–58.

93. Mastenbroek S, Twisk M, van Echten-Arends J, et al. In vitro fertilization with preimplantation genetic screening. N Engl J Med 2007; 357: 9–17.

94. Mastenbroek S, Twisk M, van der Veen F, Repping S. Preimplantation genetic screening: a systematic review and meta-analysis of RCTs. Hum Reprod 2011; 17: 454–66.

95. Pehlivan T, Rubio C, Rodrigo L, et al. Impact of preimplantation genetic diagnosis on IVF outcome in implantation failure patients. Reprod Biomed Online 2002; 6: 232–7.

96. Munné S, Sandalinas M, Escudero T, et al. Improved implantation after preimplantation genetic diagnosis of aneuploidy. Reprod Biomed Online 2003; 7: 91–7.

97. Taranissi M, El-Toukhy T, Verlinsky Y. Influence of maternal age on the outcome of PGD for aneuploidy screening in patients with recurrent implantation failure. Reprod Biomed Online 2005; 10: 628–32.

98. Blockeel C, Schutyser V, De Vos A, et al. Prospective, randomized controlled trial of PGS in IVF/ICSI patients with poor implantation. Reprod Biomed Online 2008; 17: 848–54.

99. Harper J, Coonen E, De Rycke M, et al. What next for preimplantation genetic screening (PGS)? A position statement from the ESHRE PGD consortium steering committee? Hum Reprod 2010; 25: 821–3.

100. Gardner DK, Schoolcraft WB. No longer neglected: the human blastocyst. Hum Reprod 1998; 13: 3289–92.

101. Cruz JR, Dubey AK, Patel J, et al. Is blastocyst transfer useful as an alternative treatment for patients with multiple in vitro fertilization failures? Fertil Steril 1999; 72: 218–20.

102. Guerif F, Bidault R, Gasnier O, et al. Efficacy of blastocyst transfer after implantation. Reprod Biomed Online 2004; 9: 630–6.

103. Barrenetxea G, De Laurruzea AL, Ganzabal T, et al. Blastocyst culture after repeated failure of cleavage-stage embryo transfers: a comparison of day 5 and day 6 transfers. Fertil Steril 2005; 83: 49–53.

104. Levitas E, Lunenfeld E, Har-Vardi I, et al. Blastocyst-stage embryo transfer in patients who failed to conceive in three or more day 2–3 embryo transfer cycles: a prospective, randomized study. Fertil Steril 2004; 81: 567–71.

105. Schoolcraft WB, Gardner DK, Lane M, et al. Blastocyst culture and transfer: analysis of results and parameters affecting outcome in two in vitro fertilization programs. Fertil Steril 1999; 72: 604–9.

106. Menezo YJ, Sakkas D, Janny L. Co-culture of the early human embryo: factors affecting human blastocyst formation in vitro. Microsc Res Tech 1995; 32: 50–6.

107. Wiemer KE, Hoffman DI, Maxson WS, et al. Embryonic morphology and rate of implantation of human embryos following coculture on bovine oviductal epithelial cells. Hum Reprod 1994; 61: 105–10.

108. Wiemer KE, Garrisi J, Steuerwald N, et al. Beneficial aspects of co-culture with assisted hatching when applied to multiple-failure in vitro fertilization patients. Hum Reprod 1996; 11: 2429–33.

109. Hu Y, Maxson WS, Hoffman DI, et al. Coculture of human embryos with buffalo rat liver cells for women with decreased prognosis in in vitro fertilization. Am J Obstet Gynecol 1997; 177: 358–63.

110. Bongso A, Ng SC, Sathananthan H, et al. Improved quality of human embryos when co-cultured with human ampullary cells. Hum Reprod 1989; 4: 706–13.

111. Yeung WS, Lau EY, Chan ST, Ho PC. Coculture with homologous oviductal cells improved the implantation of human embryos – a prospective randomized control trial. J Assist Reprod Genet 1996; 13: 762–27.

112. Plachot M, Antoine JM, Alvarez S, et al. Granulosa cells improve human embryo development in vitro. Hum Reprod 1993; 8: 2133–40.

113. Quinn P, Margalit R. Beneficial effects of coculture with cumulus cells on blastocyst formation in a prospective trial with supernumerary human embryos. J Assist Reprod Genet 1996; 13: 9–14.

114. Fabbri R, Porcu E, Marsella T, et al. Human embryo development and pregnancies in an homologous granulosa cell coculture system. J Assist Reprod Genet 2000; 17: 1–12.

115. Carrell DT, Peterson CM, Jones KP, et al. A simplified coculture system using homologous, attached cumulus tissue results in improved human embryo morphology and pregnancy rates during in vitro fertilization. J Assist Reprod Genet 1999; 16: 344–9.

116. Cross JC, Werb Z, Fisher SJ. Implantation and the placenta: key pieces of the development puzzle. Science 1994; 266: 1508–17.

117. Liu H-C, He Z-H, Mele CA, et al. Human endometrial stromal cells improve embryo quality by enhancing the expression of insulin-like growth factors and their receptors in cocultured human preimplantation embryos. Fertil Steril 1999; 71: 361–7.

118. Tazuke SI, Giudice L. Growth factors and cytokines in the endometrium, embryonic development, and maternal embryonic interactions. Semin Reprod Endocrinol 1996; 14: 231–45.

119. Jayot S, Parneix I, Verdaguer S, et al. Coculture of embryos on homologous endometrial cells in patients with repeated failures of implantation. Fertil Steril 1995; 63: 109–14.

120. Nieto NS, Watkins WB, Lopata A, et al. The effects of coculture with autologous cryopreserved endometrial cells on human in vitro fertilization and early embryo morphology: a randomized study. J Assist Reprod Genet 1996; 13: 386–9.

121. Simon C, Mercader A, Garcia-Velaso J, et al. Coculture of human embryos with autologous human endometrial epithelial cells in patients with implantation failure. J Clin Endocrinol Metab 1999; 84: 2638–46.

122. Eyheremendy V, Raffo FGE, Papayannis M, et al. Beneficial effect of autologous endometrial cell coculture in patients with repeated implantation failure. Fertil Steril 2010; 93: 769–73.

123. Spandorfer SD, Barmat LI, Navarro J, et al. Importance of the biopsy date in autologous endometrial cocultures for patients with multiple implantation failures. Fertil Steril 2002; 77: 1209–13.

124. Urman B, Balaban B. Is there a place for co-cultures in the era of sequential media? Reprod Biomed Online 2005; 10: 492–6.

125. Dominquez F, Gadea B, Mercadez A, et al. Embryologic outcome and secretome profile of implanted blastyocysts obtained after coculture in human endometrial epithelial cells versus the sequential system. Fertil Steril 2010; 93: 774–82.

126. Kattal, N, Cohen J, Barmat LI. Role of coculture in human in vitro fertilization: a meta-analysis. Fertil Steril 2008; 90: 1069–76.

127. Lass A, Ellenbogen A, Croucher C, et al. The effect of salpingectomy on ovarian response to superovulation in an in vitro fertilization embryo transfer program. Fertil Steril 1998; 70: 1035–8.

128. Verhulst G, Vandersteen N, Van Steirteghem AC, Devroey P. Bilateral salpingectomy does not compromise ovarian stimulation in an in vitro fertilization/embryo transfer program. Hum Reprod 1994; 9: 624–8.

129. Van Voorhis BJ, Sparks AE, Syrop CH, Stovall DW. Ultrasound-guided aspiration of hydrosalpinges is associated with improved pregnancy and implantation rates after in vitro fertilization cycles. Hum Reprod 1998; 13: 736–9.

130. Kontoravdis A, Makrakis E, Pantos K, et al. Proximal tubal occlusion and salpingectomy result in similar improvement in in vitro fertilization outcome in patients with hydrosalpinx. Fertil Steril 2006; 86: 1642–9.

131. Raziel A, El RR, Wardimon J, Arad D, et al. Ultrasono-graphic diagnosis of post salpingectomy interstitial pregnancy. Case report and review of the literature. Acta Obstet Gynecol Scand 1989; 68: 85–6.

132. Fisch B, Peled Y, Kaplan B, et al. Abdominal pregnancy following in vitro fertilization in a patient with previous bilateral salpingectomy. Obstet Gynecol 1996; 88: 642–3.

133. Cohen J, Malter H, Elsner C, et al. Immunosuppression supports implantation of zona pellucida dissected human embryos. Fertil Steril 1990; 53: 662–5.

134. Kemeter P, Feichtinger W. Prednisolone supplementation to Clomid and/or gonadotrophin stimulation for in vitro fertilization – a prospective randomized trial. Hum Reprod 1986; 1: 441–4.

135. Catt JW, Ryan JP, Saunders DM, O'Neill C. Shortterm corticosteroid treatment does not improve implantation for embryos derived from subzonal insertion of sperm. Fertil Steril 1991; 61: 565–6.

136. Slotnik RN, Ortega JE. Monoamniotic twinning and zona manipulation: a survey of U.S. IVF centers correlating zona manipulation procedures and high-risk twinning frequency. J Assist Reprod Genet 1996; 13: 381–5.

137. Herschlag A, Paine T, Cooper GW, et al. Monozygotic twinning associated with mechanical assisted hatching. Fertil Steril 1999; 71: 144–6.

138. Schacter M, Raziel A, Friedler S, et al. Monozygotic twinning after assisted reproductive techniques: a phenomenon independent of micromanipulation. Hum Reprod 2001; 16: 1264–9.

139. Schieve LA, Meikle SF, Peterson HB, et al. Does assisted hatching pose a risk for monozygotic twinning in pregnancies conceived through in vitro fertilization? Fertil Steril 2000; 74: 288–94.

140. Harper JC, Coonen E, Handyside AH, et al. Mosaicism of autosomes and sex chromosomes in morphologically normal, monospermic preimplantation human embryos. Prenat Diagn 1995; 15: 41–9.

141. Munné S, Lee A. Rosenwaks Z, et al. Diagnosis of major chromosome aneuploidies in human preimplantation embryos. Hum Reprod 1993; 8: 2185–91.

142. Reubinoff BE, Shushan A. Preimplantation diagnosis in older patients. To biopsy or not to biopsy? Hum Reprod 1996; 11: 2071–8.

143. Harper JC, Coonen E, Ramaekers FC, et al. Identification of the sex of human preimplantation embryos in two hours using an improved spreading method and fluorescent in situ hybridization (FISH) using directly labeled probes. HumReprod 1994; 9: 721–4.

144. Coulam CB, Krysa LW, Bustillo M. Intravenous immunoglobulin for in vitro fertilization failure. Hum Reprod 1994; 9: 2265–9.

145. Sher G, Feinman M, Zouves C, et al. High fecundity rates following in vitro fertilization and embryo transfer in antiphospholipid antibody seropositive women treated with heparin and aspirin. Hum Reprod 1994; 9: 2278–83.

146. Birdenfeld A, Mukaida T, Minichiello L, et al. Incidence of autoimmune antibodies in failed embryo transfer cycles. Am J Reprod Immunol 1994; 31: 65–8.

147. Coulam CB, Kaider BD, Kaider AS, et al. Antiphospholipid antibodies associated with implantation failure after IVF/ET. J Assist Reprod Genet 1997; 14: 603–8.

148. Denis AL, Guido M, Adler RD, et al. Antiphospholipid antibodies and pregnancy rates and outcome in in vitro fertilization patients. Fertil Steril 1997; 67: 1084–90.

149. Qublan HS, Eid SS, Ababneh HA, et al. Acquired and inherited thrombophilia: implication in recurrent IVF and embryo transfer failure. Hum Reprod 2006; 21: 2694–8.

150. Martinelli I, Taioli E, Ragni G, et al. Embryo implantation after assisted reproductive procedures and maternal thrombophilia. Haematologica 2003; 88: 789–93.

151. Alikani M, Cohen J, Tomkin G, et al. Human embryo fragmentation in vitro and its implications for pregnancy and implantation. Fertil Steril 1999; 71: 836–42.

152. Cohen J, Scott R, Schimmel T, et al. Birth of infant after transfer of anucleate donor oocyte cytoplasm into recipient eggs. Lancet 1997; 350: 186–7.

153. Schoolcraft WB, Surrey ES, Gardner DK. Embryo transfer: techniques and variables affecting success. Fertil Steril 2001; 76: 863–70.

154. Anderson RE, Nugent NL, Gregg AT, et al. Transvaginal ultrasound-guided embryo transfer improves outcome in patients with previous failed in vitro fertilization cycles. Fertil Steril 2002; 77: 769–75.

155. Liu HC, Tseng L. Estradiol metabolism in isolated human endometrial epithelial gland and stromal cells. Endocrinology 1979; 104: 1674–81.

48

Ultrasonography in assisted reproduction

Ilan Tur-Kaspa and Laurel Stadtmauer

INTRODUCTION

Can we imagine assisted reproductive technique (ART) today without imaging? Ultrasound has become the most widely used and important tool in the diagnosis and treatment of infertility. When a patient presents with the complaint of infertility, ultrasound evaluation is one of the first steps in the evaluation of infertility. This initial ultrasound exam will immediately affect the management of the patient. It allows us to diagnose adnexal pathology such as polycystic ovarian syndrome (PCOS), endometrioma, or other ovarian cysts, as well as hydrosalpinges. Measuring the antral follicle count (AFC) is one of the best predictors for estimating ovarian reserve. Congenital uterine anomalies, fibroids, as well as intracavitary abnormalities may be diagnosed in the uterus. When ART treatment begins, ultrasound is used in almost any interaction with the patients. This will be for monitoring of follicular development and endometrial response as well as ultrasound guidance for oocyte retrieval and embryo transfer (ET).

Passing high-frequency sound waves through tissue and reading the echoes produce ultrasound images. Real time images as well as manipulation of still images can be performed. Three-dimensional (3D) ultrasound allows better imaging as well as more accurate volume rendering. It can be used in the multiplanar display, volume rendering, or surface rendering modes. It has become a gold standard for the diagnosis of uterine anomalies and may assist in more accurate follicular monitoring measurements. Doppler modalities of ultrasound allow identification of the direction and magnitude of blood flow and calculation of velocity.

This chapter is aimed to review how 2D and 3D ultrasound are used to maximize ART outcome, starting from the initial evaluation of the infertile patient and continuing during an IVF treatment. When we see better, we do ART better.

ULTRASOUND OF THE OVARY: EVALUATION OF THE INFERTILE WOMAN AND ART MONITORING

The ovaries are composed of germ cells, stromal cells, and epithelium. The antral follicles are visible as small cysts. Follicles grow in two stages, the gonadotropin-independent and gonadotropin-dependent stages and the recruitment occurs over three months. Primordial follicles consist of the oocyte with a thin layer of granulosa and stromal cells, which cannot be seen on ultrasound. The gonadotropin-dependent stage can be visualized on ultrasound. As a follicle grows, it develops follicular fluid, which can be seen by ultrasound. Antral follicles are visible and measure from 2 to 10 mm and represent the pool of follicles that may be recruited in the follicular phase for ovulation. These follicles reach a diameter of 17–24 mm prior to ovulation. Ovarian blood flow in an ovulatory cycle is constant up to the point of ovulation. Ovarian flow velocity tends to increase at and immediately after ovulation (1). After ovulation a corpus luteum (CL) is frequently seen during the secretory phase of the cycle. It is well vascularized and may have the appearance of a "ring of fire" from the vascularity as seen by power Doppler. A normal CL has a variety of sonographic appearances. Most commonly, the CL appears as a round anechoic intraovarian or exophytic ovarian cystic mass with a homogeneous, thick, moderately echogenic wall, which may be highly vascular with a low-resistance arterial waveform (Fig. 48.1) (2). CL blood flow is characterized by low impedance and high flow pattern. Hemorrhage into a CL can create a sonographic pattern of internal echoes similar to a hemorrhagic follicular cyst (Fig. 48.2) and rupture of the cyst can result in hemorrhage or clot surrounding the ovary or within the peritoneal cavity.

Ovarian Reserve

Age has a significant impact on follicle number and oocyte quality, given the women were born with a fixed number of oocytes. The peak number of five million primordial follicles occurs prior to birth at about 20 weeks gestation, and decrease throughout life mainly by atresia. At birth there are about one million oocytes, and at puberty approximately 250,000 oocytes. The exponential loss of follicles accelerates at 37–38 years (only about 25000), and leads to full depletion of the oocytes up to menopause at average age of 51years (3). Retrieval of 10–100 of oocytes with multiple IVF cycles does not seem to significantly affect this age-related follicular loss.

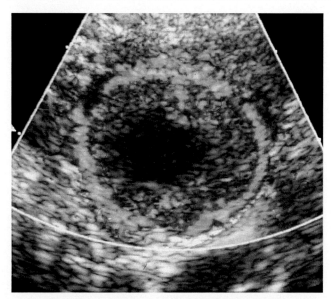

Figure 48.1   Corpus luteum cyst – the "ring of fire."

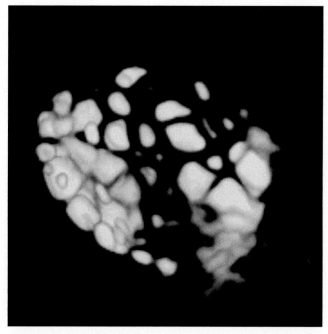

Figure 48.3   Antral follicle count of the ovary by 3D ultrasound.

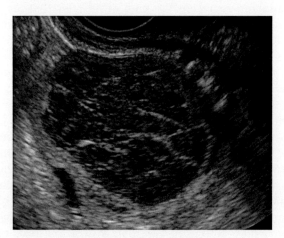

Figure 48.2   Hemorrhagic cyst.

Blood tests for estimating ovarian reserve include day 3 FSH and estradiol (E2) levels as well as anti-Müllerian hormone (AMH) and inhibin B (4–6). With ultrasound, the ovarian reserve can be assessed by measuring antral follicle counts (AFC) with or without the ovarian volumes. AFCs are typically made by counting the number of follicles measuring 2–10 mm in both ovaries and can be estimated by 2D or 3D ultrasound. 3D AFC is more reproducible and accurate but the method is less standardized and 3D technology may not be freely available for all reproductive endocrinologists (7). Figure 48.3 shows a 3D antral follicle count. AFC of >12 is mandatory for the definition of polycystic ovaries. Both AFC and AMH predict similarly ovarian reserve and the response to treatment, but ultrasound is the only method so far that allows a direct assessment of each ovary separately. Identification of participants who are likely to respond poorly during IVF treatment is clinically relevant as the couple can be counseled regarding cycle cancellation and lower chance of success. Pretreatment AFC and AMH were found to be the most significant predictors of the number of oocytes retrieved especially

for low and high responders in multiple studies including a meta-analysis by Hendricks et al. (8–12). These studies showed AFC and AMH demonstrated similar predictive power based on receiver operating curve (ROC) analysis and correlated with oocyte number better than other parameters, such as FSH or age. However, all these parameters correlate less well with pregnancy outcomes, which is the more important outcome for the patient than oocyte number. The validity of AFC for ovarian reserve comes from studies showing a direct correlation with the number of nongrowing follicles viewed on histological sections (13). On the other hand, ovarian volume, vascularity, and perfusion had no significant value in predicting poor ovarian response and are inferior to AFC (14).

The hypothesis that aneuploidy is negatively associated with the quantity of oocytes in the ovary is poorly supported by studies showing decreased AFC in women with spontaneous abortions after IVF. The conclusions are not supported by all studies possibly because some lack power and it may depend on the mechanism of diminished ovarian reserve. In many women with low AFC, especially at a young age, there is a decrease in quantity but not in quality of the oocytes.

Ovarian Cysts

Ultrasound is the best method for evaluating the ovaries for cysts, and it is a mandatory step in the initial evaluation of the infertile woman. The most common ovarian cysts seen in infertility patients are simple functional cysts, hemorrhagic cysts, endometrioma, and dermoid cysts. Functional cysts are the most common cystic masses seen in the reproductive age group. These cysts tend to stay less than 3–8 cm in diameter and regress after 1–2 cycles. They are usually either follicular cysts or luteal cysts. If they are small (<3 cm) and not hormonally active, they do not need to be treated before ART. However, patients with large simple ovarian cysts may have lower response to stimulation and ovarian cyst aspiration under ultrasound guidance, with local or IV sedation, immediately prior to ovarian stimulation, has been shown to be beneficial (15).

An endometrioma is also a common finding in the infertile patient and is a sign of the presence of endometriosis in other areas (16,17). The typical endometrioma is a unilocular cyst with homogeneous low-level internal echogenicity (ground glass echogenicity) of the cyst fluid (Fig. 48.4). With respect to endometrioma, a correct diagnosis is important for infertility with possible need for ART. Transvaginal ultrasonography is the imaging of choice to differentiate ovarian endometrioma from other adnexal masses (18,19). Studies show that an endometrioma is associated with lower response to ovarian stimulation; however, removing the endometrioma can also affect ovarian response and may significantly diminish ovarian reserve as the base of the ovary is usually burned and the cyst wall is stripped with damage of follicles (20). Some studies show that previous or present ovarian endometriosis does not impair success rates at IVF and that ovarian surgery for endometriosis does not result in improved ART outcome, but, on the contrary, may compromise ovarian reserve (21–25). IVF outcome in women with a diagnosis of ovarian endometriosis has been addressed in numerous studies and summarized by a meta-analysis showing reduced pregnancy rates (PRs) after IVF (26). Intervention studies investigating the effectiveness of laparoscopic removal of ovarian endometriosis as a tool to improve subsequent IVF results show mainly negative results. Several reports showed that the outcome of IVF in patients previously submitted to laparoscopic stripping of endometrioma was similar to that of endometriosis-free controls (27–31). In line with results of Wong et al (32), a more recent meta-analysis showed that the outcome of IVF was similar in patients with in situ ovarian endometrioma as in endometriosis-free women and that removing endometrioma was not harmful (26). If an endometrioma is seen during oocyte retrieval, it should not be aspirated as there is a high risk of ovarian infection and surgery pre-IVF should be considered in cases of follicle inaccessibility due to the size or position of the endometrioma.

Dermoid cysts can present as solid hyperechoic heterogeneous masses with a mixed pattern of solid and cystic areas. They may contain calcifications, fat, and hair. They should be removed prior to IVF if they are causing pain or if there is a question of malignancy. Puncture during oocyte retrieval should be avoided due to high risk of peritonitis (33).

Polycystic Ovary (PCO)

Ultrasound is one of the criteria for the diagnosis of polycystic ovarian syndrome (PCOS) based on the Rotterdam

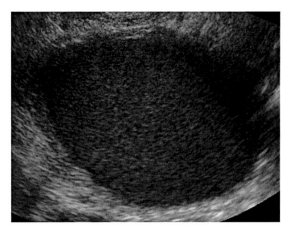

Figure 48.4 Endometrioma.

Consensus conference. Current data suggest that polycystic ovaries detected by transvaginal ultrasonography may be found in approximately 75% of women with a clinical diagnosis of PCOS (34,35). However, it is not a rule that all women with polycystic ovaries will demonstrate the clinical and biochemical features of PCOS, oligomenorrhea, and/or hyperandrogenism (36). Polycystic ovaries per se, even without PCOS, constitute a risk factor for the development of ovarian hyperstimulation syndrome (OHSS) and the stimulation protocol chosen should reflect this and should be aimed at reducing the risk of OHSS (37).

Transvaginal ultrasound (TVS) is a highly sensitivity method for identification of PCO and the transvaginal definition is based on the presence of >12 small follicles in a single ovary (38). Comparisons between transabdominal and transvaginal ultrasound do not find significant differences in the detection rate of PCO (39). The 3D ultrasound and the use of color and pulsed Doppler ultrasound showing increased ovarian blood flow are techniques that further enable the identification of PCO, but are not mandatory for the diagnosis (40). No other imaging modality, such as magnetic resonance imaging (MRI) for the visualization of the ovaries are needed for the diagnosis of PCO, and should not be used as routine examination (41).

The diagnosis of polycystic ovaries has been revised recently (42). The most commonly used criteria today are those proposed by Dewailly and colleagues with a string of pearls pattern (43) and reaffirmed in the Rotterdam 2003 consensus (44,45). Polycystic ovaries can be established when at least one ovary demonstrates an ovarian volume of greater than 10 cm³ or 12 or more follicles measuring 2–9 mm in diameter (small antral follicles) arranged peripherally with a dense core of ovarian stroma. The optimal time to perform this assessment in regularly menstruating women is within the third to the fifth day of the menstrual cycle. The subjective appearance of an increased stromal volume or echogenicity is not included in the definition. The presence of a single polycystic ovary is sufficient to provide the diagnosis (Fig. 48.5).

Ultrasound Monitoring of Ovarian Stimulation: - 2D and 3D SonoAVC

Ultrasound monitoring of follicle growth during gonadotropin stimulation was first performed in 1978 (46) showing a linear relationship between follicle size and E2 levels. Since 1983, once TVS was used for oocyte retrieval, it has been used routinely for monitoring follicle growth for ovulation induction with clomiphene citrate, gonadotropins, and for ART. Gonadotropins cause growth of the cohort of follicles at various stages of development and monitoring with serial ultrasound and serum E2 is an imperative step to reduce the risks of OHSS and multiple births. Follicle size in 2D is best estimated by calculating the mean of the maximum follicular diameter in three planes, but is more commonly done in

two planes. Follicular growth of 1–3 mm per day is expected once the dominant follicle(s) measure greater than 12 mm. Measuring baseline antral follicle count (AFC) on day 2–3 of the cycle, before beginning ovarian stimulation, is an excellent tool to predict the ovarian response. This can be done by 2D or 3D ultrasound, with or without SonoAVC.

A new automated ultrasound application, sonography-based Automated Volume Calculation (SonoAVC, GE medical systems) was developed to be used for follicular monitoring during controlled ovarian hyperstimulation (47). The lower size limit of follicles that SonoAVC can detect is 1–2 mm. The technique involves 3D manipulation. First, the multiplanar view is used to ensure that the ovary is centrally placed and the render mode is selected to generate a 3D volume of interest box. At this point SonoAVC is implemented. The individual follicles identified are then displayed with a specific color and shown together with their dimensions and relative sizes. Post-processing is required in almost all cases to manually identify those antral follicles that have been missed in the initial automated analysis and these are easily added (48) (Fig. 48.6). The total number of follicles is recorded together with the mean diameter of each follicle calculated using the relaxed sphere technique (49,50). The volume calculation is based on a voxel count within the identified hyperechoic structure and represents a true measure of follicular volume regardless of its shape.

There have been studies verifying the SonoAVC technique. Deutch et al. (51) using an ultrasound phantom showed <0.02 ml error comparing the spheres of known volume with a hyperechoic matrix. Rousian et al. (52) showed that the SonoAVC system underestimated the volume by a mean difference of −0.63 ml in their study, which used larger volumes of spheres than the previous

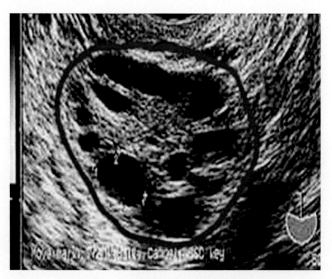

Figure 48.5   Polycystic-appearing ovary.

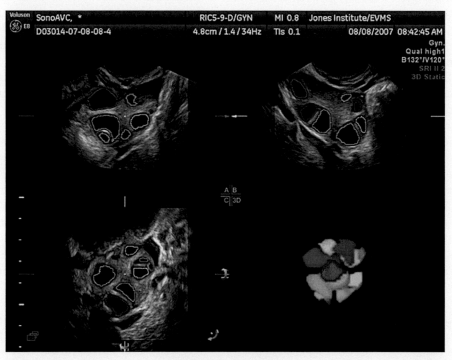

Figure 48.6   SonoAVC.

study. All published studies (53–55) looking at correlation between the number and size of follicles in stimulated ovaries have demonstrated an excellent correlation between SonoAVC and true follicle volume showing the accuracy system for the stimulated ovary. There is also a relationship between the follicular volume calculation and final oocyte maturation and likelihood of collecting mature eggs.

However, no studies have shown differences in IVF outcomes using this technique (55–57). The advantages of SonoAVC may be a time decrease during the ultrasound as the ovarian volumes are saved and less discomfort for the patients. However, there is time required for manual assessment of the 3D data, which should be added to the time in scanning and the technique needs to be learned and reproducibility documented. Rodriguez-Fuentes analyzed the impact of SonoAVC on time and the clinical outcome of IVF treatment. They found reduced time saving of four minutes per case after including the post-processing time (57). Their study has shown that SonoAVC provides different results from those of 2D ultrasound imaging when the size of the follicle is considered. It may also be possible to visualize the cumulus oophorus in the ovarian follicle prior to aspiration and this correlates with the number of retrieved mature oocytes.

ULTRASOUND OF THE UTERUS: EVALUATION OF THE INFERTILE WOMAN AND ART MONITORING

Ultrasound assessment of the endometrium and the myometrium of the uterus is important in maximizing implantation both in natural pregnancies and in IVF. Endometrial thickness and pattern varies throughout the menstrual cycle and is the parameter reviewed in most studies (58,59). The endometrium is thin immediately after menstruation (2–5 mm), thickens during the proliferative phase, is trilaminar before ovulation, and is thick and echogenic in the secretory phase of the cycle. Figure 48.7 shows the typical preovulatory endometrium. A small amount of endometrial fluid (0.5–1.0 mm film in the middle of the cavity), thought to be mucus, can be seen before ovulation and it rapidly disappears. However, significant endometrial fluid at the time of ET, usually visible with hydrosalpinges, is associated with poor prognosis and freezing all the embryos should be considered (60).

Other assessment of the uterus besides the endometrium includes obtaining the size and position of the uterus and the presence of uterine fibroids or adenomyosis. Assessment of the uterine cavity for fibroids, polyps, adhesions, and Müllerian anomalies is mandatory before ART. Uterine imaging is therefore essential in the diagnosis of infertility. These techniques include conventional hysterosalpingography (HSG), 2D ultrasound, 3D ultrasound, and sonohysterography (SHG). MRI may be considered only rarely for special cases.

Transvaginal ultrasound parameters of the endometrium have long been considered implantation markers in IVF (59,61). Ultrasound examination of the endometrium in a natural or mock cycle supplemented with estrogen and progesterone provides a noninvasive way to evaluate the endometrial development and receptivity before ET (62). Synchronization between the endometrial and embryo development is essential for successful implantation.

Sonohysterography (SHG)

SHG, Hysterosonogram, or saline infusion sonography are different names for a minimally invasive office technique used for the evaluation of intrauterine abnormalities. By injecting saline into the uterus, the fluid contrast enhances the visualization of the uterine cavity and filling defects such as, polyps, submucosal fibroids, adhesions, and uterine anomalies (Fig. 48.8). (63–71). Randolph et al. were the first to perform transabdominal ultrasound scan during saline infusion (63). The main uses for SHG are for abnormal uterine bleeding, screening of the uterine cavity prior to ART, and habitual abortion. Contrast media may be also used for injection, such as saline mixed with air or Echovist® (Schering AG, Germany).

The American College of Obstetricians and Gynecologists (ACOG) published in December 2008, ACOG Technology Assessment on Sonohysterography (SHG), prepared

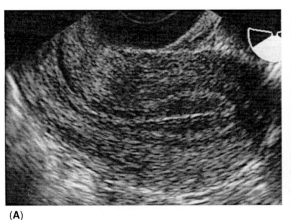

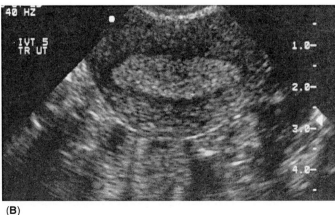

(A)   (B)

Figure 48.7   (**A**) Endometrium in proliferative phase. (**B**) Endometrium in secretory phase.

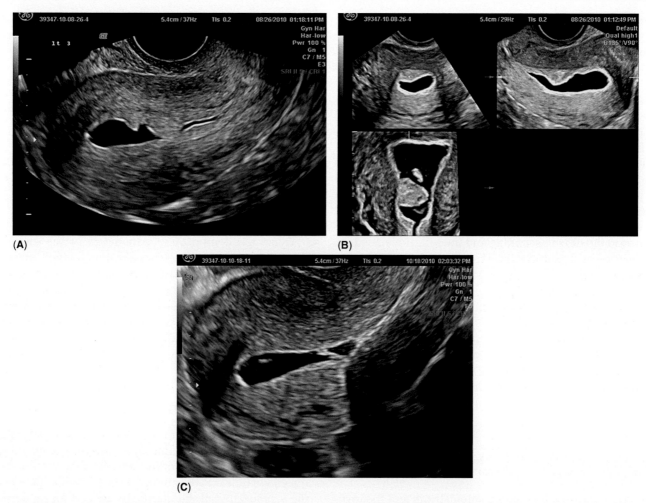

Figure 48.8   Sonohysterography (SHG). (**A**) Uterine polyps by 2D SHG. (**B**) Uterine polyps by 3D SHG. (**C**) Intrauterine adhesions.

in collaboration with the American Institute of Ultrasound in Medicine (AIUM), the Society for Reproductive Endocrinology and Infertility (SREI), an affiliate of the American Society for Reproductive Medicine (ASRM), and with the American College of Radiology (ACR) (72). It described the procedure, indications, and contraindications, and its appropriate documentation. The method for SHG according to AIUM and ACOG (73) are the following: Prior to SHG a preliminary routine TVS is performed with measurements of the endometrium, uterus, and the ovaries and evaluation for fluid in cul-de-sac. After cleansing the external os, the cervical canal and/or uterine cavity should be catheterized using aseptic technique, and appropriate sterile fluid (saline or water for injection) should be instilled slowly (emphasize by the authors) by manual injection under real-time sonographic imaging. Documentation should include images of the endometrial and cervical canals in at least two planes. SHG should be done between days 5–10 of the menstrual cycle. A recent randomized control trial (RCT) answered one of the most common questions with regards to SHG: Should the catheter be placed in the cervix or in the lower part of the uterine cavity (64). Intracervical catheter placement resulted in significantly less pain during SHG and also requires half the saline volume to perform. Therefore, intracervical balloon placement should be preferred for SHG. SHG had been described also

with gel instillation. (73,74) Evaluating the pelvic anatomy with 3D pelvic ultrasound by saline intraperitoneal sonogram (SIPS) has also been described recently (75).

Suspected abnormalities seen on TVS, including focal or diffuse endometrial thickening, and suboptimal images by 2D are enough to recommend further evaluation with SHG. Studies comparing findings on SHG with 2D and 3D ultrasound, HSG, and hysteroscopy show excellent predictive value of SHG (67,68). One study comparing SHG with hysteroscopy showed 88% sensitivity, 100% specificity, and 100% positive predictive value (PPV) and 92% negative predictive value (NPV) for the detection of abnormality (70). The advantages of SHG over HSG are that it can detect adnexal pathology such as PCOS or ovarian cysts at the same time. Infertility patients have a lower rate of intracavitary lesions than patients with abnormal uterine bleeding and higher rate of uterine anomalies. In a prospective study of 600 infertility patients by Tur-Kaspa et al. (71), 20% were found to have cavitary abnormalities including arcuate uterus (15%), polyps (13%), submucosal fibroids (3%), and adhesions (1%). This prospective study compared the incidence of uterine cavity anomalies in patients referred for infertility or abnormal bleeding group, showed that more patients in the bleeding group had intracavitary abnormalities such as polyps, fibroids, and adhesions as well as intramural abnormalities, and the infertility group had more congenital uterine anomalies. Uterine anomalies are associated with an increased risk of infertility, miscarriage, premature birth, fetal loss, malpresentation, and cesarean section (76–78).

Acquired Uterine Abnormalities (Uterine Fibroids, Adenomyosis, Polyps, and Adhesions)

Assessment of uterine fibroids has been most commonly achieved using ultrasonography. For intramural fibroids, TVS is excellent for diagnosis, while for submucosal fibroids, SHG is better at showing the cavity involvement. Using 3D ultrasound with the multiplanar display, especially the coronal views, allows precise localization of a myoma with respect to the endometrial cavity and has been shown to have the accuracy of hysteroscopy and better than 2D ultrasound (79). This localization of uterine myomas assists in determining the surgical approach (hysteroscopic resection or abdominal myomectomy). The 3D multiplanar display is also useful in some cases for differentiating adnexal lesions close to the uterus from lesions within or originating from the uterus; this obviates MRI in selected cases (80,81). Studies looking at uterine fibroids show that the number of fibroids is underestimated by ultrasound compared to those found at surgery even when 3D is used (82) Use of 3D ultrasound and 3D SHG for determining the position of the fibroids can be visualized in Figure 48.9. A normal trilaminar appearance of proliferative endometrium at mid-cycle has been shown to have a PPV of 85–95% of normal endometrial cavity and ruling out polyps, synechiae, fibroids, and Müllerian anomalies (83).

It is important to make the diagnosis of fibroids and to identify the women that would benefit from a myomectomy. Recent systematic review confirmed that ART outcomes are decreased in women with submucosal fibroids, and hysteroscopic removal improves significantly the outcome (84). A meta-analysis study showed a significantly lower PR if submucosal fibroids are present; RR 0.32 (0.12–0.85), and that removal of submucosal fibroids improves clinical PRs with a RR 2.03 (1.08–3.83). (85). Subserosal fibroids do not affect fertility, and removal does not confer benefit. Intramural fibroids appear to decrease fertility, but the results of myomectomy are unclear, and recent two RCTs failed to demonstrate clear benefits (84).

Adenomyosis can be found in most infertile women with endometriosis. On ultrasound it appears as asymmetry and thickening of the uterine walls with loss of endometrium–myometrium border and hypoechogenic nodules in the myometrium. It needs to be distinguished from fibroids (86). Whether adenomyosis in itself is a cause of infertility is controversial.

Endometrial polyps may be found in about 15% of the infertile women (71,87). The benefit of polypectomy leading to higher PRs than hysteroscopy and polyp biopsy was shown in a prospective randomized study (88). Improvement is also shown in retrospective data (89).

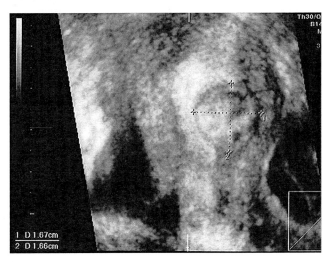

Figure 48.9   3D ultrasound of uterine fibroid with submucosal component.

Based on these studies, polyps diagnosed prior to IVF should be removed. Polyps of <1.5 cm can be removed hysteroscopically even during stimulation, as shown in a retrospective study (90). The management of polyps seen during the course of IVF should be individualized given the number of embryos created, the previous reproductive history of the patient, and the individual clinics' success rates for their ART program (91).

Congenital Uterine Anomalies

Müllerian anomalies are congenital defects in the development of the uterus and upper vagina. It has been demonstrated that conventional 2D ultrasound imaging is a good screening tool for the detection of congenital uterine anomalies and has a high sensitivity for some anomalies (92). However, the ability of 2D ultrasound to distinguish between different types of uterine abnormalities is limited and operator dependent. In addition, both routine 2D ultrasound and HSG lack the specificity for differentiating arcuate, bicornuate, and septate uterus. Precise classification of a uterine anomaly is of clinical importance because the need for intervention and the type of intervention depends on this distinction. There is prognostic significance to this classification as uterine anomalies vary with respect to obstetrical and gynecologic complications.

3D volume imaging techniques are commonplace in computed tomography (CT) and MRI. Practitioners in these modalities are familiar with the volume or multiplanar environment and recognize its clinical value (93). MRI is especially accurate in the diagnosis of uterine anomalies but its main disadvantages include high cost and limited availability. With 3D ultrasound, a volume of ultrasonographic data is acquired and stored. The stored data can be reformatted and analyzed in numerous ways; navigation through the saved volume can demonstrate innumerable arbitrary planes. In the multiplanar display, three perpendicular planes are displayed simultaneously.

Correlation between these three planes is used to confirm a given desired plane, such as the mid-sagittal or mid-coronal plane. The optimal time to examine patients for the presence of uterine anomalies is the luteal phase of the cycle when the endometrium is thick and echogenic and the cavity can be clearly differentiated from the surrounding myometrium. The most important advantage of 3D ultrasound over HSG is the ability to visualize both the uterine cavity and myometrium. It provides complete information about the nature and extent of uterine masses and congenital anomalies. A number of studies have shown complete agreement and accuracy between the congenital uterine anomaly seen on 3D ultrasound with that of HSG or hysteroscopy and laparoscopy as the gold standards (94,95).

There is a large difference in the incidence of uterine anomalies in the population of infertile women varying from 6% in some studies to 66% in others (96–98). Figure 48.10 shows the 3D visualization of the most common anomaly, the septate uterus.

Monitoring Endometrial Thickness during ART Cycle

Endometrial thickness and pattern on the day of human chorionic gonadotropin (hCG) trigger is one of the commonest parameters used in ART. Endometrial pattern can be classified as type A, a multilayered triple-line endometrium consisting of a hyperechogenic outer and central lines shown in Figure 48.7A, type B, an intermediate isoechogenic pattern with a non-prominent central line, and type C, which is an entirely homogeneous endometrium (Fig. 48.7B). Most commonly the endometrium is described as "triple line" or "homogeneous" (99).

There is a controversy regarding the value of measuring endometrial thickness in predicting pregnancy during IVF treatment (58,59). Endometrial thickness is measured from outside to outside in an anterior–posterior view at the widest point. Patients with a thin endometrium following ovarian stimulation have a significantly lower PR. A triple layer endometrial pattern and an endometrial thickness greater than 7 mm have been proposed as markers of endometrial receptivity but have yielded a high percentage of false–positive results (100). Low dose aspirin (101,102) and vaginal Sildenafil (Viagra) (103) have been used to treat patients with thin endometrium. The underlying assumption is that patients with thin endometrium would have suboptimal endometrial blood flow and may have scar tissue with the ability of aspirin or Viagra to increase the endometrial blood flow and development. However, studies are not consistently showing increased uterine receptivity and IVF success and are based on small numbers. No consensus has been reached with regard to the minimum endometrial thickness required for successful pregnancy. Pregnancies did not occur when the endometrial thickness was less than 7 mm (104) However, other studies found that a minimum endometrial thickness of 6 mm is acceptable for implantation (105–108). Sundström reported a successful pregnancy with an endometrial thickness as little as 4 mm, hence this still remains controversial (109). In a recent study (110), the thinnest endometrial lining for successful ongoing pregnancy was 5.8 mm and maximum number of conceptions occurred when the thickness was 8–10 mm. With increasing endometrial thickness (>14 mm), a high miscarriage rate was reported by Weissman et al. (111). An excessively thick endometrium may start in a previous cycle, so therefore ovarian stimulation should not be started following menstruation if the endometrial thickness is greater than 6 mm. Increased preclinical or biochemical miscarriages are also seen with endometrial thicknesses 6–8 mm verses 9 mm or greater (112). These findings correlate well with the recent report on increased pregnancy loss with low endometrial volume on the day of the first pregnancy test (14–18 days after oocyte retrieval) (113).

A good blood supply to the endometrium is usually considered to be an essential requirement for implantation and the assessment of endometrial blood flow in IVF treatment with Doppler has been studied. Assessment of endometrial blood flow adds a physiological dimension to the anatomical ultrasound parameters and has drawn a lot of attention in recent years. However, Doppler studies of uterine arteries do not reflect the actual blood flow to the endometrium. Endometrial and sub-endometrial blood flows can be more objectively and reliably measured with three-dimensional power Doppler ultrasound. With Doppler, an elevated pulsatility index of the uterine arteries is associated with low implantation and PRs (114); an adequate Doppler velocimetry of the uterine arteries is only slightly specific for predicting gestation. The absence of color Doppler mapping at endometrial and sub-endometrial levels is relied to a significant decrease in implantation rate, whereas the PR increases when vessels can be depicted reaching the sub-endometrial halo and the endometrium.

Endometrial volume can now be reliably determined by 3D ultrasound (115) and may improve the predictive value of endometrial thickness (116). Endometrial volume of <2.5 ml is predictive of low PR or pregnancy loss,

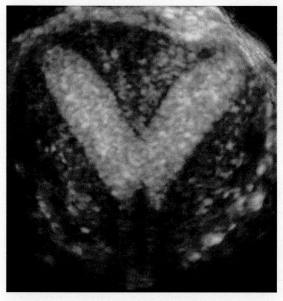

Figure 48.10   Congenital uterine anomalies - septate uterus.

but it is not found to be predictive of pregnancy if the endometrium attains at least 2.5 ml (117,118). It was found that endometrial and sub-endometrial vascularity was comparable for patients with thin and normal endometrium but was significantly lower for patients with low volume endometrium when compared with those with normal volume endometrium. Mercé et al. (114) concluded that 3D ultrasound and power Doppler angiography is a useful examination to assess endometrial receptivity in IVF/ICSI and endometrial transfer cycles. Doppler in 2D has not been shown to benefit for fertility at this time in studies with large numbers.

Several studies have suggested that a premature secretory endometrial pattern is introduced by an advanced progesterone rise, and this premature conversion has an adverse effect on PRs. The reason that no-triple-line endometrial pattern is observed prior to ovulation in some women is not known and cannot be explained by higher progesterone levels. In the study for Ng et al. (119) three patients with calcifications in the uterus and two with fluid in the endometrial cavity on the day of hCG did not conceive. These are poor prognosticating factors in the success of IVF and freezing all the embryos until an evaluation of the uterine cavity may be recommended.

ULTRASOUND OF THE FALLOPIAN TUBES

Fallopian Tube Patency

Normal fallopian tubes are usually not visualized by ultrasound. Evaluating tubal patency is a crucial step in the work up for infertility and making a diagnosis of hydrosalpinx is important prior to IVF. Tubal occlusion is seen in approximately 20% of women with infertility (120). The traditional gold standard for tubal evaluation is laparoscopy with chromopertubation (121) or HSG, and both have advantages and disadvantages.

Richman et al. were the first to describe in 1984 the use of transabdominal ultrasound for the diagnosis of tubal patency with saline contrast (122). After transcervical installation of saline, the cul-de-sac was evaluated for the appearance of free fluid. If free fluid was visualized then it was concluded that at least one of the tubes were patent. Since the development of this first technique, significant advances have been made in both ultrasound technology, including the advent of transvaginal sonography and the three-dimensional volume sonography. Furthermore, new techniques such as contrast enhancement have increased the ability to ultrasonographically visualize the fallopian tubes (123).

For infertility patients, tubal patency may be determined during SHG by using the following methods: During the preliminary ultrasound, the posterior cul-de-sac and pelvis should be evaluated for the presence of free fluid. If none is present before injection of fluid and it is present after fluid injection, then one can state that at least one tube is patent. Additionally, contrast material or a small amount of air injected with the fluid may be used with concurrent real-time sonographic imaging of

the cornua, adnexa, and cul-de-sac to assess tubal patency with recent studies showing good correlation with HSG.

The ultrasonographic evaluation of tubal patency is referred to as hysterosalpingo contrast sonography (HyCoSy). HyCoSy can be performed using air mixed with saline or Galactose-based microbubbles solution, Echovist 200 (124). HyCoSy is usually performed by injecting a small amount of contrast agent into the uterus via an intracervical balloon catheter. During the instillation process a TVS is performed to assess for tubal flow of contrast material and/or accumulation of contrast material in the pouch of Douglas (125).

There are numerous advantages to HyCoSy. HyCoSy allows for the evaluation of both the fallopian tubes and the uterus. If intrauterine pathology is detected it is relatively easy to differentiate between uterine polyps and myomas (126). HyCoSy is fairly well tolerated by patients and can usually be performed in less than 20 minutes (127). Several studies have shown that for the diagnosis of tubal patency, HyCoSy is comparable to X-ray HSG (128–130). In addition, numerous authors have found that results obtained with HyCoSy agree with the results obtained with laparoscopic chromopertubation in approximately 75% to 88.7% of the time (131–134). These findings along with the availability of positive contrast agents have lead to the increased use of HyCoSy in Europe. However, Echovist is not registered in the United States.

Agitated saline is used in lieu of commercially manufactured contrast material in the United States (Fig. 48.11). Agitated saline is produced by placing 19 cc of saline and 1 cc of air in a 20 mL syringe. The syringe is then vigorously shaken and the mixture is injected into the uterus using a balloon catheter (131). Care should be taken with this technique to insure the air alone is not accidentally injected into the uterus. A multicenter study (n = 24 women; 47 tubes) with Fem Ject Saline-Air Device

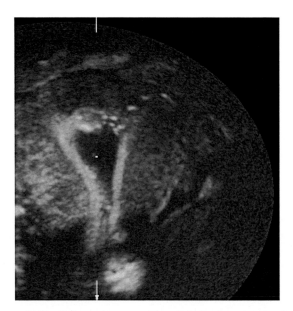

Figure 48.11   Saline sonogram with agitated saline showing tubal patency.

was attached to the FemVue Catheter and a continuous sterile saline-air train was delivered to each tube during sonographic observation (135). Sonographic criteria for tubal patency were bubbles entering the fallopian tube without production of a hydrosalpinx or exit of bubbles into the peritoneal cavity. The results showed that tubal patency was confirmed in 89% of the tubes.

While HyCoSy can be a useful screening tool, there are several factors that decrease its utility. The fallopian tubes often follow a tortuous course and it may be difficult to follow the passage of contrast through the entire length of the fallopian tube. In addition, it is almost impossible to obtain an entire view of the fallopian tube on one 2D ultrasound image and it is difficult to image the distal ends of the tubes, if there are no hydrosalpinges. Therefore, 2D HyCoSy requires significant skill on the part of the ultrasonographer. There is also a significant learning curve associated with 2D HyCoSy (136). If positive contrast media is used, it can be challenging to differentiate the echogenicity of the contrast material from the surrounding bowel. Therefore, the visualization of true spill from the fimbriated end of the fallopian tube remains difficult. Moreover, tubal pathology such as mucosal folds or salpingitis isthmica nodosa cannot be evaluated using HyCoSy. Nevertheless, HyCoSy is an excellent tool for the assessment of tubal patency when performed by an experienced sonographer, and in many centers, especially in Europe, it serves as the first test for the evaluation of tubal patency.

Doppler and 3D Ultrasound

The use of color Doppler with 2D HyCoSy has been shown to increase the ability to diagnose true tubal occlusion and help differentiate between the contrast material that has spilled out of the tube and the surrounding bowel. The accuracy color Doppler mapping for tubal patency compared to HSG and laparoscopy was with sensitivity of 76% with a specificity of 81% and a PPV and NPV of 66% and 89%, respectively (137). This technique was never incorporated in the routine evaluation of the infertile women.

The ability of 3D ultrasound to depict entire volumes of tissue makes it ideal for HyCoSy. Using 3D ultrasound, a volume of the entire fallopian tube can be obtained. The volume can then be manipulated and the tube can be followed throughout its entire length. In addition, 3D color power Doppler can be used to depict the flow of contrast material through the entire length of the fallopian tube (138). 3D HyCoSy with color power Doppler has been shown to increase the ability to depict free spillage of contrast material from the fimbrial end of the fallopian tube. One study demonstrated that free spill of contrast material was seen 91% of the time with 3D HyCoSy and only 46% of the time with 2D HyCoSy (139). In addition 3D-HyCoSy with color power Doppler seems to be accurate as it was found to agree with laparoscopy with chromopertubation 99% of the time.

The region of interest is selected by placing the 3D ultrasound box over the parametrium. Then the probe is held in place as the contrast is instilled into the uterus and tubes. The ultrasound machine automatically sweeps the predefined area of interest and acquires all the images. As a result, 3D HyCoSy is less operator dependent, easier to perform, and has less of a learning curve than 2D HyCoSy. Moreover, 2D HyCoSy can only be evaluated in real time (unless the examination is taped). On the other hand, 3D HyCoSy can be evaluated anytime by simply reviewing the saved volumes. Consequently, the volumes can be reinterpreted, if necessary, to evaluate different angles or answer.

Hydrosalpinges and ART Outcomes

Hydrosalpinges decrease IVF PRs by 50% (140). A prophylactic salpingectomy or tubal ligation is recommended to improve PRs. Even hysteroscopic tubal occlusion had been suggested for some patients (141). If a hydrosalpinx appears during stimulation, ultrasound-guided aspiration of hydrosalpinges at oocyte collection can be an option. A randomized, blinded study showed that 30% of the fallopian tubes in the aspiration group re-accumulated by 14 days after the aspiration. (142). This study implies that the window of opportunity may be present at oocyte aspiration, but not significantly earlier and even then, there may be re-accumulation by the transfer. Aboulghar et al. (143) reported that aspiration one month prior to retrieval did not improve pregnancy rates. If a hydrosalpinx develops during stimulation, an alternative option is to freeze all embryos and perform a salpingectomy later.

ULTRASOUND-GUIDED IVF PROCEDURES: OOCYTE RETRIEVAL AND EMBRYO TRANSFER

Laparoscopy was the first technique used for oocyte retrieval. The ultrasound-guided follicular aspiration was first described in the early 1980s by a Danish group, Lenz and Lauritsen, using abdominal ultrasound (144). TVS-guided oocyte retrieval is the current standard of care since the late 1980s and is associated with very few complications. It is usually performed under sedation with a 17-gauge needle. This size needle is optimal as it is thick enough to avoid deviating from the puncturing line and not too narrow to avoid harming the oocyte-cumulus complex. Thinner needles and lower pressure should be used for the in-vitro maturation technique of aspiration of immature eggs and smaller follicles. The tip of the needle is echogenic and can be visualized at all times and is aligned with the ultrasound beam. Care should be made to avoid blood vessels, bowel, or bladder, especially the internal iliac vein and artery. The current standard of care for oocyte retrieval is transvaginal aspiration under ultrasound guidance and there are no RCTs comparing the techniques of transabdominal versus transvaginal approaches. Flushing of follicles has not been shown to make a difference in oocyte yield, is known to take more time, and should not be routinely performed.

ET is a critical step in ART and can be performed with or without ultrasound guidance. However, recent

Cochrane reviews demonstrated a significant difference between "ultrasound-guided" and "clinical touch" methods (145–149). The ultrasound-guided ET significantly improved clinical PR (OR 1.49, CI 1.29–1.72, p < 0.00001). There were no statistical differences for ectopic pregnancy, miscarriage, or multiple gestation rates. Ultrasound guidance of the transfer catheter resulted in higher PRs in all but one of the studies identified; this difference was significant in five of the eight studies. The one study, which did not show any difference, varied from the others in several ways. First, a single operator performed all of the procedures – an overall benefit of ultrasound guidance among multiple practitioners does not rule out the possibility of no difference for individuals. Second, there were two unplanned interim analyses involving the investigators rather than a separate statistical or data and safety monitoring board, a process which is somewhat unorthodox for clinical trials. The Cochrane review (148) also compared the incidence of retained embryos for ultrasound versus clinical touch (3.2–10%). In one study the catheter touched the top of the uterus in 35% of the transfers and the reduction of retained embryos occurred by ultrasound guidance with mid-uterine ET. Retained embryos lead to an increased risk of blood on the catheter. Blood on the catheter decreased PR by 3.2–10%. The majority of programs are using ultrasound guidance and our experience has shown improvement.

The advantages of ultrasound guidance are that the physician can avoid touching the fundus with the catheter and can reduce the incidence of difficult transfers by allowing the direction of the catheter along the contour of the cavity and make sure the embryos are placed properly. Several transfer catheters with echogenic tips have been produced, which make it easier to visualize the placement, but without significant increase in pregnancy rates (Fig. 48.12). A few studies on comparing 2D versus 3D ultrasound guidance (150,151) show a possible advantage of 3D in monitoring catheter placement but this is not commonly used.

ULTRASOUND FOR THE DIAGNOSIS AND TREATMENT OF ART COMPLICATIONS AND OUTCOME

Ultrasound for the Diagnosis and Treatment of Ovarian Hyperstimulation Syndrome (OHSS)

OHSS is a serious iatrogenic condition that arises in women undergoing ovulation induction with fertility medication, and occurs during the luteal phase of the ovulatory cycle after hCG trigger, peaking usually three to seven days later or during early pregnancy. The incidence of severe OHSS ranges from 0.5% to 5% with increased risks in women with PCOS, thin, young women and women using long luteal agonist protocols with high E2 levels (152–157). Preventing OHSS is crucial in ART treatment and is described in another chapter. It is characterized by vascular endothelial growth factor (vEGF) overexpression, ovarian enlargement, and pelvic discomfort. In more severe cases, abdominal distention, nausea and vomiting, and ascites also may occur. In the most severe cases, third spacing of fluid can be accompanied by hemoconcentration, ascites, and pleural effusions. Patients may develop oliguria, tachypnea, and blood clots. The ovaries can grow to more than 5–10 cm in diameter, predisposing them to torsion. Acute pelvic pain in these patients can result from rapid enlargement of a follicle, stretching of the ovarian capsule, hemorrhage into or rupture of a follicle, or ovarian torsion. Sonographic findings in patients with OHSS include markedly enlarged multicystic ovaries (Fig. 48.13). Doppler evaluation may be performed in symptomatic patients to help assess for torsion, although the presence of blood flow does not exclude the diagnosis. Drainage of the ascites for improvement of symptoms is done in either the abdominal or the vaginal approach under ultrasound guidance. In contrast to the conservative approach of hospitalizing all patients with severe OHSS, early intervention with outpatient repeated transvaginal paracentesis under ultrasound guidance has become the standard of care in many leading U.S. centers (152–154). Besides studies showing the lack of significant complications with this approach, recent cost-benefit analysis confirmed the significant savings obtained (155).

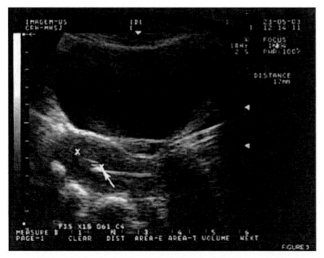

Figure 48.12 Embryo transfer under ultrasound guidance.

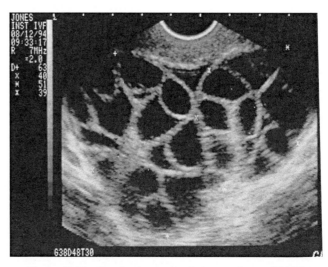

Figure 48.13 Ovarian hyperstimulation syndrome (OHSS).

Early Pregnancy Complications and Multiple Pregnancies

Ultrasound is essential for the diagnosis of clinical pregnancy, for position of the pregnancy, and the number of sacs and fetuses. The emphasis has been on reducing the number of embryos transferred to reduce the risk of multiple births. In a normally developing pregnancy a blastocyst implants by 23 days of menstrual age. The first structure identified by TVS is the gestational sac (GS) as a spherical, fluid-filled cavity surrounded by an echogenic rim. A double decidual sac sign is a reliable signal of an intrauterine pregnancy (IUP). There is a correlation between sac size and hCG level and gestational age, but there is variability and it is helpful to monitor sequential sonographic milestones. The first structure inside the GS is the yolk sac (YS), followed by the embryo. The YS is a spherical, echogenic ring-like formation with a sonolucent center and its presence confirms a true IUP with 100% PPV. The confirmation of YS is necessary by 37–40 menstrual days or six weeks gestation. Fetal heart rate is visible from six weeks and two days gestation based on embryo transfer dates. It is seen as a linear echodensity next to the yolk sac. The embryo or fetal pole is measured along its long axis and is called a "crown-rump length" (CRL). Sub-chorionic hematoma, a fluid collection between the chorionic membrane and deciduas, is very common with ART pregnancies and is associated with abnormal placentation and higher risks of miscarriages. Discriminatory values should be used with caution as they are a range rather than a specific cutoff value (158).

When compared to natural conception, ART increases the chance of multiple gestations. Twinning should be classified as either monozygotic (a single ovum divides into two embryos) or dizygotic (two separate ova) and dichorionic/diamniotic, mono-chorionic/diamniotic or mono-chorionic/mono-amniotic. The type of twinning affects the chances of maternal and fetal morbidity and mortality.

A pregnancy of unknown location may require serial ultrasounds. Ultrasonography is the primary diagnostic modality for ectopic pregnancy. The visualization of a fluid-filled sac outside the uterine cavity that contains an embryo or a yolk sac is definitive for ectopic pregnancy. An adnexal mass with the "tubal ring" is also highly predictive. The presence of an IUP in an asymptomatic patient conceived by IVF should not exclude the diagnosis of a concurrent ectopic called heterotrophic pregnancy, so evaluation of the adnexa should be done in all circumstances. In the case of heterotrophic pregnancy, methotrexate injection is unacceptable and laparoscopic surgery or aspiration of the gestational sac and injection with potassium chloride under transvaginal sonography can be done.

CONCLUSIONS

Modern ART and infertility treatments cannot be imagined today without ultrasound imaging, and advances in both fields have occurred simultaneously. Using advanced ultrasound techniques for the assessment of uterine cavity and tubal patency should eliminate almost completely women fear of pain from such procedures (159). The use of 3D visualization of the pelvic structures is the most striking advancement in the use of ultrasound in ART. As costs decrease, accessibility will increase. The future will bring smaller and portable ultrasounds for increased access in underserved communities as well as more standardization and increased automation with savings in time and possible improved outcomes. The reduction in OHSS and in multiple gestations is one of the key concerns of ART treatments and with recent advances in IVF as well as ultrasound guidance, success of mild stimulation and an elective single embryo transfer can be maximized. With modern ultrasound usage, we can see better, and do ART better.

REFERENCES

1. Jokubkiene L, Sladkevicius P, Rovas L, Valentin L. Assessment of change in volume and vascularity of the ovaries during the normal menstrual cycle using three-dimensional power Doppler ultrasound. Hum Reprod 2006; 21: 2661–8.
2. Durfee SM, Frates MC. Sonographic spectrum of the corpus luteum in early pregnancy: gray-scale, color, and pulsed Doppler appearance. J Clin Ultrasound 1999; 27: 55–9.
3. Faddy MJ, Gosden RG, Gougeon A, Richardson SJ, Nelson JF. Accelerated disappearance of ovarian follicles in mid-life: implications for forecasting menopause. Hum Reprod 1992; 7: 1342–6.
4. Muasher SJ, Oehninger S, Simonetti S, et al. The value of basal and/or stimulated serum gonadotropin levels in prediction of stimulation response and in vitro fertilization outcome. Fertil Steril 1988; 50: 298–307.
5. Broekmans FJ, Knauff EA, Te Velde ER, Macklon NS, Fausser BC. Female reproductive ageing: current knowledge and future trends. Trends Endocrinol Metab 2007; 18: 58–65.
6. Broekmans FJ, Kwee J, Hendriks DJ, Mol BW, Lambalk CB. A systematic review of tests predicting ovarian reserve and IVF outcome. Hum Reprod Update 2006; 12: 685–718.
7. Jayaprakasan K, Hilwah N, Kendall NR, et al. Does 3D ultrasound offer any advantage in the pretreatment assessment of ovarian reserve and prediction of outcome after assisted reproduction treatment? Hum Reprod 2007; 22: 1932–41.
8. Broer SL, Mol BWJ, Hendriks D, Broekmans FJM. The role of antimullerian hormone in prediction of outcome after IVF: comparison with the antral follicle count. Fertil Steril 2009; 705–14.
9. Hazout A, Bouchard P, Seifer DB, Aussage P, Junca AM. Cohen-Bacrie P. Serum antimüllerian hormone/müllerian-inhibiting substance appears to be a more discriminatory marker of assisted reproductive technology outcome than follicle-stimulating hormone, inhibin B, or estradiol. Fertil Steril 2004; 82: 1323–9.
10. Johnson NP, Bagrie EM, Coomarasamy A, et al. Ovarian reserve tests for predicting fertility outcomes for assisted reproductive technology: the International Systematic Collaboration of Ovarian Reserve Evaluation protocol for a systematic review of ovarian reserve test accuracy. BJOG 2006; 113: 1472–80.
11. Riggs RM, Duran EH, Baker MW, et al. Assessment of ovarian reserve with antimullerian hormone: a

comparison of the predictive value of antimullerian hormone, follicle-stimulating hormone, inhibin B and age. Am J Obstet Gynecol 2008; 199: 202e1–8.

12. Hendriks DI, Mol BW, Bancsi LF, Te Velde ER, Broekmans FI. Antral follicle count in the prediction of poor ovarian reserve and IVF outcome after in vitro fertilization: a meta-analysis and comparison with basal FSH level. Fertil Steril 2005; 83: 291–310.

13. Hansen KR, Hodnett GM, Knowlton N, Craig LB. Correlation of ovarian reserve tests with histologically determined primordial follicle number. Fertil Steril 2011; 95: 855–64.

14. Jayaprakasan K, Al-Hasie H, Jayaprakasan R, et al. The three-dimensional ultrasonographic ovarian vascularity of women developing poor ovarian response during assisted reproduction treatment and its predictive value. Fertil Steril 2009; 92: 1862–9.

15. Firouzabadi RD, Sekhavat L, Javedani M. The effect of ovarian cyst aspiration on IVF treatment with GnRH. Arch Gynecol Obstet 2010; 281: 545–9.

16. Okaro E, Condous G, Khalid A, et al. The use of ultrasound-based 'soft markers' for the prediction of pelvic pathology in women with chronic pelvic pain, can we reduce the need for laparoscopy? BJOG 2006; 113: 251–6.

17. Raine-Fenning N, Jayaprakasan K, Deb S. Three –dimensional ultrasonographic characteristics of endometriomata. Ultrasound obstet Gynecol 2008; 31: 718–24.

18. Asch E, Levine D. Variations in appearance of endometriomas. J Ultrasound Med 26: 993–1002.

19. Kumfer MC, Schwimer SR, Lebovic J. Transvaginal sonographic appearance of endometriomas: spectrum of findings. J Ultrasound Med 1992; 11: 129–33.

20. Somigliana E, Vercellini P, Viganó P, Ragni G, Crosignani PG. Should endometriomas be treated before IVF-ICSI cycles? Hum Reprod Update 2006; 12: 57–64.

21. Garcia-Velasco JA, Somigliana E. Management of endometriomas in women requiring IVF: to touch or not to touch. Hum Reprod 2009; 24: 496–501.

22. Aboulghar MA, Mansour RT, Serour GI, Al-Inany HG, Aboulghar MM. The outcome of in vitro fertilization in advanced endometriosis with previous surgery: a case-controlled study. Am J Obstet Gynecol 2003; 188: 371–5.

23. Suzuki T, Izumi S, Matsubayashi H, et al. Impact of ovarian endometrioma on oocytes and pregnancy outcome in in vitro fertilization. Fertil Steril 2005; 83: 908–13.

24. Gupta S, Agarwal A, Agarwal R, Loret de Mola JR. Impact of ovarian endometrioma on assisted reproduction outcomes. Reprod Biomed Online 2006; 13: 349–60.

25. Matalliotakis IM, Cakmak H, Mahutte N, et al. Women with advanced-stage endometriosis and previous surgery respond less well to gonadotropin stimulation, but have similar IVF implantation and delivery rates compared with women with tubal factor infertility. Fertil Steril 2007; 88: 1568–72.

26. Barnhart K, Dunsmoor-Su R, Coutifaris C. Effect of endometriosis on in vitro fertilization. Fertil Steril 2002; 77: 1148–55.

27. Huang HY, Lee CL, Lai YM, et al. The outcome of in vitro fertilization and embryo transfer therapy in women with endometriosis failing to conceive after laparoscopic conservative surgery. J Am Ass Gynecol Laparosc 1997; 4: 299–303.

28. Yazbeck C, Madelenat P, Sifer C, Hazout A, Poncelet C. Ovarian endometriomas: Effect of laparoscopic cystectomy on ovarian response in IVF-ET cycles. Gynecol Obstet Fertil 2006; 34: 808–12.

29. Duru NK, Dede M, Acikel CH, et al. Outcome of in vitro fertilization and ovarian response after endometrioma stripping at laparoscopy and laparotomy. J Reprod Med 2007; 52: 805–9.

30. Canis M, Pouly JL, Tamburro S, et al. Ovarian response during IVF-embryo transfer cycles after laparoscopic ovarian cystectomy for endometriotic cysts of >3 cm in diameter. Hum Reprod 2001; 16: 2583–6.

31. Donnez J, Wyns C, Nisolle M. Does ovarian surgery for endometriomas impair the ovarian response to gonadotropin? Fertil Steril 2001; 76: 662–5.

32. Wong BC, Gillman N, Oehninger S, Gibbons WE, Stadtmauer LA. Results of in-vitro fertilization on patients with endometriomas - is surgical removal beneficial? Am J Obstet and Gynecol 2004; 191: 597–607.

33. Caspi B, Weissman A, Zalel Y, et al. Ovarian stimulation and in vitro fertilization in women with mature cystic teratomas. Obstet Gynecol 1998; 92: 979–81.

34. Amer SA, Li TC, Bygrave C, et al. An evaluation of the inter-observer and intra-observer variability of the ultrasound diagnosis of polycystic ovaries. Hum Reprod 2002; 17: 1616–22.

35. Ardaens Y, Robert Y, Lemaitre L, Fossati P, Dewailly D. Polycystic ovarian disease: contribution of vaginal endosonography and reassessment of ultrasonic diagnosis. Fertil Steril 1991; 55: 1062–8.

36. Adams J, Polson DW, Franks S. Prevalence of polycystic ovaries in women with anovulation and idiopathic hirsutism. BMJ 1986; 293: 355–9.

37. McDougall MJ, Tan SL, Jacobs HS. IVF and the ovarian hyperstimulation syndrome. Hum Reprod 1992; 5: 597–600.

38. Fox R, Corrigan E, Thomas PE, Hull MG. The diagnosis of polycystic ovaries in women with oligo-amenorrhea: predictive power of endocrine tests. Clin Endocrinol Oxf 1991; 34: 127–31.

39. Farquhar CM, Birdsall M, Manning P, Mitchell JM. Transabdominal versus transvaginal ultrasound in the diagnosis of polycystic ovaries in a population of randomly selected women. Ultrasound Obstet Gynecol 1994; 4: 54–9.

40. Kyei-Mensah A, Moconochie N, Zaidi J, et al. Transvaginal three-dimensional ultrasound: reproducibility of ovarian and endometrial volume measurements. Fertil Steril 1996; 5: 718–22.

41. Faure N, Prat X, Bastide A, Lemay A. Assessment of ovaries by magnetic resonance imaging in patients presenting with polycystic ovarian syndrome. Hum Reprod 1989; 4: 468–72.

42. Balen AH, Laven JS, Tan SL, Dewailly D. Ultrasound assessment of the polycystic ovary: international consensus definitions. Hum Reprod Update 2003; 9: 505–14.

43. Jonard S, Robert Y, Cortet-Rudelli C, et al. Ultrasound examination of polycystic ovaries: is it worth counting the follicles? Hum Reprod 2003; 18: 598–603.

44. Rotterdam ESHRE/ASRM-Sponsored PCOS Consensus Workshop Group. Revised 2003 consensus on

diagnostic criteria and long-term health risks related to polycystic ovary syndrome. Fertil Steril 2004; 81: 19–25.

45. Rotterdam ESHRE/ASRM-Sponsored PCOS Consensus Workshop Group. Revised 2003 consensus on diagnostic criteria and long-term health risks related to polycystic ovary syndrome. Hum Reprod 2004; 19: 41–7.

46. Hackeloer BJ, Robinson HP. Ultrasound examination of the growing ovarian follicle and of the corpus luteum during the normal physiologie menstrual cycle. Geburtshilfe Frauenheilkd 1978; 38: 163–8.

47. Ata B, Tulandi T. Ultrasound automated volume calculation in reproduction and in pregnancy. Fertil Steril 2011; 95: 2163–70.

48. Deb S, Jayaprakasan K, Campbell BK, et al. The intraobserver and interobserver reliability of automated antral follicle counts made using three-dimensional ultrasound and Sono-AVC. Ultrasound Obstet Gynecol 2009; 33: 477–83.

49. Raine-Fenning N, Jayaprakasan K, Clewes J, et al. SonoAVC: a novel method of automatic volume calculation. Ultrasound Obstet Gynecol 2008; 31: 691–696.

50. Raine-Fenning N, Jayaprakasan K, Chamberlain S, et al. Automated measurements of follicle diameter: a chance to standardize? Fertil Steril 2009; 91: 1469–72.

51. Deutch TD, Joergner I, Matson DO, et al. Automated assessment of ovarian follicles using a novel three-dimensional ultrasound software. Fertil Steril 2009; 92: 1562–8.

52. Rousian M, Verwoerd-Dikkeboom CM, Koning AH, et al. Early pregnancy volume measurements: validation of ultrasound techniques and new perspectives. BJOG 2009; 116: 278–85.

53. Lamazou F, Arbo E, Salama S, et al. Reliability of automated volumetric measurement of multiple growing follicles in controlled ovarian hyperstimulation. Fertil Steril 2010; 94: 2172–21767.

54. Raine-Fenning N, Jayaprakasan K, Chamberlain S, et al. Automated measurements of follicle diameter: a chance to standardize? Fertil Steril 2009; 91: 1469–72.

55. Salama S, Arbo E, Lamazou F, et al. Reproducibility and reliability of automated volumetric measurement of single preovulatory follicles using SonoAVC. Fertil Steril 2010; 93: 2069–73.

56. Raine-Fenning N, Deb S, Jayaprakasan K, et al. Timing of oocyte maturation and egg collection during controlled ovarian stimulation: a randomized controlled trial evaluating manual and automated measurements of follicle diameter. Fertil Steril 2010; 94: 184–8.

57. Rodriguez-Fuentes A, Hernandez J, Garcia-Guzman R, et al. Prospective evaluation of automated follicle monitoring in 58 in vitro fertilization cycles: follicular volume as a new indicator of oocyte maturity. Fertil Steril 2010; 93: 616–20.

58. Casper RF. It's time to pay attention to the endometrium. Fertil Steril 2011; 96: 519–21.

59. Paulson RJ. Hormonal induction of endometrial receptivity. Fertil Steril 2011; 96: 530–5.

60. Chien LW, Au HK, Xiao J, Tzeng CR. Fluid accumulation within the uterine cavity reduces pregnancy rates in women undergoing IVF. Hum Reprod 2002; 17: 351–6.

61. Friedler S, Schenker JG, Herman A, et al. The role of ultrasonography in the evaluation of endometrial receptivity following assisted reproductive treatments: a critical review. Hum Reprod Update 1996; 2: 23–35.

62. Killick SR. Ultrasound and the receptivity of the endometrium. Reprod BioMed Online 2007; 15: 63–7.

63. Randolph JF Jr, Ying YK, Maier DB, et al. Comparison of real-time ultrasonography, hysterosalpingography, and laparoscopy/hysteroscopy in the evaluation of uterine abnormalities and tubal patency. Fertil Steril 1986; 46: 828–32.

64. Spieldoch RL, Winter TC, Schouweiler C, et al. Optimal catheter placement during sonohysterography: a randomized controlled trial comparing cervical to uterine placement. Obstet Gynecol 2008; 111: 15–21.

65. Parsons AK, Lense JJ. Sonohysterography for endometrial abnormalities: preliminary results. 1993; 21: 87–95.

66. Kim AH, McKay H, Keltz MD, et al. Sonohysterographic screening before in vitro fertilization. Fertil Steril 1998; 69: 841–4.

67. Cullinan JA, Fleischer AC, Kepple DM, Arnold AL. Sonohysterography: a technique for endometrial evaluation. Radiographics 1995; 15: 501–14; discussion: 15–6.

68. de Kroon CD, de Bock GH, Dieben SW, Jansen FW. Saline contrast hysterosonography in abnormal uterine bleeding: a systematic review and meta-analysis. BJOG 2003; 110: 938–47.

69. Brown SE, Coddington CC, Schnorr J, et al. Evaluation of outpatient hysteroscopy, saline infusion hysterosonography, and hysterosalpingography in infertile women: a prospective, randomized study. Fertil Steril 2000; 74: 1029–34.

70. Soares SR, Barbosa dos Reiss, Camargos AF. Diagnostic accuracy of sonohysterography, transvaginal sonography, and hysterosalpingography in patients with uterine cavity diseases. Fertil Steril 2000; 73: 406–11.

71. Tur-Kaspa I, Gal M, Hartman M, Hartman J, Hartman A. A Prospective Evaluation of Uterine Abnormalities by Saline Infusion Sonohysterography (SIS) in 1009 Women with Infertility or Abnormal Uterine Bleeding. Fertil Steril 2006; 86: 1731–5.

72. American College of Obstetricians and Gynecologists. ACOG technology assessment in obstetrics and gynecology no. 5: sonohysterography. Obstet Gynecol 2008; 112: 1467–9.

73. Werbrouck E, Veldman J, Lut J, et al. Detection of endometrial pathology using saline infusion sonography versus gel instillation sonography: a prospective cohort study. Fertil Steril 2011; 95: 285–8.

74. de Ziegler D. Contrast ultrasound: a simple-to-use phase-shifting medium offers saline infusion sonography–like images. Fertil Steril 2009; 92: 369–7.

75. Shah AA, Walmer DK. A feasibility study to evaluate pelvic peritoneal anatomy with a saline intraperitoneal sonogram (SIPS). Fertil Steril 2010; 94: 2766–8.

76. Rock JA, Schlaff WD. The obstetric consequences of uterovaginal anomalies. Fertil Steril 1985; 43: 681.

77. Ludmir J, Samuels P, Brooks S. Pregnancy outcome of patients with uncorrected uterine anomalies managed in a high risk obstetric setting. Obstet Gynecol 1990; 75: 906.

78. Valdes C, Malini S, Malinak LR. Ultrasound Evaluation of female genital tract anomalies: a review of 64 cases. Am J Obstet Gynecol 1984; 149: 285–90.

79. Salim R, Lee C, Davies A, et al. A comparative study of three-dimensional saline infusion sonohysterography and diagnostic hysteroscopy for the classification of submucosal fibroids. Hum Reprod 2005; 20: 253–7.

80. Sheth S, Macura K. Sonography of the uterine myometrium: myomas and beyond. Ultrasound Clin 2007; 2: 267–95.

81. Mayer DP, Shipilov V. Ultrasonography and magnetic resonance imaging of uterine fibroids. Obstet Gynecol Clin North Am 1995; 22: 667–725.

82. Stadtmauer L, Armstrong M, Oehninger S. Efficacy of 40 cases of robot-assisted laparoscopic myomectomy in women with symptomatic fibroids and infertility [abstract]. J Min Invasive Surg 2010.

83. Van Voorhis BJ. Ultrasound assessment of the uterus and fallopian tube in infertile women. Semin Reprod Med 2008; 26: 232–40.

84. Pritts EA, Parker WH, Olive DL. Fibroids and infertility: an updated systematic review of the evidence. Fertil Steril 2011; 91: 1215–23.

85. Pritts EA. Fibroids and infertility: a systemic review of the evidence. Obstet Gynecol Survey 2001; 56: 483–91.

86. Dueholm M. Transvaginal ultrasound for diagnosis of adenomyosis: a review. Best Prac Res Clin Obstet Gynaecol 2006; 20: 569–82.

87. Afifi K, Anand S, Nallapeta S, Gelbaya TA. Management of endometrial polyps in subfertile women: a systematic review. Euro J Obst Gynecol Reprod Biol 2010; 151: 117–21.

88. Perez-Medina T, Bajo-Arenas J, Salazar F, et al. Endometrial polyps and their implication in the pregnancy rates of patients undergoing intrauterine insemination: a prospective, randomized study. Hum Reprod 2005; 20: 1632–5.

89. Starnatellos I, Apostolides A, Stamatopoulos P Bontis J. Pregnancy rates after hysteroscopic polypectomy depending on the size or number of the polyps. Arch Gynecol Obstet 2008; 277: 395–9.

90. Madani T, Ghaffari F, Kiani K, Hosseini F. Hysteroscopic polypectomy without cycle cancellation in IVF cycles. Reprod Biomed Online 2009; 18: 412–15.

91. Afifi K, Anand S, Nallapeta S, Gelbaya TA. Management of endometrial polyps in subfertile women: a systematic review. Euro J Obst Gynecol Reprod Biol 2010; 151: 117–21.

92. Valdes C, Malini S, Malinak LR. Ultrasound Evaluation of female genital tract anomalies: a review of 64 cases. Am J Obstet Gynecol 1984; 149: 285–90.

93. Balen FG, Allen CH, Gardener JE, Siddle NC, Lees WR. 3D reconstruction of ultrasound images of the uterine cavity. B J Radiol 1993; 66: 588.

94. Jurkovic D, Geipel A, Gruboeck K, Taylor A, Nicolaides KH. Ultrasound screening for congenital uterine anomalies. Br J Obstet Gynaecol 1997; 104: 1320–1.

95. Jurkovic D. Three-dimensional ultrasound in gynecology: a critical evaluation. Ultrasound Obstet Gynecol 2002; 19: 109–17.

96. Raga F, Bonilla Musoles F, Blanes J, Osborne N. Congenital uterine anomalies: diagnostic accuracy of three-dimensional ultrasound. Fertil Steril 1996; 65: 523–8.

97. Meng-Hsing W, Chao-Chin H, Ko-En H. Detection of congenital mullerian duct anomalies using three-dimensional ultrasound. J Clin Ultrasound 1997; 25: 487–92.

98. Kupesic S, Kurjak A, Septate U. Detection and prediction of obstetrical complications by different forms of ultrasonography. J Ultrasound Med 1998; 17: 631–6.

99. Smith B, Proter R, Ahuja K, Craft I. Ultrasonic assessment of endometrial changes in stimulated cycles in an in vitro fertilization and embryo transfer program. J IVF ET 1984; 1: 233–8.

100. Frielder S, Schenker JG, Herman A, et al. The role of ultrasonography in the evaluation of endometrial receptivity following assisted reproductive treatments: a critical review. Hum Reprod Update 1996; 2: 323–36.

101. Weckstein LN, Jacobson A, Galen D, Hampton K, Hammel J. Low-dose aspirin for oocyte donation recipients with a thin endometrium: Prospective, randomized study. Fertil Steril 1997; 68: 927–30.

102. Yao-Yuan H, Horng-Der T, Chi-Chen C, Hui-Yu L, Ching-Lun C. Low-Dose Aspirin for Infertile Women with Thin Endometrium Receiving Intrauterine Insemination: A Prospective, Randomized Study. J Assist Reprod Genet 2000; 17: 174–7.

103. Sher G, Fisch JD. Effect of vaginal sildenafil on the outcome of in vitro fertilization (IVF) after multiple IVF failures attributed to poor endometrial development. Fertil Steril 2002; 78: 1073–6.

104. Oliveira JB, Baruffi RL, Mauri AL, et al. Endometrial ultrasonography as a predictor of pregnancy in an in-vitro fertilization program after ovarian stimulation and gonadotropin-releasing hormone and gonadotropins. Hum Reprod 1997; 12: 2515–18.

105. Gonen Y, Casper RF. Prediction of implantation by the sonographic appearance of the endometrium during controlled ovarian stimulation for in vitro fertilization (IVF). J In vitro Fert Embryo Transfer 1990; 7: 146–52.

106. Gonen Y, Casper RF, Jacobson W, Blankier J. Endometrial thickness and growth during ovarian stimulation: A possible predictor of implantation in in vitro fertilization. Fertil Steril 1989; 52: 446–50.

107. Shapiro H, Cowell C, Casper RF. The use of vaginal ultrasound for monitoring endometrial preparation in a donor oocyte program. Fertil Steril 1993; 59: 1055–8.

108. Coulam CB, Bustillo M, Soenksen DM, Britten S. Ultrasonographic predictors of implantation after assisted reproduction. Fertil Steril 1994; 62: 1004–10.

109. Sundström P. Establishment of a successful pregnancy following in-vitro fertilization with an endometrial thickness of on more than 4 mm. Hum Reprod 1998; 13: 1550–2.

110. Al-Ghamdi A, Coskun S, Al-Hassan S, Al-Rejjal R, Awartani K. The correlation between endometrial thickness and outcome of in vitro fertilization and embryo transfer (IVF-ET) outcome. Reprod Biol Endocrinol 2008; 6: 37.

111. Weissman A, Gotlieb L, Casper RF. The detrimental effect of increased endometrial thickness on implantation and pregnancy rates and outcome in an in vitro fertilization program. Fertil Steril 1999; 71: 147–9.

112. Dickey RP, Olar TT, Taylor SN, Curole DN, Matulich EM. Relationship of endometrial thickness and pattern to fecundity in ovulation. induction

cycles: effect of clomiphene citrate alone and with human menopausal gonadotropin. Fertil Steril 1993; 59: 756–60.

113. Zohav E, Orvieto R, Anteby EY, et al. Low endometrial volume may predict early pregnancy loss in women undergoing in vitro fertilization. J Assist Reprod Genet 2007; 24: 259–61.

114. Mercé LT, Barco MJ, Bau S, Troyano J. Are endometrial parameters by three-dimensional ultrasound and power Doppler angiography related to in vitro fertilization/embryo transfer outcome? Fertil Steril 2008; 89: 111–17.

115. Aga R, Bonilla-Musoles F, Casan EM, et al. Assessment of endometrial volume by three-dimensional ultrasound prior to embryo transfer: clues to endometrial receptivity. Hum Reprod 1999; 14: 2851–4.

116. Tur-Kaspa I, Segal S, Zohav E. The ART of imaging: three dimensional (3D) ultrasound and ART. In: Revelli A, Tur-Kaspa I, Holte JG, Massobrio M, eds. Biotechnology of Human Reproduction. New York: The Parthenon Publishing Group, 2003: 363–73.

117. Ng EHY, Chan CCW, Tang OS, et al. The role of endometrial and subendometrial vascularity measured by three-dimensional power Doppler ultrasound in the prediction of pregnancy during frozen-thawed embryo transfer cycles. Hum Reprod 2006; 21: 1612–17.

118. Yaman C, Ebner T, Spmmergrubber M, et al. Role of three dimensional ultrsonographic measurement of endometrium volume as a predictor of pregnancy outcome in an IVF-ET program. A preliminary study. Fertil Steril 2000; 74: 797–801.

119. Ng EHY, Chan CCW, Tang OS Yeung WSB, Pak CH. Changes in endometrial and subendometrial blood flow in IVF. RBM Online 2009; 18: 269–75.

120. Hoffman L, Chan K, Smith B, Okolo S. The value of saline salpingosonography as a surrogate test of tubal patency in low-resource settings. Int J Fertil Womens Med 2005; 50: 135–9.

121. Radic V, Canic T, Valetic J, Duic Z. Advantages and disadvantages of hysterosonosalpingography in the assessment of the reproductive status of uterine cavity and fallopian tubes. Eur J Radiol 2005; 53: 268–73.

122. Richman TS, Viscomi GN, deCherney A, Polan ML, Alcebo LO. Fallopian tubal patency assessed by ultrasound following fluid injection. Work in progress. Radiology 1984; 152: 507–10.

123. Sankpal RS, Confino E, Matzel A, Cohen LS. Investigation of the uterine cavity and fallopian tubes using three-dimensional saline sonohysterosalpingography. Int J Gynaecol Obstet 2001; 73: 125–9.

124. Balen FG, Allen CM, Siddle NC, Lees WR. Ultrasound contrast hysterosalpingography–evaluation as an outpatient procedure. Br J Radiol 1993; 66: 592–9.

125. Dietrich M, Suren A, Hinney B, Osmers R, Kuhn W. Evaluation of tubal patency by hysterocontrast sonography (HyCoSy, Echovist) and its correlation with laparoscopic findings. J Clin Ultrasound 1996; 24: 523–7.

126. Randolph JF Jr, Ying YK, Maier DB, Schmidt CL, Riddick DH. Comparison of real-time ultrasonography, hysterosalpingography, and laparoscopy/hysteroscopy in the evaluation of uterine abnormalities and tubal patency. Fertil Steril 1986; 46: 828–32.

127. Tufekci EC, Girit S, Bayirli E, Durmusoglu F, Yalti S. Evaluation of tubal patency by transvaginal sonosalpingography. Fertil Steril 1992; 57: 336–40.

128. Heikkinen H, Tekay A, Volpi E, Martikainen H, Jouppila P. Transvaginal salpingosonography for the assessment of tubal patency in infertile women: methodological and clinical experiences. Fertil Steril 1995; 64: 293–8.

129. Deichert U, Schleif R, van de Sandt M, Juhnke I. Transvaginal hysterosalpingo-contrast-sonography (Hy-Co-Sy) compared with conventional tubal diagnostics. Hum Reprod 1989; 4: 418–24.

130. Schlief R, Deichert U. Hysterosalpingo-contrast sonography of the uterus and fallopian tubes: results of a clinical trial of a new contrast medium in 120 patients. Radiology 1991; 178: 213–15.

131. Chenia F, Hofmeyr GJ, Moolla S, Oratis P. Sonographic hydrotubation using agitated saline: a new technique for improving fallopian tube visualization. Br J Radiol 1997; 70: 833–6.

132. Stern J, Peters AJ, Coulam CB. Color Doppler ultrasonography assessment of tubal patency: a comparison study with traditional techniques. Fertil Steril 1992; 58: 897–900.

133. Hamilton JA, Larson AJ, Lower AM, Hasnain S, Grudzinskas JG. Evaluation of the performance of hysterosalpingo contrast sonography in 500 consecutive, unselected, infertile women. Hum Reprod 1998; 13: 1519–26.

134. Kiyokawa K, Masuda H, Fuyuki T, et al. Three-dimensional hysterosalpingo-contrast sonography (3D-HyCoSy) as an outpatient procedure to assess infertile women: a pilot study. Ultrasound Obstet Gynecol 2000; 16: 648–54.

135. Parsons AK, Shapiro DB, Miller CE, et al. FemView™ Sono Tubal Evalution System for selective sonohysterosalpingography in the office setting. Fertil Steril 2010; 94(Suppl): S78.

136. Kalogirou D, Antoniou G, Botsis D, et al. Is color Doppler necessary in the evaluation of tubal patency by hysterosalpingo-contrast sonography. Clin Exp Obstet Gynecol 1997; 24: 101–3.

137. Sladkevicius P, Ojha K, Campbell S, Nargund G. Three-dimensional power Doppler imaging in the assessment of Fallopian tube patency. Ultrasound Obstet Gynecol 2000; 16: 644–7.

138. Chan CC, Ng EH, Tang OS, Chan KK, Ho PC. Comparison of three-dimensional hysterosalpingo-contrast-sonography and diagnostic laparoscopy with chromopertubation in the assessment of tubal patency for the investigation of subfertility. Acta Obstet Gynecol Scand 2005; 84: 909–13.

139. Kupesic S, Plavsic B. 2D and 3D hysterosalpingo-contrast-sonography in the assessment of uterine cavity and tubal patency. Eur J Obster Gynecol Reprod Biol 2007; 133: 64–9.

140. Johnson NP, Mak W, Sowter MC. Surgical treatment for tubal disease in women due to undergo in Vitro fertilization. Cochrane Database Syst Rev 2004; 3: CD002125.

141. Mijatovic V, Dreyer K, Emanuel MH, Schats R, Hompes PG. Essure® hydrosalpinx occlusion prior to IVF-ET as an alternative to laparoscopic salpingectomy. Eur J Obstet Gynecol Reprod Biol 2012; 161: 42–5.

142. Hammadieh N, Coomarasamy A, Ola Bk, et al. Ultrasound-guided hydrosalpinx aspiration during oocyte collection improves pregnancy outcome in

IVF:a randomized controlled trial. Hum Reprod 2008; 23: 1113–17.

143. Aboulghar MA, Mansour RT, Serour GI. Spontaneous intrauterine pregnancy following salpingectomy for a unilateral hydrosalpinx. Hum Reprod 2002; 17: 1099–100.

144. Lenz S, Lauritsen JG. Ultrasonically guided percutaneous aspiration of human follicles under local anesthesia: a new method of collecting oocytes for in vitro fertilization. Fertil Steril 1982; 38: 673–7.

145. Mirkin S, Jones EL, Mayer JF, et al. Impact of transabdominal ultrasound guidance on performance and outcome of transcervical uterine embryo transfer. JARG 2003; 20: 318–22.

146. Anderson RE, Nugent NL, Gregg AT, Nunn SL, Behr BR. Transvaginal ultrasound-guided embryo transfer improves outcome in patients with previous failed in vitro fertilization. Fertil Steril 2002; 77: 769–75.

147. Buckett WM. A meta-analysis of ultrasound-guided versus clinical touch embryo transfer. Fertil Steril 2003; 80: 1037–41.

148. Brown JA, Buckingham K, Abou-Setta A, Buckett W. Ultrasound versus 'clinical touch' for catheter guidance during embryo transfer in women. Cochrane Database Syst Rev 2007; 1: CD006107.

149. Derks RS, Farquhar C, Mol BW, Buckingham K, Heineman JM. Techniques for preparation prior to embryo transfer. Cochrane Database Syst Rev 2009; 7: CD007682.

150. Gergely RZ, DeUgarte CM, Danzer H, et al. Three dimensional/four dimensional ultrasound-guided embryo transfer using the maximal implantation potential point. Fertil Steril 2005; 84: 500–3.

151. Letterie GS. Three-dimensional ultrasound-guided embryo transfer: a preliminary study. Am J Obstet Gynecol 2005; 192: 1983–8.

152. Shrivastav P, Nadkarni P, Craft I. Day care management of severe ovarian hyperstimulation syndrome avoids hospitalization and morbidity. Hum Reprod 1994; 9: 812–14.

153. Fluker MR, Copeland JE, Yuzpe AA. An ounce of prevention: outpatient management of the ovarian hyperstimulation syndrome. Fertil Steril 2000; 73: 821–4.

154. Smith LP, Hacker MR, Alper MM. Patients with severe ovarian hyperstimulation syndrome can be managed safely with aggressive outpatient transvaginal paracentesis. Fertil Steril 2009; 92: 1953–9.

155. Csokmay JM, Yauger BJ, Henne MB, et al. Cost analysis model of outpatient management of ovarian hyperstimulation syndrome. with paracentesis: "Tap early and often" versus hospitalization. Fertil Steril 2010; 93: 167–73.

156. Aboulghar MA, Mansour RT. Ovarian hyperstimulation syndrome: classifications and critical analysis of preventive measures. Hum Reprod Update 2003; 9: 275–89.

157. Delvigne A, Dubois M, Batteu B, et al. The ovarian hyperstimulation in in-vitro fertilization: a Belgian multicenter study.II. Multiple discriminant analytes for risk prediction. Hum Reprod 1993; 8: 1361–6.

158. Jauniaux E, Johns J, Burton GJ. The role of ultrasound imaging in diagnosing and investigating early pregnancy failure. Ultrasound Obstet Gynecol 2005; 25: 613–24.

159. Tur-Kaspa I. Fear no pain: uterine cavity and tubal patency assessment tests should be pain free. Ultrasound Obstet Gynecol 2012; 39: 247–251.

49

Sperm recovery techniques: Clinical aspects

Herman Tournaye and Patricio Donoso

In the past 10–20 years, several changes have taken place in clinical andrology. Gradually, empirical treatments have been replaced by techniques of assisted reproduction – intrauterine insemination (IUI), in vitro fertilization (IVF), and intracytoplasmic sperm injection (ICSI). Especially the introduction of ICSI in 1992 (1,2) has completely changed the clinical approach toward male infertility by offering a novel opportunity for parenthood to azoospermic men. A single spermatozoon can be injected into an oocyte and result in normal fertilization, embryonic development, and implantation. Not only ejaculated spermatozoa can be used; epididymal or testicular spermatozoa too can be used for ICSI. Testicular spermatozoa can be retrieved in some patients with nonobstructive azoospermia (NOA) because of the persistence of isolated foci of active spermatogenesis. The first pregnancies using epididymal and testicular spermatozoa in men with obstructive azoospermia (OA) and NOA were published in 1993 and 1995, respectively (3–6). Surgical retrieval of spermatozoa for ICSI has currently become a routine technique in clinical andrology. Several techniques are available to retrieve epididymal or testicular spermatozoa. Although there is no real method of choice, some guidelines may be given to make the best choice for a specific clinical setting. ICSI has also reinforced the role of nonsurgical techniques to retrieve sperm in men suffering from anejaculation.

AZOOSPERMIA: WHAT'S IN A NAME?

Most azoospermic patients suffer from primary testicular failure (60%) (7,8). Because these patients do not show any clinical sign of obstruction, often they are referred to as patients with NOA. However, in a few cases, azoospermia without any obstruction is the result of a hypogonadotropic hypogonadism, i.e., a lack of adequate hormonal stimulation to support spermatogenesis. These patients have an early maturation arrest in spermatogenesis. Treatment with follicle-stimulating hormone (FSH) and human chorionic gonadotropin (hCG) will restore spermatogenesis and they do not, in the first instance, need assisted reproduction (9). In general, these patients are not referred to as suffering from NOA.

Azoospermic patients with primary testicular failure show a germ cell aplasia (Sertoli-cell-only), maturation arrest, or tubular sclerosis and atrophy at their testicular histopathology.

Germ cell aplasia may be iatrogenic as it may result from irradiation or chemotherapy, or may be congenital: Because of a genetic disorder such as Klinefelter's syndrome or a deletion on the long arm of the Y-chromosome. In many cases, however, the cause of germ cell aplasia remains unknown. Many patients with primary testicular dysfunction, however, are now assumed to have testicular dysgenesis syndrome, a congenital developmental disorder causing spermatogenic failure, maldescence of the testis (cryptorchidism), and eventually hypospadias in more severe forms of the spectrum of this disorder (10). They also have a higher risk to develop testis carcinoma (10).

Men with NOA may also show maturation arrest at testicular histology. Maturation arrest may be caused by viral orchitis, irradiation, and/or chemotherapy and Yq-deletions. Other causes include systemic illness or exposure to gonadotoxins, but here too, idiopathic maturation arrest is most common. Again, testicular dysgenesis syndrome may explain some of these cases.

Fewer men with NOA will show tubular sclerosis and atrophy at their testicular histology. This may be the result of testicular torsion, vascular injury, or infection, but is also a common finding in Klinefelter's patients.

Many studies on assisted reproductive techniques (ART) with testicular spermatozoa or spermatids use inadequate definitions often based on the absence or presence of clinical signs of obstruction. According to WHO guidelines for ART, the diagnosis of "nonobstructive azoospermia" should be made according to the histopathological findings, rather than on the basis of clinical indicators such as FSH levels or testicular size (11,12). Testicular failure is found in a third of normogonadotropic azoospermic men with normally sized testes; on the other hand, small testicular size or elevated FSH does not preclude normal spermatogenesis. Whenever testicular biopsy shows a normal spermatogenesis or a mild hypospermatogenesis, an obstruction of the excretory ducts is present. In a substantial subgroup of these men, however, no clinical signs of obstruction will be present. An accurate distinction between these two types of azoospermia is particularly relevant since spermatozoa can be retrieved in almost all patients with OA and mild hypospermatogenesis but only in up to 50% of unselected patients with NOA when no preliminary selection of patients on the basis of histopathology has been performed (13).

DOES MY PATIENT NEED SURGICAL SPERM RECOVERY?

In patients with obstructive azoospermia, fertility can be restored by surgical correction, i.e., vasoepididymostomy, vasovasostomy or perurethral prostatic resection. When surgery has failed or is not indicated, e.g., patients with congenital bilateral absence of the vas deferens (CBAVD), surgical sperm recovery procedures are indicated.

Most methods described for surgical sperm recovery are simple techniques. However, in some patients with azoospermia even these simple techniques are not indicated. When after appropriate analysis the diagnosis of azoospermia is made, an appropriate clinical workup is necessary to define the exact cause of the azoospermia and to define the best treatment option. If azoospermia is the result of a primary testicular failure caused by hormonal deficiency, such as hypogonadotropic hypogonadism, then hormone replacement therapy must be proposed.

Often the diagnosis of azoospermia is made without centrifugating the semen. Centrifugation at 1800xG for at least five minutes may reveal spermatozoa in the pellet, which may be used for ICSI.(14) In a series of 49 patients with NOA it was shown that spermatozoa could be recovered from the ejaculate for ICSI in 35% of patients.(14) In cases of NOA it may therefore be worthwhile to perform centrifugation of an ejaculate before embarking on a surgical recovery procedure to retrieve spermatozoa. Only when no spermatozoa are found in the pellet after centrifugation or when only immotile nonviable spermatozoa are found, is surgical sperm recovery indicated to avoid performing ICSI with spermatozoa with DNA damage.

ANEJACULATION DOES NOT EQUAL AZOOSPERMIA

Surgical sperm retrieval methods have been proposed as a means for obtaining spermatozoa for assisted reproduction in men with anejaculation, i.e., the absence of antegrade or retrograde ejaculation. However, given the efficiency of assisted ejaculation in these men, surgical methods are only to be considered when penile vibrostimulation or electroejaculation (EEJ) has failed.

Epididymal or testicular sperm recovery procedures are often proposed to anejaculatory patients because no penile vibrostimulation or EEJ is available.(15) When these first-line recovery methods are unavailable, it is even preferable to refer anejaculatory patients, especially patients with spinal cord injuries, to specialized services where assisted ejaculation can be performed and semen can be cryopreserved. Vibro- or electrostimulation are noninvasive techniques that may be performed without

any anesthesia in paraplegic men. EEJ is now a well-established method for procuring sperm from spinal cord–injured men.(16) Since scrotal hematoma may take a long time to heal in such men, surgical sperm retrieval techniques are indicated only where these noninvasive techniques fail to produce an ejaculate that may be used for ICSI. Even here, vas deferens aspiration may be preferable because of its low risk of iatrogenic obstruction (17,18). The ejaculates, even when oligoasthenoteratozoospermic, can be cryopreserved for later use. Testicular sperm retrieval must be considered only where primary testicular failure is present in an anejaculatory patient or when techniques of assisted ejaculation have failed to produce an ejaculate that can be used for ICSI.

It is preferable in such patients to refrain from epididymal sperm aspiration techniques because of their higher risk of iatrogenic epididymal obstruction.

Psychogenic anejaculation may be encountered unexpectedly during treatments with ARTs, for example, ICSI. Here too, assisted ejaculation may be useful, rather than surgical methods, to obtain spermatozoa if treatment by sildenafil citrate has failed to overcome the problem of an acute erectile dysfunction (19). In some anejaculatory patients, prostatic massage, a simple alternative noninvasive method, can be used to obtain spermatozoa for ART (20).

EJACULATION INDUCED BY PENILE VIBRATORY STIMULATION AND ELECTROEJACULATION

Anejaculation may be psychogenic or may result from spinal cord injury or retroperitoneal lymph node dissection. These causes represent almost 95% of etiologies. Diabetic neuropathy, multiple sclerosis, Parkinson's disease, and aortoiliac, colorectal, or bladder neck surgery are less encountered causes. Occasionally anejaculation is drug associated: antidepressive, antipsychotic, and antihypertensive medication may induce anejaculation.

Given the low efficiency of medical treatments for inducing ejaculation in anejaculatory men, penile vibratory stimulation (PVS, Fig. 49.1 and protocol 2 in appendix) and EEJ (Fig. 49.2 and protocol 1 in appendix) may be considered as the first-line treatments for anejaculation (21).

PVS is recommended because it is still less invasive and less expensive than EEJ and because semen quality has been reported to be much better after PVS than after EEJ, especially in men with spinal cord injury (22). PVS will restore ejaculation in half of the anejaculatory patients when a high amplitude (at least 2.5 mm amplitude) is used (22). The amplitude of a vibrator is the distance over which the vibrating part is moving up and down. The frequency of vibration should be around 100 Hertz.

Each patient scheduled for PVS should undergo a complete neurological and uroandrological examination. PVS needs an intact spinal cord up to the lumbosacral level. In spinal cord–injured men, PVS is less successful in case of lower cord lesions. When the patient has a transection at T6 or higher, an increase in blood pressure because of autonomic dysreflexia may occur during a PVS procedure. Close monitoring of the blood pressure is thus indicated. Whenever acute hypertension develops, 10 to 20 mg nifedipine should be administered sublingually. In spinal cord–injured patients with a history of autonomic dysreflexia, 10 mg nifedipine should be given preventively about 15 minutes before starting PVS.

The patient is instructed to drink 500 ml water containing 600 mg sodium bicarbonate on the morning of the procedure, to alkalinize the urine.

After emptying, the bladder is washed with a buffered sperm preparation medium. About 50 ml of this medium is left in the bladder. The vibrating part of the vibrator is placed on the posterior glans penis and frenulum. The position can be slowly changed to find a reactive trigger point. When no ejaculation is obtained within 10 minutes, the procedure should be discontinued. Although less frequent than with EEJ, retrograde ejaculation may occur during PVS. Flushing, goose skin, and spasms of the abdominal muscles and legs may indicate ejaculation. In general, spermatozoa can be obtained in approximately 55% of men, however, in spinal cord–injured men with lesions above T11, the retrieval rate will be reaching 88% (15).

High amplitude penile vibrostimulators have become affordable and therefore couples, infertile because of anejaculation, can use PVS at home for attempting pregnancy or to improve semen quality by regular ejaculation. Home-use PVS may be not indicated in spinal cord–injured men with lesions above T6 because of the risk of autonomic dysreflexia.

EEJ is the treatment of choice if PVS fails. EEJ is a technique initially introduced to obtain spermatozoa from endangered species. In the late eighties the technique was introduced successfully in the clinic too (23). Patients should receive the same workup and preparation as for PVS.

For EEJ, patients with no spinal cord injury or patients with incomplete spinal cord lesions need general anesthesia. Sympathicolytic agents should not be used during anesthesia. As for PVS, spinal cord–injured men with lesions at T6 or above must be closely monitored for autonomic dysreflexia and pretreated whenever indicated (see above).

The patient is placed in lateral decubitus. Because of the risk of rectal burning by the heating of the EEJ probe, it is recommended to use equipment with a built-in temperature sensor.

The EEJ probe is introduced in the rectum with the electrodes facing the prostate. In spinal cord–injured men it may be recommended to perform a preliminary digital rectal examination and an anoscopy. A repetitive electrical stimulus of maximum five volts is applied for about two to fours seconds each stimulus. When no ejaculation, either antegrade or retrograde, is obtained, the voltage may be gradually increased. With a few exceptions, ejaculation occurs at voltages lower than 20 V. During the stimulation an assistant collects the antegrade fraction. After the procedure, anoscopy is repeated to ensure no rectal lesions occurred. The patient is placed in lithotomy position and the bladder is washed to recover any retrograde fraction. In 80–95% of patients spermatozoa can be recovered (23,15). According to the quality of the specimen obtained, either IUI or assisted reproduction by ICSI can be performed. In anejaculatory men, and especially in spinal cord–injured men, both semen quality and sperm function may be deteriorated because of accumulation of reactive oxygen species, denervation, male accessory gland infection, postinfectious partial obstruction, or postinfectious primary testicular failure. Therefore, the introduction of ICSI has dramatically changed the perspective of patients suffering from anejaculation (15,24). Indeed, in combination with ICSI, spinal cord–injured men can father their genetically own children even when sperm quality is

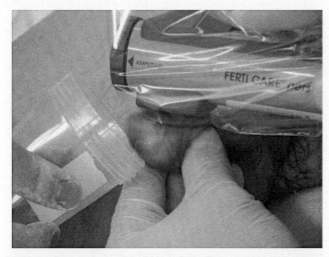

Figure 49.1 Penile vibrostimulation (PVS). The vibrator should deliver a high peak-to-peak amplitude of at least 2.5 mm and a frequency of about 100 Hz. The vibrating part is applied to the posterior glans penis and frenulum.

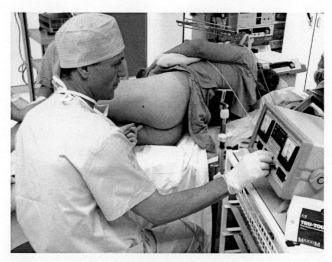

Figure 49.2 Electroejaculation (EEJ). The patient is in lateral decubitus and a stimulatory probe is gently introduced in the rectum with the electrodes facing the prostate.

limited. In a small retrospective study prostatic massage, EEJ and testicular sperm extraction were compared in terms of establishing a pregnancy by ICSI. It was shown that the three techniques resulted in similar pregnancy and live birth rates (20). A recent study showed that spinal cord–injured men who had ICSI with sperm obtained either after PVS or after EEJ had similar take-home baby rates compared to non–spinal cord–injured men (25).

METHODS FOR RETRIEVING EPIDIDYMAL OR TESTICULAR SPERMATOZOA

If no motile spermatozoa can be obtained from the ejaculate after centrifugation, a sperm retrieval procedure has

to be performed. At present, different methods are available to obtain spermatozoa from the vas deferens, epididymis, or testicular mass (26,27). The method of choice will depend on the type of azoospermia (nonobstructive or obstructive), surgical skills, and the techniques available in a given setting. If sperm has to be retrieved on an outpatient basis, techniques should be adopted that are compatible with local or locoregional anesthesia.

In case of obstructive azoospermia, several methods are available. Figure 49.3 shows the algorithm currently used in our setting. If OA is expected but either the cause or the site of the obstruction is unknown, a scrotal exploration must be performed. A scrotal exploration may not

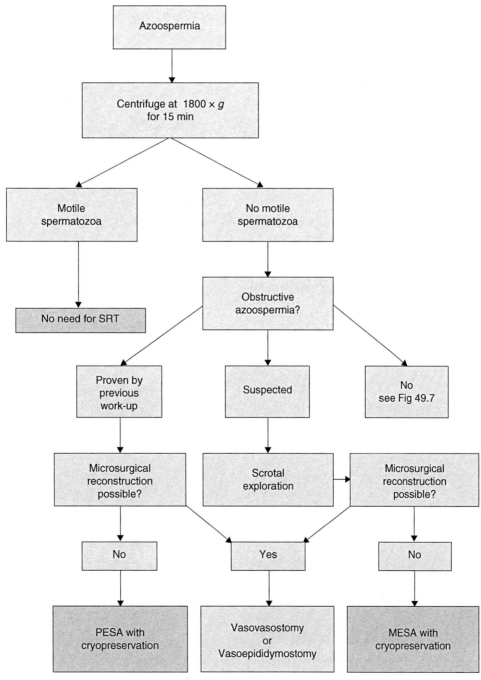

Figure 49.3 Treatment algorithm for patients with obstructive azoospermia.

only reveal the cause and site of the obstruction and confirm the diagnosis of OA, but also provide the possibility of performing reconstructive surgery. If no surgical correction is feasible then microsurgical epididymal sperm aspiration (MESA) is performed during scrotal exploration (Fig. 49.4, protocol 7 in appendix). The epididymal spermatozoa that are obtained can be easily cryopreserved for later use (28). A meta-analysis showed no difference in fertilization (RR 1.02; 95% CI: 0.96–1.08) or implantation rates (RR 1.17; 95% CI: 0.86–1.59) after fresh versus frozen–thawed epididymal sperm were used. Although a significantly higher clinical pregnancy rate was observed (RR 1.20; 95% CI: 1.0 –1.42), no difference was found on ongoing pregnancy rates (RR 1.17; 95% CI: 0.96–1.43) (29).

If, however, previous workup has shown that microsurgical reconstruction is not possible, then a percutaneous epididymal sperm aspiration (PESA) may be performed (Fig. 49.5, protocol 3 in appendix). Although there have been some concerns that this blind method may cause epididymal damage and fibrosis (30), this issue is not important where reconstruction is not possible. When epididymal sperms are to be used for ICSI, spermatozoa with low levels of DNA damage, i.e., motile spermatozoa should be obtained so as to not jeopardize the success rate of the coincident ICSI cycle. Epididymal sperm may accumulate DNA damage over time: The study by Ramos reported that about 17% of sperm obtained from the epididymis by MESA shows DNA damage as demonstrated by TUNEL assay. The DNA damage rate was only 9.3% for sperm recovered from the testis and 6.2% in fresh sperm obtained from sperm donors (31). Consequently, in men with very high levels of DNA-damage in their ejaculated spermatozoa, the use of testicular spermatozoa has been advocated in a small study to improve the pregnancy rate after ICSI (32). However, in the motile fractions of the surgically recovered sperm the final DNA damage rate was less than 1% and comparable to that of donor

sperm (31). When motile spermatozoa are used, no differences in fertilization rate or live birth rates are observed between epididymal and testicular sperm used for ICSI (29). After PESA, epididymal sperm may not always be obtained (33). In this case, testicular spermatozoa may be obtained either by fine needle aspiration (FNA) or by open testicular biopsy of the testis (Fig. 49.6, protocols 4 and 5 in appendix). Both methods are similar in terms of outcome in obstructive azoospermia, but the numbers of sperm obtained after open biopsies are much higher (34). For this reason, open testicular biopsy may be preferred whenever cryopreservation is desired. Alternative methods of testicular aspiration have been described yielding higher numbers of spermatozoa (27,35). In these aspiration techniques, either needles with a larger diameter are used to obtain tissue cylinders or seminiferous tubules

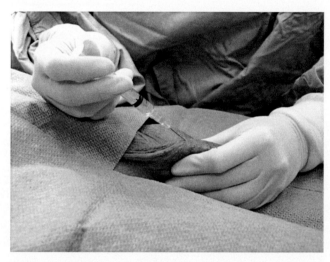

Figure 49.5 Percutaneous epididymal sperm aspiration (PESA). The epididymis is palpated and epididymal fluid is collected after a blind percutaneous puncture with a 19- or 21-gauge needle.

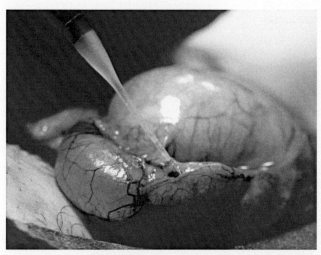

Figure 49.4 Microsurgical epididymal sperm aspiration (MESA). The epididymis is exposed and epididymal fluid is collected after a micro-incision in a dilated tubule.

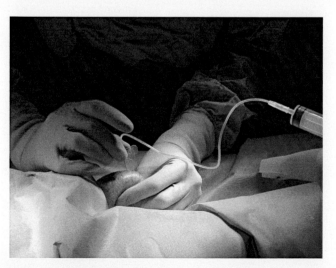

Figure 49.6 Fine needle aspiration (FNA) of the testis. Using a fine 21-gauge butterfly needle filled with a minute volume of sperm preparation medium, the testicular mass is punctured and an aspirate is collected.

are pulled out by microforceps after puncturing or incising the tunica albuginea (27). Compared with FNA, these alternative methods are less patient friendly and need local or locoregional anesthesia. Sometimes they even need to be combined with a small incision by a sharp blade in the scrotal skin. Their main advantage is that cryopreservation is easy and efficient because of the higher numbers of sperm obtained.

Figure 49.7 shows our current algorithm for patients with NOA willing to undergo ICSI treatment.

For men with OA who need surgical sperm recovery for ICSI, both patient and surgeon can decide which approach will be used. When cryopreservation is required, then PESA is the method of choice, followed by testicular sperm extraction (TESE) whenever the former approach fails. These two techniques yield high numbers of sperm necessary for cryopreservation.

When a minimally invasive technique is preferred ("no-scar technique"), then again PESA is the first-choice method, followed by FNA whenever PESA fails to recover motile spermatozoa.

TESE is the most frequently used technique for NOA with an average sperm retrieval rate of 50% (36). Although testicular volume and serum FSH are routinely assessed in azoospermic men, these parameters are often used in studies on prediction either as a stand-alone parameter or in combination with other parameters. Unfortunately, their predictive power remains limited and is subject to the heterogeneity of the population of NOA patients studied (37–39). There exists still some

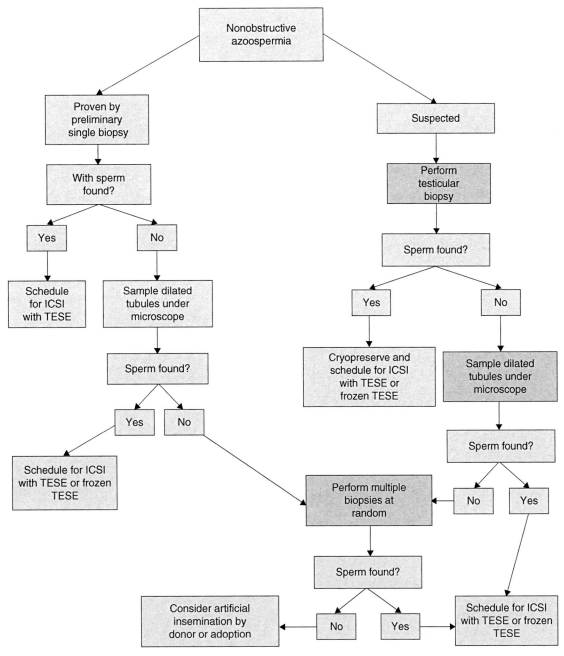

Figures 49.7 Treatment algorithm for patients with nonobstructive azoospermia (NOA).

controversy about the role of non-routine assessments such as inhibin-B for predicting successful sperm recovery (40–42). Recently other non-routine markers, e.g., leptin have been described as being useful in the prediction of sperm recovery after TESE (43). Since a single parameter has a low sensitivity for predicting TESE outcome, predictive models have been published combining several parameters (44). At present it remains unclear whether such predictive models can be applied on a population of patients, other than the one they originated from and thus prediction may remain difficult due to patient heterogeneity.

Apart from clinical parameters and hormonal tests, Doppler ultrasound of the testis has also been proposed as a method to predict successful recovery. But even such testicular vascularity assessment has a sensitivity not exceeding 50% (45). Doppler ultrasound has also been proposed as a tool to recover better quality spermatozoa for ICSI (46).

The most invasive predictive strategy for TESE is "testicular mapping." According to an organized pattern, the testis is aspirated in different locations, followed by a cytological examination of these aspirates. But again the sensitivity of this approach is below 50%. A mapping study by Bettella et al. reported that in 70 patients with a Sertoli-cell-only pattern at testicular histology, mapping did not show any sperm; however, during a subsequent TESE procedure sperm were recovered in 41% of these patients (47). To date, only histopathology has shown to predict the probability of finding sperm with both acceptable sensitivity and specificity in subgroups of NOA men (37,48).

Although only applicable to few patients, Yq deletion testing provides a robust prediction: testicular sperm recovery fails in all azoospermic men with azoospermia factor B (AZFb) deletions (49).

The appropriate number of biopsies to be taken remains controversial. Although single testicular biopsy was initially proposed as the best approach (50–52), it is currently recommended to take multiple samples from different sites of the testis since a patchy distribution of spermatogenesis throughout the testis has been identified (36,53,54). In addition it has been shown that TESE with multiple biopsies results in a higher chance of finding motile spermatozoa (54). Care should be taken to take small tissue pieces and to avoid cutting the arterioles as much as possible to avoid causing too much devascularization. The retrieval of testicular spermatozoa in difficult cases may be facilitated by using erythrocyte lysing buffer (55) and enzymatic digestion (56). Some authors have reported that scheduling the testicular recovery procedure one day before the ovum pickup (57) or the use of motility stimulants, for example, pentoxifylline, may facilitate the retrieval of motile spermatozoa from the tissue (58).

Concerning the best location to perform the biopsy two small descriptive studies reported opposite results (54,59). Hauser et al. (54) found no differences on the sperm retrieval rate between three testicular sites, whereas Witt et al. concluded that the midline portion of the testis enabled the highest retrieval rate (59).

If a preliminary single biopsy has shown focal spermatogenesis with testicular spermatozoa present, the patient and his partner may be scheduled for ICSI with a TESE performed on the day of the oocyte retrieval. Vernaeve et al. reported to find sperm in up to 78% of patients in whom TESE had been previously successful (60).

When a preliminary single biopsy has not shown the presence of testicular spermatozoa, a testicular sperm retrieval procedure with multiple biopsies has to be proposed (Figure 49.8, protocol 6 in appendix) (61,54). Because multiple biopsies may lead to extensive fibrosis and devascularization, (62,63) multiple excisional biopsies may be taken under an operating microscope at x40 and x80 magnification (64). This microsurgical approach aims at sampling the more distended tubules to limit testicular damage. Micro-TESE may be very useful in cases of Sertoli-cell-only syndrome with focal spermatogenesis, but is useless in cases with maturation arrest where there is generally no difference in diameter of tubules with or without focal spermatogenesis. The technique is more time consuming than conventional TESE and may be influenced by the surgeon's case volume (65).

When sperm are found, the samples may be frozen for later use with ICSI. If only a few spermatozoa are available or only a tiny amount of tissue is cryopreserved with only a few spermatozoa observed, we ask the patient to be on standby on the day of oocyte retrieval in case no spermatozoa can be observed after thawing. In the study by Verheyen et al. the frozen–thawed suspensions could not be used in 20 out of 97 cycles (20.6%) despite extensive search for motile sperm (66). However, a backup fresh retrieval was successfully carried out in 14 cycles. Donor semen backup should also be discussed prior to treatment (66).

A special subgroup of NOA is Klinefelter's syndrome patients accounting for 11% of men with azoospermia.

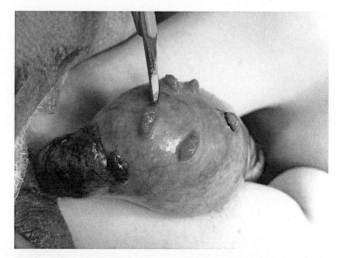

Figure 49.8 Multiple testicular sampling by open excisional testicular biopsy (TESE). Small tissue specimens are taken from the testicular mass while avoiding vascular injuries when incising the tunica albuginea.

Again, in half of these patients spermatozoa may be recovered for ICSI (range 16–60%) (67,68).

Pregnancies have been obtained after ICSI with testicular spermatozoa from 47, XXY non-mosaic Klinefelter's syndrome (67,69–71). Age represents an important parameter to predict sperm recovery in this group of patients as shown by Okada et al. with a cut-off value of 35 years (72). Preimplantation genetic diagnosis should be discussed because of the risk of aneuploidy in the embryos obtained in these patients (73–75). Staessen et al. (75) found that 46% of the embryos were chromosomally abnormal with a significant increase in sex and autosomal chromosome abnormalities.

Oncological patients are another subgroup. Patients undergoing a potentially sterilizing chemotherapy must bank their semen before starting any treatment. However, they may be azoospermic at the time of cancer diagnosis because of spermatogenic depression due to factors related to the malignancy. Yet these patients may be offered sperm recovery and banking before starting chemotherapy by vasal or epididymal sperm aspiration during orchiectomy (76) or testicular sperm extraction (onco-TESE) (77,78).

Whenever no semen was banked before starting for chemotherapy, patients with post-chemotherapy azoospermia may benefit from testicular sperm extraction too (79–82). Hsiao et al. (82) reported to have retrieved sperm in 37% of patients using Micro-TESE technique.

Less invasive methods have been proposed to obtain testicular spermatozoa from patients with NOA, i.e., testicular aspiration (TESA). The main advantages of this technique are simplicity, low cost, being minimally invasive, and that it produces less postoperative pain compared to TESE under local anesthesia (26). However, multiple prospective controlled studies have shown a lower recovery rate than with excisional biopsies (26,83–86). An additional disadvantage is that frequently there are no supernumerary spermatozoa to cryopreserve because of the limited number retrieved (26,83). Furthermore, in patients with a history of cryptorchidism, testicular aspiration is contraindicated. These patients have a higher risk of developing a testicular cancer from carcinoma in-situ cells and an excisional biopsy must therefore be performed to verify for carcinoma in-situ (87). TESA has also been used as a mapping technique prior to TESE aiming to identify the areas in which sperm are present (88,89), resulting in a high retrieval rate (95% of the cycles). However, as mentioned above, this approach has a low sensitivity (47). The main complications of testicular retrieval techniques are hematoma, fibrosis, and testicular atrophy. Microdissection TESE appears to be the safest technique regarding postoperative complications followed by TESA. Studies in animal models have however raised concerns on the possible long-term consequences of TESA because of an increased disturbance of the tubular architecture compared to TESE. Furthermore, the fact that conventional TESE performed by a skilled surgeon achieves high rates of sperm retrieval even after two or three repeated biopsies reinforces this strategy as a safe procedure (90,91).

A SUCCESSFUL TESTICULAR SPERM RECOVERY: WHAT'S NEXT?

In patients with normal spermatogenesis pregnancy rates after ICSI using testicular spermatozoa are comparable to those obtained after ICSI using epididymal spermatozoa (92). OA has a significantly higher fertilization (RR1.18; 95% CI 1.13–1.23) and clinical pregnancy rates (RR 1.36; 95% CI: 1.10 –1.69) compared to NOA (29). This meta-analysis did not include a large study published earlier reaching the same conclusion: lower fertilization, implantation, and pregnancy rates in NOA compared to OA (93). The reasons for these findings are unclear, but are possibly associated with meiosis defects in NOA (94). There was no difference in either implantation or miscarriage rates between these two groups. When fresh and frozen–thawed epididymal sperm cycles were compared, no significant difference was observed in fertilization or implantation rates; however, a significantly higher clinical pregnancy rate was reported for fresh cycles (RR 1.20; 95% CI: 1.0 –1.42) (29).

In azoospermic men with primary testicular failure, significant differences do exist between various reports mainly because of differences in patient selection, sample size of the study, and definition of NOA (11,35,95). Limited evidence is available concerning the influence of the sperm retrieval technique on the pregnancy rate.

Although it has been suggested that TESA results in higher implantation and pregnancy rates compared to TESE because of a lesser degree of spermatogenetic impairment in these patients (91), others found no significant difference on the fertilization, implantation, and clinical pregnancy rates between TESA and TESE (96).

Preimplantation genetic aneuploidy screening (PGS) has been proposed as a way to improve embryo selection in azoospermic men because of a higher frequency of aneuploid and mosaic embryos (97). PGS could be particularly important under the framework of a single embryo transfer policy, where a higher chance of selecting a chromosomally abnormal embryo was reported when morphological criteria had solely been used.(98). Nevertheless, extensive evidence from RCTs has shown a null effect of PGS in other indications such as advanced maternal age (99).

Few data are available about the pregnancy outcome and the neonatal data of children born after ICSI with testicular sperm in patients with NOA.(100,101) Although based on small sample sizes, these data have not shown any difference between pregnancies after the use of testicular sperm from nonobstructive azoospermic men compared to obstructive azoospermic men. A large study including the follow-up of 724 children born after ICSI using non-ejaculated sperm showed no significant differences on neonatal health, major anomalies, and chromosomal aberrations in comparison to the children born after ICSI with ejaculated(102).

Patients should thus be counseled that treating sterility because of NOA has many limitations: First, there are limitations in the chances to recover testicular spermatozoa and second, there are limitations in the outcome after ICSI itself.

APPENDICES

Protocol 1: Electroejaculation

Indication

Anejaculation refractory to penile vibrostimulation (see below)

Patient Preparation

In spinal cord–injured men a preliminary microbiological examination of the urine has to be performed. No rectal preparation (such as clysma)! Fluid intake should be restricted to 500 ml in the 12 hours preceding the procedure.

The patient has to empty the bladder before EEJ. In spinal cord–injured men with lesions at T6 or higher, monitoring of blood pressure is mandatory. Nifedipine 10 to 20 mg may be given for preventing autonomic dysreflexia related hypertension.

Patient wears a top only. He is placed at lithotomy position. Penal region cleansed with antiseptic solution (for example, HAC, Zeneca: Hospital antiseptic concentrate. Contains chlorhexidine).

The EEJ Procedure

The tip of a Nelaton bladder catheter is dipped into sterile liquid mineral oil as used in IVF. After instillation of 10 ml of sperm preparation medium into the urethra, the catheter is gently introduced into the bladder. The bladder is emptied and the urinary pH is measured. The bladder is then washed with 200 ml medium. After emptying, 50 ml of the medium is left in the bladder for collecting retrograde-ejaculated sperm. The patient is put into lateral decubitus. In spinal cord–injured men, an assistant should control leg spasm during the procedure.

Electrostimulation is performed using equipment with a built-in temperature sensor. After digital rectal examination and anoscopy, a standard probe is gently inserted into the rectum. Care is taken to orientate the electrodes anteriorly. Electrostimulations are repeated, each stimulation lasting for two to four seconds. Baseline voltage should be five volts and voltage can be increased or maintained according to the patient's reaction. In case of acute hypertension in patients with spinal cord lesions at T6 or higher, the procedure must be discontinued until blood pressure is again under control.

An assistant collects the antegrade fraction in a sterile container containing buffered sperm washing medium. The pendulous and bulbar urethra are continuously massaged by the assistant during the procedure. With the aid of a 1 ml syringe, ejaculated drops are flushed into the container. When no antegrade ejaculation is observed, indirect signs such as spasms of the lower abdominal muscles and legs and the appearance of goose bumps may indicate (retrograde) ejaculation. When ejaculation discontinues, the probe is removed and anoscopy is performed again to check for rectal lesions.

Then the patient is put again in lithotomy position. The bladder is re-catheterized and the emptied into a sterile container to collect any retrograde fraction. The bladder is flushed with 100 ml of medium until the flushing medium remains clear.

The collected fractions are transported to the andrology laboratory for identification of spermatozoa and further preparation. Centrifugation of the retrograde suspension may be necessary or open biopsy under local anesthesia should be performed.

Dressing After

Disposable underpants

Patient Care Post Operation

None

Requirements

- A runner
- Two assistants
- Seager Model 14 Electroejaculator (Dalzell Medical System, The Plains, VA, USA)
- Anoscope
- Manual manometer
- Nelaton catheter ch 14 (Cat.nr.110)
- Ph indicator strip (Merck, Germany)
- Mineral oil (Sigma)
- Cleaning solution (3.5% HAC)
- Syringe 50 cc (BS-50 ES Terumo)
- Syringe Norm-Ject Cook1 ml (K-ATS-1000)
- 100 ml Modified Earle's Balanced Salt Solution with HEPES, 0.4 Heparin Novo, and 2.25% Human Serum Albumin
- Gauze squares 10 × 10

Protocol 2: Penile Vibrostimulation

Indication

Anejaculation

Patient Preparation

As for EEJ

The PVS Procedure

Patient empties his bladder before PVS and the urinary pH is measured. Penile vibrostimulation is performed using high-amplitude equipment.

The antegrade fraction is collected into a sterile container containing buffered sperm washing medium. When no ejaculation occurs after five minutes, PVS is discontinued.

Then the patient is put again in lithotomy position. When no antegrade ejaculation is observed, but indirect signs are present (goose bumps, muscular spasms), the bladder is catheterized and emptied into a sterile container to collect any retrograde fraction (see above). The collected specimens are transported to the andrology laboratory for identification of spermatozoa and further preparation.

When PVS fails to induce ejaculation, EEJ has to be performed.

Patient Care Post Operation

None

Requirements

> FertiCare Personal vibrostimulator (Multicept ApS, Denmark)
> Manual sphygmomanometer
> Ph indicator strip (Merck, Germany)
> Cleaning solution (3.5% HAC)
> Syringe Norm-Ject Cook1 ml (K-ATS-1000)
> 50 ml Modified Earle's Balanced Salt Solution with HEPES, 0.4 Heparin Novo, and 2.25% Human Serum Albumin.

Protocol 3: Percutaneous Epididymal Sperm Aspiration (PESA)

Indication

All cases of OA with normal spermatogenesis, for example, congenital absence of the vas deferens, failed vasectomy reversal. (CBAVD patients: read caveat in MESA section; protocol 7).

Patient Preparation

The man is given hibitane soap, to wash the area the night before and the morning of the operation. He is also asked to shave the area.

Meperidine hydrochloride 1 mg/kg IM and midazolam 2.5 mg IM may be given.

Patient has to empty the bladder before surgery.

Patient is fully draped with the operation site obscured to the patient. Patient wears a top only. Operation site cleansed with antiseptic solution (for example, HAC, Zeneca: hospital antiseptic concentrate. Contains chlorhexidine). Penis held up out of the way with a swab fixed underneath the drape. A drape with a small hole of 5 cm in diameter in the middle covers the operation site. The testes are gently pulled through to be in the field of the procedure. Local anesthetic– 1–2 ml of 2% lidocaine (without epinephrine) – is injected in the spermatic cord to obtain locoregional anesthesia and into the scrotal skin.

The PESA Procedure

A 19 or 21 G needle is used. Attached is a 10 ml syringe. The epididymis is held firmly between two fingers of one hand and the needle is inserted with the other hand perpendicular to the epididymis. The needle is inserted into the epididymal mass and then gently withdrawn under slight suction. Care is taken not to move the needle to minimize contamination with blood and prevent epididymal damage. The embryologist/nurse brings a 1.5 ml Eppendorf micro test tube filled with culture medium. The needle is placed in the micro test tube and rinsed several times with the medium. The micro test tube is then passed to the embryologist for identification of spermatozoa. Centrifugation of the suspension may be necessary. The procedure can be repeated if not enough sperm are retrieved. However, if after two aspirations there is no success, then an aspiration of the testis or open biopsy under local anesthetic should be performed.

Dressing After

Gauze squares and disposable underpants.

Patient Care Post Operation

The man is told that there may be some pain, but it should be minimal. Acetomiphen (paracetamol) can be taken. If more is required then he should contact the clinic.

Requirements

> A runner
> Drape with central hole
> Non-iodine cleaning solution
> Syringe 10 cc (BS-10 ES Terumo)
> Micro test tube 1.5 ml (Eppendorf 3810)
> (to be washed and sterilized first)
> with medium Modified Earle's Balanced Salt Solution + HEPES + 0.4 Heparin Novo + 2.25% Human Serum Albumin
> Gauze squares 10 × 10 (35813 Hartmann)

Protocol 4: Fine Needle Aspiration (FNA) of Testis for Sperm Retrieval

Indication

All cases of OA with normal spermatogenesis, for example, congenital absence of the vas deferens, failed vasectomy reversal. (CBAVD patients: read caveat in MESA section; protocol 7).

Patient Preparation

As for PESA (see protocol 3).

The FNA Procedure

A 21G 3/4" butterfly needle is used. Attached is a 20 ml syringe. A small amount of culture medium is drawn up into the tubing and the majority expelled, until only about 1–2 mm is left in the butterfly tubing. There may be no air in the fluid. The butterfly needle is inserted perpendicular to the testis, and a little away from the site of insertion of the needle used to inject the local anesthetic as there is usually some blood at that site. The testis is held firmly in one hand, and the butterfly needle is inserted with the other. Care is taken not to move the butterfly needle to minimize contamination with blood and prevent testicular damage. The patient may feel some pain only when the needle enters the tunica. The operator or assistant now "pumps" five to 10 times on the 20 ml syringe to generate suction to aspirate sperm. It is important to keep a slight negative pressure to make sure the aspirate is not pushed back into the testis. This is done by ensuring the plunger does not return all the way to the end. The butterfly needle tubing is then occluded near the needle and the butterfly subsequently removed with a smooth sharp movement to minimize tissue trauma and contamination with blood. Occluding the tubing prevents aspirating blood from the skin surface. With the tubing still occluded, the 20 ml syringe (must have rubber stop that should never be in contact with the medium) is removed and a 1 ml syringe with the plunger partially withdrawn is attached. Otherwise the 20 ml syringe may be used.

The embryologist/nurse brings a dish with nine droplets of culture medium placed (one central droplet surrounded by eight droplets). The butterfly needle is placed in a droplet of culture medium, and the butterfly needle tubing released, thereby removing the negative pressure. A small amount of the aspirate and the culture medium in the butterfly needle is then injected into each droplet in turn. Usually about three to five droplets will be used in this way. Fractionating the aspirate containing red blood cells will improve subsequent visualization under the microscope. The dish is then passed to the embryologist for identification of spermatozoa. The procedure can be repeated if not enough sperm are retrieved initially. However, if after three aspirations there is no success, then an open biopsy under local anesthetic should be performed.

Dressing After

As for PESA (see protocol 3).

Patient Care Post Operation

As for PESA (see protocol 3).

Requirements

A runner
Drape with central hole
Non-iodine cleaning solution
Syringe 20 cc (BS-20 ES Terumo)
Surflo winged infusion set
CE 0197 21G × 3/4" (SV-21BL Terumo)
Flushed with medium
(Modified Earle's balanced salt solution + HEPES + 0.4 Heparin Novo + 2.25% human serum albumin)
Syringe 1 cc (Air-Tite K-ATS-1000 Cook)
Gauze squares 10 × 10 (35813 Hartmann)
To transport sperm
Tissue culture dishes (3200 Falcon Becton Dickinson)

With droplets medium (modified Earle's balanced salt solution + HEPES + 0.4 Heparin Novo + 2.25% human serum albumin)

Protocol 5: Open Testicular Biopsy under Local Anesthesia

Indication

Patients with OA with normal spermatogenesis who wish to have testicular sperm cryopreserved. (CBAVD patients: read caveat in MESA section; protocol 7).

Patient Preparation

As for PESA (see protocol 3).

Procedure

Approximately 5 ml lidocaine (2%) is injected into the skin and the underlying layers up to the tunica albuginea. The testis is fixed in the left hand and a 1–2 cm incision is then made into the scrotum and down through the tissue made edematous by the lignocaine to the tunica. The testis must remain fixed so that the alignment of the scrotal incision with the incision into the tunica is not lost. With the sharp point of the blade, the tunica is opened and the incision slightly extended. Under gentle pressure with the left hand testicular tissue will protrude through the incision. By the use of a curved pair of Mayo scissors a small sample is excised and placed into a petri dish filled with sperm preparation medium, for example, Earle's. Selective hemostasis with diathermy is performed since intratesticular bleeding may cause discomfort and fibrosis.

The testicular tissue is rinsed in the medium and then placed into another petri dish filled with medium. After hemostasis the tunica is closed with 3.0 vicryl. The skin is closed with interrupted 3.0 vicryl sutures. A clean gauze swab covers the suture site and disposable underpants are given for support.

Patient Care Post Operation

As for PESA (see protocol 3).

The patient is told that the sutures will dissolve. There is increased risk of hematoma. The patient should report undue bruising or pain that is not alleviated with paracetamol.

Requirements

An assistant and a runner
Monopolar pencil with needle and Cord (E 2502 Valleylab)
Tube holder (1×) (708130 Mölnlycke)
To fix cords on drape (pencil cord off foot end)
Needle holder Mayo-Hegar (20-642-16 Martin)
Straight Mayo scissors (11 180 15 Martin)
Adlerkreutz pincet (12-366-15 Martin)
Allis forceps (30-134-15 Martin)

Kryle forceps (13-341-14 Martin)
Micro Adson pincet (2×) (12-404-12 Martin)
Micro Adson pincet (2×) (12-406-12 Martin)
Adson pincet (31-09770 Leibinger)
Adson pincet (31-09772 Leibinger)
Metzenbaum scissors (11-264-15 Martin)
Metzenbaum scissors (11-939-14 Martin)
Knife handle with blades nr 15 (0505 Swann-Morton)
Swabs 10 X 10 (35813 Hartmann)
Vicryl 3/0
(JV 497 Ethicon Johnson/Johnson)
Tissue culture dishes 2× (3102 Falcon Becton Dickinson)
With medium (modified Earle's balanced salt solution + Hepes + 0.4 Heparin Novo + 2.25% Human Serum Albumin)
Local anesthesia
Syringe 20 cc CE 0197 (BS-20 ES Terumo)
Needle 18 G (NN 1838 S Terumo)
Needle 26 G (NN 2613 R Terumo)
Xylocaine 2% (Astra Pharmaceuticals)

Protocol 6: Testicular Biopsy under General Anesthesia

Indication

All cases of NOA (primary testicular failure). When testicular biopsy is performed in such patients, a preliminary screening for deletions of the Yq region of the Y-chromosome is preferable in the male partner, since deletions may be found in about 5–10% of patients with unexplained primary testicular failure. Before undertaking the procedure it is important to identify the best testis to explore. This is done by reading any previous histology reports, feeling the testis for size and consistency. If the testis is high or retracted, then the chance of retrieving spermatozoa is lower.

Patient Preparation

As for PESA (see protocol 3).

Procedure

Biopsies Taken at Random As for under local anesthetic(see protocol 4). The main difference is that a larger scrotal incision is made, and the testis is delivered.

If no sperm are observed in the wet preparation, multiple small incisions can be made and biopsies taken accordingly. The incisions must avoid the arterial blood supply. The contralateral testis may be explored as well.

Biopsies Taken With Operating Microscope (Microtese) After scrototomy the tunica albuginea is opened longitudinally with the sharp point of the blade avoiding the arterial blood supply. Then the testicular pulpa containing the tubuli seminiferi is exposed to a 40–80 × magnification using an operating microscope. Care is taken to keep the tubuli wet by a constant drip of saline. Distended tubules are spotted and sampled by microscissors avoiding the arterial blood supply.

The tiny samples are placed into a petri dish filled with sperm preparation medium, for example, Earle's. The testicular samples are rinsed in the medium and then placed into another petri dish filled with medium. After controlling hemostasis the tunica is closed with a continuous 7.0 ethilon suture. The skin is closed with interrupted 3.0 vicryl sutures. A clean gauze swab covers the suture site and disposable underpants are given for support.

Patient Care Post Operation

See open biopsy under local anesthesia.

Protocol 7: Microsurgical Epididymal Sperm Aspiration (MESA)

Indication

Patients with OA with normal spermatogenesis who wish to have epididymal sperm cryopreserved. The main drawback of MESA is that it is an invasive and expensive procedure requiring a basic knowledge of epididymal anatomy and of microsurgical techniques. However, the major benefit of this procedure is its diagnostic power: A full scrotal exploration can be performed and whenever indicated a vasoepididymostomy may be performed concomitantly. Furthermore the number of spermatozoa retrieved is high, which facilitates cryopreservation.

Caveat

When MESA is performed in CBAVD patients, a preliminary screening for mutations of the cystic fibrosis (CF) gene is mandatory in both the male CBAVD patient and his partner, since mutations are found in 60–70% of CBAVD patients without congenital renal malformations. If the female partner is found to be a carrier of a CF gene mutation, preimplantation genetic diagnosis (PGD) should be proposed. Even where only the man is a carrier of a CF-mutation, the couple has to be informed of the risk of having a boy with a genital CF phenotype– with CBAVD.

Patient Preparation

as for PESA (see protocol 3).

MESA Procedure

MESA can be performed during any scrotal exploration taking place even long before the ICSI treatment is scheduled or in a satellite center, for example, by a surgeon not involved in assisted reproduction.

Using an operating microscope, the epididymis is carefully dissected and after hemostasis, using bipolar coagulation, a distended epididymal tubule is longitudinally opened by microscissors through a small opening in the serosa. The proximal corporal or distal head region of the epididymis is opened first. The epididymal fluid is aspirated by means of a disposable tip from an intravenous cannula mounted on a 1 ml syringe filled with 0.1 ml HEPES-buffered Earle's medium supplemented with

0.4% human serum albumin. The aspirated epididymal fluid is then transferred into a Falcon test tube, filled with 0.9 ml of this Earle's medium. When motile spermatozoa, as assessed by preoperative microscopic examination of the aspirates, are recovered, no further epididymal incision is made and a maximum of fluid is aspirated. If microscopic assessment does not show any motile sperm cells, a more proximal incision is made until motile sperm cells are found. In some instances centrifugation (1800 × g, 5 min) of the epididymal aspirates is needed to observe spermatozoa under the microscope. In cases where no motile spermatozoa are recovered, a testicular biopsy is taken for sperm recovery (see below). The sperm suspension is further prepared and kept in the incubator until the moment of intracytoplasmic injection or cryopreservation.

Patient Care Post Operation

Same as for TESE under general anesthesia (see protocol 6).

Requirements

An assistant and a runner
Needle holder Mayo-Hegar (20-642-16 Martin)
Straight Mayo scissors (11 180 15 Martin)
Monopolar pencil and cord (E 2502 Valleylab)
Bipolar pincet and cord (4055 Valleylab)
Tube holders (2X) (708130 Mölnlycke)
to fix cords on drape (bipolar cord off head end, pencil cord off foot end)
Microscissors (OP 5503 V-Mueller)
Micro needle holder (GU 8170 V-Meuller)
Jeweler's forceps (3X) (E 1947 Storz)
(72 BD 330 Aesculaep)
Curved blunt scissors (11 939 14 Martin)
1 cc syringe (4X) (Air-tite K-ATS-1000 Cook)
with or 22 ga medicut (8888 100 107 Argyle)
or Cook aspiration CT (K Sal 400 300 Cook)
Micro Adson pincet with teeth (2X) (12-406-12 Martin)
Knife handle with blades nr 15 (0505 Swann-Morton)
Knife handle with blades nr 11 (0503 Swann-Morton)
NaCl 0.9% 500 ml (B1323 Baxter)
with 2500 U.I. heparine Novo
(Heparine Novo Nordisk Pharma)
Syringes 20 cc (2×) (SS 20 ES Terumo)
with 22 ga Medicut tip (8888 100107 Argyle)
Swabs 10 × 10 (35813 Hartmann)
Tip cleaner
(Surgikos 4315 Johnson-Johnson)
Micro sponges (NDC 8065-1000-02 Alcon)
Sutures
Ethilon 9/0 (W 1769 Ethicon)
Vicryl 3/0 (JV 497 Ethicon)
Microscope
Surgical operating and diagnostic microscope Wild M 691 with 180° positioning for doctor and assistant and optical eyepiece opposite each other. (M 691 Leica)
Achromatic lens f = 200 mm (M 382162 Leica)

REFERENCES

1. Palermo G, Joris K, Devroey P, et al. Pregnancies after intracytoplasmic injection of single spermatozoon into an oocyte. Lancet 1992; 340: 17–18.
2. Van Steirteghem AC, Nagy Z, Joris H, et al. Higher fertilization and implantation rates after intracytoplasmic sperm injection. Hum Reprod 1993; 8: 1061–6.
3. Craft I, Benett V, Nicholson N. Fertilising ability of testicular spermatozoa (Letter). Lancet 1993; 342: 864.
4. Schoysman R, Vanderzwalmen P, Nijs M, et al. Pregnancy after fertilisation with human testicular spermatozoa. Lancet 1993; 342: 1237.
5. Devroey P, Liu J, Nagy Z, et al. Pregnancies alter testicular sperm extraction and intracytoplasmic sperm injection in non-obstructive azoospermia. Hum Reprod 1995; 10: 1457–60.
6. Tournaye H, Camus M, Goosens A, et al. Recent concepts in the management of infertility because of non-obstructive azoospermia. Hum Reprod 1995; 10(Suppl 1): 115–19.
7. Jarow JP, Espeland MA, Lipshultz LI. Evaluation of the azoospermic patients. J Urol 1989; 142: 62.
8. Matsumiya K, Namiki M, Takahara S., et al. Clinical study of azoospermia. Int J Androl 1994; 17: 140–2.
9. Burgues S, Calderon MD. Subcutaneous self-administration of highly purified follicle stimulating hormone and human chorionic gonadotrophin for the treatment of male hypogonadotrophic hypogonadism. Spanish Collaborative Group on male hypogonatrophic hypogonadism. Hum Reprod 1997; 12: 980–6.
10. Skakkebaek NE. Testicular dysgenesis syndrome. Horm Res 2003; 60(Suppl 3): 49.
11. Tournaye H, Camus M, Vandervorst M, et al. Surgical sperm retrieval for intracytoplasmic sperm injection. Int J Androl 1997; 20(Suppl3): 69–73.
12. Tournaye H. Gamete source and manipulation. In: Vayena E, Rowe PJ, David P, Griffin PD, eds. Current practices and controversies in assisted reproduction. Oxford University Press, 2002.
13. Tournaye H, Liu J, Nagy Z, et al. Correlation between testicular histology and outcome after intracytoplasmic sperm injection using testicular sperm. Hum Reprod 1996; 11: 127–32.
14. Ron-El R, Strassburger D, Friedler S, et al. Extended sperm preparation: an alternative to testicular sperm extraction in non-obstructive azoospermia. Hum Reprod 1997; 12: 1222–6.
15. Kafetsoulis A, Brackett N, Ibrahim E, Attia G, Lynne C. Current trends in the treatment of infertility in men with spinal cord injury. Fertil Steril 2006; 86: 781–9.
16. O'Kelly F, Manecksha R P, Cullen I M, et al. Electroejaculatory stimulation and its implications for male infertility in spinal cord injury: a short history through four decades of sperm retrieval (1975–2010). J Urology 2011; 77: 6.
17. Hirsh A, Mills C, Tan SL, et al. Pregnancy using spermatozoa aspirated from the vas deferens in a patient with ejaculatory failure due to spinal injury. Hum Reprod 1993; 8: 89–90.
18. Hovatta O, Reima I, Foudila T, et al. Vas deferens aspiration and intracytoplasmic sperm injection of frozen-thawed spermatozoa in a case of anejaculation in a diabetic man. Hum Reprod 1996; 11: 334–5.

19. Tur-Kaspa I, Segal S, Moffa F, Massobrio M, Meltzer S. Viagra for temporary erectile dysfunction during treatments with assisted reproductive technologies. Hum Reprod 1999; 14: 1783–4.

20. Engin-Ustun Y, Korkmaz C, Duru NK, Baser I. Comparison of three sperm retrieval techniques in spinal cord-injured men: pregnancy outcome. Gynecol Endocrin 2006; 22: 252–5.

21. Kamischke A, Nieschlag E. Update on medical treatment of ejaculatory disorders. Int J Androl 2002; 25: 333–44.

22. Brackett N. Semen retrieval by penile vibratory stimulation in men with spinal cord injury. Hum Reprod Update 1999; 5: 216–22.

23. Halstead LS, Vervoort S, Seager S. Rectal probe electrostimulation in the treatment of anejaculatory spinal cord injured men. Paraplegia 1987; 25: 120–9.

24. Seager SW, Halstead LS. Fertility options and success after spinal cord injury. Urol Clin North Am 1993; 20: 543–8.

25. Kathiresan AS, Ibrahim E, Aballa TC, et al. Comparison of in vitro fertilization/intracytoplasmic sperm injection outcomes in male factor infertility patients with and without spinal cord injuries. Fertil Steril 2011; 96: 562–6.

26. Tournaye H. Surgical sperm recovery for intracytoplasmic sperm injection: which method is to be preferred? Fertil Steril 2011; 96: 562–6.

27. Shah R. Surgical sperm retrieval: techniques and their indications. Indian J Urol 2011; 27: 102–9.

28. Tournaye H, Merdad T, Silber S. No differences in outcome after intracytoplasmic sperm injection with fresh or with frozen-thawed epididymal sperm. Hum Reprod 1999; 14: 101–6.

29. Nicopoullos J, Gilling-Smith C, Almeida P, et al. Use of surgical sperm retrieval in azoospermic men: a meta-analysis. Fertil Steril 2004; 82: 691–701.

30. Girardi SK, Schlegel P. MESA: review of techniques, preoperative considerations and results. J Androl 1996; 17: 5–9.

31. Ramos L, Kleingeld P, Meuleman E, et al. Assessment of DNA fragmentation of spermatozoa that were surgically retrieved from men with obstructive azoospermia. Fertil Steril 2002; 77: 233–7.

32. Greco E, Scarselli F, Iacobelli M, et al. Efficient treatment of infertility due to sperm DNA damage by ICSI with testicular spermatozoa. Hum Reprod 2005; 20: 226–30.

33. Gorgy A, Meniru GI, Bates S, Craft IL. Percutaneous epididymal sperm aspiration and testicular sperm aspiration for intracytoplasmic sperm injection under local anesthesia. Assist Reprod Rev 1998; 8: 79–93.

34. Tournaye H, Clasen K, Aytoz A, et al. Fine needle aspiration versus open biopsy for testicular sperm recovery: a controlled study in azoospermic patients with normal spermatogenesis. Hum Reprod 1998; 13: 901–4.

35. Morey AF, Deshon GE Jr, Rozanski TA, Dresner ML. Technique of biopty gun testis needle biopsy. Urology 1993; 42: 325–6.

36. Donoso P, Tournaye H, Devroey P. Which is the best sperm retrieval technique for non-obstructive azoospermia? a systematic review. Hum Reprod Update 2007; 13: 539–49.

37. Tournaye H, Verheyen G, Nagy P, et al. Are there any predictive factors for successful testicular sperm recovery? Hum Reprod 1997; 12: 80–6.

38. Ezeh UIO, Moore HDM, Cooke ID. Correlation of testicular sperm extraction with morphological, biophysical and endocrine profiles in men with azoospermia due to primary gonadal failure. Hum Reprod 1998; 13: 3066–74.

39. Mitchell V, Robin G, Boitrelle F, et al. Correlation between testicular sperm extraction outcomes and clinical, endocrine and testicular histology parameters in 120 azoospermic men with normal serum FSH levels. Int J Androl 2011; 344: 299–305.

40. Tunc L, Kirac M, Gurocak S, et al. Can serum inhibin B and FSH levels, testicular histology and volume predict the outcome of testicular sperm extraction in patients with non-obstructive azoospermia? Int Urol Nephrol 2006; 38: 629–35.

41. Ballesca JL, Balasch J, Calafell JM, et al. Serum inhibin B determination is predictive of successful testicular sperm extraction in men with non-obstructive azoospermia. Hum Reprod 2000; 15: 1734–8.

42. Vernaeve V, Tournaye H, Schiettecatte J, et al. Serum inhibin B cannot predict testicular sperm retrieval in patients with non-obstructive azoospermia. Hum Reprod 2002; 17: 971–6.

43. Ma Y, Chen B, Wang H, Hu K, Huang Y. Prediction of sperm retrieval in men with non-obstructive azoospermia using artificial neural networks: leptin is a good assistant diagnostic marker. Hum Reprod 2011; 262: 294–8.

44. Boitrelle F, Robin G, Marcelli F, et al. A predictive score for testicular sperm extraction quality and surgical intra-cytoplasmic sperm injection outcome in non-obstructive azoospermia: a retrospective study. Hum Reprod 2011; 26: 3215–21.

45. Har-Toov J, Eytan O, Hauser R, et al. A new power Doppler ultrasound guiding technique for improved testicular sperm extraction. Fertile Steril 2004; 81: 430–4.

46. Herwig R, Tosun K, Pinggera GM, et al. Tissue perfusion essential for spermatogenesis and outcome of testicular sperm extraction (TESE) for assisted reproduction. J Assist Reprod Genet 2004; 21: 175–80.

47. Bettella A, Ferlin A, Menegazzo M, et al. Testicular fine needle aspiration as a diagnostic tool in non-obstructive azoospermia. Asian Journal Andrology 2005; 7: 289–94.

48. Ezeh UI, Taub NA, Moore HD, Cooke ID. Establishment of predictive variables associated with testicular sperm retrieval in men with non-obstructive azoospermia. Hum Reprod 1999; 144: 1005–12.

49. Brandell R.A, Mielnik A, Liotta D, et al. AZFb deletions predict the absence of spermatozoa with testicular sperm extraction: Preliminary report of a prognostic genetic test. Hum Reprod 1998; 13: 2812–15.

50. Silber S, Nagy Z, Devroey P, Tournaye H, Van Steirteghem AC. Distribution of spermatogenesis in the testicles of azoospermic men: the presence or abscence of spermatids in the testes of men with germinal failure. Hum Reprod 1997; 12: 2422–8.

51. Roosen-Runge EC. Quantitative investigations on human testicular biopsies. I Normal testis. Fertil Steril 1956; 7: 1222–6.

52. Steinberg E, Tjioe DY. A method for quantitative analysis of human seminiferous epithelium. Fertil Steril 1968; 19: 960–7.

53. Gil-Salom M, Minguez Y, Rubio C, et al. Efficacy of intracytoplasmic sperm injection using testicular spermatozoa. Hum Reprod 1995; 10: 3166–70.

54. Hauser R, Botchan A, Amit A, et al. Multiple testicular sampling in non-obstructive azoospermia-is it necessary? Hum Reprod 1998; 13: 3081–5.

55. Nagy P, Verheyen G, Tournaye H, Devroey P, Van Steirteghem A. An improved treatment procedure for testicular biopsy offers more efficient sperm recovery: case series. Fertil Steril 1997; 68: 376–9.

56. Crabbé E, Verheyen G, Tournaye H, Van Steirteghem A. The use of enzymatic procedures to recover testicular sperm. Hum Reprod 1997; 12: 1682–7.

57. Angelopoulos T, Adler A, Krey L, et al. Enhancement or initiation of testicular sperm motility by in vitro culture of testicular tissue. Fertil Steril 1999; 71: 240–3.

58. Tasdemir I, Tasdemir M, Tavukcuoglu S. Effect of pentoxifylline on immotile testicular spermatozoa. J Assisted Reprod Genet 1998; 15: 90–2.

59. Witt MA, Richard JR, Smith SE, Rhee EH, Tucker MJ. The benefit of additional biopsy sites when performing testicular sperm extraction in non-obstructive azoospermia. Fertil Steril 1997; 67: S79–80.

60. Vernaeve V, Verheyen G, Goossens A, et al. How successful is repeat testicular sperm extraction in patients with azoospermia? Hum Reprod 2006; 21: 1551–4.

61. Tournaye H, Camus M, Goossens A, et al. Recent concepts in the management of infertility because of non-obstructive azoospermia. Hum Reprod 1995(Suppl1); 10: 115–19.

62. Schlegel P, Su LM. Physiological consequences of testicular sperm extraction. Hum Reprod 1997; 12: 1688–92.

63. Ron-El R, Strauss S, Friedler S, et al. Serial sonography and colour flow Doppler imaging following testicular and epididymal sperm extraction. Hum Reprod 1998; 13: 3390–3.

64. Schlegel PN, Li PS. Microdissection TESE: sperm retrieval in non-obstructive azoospermia. Hum Reprod Update 1998; 4: 439.

65. Ishikawa T, Nose R, Yamaguchi K, et al. Learning curves of microdissection testicular sperm extraction for nonobstructive azoospermia. 2010; 94: 1008–11.

66. Verheyen G, Vernaeve V, Van Landuyt L, et al. Should diagnostic testicular sperm retrieval followed by cryopreservation for later ICSI be the procedure of choice for all patients with non-obstructive azoospermia? Hum Reprod 2004; 19: 2822–30.

67. Tournaye H, Camus M, Vandervorst M, et al. Sperm retrieval for ICSI. Int J Andrology 1997; 20(Suppl 3): 69–73.

68. Tournaye H, Staessen C, Liebaers I, et al. Testicular sperm recovery in 47, XXY Klinefelter patients. Hum Reprod 1996; 11: 1644–9.

69. Fullerton G, Hamilton M, Maheshwari A. Should non-mosaic Klinefelter syndrome men be labelled as infertile in 2009? Hum Reprod 2010; 253: 588–97.

70. Palermo GD, Schlegel PN, Scott Sils E. Births after intracytoplasmic sperm injection of sperm obtained by testicular sperm extraction from men with non-mosaic Klinefelter's syndrome. N Engl J Med 1998; 338: 588–90.

71. Ron-El R, Friedler S, Strassburger D, et al. Birth of a healthy neonate following the intracytoplasmic injection of testicular spermatozoa from a patient with Klinefelter's syndrome. Hum Reprod 1999; 14: 368–70.

72. Okada H, Goda K, Yamamoto Y, et al. Age as a limiting factor for successful sperm retrieval in patients with nonmosaic Klinefelter's syndrome. Fertil Steril 2005; 84: 1662–4.

73. Staessen C, Coonen E, Van Assche E, et al. Preimplantation diagnosis for X and Y normality in embryos from three Klinefelter patients. Hum Reprod 1996; 11: 1650–3.

74. Guttenbach M, Michelmann HW, Hinney B, Engel W, Schmid M. Segregation of sex chromosomes into sperm nuclei in a man with 47, XXY Klinefelter's karyotype: A FISH analysis. Hum Genet 1997; 99: 474–7.

75. Staessen C, Tournaye H, Van Assche E, et al. Preimplantation diagnosis in 47, XXY Klinefelter patients. Hum Reprod Update 2003; 9: 319–30.

76. Rosenlund B, Sjoblom P, Tornblom M, et al. In-vitro fertilization and intracytoplasmic sperm injection in the treatment of infertility after testicular cancer. Hum Reprod 1998; 13: 414–18.

77. Baniel J, Sella A. Sperm extraction at orchiectomy for testis cancer. Fertil Steril 2001; 75: 260–2.

78. Schrader M, Muller M, Straub B, et al. Testicular sperm extraction in azoospermic patients with gonadal germ cell tumors prior to chemotherapy - a new therapy option. Urology 2003; 61: 421–5.

79. Tournaye H. Storing reproduction for oncological patients. Mol Cell Endocrinol 2000; 27: 133–6.

80. Chan PT, Palermo GD, Veeck LL, Rosenwaks Z, Schlegel PN. Testicular sperm extraction combined with intracytoplasmic sperm injection in the treatment of men with persistent azoospermia postchemotherapy. Cancer 2001; 15: 1632–7.

81. Damani MN, Masters V, Meng MV, et al. Postchemotherapy ejaculatory azoospermia: fatherhood with sperm from testis tissue with intracytoplasmic sperm injection. J Clin Oncol 2002; 15: 930–634.

82. Hsiao W, Stahl PJ, Osterberg EC, et al. Successful treatment of postchemotherapy azoospermia with microsurgical testicular sperm extraction: the Weill Cornell experience. J Clin Oncol 2011; 2912: 1607–11.

83. Hauser R, Yogev L, Paz G, et al. Comparison of efficacy of two techniques for testicular sperm retrieval in nonobstructive azoospermia: Multifocal testicular sperm extraction versus multifocal testicular sperm aspiration. J Androl 2006; 27: 28–33.

84. Rosenlund B, Kvist U, Ploen L, et al. A comparison between open and percutaneous needle biopsies in men with azoospermia. Hum Reprod 1998; 13: 1266–71.

85. Friedler S, Raziel A, Strassburger D, et al. Testicular sperm retrieval by percutaneous fine needle sperm aspiration compared with testicular sperm extraction by open biopsy in men with non-obstructive azoospermia. Hum Reprod 1997; 12: 1488–93.

86. Ezeh UIO, Moore HDM, Cooke ID. A prospective study of multiple needle biopsies versus a single open biopsy for testicular sperm extraction in men with non-obstructive azoospermia. Hum Reprod 1998; 13: 3075–80.

87. Novero V, Goossens A, Tournaye H, et al. Seminoma discovered in two males undergoing successful testicular sperm extraction for intracytoplasmic sperm injection. Fertil Steril 1996; 65: 1015–54.

88. Turek P, Givens CR, Schriock ED, et al. Testis sperm extraction and intracytoplasmic sperm injection guided by prior fine-needle aspiration mapping in

patients with nonobstructive azoospermia. Fertil Steril 1999; 71: 552–7.

89. Meng MV, Cha I, Ljung B, Turek P. Relationship between classic histological pattern and sperm findings on fine needle aspiration map in infertile men. Hum Reprod 2000; 15: 1973–7.

90. Kamal A, Fahmy I, Mansour R, et al. Outcome of repeated testicular sperm extraction and ICSI in patients with non-obstructive azoospermia. MEFSJ 2004; 9: 42–6.

91. Vernaeve V, Verheyen G, Goosens A, et al. How successful is repeat testicular sperm extraction in patients with azoospermia? Hum Reprod 2006; 21: 1551–4.

92. Nagy Z, Liu J, Janssenwillen C, et al. Comparison of fertilization, embryo development and pregnancy rates after intracytoplasmic sperm injection using ejaculated, fresh and frozen-thawed epididymal and testicular spermatozoa. Fertil Steril 1995; 63: 808–5.

93. Vernaeve V, Tournaye H, Osmanagaoglu K, et al. Intracytoplasmic sperm injection with testicular spermatozoa is less successful in men with nonobstructive azoospermia than in men with obstructive azoospermia. Fertil Steril 2003; 79: 529–33.

94. Levron J, Aviram-Goldring A, Madgar I, et al. Sperm chromosome abnormalities in men with severe male factor infertility who are undergoing in-vitro fertilization with intracytoplasmic sperm injection. Fertil Steril 2001; 76: 479–84.

95. Mercan R, Urman B, Alatas C, et al. Outcome of testicular sperm retrieval procedures in non-obstructive azoospermia: percutaneous aspiration versus open biopsy. Hum Reprod 2000; 15: 1548–51.

96. Nassar ZA, Lakkis D, Sasy M, et al. Fine needle testicular sperm aspiration: an alternative to open testicular biopsy in patients with non-obstructive azoospermia. Fertil Steril 2001; 76: S137.

97. Platteau P, Staessen C, Michiels A, et al. Comparison of the aneuploidy frequency in embryos derived from testicular sperm extraction in obstructive and non-obstructive azoospermic men. Hum Reprod 2004; 19: 1570–4.

98. Donoso P, Platteau P, Papanikolaou EG, et al. Does PGD for aneuploidy screening change the selection of embryos derived from testicular sperm extraction in obstructive and non-obstructive azoospermic men? Hum Reprod 2006; 21: 2390–5.

99. Mastenbroeck S, Twisk M, van der V, Repping S. Pre-implantation genetic screening: a systematic review and meta-analysis of RCTs. Hum Reprod Update 2011; 17: 454–66.

100. Palermo GD, Schlegel PN, Hariprashad JJ, et al. Fertilization and pregnancy outcome with intracytoplasmic sperm injection for azoospermic men. Hum Reprod 1999; 14: 741–8.

101. Vernaeve V, Bonduelle M, Tournaye H, et al. Pregnancy outcome and neonatal data on children born after ICSI with testicular sperm in obstructive and non-obstructive azoospermia. Hum Reprod 2003; 18: 2093–7.

102. Belva F, De Schrijver F, Tournaye H, et al. Neonatal outcome of 724 children born after ICSI using non-ejaculated sperm. Hum Reprod 2011; 26: 1752–8.

50

Processing and cryopreservation of testicular sperm

Kathleen Hwang, Joseph P. Alukal, Dolores J. Lamb, and Larry I. Lipshultz

HANDLING AND CRYOPRESERVATION OF TESTICULAR SPERM

The treatment of male infertility presents many unique challenges. Amongst these are the dilemmas that arise from needing to coordinate treatments for both male and female patients. These logistical issues, such as the need to time testicular sperm extraction to coincide with oocyte retrieval, can end up posing as much of a problem to practitioners as almost any cause of male or female infertility. Of course, the real impact of this dilemma is the fact that many patients with male factor infertility will have unsuccessful attempts at sperm extraction, thereby wasting the efforts of their female partner, who has by this point gone through ovarian hyperstimulation. The financial and emotional cost of this outcome can be devastating.

Amongst the tools available to practitioners to combat this dilemma, cryopreservation of testicular sperm may be the most useful. Recovery of viable spermatozoa after freeze–thawing of testicular spermatozoa (obtained via percutaneous extraction) was first described by Craft and Tsirigotis in 1995 (1). Subsequently, Romero demonstrated successful fertilization using cryopreserved spermatozoa obtained via testis biopsy; intra-cytoplasmic sperm injection (ICSI) performed using testicular spermatozoa at the time of the biopsy was unsuccessful (2). However, repeated attempts at ICSI using excess tissue that had been cryopreserved did result in fertilization. Importantly, Romero described this procedure in only two patients, both of whom were azoospermic, and pregnancy did not result in either case.

The widespread application of cryopreservation to testicular spermatozoa is the result of the work of Oates and colleagues (3). In 1997, they published their results from a series of 10 patients with nonobstructive azoospermia (NOA) who underwent testicular sperm extraction (TESE) with planned cryopreservation of testicular tissue. With subsequent thawing and usage for ICSI, their fertilization rate was 48% and clinical pregnancies with live births did occur. An acceptable fertilization rate, comparable to those found in routine cycles of IVF–ICSI using freshly obtained testis spermatozoa from patients with NOA, was consistent with the hypothesis that freeze–thaw of testis tissue was not injurious to testicular spermatozoa in any meaningful way.

Cryopreservation of testicular spermatozoa remains a commonly used and vital technique in assisted reproduction. There are several reasons for this, many of which relate to the unique treatment dilemmas posed by patients with NOA. First, the chance of unsuccessful sperm retrieval in a patient with NOA is approximately 30% (4). Obviously, an unsuccessful biopsy makes the effort undertaken by the couple to coordinate ovarian hyperstimulation and oocyte retrieval completely wasted. However, there is no way to predict the likelihood of this occurrence. Cryopreservation allows the couple to time oocyte retrieval to their convenience and only in the event of successful testis sperm extraction. Second, without cryopreservation, the couple is forced to undergo repeated testis biopsies for each desired cycle of IVF–ICSI. This assumes that couples will need repeated cycles due to: (i) failure of attempted cycles and (ii) desire for multiple children. Both these occurrences are common; if patients with NOA were required to undergo fresh testis biopsy every time they planned to undergo an IVF–ICSI cycle, there would be a far higher likelihood of failure at each cycle (again a 30% risk of unsuccessful biopsy). In addition, there is significant injury to the testis incurred with each sperm extraction (5). This injury is compounded by the fact that both androgen production and spermatogenesis are often already impaired in the patient with NOA. Taken together, these reasons help illustrate why cryopreservation of testicular sperm is so crucially important to patients with NOA.

On the other hand, there remain serious limitations to this technology as it currently exists. As many as 50% of viable sperm may be lost with each freeze–thaw cycle even in experienced hands (6); in patients with severe oligospermia or azoospermia, this can result in an unacceptable rate of loss when viable testicular spermatozoa are rare in the first place. Continued research into cryopreservative techniques allowing for better preservation of single digit numbers of cells is yielding promising results.

This chapter will serve as an update on technologies available for cryopreservation of testicular sperm. We will also outline handling techniques that are crucial to increasing the likelihood of successful sperm preservation after freeze–thaw. Finally, we outline our own technique for cryopreservation of testicular sperm, in hopes of providing a simple set of directions for anyone wishing to perform this technique for their patients.

CRYOPRESERVATION

As is expected, spermatozoa are no different from other living cells in that they do not tolerate massive changes in temperature well. Much of the physiology of cryopreservation of testis spermatozoa derives from our understanding of cryopreservation of ejaculated spermatozoa, first used to achieve pregnancy by Bunge and Sherman in 1953 (7). Freezing of donor sperm results in dehydration, ionic concentration, and loss of plasma membrane integrity; as a result, approximately 50% of sperm die during a single freeze–thaw cycle. Similar losses are encountered with a single freeze–thaw cycle performed on testicular spermatozoa (6,8–10). This is problematic given the low numbers of spermatozoa that are typically returned from testicular tissue on patients with NOA.

Inquiry into the specific causes of lethal injury to living cells undergoing cryopreservation identified several correctable factors that minimize the likelihood of failure. These include avoidance of phase transition and resultant membrane damage; optimization of cooling and warming rates, and prevention of ice formation. Finally, the usage of cryoprotectants represents an additional means of preventing lethal injury.

Phase transition describes the thermodynamic event in which a compound is transformed from one phase to another; this event declares itself through an abrupt change in the physical properties of the compound after only a small change in temperature (e.g., liquid water to ice at 0°C). Numerous animal and human studies have demonstrated that by preventing the phase transition of the surrounding media, lethal injury to sperm is prevented. Sawada first demonstrated plasma membrane damage and cell death in human spermatozoa as a result of phase transition (10); subsequent work by Leibo in 1977 demonstrated optimal freezing characteristics for both sperm and embryos (11). This work focused on the notion that slow cooling rates allow for extracellular ice formation; this phase transition dehydrates cells thereby resulting in hyperosmolarity of the intracellular environment and cell death. Conversely, rapid cooling rates resulted in intracellular ice formation, which was also lethal. More recent work by Jeyendran demonstrated that the membrane damage Sawada observed during freezing may specifically be due to lipid peroxidation in the setting of phase transition (12).

As such, the media within which spermatozoa are kept and the rate at which this media is cooled is vitally important. Mazur and Schmidt elaborated this balance in yeast, showing clearly that rapid cooling rates prevented extracellular ice formation and increased cell survival up until a rate was reached, which allowed for intracellular

ice formation (13). This optimal cooling rate varied from cell type to cell type (8). In human ejaculated sperm and testicular spermatozoa, optimal cooling is achieved with a stepwise cooling of –10°C/minute to –80°C. The sample is maintained at this temperature for 20 minutes and then stored permanently in liquid nitrogen at a temperature of –196°C (14). Warming rates are also important to cell survival; rapid warming prevents aggregation of extracellular ice crystals (8).

Finally, cryoprotectants act to protect cells from the abrupt fluid shifts involved in freezing. They can be grouped into two categories: Intracellular cryoprotectants permeate the plasma membrane of cells and prevent intracellular solute toxicity; conversely, extracellular cryoprotectants act to prevent ice formation. Commonly used intracellular cryoprotectants include glycerol and polyethylene glycol; extracellular cryoprotectants include dextran, glucose, and sucrose. The most commonly used cryoprotectant for the purposes of freezing sperm and/or spermatozoa is glycerol; many cryobanks employ egg yolk buffer containing glycerol as media for freezing specimens (15).

PROCESSING OF SPECIMENS

Methods for processing testis tissue are also vitally important to the eventual success of cryopreservation. The initial method described by Oates involves mechanical homogenization followed by repeated aspiration through a 16-gauge hypodermic needle; the resultant specimen is stored with media in polypropylene tubes (3). Non-mechanical methods for processing include ones such as that described by Salzbrunn (16). This enzymatic digestion protocol uses type IV collagenase, trypsin, and trypsin inhibitor. Obviously, both methodologies introduce the risk of extensive cellular injury. The mechanical protocols can introduce cellular injury through shearing force. Enzymatic digestion results in unintentional digestion of healthy spermatozoa. Regardless of the methodology used, minimal processing of tissue results in maximized live-cell yield after freeze–thaw (personal communication, Oates).

Much of the difficulty in processing testicular specimens derives from the paucity of spermatozoa in specimens obtained from patients with NOA. Identification of sperm within specimens is labor intensive, often resulting in only tens or hundreds of cells appropriate for freezing. Unfortunately, standard techniques for freezing ejaculated sperm and/or testicular spermatozoa have been shown to yield poor results when applied to specimens with a low number of sperms (17). As a result, significant effort has been made to develop techniques that are appropriate for poor sperm density specimens.

The most intriguing of these was described by Cohen in 1991 (18); this method employs empty hamster oocytes as a storage vessel for individual sperm. After removal of the ooplasm via a microdissection technique, individual sperms are inserted in the zona pellucida and then frozen. Excellent results with regard to eventual thawing, viability of sperm, and fertilization have been obtained. These results were confirmed by Borini in 2000 using sperm obtained via testicular sperm aspiration (TESA) (19). Despite this, due to concerns of trans-species migration of viral infection from hamsters, this technique is not employed for clinical purposes, and no human pregnancy as a result of this technique has been described.

Other methodologies for the storage of individual or low numbers of sperm include freezing of small aliquots on nylon microloops, as described by Schuster (20). This technique, which was described in 2003, was offered as a simple alternative to the empty zona pellucida technique. This experiment considered sperm motility and viability after freeze–thaw with the microloop technique; in addition, four separate cryoprotective solutions were used in an effort to ascertain whether or not a difference existed with regard to success. Ultimately, viability was poor with each solution used. Despite this, research into this technique continues, as the opportunity to individually store and then use single digit numbers of sperm would represent a significant advance in cryopreservation. The opportunity to avoid multiple freeze–thaw cycles, which are injurious to sperm, represents a meaningful step forward, especially when dealing with samples possessing minimal sperm (21). Research into other methodologies for addressing this challenge continues. In 2004, Just and colleagues reported successful freeze–thaw of human spermatozoa using the algae species *Volvox globator* as a vehicle (22). More fascinating developments in this field are sure to follow.

TECHNIQUE FOR TESTICULAR SPERM EXTRACTION AND CRYOPRESERVATION

Diagnostic biopsy and testicular sperm extraction is performed at our institution using an open window technique (23). After administration of IV conscious sedation and local anesthesia, a transverse scrotal incision is made through the scrotal skin, dartos, and tunica vaginalis. The tunica albuginea is then incised, and seminiferous tubules are extruded from the testis. These tubules are sharply dissected from the testis using Iris scissors, and then a wet preparation is prepared using modified sperm washing medium (Irvine Scientific). A portion of the tissue is set aside in Bouin's fixative for formal histologic examination. The wet preparation is then examined using phase contrast microscopy; if mature spermatozoa are identified, then additional tubules are harvested via the same incision and placed in 1 ml of test-yolk buffer (TYB, Irvine Scientific). If mature spermatozoa are not seen, additional biopsies are first taken from the ipsilateral testis and then the contralateral testis, until sperm are found. At this point, if mature spermatozoa are still not seen, we will proceed onto a microsurgical dissection where the testicular capsule is opened, and individual tubules are examined under approximately 20 to 25x magnification. This optimal magnification allows for identification of avascular regions of the testis to minimize risks of injury while allowing a complete examination of the testis.

The testis tissue is then mechanically dispersed under an inverted dissecting microscope; this is performed in a cell culture dish (BD Falcon) using fine jeweler's forceps. Fluid from the homogenized tissue is then examined for spermatozoa. Once sperm are found, the homogenate is adjusted to a total of 5 ml using equal parts of TYB with 20% egg yolk and 12% glycerol. The final volume is then partitioned into 1 ml aliquots and stored in sterile polypropylene vials. These are then frozen in liquid nitrogen using the above described protocol (stepwise cooling to –80°C in liquid nitrogen vapor followed by immersion in liquid nitrogen at –196°C, Gordinier Electronics).

FERTILITY PRESERVATION

With drastic improvements in the treatment of childhood cancers more attention has been given to the quality of life of cancer survivors. For all childhood cancers the five-year overall survival rate of adolescents has considerably improved over the past four decades from less than 50% to nearly 80%, due to improved therapies and supportive care (24). Preservation of fertility is a major concern for patients requiring treatment, such as radiation and chemotherapy that can inadvertently destroy germ cells. Whereas cryopreservation of sperm for preservation of fertility in men undergoing gonadotoxic treatment is well established, translating this effective method to adolescents has been more challenging. In adults, this obstacle is addressed with cryopreservation of sperm prior to treatment; however, the fertility status of childhood cancer survivors is now the focus of attention as a result of the overwhelming improvements in cancer treatment. Nevertheless, the solution to secondary infertility following cancer treatment is less obvious and direct in prepubescent boys.

Unfortunately, sperm banking is not universally performed in pediatric oncology centers across the world; however, it is imperative that open discussions regarding fertility are considered standard of care. These sensitive discussions not only emphasize the future but also provide an assurance that curative treatment is the aim (25). The American Society of Clinical Oncology concluded that sperm and embryo cryopreservation should be considered standard practice and be widely available (26). Cryopreservation of sperm before the initiation of gonadotoxic treatment is currently the best method of preserving fertility; however, if the young patient is unable to provide a semen sample, electroejaculation, penile vibratory stimulation, or surgical sperm extraction can be performed (27).

While alternative options remain experimental, cryopreservation of prepubertal testicular tissue has emerged as a viable and ethical strategy for preserving fertility in this patient population (28). Although a cryopreservation protocol of immature testicular tissue has not been established, using dimethyl sulfoxide (DMSO) as a permeating cryoprotectant to control slow-freezing has proven to be a promising approach to preserve human immature testicular tissue biopsies (29,30). Investigators evaluated vitrification as an alternate approach in both animal and human models, as this technique avoids ice crystal formation and potential freeze injuries (31,32), and demonstrated that this method is a feasible option and shows great promise in the emerging field of immature testicular tissue cryopreservation.

Spermatogonial stem cells are male germline stem cells capable of self-renewal and differentiation into mature spermatozoa for the sole purpose of transmission of the genome to the next generation. Germ cell transplantation was developed in rodent models and successfully performed by Brinster in 1994 (33). Microinjection of spermatogonial stem cell suspensions into the seminiferous tubules of infertile mice demonstrated a restimulation of spermatogenesis. Cryopreservation of spermatogonial stem cells before the start of any cancer therapy followed by autologous intratesticular transplantation of these cells after cure offers potential for preserving fertility (33,34).

Offering human spermatogonial stem cell autotransplantation as an option for fertility preservation to patients becomes more tangible everyday. There are institutions that recognize the realistic potential of this being a valid option for patients in the near future (34), so much so that they have begun to offer cryopreservation of testicular tissue in hope that within the next 10 years science will have solved all of the intricacies to revolutionize the ability to preserve fertility.

CONCLUSION

Cryopreservation of testicular spermatozoa remains crucially important to the treatment of patients with male infertility; coupled with IVF–ICSI, this technique allows for reasonable hope of a live pregnancy for patients with NOA, while at the same time minimizing morbidity and unnecessary procedures. Future directions for inquiry include safe and effective means for cryopreservation of specimens with limited numbers of spermatozoa, and minimization of cell death with multiple freeze–thaw cycles. With increasing awareness among pediatric oncologists and reproductive medicine specialists of fertility issues in young patients with cancer, it is crucial that an evidence-based approach to the management of these patients is developed. As these and other advances in cryopreservation are made, they will continue to directly benefit patients with severe male factor infertility.

REFERENCES

1. Craft I, Tsirigotis M. Simplified recovery, preparation and cryopreservation of testicular spermatozoa. Hum Reprod 1995; 10: 1623–6.
2. Romero J, Remohi J, Minguez Y, et al. Fertilization after intracytoplasmic sperm injection with cryopreserved testicular spermatozoa. Fertil Steril 1996; 65: 877–9.
3. Oates RD, Mulhall J, Burgess C, Cunningham D, Carson R. Fertilization and pregnancy using intentionally cryopreserved testicular tissue as the sperm source for intracytoplasmic sperm injection in 10 men with non-obstructive azoospermia. Hum Reprod 1997; 12: 734–9.
4. Mulhall JP, Burgess CM, Cunningham D, et al. Presence of mature sperm in testicular parenchyma of men with nonobstructive azoospermia: prevalence and predictive factors. Urology 1997; 49: 91–5; discussion 95–96.
5. Schlegel PN, Su LM. Physiological consequences of testicular sperm extraction. Hum Reprod 1997; 12: 1688–92.
6. Pegg DE. The history and principles of cryopreservation. Semin Reprod Med 2002; 20: 5–13.
7. Bunge RG, Sherman JK. Fertilizing capacity of frozen human spermatozoa. Nature 1953; 172: 767–8.
8. Leibo SP, Mazur P. The role of cooling rates in low-temperature preservation. Cryobiology 1971; 8: 447–52.
9. Mazur P, Leibo SP, Chu EH. A two-factor hypothesis of freezing injury. Evidence from Chinese hamster tissue-culture cells. Exp Cell Res 1972; 71: 345–55.
10. Sawada Y, Ackerman D, Behrman SJ. Motility and respiration of human spermatozoa after cooling to various low temperatures. Fertil Steril 1967; 18: 775–81.
11. Leibo SP. Fundamental cryobiology of mouse ova and embryos. Ciba Found Symp 1977: 69–96.
12. Jeyendran RS, Van der Ven HH, Kennedy W, Perez-Pelaez M, Zaneveld LJ. Comparison of glycerol and a zwitter ion buffer system as cryoprotective media for human spermatozoa. Effect on motility, penetration of zona-free hamster oocytes, and acrosin/proacrosin. J Androl 1984; 5: 1–7.
13. Mazur P, Schmidt JJ. Interactions of cooling velocity, temperature, and warming velocity on the survival of frozen and thawed yeast. Cryobiology 1968; 5: 1–17.
14. Anger JT, Gilbert BR, Goldstein M. Cryopreservation of sperm: indications, methods and results. J Urol 2003; 170(4 Pt 1): 1079–84.
15. Gilmore JA, Liu J, Gao DY, Critser JK. Determination of optimal cryoprotectants and procedures for their addition and removal from human spermatozoa. Hum Reprod 1997; 12: 112–18.
16. Salzbrunn A, Benson DM, Holstein AF, Schulze W. A new concept for the extraction of testicular spermatozoa as a tool for assisted fertilization (ICSI). Hum Reprod 1996; 11: 752–5.
17. Hewitt J, Cohen J, Mathew T, Rowland G. Cryopreservation of semen in patients with malignant disease: role of in-vitro fertilisation. Lancet 1985; 2: 446–7.
18. Cohen J, Garrisi GJ, Congedo-Ferrara TA, et al. Cryopreservation of single human spermatozoa. Hum Reprod 1997; 12: 994–1001.
19. Borini A, Sereni E, Bonu, Flamigni C. Freezing a few testicular spermatozoa retrieved by TESA. Mol Cell Endocrinol 2000; 169: 27–32.
20. Schuster TG, Keller LM, Dunn RL, Ohl DA, Smith GD. Ultra-rapid freezing of very low numbers of sperm using cryoloops. Hum Reprod 2003; 18: 788–95.
21. Rofeim O, Brown TA, Gilbert BR. Effects of serial thaw-refreeze cycles on human sperm motility and viability. Fertil Steril 2001; 75: 1242–3.
22. Just A, Gruber I, Wober M, et al. Novel method for the cryopreservation of testicular sperm and ejaculated spermatozoa from patients with severe oligospermia: a pilot study. Fertil Steril 2004; 82: 445–7.
23. Coburn M, Wheeler T, Lipshultz LI. Testicular biopsy. Its use and limitations. Urol Clin North Am 1987; 14: 551–61.
24. Cancer Facts and Figures. American Cancer Society 2008.

25. Schover LR, Brey K, Lichtin A, Lipshultz LI, Jeha S. Knowledge and experience regarding cancer, infertility, and sperm banking in younger male survivors. J Clin Oncol 2002; 20: 1880–9.

26. Lee SJ, Schover LR, Partridge AH, et al. American Society of Clinical Oncology recommendations on fertility preservation in cancer patients. J Clin Oncol 2006; 24: 2917–31.

27. Schmiegelow ML, Sommer P, Carlsen E, et al. Penile vibratory stimulation and electroejaculation before anticancer therapy in two pubertal boys. J Pediatr Hematol Oncol 1998; 20: 429–30.

28. Wyns C, Curaba M, Vanabelle B, Van Langendonckt A, Donnez J. Options for fertility preservation in prepubertal boys. Hum Reprod Update 2010; 16: 312–28

29. Wyns C, Van Langendonckt A, Wese FX, Donnez J, Curaba M. Long-term spermatogonial survival in cryopreserved and xenografted immature human testicular tissue. Hum Reprod 2008; 23: 2402–14.

30. Keros V, Hultenby K, Borgstrom B, et al. Methods of cryopreservation of testicular tissue with viable spermatogonia in pre-pubertal boys undergoing gonadotoxic cancer treatment. Hum Reprod 2007; 22: 1384–95.

31. Curaba M, Poels J, van Langendonckt A, Donnez J, Wyns C. Can prepubertal human testicular tissue be cryopreserved by vitrification? Fertil Steril 2011; 95: 2123. e9–12.

32. Gouk SS, Jason Loh YF, Kumar SD, Watson PF, Kuleshova LL. Cryopreservation of mouse testicular tissue: prospect for harvesting spermatogonial stem cells for fertility preservation. Fertil Steril 2011; 95: 2399–403.

33. Brinster RL, Avarbock MR. Germline transmission of donor haplotype following spermatogonial transplantation. Proc Natl Acad Sci USA 1994; 91: 11303–7.

34. Schlatt S, Ehmcke J, Jahnukainen K. Testicular stem cells for fertility preservation: preclinical studies on male germ cell transplantation and testicular grafting. Pediatr Blood Cancer 2009; 53: 274–80.

51

Embryo transfer technique

Ragaa Mansour

INTRODUCTION

Despite major advances in assisted reproductive techniques (ART), the implantation rates remain relatively low to allow the wide spread use of single embryo transfer. Successful implantation requires a viable embryo, a receptive endometrium, and an optimal embryo transfer (ET) technique.

Various IVF steps proceed successfully up to the ET stage in about 93% of the cases, however the clinical pregnancy rate per oocyte pick up is only about 28.9% (1). There are numerous technical aspects that affect the ET results. The variables in IVF are so numerous that makes it difficult to fix all other factors while studying one (2).

Unfortunately, most clinicians consider the ET technique a simple procedure. To them, it only means a simple task of inserting the ET catheter into the uterine cavity and delivering the embryos. However, it is not as simple as it appears and it is easier said than done (3).

The ET technique has a great impact on the IVF results. It has been proven that the pregnancy rates differ significantly among different individuals performing ET within the same IVF program (4,5). However, when the ET technique is standardized, the probability of pregnancy is not dependant on the physician performing the ET (6).

We need to standardize the protocol for the ET technique. In a survey of 80 IVF practitioners, standardization of the ET technique was considered the most important factor influencing the success rate in IVF (7). Furthermore, it was estimated that poor ET technique may account for as much as 30% of all IVF failures (8).

Extra attention and time should be given to the procedure of ET so that it will be performed meticulously (9).

ET is routinely performed using the transcervical route, which is basically a blind technique associated with multiple negative factors.

POTENTIAL NEGATIVE FACTORS ASSOCIATED WITH ET

Uterine Contractions

Initiation of uterine contractions may lead to an immediate or delayed expulsion of the embryos and has been considered a big concern in ART. In a study on cows, "artificial embryos" in the form of resin spheres impregnated with radioactive gold were traced after ET (10).

After 1.5 hours, a large proportion of the spheres were expelled from the uterus.

In human IVF, Fanchin et al. (11) noted that more uterine contractions at the time of ET were associated with a lower pregnancy rate. In a study by Woolcott and Stanger, it was observed that the embryos could move as easily toward the cervical canal as toward the Fallopian tubes (12). As a result, it is possible that the embryos may be expelled from the uterus partially or totally, after the transfer (13–15). In a study using radio-opaque dye, mimicking ET, it was found that the dye remained primarily in the uterine cavity in only 58% of cases (16). In another study using methylene blue, the dye was extruded in 42% of the cases after dummy ET (14).

Failure to Pass the Internal Cervical Os

It is crucial for a successful ET that the catheter passes through the cervical canal and internal os to enter the uterine cavity. The ET catheter, especially soft ones, can be unnoticeably curved inside the cervical canal. An important cause for failure of the catheter to pass the internal cervical os is the lack of alignment between the catheter (straight) and the utero-cervical angle (curved or acutely angulated). The acute degree of anteversion/retroversion or utero-cervical angulation and cervical stenosis are the most common reasons of difficult transfer (17,18).

In some rare cases, it may be impossible to pass the catheter inside the uterine cavity. Scaring of the lower uterine segment and cervix, distorted anatomy with fibroids, previous surgery, or congenital anomalies may lead to very difficult ET (18–20).

Cervical Mucus

Cervical mucus can seriously impair proper embryo replacement. Plugging the tip of the catheter can cause embryo retention, especially with such a small volume of culture media to inject with the embryos (21).

The mucus can also drag the embryos outside during withdrawal of the catheter. It may also interfere with implantation if the mucus is pushed or injected in the uterine cavity. In an experimental dummy ET using methylene blue, it was demonstrated that the dye was extruded at the external os in a significantly higher rate when the cervical mucus was not removed (14).

In a large study by Nabi et al. (22), the authors reported that the embryos were much more likely to be retained when the catheter contained mucus or blood. Moreover, cervical mucus may be a source of bacterial contamination with subsequent lower pregnancy rates (23,24). In a prospective randomized trial by Eskandar et al. (25), removal of cervical mucus prior to ET significantly improved the pregnancy rates. In another randomized controlled trial (RCT) by Visschers et al., this positive effect of mucus removal was not significant (26).

OPTIMIZING THE ET TECHNIQUE

Evaluation of the Uterine Cavity

To ensure proper embryo replacement it is important to evaluate the uterine cavity before starting the IVF cycle by the following:

Dummy ET

Performing dummy ET before the IVF cycle has been shown to significantly improve the pregnancy rate (27). This procedure is recommended to be performed before the start of the IVF cycle (21,27) or immediately before the actual ET. At our center we usually do both. In a retrospective study of 289 ETs there was significant difference in ongoing pregnancy rates when dummy ET was done before the IVF cycle compared to performing it at retrieval (28). During the dummy ET the length of the uterine cavity can be measured and its direction and the degree of cervico-uterine angulation can be evaluated. It is also a good test to choose the most suitable kind of catheter and discover any unanticipated difficulty such as pinpoint external as, cervical polyp or fibroids, stenosed cervix from previous surgery, or congenital anomalies. If cervical stenosis is diagnosed it is advisable to perform cervical dilatation before starting the IVF cycle (29,30). The use of cervical laminaria one month before the IVF cycle is an adequate means of cervical dilation (31).

Ultrasonographic Evaluation

The ultrasound (US) is a precise method to measure the length of the uterine cavity and the cervical canal. It is very important in evaluating the cervico-uterine angle (18,32). Ultrasonography is also essential in diagnosing the presence of fibroids and its encroachment on the uterine cavity or cervical canal.

The accuracy of measuring the uterine length using a catheter was determined with the US (33). The anthers reported a discrepancy of ≥1.5 cm in approximately 19% of the patients and ≥1 cm in 30% of the patients.

Avoiding the Initiation of Uterine Contractions

The following precautions have to be taken to avoid the initiation of uterine contractions.

Avoid Touching the Uterine Fundus

It was demonstrated that touching the uterine fundus with the catheter stimulated uterine contractions (11,34). In an experiment by Lesny et al. (34) using ultrasonically visible material, the authors demonstrated that touching the fundus with the catheter initiated strong random uterine contractions relocating the contrast material. That is probably why early sources in IVF described the optimal location for embryo placement as between 0.5 and 1.0 cm from the fundus (35,36). Not touching the fundus was ranked high as a prognostic factor for IVF success in a recent survey (37).

It is a routine procedure for some IVF specialists to place the catheter approximately 0.5 cm (38,39), or 1–1.5 cm (40) below the fundus to avoid touching.

Depositing the embryos in the mid-fundal area of the uterus improved the pregnancy rates (41–45). It was also found by another study that the position of the catheter 2 cm from the fundus was superior to 1 cm from the fundus (46).

Therefore, individual measurement of the cervical canal and uterine cavity length is extremely important. However, the use of a fixed-distance technique greatly reduced the variation in pregnancy rates among physicians (47), probably due to reducing the rate of touching the fundus.

Soft Catheters

The value of soft ET catheters has been recognized since the beginning of IVF. The ideal catheter should be soft enough to avoid any trauma to the endometrium and malleable enough to find its way through the cervical canal into the uterine cavity (18). Soft ET catheter means a combination of physical flexibility, malleability, and smoothness of the tip (8). Soft catheters usually have an outer rigid sheath which should be stopped short of the internal cervical os to benefit from the advantages of soft catheters. If the outer sheath is introduced, it will convent a "soft" catheter into "a stiff" catheter (21). The stimulus of the ET catheter passing through the internal cervical os can possibly cause the release of prostaglandins and uterine contractions (48).

Different kinds of catheters were studied and soft catheters were associated with improved pregnancy rates (8,27,49,50), and in other studies there was no significant difference (38,40,51–55). Two large prospective randomized studies have shown significantly higher ongoing clinical pregnancy rates using soft catheters as compared to rigid ones (56,57). Changing from rigid catheters to soft ones has been associated with improved pregnancy rates (42,58). It is recommended to use soft catheters for ET of embryos with assisted hatching (49). A recent meta-analysis has shown that the clinical pregnancy rates were significantly better using soft ET catheter as compared with rigid ones (59). Different soft catheters are more or less the same and the pregnancy rates associated with them are not significantly different (60).

Gentle Manipulations

Atraumatic delivery of embryos into the endometrial cavity is the prime goal of ET (21). As a rule, the ET procedure should be simple and painless, and gentle manipulations should be observed, even when introducing the vaginal speculum. Holding the cervix with a vullsellum should be avoided except in rare cases (37). On a clinical study on humans, serial blood samples were collected in time intervals of 20 seconds during the ET procedure to measure the serum oxytocin concentrations (61). When the tenaculum was used, there was a temporary elevation of oxytocin level, which remained elevated until the end of ET. In another study on humans, the use of tissue forceps to hold the cervix was found to trigger uterine contractions (62).

Applying 1–2 mL of local anesthetic (1% procaine) to the anterior lip of the cervix through a fine needle before applying the tenaculum was very acceptable to the patients and did not affect the outcome (40). Technically difficult ETs were associated with reduced pregnancy rates in a number of studies (27,63–67). Difficult manipulations initiate uterine contractions with possible embryo expulsion (11).

Uterine Relaxing Substances

Serum progesterone levels on the day of ET correlate with the frequency of uterine contractions inversely (11). Starting progesterone on the day of oocyte pick-up to relax uterine contractility at the time of ET was suggested (68,69), although it did not improve the pregnancy rates as compared to starting it on the day of ET (70). Sedation with 10 mg diazepam, 30–60 minutes before ET did not make a difference in the pregnancy rates (38).

Similarly, tocolytic agents or prostaglandin synthetase inhibitor did not have a positive effect (38). In some patients who experience severe stress and anxiety during ET, propofol anesthesia can be used and it was found to have no effect on the pregnancy rates (71). Nonsteroidal anti-inflammatory drugs to inhibit prostaglandin production (72) were given, 10 mg piroxicam, and there was a significant improvement of the implantation and pregnancy rates (73).

Removal of Cervical Mucus

Removing the cervical mucus before ET is advisable, to avoid the adverse effects mentioned previously. It can be removed by repeated gentle aspiration using 1 cm^3 syringe with its tip placed at the external cervical os or using a soft catheter. The endocervix can be cleaned of mucus using a sterile cotton swab or a small brush and then a small amount of culture media (40,63).

Vigorous cervical washing was reported in a retrospective study to improve the pregnancy rates (74), however, a prospective randomized study showed no significant difference (75). Another large multicenter study showed no significant difference (76).

Ensure that the ET Catheter Passed the Internal Cervical Os

The ultimate goal at the end of an IVF cycle is to safely deposit the embryos inside the uterine cavity. We have to

be sure that the catheter has passed the internal os and is not kinked or curved inside the cervical canal. Performing the ET under US guidance makes it easy to ensure proper passage of the catheter. For clinicians performing ET without US guidance, soft catheters can sometimes be misleading. A simple test of rotating the catheter 360° can discover kinking of the catheter if it recoils. It is advisable to perform a dummy ET to choose the most suitable kind of catheter before loading the embryos to avoid harshly navigating the cervix during the actual ET.

One of the most common causes of failure to pass the ET catheter is the pronounced curvature or angulations of the cervico-uterine angle. Proper curving of the catheter to follow the cervico uterine curvature should be done before loading the embryos in the catheter. That is why it is important to perform a dummy ET and revise the US picture of the uterus before loading the embryos. It has been reported that molding the ET catheter according to the US cervico-uterine angle improved the clinical pregnancy rate and diminished the incidence of difficult ET (32). Straightening the utero-cervical angle can be achieved with a full bladder before ET (66,77). This effect can be achieved indirectly in performing ET under US (77,78).

Sometimes just simple maneuver of the vaginal speculum can change the direction of the cervix and facilitate introduction of the ET catheter.

If the soft catheter cannot pass the cervical canal, a more rigid one should be used. Rigid catheters should be malleable to allow making the required curve to overcome the acute cervico-uterine angulations.

Using a malleable stylette to place the outer sheath correctly through the cervical canal before introducing the soft catheter did not have a negative impact on the implantation and pregnancy rates (79).

In difficult cases it may be necessary to hold the cervix with a vullsellum to stabilize the uterus during the introduction of the ET catheter. Holding the cervix with a vullsellum is painful and it should be under local a general anesthesia (40,71).

In rare cases it is very difficult or even impossible to pass the catheter. More rigid stiffer catheters have to be used (27,66). Another system that can be used in difficult cases is the coaxial catheter (19). Cannulation of a resistant internal os can be done with the outer sheath, and then the soft inner catheter can be introduced (80).

Cervical dilatation can be resorted to in cases of cervical stenosis. A short interval between cervical dilation can result in a very low pregnancy rate (63,81). Performing cervical dilatation before the IVF cycle resulted in easier ET and improved pregnancy rates (29,30).

Another helpful way in cases of cervical stenosis is to place a laminaria before the start of the IVF cycle (31), or to place the hygroscopic rods in the cervix prior to ovarian stimulation (82). Canulation of the cervix under fluoroscopic guidance and then dilatation was successfully tried in some tortuous and stenotic cervical canals (20). In the early days of IVF, the rate of difficult ET was high. In a report of 867 ET procedures, 1.3% were impossible, 3.2% were very difficult (manipulation >five minutes or cervical dilatation), and 5.6% were difficult (83). Twenty-five years after this report, the current experience of most IVF centers makes the rate of impossible and difficult ET procedures extremely low. In these rare difficult cases transmyometrial surgical ET can be used (81,84).

Surgical ET has been used successfully, achieving results comparable to the transcervical route (85).

The surgical technique is straightforward and requires no greater experience than that necessary for US-guided oocyte collection (85). The surgical ET set is composed of a metal needle (like an oocyte pick-up needle) with a stylet and an ET catheter that fits in the needle after the withdrawal of the stylet.

Prevention of Embryo Expulsion

Recently, a technique using the vaginal speculum to prevent embryo expulsion after ET was described (86). After introducing the ET catheter in the uterine cavity, the screw of the vaginal speculum is loosened so that its two valves press on the portio vaginalis of the cervix occluding the cervical canal. After waiting for one minute, the embryos are ejected and the catheter is withdrawn slowly. The speculum is kept in place pressing on the cervix for about seven more minutes and is then removed. The results of this study reported a significant improvement in the implantation and pregnancy rates.

EMBRYO TRANSFER USING US

Using US guidance for ET was reported by a number of investigators as simple and reassuring, and it significantly improved the pregnancy rates (8,50,87–93). However, other investigators found no significant difference in the pregnancy rates when ET was performed under US guidance as compared to clinical touch ET (40,94,95). An RCT by Kosmas et al. (96) showed that US-guided ET does not offer any benefit in clinical outcome. For easier identification of the catheter, some kinds have an ultrasonically visible tip (54).

The results of a meta-analysis of eight prospective randomized trials showed that the pregnancy and implantation rates were significantly better when US was used (97).

Another recent meta-analysis has reached a similar conclusion (98). A Cochrane review of 17 RCTs showed that ultrasound-guided ET increased the ongoing pregnancy rates compared with clinical touch (99). Transrectal US can be used in obese women during ET (100).

LOADING THE EMBRYOS IN THE ET CATHETER

Putting the embryos in the ET catheter should start after completing the dummy ET and making sure that the dummy catheter passed the internal os. After the dummy ET, the suitable kind of ET catheter will be selected and flushed with tissue culture medium. Then the ET catheter is filled with ET culture medium and up to 10–15 μL will be in the attached syringe. The embryos are aspirated in another 5–10 μL medium and moved in the catheter to stop away from the tip.

Using a continuous fluid column without air bubbles is recommended (21,88). The volume of fluid used for ET should be as small as possible to prevent flowing out of the embryos into the cervical canal or the fallopian tubes. A large volume (60 μL) of transfer media and a large air bubble in the catheter may result in the expulsion of the embryos (14). A continuous fluid column of 30 μL without air bubbles is recommended (21).

Two prospective randomized trials were performed to investigate the effect of the presence of air bubbles in the ET catheter, on the IVF outcome (101,102). The authors concluded that the presence of air bubbles had no negative effect. However, there is no definitive reason to support the enclosure of air spaces before and after the media containing the embryos in the ET catheter. It was suggested that the air bubbles mark the position of the embryos inside the catheter (101) and protect against loss (103) or entangling with mucus (101).

The protein concentration in the transfer media does not affect the result nor does it increase the viscosity (104). Hyaluronan-enriched transfer medium has been re`cently used in a large randomized trail and showed significant improvement in implantation and pregnancy rates (105). However, another RCT showed no beneficial effect (106). In patients with repeated IVF failures, the use of hyaluronan improved the pregnancy rate (107). Recently, a Cochrane review was performed to determine whether ET medium enriched with adherence compounds have an impact on live birth rate in ART compared to regular ET medium (108). The review included 15 studies using hyaluronic acid and the results showed no evidence of a treatment effect on live birth rate. However, effects could be found on the clinical pregnancy rate (OR 1.41, 95% CI 1.22 to 1.63; $P < 0.00001$) and multiple pregnancy rate (OR 1.86, 95% CI 1.49 to 2.31; $P < 0.00001$), with higher rates in hyaluronic acid groups.

RETAINED EMBRYOS AFTER ET

The ET catheter must be checked for retained embryos after ET. This problem occurs more frequently after a difficult ET (22), or when the catheter is filled with mucus or blood (109). It decreases the implantation rates (63,110). It is advisable to retransfer the retained embryos immediately (22,111–113).

The volume of tissue culture medium for the ET is another cause of retained embryos. It is advisable to aspirate approximately 10–15 μL of culture medium first before aspirating the embryos to ensure the presence of enough medium to push out the embryos (18). It is also important to keep the pressure on the plunger of the syringe after ejecting the embryos until complete withdrawal of the catheter 5 to avoid re-aspirating the embryos.

It is also advisable to withdraw the catheter slowly after ejecting the embryos to avoid creating negative pressure and the withdrawal of the embryos following the catheter. Leong et al. (114) reported that withdrawal of the catheter about 1 cm and brisk injection avoided retrograde flow of the transfer media along the catheter by "capillary action."

BED REST AFTER ET

Bed rest after ET was originally practiced in most IVF centers for several hours for fear of mechanical expulsion of the embryos (115–118). Different investigators have reported that there is no need for bed rest after ET (40,66,119–121). The position of the embryos was ultrasonically traced after ET immediately in a standing position (122). The authors reported that standing shortly after ET did not play a significant role in the final position of embryos. It has also been reported in a prospective controlled trial of 406 patients that immediate ambulation following the ET has no adverse effect on the pregnancy rate (123).

The so-called endometrial cavity is only a potential space and not a real cavity. The ET catheter only separates the opposed endometrial surfaces, and once the catheter is removed, the endometrial surfaces re-oppose. Then, the embryos and fluid injected into the potential space are relocated by the endometrial and myometrial peristalsis as well as the surface tension between the fluid–solid interface (122–125). It is believed that the embryos generally implant near where they were deposited (126). Dummy ET was performed using small microspheres immediately before hysterectomy. The uterine cavity was then inspected and the microspheres were found within 1 cm from the site of deposition (125). In another study by Baba et al., it was found that 26 of 32 gestational sacs, seen by US, were in the area where the air bubble was seen immediately after ET (127).

ET TECHNIQUE AS A CAUSE OF ECTOPIC PREGNANCY

The risk of ectopic pregnancy following IVF was estimated to be 5% in a multicenter study undertaken on 1163 pregnancies (128). This figure is much higher than in natural conception.

The distance from the fundus to the tip of the ET catheter was studied in relation to the ectopic rate (129). The authors reported a decrease in the ectopic rate associated with an increased distance between the fundus and the tip of the catheter. The mid-fundal technique resulted in a lower percentage of ectopic pregnancy and did not negatively affect the pregnancy rate (130).

Ectopic pregnancy was 3.9 times more frequently associated with difficult ET than with an easy procedure (131).

Another factor in the etiology of ectopic pregnancy in IVF is the size of the uterus. It was reported that the ectopic pregnancy rate was significantly higher in women with uterine cavity length less than 7 cm (132).

Finally it was found that the uterine contractions in the early luteal phase are generally cervico-fundal in origin (131) and it may be the cause for some ectopic pregnancies in IVF (21).

DESCRIPTION OF AN ET PROCEDURE

- The patient is instructed to be fasting as the need for general anesthesia may arise.
- The patient is informed of the fertilization rate, the number of embryos selected for the transfer, and if there are extra embryos for cryopreservation.
- The file of the patient is revised to see the US picture of the uterus and the comments on the previous dummy ET.
- The patient is put in the lithotomy position and the cervix is visualized using Cusco's speculum.
- The cervix and vaginal vaults are wiped with sterile gauze and tissue culture media to remove excess cervical mucus and vaginal secretions.
- The cervical mucus at the external os is aspirated gently and repeatedly using a 1 cm³ syringe.
- A dummy ET is performed using a sterile soft ET catheter. Only the soft inner catheter is introduced to pass the internal os and the rigid outer sheath is stopped short of the internal os. To make sure the soft catheter is not kinked inside the cervical canal, the catheter is rotated 360°, then left alone resting on the hand. If it recoils, it indicates that the catheter is coiled. The catheter can be withdrawn to be reintroduced again after modifying the position of the cervix by manipulating the vaginal speculum (the degree of opening and how far it is introduced). If the soft catheter cannot be introduced, a more rigid and malleable one can be tried. The rigid malleable catheter can be molded to follow the curvature of the cervico-uterine angle (directed by the US picture). Sometimes the catheter needs to be moved gently in different directions until its tip passes the internal os. The catheter curvature may need to be increased to overcome the acute angulation of the cervico-uterine angle. In almost all cases, it is possible to introduce the rightly curved rigid catheter.
- If the above maneuvers fail, the procedure is stopped and the patient is put under general anesthesia. General anesthesia is given in the form of propofol 2 mg/kg as an induction dose and anesthesia is maintained by inhalation of isoflurane 1.5% and oxygen 100% through a facemask. The previous trial is repeated with or without a vullsellum to support the cervix. As a last resort, rigid introducer may be used. In extremely rare cases nor the dummy ET catheter nor the rigid (or even metal) introducer can pass the cervical canal and enter the internal os. If this happens you can either resort to transmyometrial surgical ET, or you can cryopreserve the embryos and postpone the ET for later after doing cervical dilatation or hysteroscopic cannulation of the cervix.
- After introduction of the dummy ET catheter 40 μL ET medium containing 500 IU human chorionic gonadotropin (hCG) is injected intrauterine (133).
- The embryologist will start loading the embryos in a similar catheter that was introduced in the dummy ET.
- The ET catheter is flushed with tissue culture medium, and then filled with ET medium. About 10–15 μL of transfer medium is aspirated first in the ET catheter, and the embryos are aspirated in another 5–10 μL medium, to withdraw the embryos away from the tip of the catheter.
- The loaded ET catheter is introduced gently through the cervical canal to pass the internal os, then

advanced slowly till the mid-uterine cavity, and stopped 1–2 cm short of the uterine fundus.

- The screw of the vaginal speculum is loosened so as the two valves of the speculum press on the portio-vaginalis of the cervix. At this moment some patients experience suprapubic heaviness or discomfort. After one minute, when this complaint disappears, the embryos are ejected and pressure is kept on the plunger of the syringe while slowly withdrawing the catheter out. The speculum is kept in place for an average of about seven minutes and then removed.
- The ET catheter is returned to the laboratory to check for the presence of any retrained embryos. If found, retransfer is done immediately.

REFERENCES

1. Nygren KG, Sullivan E, Zegers-Hochschild F, et al. International Committee for Monitoring Assisted Reproductive Technology (ICMART) world report: assisted reproductive technology 2003. Fertil Steril 2011; 95: 2209–22.
2. Mains L, Van Voorhis BJ. Optimizing the technique of embryo transfer. Fertil Steril 2010; 94: 785–90.
3. Naaktgeboren N, Dieben S, Heijnsbroek I. Embryo transfer easier said than done. Fetril Steril 1998; 70: S352.
4. Karande VC, Morris R, Chapman C, Rinehart J, Gleicher N. Impact of the "physician factor" on pregnancy rates in a large assisted reproductive technology program: do too many cooks spoil the broth? Fertil Steril 1999; 71: 1001–9.
5. Harns-Stokes RM, Miller BT, Scott L, et al. Pregnancy rates after embryo transfer depend on the provider at embryo transfer. Fertil Steril 2000; 74: 80–6.
6. van Weering HG, Schats R, McDonnell J, Hompes PG. Ongoing pregnancy rates in in vitro fertilization are not dependent on the physician performing the embryo transfer. Fertil Steril 2005; 83: 316–20.
7. Salha OH, Lamb VK, Balen AH. A postal survey of embryo transfer practice in the UK. Hum Reprod 2001; 16: 686–90.
8. Cohen J. Embryo replacement technology. San Francisco 31 Annual Post Graduate Course. ASRM 1998.
9. Meldrum DR, Chetkowski R, Steingold KA, et al. Evolution of a highly successful in vitro fertilization-embryo transfer program. Fertil Steril 1987; 48: 86–93.
10. Harper MJK, Bennett JP, Rowson LEA. Movement of the ovum in the reproductive tract. Nature 1961; 190: 788.
11. Fanchin R, Righini C, Olivennes F, et al. Uterine contractions at the time of embryo transfer alter pregnancy rates after in-vitro fertilization. Hum Reprod 1998; 13: 1968–74.
12. Woolcott R, Stanger J. Potentially important variables identified by transvaginal ultrasound-guided embryo transfer. Hum Reprod 1997; 12: 963–6.
13. Poindexter AN 3rd, Thompson DJ, Gibbons WE, et al. Residual embryos in failed embryo transfer. Fertil Steril 1986; 46: 262–7.
14. Mansour RT, Aboulghar MA, Serour GI, Amin YM. Dummy embryo transfer using methylene blue dye. Hum Reprod 1994; 97: 1257–9.
15. Schulman JD. Delayed expulsion of transfer fluid after IVF/ET. Lancet 1986; 1: 44.
16. Knutzen V, Stratton CJ, Sher G, et al. Mock embryo transfer in early luteal phase, the cycle before in vitro fertilization and embryo transfer: a descriptive study. Fertil Steril 1992; 57: 156–62.
17. Garzo VG. Embryo transfer technique. Clin Obstet Gynecol 2006; 49: 117–22.
18. Mansour RT, Aboulghar MA. Optimizing the embryo transfer technique. Hum Reprod 2002; 17: 1149–53.
19. Patton PE, Stoelk EM. Difficult embryo transfer managed with a coaxial catheter system. Fertil Steril 1993; 60: 182–3.
20. Zreik TG, Dickey KW, Keefe DL, Glickman MG, Olive DL. Fluoroscopically Guided Cervical Dilatation in Patients with Infertility. J Am Assoc Gynecol Laparosc 1996; 3(Suppl 4): S56.
21. Schoolcraft WB, Surrey ES, Gardner DK. Embryo transfer: techniques and variables affecting success. Fertil Steril 2001; 76: 863–70.
22. Nabi A, Awonuga A, Birch H, Barlow S, Stewart B. Multiple attempts at embryo transfer: does this affect in-vitro fertilization treatment outcome? Hum Reprod 1997; 12: 1188–90.
23. Egbase PE, al-Sharhan M, al-Othman S, et al. Incidence of microbial growth from the tip of the embryo transfer catheter after embryo transfer in relation to clinical pregnancy rate following in-vitro fertilization and embryo transfer. Hum Reprod 1996; 11: 1687–9.
24. Moore DE, Soules MR, Klein NA, et al. Bacteria in the transfer catheter tip influence the live-birth rate after in vitro fertilization. Fertil Steril 2000; 74: 1118–24.
25. Eskandar MA, Abou-setta AM, El-Amin M, Almushait MA, Sobande AA. Removal of cervical mucus prior to embryo transfer improves pregnancy rates in women undergoing assisted reproduction. Reprod Biomed Online 2007; 14: 308–13.
26. Visschers BA, Bots RS, Peeters MF, Mol BW, van Dessel JH. Removal of cervical mucus: effect on pregnancy rates in IVF/ICSI. Reprod Biomed Online 2007; 15: 310–15.
27. Mansour R, Aboulghar M, Serour G. Dummy embryo transfer: a technique that minimizes the problems of embryo transfer and improves the pregnancy rate in human in vitro fertilization. Fertil Steril 1990; 54: 678–81.
28. Katariya KO, Bates GW, Robinson RD, Arthur NJ, Propst AM. Does the timing of mock embryo transfer affect in vitro fertilization implantation and pregnancy rates? Fertil Steril 2007; 88: 1462–4.
29. Abusheikha N, Lass A, Akagbosu F, Brinsden P. How useful is cervical dilatation in patients with cervical stenosis who are participating in an in vitro fertilization-embryo transfer program? The Bourn Hall experience. Fertil Steril 1999; 72: 610–12.
30. Prapas N, Prapas Y, Panagiotidis Y, et al. Cervical dilatation has a positive impact on the outcome of IVF in randomly assigned cases having two previous difficult embryo transfers. Hum Reprod 2004; 19: 1791–5.
31. Glatstein IZ, Pang SC, McShane PM. Successful pregnancies with the use of laminaria tents before embryo transfer for refractory cervical stenosis. Fertil Steril 1997; 67: 1172–4.
32. Sallam HN, Agameya AF, Rahman AF, Ezzeldin F, Sallam AN. Ultrasound measurement of the uterocervical

angle before embryo transfer: a prospective controlled study. Hum Reprod 2002; 17: 1767–72.

33. Shamonki MI, Spandorfer SD, Rosenwaks Z. Ultrasound-guided embryo transfer and the accuracy of trial embryo transfer. Hum Reprod 2005; 20: 709–16.

34. Lesny P, Killick SR, Tetlow RL, Robinson J, Maguiness SD. Embryo transfer–can we learn anything new from the observation of junctional zone contractions? Hum Reprod 1998; 13: 1540–6.

35. Kerin JF, Jeffrey R, Warnes GM, Cox LW, Broom TJ. A simple technique for human embryo transfer into the uterus. Lancet 1981; 2: 726–7.

36. Leeton J, Trounson A, Jessup D, Wood C. The technique for embryo transfer. Fertil Steril 1982; 14: 2417.

37. Kovacs GT. What factors are important for successful embryo transfer after in-vitro fertilization? Hum Reprod 1999; 14: 590–2.

38. Diedrich K, van der Ven H, al-Hasani S, Krebs D. Establishment of pregnancy related to embryo transfer techniques after in-vitro fertilization. Hum Reprod 1989; 4(Suppl 8): 111–14.

39. Egbase PE, Al-Sharhan M, Grudzinskas JG. Influence of position and length of uterus on implantation and clinical pregnancy rates in IVF and embryo transfer treatment cycles. Hum Reprod 2000; 15: 1943–6.

40. al-Shawaf T, Dave R, Harper J, et al. Transfer of embryos into the uterus: how much do technical factors affect pregnancy rates? J Assist Reprod Genet 1993; 10: 31–6.

41. Waterstone J, Curson R, Parsons J. Embryo transfer to low uterine cavity. Lancet 1991; 3: 1413.

42. Rosenlund B, Sjöblom P, Hillensjö T. Pregnancy outcome related to the site of embryo deposition in the uterus. J Assist Reprod Genet 1996; 13: 511–13.

43. Naaktgeboren N, Broers FC, Heijnsbroek I. Hard to believe hardly discussed, nevertheless very important for the IVF/ICSI result: embryo transfer technique can double or halve the pregnancy rate. Hum Reprod 1997; 12: 149.

44. Frankfurter D, Trimarchi JB, Silva CP, Keefe DL. Middle to lower uterine segment embryo transfer improves implantation and pregnancy rates compared with fundal embryo transfer. Fertil Steril 2004; 81: 1273–7.

45. Oliveira JB, Martins AM, Baruffi RL, et al. Increased implantation and pregnancy rates obtained by placing the tip of the transfer catheter in the central area of the endometrial cavity. Reprod Biomed Online 2004; 94: 435–41.

46. Coroleu B, Barri PN, Carreras O, et al. The influence of the depth of embryo replacement into the uterine cavity on implantation rates after IVF: a controlled, ultrasound-guided study. Hum Reprod 2002; 17: 341–6.

47. Van de Pas MM, Weima S, Looman CW, Broekmans FJ. The use of fixed distance embryo transfer after IVF/ICSI equalizes the success rates among physicians. Hum Reprod 2003; 18: 774–80.

48. Fraser IS. Prostaglandins, prostaglandin inhibitors and their roles in gynaecological disorders. Baillieres Clin Obstet Gynaecol 1992; 64: 829–57.

49. Choe JK, Nazari A, Check JH, Summers-Chase D, Swenson K. Marked improvement in clinical pregnancy rates following in vitro fertilization-embryo transfer seen when transfer technique and catheter were changed. Clin Exp Obstet Gynecol 2001; 28: 223–4.

50. Wood EG, Batzer FR, Go KJ, Gutmann JN, Corson SL. Ultrasound-guided soft catheter embryo transfers will improve pregnancy rates in in-vitro fertilization. Hum Reprod 2000; 15: 107–12.

51. Wisanto A, Janssens R, Deschacht J, et al. Performance of different embryo transfer catheters in a human in vitro fertilization program. Fertil Steril 1989; 52: 79–84.

52. Ghazzawi IM, Al-Hasani S, Karaki R, Souso S. Transfer technique and catheter choice influence the incidence of transcervical embryo expulsion and the outcome of IVF. Hum Reprod 1999; 14: 677–82.

53. De Placido G, Wilding M, Stina I, et al. The effect of ease of transfer and type of catheter used on pregnancy and implantation rates in an IVF program. J Assist Reprod Genet 2002; 19: 14–18.

54. Karande V, Hazlett D, Vietzke M, Gleicher N. A prospective randomized comparison of the Wallace catheter and the Cook Echo-Tip catheter for ultrasound-guided embryo transfer. Fertil Steril 2002; 77: 826–30.

55. Burke LM, Davenport AT, Russell GB, Deaton JL. Predictors of success after embryo transfer: experience from a single provider. Am J Obstet Gynecol 2000; 182: 1001–4.

56. van Weering HG, Schats R, McDonnell J, et al. The impact of the embryo transfer catheter on the pregnancy rate in IVF. Hum Reprod 2002; 17: 666–70.

57. McDonald JA, Norman RJ. A randomized controlled trial of a soft double lumen embryo transfer catheter versus a firm single lumen catheter: significant improvements in pregnancy rates. Hum Reprod 2002; 17: 1502–6.

58. Penzias A, Harris D, Barrett C, et al. Outcome oriented research in an IVF program: transfer catheter type affects IVF outcome [abstr]. In: Proceedings of the 53rd Annual Meeting of the American Society for Reproductive Medicine. 1997: S163.

59. Abou-Setta AM, Al-Inany HG, Mansour RT, Serour GI, Aboulghar MA. Soft versus firm embryo transfer catheters for assisted reproduction: a systematic review and meta-analysis. Hum Reprod 2005; 20: 3114–21.

60. Saldeen P, Abou-Etta A, Bergh T, Sundstrom P, Holte J. A prospective randomized controlled trial comparing two embryo transfer catheters in an ART program. Fertil Steril 2008; 90: 599–603.

61. Dorn C, Reinsberg J, Schlebusch H, et al. Serum oxytocin concentration during embryo transfer procedure. Eur J Obstet Gynecol Reprod Biol 1999; 87: 77–80.

62. Lesny P, Killick SR, Robinson J, Raven G, Maguiness SD. Junctional zone contractions and embryo transfer: is it safe to use a tenaculum? Hum Reprod 1999; 14: 2367–70.

63. Visser DS, Fourie FL, Kruger HF. Multiple attempts at embryo transfer: effect on pregnancy outcome in an in vitro fertilization and embryo transfer program. J Assist Reprod Genet 1993; 10: 37–43.

64. Choe JK, Nazari A, Check JH, Summers-Chase D, Swenson K. Marked improvement in clinical pregnancy rates following in vitro fertilization-embryo transfer seen when transfer technique and catheter were changed. Clin Exp Obstet Gynecol 2001; 28: 223–4.

65. Englert Y, Puissant F, Camus M, Van Hoeck J, Leroy F. Clinical study on embryo transfer after human in vitro fertilization. J In Vitro Fert Embryo Transf 1986; 34: 243–6.

66. Sharif K, Afnan M, Lenton W. Mock embryo transfer with a full bladder immediately before the real transfer for in-vitro fertilization treatment: the Birmingham experience of 113 cases. Hum Reprod 1995; 10: 1715–18.

67. Tomás C, Tikkinen K, Tuomivaara L, Tapanainen JS, Martikainen H. The degree of difficulty of embryo transfer is an independent factor for predicting pregnancy. Hum Reprod 2002; 17: 2632–5.

68. Fanchin R, Righini C, de Ziegler D, et al. Effects of vaginal progesterone administration on uterine contractility at the time of embryo transfer. Fertil Steril 2001; 75: 1136–40.

69. Ayoubi JM, Fanchin R, Kaddouz D, Frydman R, de Ziegler D. Uterorelaxing effects of vaginal progesterone: comparison of two methodologies for assessing uterine contraction frequency on ultrasound scans. Fertil Steril 2001; 76: 736–40.

70. Baruffi R, Mauri AL, Petersen CG, Felipe V, Franco JG Jr. Effects of vaginal progesterone administration starting on the day of oocyte retrieval on pregnancy rates. J Assist Reprod Genet 2003; 20: 517–20.

71. Al-Inany HG, Waseef M, Aboulghar MA, et al. Embryo transfer under propofol anesthesia: the impact on implantation and pregnancy rate. Middle East Fertil Soc J 2003; 8: 269.

72. Dawood MY. Nonsteroidal antiinflammatory drugs and reproduction. Am J Obstet Gynecol 1993; 169: 1255–65.

73. Moon HS, Park SH, Lee JO, Kim KS, Joo BS. Treatment with piroxicam before embryo transfer increases the pregnancy rate after in vitro fertilization and embryo transfer. Fertil Steril 2004; 82: 816–20.

74. McNamee P, Huang T, Carwile A. Significant increase in pregnancy rates achieved by vigorous irrigation of endocervical mucus prior to embryos transfer with a Wallace catheter in an IVF-ET program [abstr]. Fertil Steril 1998; 70(suppl 1): S228.

75. Sallam HN, Farrag A, Ezzeldin F, Agameya A, Sallam AN. The importance of flushing the cervical canal with cluture medium prior to embryo transfer. Fertil Steril 2000; 74(Suppl 11): S64–5.

76. Glass KB, Green CA, Fluker MR, et al. Multicenter randomized trial of cervical irrigation at the time of embryo transfer [abstr]. Fertil Steril 2000; 74(Suppl 1): S31.

77. Lewin A, Schenker JG, Avrech O, et al. The role of uterine straightening by passive bladder distension before embryo transfer in IVF cycles. J Assist Reprod Genet 1997; 14: 32–4.

78. Sundström P, Wramsby H, Persson PH, Liedholm P. Filled bladder simplifies human embryo transfer. Br J Obstet Gynaecol 1984; 91: 506–7.

79. Nielsen IK, Lindhard A, Loft A, Ziebe S, Andersen AN. A Wallace malleable stylet for difficult embryo transfer in an in vitro fertilization program: a case-control study. Acta Obstet Gynecol Scand 2002; 81: 133–7.

80. Silberstein T, Weitzen S, Frankfurter D, et al. Cannulation of a resistant internal os with the malleable outer sheath of a coaxial soft embryo transfer catheter does not affect in vitro fertilization-embryo transfer outcome. Fertil Steril 2004; 82: 1402–6.

81. Groutz A, Lessing JB, Wolf Y, et al. Comparison of transmyometrial and transcervical embryo transfer in patients with previously failed in vitro fertilization-embryo transfer cycles and/or cervical stenosis. Fertil Steril 1997; 67: 1073–6.

82. Serhal P, Ranieri DM, Khadum I, Wakim RA. Cervical dilatation with hygroscopic rods prior to ovarian stimulation facilitates embryo transfer. Hum Reprod 2003; 18: 2618–20.

83. Wood C, McMaster R, Rennie G, Trounson A, Leeton J. Factors influencing pregnancy rates following in vitro fertilization and embryo transfer. Fertil Steril 1985; 43: 245–50.

84. Kato O, Takatsuka R, Asch RH. Transvaginal-transmyometrial embryo transfer: the Towako method; experiences of 104 cases. Fertil Steril 1993; 59: 51–3.

85. Sharif K, Afnan M, Lenton W, et al. Transmyometrial embryo transfer after difficult immediate mock transcervical transfer. Fertil Steril 1996; 65: 1071–4.

86. Mansour R. Minimizing embryo expulsion after embryo transfer: a randomized controlled study. Hum Reprod 2005; 20: 170–4.

87. Lindheim SR, Cohen MA, Sauer MV. Ultrasound guided embryo transfer significantly improves pregnancy rates in women undergoing oocyte donation. Int J Gynaecol Obstet 1999; 66: 281–4.

88. Coroleu B, Carreras O, Veiga A, et al. Embryo transfer under ultrasound guidance improves pregnancy rates after in-vitro fertilization. Hum Reprod 2000; 15: 616–20.

89. Prapas Y, Prapas N, Hatziparasidou A, et al. Ultrasound-guided embryo transfer maximizes the IVF results on day 3 and day 4 embryo transfer but has no impact on day 5. Hum Reprod 2001; 16: 1904–8.

90. Tang OS, Ng EH, So WW, Ho PC. Ultrasound-guided embryo transfer: a prospective randomized controlled trial. Hum Reprod 2001; 16: 2310–15.

91. Anderson RE, Nugent NL, Gregg AT, Nunn SL, Behr BR. Transvaginal ultrasound-guided embryo transfer improves outcome in patients with previous failed in vitro fertilization cycles. Fertil Steril 2002; 77: 769–75.

92. Matorras R, Urquijo E, Mendoza R, et al. Ultrasound-guided embryo transfer improves pregnancy rates and increases the frequency of easy transfers. Hum Reprod 2002; 17: 1762–6.

93. Li R, Lu L, Hao G, et al. Abdominal ultrasound-guided embryo transfer improves clinical pregnancy rates after in vitro fertilization: experiences from 330 clinical investigations. J Assist Reprod Genet 2005; 22: 3–8.

94. Kan AK, Abdalla HI, Gafar AH, et al. Embryo transfer: ultrasound-guided versus clinical touch. Hum Reprod 1999; 14: 1259–61.

95. García-Velasco JA, Isaza V, Martinez-Salazar J, et al. Transabdominal ultrasound-guided embryo transfer does not increase pregnancy rates in oocyte recipients. Fertil Steril 2002; 78: 534–9.

96. Kosmas IP, Janssens R, De Munch L, et al. Ultrasound-guided embryo transfer does not offer any benefit in clinical outcome: a randomized controlled trial. Hum Reprod 2007; 22: 1327–34.

97. Buckett WM. A meta-analysis of ultrasound-guided versus clinical touch embryo transfer. Fertil Steril 2003; 80: 1037–41.

98. Abou-Setta AM, Mansour RT, Al-Inany HG, et al. Among women undergoing embryo transfer, is the probability of pregnancy and live birth improved with ultrasound guidance over cli nical touch alone? A systemic review and meta-analysis of prospective randomized trials. Fertil Steril 2007; 88: 333–41.

99. Brown J, Buckingham K, Abou-Setta AM, Buckett W. Ultrasound versus 'clinical touch' for catheter guidance

during embryo transfer in women. Cochrane Database Syst Rev 2010; 1: CD006107. Review.

100. Sohan K, Woodward B, Ramsewak SS. Successful use of transrectal ultrasound for embryo transfer in obese women. J Obstet Gynaecol 2004; 47: 839–40.

101. Krampl E, Zegermacher G, Eichler C, et al. Air in the uterine cavity after embryo transfer. Fertil Steril 1995; 63: 366–70.

102. Moreno V, Balasch J, Vidal E, et al. Air in the transfer catheter does not affect the success of embryo transfer. Fertil Steril 2004; 81: 1366–70.

103. Ebner T, Yaman C, Moser M, et al. The ineffective loading process of the embryo transfer catheter alters implantation and pregnancy rates. Fertil Steril 2001; 76: 630–2.

104. Menezo Y, Arnal F, Humeau C, Ducret L, Nicollet B. Increased viscosity in transfer medium does not improve the pregnancy rates after embryo replacement. Fertil Steril 1989; 52: 680–2.

105. Urman B, Yakin K, Ata B, Isiklar A, Balaban B. Effect of hyaluronan-enriched transfer medium on implantation and pregnancy rates after day 3 and day 5 transfers: a prospective randomized study. Fertil Steril 2008; 90: 604–12.

106. Karimian L, Rezazadeh VM, Baghestani AR, Moeini A. A prospective randomized comparison of two commercial embryo transfer medium in IVF/ ICSI cycles. Hum Reprod 2004; 19(Suppl 1): i52.

107. Friedler S, Schacter M, Strassburger D, et al. A randomized clinical trial comparing recombinant hyaluronan/recombinant albumin versus human tubal fluid for cleavage stage embryo transfer in patients with multiple IVF-embryo transfer failure. Hum Reprod 2007; 22: 2444–8.

108. Bontekoe S, Blake D, Heinemlan MJ, Williams EC, Johnson N. Adherence compounds in embryo transfer media for assisted reproductive technologies. Cochrane Database Syst Rev 2010; 7: CD007421.

109. Awonuga A, Nabi A, Govindbhai J, Birch H, Stewart B. Contamination of embryo transfer catheter and treatment outcome in in vitro fertilization. J Assist Reprod Genet 1998; 15: 198–201.

110. Alvero R, Hearns-Stokes RM, Catherino WH, Leondires MP, Segars JH. The presence of blood in the transfer catheter negatively influences outcome at embryo transfer. Hum Reprod 2003; 18: 1848–52.

111. Tur-Kaspa I, Yuval Y, Bider D, et al. Difficult or repeated sequential embryo transfers do not adversely affect in-vitro fertilization pregnancy rates or outcome. Hum Reprod 1998; 13: 2452–5.

112. Goudas VT, Hammitt DG, Damario MA, et al. Blood on the embryo transfer catheter is associated with decreased rates of embryo implantation and clinical pregnancy with the use of in vitro fertilization-embryo transfer. Fertil Steril 1998; 70: 878–82.

113. Leeton HC, Seifer DB, Shelden RM. Impact of retained embryos on the outcome of assisted reproductive technologies. Fertil Steril 2004; 82: 334–7.

114. Leong M, Leung C, Tucker M, Wong C, Chan H. Ultrasound-assisted embryo transfer. J In Vitro Fert Embryo Transf 1986; 36: 383–5.

115. Garcia J. Conceptus transfer. In: Jones G, Jones G, Hodgen G, Rosen-Waks Z, eds. In Vitro Fertilzation. Norfolk, Baltimore: Williams and Wilkins, 1986: 215.

116. Edwards RG, Steptoe PC, Purdy JM. Establishing full-term human pregnancies using cleaving

117. Lopata A, Johnston IW, Hoult IJ, Speirs AI. Pregnancy following intrauterine implantation of an embryo obtained by in vitro fertilization of a preovulatory egg. Fertil Steril 1980; 33: 117–20.

118. Damewood MD, Meng SG. Personal and the organization of the IVF team. In: Damewood MD, ed. The Johns Hopkins Handbook of In Vitro Fertilization and Assisted reproductive Technologies. Boston: Little, Brown and Company, 1990.

119. Botta G, Grudzinskas G. Is a prolonged bed rest following embryo transfer useful? Hum Reprod 1997; 12: 2489–92.

120. Sherif K, Afnan M, Lashen H, et al. Is bed rest following embryo transfer necessary? Fertil Steril 1998; 69: 478–81.

121. Purcell KJ, Schembri M, Telles TL, Fujimoto VY, Cedars MI. Bed rest after embryo transfer: a randomized controlled trial. Fertil Steril 2007; 87: 322–6.

122. Woolcott R, Stanger J. Ultrasound tracking of the movement of embryo-associated air bubbles on standing after transfer. Hum Reprod 1998; 13: 2107–9.

123. Bar-Hava I, Kerner R, Yoeli R, et al. Immediate ambulation after embryo transfer: a prospective study. Fertil Steril 2005; 83: 594–7.

124. Birnholz JC. Ultrasonic visualization of endometrial movements. Fertil Steril 1984; 41: 157–8.

125. de Vries K, Lyons EA, Ballard G, Levi CS, Lindsay DJ. Contractions of the inner third of the myometrium. Am J Obstet Gynecol 1990; 162: 679–82.

126. Lindholm P, Sundstrom P, Wramsby H. A model for experimental studies on human egg transfer. Arch Androl 1980; 5: 92.

127. Baba K, Ishihara O, Hayashi N, et al. Where does the embryo implant after embryo transfer in humans? Fertil Steril 2000; 73: 123–5.

128. ohen J, Mayaux MJ, Guihard-Moscato ML, Schwartz D. In-vitro fertilization and embryo transfer: a collaborative study of 1163 pregnancies on the incidence and risk factors of ectopic pregnancies. Hum Reprod 1986; 14: 255–8.

129. Pope CS, Cook EK, Arny M, Novak A, Grow DR. Influence of embryo transfer depth on in vitro fertilization and embryo transfer outcomes. Fertil Steril 2004; 81: 51–8.

130. Nazari A, Askari HA, Check JH, O'Shaughnessy A. Embryo transfer technique as a cause of ectopic pregnancy in in vitro fertilization. Fertil Steril 1993; 60: 919–21.

131. Lesny P, Killick SR, Tetlow RL, Robinson J, Maguiness SD. Uterine junctional zone contractions during assisted reproduction cycles. Hum Reprod Update 1998; 44: 440–5.

132. Egbase PE, al-Sharhan M, al-Othman S, et al. Incidence of microbial growth from the tip of the embryo transfer catheter after embryo transfer in relation to clinical pregnancy rate following in-vitro fertilization and embryo transfer. Hum Reprod. 1996; 11: 1687–9.

133. Mansour R, Tawab N, Kamal O, et al. Intrauterine injection of human chorionic gonadotropin before embryo transfer significantly improves the implantation and pregnancy rates in in vitro fertilization/intracytoplasmic sperm injection: a prospective randomized study. Fertil Steril 2011; 96: 1370–4.

52

Cycle regimes for frozen–thawed embryo transfer

Ingrid Granne and Tim Child

Ovarian stimulation commonly results in the generation of more embryos than are necessary for the fresh embryo transfer. Therefore, cryopreservation and subsequent replacement of frozen–thawed embryos is an integral part of assisted reproductive technique (ART) programs. Frozen embryo replacement (FER) cycles contribute to around 25% of all births achieved by ART (1). The clinical pregnancy rate associated with FER varies widely. This is at least in part because clinics have varying protocols as to the quality of the embryos that are cryopreserved after a fresh cycle, the day of development at which the embryo is frozen and the technique (slow freezing or vitrification) that is used for cryopreservation.

Multiple pregnancy remain one of the most significant risks of ART. Studies have shown that elective single embryo transfer dramatically reduces the rate of multiple pregnancy (2). Most importantly, there is increasing evidence that single embryo transfer followed by subsequent FER, if pregnancy does not occur, can lead to a cumulative live birth rate per oocyte retrieval equivalent to double embryo transfer. This enables countries with single embryo transfer policies and clinics aiming to reduce their multiple pregnancy rate to achieve similar live birth rates to those performing multiple embryo transfer (2–5). Importantly, there is evidence that a policy of culturing embryos to the blastocyst stage, transferring a single embryo, and cryopreserving surplus embryos is acceptable to patients (6,7).

FROZEN EMBRYO REPLACEMENT PROTOCOLS

It is vital that a frozen–thawed embryo is replaced during the window of endometrial receptivity and that there is synchronization between embryo and endometrial development. There have been a number of different protocols developed to achieve this; replacement during a natural ovulatory cycle, hormone (estrogen and progesterone) replacement cycles (with or without prior downregulation), and ovulation induction cycles.

There is evidence that endometrial receptivity may be negatively affected by ovarian stimulation (8,9). Although most clinicians would advise the use of fresh embryo transfer over FER cycles, both a retrospective study and a recent randomized controlled trial (RCT) have suggested that there may be an advantage to freezing all blastocysts in the fresh cycle and replacing them in a natural or downregulated cycle (10,11). The finding of significantly improved pregnancy rates in a cryopreserved blastocyst cycle compared to the fresh cycle may be due to the improved endometrial receptivity and endometrial-embryo synchronization.

Natural FER Cycles

In natural FER cycles, embryo transfer is usually timed using a combination of ultrasound monitoring to confirm follicular development and daily urinary luteinizing hormone (LH) urine dipsticks to detect the LH surge. Natural cycle FER is becoming an increasingly common approach. The major advantage to replacement of embryos in a woman's natural ovulatory cycle is that no medication is required and the time taken to complete the cycle is short. However, there will be a significant proportion of women for whom this approach will not be suitable, for example, women with anovulatory polycystic ovary syndrome.

Some clinics advocate the use of human chorionic gonadotropin (HCG) to trigger ovulation and aid in the timing of embryo replacement. A small RCT has shown that the use of an HCG trigger (compared to ultrasound and LH monitoring) decreases the number of monitoring visits required in the natural cycle FER with no difference in pregnancy rate (12). However, if urinary LH testing is undertaken, multiple visits for ultrasound monitoring should be unnecessary. A further RCT contradicted these findings and was terminated after interim analysis because of a significantly increased ongoing pregnancy rate in the group having embryo transfer timed to the LH surge compared to those randomized to an HCG trigger (13). No RCTs have addressed the question of luteal phase progesterone supplementation in natural cycle FER but a recent large retrospective study showed no benefit to luteal phase support in HCG triggered natural cycles (14).

Hormone Replacement Cycles

One possible advantage of medicated FER cycles is that it allows flexibility as to the timing of embryo transfer that may suit both the patient and the clinic. A number of different protocols exist for artificial cycles. First, ovarian downregulation can be achieved by the use of a gonadotropin-releasing hormone (GnRH) agonist, after which sequential estrogen with the subsequent addition of progesterone is used. A simpler regime commencing estrogen on day 1 of the cycle (which prevents follicular recruitment) with the addition of progesterone later but without the use of a GnRH agonist is also commonly followed.

Four randomized studies have evaluated the use of a GnRH analogue and subsequent hormone replacement compared to using estrogen and progesterone alone. A recent meta-analysis of that data showed no statistical difference in pregnancy rates (15), however, the only study to report live birth rates did show a statistically significant increase in the group who underwent downregulation prior to estrogen and progesterone supplementation (16). In that study, ovarian activity was not monitored and the authors concluded that in medicated cycles, when embryo replacement was timed with endometrial thickness alone, ovarian activity should either be monitored or suppressed. In the meta-analysis of studies comparing estrogen and progesterone with and without a GnRH analogue, there were no significant differences in cycle cancellation, endometrial thickness, or miscarriage rate.

HORMONE PREPARATIONS IN FER CYCLES

In artificial cycles a number of preparations of both estrogen and progesterone have been used. Commonly, estrogen is administered in either tablet form or via transdermal patches. There are no randomized studies comparing the preparation, dose, or route of estrogen preparations in frozen–thawed cycles. Progesterone is commonly administered as a tablet, pessary (rectal or transvaginal), or by intramuscular injection. Two RCTs have compared different progesterone preparations in non-downregulated medicated cycles. No difference in pregnancy rates were identified using vaginal pessaries versus intramuscular progesterone (17), or comparing vaginal micronized tables and vaginal progesterone gel (18).

Regimes differ in the length of time progesterone is given prior to embryo transfer although there are no RCTs addressing this issue. In the case of day 2 or day 3 cryopreserved embryos, most retrospective studies have commenced progesterone three days prior to embryo transfer (19), whilst in the case of blastocysts transfer, high pregnancy rates have been reported replacing embryos after five days of progesterone (20). Although there are no studies as to the optimal duration of continued progesterone support in pregnancy, most clinics advise patients to continue progesterone treatment for between eight and 12 weeks, by which time placental progesterone production is adequate.

It has been hypothesized that HCG may have a beneficial effect on the secretory endometrium stimulating cytokines and proteins that are important in the implantation process. However, in an RCT of HCG supplementation versus no treatment in non-downregulated hormonally induced cycles, no significant difference in the pregnancy rate was identified (21). The question as to the benefit of glucocorticoids in FER cycles has been addressed by two RCTs. Neither study identified any benefit in terms of implantation or clinical pregnancy rate (22,23).

Efficacy of Natural Cycle vs. Hormone Replacement in Frozen–Thawed Embryo Transfers

Whilst a number of retrospective studies comparing estrogen and progesterone (with no prior downregulation) with natural cycles showed a higher pregnancy rate in the natural cycle group (24,25), a number of non-randomized controlled trials and one RCT (26) showed no significant difference. No RCTs have been published that compare natural cycle with a downregulated hormone replacement cycle in women with regular menstrual cycles. One such study is currently recruiting (trial number NCT00843570 registered at clinicaltrial.gov) and an interim analysis of 60 recruits (in each arm of the study) has shown no difference in pregnancy or live birth rates. A number of retrospective studies have shown no difference in implantation, pregnancy, or live birth rates (27,28).

Stimulation Regimes for FER

An alternate approach to endometrial preparation for FER cycles is to use low dose ovarian stimulation. One RCT of 199 women compared the use of 150 IU FSH on day 6, 8, and 10 of the menstrual cycle to estrogen and progesterone endometrial preparation (with no prior downregulation). No differences were identified in implantation or pregnancy rate, cancellation rate, or endometrial thickness (29). Clomiphene citrate has also been used for stimulation but the only RCT using this intervention showed no benefit over estrogen and progesterone, used with or without a GnRH analogue (30). Ovulation induction cycles have no benefit in terms of pregnancy rate. In addition, they require increased monitoring, are relatively expensive, and do not have the advantage of flexibility with regard to the timing of embryo replacement. Thus few centers now use this regime.

THE USE OF ULTRASOUND-GUIDED EMBRYO TRANSFER IN FER CYCLES

As with fresh embryo transfer there is evidence that ultrasound-guided transfer increases the pregnancy rate when compared to the "clinical touch" technique (31). A recent systematic review (although not differentiating between fresh and frozen cycles) has confirmed the benefit of ultrasound guidance (32).

ENDOMETRIAL THICKNESS AND QUALITY IN FER CYCLES

Ultrasound has been used to relate treatment outcome of FER cycles to both endometrial thickness and morphology at the time of embryo transfer. Several studies have failed to identify a difference between conception and non-conception cycles in both natural and medicated cycles (33,34). However, a recent large retrospective study of medicated (non-downregulated) FER cycles found that implantation and pregnancy rates were significantly lower when the endometrial thickness was less than 7 mm or greater than 14 mm (35). Although in fresh

IVF cycles the presence of a triple line has been shown to be associated with an increased clinical pregnancy rate, in FER cycles no such association has been identified (34,36). However a non-homogenous hyperechogenic endometrial echo three days after frozen embryo transfer has been shown by one group to be associated with a reduced pregnancy rate (37). Several studies have evaluated endometrial blood flow parameters in FER cycles. One group has reported a decreased mean uterine artery pulsatility index in conception cycles compared to those in which pregnancy did not occur (34). No differences have been identified in three-dimensional sub-endometrial blood flow parameters in natural- or clomiphene-induced cycles (36).

THE DEVELOPMENTAL STAGE OF THE EMBRYO AT THE TIME OF FREEZING

Cryopreservation has been successfully achieved at the zygote, cleavage, and blastocyst stage of development. There are no RCTs comparing clinical pregnancy or live birth rates at each of these possible stages of cryopreservation.

Pronuclear vs. Cleavage Stage Freezing

If cryopreservation takes place at the pronuclear (2PN) stage, all of the embryos are usually frozen. At this stage the temperature-sensitive spindles are not present and the nuclear material is protected by the pronuclear membrane and survival rates of 70–80% can be anticipated (38–40).

Once thawed, zygotes are usually cultured overnight prior to transfer as it is known that day 1 transfer may be suboptimal (41). Pronuclear-stage cryopreservation is used extensively in countries where the law does not allow culture of more than three embryos beyond the 2PN stage. In most other countries, cryopreservation at this stage is often undertaken for medical reasons, for example, in women at very high risk of ovarian hyperstimulation syndrome or in women undergoing IVF for fertility preservation prior to chemotherapy. Although clinics apply different protocols, if a good number of zygotes have been cryopreserved a number of embryos are often thawed and cultured to day 3 or 5 prior to transfer to aid embryo selection.

In the day 2 embryo, the number of blastomeres appears to be related to the implantation potential of the embryo, those with four cells having a significantly higher implantation rate than those with two cells. On day 3, the data is inconsistent. Studies have shown significantly fewer embryos surviving intact on day 3 compared to day 2 (42,43). However, retrospective studies comparing day 2 and 3 frozen–thawed embryo transfers have shown similar (43) or improved (44) pregnancy rates with day 3 transfer. Comparing 2PN and cleavage stage cumulative pregnancy rates, RCTs have shown conflicting results, one study showing similar pregnancy rates with 2PN or cleavage stage freezing (45), another showing an increase in clinical pregnancy rates in the group randomized to 2PN freezing (38).

Cleavage Stage vs. Blastocyst Freezing

In the context of fresh IVF treatment, it has been shown that blastocyst transfer increases the live birth rate compared to cleavage stage transfer. One consequence of blastocyst transfer is that the number of embryos available for cryopreservation is reduced (46). Historically, blastocysts were cryopreserved using slow freezing techniques. This was generally less successful than zygote or cleavage stage freezing. However, the development of vitrification techniques has radically changed the potential of blastocyst cryopreservation. Post-thaw survival of vitrified blastocysts is in the range of 80–100% (47,48). Clinical pregnancy rates, even from single embryo transfer of frozen–thawed embryos may be as high as 35–40% (49,50). Of course the majority of ART patients will not have supernumerary high quality blastocysts suitable for vitrification and therefore these success rates will only be seen in a small percentage of the overall ART population.

EFFECT OF EMBRYO QUALITY AT THE TIME OF FREEZING

Clinics often have very different protocols determining the quality of embryos they choose to cryopreserve. The policy adopted by an individual clinic as to the threshold of embryo quality they agree to cryopreserve will play a large part in the success rates of their FER cycles. For example, if only top quality blastocysts are cryopreserved, the overall pregnancy rates will be significantly higher than a clinic with a policy of freezing all surplus cleavage stage embryos.

Pronuclear Stage Embryo Quality

Features of 2PN embryos have been suggested as viability markers that may assist in the decision as to which zygotes to freeze (51–54). However, the effectiveness of these criteria has been questioned and most centers, if freezing at 2PN, will cryopreserve all zygotes (55). One study has shown that cryopreserved and fresh 2PN embryos have the same implantation potential (56); however, other authors have shown a decreased implantation potential even when the thawed zygote remained intact (54). Particular morphological features including nucleolar precursor body patterns and the presence of a cytoplasmic halo have been found to correlate most highly with implantation rates in both fresh and frozen cycles (57).

Cleavage Stage Embryo Quality

Evaluation of cleavage stage embryo quality is more reliable than at the 2PN stage because significant variability between embryos is evident at this stage. At the cleavage stage the number and regularity of blastomeres along with the speed of cleavage can be observed. In addition, the appearance of the membrane and cytoplasm, and the level of cellular fragmentation can be assessed. The loss of blastomeres after thawing has been shown to decrease the implantation potential of cleavage stage embryos whilst minimal fragmentation (0–30%) was found to have no effect (58).

Blastocyst Quality

Embryos may reach the blastocysts stage on day 5 or day 6 of development. A number of studies have shown conflicting results as to whether the rate of blastocyst formation affects the treatment outcome. A recent meta-analysis has shown that there is a significant increase in the clinical pregnancy and live birth rate when day 5 rather than day 6 frozen–thawed blastocysts are transferred. However, this difference was no longer seen where the day 5 and day 6 embryos had the same morphological quality (59). Morphological grading of blastocysts is also related to outcome. In a large series of nearly 1500 frozen–thawed embryo transfers, the chance of a clinical pregnancy and live birth was significantly reduced after the transfer of lower morphological quality blastocysts. This was found to be the case in each of the age groups studied (22–33, 34–37, and 38–45 years). Age was also found to be independent of morphological quality as a predictor of pregnancy (60).

ZONA PELLUCIDA BREACHING

It is thought that the process of cryopreservation may cause hardening of the zona pellucida (61) and therefore it has been suggested that assisted hatching may be beneficial in FER cycles. A recent meta-analysis of six RCTs evaluating assisted hatching in FER cycles in non-poor prognosis patients showed that there was a significant increase in the clinical pregnancy rate with the use of assisted hatching (62).

REFREEZING OF THAWED EMBRYOS

There are a number of reports of successful live births after the transfer of embryos that have been frozen and thawed more than once (63). Perinatal outcomes appear to be reassuring (64). Although the routine use of multiple freeze thaws is not recommended because of the potential stress of cryopreservation, it may be of value in particular circumstances. If, for example, embryos have been frozen at 2PN for fertility preservation, the decision may be made to thaw a number of zygotes to try and reach the blastocyst stage. If at the end of this process there are surplus good quality blastocysts, these could be vitrified for future use.

SAFETY AND FOLLOW UP OF CHILDREN BORN AFTER FER CYCLES

The safety of embryo cryopreservation has been questioned. Concerns have been raised regarding its effects on embryonic gene expression, embryo metabolism, as well as the potential negative effects of cryoprotectants (65). There is currently no long-term follow-up data regarding outcomes of children born after either slow freezing or vitrification of embryos. However, with regard to slow-freezing there is no difference in obstetric outcome or congenital malformation comparing frozen or fresh IVF cycles (66). In addition, there is no evidence of an increase in the prevalence of chronic diseases (67). Given that vitrification is a relatively new technique, less data is available. It is essential that continuing long-term follow-up studies of all cryopreservation techniques are carried out.

REFERENCES

1. Nygren KG, Sullivan E, Zegers-Hochschild F, et al. International Committee for Monitoring Assisted Reproductive Technology (ICMART) world report: assisted reproductive technology 2003. Fertil Steril 2011; 95: 2209–22; 22e1–17.
2. Thurin A, Hausken J, Hillensjo T, et al. Elective single-embryo transfer versus double-embryo transfer in in vitro fertilization. N Engl J Med 2004; 351: 2392–402.
3. Tiitinen A, Halttunen M, Harkki P, Vuoristo P, Hyden-Granskog C. Elective single embryo transfer: the value of cryopreservation. Hum Reprod 2001; 16: 1140–4.
4. Pandian Z, Bhattacharya S, Ozturk O, Serour G, Templeton A. Number of embryos for transfer following in-vitro fertilisation or intra-cytoplasmic sperm injection. Cochrane Database Syst Rev 2009; 2: CD003416.
5. McLernon DJ, Harrild K, Bergh C, et al. Clinical effectiveness of elective single versus double embryo transfer: meta-analysis of individual patient data from randomised trials. BMJ 2010; 341: c6945.
6. Csokmay JM, Hill MJ, Chason RJ, et al. Experience with a patient-friendly, mandatory, single-blastocyst transfer policy: the power of one. Fertil Steril 2011; 96: 580–4.
7. Martini S, Van Voorhis BJ, Stegmann BJ, et al. In vitro fertilization patients support a single blastocyst transfer policy. Fertil Steril 2011; 96: 993–7.
8. Haouzi D, Assou S, Dechanet C, et al. Controlled ovarian hyperstimulation for in vitro fertilization alters endometrial receptivity in humans: protocol effects. Biol Reprod 2010; 82: 679–86.
9. Haouzi D, Assou S, Mahmoud K, et al. Gene expression profile of human endometrial receptivity: comparison between natural and stimulated cycles for the same patients. Hum Reprod 2009; 24: 1436–45.
10. Zhu D, Zhang J, Cao S, et al. Vitrified-warmed blastocyst transfer cycles yield higher pregnancy and implantation rates compared with fresh blastocyst transfer cycles—time for a new embryo transfer strategy? Fertil Steril 2011; 95: 1691–5.
11. Shapiro BS, Daneshmand ST, Garner FC, et al. Evidence of impaired endometrial receptivity after ovarian stimulation for in vitro fertilization: a prospective randomized trial comparing fresh and frozen-thawed embryo transfer in normal responders. Fertil Steril 2011; 96: 344–8.
12. Weissman A, Horowitz E, Ravhon A, et al. Spontaneous ovulation versus HCG triggering for timing natural-cycle frozen-thawed embryo transfer: a randomized study. Reprod Biomed Online 2011; 23: 484–9.
13. Fatemi HM, Kyrou D, Bourgain C, et al. Cryopreserved-thawed human embryo transfer: spontaneous natural cycle is superior to human chorionic gonadotropin-induced natural cycle. Fertil Steril 2010; 94: 2054–8.

14. Kyrou D, Fatemi HM, Popovic-Todorovic B, et al. Vaginal progesterone supplementation has no effect on ongoing pregnancy rate in hCG-induced natural frozen-thawed embryo transfer cycles. Eur J Obstet Gynecol Reprod Biol 2010; 150: 175–9.

15. Ghobara T, Vandekerckhove P. Cycle regimens for frozen-thawed embryo transfer. Cochrane Database Syst Rev 2008; 1: CD003414.

16. El-Toukhy T, Taylor A, Khalaf Y, et al. Pituitary suppression in ultrasound-monitored frozen embryo replacement cycles. A randomised study. Hum Reprod 2004; 19: 874–9.

17. Lightman A, Kol S, Itskovitz-Eldor J. A prospective randomized study comparing intramuscular with intravaginal natural progesterone in programmed thaw cycles. Hum Reprod 1999; 14: 2596–9.

18. Lan VT, Tuan PH, Canh LT, Tuong HM, Howles CM. Progesterone supplementation during cryopreserved embryo transfer cycles: efficacy and convenience of two vaginal formulations. Reprod Biomed Online 2008; 17: 318–23.

19. Nawroth F, Ludwig M. What is the 'ideal' duration of progesterone supplementation before the transfer of cryopreserved-thawed embryos in estrogen/progesterone replacement protocols? Hum Reprod 2005; 20: 1127–34.

20. Lelaidier C, de Ziegler D, Freitas S, et al. Endometrium preparation with exogenous estradiol and progesterone for the transfer of cryopreserved blastocysts. Fertil Steril 1995; 63: 919–21.

21. Ben-Meir A, Aboo-Dia M, Revel A, et al. The benefit of human chorionic gonadotropin supplementation throughout the secretory phase of frozen-thawed embryo transfer cycles. Fertil Steril 2010; 93: 351–4.

22. Bider D, Amoday I, Yonesh M, et al. Glucocorticoid administration during transfer of frozen-thawed embryos: a prospective, randomized study. Fertil Steril 1996; 66: 154–6.

23. Moffitt D, Queenan JT Jr, Veeck LL, et al. Low-dose glucocorticoids after in vitro fertilization and embryo transfer have no significant effect on pregnancy rate. Fertil Steril 1995; 63: 571–7.

24. Morozov V, Ruman J, Kenigsberg D, Moodie G, Brenner S. Natural cycle cryo-thaw transfer may improve pregnancy outcome. J Assist Reprod Genet 2007; 24: 119–23.

25. Loh SK, Leong NK. Factors affecting success in an embryo cryopreservation programme. Ann Acad Med Singapore 1999; 28: 260–5.

26. Cattoli M, Ciotti PM, Seracchioli R, et al. A randomized prospective study on cryopreserved-thawed embryo transfer: natural verses hormone replacement cycles. Abstracts of the 10th Annual Meeting of ESHRE. Brussels 1994; 5: 956–60.

27. Gelbaya TA, Nardo LG, Hunter HR, et al. Cryopreserved-thawed embryo transfer in natural or down-regulated hormonally controlled cycles: a retrospective study. Fertil Steril 2006; 85: 603–9.

28. Queenan JT Jr, Veeck LL, Seltman HJ, Muasher SJ. Transfer of cryopreserved-thawed pre-embryos in a natural cycle or a programmed cycle with exogenous hormonal replacement yields similar pregnancy results. Fertil Steril 1994; 62: 545–50.

29. Wright KP, Guibert J, Weitzen S, et al. Artificial versus stimulated cycles for endometrial preparation prior to frozen-thawed embryo transfer. Reprod Biomed Online 2006; 13: 321–5.

30. Loh SKE, Ganesan G, Leong NK. Clomid verses hormone endometrial preperation in FET cycles. Abstract book of the 17th World Congress in Fertility and Sterility (IFFS). Melbourne, Australia, 25–30 November 2001: 3. 2001.

31. Coroleu B, Barri PN, Carreras O, et al. The usefulness of ultrasound guidance in frozen-thawed embryo transfer: a prospective randomized clinical trial. Hum Reprod 2002; 17: 2885–90.

32. Brown J, Buckingham K, Abou-Setta AM, Buckett W. Ultrasound versus 'clinical touch' for catheter guidance during embryo transfer in women. Cochrane Database Syst Rev 2010; 1: CD006107.

33. Check JH, Dietterich C, Graziano V, Lurie D, Choe JK. Effect of maximal endometrial thickness on outcome after frozen embryo transfer. Fertil Steril 2004; 81: 1399–400.

34. Coulam CB, Bustillo M, Soenksen DM, Britten S. Ultrasonographic predictors of implantation after assisted reproduction. Fertil Steril 1994; 62: 1004–10.

35. El-Toukhy T, Coomarasamy A, Khairy M, et al. The relationship between endometrial thickness and outcome of medicated frozen embryo replacement cycles. Fertil Steril 2008; 89: 832–9.

36. Ng EH, Chan CC, Tang OS, Yeung WS, Ho PC. The role of endometrial and subendometrial vascularity measured by three-dimensional power Doppler ultrasound in the prediction of pregnancy during frozen-thawed embryo transfer cycles. Hum Reprod 2006; 21: 1612–17.

37. Check JH, Dietterich C, Nazari A, et al. Non-homogeneous hyperechogenic echo pattern three days after frozen embryo transfer is associated with lower pregnancy rates. Clin Exp Obstet Gynecol 2005; 32: 15–18.

38. Senn A, Vozzi C, Chanson A, De Grandi P, Germond M. Prospective randomized study of two cryopreservation policies avoiding embryo selection: the pronucleate stage leads to a higher cumulative delivery rate than the early cleavage stage. Fertil Steril 2000; 74: 946–52.

39. Veeck LL. Does the developmental stage at freeze impact on clinical results post-thaw? Reprod Biomed Online 2003; 6: 367–74.

40. Queenan JT Jr, Veeck LL, Toner JP, Oehninger S, Muasher SJ. Cryopreservation of all prezygotes in patients at risk of severe hyperstimulation does not eliminate the syndrome, but the chances of pregnancy are excellent with subsequent frozen-thaw transfers. Hum Reprod 1997; 12: 1573–6.

41. Jaroudi K, Al-Hassan S, Sieck U, et al. Zygote transfer on day 1 versus cleavage stage embryo transfer on day 3: a prospective randomized trial. Hum Reprod 2004; 19: 645–8.

42. Hartshorne GM, Wick K, Elder K, Dyson H. Effect of cell number at freezing upon survival and viability of cleaving embryos generated from stimulated IVF cycles. Hum Reprod 1990; 5: 857–61.

43. Salumets A, Tuuri T, Makinen S, et al. Effect of developmental stage of embryo at freezing on pregnancy outcome of frozen-thawed embryo transfer. Hum Reprod 2003; 18: 1890–5.

44. Sifer C, Sellami A, Poncelet C, et al. Day 3 compared with day 2 cryopreservation does not affect embryo survival but improves the outcome of frozen-thawed embryo transfers. Fertil Steril 2006; 86: 1537–40.

45. Horne G, Critchlow JD, Newman MC, et al. A prospective evaluation of cryopreservation strategies in a two-embryo transfer programme. Hum Reprod 1997; 12: 542–7.

46. Blake DA, Farquhar CM, Johnson N, Proctor M. Cleavage stage versus blastocyst stage embryo transfer in assisted conception. Cochrane Database Syst Rev 2007; 4: CD002118.

47. Kader AA, Choi A, Orief Y, Agarwal A. Factors affecting the outcome of human blastocyst vitrification. Reprod Biol Endocrinol 2009; 7: 99.

48. Youssry M, Ozmen B, Zohni K, Diedrich K, Al-Hasani S. Current aspects of blastocyst cryopreservation. Reproductive BioMedicine Online 2008; 16: 311–20.

49. Berin I, McLellan ST, Macklin EA, Toth TL, Wright DL. Frozen-thawed embryo transfer cycles: clinical outcomes of single and double blastocyst transfers. J Assist Reprod Genet 2011; 28: 575–81.

50. Yanaihara A, Yorimitsu T, Motoyama H, Ohara M, Kawamura T. Clinical outcome of frozen blastocyst transfer; single vs. double transfer. J Assist Reprod Genet 2008; 25: 531–4.

51. Scott LA, Smith S. The successful use of pronuclear embryo transfers the day following oocyte retrieval. Hum Reprod 1998; 13: 1003–13.

52. Garello C, Baker H, Rai J, et al. Pronuclear orientation, polar body placement, and embryo quality after intracytoplasmic sperm injection and in-vitro fertilization: further evidence for polarity in human oocytes? Hum Reprod 1999; 14: 2588–95.

53. Tesarik J, Greco E. The probability of abnormal preimplantation development can be predicted by a single static observation on pronuclear stage morphology. Hum Reprod 1999; 14: 1318–23.

54. Hammitt DG, Sattler CA, Manes ML, Singh AP. Selection of embryos for day-3 transfer at the pronuclear-stage and pronuclear-stage cryopreservation results in high delivery rates in fresh and frozen cycles. J Assist Reprod Genet 2004; 21: 271–8.

55. James AN, Hennessy S, Reggio B, et al. The limited importance of pronuclear scoring of human zygotes. Hum Reprod 2006; 21: 1599–604.

56. Miller KF, Goldberg JM. In vitro development and implantation rates of fresh and cryopreserved sibling zygotes. Obstet Gynecol 1995; 85: 999–1002.

57. Senn A, Urner F, Chanson A, et al. Morphological scoring of human pronuclear zygotes for prediction of pregnancy outcome. Hum Reprod 2006; 21: 234–9.

58. Edgar DH, Bourne H, Jericho H, McBain JC. The developmental potential of cryopreserved human embryos. Mol Cell Endocrinol 2000; 169: 69–72.

59. Sunkara SK, Siozos A, Bolton VN, et al. The influence of delayed blastocyst formation on the outcome of frozen-thawed blastocyst transfer: a systematic review and meta-analysis. Hum Reprod 2010; 25: 1906–15.

60. Goto S, Kadowaki T, Tanaka S, et al. Prediction of pregnancy rate by blastocyst morphological score and age, based on 1,488 single frozen-thawed blastocyst transfer cycles. Fertil Steril 2011; 95: 948–52.

61. Carroll J, Depypere H, Matthews CD. Freeze-thaw-induced changes of the zona pellucida explains decreased rates of fertilization in frozen-thawed mouse oocytes. J Reprod Fertil 1990; 90: 547–53.

62. Martins WP, Rocha IA, Ferriani RA, Nastri CO. Assisted hatching of human embryos: a systematic review and meta-analysis of randomized controlled trials. Hum Reprod Update 2011; 17: 438–53.

63. Kumasako Y, Otsu E, Utsunomiya T, Araki Y. The efficacy of the transfer of twice frozen-thawed embryos with the vitrification method. Fertil Steril 2009; 91: 383–6.

64. Murakami M, Egashira A, Murakami K, Araki Y, Kuramoto T. Perinatal outcome of twice-frozen-thawed embryo transfers: a clinical follow-up study. Fertil Steril 2011; 95: 2648–50.

65. Winston RM, Hardy K. Are we ignoring potential dangers of in vitro fertilization and related treatments? Nat Cell Biol 2002; (4 Suppl): s14–18.

66. Wennerholm UB, Soderstrom-Anttila V, Bergh C, et al. Children born after cryopreservation of embryos or oocytes: a systematic review of outcome data. Hum Reprod 2009; 24: 2158–72.

67. Wennerholm UB, Albertsson-Wikland K, Bergh C, et al. Postnatal growth and health in children born after cryopreservation as embryos. Lancet 1998; 351: 1085–90.

53

Anesthesia and in vitro fertilization

Shmuel Evron and Tiberiu Ezri

INTRODUCTION

Transvaginal ultrasound-guided oocyte aspiration is a major step for successful in vitro fertilization (IVF) process. Although considered a minor surgical procedure, it might be very painful and associated with fear and anxiety (1). Pain is naturally subjective and intermittent in character (2); therefore, it is difficult to assess efficacy of various techniques for analgesia. The pain is caused by punctures and traction on the vaginal wall, ovarian capsule, and ligaments. In the last decade, there has been a great worldwide expansion of the assisted reproductive techniques (ART). According to the Society of Assisted Reproductive Technique (SART) 2009 report, a total of 142,241 IVF cycles were performed in the United States (3). The European Society of Human Reproduction and Embryology (ESHRE) has reported on 367,000 IVF procedures performed in Europe in 2004 (4).

In the past, oocyte retrieval was done laparoscopically with general anesthesia requiring a hospital setting. Pregnancy rates in the laparoscopy era were low as compared to present techniques (5). Development of ultrasonic-guided oocyte aspiration and newer anesthetic techniques and drugs allowed the performance of this procedure outside the hospital and under different modes of anesthesia, other than general, and without the obligatory presence of an anesthesiologist, radically reducing the cost of the procedure. There are many effective analgesic options available today with consideration of patient safety and comfort, fast postoperative recovery, and successful outcome of the entire IVF procedure. The analgesic agent should be potent, short acting, easy to administer, nontoxic, and inexpensive. However, there has always been a concern regarding the potential adverse effects of analgesic agents on embryonic development and reproductive outcome (6–9).

The anesthetic options available today for the transvaginal ultrasound-guided oocyte retrieval (TUGOR) are conscious sedation and local anesthesia, epidural, spinal, and general anesthesia; and acupuncture which has been gaining more acceptance currently (10). The most commonly used method is conscious sedation that provides analgesia, sedation, and amnesia and enables full patient cooperation. According to the Cochrane review of 2010 (11), conscious sedation is used in 84% of IVF clinics in the United Kingdom (12) and in 95% of IVF clinics

in the United States (13). Another survey from the United Kingdom (14) showed that 48% of IVF clinics used conscious sedation, 29% general anesthesia, 12% sedation with regional anesthesia, and 2% used regional anesthesia. The current standard of care for the various methods of pain relief has not been defined. This was shown by a recent Cochrane review (11) identifying 390 reports of which only 12 papers were included. It was concluded that no one particular pain relief method or delivery system appeared advantageous over the other and no significant differences were found in regard to pregnancy rate or patient satisfaction.

ANESTHETIC TECHNIQUE FOR OOCYTE RETRIEVAL

Conscious Sedation

With this technique, patient consciousness is minimally depressed, and the patient is able to respond to verbal commands and cooperate (15) while receiving appropriate analgesia and some form of amnesia with patent airway throughout the surgical process. The drugs used are easily delivered, well tolerated with minimal immediate or long-term side effects, when dispensed properly, especially in motivated and cooperative patients (13). The margin of safety of these drugs should be wide enough to render loss of consciousness unlikely (16). To cope with changing patient requirements for pain relief, a patient controlled analgesia (PCA) device has been developed, which facilitates a patient's degree of control over pain relief, with increased satisfaction (17). This technique may not be appropriate for patient with marked obesity or underlying cardiorespiratory diseases. Conscious sedation is a widely accepted technique. It is used in 95% of IVF clinics in the United States (13), 84% of IVF clinics in the United Kingdom, (12) and 50% of the IVF centers in Germany (18). Additional techniques practiced in the United States as reported (13) by SART include: general anesthesia, regional and local anesthesia (which require personnel trained in anesthesia). The most popular agent used is propofol or its combination with midazolam and fentanyl. Personnel not trained in anesthesia preferred the midazolam–meperidine combination. The complication rate and recovery time for both groups was similar (90–120 minutes), but the cost of drugs used by anesthesiologists was higher. Monitoring of the patient's condition during conscious sedation should include the standard American Society of Anesthesiology (ASA) monitors to record blood pressure, heart rate, oxygen saturation, heart electrical activity (electrocardiogram), end tidal CO_2 and respiratory rate.

Administration of conscious sedation should be started only after obtaining verbal and written patient consent. Peripheral venous cannulation is performed, and the patient is connected to the standard ASA monitors. According to Ditkoff et al. (13), the non-anesthesiologists providing sedation for IVF mainly used meperidine and midazolam, while 90% of the anesthesiologists preferred using midazolam and/or propofol plus fentanyl. To prevent the local burning sensation caused by propofol injection, pretreatment of 1 mg/kg lidocaine administration may be helpful. For achievement of pain control during the transvaginal ovarian puncture and for postoperative analgesia (preemptive analgesia), fentanyl has to be administered before the beginning of the noxious stimulus in repetitive boluses of 25 mcg up to a total dose of 50–100 mcg (19). With completion of the surgical procedure, all drug boluses and infusions are stopped leading to patient recovery in a few minutes. Careful standard ASA monitoring of such patients by an experienced anesthesiologist is paramount for patient safety and assistance in accomplishing the surgical procedure.

A Cochrane review published in 2010 (11) assessed the efficacy of conscious sedation and analgesia versus alternative methods on pregnancy outcomes and pain relief. Out of 390 eligible papers, only 12 met the selection criteria (randomized controlled trials; RCTs). There were no significant differences in the pregnancy rate or patient satisfaction. There were conflicting results concerning pain sensation and treatment due to methodological variability in terms of anesthesia mode or the dose and type of the drug used. Therefore, a meta-analysis was not done. In terms of pregnancy rate, three trials compared alfentanil (opioid) IV conscious sedation plus paracervical block (PCB) with electroacupuncture (EA) plus PCB (20–22).

Intraoperative pain control was assessed in 11 trials and postoperative pain control in five trials (23). Patients who received sedation in addition to PCB reported lower pain scores, as compared to those who received PCB with placebo. The response to pain in oocyte retrieval during conscious sedation was higher when compared to general anesthesia, but postoperative abdominal pain was significantly lower in the sedation group than in the general anesthesia group (24). Four trials have compared the intraoperative pain control with sedatives/analgesics administered by patient controlled analgesia (PCA), as compared with physician-controlled administration (11). Less pain perception was reported by patients in the physician-controlled group. When comparing pain perception during needle puncture under conscious sedation versus placebo group (25), there was a significant greater pain perception in the placebo group. Lok et al. (26), in an RCT, compared the fertility outcomes and anesthetic parameters in two groups – a PCA group, who received propofol with alfentanil, and a second

patient group, who received intravenous pethidine with diazepam, plus additional doses of pethidine administered by the anesthesiologist. Levels of sedation, cooperation, and fertility outcomes were similar. Pain scores were higher throughout the procedure in the PCA group, although their future preference for this mode of analgesia was higher. Recently, Edwards et al. (27) reported on 4342 patients in the United Kingdom who were administered propofol TCI – target controlled infusion and alfentanil boluses by non-anesthetists during oocyte retrieval. The nonphysician sedationists were specially trained by an institutional program to deliver sedation. No episode of transient apnea occurred, although direct anesthesiologist assistance was necessary in 15 occasions. In only 1% of patients was the procedure unpleasant.

Complications of conscious sedation

In the 2006 Cochrane review (23), no serious adverse effects or oocyte retrieval procedure cancellations were reported. The rate of postoperative nausea and vomiting was similar in all conscious sedation groups. In another trial (28) that compared propofol with midazolam, two patients in the propofol group were unable to complete the study. One patient fainted when sitting up, and the other did not respond after additive alfentanil administration.

Drugs Used in Conscious Sedation

Midazolam (a benzodiazepine) is probably the most commonly used drug in conscious sedation because of its sedative and anxiolytic effects (29). Additionally, it has anticonvulsant, amnesic (anterograde amnesia), and mild muscle relaxation effects. When combined with opioids, mainly fentanyl, the synergistic effect may enhance sedation, perhaps leading to respiratory depression or even apnea; therefore, reduced doses of both drugs are mandatory. Although minimal concentrations are found in the follicular fluid, it has no detrimental effects on fertilization in animal or human studies (30–32). All adverse effects can be reversed by Anexate (flumazenil).

Opioids (meperidine, fentanyl, alfentanil, and remifentanil) are narcotic agents widely used for general anesthesia and conscious sedation, mainly for their potent analgesic effect. Remifentanil is a potent synthetic opioid with fast action and short elimination time and is known for its ease of administration because of its flexibility during general anesthesia and conscious sedation (33,34). In high doses or rapid administration, opioids may cause respiratory depression, bradycardia, and muscle rigidity. Apnea or stiff chest may necessitate manual ventilation or administration of naloxone or succinylcholine for muscle relaxation followed by tracheal intubation. Other opioids' adverse effects are nausea, vomiting, and pruritus. As mentioned above, they have a synergistic effect when combined with benzodiazepines, which necessitates a reduction of the administered doses. All adverse effects can be reversed by naloxone administration.

Propofol is a useful induction and analgesic agent with fast onset and short elimination time (27). It is used for general anesthesia and conscious sedation (27). Its administration is associated with decreased postoperative nausea and vomiting, especially when used alone. When administered through a peripheral vein it causes local burning pain. To mitigate this effect, a prior injection of intravenous lidocaine and slow administration of propofol may relieve this discomfort. Egg allergy is a contraindication to its administration. The use of propofol in conscious sedation for oocyte retrieval necessitates an anesthesiologist or personnel skilled in airway management (27); in dose-dependent administration, it may cause respiratory and myocardial depression. The use of propofol in combination with fentanyl or alfentanil in such a setting was found to be beneficial (35). The amount of propofol recovered in the follicular fluid is dose-dependent (9,36). When compared with thiopental administration, there were no differences regarding fertilization, cleavage, implantation, or abortion rates (37,38).

Ketamine is an old induction agent used in general anesthesia and as a sedative and analgesic agent in conscious sedation. It belongs to the phencyclidine family of drugs which cause, through their central neurological action, dissociative anesthesia (a cataleptic condition with patient eyes open with slow nystagmic gaze). It was considered an ideal anesthetic agent due to several properties required for general anesthesia, such as analgesia, loss of consciousness, and anterograde amnesia without depressant effects on the cardiorespiratory systems or the laryngeal reflexes. However, this drug has not became widely popular because of postoperative psychological adverse effects in 5–30% of the patients, such as illusions, vivid dreaming, and feelings of excitement or fear that may last for several hours (39). When combined with midazolam, it was found to be a good alternative to general anesthesia with propofol and midazolam in a prospective trial involving 50 women (24). The results measured included pregnancy outcomes, postoperative pain perception, and patient satisfaction. Another laboratory finding, associated with ketamine administration and with unclear impact on IVF, was an increase of prolactin and beta-endorphin levels (40).

General Anesthesia

General anesthesia (GA) is the second most common technique for transvaginal oocyte retrieval and the most common technique for laparoscopic zygote or gamete intrafallopian transfer (ZIFT/GIFT) (41). In the early days of ART, it was considered the technique of choice (24,42). General anesthesia is induced and maintained in a hospital setting by specially trained personnel using either intravenous or inhalational agents. The intravenous agents include rapid induction ones, narcotics, and sedatives. The inhalational gases include nitrous oxide (N_2O) and vapors of volatile liquids, such as isoflurane, desflurane, and sevoflurane. Ventilation during GA can be maintained as spontaneous ventilation through face mask or laryngeal mask airway or may necessitate mechanical ventilation through endotracheal tube or laryngeal mask airway. Drawbacks of GA are prolonged recovery, drowsiness, nausea, and vomiting and possible detrimental effects on reproduction. Early studies reported detrimental effects of GA on fertilization and cleavage rate (43–45). Studies using halogenated fluorocarbons with nitrous oxide showed decreased fertilization and number of oocytes collected (46). Vincent et al. (47) showed that administration of propofol with N_2O was associated with lower pregnancy rate when compared with isoflurane for laparoscopic pronuclear stage transfer (PROST).

Administration of opioids during GA was shown to have many advantages (41). The combination of propofol with remifentanil or isoflurane was associated with higher oocyte retrieval rates than sedation with midazolam, diazepam, or propofol. Also, with the ease of GA, more oocytes can be retrieved, including immature oocytes from small follicules, with a lower fertilization rate. The use of isoflurane has been shown to inhibit mouse embryo development contrary to the use of GA with nitrous oxide and narcotics (26). When comparing fertilization and cleavage rates of mature oocytes following GA versus intravenous sedation, there were no significant differences in the first or last collected oocytes. Since there was a trend toward lower fertilization rate with prolonged GA drugs (46), the recommendation, therefore, was to minimize anesthetic drug exposure (36). Our personal experience in anesthesia for TUGOR (unpublished data) includes 1500 patients, who were given balanced GA (without premedication), with a preinduction dose of 1 mg of midazolam or 20 mg propofol followed by 50 mcg of fentanyl, keeping spontaneous ventilation with face mask and anesthesia maintenance with 50% O_2/N_2O inhalation with repetitive doses of 20–40 mg propofol. Postoperative analgesia is provided with nonsteroidal anti-inflammatory medications (NSAIDs) until discharge from hospital within one to two hours.

Drugs Used in General Anesthesia

Drugs used in general anesthesia that have been mentioned already include: propofol, ketamine, opioids, benzodiazepines, and volatile gases. The use of nitrous oxide (N_2O) for sedation or general anesthesia is controversial as it inactivates methionine synthetase, diminishing the amount of thymidine needed for DNA production and so becoming deleterious on mouse embryos (48) and human pregnancy outcomes (49). Another study (31) had not shown such detrimental effects on IVF outcomes. It was speculated that the inactivation of methionine synthetase progressed slowly in the human liver reducing the N_2O effects, and additionally, its low solubility, short exposure time, and the transfer of oocytes to a rich O_2/CO_2 media also minimized these harmful effects (50).

Regional Anesthesia

Regional or neuraxial anesthesia is an effective method used for TUGOR. This can be achieved by injection of local anesthetics into the epidural or spinal space. With the use of different doses and in various patient positions, the specific region to be anesthetized, i.e., the vaginal wall and/or pelvic floor can be chosen, but not affecting the lower extremities. Neuraxial anesthesia has the advantage of minimal local anesthetic absorption, and therefore, minimal follicular accumulation (51).

When compared with intravenous sedation using propofol and nitrous oxide, no advantages have been shown (52). Epidural anesthesia has been shown to be effective and safe for the GIFT procedure (53). Adverse effects of epidural anesthesia are spinal headache, urinary retention, and accidental intravascular injection of local anesthetics. A high spinal block can cause respiratory depression. Local infection, coagulopathy, increased intracranial pressure, and patient refusal are contraindications for epidural or spinal anesthesia. Spinal anesthesia was used in the past for laparoscopic oocyte retrieval (54) and for TUGOR (55). Tsen et al. (56) compared the effects of an additional 25 mcg of fentanyl to bupivacaine or lidocaine intraspinal administration. In the bupivacaine group, the time to discharge and first micturition was 30 minutes longer.

PCB is another mode of regional anesthesia accomplished by local anesthetic (150–200 mg of lidocaine) injection in both sides of the cervical os below the entrance of the uterine artery branches (57). Three RCTs have compared the effects of PCB when combined with conventional analgesics to PCB plus electroacupuncture (20–22). There were no significant differences regarding clinical pregnancy rates but the intraoperative analgesic scores were lower in the group with conventional analgesics with PCB.

Alternative and Non-Pharmacological Anesthesia

Acupuncture has a prominent place in Chinese medicine since thousands of years and it has garnered a growing awareness in the western countries as a modality for successful treatment in chronic pain, nausea and vomiting, fibromyalgia, and drug addiction (58,59) and is increasingly used as an adjunct in fertility treatment and pregnancy. As to the mechanism of action, there are no consistent or comprehensive explanations and sometimes only the Chinese medical theory can be appreciated. Acupuncture has been shown to increase the endorphin and cortical activity (58,60). It has a central sympatholytic activity and may contribute to the decrease of uterine artery impedance and the increase of uterine blood flow (61) and myometrial activity (62) which, in turn, may explain the increased rate of implantation that was reported in several studies. However, although consumer demand is increasing, to endorse this modality of treatment in general medical practice, properly conducted studies with standardization of the method should be carried out.

Paules et al. (63), in a RCT compared a group of patients receiving acupuncture treatment shortly before and after embryo transfer with a control group receiving no acupuncture. An increased clinical pregnancy rate in the acupuncture group was observed (42.5% vs. 26.3%, p = 0.03). Stener-Victorin et al. (20) have compared in a RCT, patients undergoing IVF using electroacupuncture (needles inserted into the abdominal muscles and forearm) versus intravenous alfentanil, both groups receiving PCB. There were no significant differences with regard to pain perception or nausea. The acupuncture group had significantly higher pregnancy, implantation, and take-home-baby rates. Auricular electroacupuncture has proven to be effective by reducing analgesic requirement during IVF treatment (64,65).

Three meta-analyses have now been published concerning the effects of acupuncture on IVF outcome (66–68). The meta-analysis published by Manheimer et al. (66) indicated that acupuncture at the time of embryo transfer improved the clinical pregnancy rates. In the other two meta-analyses (67,68), no beneficial effects of acupuncture had been shown on clinical pregnancy rate or live birth rates. The authors of all meta-analyses indicated bias effects as a result of the heterogeneity of the trials reviewed, the use of sham acupuncture (use of non-selected points) as control or lack of control, the timing of acupuncture use, and the heterogeneity of procedures. However, acupuncture is devoid of toxicity and may be appropriate in view of a patient's intolerance or contraindication for conventional anesthesia.

CONCLUSION

Anesthesia or sedation for oocyte retrieval are relatively safe although they cannot be provided in a state-of-the-art manner without trained anesthesia personnel. The anesthetic agents must be short acting and easy to administer and have minimal side effects and little penetration to the follicle without detrimental effect on the oocyte or the implantation. The majority of anesthetic agents are safe. There is a controversy with the use of nitrous oxide and inhalatory agents. There is as yet insufficient evidence to determine the effect of various methods of pain relief when compared with conscious sedation and analgesia used during oocyte retrieval. Future studies are needed using standardized practices and policies to determine pain assessment, timing of drug administration, and evaluation of perioperative complications, such as respiratory and cardiovascular adverse effects.

REFERENCES

1. Tang J, Gibson SJ. A psychophysical evaluation of the relationship between trait anxiety, pain perception, and induced state anxiety. J Pain 2005; 6: 612–19.
2. Zelcer J, White PF, Chester S, et al. Intraoperative patient-controlled analgesia: an alternative to physician administration during outpatient monitored anesthesia care. Anesth Analg 1992; 75: 41–4.

3. Clinical summary report. SART member clinics, 2009. [cited 2011 May 31]; [about __PM/AM]. [Available from: https://www.sartcorsonline.com/rptCSR_PublicMult-Year.ASPX?ClinicPKID=0]

4. Andersen AN, Goossens V, Ferraretti AP, et al. Assisted reproductive technology in Europe, 2004: results generated from European registers by ESHRE. Hum Reprod 2008; 23: 756–71.

5. Tanbo T, Henriksen T, Magnus O, Abyholm T. Oocyte retrieval in an IVF program. A comparison of laparoscopy and vaginal ultrasound-guided follicular puncture. Acta Obstet Gynecol Scand 1988; 67: 243–6.

6. Wikland M, Evers H, Jacobsson AH, et al. The concentration of lidocaine in follicular fluid when used for paracervical block in a human IVF-ET programme. Hum Reprod 1990; 5: 920–3.

7. Coetsier T, Dhont M, DeSutter P, et al. Propofol anesthesia for ultrasound guided oocyte retrieval: accumulation of the anesthetic agent in follicular fluid. Hum Reprod 1992; 7: 1422–4.

8. Soussis I, Boyd O, Paraschos T, et al. Follicular fluid levels of midazolam, fentanyl, and alfentanil during transvaginal oocyte retrieval. Fertil Steril 1995; 64: 1003–7.

9. Christians F, Janssenswillen C, Verborgh C, et al. Propofol concentration in follicular liquid during general anesthesia for transvaginal oocyte retrieval. Hum Reprod 1999; 14: 345–8.

10. Rowe T. Acupuncture and reproduction. J Obstet Gynaecol Can 2010; 32: 1023–4.

11. Kwan I, Bhattacharya S, Knox F, McNeil A. The cochrane collaboration. conscious sedation and analgesia for oocyte retrieval during in vitro fertilization procedures (review). Cochrane Libr 2010; 11: 1–25.

12. Elkington NM, Kehoe J, Acharya U. Intravenous sedation in assisted conception unit: a UK survey. Hum Fertil 2003; 6: 74–6.

13. Ditkoff EC, Plumb J, Selick A, Sauer MV. Anesthesia practices in the United States common to in vitro fertilization (IVF) centers. J Assist Reprod Genet 1997; 14: 145–7.

14. Bokhari A, Pollard BJ. Anaesthesia for assisted conception: a survey of UK practice. Eur J Anaesthesiol 1999; 16: 225–230.

15. White DC. Anaesthesia: a privation of the senses. In: Rosen M, Lunn JN, eds. Conscious Awareness and Pain in General Anaesthesia. London: Butterworth, 1987: 5.

16. Skelly AM. Analgesia and sedation. In: Watkinson A, Adams A, eds. Interventional Radiology. Oxford: Radcliffe Medical Press, 1996: 3–11.

17. Dell RG, Cloote AH. Patient-controlled sedation during transvaginal oocyte retrieval: an assessment of patient acceptance of patient-controlled sedation using a mixture of propofol and alfentanil. Eur J Anaesthesiol 1998; 15: 210–15.

18. Rjosk HK, Haeske-Seeberg H, Seeberg B, Kreuzer E. IVF and GIFT. Brgebnisse in Deuchland 1993. Fertilitaet 1995; 11: 48–54; German.

19. Dershwitz M. Intravenous and inhalation anesthetics. In: William HE, ed. Clinical Anesthesia Procedures of the Massachusetts General Hospital. 6th edn. Philadelphia: Lippinkott Williams and Wilkins, 2002: 156–8.

20. Stener-Victorin E, Waldenstrom U, Nilsson L, et al. A prospective randomized study of electro-acupuncture versus alfentanil as anaesthesia during oocyte aspiration in in-vitro fertilization. Hum Reprod 1999; 14: 2480–4.

21. Stener-Victorin E, Waldenstrom U, Wikland M, et al. Electro-acupuncture as a peroperative analgesic and its effect on implantation rate and neuropeptide Y concentrations in follicular fluid. Hum Reprod 2003; 18: 1454–60.

22. Humaidan P, Stener-Victorin E. Pain relief during oocyte retrieval with a new short duration electro-acupuncture technique – an alternative to conventional analgesic methods. Hum Reprod 2004; 19: 1367–72.

23. Kwan I, Bhattacharya S, Knox F, McNeil A. Conscious sedation and analgesia for oocyte retrieval during IVF procedures: a cochrane review. Hum Reprod 2006; 21: 1962–79.

24. Ben-Shlomo I, Moskovich R, Katz Y, Shalev E. Midazolam/ketamine sedative combination compared with fentanyl/propofol/isoflurane anaesthesia for oocyte retrieval. Hum Reprod 1999; 14: 1757–9.

25. Ramsewak SS, Kumar A, Welsby R, et al. Is analgesia required for transvaginal single – follicle in in vitro fertilization? a double-blind study. J In Vitro Fertil Embryo Transf 1990; 7: 103–6.

26. Lok IH, Chan MT, Chan DL, et al. A prospective randomized trial comparing patient-controlled sedation using propofol and alfentanil and physician-administered sedation using diazepam and pethidine during transvaginal ultrasound-guided oocyte retrieval. Hum Reprod 2002; 17: 2101–6.

27. Edwards JA, Kinsella J, Shaw A, et al. Sedation for oocyte retrieval using target controlled infusion of propofol and incremental alfentanil delivered by nonanesthetists. Anaesthesia 2010; 65: 453–61.

28. Cook LB, Lockwood GG, Moore CM, Whitman JC. True patient-controlled sedation. Anaesthesia 1993; 48: 1039–44.

29. Trout S, Vallerand A, Kemmann E. Conscious sedation for in vitro fertilization. Fertil Steril 1998; 69: 799–808.

30. Swanson R, Leavitt M. Fertilization and mouse embryo development in the presence of midazolam. Anesth Analg 1992; 74: 549–54.

31. Schell VL, Ataya G, Sacco A, et al. Midazolam at physiological levels does not adversely affect mouse in vitro fertilization, embryo development and cleavage rate. [Abstract]. Proc 45th Meeting of the American Fertility Society. San Francisco, CA; Birmingham, Al, American Fertility Society; 11-16 November 1989; 109.

32. Chapineau J, Brazin JE, Terrisse MP, et al. Assay for midazolam in liquor folliculi during in vitro fertilization under anesthesia. Clin Pharm 1993; 12: 770–3.

33. Hammadeh M, Wilhelm W, Huppert A, et al. Effects of general anaesthesia vs. sedation on fertilization cleavage and pregnancy rates in an IVF program. Arch Gynecol Obstet 1999; 203: 56–9.

34. Arndt M, Kreienmeyer J, Vagts DA, Noldge-Schomburg GH. Remifentanil Analgesia for aspiration of follicles for oocyte retrieval. Anaesthesiol Reanim 2004; 29: 69–73; German.

35. Elkington N, Kehoe J, Acharya U. Recommendations for good practice for sedation in assisted conception. Hum Fertil (Camb) 2003; 6: 77–88.

36. Coetsier T, Dhont M, De Sutter P, et al. Propofol anaesthesia for ultrasound-guided oocyte retrieval: accumulation of the anaesthetic agent in follicular fluid. Hum Reprod 1992; 7: 1422–4.

37. Ben Shlomo I, Moskovich R, Golan J, et al. The effect of propofol anaesthesia on oocyte fertilization and early embryo quality. Hum Reprod 2000; 15: 2197–9.

38. Huang HW, Huang FJ, Kung F, et al. Effects of induction anesthetic agents on outcome of assisted reproductive technology: a comparison of propofol and thiopental sodium. Chang Gung Med J 2000; 23: 513–19.

39. Garfield JM, Garfield FB, Stone JG, et al. A comparison of psychologic responses to ketamine and thiopental-nitrous oxide-halothane anesthesia. Anesthesiology 1972; 36: 329–38.

40. Sterzik K, Nitsch CD, Korda P, et al. The effect of different anesthetic procedures on hormone levels in women. Studies during an in vitro fertilization-embryo transfer (IVF-ER) program. Anaesthesist 1994; 43: 738–42; German.

41. Jennings J, Moreland K, Petersen CM. In vitro fertilisation: a review of drug therapy and clinical management. Drugs 1996; 52: 313–43.

42. Christians F, Janssenswillen C, Van Steirteghem AC, et al. Comparison of assisted reproductive technology performance after oocyte retrieval under general anaesthesia (propofol) versus paracervical local anaesthesia block: a case-controlled study. Hum Reprod 1998; 13: 2456–60.

43. van der Ven H, Dietrich K, Al-Hasani S, et al. The effect of general anaesthesia on the success of embryo transfer following human in-vitro fertilization. Hum Reprod 1988; 3(Suppl): 81–3.

44. Boyers SP, Lavy G, Russell JB, et al. A paired analysis of in vitro fertilization and cleavage rate of first- versus last-exposed preovulatory human oocytes exposed to varying intervals of 100% CO_2 pneumoperitoneum and general anesthesia. Fertil Steril 1987; 48: 969–74.

45. Hayes MF, Sacco AG, Savoy-Moore RT, et al. Effect of general anesthesia on fertilization and cleavage of human oocytes in vitro. Fertil Steril 1987; 48: 975–81.

46. Jensen JT, Boyers SP, Grunfeld LH, et al. Anesthesia exposure may affect fertilization rates in human oocytes collected by ultrasound aspiration. Presented at the Fifth World Congress on In Vitro Fertilization and Embryo Transfer. Norfolk, VA, 1987: 48.

47. Vincent R, Syrop C, Van Voorhis B, et al. An evaluation of the effect of anesthetic technique on reproductive success after laparoscopic pronuclear stage transfer. Anesthesiology 1995; 82: 352–8.

48. Warren JR, Shaw B, Steinkampf MP. Effects of nitrous oxide on preimplantation mouse embryo cleavage and development. Biol Reprod 1990; 43: 158–61.

49. Gonen O, Shulman A, Ghetler Y, et al. The impact of different types of anesthesia on in vitro fertilization-embryo transfer treatment outcome. J Assist Reprod Genet 1995; 12: 678–82.

50. Rosen M, Roizen M, Egar E, et al. The effect of nitrous oxide in vitro fertilization success rate. Anesthesiology 1987; 67: 42–4.

51. Kogosowsky A, Lessing JB, Amit A, et al. Epidural block: a preferred method of anesthesia for ultrasonically guided oocyte retrieval. Fertil Steril 1987; 47: 166–8.

52. Botta G, D'Angelo A, Giovanni D, et al. Epidural anesthesia in an in vitro fertilization and embryo transfer program. J Assist Reprod Genet 1995; 12: 187–90.

53. Chung P, Timothy Y, Mayer J, et al. Gamete intrafallopian transfer; comparison of epidural vs. general anesthesia. J Reprod Med 1998; 43: 681–6.

54. Endler G, Magyar D, Hayes M, Moghissi K. Use of spinal anesthesia in laparoscopy for in vitro fertilization. Fertil Steril 1985; 43: 809–10.

55. Martin R, Tsen L, Tzeng G, et al. Anesthesia for in vitro fertilization: the addition of fentanyl to 1.5% lidocaine. Anesth Analg 1999; 88: 523–6.

56. Tsen L, Schultz R, Martin R, et al. Intrathecal low-dose bupivacaine versus lidocaine for in vitro fertilization procedures. Reg Anesth Pain Med 2000; 26: 52–6.

57. Ng EHY, Tang OS, Chui DKC, Ho PC. Comparison of two different doses of lidocaine used in paracervical block during oocyte collection in an IVF programme. Hum Reprod 2000; 15: 2148–51.

58. Andersson S, Lundberg T. Acupuncture – from empiricism t o science: functional background to acupuncture effects in health and disease. Med Hypothesis 1995; 45: 271–81.

59. Manheimer E, White A, Berman B, et al. Meta-analysis: acupuncture for low back pain. Ann Intern Med 2005; 142: 651–63.

60. Wu MT, Sheen JM, Chuang KH, et al. Neuronal specificity of acupuncture response: a fMRI with electroacupuncture. Neuroimage 2002; 16: 1028–37.

61. Stener-Victorin E, Waldenstrom U, Andersson SA, Wilkand M. Reduction of blood flow impedance in uterine arteries of infertile women with electro-acupuncture. Hum Reprod 1996; 11: 1314–17.

62. Kim J, Shin K, Na C. Effect of acupuncture on uterine motility and cyclooxygenase-2 in pregnant rats. Gynecol Obstet Invest 2000; 50: 225–30.

63. Paules WE, Zhang M, Strehler E, et al. Influence of acupuncture on the pregnancy rate in patients who undergo assisted reproduction therapy. Fertil Steril 2002; 77: 721–4.

64. Humaidan P, Brock K, Bungum L, Stener-Victoria E. Pain relief during oocyte retrieval – exploring the role of different frequencies of electro-acupuncture. Reprod Biomed Online 2006; 13: 120–5.

65. Sator-Katzenschlager SM, Wolfler MM, Kozek-Langenecker SA, et al. Articular electro-acupuncture as an additional perioperative analgesic method during oocyte aspiration in IVF treatment. Hum Reprod 2006; 21: 2114–20.

66. Manheimer E, Zhang G, Udoff L, et al. Effects of acupuncture on rates of pregnancy and live birth among women undergoing in vitro fertilisation: systemic review and meta-analysis. BMJ 2008; 336: 545–9.

67. El-Toukhy T, Sunkara SK, Khairy M, et al. A systemic review and meta-analysis of acupuncture in in vitro fertilisation. BJOG 2008; 115: 1203–13.

68. Cheong Y, Nardo LG, Rutherford T, Ledger W. Acupuncture and herbal medicine in in vitro fertilisation: a review of the evidence for clinical practice. Hum Fertility 2010; 13: 3–12.

54

Medical considerations of single embryo transfer

Outi Hovatta

HEALTHIER IVF CHILDREN FOLLOWING SINGLE EMBRYO TRANSFER

The health of children born after IVF has been followed up since the beginning of the clinical infertility treatment. In the beginning, the numbers of children were small, but then national and international registers were established. Accumulated data showed that children born as a result of IVF had a higher risk of abnormalities when compared to conventionally born children as described in a review article by Edwards and Ludwig (1). The risk ratio of having some abnormality was 1.2 to 1.4 in the reviewed literature.

There are many possible causes for such abnormalities. Parental factors are the most likely ones (1), but multiple pregnancies and their consequences have appeared to be the most common one.

RISKS OF MULTIPLE PREGNANCIES FOR THE CHILDREN

The increased risk of premature births even among twin pregnancies, not to mention triplets and higher order multiple pregnancies was the main cause of morbidity and mortality also among IVF children. This became very clear in a Swedish nationwide analysis of all IVF 5856 children born in 1982–1995 in this country (2). Data regarding all the IVF children born were compared to the children born in the general population during the same time (1,505,724 children), using Swedish Medical Birth Registry and the Registry of Congenital Malformations. There were 27% multiple births after IVF but only 1% in the control population. The rate of preterm births was 30.3% among the IVF infants, while it was only 6.3% in the control population. The percentage of low birth weight (<2500 g) infants after IVF was 27.4, while it was 4.6% among the control infants. The perinatal mortality was 1.9% in the IVF group and 1.1% in the controls. The high frequency of multiple births and maternal characteristics were regarded as the main factors for adverse outcome, and not the IVF technique itself.

A closer analysis of the abnormalities among the IVF children was very alarming. (3) From the same population of Swedish IVF children that is, in the 2060 twins out of 5680 IVF children, it became clear that the risk of particularly a neurological diagnosis was significantly higher than that among the control children. It did not differ from the risk of control twins. The most common neurological diagnosis was cerebral palsy, for which IVF children had an increased risk of 3.7 (2.0 – 6.6). The risk for IVF singletons was 2.8 (1.3 – 5.8). Also the risk of developmental delay was fourfold among the IVF children.

After these results, the Swedish IVF clinics have been allowed to transfer only one embryo at a time, in exceptional cases, two.

In Denmark, a large register study including all 8602 infants born after IVF and intra-cytoplasmic sperm injections between 1995 and 2000 was carried out (4). The cohort included 3438 twins and 5164 singletons. A significantly increased risk of premature delivery was found between twins and singletons. The was tenfold increase among all births before 37 completed weeks, and 7.4-fold increased in births before 32 completed weeks. The stillbirth rate was doubled in twins (13.1/1000) when compared to that in singletons (6.6/1000).

In addition to premature births, also congenital anomalies are more common in twin pregnancies (5). A 2.3-fold higher prevalence of major malformation (9.3%) was found among IVF infants when compared to control infants. Of the IVF infants with malformation, 70% were born from twin or triplet pregnancies (6). Congenital heart disease is more common among twins than among singletons (7,8). In the large Danish register study (4), the total malformation rate (minor + major, 73.7/100) was significantly higher than that in singletons (55.0/1000). Patent ductus arteriosus, typical of premature birth, was very common among twins. An increased risk of anencephaly among twin infants born after assisted reproduction was also found (9). Other perinatal complications typical of twin pregnancies occurred as well in IVF twin pregnancies.

One of the causes why IVF singleton pregnancies also have more growth retardation and other perinatal problems is the vanishing twin syndrome, which is actually a consequence of an IVF twin pregnancy (10–12).

Risk of premature birth is further enhanced in other conditions predisposing to prematurity, such as uterine malformations. Twin pregnancies should not be induced among individuals who have any known increased risk factor of premature delivery.

MULTIPLE PREGNANCIES ARE ALSO RISKY FOR THE MOTHERS

Multiple pregnancies are not risk-free for the mother, either. The risk of preeclampsia, gestational hypertension, placental abruption, and placenta praevia is higher among twin pregnancies (13–15). It causes consequences for the mothers' health.

Impaired glucose tolerance and pregnancy-induced diabetes (16) are more common during multiple pregnancies. Diabetic mother's pregnancy is always a high-risk condition, both for the mother and the fetus, and all the possible actions should be taken into account to diminish such risks (17). Obesity further increases the risks of gestational diabetes and hypertension (18). Increasing the risk of diabetic complications by inducing a twin pregnancy with transferring more than one embryo is not acceptable. For a diabetic woman, elective single embryo transfer (SET) is always indicated irrespective of the embryo quality. The same regards all other chronic disorders. A noncomplicated singleton pregnancy after kidney transplantation and SET was reported (19).

Turner's syndrome is a medical situation in which the majority of the women need donated oocytes (20,21). These women often have cardiac anomalies and hypertension, and it is not justified to make these pregnancies more risky by transferring more than one embryo at a time. The most dangerous complication among Turner women is aortic dissection, and several cases have occurred during pregnancy (22). In Turner's syndrome, elective SET only can be accepted.

Oocyte donation is a situation in which the pregnancy rates are relatively high. Elective SET gives excellent pregnancy rates in oocyte donation (23,24). Elective SET is further motivated in this group of women because they have an increased risk of hypertension in pregnancy (25).

The likelihood of operative delivery with possible complications is higher in multiple pregnancies (4), which is another maternal indication not to transfer more than one embryo at a time (26).

ELECTIVE SET AS A METHOD TO AVOID MULTIPLE PREGNANCIES

During the early days of IVF, the evolving embryo culture techniques did not allow high pregnancy rates. In early statistics the pregnancy rate per SET was clearly lower than that after transfer of more than one embryo. This urged clinicians to try to improve the treatment results by transfer of multiple embryos. The consequence was the well-known increase in multiple pregnancies. However, pediatricians who saw the increase in complications caused by this new epidemic of multiple births alarmed the IVF community relatively early. They were particularly active in Northern Europe. In Finland, we started elective SETs in mid 1990s. We then analysed the pregnancy rates after SET during one year in two IVF units in Helsinki (27). These results demonstrated very clearly the difference between nonelective and elective SET. If only one embryo was available for transfer, the pregnancy rate was 20% per transfer, but if an elective SET was carried out in this nonselected patient population, a pregnancy rate of 29.7% was achieved. It was similar to that in the two-embryo transfer, that is, 29.4%.

That elective SET results in much better pregnancy rates than nonelective ones, and that such pregnancy rate is similar to that achieved in transfer of two embryos when top or good quality embryos were available, was soon demonstrated in two prospective randomized trials. Gerris et al. (28) randomized 53 couples with a female partner <34 years and who had at least two top quality embryos for elective SET or two-embryo transfer. The pregnancy rate after elective SET was 42.3%, and that among the couples with double embryo transfer was 48.1% with 30% twins. We carried out a multicenter study in Finland (29) in which 144 couples with good quality embryos were randomized to elective SET or double embryo transfer. The pregnancy rate per transfer was 32.4% in the SET group and 47.1% in the double ET group. The difference was not statistically significant. The cumulative pregnancy rates after frozen embryo transfers were 47.3% in the SET and 58.6% in the double embryo transfer groups. After double embryo transfer, there were 39% twins.

A large North European multicenter study was then carried out (30). Couples where the female partner was younger than 36 years and who had at least two good quality embryos, were randomized to receiving either two embryos or first a single fresh embryo and then a frozen–thawed single embryo. A pregnancy resulting in at least one live birth was encountered in 142 of the 331 women (42.9%) who received two fresh embryos, and in 128 women (38.8%) who received first one fresh and then one frozen embryo. The pregnancy rate after SETs was lower, but not substantially lower than that after double embryo transfer. But there was a highly significantly (p < 0.001) lower twinning rate after SET (0.8%) compared to that after double embryo transfer (33.1%).

That pregnancy outcome was not affected when blastocysts were transferred, as shown in an analysis of couples undergoing single blastocyst transfer (n = 52, live birth rate 53.8%) or a double blastocysts transfer (n = 187, live birth rate 54.4%). In single blastocyst transfer, the twin rate was 3.1%, while it was 51% in double blastocyst transfer (31).

Effective and active cryopreservation policy particularly in connection with SET increases the pregnancy rates per oocyte retrieval (32). Elective SET reduces multiple pregnancies also in frozen embryo transfers (33).

Elective SET has proved to be a method using which multiple pregnancies can be reduced without decreasing the overall pregnancy rates (34). In real life, it has not only been equally effective but also been economically substantially cheaper than double embryo transfer with all its complications (35,36). In nonselected population, SET has resulted in lower pregnancy rate than double embryo transfer. Hence, some criteria have been used to select the couples for elective SET (37). Effective cryopreservation methods have probably greatly reduced the need of strict selection (38,39). All the obtained embryos can be transferred, anyway, but a longer time may be required for achieving a pregnancy.

There is now data from Sweden and Belgium, which have a law and guideline for regular SET, that the pregnancy rates have remained similar in these countries, while the rate was multiple pregnancies have dropped significantly (40,41). After the latest published Swedish data, which covers all the cycles in Sweden, a similar follow up has continuously been collected by the Swedish Authorities, and the pregnancy rate has remained constant during the many years' time with SET, and the twin rate has remained in some 5%. But at the same time, the proportion of children weighing less than 2500 g, or born prematurely, has significantly decreased, hence bringing better health for the infants (PO Karlström, personal communication).

OPTIMIZING CRITERIA FOR SET

To achieve equal pregnancy rates within the same time between single and double embryo transfers, some kind of selection has been made to balance the likelihood of pregnancy and to minimize the risk of twins (37). The criteria presented in all the above-mentioned articles include the age of the female partner, the number of earlier unsuccessful cycles, and embryo quality. In Sweden, these criteria have in most clinics become stricter during the period in which SET has been practiced. The National Board of Health and Welfare in Sweden has collected statistics from all IVF clinics (41), and the units by themselves have agreed upon criteria using which a twin rate of <5%, and unchanged pregnancy rate can be achieved. The recommended criteria for elective SET at that time were: The age of the woman <40 years, not more than three failed ART cycles, and at least two good quality embryos. Regarding cleavage stage embryos, the criteria are: Less than 20% fragmentation, the embryo fills an even zona, no multinuclear blastomeres, four cells on day 2, and eight cells on day 3. An exception of one of these parameters still counts a good quality embryo. Early cleavage is an additional sign urging SET. At blastocyst stage, an expanded blastocyst on day 5 is of good quality. In frozen embryo transfers, intact embryo after thawing indicates for SET. But there are now also more advanced systems for embryo selection. A computer-assisted scoring system proved to be better than the conventionally used one (42). Using gene expression or biochemical information from the cumulus cells may become more widely used (43,44). Glucose consumption by an embryo may be measured (45).

CONCLUSIONS

Multiple pregnancies, including twins, cause high risks for the health of the infants and the mothers. The risks are largely caused by the high incidence of premature birth, but also congenital anomalies are increased among twins. Twin pregnancies can be almost completely avoided by carrying out elective SET. Even though there are no big differences in cumulative pregnancy rates

between the first fresh and the following frozen–thawed ones transferred one at a time, or the same done with frozen transfer in spite of the embryo quality, many teams still search for optimal quality of embryos giving the highest possible pregnancy rate as soon as possible. A twin rate <5% can be achieved if a single good quality embryo is transferred to a woman under <40 years during her three first ART cycles, and she has at least two good quality embryos, and two for the rest. But actually the cumulative pregnancy rate among women over 40 years is similar if she cumulatively receives all her embryos either one or two at a time. And if the embryo is intact after thawing, a single frozen embryo should be transferred.

Irrespective of the woman's age, number of earlier cycles, or embryo quality, a SET should be carried out in situations with known high risk of premature birth, such as uterine abnormalities. The same regards maternal contraindications for multiple pregnancies, such as diabetes, hypertension, or Turner's syndrome.

REFERENCE

1. Edwards RG, Ludwig M. Are major defects in children conceived in vitro due to innate problems in patients or to induced genetic damage? Reprod Biomed Online 2003; 7: 131–82.
2. Bergh T, Ericson A, Hillensjö T, Nygren KG, Wennerholm UB. Deliveries and children born after in-vitro fertilisation in Sweden 1982–95: A retrospective cohort study. Lancet 1999; 354: 1579–85.
3. Strömberg B, Dahlquist G, Ericson A, Finnström O, Köster M. Stjernqvist K.Neurological sequelae in children born after in-vitro fertilisation: A population-based study. Lancet 2002; 359: 461–5.
4. Pinborg A, Loft A, Nyboe Andersen A. Neonatal outcome in a Danish national cohort of 8602 children born after in vitro fertilization or intracytoplasmic sperm injection: the role of twin pregnancy. Acta Obstet Gynecol Scand 2004; 83: 1071–8.
5. Sperling L, Kiil C, Larsen LU, et al. Detection of chromosomal abnormalities, congenital abnormalities and transfusion syndrome in twins. Ultrasound Obstet Gynecol 2007; 29: 517–26.
6. Merlob P, Sapir O, Sulkes J, Fisch B. The prevalence of major congenital malformations during two periods of time, 1986–1994 and 1995–2002 in newborns conceived by assisted reproduction technology. Eur J Med Genet 2005; 48: 5–11.
7. Caputo S, Russo MG, Capozzi G, et al. Congenital heart disease in a population of dizygotic twins: an echocardiographic study. Int J Cardiol 2005; 102: 293–6.
8. Hajdu J, Beke A, Marton T, et al. Congenital heart diseases in twin pregnancies. Fetal Diagn Ther 2006; 21: 198–203.
9. Ben-Ami I, Vaknin Z, Reish O, et al. Is there an increased rate of anencephaly in twins? Prenat Diagn 2005; 25: 1007–10.
10. Spellacy WN. Antepartum complications in twin pregnancies. Clin Perinatol 1988; 15: 79–86.
11. Pinborg A, Lidegaard O, Freiesleben NC, Andersen AN. Vanishing twins: a predictor of small-for-gestational age in IVF singletons. Hum Reprod 2007; 22: 2707–14; Epub.

12. Sazonova A, Källen K, Thurin-Kjellberg A, Wennerholm UB, Bergh C. Factors affecting obstetric outcome of singletons born after IVF. Hum Reprod 2011; 26: 2878–86

13. Duckitt K, Harrington D. Risk factors for pre-eclampsia at antenatal booking: systematic review of controlled studies. BMJ 2005; 12: 330–565.

14. Erez O, Vardi IS, Hallak M, et al. Preeclampsia in twin gestations: association with IVF treatments, parity and maternal age. J Matern Fetal Neonatal Med 2006; 19: 141–6.

15. Allen VM, Wilson RD, Cheung A. Genetics committee of the society of obstetricians and gynaecologists of Canada (SOGC); reproductive endocrinology infertility committee of the society of obstetricians and gynaecologists of Canada (SOGC). pregnancy outcomes after assisted reproductive technology. J Obstet Gynaecol Can 2006; 28: 220–50.

16. Adler Levy Y, Lunenfeld E, Levy A. Obstetric outcome of twin pregnancies conceived by in vitro fertilization and ovulation induction compared with those conceived spontaneously. Eur J Obstet Gynecol Reprod Biol 2007; 133: 173–8.

17. Hod M, Jovanovic L. Improving outcomes in pregnant women with type 1 diabetes. Diabetes Care 2007; 30: e62.

18. Dokras A, Baredziak L, Blaine J, Syrop C, VanVoorhis BJ. Sparks A.Obstetric outcomes after in vitro fertilization in obese and morbidly obese women. Obstet Gynecol 2006; 108: 61–9.

19. Nouri K, Bader Y, Helmy S, et al. Live birth after in vitro fertilization and single embryo transfer in a kidney transplant patient: a case report and review of the literature. J Assist Reprod Genet 2011; 28: 351–3.

20. Foudila T, Söderström-Anttila V, Hovatta O. Turner's syndrome and pregnancies after oocyte donation. Hum Reprod 1999; 14: 532–5.

21. Hovatta O. Pregnancies in women with Turner's syndrome. Ann Med 1999; 31: 106–10.

22. Bondy CA. Turner syndrome study group.care of girls and women with turner syndrome: a guideline of the turner syndrome study group. J Clin Endocrinol Metab 2007; 92: 10–25.

23. Söderström-Anttila V, Vilska S, Mäkinen S, Foudila T, Suikkari AM. Elective single embryo transfer yields good delivery rates in oocyte donation. Hum Reprod 2003; 18: 1858–63.

24. Söderström-Anttila V, Vilska S. Five years of single embryo transfer with anonymous and non-anonymous oocyte donation. Reprod Biomed Online 2007; 15: 428–33.

25. Söderström-Anttila V, Tiitinen A, Foudila T, Hovatta O. Obstetric and perinatal outcome after oocyte donation: comparison with in-vitro fertilization pregnancies. Hum Reprod 1998; 13: 483–90.

26. De Sutter P. Single embryo transfer (set) not only leads to a reduction in twinning rates after IVF/ICSI, but also improves obstetrical and perinatal outcome of singletons. Verh K Acad Geneeskd Belg 2006; 68: 319–27.

27. Vilska S, Tiitinen A, Hydén Granskog C, Hovatta O. Elective transfer of one embryo results in an acceptable pregnancy rate and eliminates the risk of multiple birth. Hum Reprod 1999; 14: 2392–5.

28. Gerris J, De Neubourg D, et al. Prevention of twin pregnancy after in-vitro fertilization or intracytoplasmic sperm injection based on strict embryo criteria: a prospective randomized clinical trial. Hum Reprod 1999; 14: 2581–7.

29. Martikainen H, Tiitinen A, Tomás C, et al. Finnish ET study group.one versus two embryo transfer after IVF and ICSI: a randomized study. Hum Reprod 2001; 16: 1900–3.

30. Thurin A, Hausken J, Hillensjö T, et al. Elective single-embryo transfer versus double-embryo transfer in in vitro fertilization. N Engl J Med 2004; 351: 2392–402.

31. Styer AK, Wright DL, Wolkovich AM, Veiga C, Toth TL. Single-blastocyst transfer decreases twin gestation without affecting pregnancy outcome. Fertil Steril 2007; 330: 549–50

32. Tiitinen A, Hydén-Granskog C, Gissler M. What is the most relevant standard of success in assisted reproduction? The value of cryopreservation on cumulative pregnancy rates per single oocyte retrieval should not be forgotten. Hum Reprod 2004; 19: 2439–41.

33. Hydén Granskog C, Unkila et al. Single embryo transfer is an option in frozen embryo transfer. Hum Reprod 2005; 20: 2935–8.

34. Tiitinen A, Unkila Kallio L, et al. Impact of elective single embryo transfer on the twin pregnancy rate. Hum Reprod 2003; 18: 1449–53.

35. Gerris J, De Sutter P, De Neubourg D, et al. A real-life prospective health economic study of elective single embryo transfer versus two-embryo transfer in first IVF/ICSI cycles. Hum Reprod 2004; 19: 917–23.

36. Fiddelers AA, Severens JL, Dirksen CD, et al. Economic evaluations of single- versus double-embryo transfer in IVF. Hum Reprod Update. 2007; 13: 5–13.

37. van Montfoort AP, Fiddelers AA, Land JA, et al. ESET irrespective of the availability of a good-quality embryo in the first cycle only is not effective in reducing overall twin pregnancy rates. Hum Reprod 2007; 22: 1669–74.

38. Sundström P, Saldeen P. Cumulative delivery rate in an in vitro fertilization program with a single embryo transfer policy. Acta Obstet Gynecol Scand 2009; 88: 700–6.

39. Veleva Z, Karinen P, Tomás C, Tapanainen JS, Martikainen H. Elective single embryo transfer with cryopreservation improves the outcome and diminishes the costs of IVF/ICSI. Hum Reprod 2009; 24: 1632–9.

40. Van Landuyt L, Verheyen G, et al. New Belgian embryo transfer policy leads to sharp decrease in multiple pregnancy rate. Reprod Biomed Online 2006; 13: 765–71.

41. Karlström PO, Bergh C. Reducing the number of embryos transferred in Sweden-impact on delivery and multiple birth rates. Hum Reprod 2007; 22: 2202–7.

42. Paternot G, Debrock S, D'Hooghe T, Spiessens C. Computer-assisted embryo selection: a benefit in the evaluation of embryo quality? Reprod Biomed Online 2011; 23: 347–54.

43. Assou S, Haouzi D, De Vos J, Hamamah S. Human cumulus cells as biomarkers for embryo and pregnancy outcomes. Mol Hum Reprod 2010; 16: 531–8.

44. Gebhardt KM, Feil DK, Dunning KR, Lane M, Russell DL. Human cumulus cell gene expression as a biomarker of pregnancy outcome after single embryo transfer. Fertil Steril 2011; 96: 47–52.

45. Gardner DK, Wale PL, Collins R, Lane M. Glucose consumption of single post-compaction human embryos is predictive of embryo sex and live birth outcome. Hum Reprod 2011; 26: 1981–6.

55

Endometriosis and ART

Marli Amin, Andy Huang, and Alan H. DeCherney

INTRODUCTION

Endometriosis, as a clinical entity, has been recognized and intensely investigated for well over 100 years. Despite the accumulation of an enormous amount of information, uncertainty still exists regarding etiologies, clinical consequences, and treatment efficacy. The two most common complaints leading to a diagnosis of endometriosis are pelvic pain and infertility. The advancement of innovative medical and surgical approaches, such as gonadotropin-releasing hormone (GnRH) agonists and laparoscopically guided laser ablation, have proven quite effective in improving many of the symptoms associated with endometriosis. It does appear that assisted reproductive technique (ART) is becoming an indispensable asset in providing affected couples with viable pregnancies, and with the accumulation of randomized trials, the role of both long and short GnRH protocols is becoming clear.

ENDOMETRIOSIS AND INFERTILITY

There is little debate that the extensive anatomical distortion and tubal obstruction, frequently attributed to severe endometriosis, does impair fertility. Less clear is the reported association between minimal or mild endometriosis and infertility, in the absence of any mechanical disruption. Although there is no conclusive evidence that minimal to moderate endometriosis actually causes infertility, several studies dating back to the 1930s have suggested that there is at least an association between the two (1). In the 1970s, three studies retrospectively compared the incidence of endometriosis in women undergoing laparoscopy for infertility or voluntary sterilization (2–4). The incidences of endometriosis ranged from 21% to 48% in infertile women, while endometriosis was noted in only 1.3–5% of fertile women undergoing tubal ligation. More recent studies (5,6) including one prospective investigation (7) have demonstrated that among women undergoing insemination with donor sperm due to severe male factor infertility, those with coexisting endometriosis had markedly fewer conceptions per exposure than women who did not have the disease. Another recent prospective double-blind study (8), which looked specifically at women with mild endometriosis compared to women without endometriosis, was able to show a trend toward higher pregnancy rates in women without the disease. The results, however, did not reach statistical significance. This may be attributable to the fact that the number of patients enrolled did not meet the study's power calculation.

Although the above studies were methodologically imperfect and far from conclusive, virtually every area within the reproductive process has been intensely investigated, in an attempt to describe a causal relationship between endometriosis and infertility. The results of several tangential lines of investigation have added to the confusion, as studies are frequently in direct contradiction to one another. Investigators have suggested that women with mild to moderate endometriosis have a higher incidence of endocrine abnormalities, (9) anovulation, (10) corpus luteum insufficiency, (11) hyperprolactinemia, (12) luteinized unruptured follicle syndrome, (13) and spontaneous abortions (14). However, other well organized, prospective studies have found most of these factors to be either normal or lacking in clinical significance (15–20).

Immune dysfunction in endometriosis has become the focus of more recent efforts, as it is hypothesized that immunity plays a role in the pathogenesis of the disease. Several immunologic abnormalities, which could potentially impair fertility, have been identified. Researchers have reported increased B-cell activity, with the production of specific antibodies against endometrial antigens, T-cell and macrophage dysfunction, and nonspecific polyclonal B-cell activation. In addition, some have reported increased production of cytokines and eicosanoids in the peritoneal fluid and sera, which may affect sperm motility and velocity, acrosome reactivity, sperm penetration, embryo implantation, and early development (15,21). As with other factors, many conflicting reports have emerged. Furthermore, it is not at all clear which is the cause and which the effect, or what role each abnormality actually plays in the pathogenesis of endometriosis-associated infertility.

Many investigators have proposed that endometriosis is actually caused by an interplay between environmental and genetic factors. Many have also suggested that certain genetic polymorphisms associated with endometriosis could be predispose a woman to infertility. In a review of the advances in the genetics of endometriosis,

Dun et al. (22) reviewed the most commonly studied genes thought to be associated with endometriosis. Over 18 genes were implicated, with most relating to xenobiotic metabolism, steroid action and receptors, and inflammatory and angiogenic factors.

A direct association between these genetic polymorphisms and endometriosis-associated infertility has yet to be shown though.

As stated, one argument that has been proposed against a causal relationship between endometriosis and infertility is in the outright failure of medical or surgical treatment to significantly improve pregnancy success in these patients. The use of medical treatments, otherwise successful in alleviating the nonreproductive symptoms of endometriosis, has failed to demonstrate a reasonable improvement in fertility (23). Most studies investigating the effect of surgical ablation of endometriotic lesions, by any one of a number of techniques, have failed to show an increased fecundity. One recent randomized study, however, did show an improved rate of pregnancy for women with minimal/mild endometriosis treated with ablation of endometriotic lesions, when compared with a control group receiving diagnostic laparoscopy alone (24). However, this study has been criticized for having a lower fecundity rate among untreated patients than would normally be expected, for notifying patients of their treatment status, and for following pregnancies to only 20 weeks. Subsequently, another randomized study, which looked at actual birth rates, failed to demonstrate a reproductive benefit for patients whose lesions were ablated, but had lower power than the first study (25). When the results were combined, no significant statistical heterogeneity was noted and the increased chance of achieving pregnancy after surgery was found to be only 8.6% (95% confidence interval [CI] 2.1, 15) (26). Thus, surgically ablating visible endometriosis lesions only potentially benefits pregnancy outcomes minimally. With regard to endometriomas, a recent Cochrane review of four trials concluded that surgery (aspiration or cystectomy) versus expectant management showed no evidence of a benefit for clinical pregnancy with either technique (27).

OVULATION INDUCTION AND INSEMINATION

Controlled ovarian hyperstimulation (COH), in combination with intrauterine insemination (IUI), has proven to be a cost-effective and appropriate first-line treatment for many infertility diagnoses (28). However, it is not entirely clear that this approach is as effective for patients with endometriosis. Deaton et al. (29) demonstrated increased fecundity in patients treated with clomiphene citrate and IUI. However, Fedele and colleagues (30) reported that the increased conception rate with COH and IUI did not follow with a significantly different pregnancy rate at six months. Furthermore, a retrospective comparison of COH and IUI reported per-cycle pregnancy rates of 6.5%, 11.8%, and 15.3% for endometriosis, male factor, and unexplained infertility, respectively (31). Similarly, although with more optimistic results, a prospective, observational study reported pregnancy rates of 16.3%

and 33.6% following COH/IUI in patients with endometriosis and unexplained infertility, respectively (32). In a meta-analysis, Hughes (33) reported that a diagnosis of endometriosis decreased the per-cycle COH/IUI conception rate by half. Also, a later prospective, randomized study reported live birth rates of 11% and 2% for endometriosis patients undergoing COH/IUI and no treatment, respectively (34). While this demonstrates a live birth odds ratio (OR) of 5.5 for the treatment group, the actual percentage of live births after treatment remains relatively low. Failure of COH/IUI has recently been correlated with advanced endometriosis. A retrospective study of 92 patients found that more than one-third of patients failing to conceive after four ovulatory cycles of clomiphene citrate had stage III or IV disease, an endometrioma, pelvic adhesions, and/or tubal disease (35). Most recently, however, a retrospective, controlled cohort study of 259 COH/IUI cycles found no difference in cycle pregnancy rate and cumulative live birth rate between women with surgically treated minimal to mild endometriosis and women with unexplained infertility, indicating potentially improved outcomes after surgical treatment (36).

The advent of aromatase inhibitors has added to the armamentarium of therapeutic modalities for the treatment of endometriosis. With its efficacy in treating the endometriosis-associated pain, more formally established (37,38) studies are underway to evaluate its utility in ovulation induction. Most recently, Wu et al. (39) found that a third-generation aromatase inhibitor was able to achieve a reasonable pregnancy rate, with a thicker endometrium but fewer ovulatory follicles, when randomized and compared with clomiphene citrate.

The use of GnRH antagonists in intrauterine insemination cycles with COH has also been studied. A recent randomized, double blinded, placebo-controlled trial showed no difference in live birth rates for women with minimal or mild endometriosis when comparing women who were treated with GnRH antagonist to those who received a placebo (40).

ENDOMETRIOSIS AND ART

Treatment strategies for the infertile couple must be based on the specific situation. For the young women with only minimal or mild endometriosis, expectant management may be the most appropriate course. However, for women approaching the end of their reproductive age, the chances of conceiving drop precipitously. In these women, intervention, in the form of COH/IUI or in vitro fertilization (IVF) may be warranted more expeditiously (41). The lower cost and low complication rate of ovulation induction and IUI make the combination an attractive first step. However, for women with severe endometriosis or tubal disease, or when male factor or a combination of etiologies is involved, assisted reproduction such as IVF may be pursued sooner. In addition, IVF offers the added benefit of being able to directly observe key events in the conception process, such as the assessment of gamete quality, the observation of fertilization, and the evaluation of early embryo development. As a result, the increasing use of ART in the treatment of endometriosis-associated infertility may help to answer some of the questions regarding this elusive association.

It is thought that the use of IVF–ET (embryo transfer) in the infertile patient with endometriosis removes critical steps in reproduction, such as fertilization and early embryo development, from an in vivo environment that some have suggested is hostile to these processes. Thus, it has been anticipated that endometriosis patients will have IVF outcomes approaching those of other infertility etiologies. Recent studies, however, confirm that endometriosis patients, particularly those with moderate to severe disease, had lower pregnancy rates (42,43). Certainly, the development of GnRH agonists and transvaginal oocyte retrieval has been associated with increased success in the use of IVF for endometriosis-associated infertility. However, the value of reported ART results must be considered along with the understanding that there is great clinical and laboratory variability among centers, leading to a wide range of reported pregnancy rates. Furthermore, most studies are retrospective and observational and are therefore of limited value in reaching definitive conclusions regarding therapy efficacy. Barnhart et al. (44) performed a meta-analysis on the studies evaluating the effects of endometriosis on the outcomes of ARTs. They evaluated a total of 22 articles and concluded that overall, patients with endometriosis had lower pregnancy rates, decreased fertilization and implantation rates, and a decreased number of oocytes retrieved compared to controls of tubal factor infertility (Fig. 55.1).

COH and Oocyte Retrieval

As the practice of assisted reproduction has evolved over the past three decades, so has the efficacy of IVF in the treatment of endometriosis. With regard to the effect of endometriosis on COH and oocyte retrieval, an obvious divide exists between earlier studies, using clomiphene citrate with laparoscopic oocyte retrieval, and more recent

investigations benefiting from the development of GnRH agonists and ultrasound-guided transvaginal retrieval. Earlier studies did in fact report a reduced oocyte yield in patients with endometriosis undergoing IVF. In one small study, Chillik and colleagues (45) compared patients with either no endometriosis, mild to moderate endometriosis, or severe disease, and reported that oocyte yield was reduced in those patients of advanced stage. Oehninger et al. (46) reported a similar effect on oocyte retrieval for patients with stage III or IV endometriosis. Both studies suggested that oocyte yield was impaired in this group of patients due to technical difficulties at the time of laparoscopic oocyte retrieval. Alternatively, other researchers have reported decreased folliculogenesis in patients with endometriosis (47–50). Furthermore, Dlugi and colleagues (51), and more recently, Somigliana and colleagues (52) reported a significantly lower number of preovulatory follicles in patients with endometriomas, when compared to patients with hydrosalpinges.

Several contemporary studies utilizing GnRH agonists and transvaginal retrieval have not confirmed that endometriosis has a significant effect on oocyte yield. Dmowski et al. (53) retrospectively analyzed 237 IVF cycles and found no difference in either folliculogenesis or in the number of oocytes obtained for women with or without endometriosis. In a case–control study comparing 65 cycles of IVF for women with endometriosis, to 98 cycles of IVF in patients with tubal infertility, Bergendal et al. (54) found no difference in folliculogenesis or oocyte retrieval. Several recent studies have further concluded that there is no difference in the number of oocytes obtained in patients with mild to moderate endometriosis, when compared to patients with more severe disease (55–58). Barnhart et al. demonstrated a lower number of oocytes retrieved (OR = 0.82, 95% CI 0.75–0.90) for patients with endometriosis when compared to patients with tubal factor (44).

The improvement in IVF outcomes, brought about by the development of GnRH agonists, is largely undisputed.

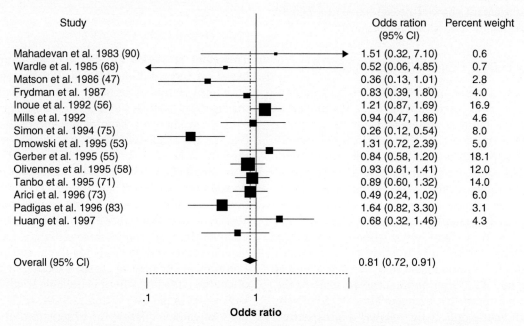

Figure 55.1 Unadjusted meta-analysis of odds of pregnancy in endometriosis patients versus tubal factor controls. *Source*: From Ref. 44.

Olivennes and colleagues (58) reported a significantly improved clinical pregnancy rate for patients treated with GnRH agonists, when compared with standard, gonadotropin-only, ovarian-stimulation protocols (Fig. 55.1). Other investigations have reported similar results (59). Long-term GnRH agonist suppression has been thought to repress further endometriotic lesions and improve IVF outcome for patients with endometriosis. Dicker and associates, (60) as well as Rickes et al. (61) reported a significantly higher clinical pregnancy rate after six months of GnRH agonist therapy, compared with ovarian stimulation with gonadotropins alone. Chedid et al. (62) also investigated the use of a three-month and a three-week GnRH agonist downregulation protocol and reported a significantly increased oocyte yield, when compared with controls receiving only gonadotropins. Although they noted an improved pregnancy rate, it did not reach statistical significance.

Nakamura and colleagues (63) compared GnRH agonist suppression for 60 days with a shorter, mid-luteal downregulation, prior to ovulation induction. They reported pregnancy rates of 67% and 27%, for longer and shorter protocols, respectively. Marcus and Edwards (64) also reported a significantly higher pregnancy rate for patients treated with longer GnRH agonist protocols (Table 55.1), although they used different GnRH agonists for the two groups and assigned patients based on their refusal to accept the longer regimen. Surrey et al. (65) investigated a three-month course of GnRH agonist therapy prior to IVF–ET, and found the agonist therapy to be associated with a significantly higher ongoing pregnancy rate. Conversely, Chedid and colleagues (62) found no difference between long and short GnRH agonist administrations.

The use of continuous oral contraceptive pills prior to assisted reproduction treatment has also been examined. De Ziegler et al. (66) found that six to eight weeks of continuous use of oral contraceptive pills before IVF-ET for patients with endometriosis had similar outcomes to age-matched controls without endometriosis.

Recent studies have also analyzed the use of GnRH antagonist protocols for IVF in patients with endometriosis. A recent prospective randomized trial compared GnRH agonist and antagonist protocols for women with mild to moderate endometriosis (67). This study showed similar implantation and clinical pregnancy rates for patients treated with both GnRH agonist and antagonist protocols. Patients treated with a GnRH agonist, however, had a significantly higher number of additional embryos available for cryopreservation, making the cumulative fecundity rate higher with the agonist protocol.

For now, it appears that endometriosis patients respond to ovarian stimulation in a manner that is similar to other infertility etiologies. Although standard gonadotropin stimulation protocols work reasonably well, the addition of longer GnRH agonist downregulation or the use of continuous oral contraceptive pills may increase IVF success and should be considered on a case-by-case basis.

Fertilization and Early Embryo Development

It is unclear as to the degree to which endometriosis is a detriment to the process of fertilizing oocytes in vitro, as several investigations have now reported significantly impaired fertilization rates for these patients. One early

Table 55.1   Comparison of IVF-ET Outcomes for Women with and without Endometriosis

Study	Group	Number of cycles	Clinical pregnancies (% cycle)	Study	Group	Number of cycles	Clinical pregnancies (% cycle)
Mahadevan (89)	I–IV	14	14	Inoue (56)	I	111	40
	Tubal	261	10		II	78	42
Wardle (68)	I–IV	17	6		III	51	47
	Tubal	47	11		IV	69	42
					Other	372	44
Chillik (45)	I/II	10	60		I–IV	360	29
	III/IV	14	7	Olivennes (58)	Tubal	160	36
Matson (47)	I	24	13				
	II	37	14	Geber (55)	I/II	100	29
	III	36	6		III/IV	29	52
	VI	57	2		Tubal	1139	41
	Tubal	40	18	Dmowski (53)	I/II	89	25
Sharma (90)	I/II	135	16		III/IV	30	30
	III/IV	141	8		Other	118	21
	Tubal	994	13	Arici (73)	I/II	43	12
Oehninger (46)	I/II	191	24		III/IV	46	15
	III/IV	35	20		Tubal	147	24
Yovich (48)	I/II	61	13	Bergendal (54)	I–IV	65	28
	III/IV	93	3		Tubal	98	30
	Tubal	49	14	Pal (57)	I/II	45	44
					III/IV	39	33

study noted fertilization rates per oocyte of 33%, 63%, and 68% for patients with endometriosis, unexplained infertility, and tubal infertility, respectively, (68) while another reported a marked impairment in fertilization with the presence of an endometrioma (51). Bergendal et al. (54) reported fertilization rates of 60% and 78% for patients with endometriosis and tubal factor, respectively (p <0.0001). Other investigators have reported significantly lower fertilization success for stage III or IV endometriosis, when compared with stages I or II (57,58). With regard to early embryo development, researchers have reported fewer embryos reaching the 4-cell stage at 48 hours, (69) a reduced number of blastomeres at 72 hours, (70) and lower cleavage rates when endometriosis is compared with tubal-factor or unexplained infertility (71). Furthermore, Brizek and colleagues (72) retrospectively analyzed video records of 235 embryos and found a statistically significant increase in the incidence of aberrant nuclear and cytoplasmic morphology within embryos from patients with endometriosis.

Conversely, there have been several large studies that have failed to detect an impairment in fertilization. Dmowski et al. (53) analyzed 237 cycles and found no difference in either the fertilization rate or the early cleavage rate among patients with endometriosis or tubal-factor infertility. Another case–control study, also comparing endometriosis with tubal factor, found no evidence of either impaired fertilization or a decrease in embryo quality (73). In comparing the effect of progressive endometriosis stages on fertilization and embryo development, Inoue and colleagues (56) found no difference in either the fertilization rate or the embryo transfer rate for 309 patients with stage I–IV endometriosis. Furthermore, Bergendal et al, (54) although reporting impaired fertilization for women with endometriosis, noted no difference in either the cleavage rate or the morphologic embryo score, when compared with tubal infertility.

As it remains, the question of a significant effect by endometriosis on fertilization and in vitro embryo development has yet to be answered. Barnhart et al. (44) showed an overall decrease in fertilization rate when all endometriosis patients were compared to patients with tubal infertility, but when stratified by stage of disease, patients with severe endometriosis actually had an increase in fertilization rates. However, more recent studies have shown that any impaired fertilization has little or no effect on the ultimate outcome of IVF, as pregnancy rates for patients with endometriosis are comparable with other etiologies. Most recently, Suzuki et al. (74) found that endometriosis affects oocyte number but not embryo quality or pregnancy outcome, irrespective of the presence of an ovarian endometrioma. Perhaps the clinical insignificance of impaired fertilization is due to the fact that improved ovarian stimulation and oocyte-recovery techniques have led to a surplus of available oocytes for fertilization. An increased oocyte yield can readily sustain a slight decrease in fertilization capacity to produce enough embryos for implantation. It is unclear what role, if any, intracytoplasmic sperm injection (ICSI) may play in the fertilization of oocytes from women with endometriosis.

Implantation, Pregnancy, and Loss

Assuming a minimum number of good-quality embryos are available for transfer, a successful live birth is dependent on adequate implantation and a low rate of spontaneous abortion. However, as a result of the transfer of multiple embryos, a lower rate of implantation has not necessarily translated into a low pregnancy rate. Although a few contemporary studies have in fact reported reduced implantation rates, most have failed to demonstrate a correspondingly low pregnancy rate for patients with endometriosis. Some early studies have shown a decrease in the implantation rate with a subsequent decrease in the pregnancy rate (46,47,65). In a small study, Chillik and colleagues (45) reported a significantly lower implantation and pregnancy rate for patients with stage III or IV endometriosis when compared to patients with tubal factor or endometriosis of a lesser severity. Matson and Yovich (47) demonstrated pregnancy rates of 18%, 13%, 14%, 6%, and 2%, for patients with tubal factor, and stage I–IV endometriosis, respectively. Arici et al., (73) in a case–control study of 284 IVF cycles, reported a significantly lower implantation rate of 3.9% for patients with endometriosis, compared with 8.1% and 7.2% for tubal infertility and unexplained infertility, respectively. They also demonstrated a trend toward a lower pregnancy rate in patients with endometriosis, although this did not reach significance. More recent studies have taken this finding and added live birth and cumulative pregnancy rates. Omland et al. (43) found the live birth rate after transfer of two embryos to be 66.0% compared with 78.8% for unexplained etiology of infertility. Kuivasaari et al. (42) found a significantly lower cumulative pregnancy rate after one to four IVF/ICSI treatments in women with stage III/IV endometriosis compared to women with stage I/II endometriosis and a control of women with tubal infertility.

While Simon and colleagues (75) also reported lower implantation and pregnancy rates for patients with endometriosis versus tubal infertility, they added a dimension to the data by analyzing the outcomes of oocyte donation from donors with and without endometriosis. They reported comparable implantation and pregnancy rates for women with and without endometriosis, who received oocytes from donors without endometriosis. However, patients who received oocytes from endometriotic ovaries had significantly lower implantation rates. Another study reported on 239 oocyte donor cycles and found that the presence of endometriosis in the recipient had no effect on implantation or pregnancy rates, regardless of the disease stage (76). From this, it has been suggested that an endometriosis-associated impairment of implantation results from a compromise to the potential of the oocyte or early embryo, and not to the endometrium itself.

Several large investigations have failed to demonstrate either an impaired implantation rate or a lower pregnancy rate for patients with endometriosis, comparing stage by stage or with other infertility etiologies (54–58). Geber and colleagues (55) reported pregnancy rates in 140 cycles of 40% and 45% for patients with endometriosis or tubal infertility, respectively. Olivennes et al. noted similar pregnancy rates of 29% for endometriosis and 36% for tubal factor, (58) while another study reported 28% and 30%, respectively (54). Inoue et al. (56), in a study of 681 women with and without endometriosis, found no difference in the IVF conception rate between the two groups. Several comparisons within endometriosis stages have reported similar pregnancy rates despite increasing disease severity (46,53,55,73). Pal and colleagues (57) analyzed (77) IVF cycles in endometriosis patients with either stage I–II or stage III–IV disease. Although they reported a lower fertilization rate for patients with stage III or IV endometriosis, clinical pregnancy rates did not differ significantly between the two groups. In his meta-analysis, Barnhart et al. (44) calculated that the adjusted OR of achieving pregnancy compared with the group of controls was 0.56, 0.79, and 0.46, respectively, for overall patients, stage I/II, and stage III/IV patients, respectively (Table 55.2).

A few studies have associated endometriosis with increased pregnancy loss during IVF cycles. Oehninger and colleagues (46) noted a higher miscarriage rate following IVF among patients with stage III or IV endometriosis, when compared to those with less severe disease. Yanushpolsky et al. (69) reported, along with a diminished oocyte yield and poor embryo quality, a significantly higher early pregnancy loss when endometriomas were aspirated at the time of oocyte retrieval. However, another large study comparing patients with aspirated endometriomas to others with endometriosis found no difference in oocyte yield, embryo quality, pregnancy rate, or miscarriage (78). Furthermore, most studies have not reported a significant endometriosis-associated increase in pregnancy loss (54,55).

Endometriosis may also be associated with late pregnancy complications, such as preterm birth. Stephansson et al. (79) showed that compared with women without endometriosis, women with endometriosis had a higher risk of preterm birth, with an adjusted OR of 1.33. Conversely, Fernando et al. (80) showed an increased risk in preterm birth only when endometrioma were present. Women with endometriosis, but without endometrioma, did not show an increased risk for preterm birth when compared to women without endometriosis.

Endometriosis and Gamete Intrafallopian Transfer

There are limited data concerning the effect of endometriosis on gamete intrafallopian transfer (GIFT). Guzick and colleagues, (81) in a retrospective, case–control study, reported significantly different pregnancy rates of 32% and 47% for patients with or without endometriosis, respectively. Another study analyzed GIFT outcomes in patients with endometriosis and found decreased folliculogenesis and a lower oocyte yield with more severe disease, although the clinical pregnancy rate did not differ between patients with different stages of the disease or with other infertility etiologies (50).

In an early observational study, Yovich and Matson (82) reported a significantly higher pregnancy rate for patients with severe endometriosis treated with GIFT than for those undergoing IVF. Another study, however, failed to find a difference between the two (83) as with much of the ART data concerning endometriosis, no prospective, randomized studies exist comparing GIFT with IVF. With a lack of compelling evidence and an impressive success rate for IVF, it is difficult to assess the role of the more invasive GIFT procedure in initial attempts at assisted reproduction for patients with endometriosis.

Surgery and ART

As stated earlier, the data are conflicting regarding the effect of surgery on fertility in patients with endometriosis. Unfortunately, there have been no prospective, randomized studies investigating the effect of surgery for endometriosis on ART outcome. One retrospective study compared IVF with repeat surgery for patients with stage III or IV endometriosis (84). Recently, however, a Cochrane Review of two randomized trials comparing the effectiveness of laparoscopic surgery in the treatment of subfertility associated with endometriosis versus other treatment modalities or placebo found that use of laparoscopic surgery may improve the chance of pregnancy by an OR of 1.6 (85). Pregnancy rates were reported as 70% over two cycles of IVF compared with 24% for the nine months following surgery. There are no similar randomized studies evaluating the effects of surgery on severe disease. A nonrandomized study (26) demonstrated that

Table 55.2 Comparing Stage III–IV Disease with Stage I–II Disease: Results of Bivariate Analysis and Multiple Logistic Regression Comparing Endometriosis Endo Patients with Stage III–IV Disease with Patients with Stage I–II Disease

Outcome	Endo III–IV	Endo I–II	P	Crude OR (95 %CI)	Adjusted OR (95 %CI)
Pregnancy rate	13.84	21.12	<0.001	0.60 (0.42–0.87)	0.64 (0.34–1.17)
Fertilization rate	74.47	58.38	<0.001	1.11 (1.09–1.13)	Not interpretable
Implantation rate	10.23	11.31	0.003	0.93 (0.89–0.98)	0.21 (0.15–0.32)
Mean oocyte count	6.70	8.19	<0.001	0.83 (0.78–0.87)	0.31 (0.24–0.39)
Peak E$_2$	1447.74	5813.38	<0.001	N/A	N/A

Note: Total number of observations: 699.
[a]Adjusted for publication date and age.
Abbreviations: N/A, not applicable; OR, odds ratio.
Source: From Ref. 44.

the cumulative probability of pregnancy in 216 infertile patients with severe disease two years after surgery was significantly increased.

In another study, Garcia-Velasco et al. reported no difference in fertilization, implantation, or pregnancy rates for patients who had undergone removal of an endometrioma, as compared to patients with suspected endometriomas that were not removed (77). A meta-analysis (86) of five studies agreed with these results by concluding that surgical management of endometriomas has no significant effect on IVF pregnancy rates and ovarian response to stimulation compared with no treatment. In another recent randomized study comparing minimal and severe endometriosis with treatment modality, there was a significant difference in the cumulative probability of pregnancy rates between operative laparoscopy and expectant of GnRH analog treatment in patients with minimal disease. With severe disease, however, severity of disease, the number of endometriomata, their size, and unilateral or bilateral existence did not significantly affect the estimated cumulative pregnancy rates (87). Until better data are available, however, no definitive conclusions can be drawn regarding the role of surgery for endometriosis prior to ART. In fact, one recent study (88) finds that in the absence of tubal occlusion or severe male factor infertility, laparoscopy may still be considered for the treatment of endometriosis even after multiple failed IVF cycles.

Future Directions

Some researchers have suggested that endometriosis is associated with impaired folliculogenesis and a decreased oocyte yield. Although the data are conflicting, it is possible that the introduction of aromatase inhibitors may represent another large step forward in improving ovarian stimulation protocols and increasing IVF success. Further study of GnRH antagonists may also show a benefit for patients with endometriosis. Furthermore, the use of donor oocytes has been suggested to improve efficacy in patients with endometriosis. As ovarian hyperstimulation protocols become more tolerable, and as oocyte cryopreservation becomes efficacious and efficient, it is possible that an increased number of women with endometriosis who have failed standard IVF will benefit from donation.

There is evidence for and against an endometriosis-associated impairment of oocyte fertilization in vitro. One of the tremendous benefits of fertilizing an oocyte in vitro is the ability to assess the process on a case-by-case basis. For patients with endometriosis who are experiencing fertilization difficulty, it is likely that ICSI will prove to be a valuable addition to the technology of assisted reproduction for this disease. Indeed, ICSI has proven to be of tremendous worth in achieving pregnancy in couples with male factor infertility. Minguez et al. (87) analyzed 980 cycles of ICSI for couples with male factor infertility, of which 101 cycles were also complicated by endometriosis. They found no significant difference in fertilization, implantation, or pregnancy rates with coexisting endometriosis.

Finally, there is an increasing interest in the prolongation of in vitro embryo maturation, with many investigators studying the efficacy of blastocyst development and implantation. An endometriosis-associated detriment to implantation may be responsible for some IVF failures. Although reports are conflicting, some have suggested an impaired early embryo development in patients with endometriosis. It is possible that the practice of in vitro maturation to the blastocyst stage in these patients may allow for the transfer of a more selected group of healthier embryos, thus improving the implantation rate. It is anticipated that the improvements from this approach will eventually raise the implantation rate to a point at which it will become routine to transfer no more than one or two embryos at a time, thereby significantly lowering the incidence of multiple pregnancies. Furthermore, the adoption of various techniques in embryo manipulation, such as assisted hatching, may also have a positive effect on the implantation rate for these patients.

CONCLUSION

It is important to stress the heterogeneous nature of the data that has been reviewed. Laboratory and clinical practices vary greatly from center to center, as do the corresponding IVF success rates. Randomized, prospective studies designed to answer key questions about the optimum algorithmic approach to the treatment of endometriosis-associated infertility simply do not exist. With the evidence evaluated as a whole, it does appear that IVF outcomes have improved significantly for endometriosis patients with the adoption of GnRH agonists and transvaginal oocyte retrieval.

Although ART procedure alterations are site-specific, the vast majority of endometriosis patients undergo the same treatment protocol as for those patients with tubal factor or unexplained infertility. There is, to date, no compelling evidence that endometriosis patients benefit from significant alterations from standard ART protocols or procedures, with the notable exception of prolonged GnRH agonist downregulation. Until large, randomized, prospective studies have answered questions regarding the optimum length of downregulation, the use of in vitro maturation or manipulation, the role of autoantibodies and immunosuppression, and other controversies, it is likely that patients with endometriosis will continue to undergo the same treatment protocol as everyone else. At the very least, it can be said that ART represents a tremendous advancement for women who, for whatever reason, have been unable to achieve pregnancy. For the patient with endometriosis, evolving options in pharmacotherapy and assisted reproduction may finally offer the blessing of a pain-free and reproductive life.

REFERENCES

1. Counseller VS. Endometriosis: A clinical and surgical review. Am J Obstet Gynecol 1938; 36: 877–88.
2. Hasson HM. Incidence of endometriosis in diagnostic laparoscopy. J Reprod Med 1976; 16: 135–8.

3. Strathy JH, Molgaard CA, Coulam CB, Melton LJ. Endometriosis and infertility: A laparoscopic study of endometriosis among fertile and infertile women. Fertil Steril 1982; 38: 667–72.

4. Drake TS, Grunert GM. The unsuspected pelvic factor in the infertility investigation. Fertil Steril 1980; 34: 27–31.

5. Hammond MG, Jordan S, Sloan CS. Factors affecting pregnancy rates in a donor insemination program using frozen semen. Am J Obstet Gynecol 1986; 155: 480–5.

6. Yeh J, Seibel MM. Artificial insemination with donor sperm: A review of 108 patients. Obstet Gynecol 1987; 70: 313–16.

7. Jansen RPS. Minimal endometriosis and reduced fecundibility: Prospective evidence from an artificial insemination by a donor program. Fertil Steril 1986; 46: 141–3.

8. Matorras R, Corcostegui B, Esteban J, et al. Fertility in women with minimal endometriosis compared with normal women was assessed by means of a donor insemination program in unstimulated cycles. Am J Obstet Gynecol 2010; 203: 345.e1–6.

9. Bancroft K, Vaughan-Williams CA, Elstein M. Pituitary–ovarian function in women with minimal or mild endometriosis and otherwise unexplained infertility. Clin Endocrinol 1992; 36: 177–81.

10. Matorras R, Rodriguez F, Perez C, et al. Infertile women with and without endometriosis: A case control study of luteal phase and other infertility conditions. Acta Obstet Gynecol Scand 1996; 75: 826–31.

11. Pittaway DE, Maxson W, Daniell J, Herbert C, Wentz AC. Luteal phase defects in infertility patients with endometriosis. Fertil Steril 1983; 39: 712–13.

12. Hirschowitz JS, Soler NG, Wortsman J. The galactorrhea-endometriosis syndrome. Lancet 1978; 1: 896–8.

13. Mio Y, Toda T, Harada T, Terakawa N. Luteinized unruptured follicle in the early stages of endometriosis as a cause of unexplained infertility. Am J Obstet Gynecol 1992; 167: 271–3.

14. Wheeler JM, Johnston BM, Malinak LR. The relationship of endometriosis to spontaneous abortion. Fertil Steril 1983; 39: 656–60.

15. Burns WN, Schenken RS. Pathophysiology of endometriosis-associated infertility. Clin Obstet Gynecol 1999; 42: 586–610.

16. Thomas EJ, Lenton EA, Cooke ID. Follicle growth patterns and endocrinological abnormalities in infertile women with minor degrees of endometriosis. Br J Obstet Gynaecol 1986; 93: 852–8.

17. Kusuhara K. Luteal function in infertile patients with endometriosis. Am J Obstet Gynecol 1992; 167: 274–7.

18. Matalliotakis I, Panidis D, Vlassis G, et al. PRL, TSH and their response to the TRH test in patients with endometriosis before, during, and after treatment with danazol. Gynecol Obstet Invest 1996; 42: 183–6.

19. Pittaway DE, Vernon C, Fayez JA. Spontaneous abortions in women with endometriosis. Fertil Steril 1988; 50: 711–15.

20. Matorras R, Rodriguez F, Gutierrez de Teran G, et al. Endometriosis and spontaneous abortion rate: A cohort study in infertile women. Eur J Obstet Gynecol Reprod Biol 1998; 77: 101–5.

21. Senturk LM, Arici A. Immunology of endometriosis. J Reprod Immunol 1999; 43: 67–83.

22. Dun EC, Taylor RN, Wieser F. Advances in the genetics of endometriosis. Genome Medicine 2010; 2: 75.

23. Hughes E, Fedorkow DM, Collins J, Vandekerckhove P. Ovulation suppression versus placebo in the treatment of endometriosis. In: Lilford R, Hughes E, Vandekerckehove P, eds. Subfertility Module of the Cochrane Database of Systematic Reviews. Oxford: The Cochrane Collection, 1997.

24. Marcoux S, Maheux R, Berube S. The Canadian Collaborative Group on Endometriosis. Laparoscopic surgery in infertile women with minimal or mild endometriosis. N Engl J Med 1997; 336: 217–22.

25. Gruppo Italiano per lo Studio dell'Endometriosi. Ablation of lesions or no treatment in minimal–mild endometriosis in infertile women: A randomized trial. Hum Reprod 1999; 14: 1332–4.

26. Al-Inany HG, Crosignani PG, Vercellini P. Evidence may change with more trials: Concepts to be kept in mind [letters]. Hum Reprod 2000; 15: 2447–8.

27. Benschop L, Farquhar C, van der Poel N, Heineman MJ. Interventions for women with endometrioma prior to assisted reproductive technology. Cochrane Dateabase of SystemicReviews 2010:CD008571.DOI:10.1002/14651858. CD008571.pub2.

28. Guzick DS, Carson SA, Coutifaris C, et al. Efficacy of superovulation and intrauterine insemination in the treatment of infertility. N Engl J Med 1999; 340: 177–83.

29. Deaton JL, Gibson M, Blackmer KM, et al. A randomized, controlled trial of clomiphene citrate and intrauterine insemination in couples with unexplained infertility or surgically corrected endometriosis. Fertil Steril 1990; 54: 1083–8.

30. Fedele L, Parazzini F, Radici E, et al. Buserelin acetate versus expectant management in the treatment of infertility associated with mild endometriosis: A randomized clinical trial. Fertil Steril 1992; 58: 28–31.

31. Nuojua-Huttunen S, Tomas C, Bloigu R, Tuomivaara L, Martikainen H. Intrauterine insemination treatment in subfertility: An analysis of factors affecting outcome. Hum Reprod 1999; 14: 698–703.

32. Omland A, Tanbo T, Dale PO, Abyholm T. Artificial insemination by husband in unexplained infertility compared with infertility associated with peritoneal endometriosis. Hum Reprod 1998; 13: 2602–5.

33. Hughes EG. The effectiveness of ovulation induction and intrauterine insemination in the treatment of persistent infertility: A meta-analysis. Hum Reprod 1997; 12: 1865–72.

34. Tummon IS, Asher LJ, Martin JS, Tulandi T. Randomized controlled trial of superovulation and insemination for infertility associated with minimal or mild endometriosis. Fertil Steril 1997; 68: 8–12.

35. Capelo F, Kumar A, Steinkampf M, Azziz R. Laparoscopic evaluation following failure to achieve pregnancy after ovulation induction with clomiphene citrate. Fertil Steril 2003; 80: 1450–3.

36. Werbrouck E, Spiessens C, Meuleman C, D'Hooghe T. No difference in cycle pregnancy rate and in cumulative live-birth rate between women with surgically treated minimal to mild endometriosis and women with unexplained infertility after controlled ovarian hyperstimulation and intrauterine insemination. Fertil Steril 2005; 86: 566–71.

37. Karaer O, Oruc S, Koyuncu FM. Aromatase inhibitors: Possible future applications. Acta Obstet Gynecol Scand 2004; 83: 699–706.

38. Attar E, Bulun S. Aromatase inhibitors: the next genera-
     tion of therapeutics for endometriosis? Fertil Steril
     2006; 85: 1307–18.
39. Wu HH, Wang NM, Cheng ML, Hsieh JN. A randomized
     comparison of ovulation induction and hormone pro-
     file between the aromatase inhibitor anastrozole and
     clomiphene citrate in women with infertility. Gynecol
     Endocrinol 2007; 23: 76–81.
40. Cantineau AEP, Cohlen BJ, Klip H, Heineman MJ. Dutch
     IUI Study Group Collaborators. The addition of GnRH
     antagonists in intrauterine insemination cycles with
     mild ovarian hyperstimulation does not increase live
     birth rates – a randomized, double-blinded, placebo-
     controlled trial. Hum Reprod 2011; 26: 1104–11.
41. The Practice Committee of the American Society of
     Reproductive Medicine. Endometriosis and infertiity.
     Fertil Steril 2006; 86: S156–60.
42. Kuivasaari P, Hippelainen M, Anttila M, Heinonen S.
     Effect of endometriosis on IVF/ICSI outcome: Stage III/
     IV endometriosis worsens cumulative pregnancy and
     live-born rates. Hum Reprod 2005; 20: 3130–5.
43. Omland AK, Abyholm T, Fedorcsak P, et al. Preg-
     nancy outcome after IVF and ICSI in unexplained,
     endometriosis-associated and tubal factor infertility.
     Hum Reprod 2005; 20: 722–7.
44. Barnhart K, Dunsmoor-Su R, Coutifaris C. Effect of
     endometriosis on in vitro fertilization. Fertil Steril
     2002; 77: 1148–55.
45. Chillik CF, Acosta AA, Garcia JE, et al. The role of
     in vitro fertilization in infertile patients with endome-
     triosis. Fertil Steril 1985; 44: 56–61.
46. Oehninger S, Acosta AA, Kreiner D, et al. In vitro fertil-
     ization and embryo transfer IVF/ET: An established
     and successful therapy for endometriosis. J In Vitro
     Fert Embryo Transf 1988; 5: 249–56.
47. Matson PL, Yovich JL. The treatment of infertility
     associated with endometriosis by in vitro fertilization.
     Fertil Steril 1986; 46: 432–4.
48. Yovich JL, Matson PL, Richardson PA, Hilliard C. Hor-
     monal profiles and embryo quality in women with
     severe endometriosis treated by in vitro fertilization
     and embryo transfer. Fertil Steril 1988; 50: 308–13.
49. Yovich JL, Matson PL. The influence of infertility etiol-
     ogy on the outcome of IVF–ET and GIFT treatments. Int
     J Fertil 1990; 35: 26–33.
50. Chang MY, Chiang CH, Hsieh TT, Soong YK, Hsu KH.
     The influence of endometriosis on the success of gam-
     ete intrafallopian transfer GIFT. J Assist Reprod Genet
     1997; 14: 76–82.
51. Dlugi AM, Loy RA, Dieterle S, Bayer SR, Seibel MM.
     The effect of endometriomas on in vitro fertilization
     outcome. J In Vitro Fert Embryo Transf 1989; 6: 338–41.
52. Somigliana E, Infantino M, Benedetti F, et al. The pres-
     ence of ovarian endometriomas is associated with a
     reduced responsiveness to gonadotropins. Fertil Steril
     2006; 86: 192–6.
53. Dmowski WP, Rana N, Michalowska J, et al. The effect
     of endometriosis, its stage and activity, and of autoanti-
     bodies on in vitro fertilization and embryo transfer suc-
     cess rates. Fertil Steril 1995; 63: 555–62.
54. Bergendal A, Naffah S, Nagy C, et al. Outcome of IVF in
     patients with endometriosis in comparison with tubal-
     factor infertility. J Assist Reprod Genet 1998; 15: 530–4.
55. Geber S, Paraschos T, Atkinson G, Margara R, Winston
     RM. Results of IVF in patients with endometriosis: The
     severity of the disease does not affect outcome, or
     the incidence of miscarriage. Hum Reprod 1995; 10:
     1507–11.
56. Inoue M, Kobayashi Y, Honda I, Awaji H, Fujii A. The
     impact of endometriosis on the reproductive outcome
     of infertile patients. Am J Obstet Gynecol 1992; 167:
     278–82.
57. Pal L, Shifren JL, Isaacson KB, et al. Impact of varying
     stages of endometriosis on the outcome of in vitro
     fertilization–embryo transfer. J Assist Reprod Genet
     1998; 15: 27–31.
58. Olivennes F, Feldberg D, Liu HC, et al. Endometriosis:
     A stage by stage analysis – the role of in vitro fertiliza-
     tion. Fertil Steril 1995; 64: 392–8.
59. Oehninger S, Brzyski RG, Muasher SJ, Acosta AA, Jones
     GS. In vitro fertilization and embryo transfer in patients
     with endometriosis: Impact of a gonadotrophin releas-
     ing hormone agonist. Hum Reprod 1989; 4: 541–4.
60. Dicker D, Goldman JA, Levy T, Feldberg D, Ashkenazi J.
     The impact of long-term gonadotropin-releasing hor-
     mone analogue treatment on preclinical abortions in
     patients with severe endometriosis undergoing in vitro
     fertilization–embryo transfer. Fertil Steril 1992; 57:
     597–600.
61. Rickes D, Nickel I, Kropf S, Kleinstein J. Increased preg-
     nancy rates after ultralong postoperative therapy with
     gonadotropin-releasing hormone analogs in patients
     with endometriosis. Fertil Steril 2002; 78: 757–62.
62. Chedid S, Camus M, Smitz J, Van Steirteghem AC,
     Devroey P. Comparison among different ovarian stim-
     ulation regimens for assisted procreation procedures
     in patients with endometriosis. Hum Reprod 1995; 10:
     2406–11.
63. Nakamura K, Oosawa M, Kondou I, et al. Metrodin
     stimulation after prolonged gonadotropin releasing
     hormone agonist pretreatment for in vitro fertilization
     in patients with endometriosis. J Assist Reprod Genet
     1992; 9: 113–17.
64. Marcus SF, Edwards RG. High rates of pregnancy after
     long-term down-regulation of women with severe endo-
     metriosis. Am J Obstet Gynecol 1994; 171: 812–17.
65. Surrey ES, Silverberg KM, Surrey MW, Schoolcraft WB.
     Effect of prolonged gonadotropin-releasing hormone
     agonist therapy on the outcome of in vitro fertilization–
     embryo transfer in patients with endometriosis. Fertil
     Steril 2002; 78: 699–704.
66. de Ziegler D, Gayet V, Aubriot PF, et al. Use of oral
     contraceptives in women with endometriosis before
     assisted reproduction treatment improves outcomes.
     Fertil Steril 2010; 94: 2796–9.
67. Recai P, Onalan G, Kaya C. GnRH agonist and antago-
     nist protocols for stage I-II endometriosis and endome-
     trioma in in vitro fertilization/intracytoplasmic sperm
     injection cycles. Fertil Steril 2007; 88: 832–8.
68. Wardle PG, Mitchell JD, McLaughlin EA, et al. Endome-
     triosis and ovulatory disorder: Reduced fertilisation in
     vitro compared with tubal and unexplained infertility.
     Lancet 1985; 2: 236–9.
69. Yanushpolsky EH, Best CL, Jackson KV, et al. Effects of
     endometriomas on ooccyte quality, embryo quality,
     and pregnancy rates in in vitro fertilization cycles:
     A prospective, case-controlled study. J Assist Reprod
     Genet 1998; 15: 193–7.
70. Pellicer A, Oliveira N, Ruiz A, Remohi J, Simon C.
     Exploring the mechanisms of endometriosis-related

infertility: An analysis of embryo development and implantation in assisted reproduction. Hum Reprod 1995; 10(Suppl 2): 91–7.

71. Tanbo T, Omland A, Dale PO, Abyholm T. In vitro fertilization/embryo transfer in unexplained infertility and minimal peritoneal endometriosis. Acta Obstet Gynecol Scand 1995; 74: 539–43.

72. Brizek CL, Schlaff S, Pellegrini VA, Frank JB, Worrilow KC. Increased incidence of aberrant morphological phenotypes in human embryogenesis – an association with endometriosis. J Assist Reprod Genet 1995; 12: 106–12.

73. Arici A, Oral E, Bukulmez O, et al. The effect of endometriosis on implantation: Results from the Yale University in vitro fertilization and embryo transfer program. Fertil Steril 1996; 65: 603–7.

74. Suzuki T, Izumi SI, Matsubayashi H, et al. Impact of ovarian endometrioma on oocyte and pregnancy outcome in in vitro fertilization. Fertil Steril 2005; 83: 908–13.

75. Simon C, Gutierrez A, Vidal A, et al. Outcome of patients with endometriosis in assisted reproduction: Results from in vitro fertilization and oocyte donation. Hum Reprod 1994; 9: 725–9.

76. Sung L, Mukherjee T, Takeshige T, Bustillo M, Copperman AB. Endometriosis is not detrimental to embryo implantation in oocyte recipients. J Assist Reprod Genet 1997; 14: 152–6.

77. Garcia-Velasco JA, Mahutte NG, Corona J, et al. Removal of endometriomas before in vitro fertilization does not improve fertility outcomes: A matched, case-control study. Fertil Steril 2004; 81: 1194–7.

78. Isaacs JD Jr, Hines RS, Sopelak VM, Cowan BD. Ovarian endometriomas do not adversely affect pregnancy success following treatment with in vitro fertilization. J Assist Reprod Genet 1997; 14: 551–3.

79. Stephansson O, Kieler H, Granath F, Falconer H. Endometriosis, assisted reproduction technology, and risk of adverse pregnancy outcome. Hum Reprod 2009; 24: 2341–7.

80. Fernando S, Breheny VS, Jaques AM, et al. Preterm birth, ovarian endometriomata, and assisted reproduction technologies. Fertil Steril 2009; 91: 325–30.

81. Guzick DS, Yao YA, Berga SL, et al. Endometriosis impairs the efficacy of gamete intrafallopian transfer: Results of a case-control study. Fertil Steril 1994; 62: 1186–91.

82. Yovich JL, Matson PL. The influence of infertility etiology on the outcome of IVF–ET and GIFT treatments. Int J Fertil 1986; 35: 26–33.

83. Tanbo T, Dale PO, Abyholm T. Assisted fertilization in infertile women with patent fallopian tubes. A comparison of in vitro fertilization, gamete intrafallopian transfer, and tubal embryo stage transfer. Hum Reprod 1990; 5: 266–70.

84. Pagidas K, Falcone T, Hemmings R, Miron P. Comparison of reoperation for moderate stage III and severe stage IV endometriosis-related infertility with in vitro fertilization–embryo transfer. Fertil Steril 1996; 65: 791–5.

85. Jacobson T, Barlow D, Koninckx P, Olive D, Farquhar C. Laparoscopic surgery for subfertility associated with endometriosis Cochrane Review. In: The Cochrane Library. Chichester, UK: John Wiley and Sons, 2004: 1.

86. Tsoumpou I, Kyrgiou M, Gelbaya TA, Nardo LG. The effect of surgical treatment for endometrioma on in vitro fertilization outcomes: a systematic review and meta-analysis. Fertil Steril 2009; 92: 75–87.

87. Minguez Y, Rubio C, Bernal A, et al. The impact of endometriosis in couples undergoing intracytoplasmic sperm injection because of male infertility. Hum Reprod 1997; 12: 2282–5.

88. Littman E, Giudice L, Lathi R, et al. Role of laparoscopic treatment of endometriosis in patients with failed in vitro fertilization cycles. Fertil Steril 2005; 84: 1574–8.

89. Mahadevan MM, Trounson AO, Leeton JF. The relationship of tubal blockage, infertility of unknown cause, suspected male infertility, and endometriosis to the success of in vitro fertilization and embryo transfer. Fertil Steril 1983; 40: 755–62.

90. Sharma V, Riddle A, Mason BA, Pampiglione J, Campbell S. An analysis of factors influencing the establishment of a clinical pregnancy in an ultrasound-based ambulatory in vitro fertilization program. Fertil Steril 1988; 49: 468–78.

56

PCOS and assisted reproduction

Susie Nicholas, Christopher Brewer, Thomas H. Tang, and Adam H. Balen

INTRODUCTION

Polycystic ovary syndrome (PCOS) is a common polygenic multifactorial condition, affecting a wide population. Historically, the classic combination of symptoms was first described in 1935 by Stein and Leventhal (1), who recognized that enlarged ovaries, amenorrhea, infertility, and hirsutism could be collated together. This collection of symptoms has been widely researched and many conclusions made, yet it continues to pose a difficult condition to treat. PCOS is now recognized as a spectrum disorder ranging from ultrasound features of polycystic ovarian morphology (2) to anovulatory infertility. Obesity, hyperandrogenemia, and insulin resistance are all key factors that influence the expression and symptoms of the condition (3–5).

PCOS poses an interesting problem for assisted reproduction. Anovulation is common among women with PCOS and accounts for 80–90% of WHO group II anovulatory subfertility. Treatment has centered on weight management and lifestyle modification followed by ovulation induction with clomiphene citrate (6). The cumulative pregnancy rate with clomiphene after six months of treatment is between 40% and 50% (7,8). Women who remain anovulatory can be stimulated with low dose gonadotropins. Ovarian diathermy has been suggested as an effective alternative in ovulation induction (9). For those who remain refractory to these treatments or with coexisting pathologies, assisted reproductive techniques (ARTs) can be employed within a closely supervised setting to produce the desired outcome of pregnancy with the challengingly sensitive polycystic ovary (PCO) (10).

DIAGNOSIS AND PREVALENCE

The classification of PCOS has been accepted and simplified through the Rotterdam consensus workshop in 2003 (11). No single diagnostic criterion is sufficient for the clinical diagnosis of PCOS. Two of the following are required:

1. oligo and/or anovulation,
2. clinical and/or biochemical signs of hyperandrogenism, and
3. polycystic ovary morphology on ultrasound.

Exclusion of other etiologies (such as congenital adrenal hyperplasia, androgen-secreting tumor, and Cushing's syndrome) must be elucidated by appropriate investigation as indicated.

With the advancing technology and imaging of transvaginal ultrasound, the consensus went further in defining PCO morphology (12). Twelve or more follicles measuring 2–9 mm or increased ovarian volume over $10\,cm^3$ offers the best specificity (99%) and sensitivity (75%) for the diagnosis of PCOS (13). The distribution of follicles and description of the stroma are not required. Jonard et al. reported a significant increase in 2–5 mm follicles with no change in 6–9 mm follicle number compared with controls. This prompted a hypothesis that the hyperandrogenic microenvironment resulted from an increased recruitment of growing follicles followed by their arrest at 6–9 mm (13). Since the Rotterdam consensus, there has been further debate about the definitions of both the syndrome and the morphology of the PCO. Yet it is beyond the scope of this chapter to expand on these challenging controversies.

The prevalence of PCOS is determined by the diagnostic criteria used within the study, ethnic origin, and the population of women studied. Michelmore et al., (14) who included US morphology and menstrual disturbance, revealed a prevalence of 26% in 230 volunteers. Further population studies have confirmed a common finding of PCO in 21–23%; although a significant proportion (25%) were without any clinical features of PCOS (2). The highest reported prevalence of PCO is 52% in South Asians living within Britain (15) with menstrual irregularities in 49.1%. South Asians with anovulatory PCOS have greater insulin resistance and severity of symptoms compared with their Caucasian counterparts (16). However, Knochenhauer et al., who did not use ultrasound features, did not find a significant difference between black and white women within a U.S. population (3.4% vs. 4.7%) and the lower prevalence related to the use of the older NIH definition for the syndrome (17).

REPRODUCTIVE HEALTH IN PCOS

In addition to anovulation there may be other factors that contribute to subfertility in women with PCOS including the effects of obesity, metabolic, inflammatory, and endocrine abnormalities on oocyte quality and fetal development. Oocytes from polycystic ovaries may exhibit reduced developmental competence with a reduced ability to complete meiosis, achieve fertilization, and develop into a normal embryo. Ovarian hyperandrogenism and hyperinsulinemia may promote premature granulosa cell luteinization; furthermore, paracrine dysregulation of growth factors may disrupt the intrafollicular environment, alter granulosa cell–oocyte interactions, and impair cytoplasmic and/or nuclear maturation of oocytes (18). There is variability, however, and oocyte quality, fertilization, and implantation rates in women with PCOS may be normal (19).

PCOS is associated with metabolic disturbances that include impaired insulin signaling and glucose metabolism in ovarian follicles (20). It is likely that the metabolic lesion in the follicle precipitates an altered metabolic milieu throughout oogenesis, which may have downstream consequences for oocyte energy generation. This may lead to reduced expression of genes encoding oxidative phosphorylation (21). Altered expression of key genes associated with chromosome alignment and segregation has also been attributed to hyperandrogenemia (22). Indeed it has been shown that differences in metabolism exist in oocytes derived from women with PCOS and this is associated with chromosomal predivision, that is premature separation of sister chromatids (23). During early pregnancy the embryo may be exposed to androgen excess in utero, which may have long-term effects particularly on female offspring. Fetal hyperandrogenism may disturb epigenetic programming, in particular those genes regulating reproduction and metabolism (24,25). It is also possible that transgenerational effects may be related to the potential influences of hyperinsulinemia and its effect on the intrauterine environment.

In a meta-analysis in which pregnancy outcomes in women with PCOS were compared with controls, women with PCOS demonstrated a significantly higher risk of developing gestational diabetes mellitus (GDM) [odds ratio (OR) 2.94; 95% confidence interval (CI): 1.70–5.08], pregnancy-induced hypertension (OR 3.67; 95% CI: 1.98–6.81), pre-eclampsia (OR 3.47; 95% CI: 1.95–6.17), and preterm birth (OR 1.75; 95% CI: 1.16–2.62). Their babies had a significantly higher risk of admission to a neonatal intensive care unit (OR 2.31; 95% CI: 1.25–4.26) and a higher perinatal mortality (OR 3.07; 95% CI: 1.03–9.21), unrelated to multiple births (26). In addition, GDM may also result in fetal macrosomia. Obesity in its own right is associated with several adverse pregnancy outcomes, including spontaneous miscarriage, pre-eclampsia, gestational diabetes, congenital anomalies (e.g., cardiac and spina bifida), and fetal macrosomia (27).

HYPERANDROGENEMIA

Hyperandrogenism, in conjunction with hyperinsulinemia, is a cardinal feature of PCOS. It is plausible that the follicular microenvironment is related to oocyte quality. Teissier et al. showed that follicular testosterone levels were significantly elevated in PCOS, especially in the meiotically incompetent oocytes (28). High androgen levels may therefore contribute to the lower fertilization rate among the oocytes retrieved from a PCO.

Conversely, a positive correlation exists between testosterone concentration and the number of antral follicles (2–5 mm in diameter). Pretreatment with an aromatase inhibitor increases the ovarian androgen level, improving ovarian response in the low responder within an in vitro fertilization (IVF) treatment (29). Increased androgen levels therefore result in an increased recruitment of primordial follicles from the resting pool.

On the day of administration of human chorionic gonadotropin (hCG), the PCOS subject will have a higher estradiol concentration. This may, in part, be explained by an increase in androgen substrates and aromatase activity (30). Under in vitro conditions, granulosa cells from a PCO exhibit an increased response to FSH stimulation to size matched controls (31,32), potentially from the higher number of FSH receptors attributed to the stimulatory effects of androgen on FSH receptor synthesis (33). Androgen enhances the production of ovarian steroids in response to gonadotropin stimulation while promoting the expression of insulin-like growth factor-1 (IGF-1) and IGF-1 receptor gene expression in the growing follicles up to the small antral stage (34).

Serum androgen levels rise during ovarian stimulation and are higher in PCOS patients. The higher levels are suggested to negatively impact on pregnancy outcome (35,36). A negative correlation exists between androgen concentration and uterine placental protein (PP14, also known as glycodelin) (37) in women with PCOS and recurrent miscarriage. Glycodelin is an important secretory protein from the endometrium and is a marker of endometrial receptivity (38). They are increased in successful conception IVF cycles. Androstenedione causes a dose-dependent reduction in glycodelin and endometrial cell proliferation, (39) which is inhibited by administration of an antiandrogen, cyproterone. A reduction in sex hormone-binding globulin in the endometrial stroma in PCOS increases the bioavailability of androgens (40). With an overall increase in expression of endometrial androgen receptors, high levels of estrogen and androgen upregulate this expression, while progesterone has the opposite effect (41). Alpha-v Beta-3 integrin, a cell adhesion molecule, is suppressed at the time of implantation by high androgen levels further reflecting endometrial reduced receptivity (42).

OBESITY

Central obesity is a major factor influencing outcomes of both treatment of symptoms and infertility in women with PCOS. Obesity is seen in 38–66% of those with PCOS, with body mass index (BMI) correlating with severity of the phenotypical features. Clinical pregnancy rates (CPRs) are significantly lower in the obese in both natural and assisted conception cycles (43–45). Jungheim et al. have shown in a retrospective cohort that a BMI >40 kg/m² in women with PCOS who undergo IVF significantly reduced the CPR (32% vs. 72%, relative risk 0.44) (46). This also translated to a reduced live birth rate although failed to reach significance (32% vs. 60%) (47). A reduced fertilization rate, fewer oocytes, and reduced peak estradiol level highlight the impaired follicular and oocyte response in the morbidly obese. Other problems related to obesity include miscarriage and cancellation of assisted reproductive cycles (48). Fedorcsak et al. (49) concluded that obesity, independent of insulin resistance, is associated with the increase in miscarriage, gonadotropin resistance, and reduction in oocyte number. Dokras et al. found a 25.3% IVF cycle cancellation rate (BMI > 40) compared with 10.9% in those with a normal BMI (OR 2.73, 95% CI 1.49–5) (50).

An increased follicle-stimulating hormone (FSH) requirement is needed in the obese to stimulate the ovary but once the threshold has been reached, the subsequent response can be dramatic leading to an uncontrolled response and a risk of ovarian hyperstimulation syndrome (OHSS) (51,52). This may be related in part to insulin resistance.

We should not purely focus on conception as the main problem of the obese. As the epidemic of obesity gains velocity, the importance of maternal health should remain paramount. The triennial CEMACH report on "Saving mother's lives" is sobering with obesity implicated in 22% of maternal deaths in the United Kingdom (53). Both obesity and PCOS increase the risk of developing GDM, pre-eclampsia, and preterm birth. Obesity also increases the need for operative delivery with the ensuing problems of wound infection and venous thromboembolism. Targeted preconceptional counseling is paramount in reducing the spiraling problems related to obesity, fertility, and childbirth. The national guidance of needing to obtain a BMI of less than 30 to be eligible for national health service (NHS) fertility treatment within the United Kingdom goes a small way in promoting these salient facts.

OVARIAN STIMULATION RESPONSE IN PCOS

Ovulation induction for women with polycystic ovaries requires a different approach to that for women with normal ovaries. The response is often initially slow but then may spiral rapidly to a picture of over-response, with a significant risk of ovarian hyperstimulation and cyst formation (54,55). Theoretically one would expect an altered response in the multifollicular recruitment required for conventional IVF and indeed this has been illustrated in a number of studies (55).

Dor et al. showed a significant increase in oocyte number recovered per cycle when compared with tubal factor infertility (10.6 ± 6.1 vs. 5.4 ± 2.9 $p < 0.004$) but a lower fertilization rate (40.4% vs. 67.6%, $p < 0.001$) (56). Mac-Dougall et al. compared ultrasonographic PCO patients with matched controls (57). PCO patients needed significantly less human menopausal gonadotropin (hMG) but still reached a significantly higher estradiol level on the ovulation trigger day with hCG (5940 vs. 4370 pmol/l, $p < 0.001$). More oocytes were retrieved (9.3 vs. 6.8, $p = 0.003$) but fertilization rates were reduced (52.8% vs. 66.1%, $p = 0.007$). The pregnancy rate per transfer favored

the PCO group (25.4% vs. 23%) although live birth rate was similar. Kodama et al. demonstrated a higher incidence of embryo transfer cancellation due to failed fertilization and OHSS (58). A recent meta-analysis confirmed these findings despite a wide range of demographics and regimens being included (59).

Despite comparable pregnancy rates, the miscarriage rate in women with PCOS following IVF remains high compared with women with normal ovaries (35.8% vs. 23.6%, $p = 0.0038$) (60,61). This unwanted outcome is proportional to BMI, increased waist-hip ratio, and insulin resistance. Fedorcsak et al. (62) reported a relative risk of 1.77 of miscarriage for women with a BMI over 25 kg/m² before six weeks gestation.

Several explanations exist for the excessive response of the PCO to ovarian stimulation. Women with PCOS have an increased number of antral follicles (63,64). Contrary to earlier theories, these follicles are not atretic but rather there is an increased cohort of selectable antral follicles sensitive to exogenous gonadotropins. Anti-Müllerian hormone (AMH), a dimeric glycoprotein produced from the granulosa cells of the preantral and antral follicles, is elevated in PCOS (65). An increased stockpile of antral follicles is contributed to by an increase in recruitment of primordial follicles from the resting pool (66,67). There is a spectrum of response, with some responding easily to treatment and others with higher AMH levels, who may exhibit more symptoms such as amenorrhea and insulin resistance. Circulating insulin, IGF, and androgen concentrations are all implicated in the higher rate of recruitment (68–70).

OVARIAN HYPERSTIMULATION SYNDROME

OHSS is the most serious iatrogenic complication of IVF treatment (71). In the most severe cases hypovolemia, thromboembolism, hemoconcentration, ascites, hydrothorax, pericardial effusion, or adult respiratory distress syndrome can occur. Patients with PCOS undergoing IVF treatment are at a higher risk (72) but the incidence is hard to quantify, ranging from 10% to 18% (57,58). The documentation of OHSS as a study endpoint has historically been neglected as shown by a meta-analysis in this high risk population (59). Higher estradiol concentrations and oocyte number occur in those who develop OHSS (73). The cardinal feature of the pathogenesis of OHSS is an increased capillary permeability (74).

Vascular endothelial growth factor (VEGF) is a potent angiogenic endothelial cell mitogen and a key mediator of OHSS (75). Serum and follicular levels are higher in PCOS subjects and those who develop OHSS on the day of egg collection (76). Estradiol and VEGF levels positively correlate on the day of hCG administration, with VEGF being the best predictor of OHSS (77). Furthermore, OHSS is more common in a successful pregnancy cycle or IVF cycle using HCG for luteal support (71). Herr et al. demonstrate the direct effect of hCG on the expression of VEGF mRNA within human luteinized granulosa cells (78). The expression is higher in OHSS subjects compared with controls (79). Miele et al. demonstrated that insulin and

IGF-1 increase VEGF mRNA expression (80). The synergistic effect of insulin with gonadotropin and hCG is confirmed by Agrawal et al. (81). More recently, Stanek et al. confirmed the effects of insulin and IGF on VEGF production in PCOS and non-PCOS women (82).

SUPEROVULATION STRATEGIES

Pituitary desensitization with a gonadotropin-releasing hormone (GnRH) agonist has become a universal concept within assisted conception regimens. Reversible hypogonadotropic hypogonadism allows enhanced control of follicular development and improved pregnancy rates in IVF cycles (83,84). Suppression of endogenous luteinizing hormone (LH) by GnRH agonists may be advantageous for the sensitive polycystic ovary, allowing follicular development to occur without the adverse effects of high LH concentrations (85). These oocytes appear to fertilize better than those obtained in cycles without pituitary desensitization.

Few studies exist that compare the duration of treatment with GnRH analogues in women with and without PCOS in IVF cycles (86). A prolonged pituitary desensitization (30 days rather than 15) avoids the initial surge of gonadotropins and the resultant ovarian steroid release seen with shorter treatments. Androgen levels may be reduced and an increase in exogenous gonadotropin dosage is not required. Although pregnancy rates are not improved, ovarian hyperstimulation is reduced (87). Unfortunately there are too few specific randomized controlled comparisons for women with PCOS.

The pros and cons of different gonadotropin preparations have been debated for years. After the initial use of hMG and then the highly purified urinary FSH came the recombinant preparations of FSH (rFSH), LH, and hCG. Overall there appears to be little difference in outcomes when all studies are combined (88).

The newer preparations provide greater flexibility with doses such that low doses with small incremental increases may be administered, thereby minimizing the risk of OHSS and at the same time maintaining satisfactory pregnancy rates (89). Teissier et al. demonstrated that women with PCOS undergoing IVF using hMG compared with rFSH have a higher testosterone and estradiol level due to higher LH (90). A meta-analysis has shown no difference in outcome between hMG and rFSH when used in conjunction with a long GnRH agonist protocol (91). There was no significant difference in number of oocytes retrieved, live birth rates, miscarriage, multiple pregnancy, or OHSS. This was confirmed by Anderson et al. with respect to pregnancy outcomes (92). As new products are marketed, Al-Inany et al. suggest caution in their meta-analysis concluding that not all human-derived FSH products are inferior to rFSH. They conclude that Fostimon is superior to Metrodin, which in any case, is no longer available (93).

The more recent introduction of regimens using a GnRH antagonist for pituitary suppression holds promise for PCOS patients. GnRH antagonists do not activate the GnRH receptors and produce a rapid suppression of gonadotropin secretion within hours. This offers the potential for shorter treatments compared with the long

protocol using a GnRH agonist (94). A Cochrane Review comparing a GnRH antagonist regimen to the long protocol GnRH agonist includes 27 randomized controlled trials (RCTs). A significant reduction in the incidence of severe OHSS was demonstrated (OR 0.61, 95% CI 0.42–0.89); however, the clinical pregnancy and live birth rates were also significantly lower (OR 0.84, 95% CI 0.72–0.97 and OR 0.81, 95% CI 0.69–0.98, respectively) (95). Consideration has recently been given to use of a GnRH antagonist within an ovulation induction protocol to reduce the risk of premature luteinization. Although a small improvement was seen in live birth rate, this was not significant (96).

In another study, patients with PCOS undergoing IVF in a GnRH antagonist protocol were found to have an earlier follicular growth and higher estradiol concentration during rFSH stimulation compared with those on a long GnRH agonist regimen (97). Despite a shorter stimulation phase, the number of oocytes, fertilization, CPRs were not different but the risk of OHSS was significantly lower. This is consistent with results of early trials (98,99) and the meta-analysis conducted by Griesinger et al. who concluded for PCOS the clinical outcome is the same irrespective of the protocols apart from a reduction in OHSS (100). Lainas et al. again revisited this concept in an RCT confirming similar ongoing pregnancy rates between the two protocols (101). Despite this reduction in those experiencing OHSS, overall there remains a significant majority with OHSS who have PCOS, even using an antagonist protocol (65.2% vs. 8.1%; $p < 0.05$) (102).

Native GnRH or GnRH agonist can displace the antagonist from the pituitary GnRH receptors. This realizes the potential to use a GnRH agonist as the final trigger for the LH surge, and subsequent oocyte maturation (103). Itskovitz-Eldor et al. demonstrated a rapid rise in LH after administration of a GnRH agonist, with a peak in levels four hours after injection (104). This trigger is potentially more physiological, with a lower risk of OHSS, due to the shorter half-life of LH (60 minutes vs. 32–34 hours). Fauser et al. have produced comparable data between an agonist trigger and HCG, with respect to number of oocytes retrieved, quality of embryos, implantation and pregnancy rates (105). This is supported by more recent studies (106,107). Unfortunately this is not supported in a Cochrane Review by Youssef et al. (108) who demonstrated an inferior live birth rate (OR 0.44, 95% CI 0.29–0.68), but the reduction in OHSS is certainly an advantage.

A multicenter, double blind study revealed that recombinant human LH can be as effective as hCG in inducing the final follicular maturation in IVF treatment with a lower incidence of OHSS (109). The clinical application within ART has yet to be fully elucidated.

Currently we recommend an antagonist protocol for women with PCOS or PCO who require IVF.

INSULIN RESISTANCE AND METFORMIN

Insulin resistance is a key factor coupled with hyperandrogenemia in the pathophysiology of PCOS. Insulin resistance is thought to arise from aberrant phosphorylation of tyrosine and serine residues on the insulin receptor resulting in increasing insulin resistance and compensatory hyperinsulinemia. As insulin binds IGF-1 receptors, it augments the response of theca cells to LH resulting in disordered steroidogenesis and excess androgen production. Hyperinsulinemia results in reduced hepatic synthesis of SHBG and insulin-like growth factor binding protein-1 (IGFBP-1). In turn this increases the bioavailability of both androgens and IGF1 and 2, which are important regulators of ovarian follicular maturation and steroidogenesis (110–113). Insulin resistance has been stipulated as a risk factor for cardiovascular disease in high-risk populations such as those with PCOS (114,115). Measurement of insulin resistance in this population is best screened for using a traditional oral glucose tolerance test or Hemoglobin A1c (HbA1c) (116).

With hyperinsulinemia being well recognized in women with PCOS, it is reasonable to assume that the use of insulin sensitizing drugs should improve many aspects of the syndrome, with respect to both metabolic and reproductive function. Metformin, an oral biguanide, is the most widely researched in this category. Metformin reduces hepatic gluconeogenesis, increasing peripheral glucose utilization and mediating receptor kinase activity within numerous cells including the theca and granulosa cells. A recent systematic review of insulin sensitizing agents concluded that metformin as a first line agent in ovulation induction was less effective than clomiphene with lower ovulation and pregnancy rates (OR = 0.63, 95% CI 0.43–0.92) (113). Those patients with clomiphene resistance, however, did benefit from adjunctive metformin. Interestingly it was the nonobese PCOS women who had the biggest improvement in effect.

The use of metformin as an adjunct within the context of IVF has also been explored. Five RCTs exist to answer this question (117–121). Four of these use the long protocol with a GnRH agonist for downregulation. The total dose and duration of metformin use is not standardized, ranging from 500 mg twice a day to 850 mg three times a day taken for up to 16 weeks usually up to hCG trigger. Fleming et al. (122) demonstrated that a protracted treatment of metformin over four months may decrease the antral follicle count and AMH levels; however, this was not shown to improve the number of oocytes retrieved or fertilization rates (120). Tang et al. reported a significant improvement in live birth rates for those taking metformin over a much shorter period of time (from the commencement of GnRH agonist to the day of hCG in a long protocol), with rates of 32.7% versus 12.2% in the placebo arm (117). The lower than expected birth rate in the placebo group is difficult to explain and may be secondary to subtle effects on oocyte/embryo quality or endometrial development. Kjotred et al. corroborated the findings of Tang by suggesting that the live birth rate may be improved in the lean women with PCOS (121). A further study of 112 women with a BMI <28 kg/m2 showed that the live birth rate was also higher when metformin was given over 12 weeks (48.6% vs. 32.0%; 95% CI 1.1–32.2, $p = 0.0383$) (123). Another study looking at

134 women with polycystic ovaries but without the syndrome failed to show an advantage (124).

The consistent advantage of using metformin appears to be a reduction in OHSS, with an OR of 0.27 (95% CI 0.16–0.47, $p = 0.000044$) in a recent Cochrane Review (110). The use of GnRH antagonists in IVF protocols also reduces the risk of OHSS. Doldi et al. presented their findings of a reduction in OHSS from 15% with placebo to 5% with metformin (121). Although promising, this study was inadequately powered to show a significant improvement. A prospective RCT is underway within our own unit to attempt to answer this question (ISRCTN 21199799).

Metformin has been observed to reduce serum testosterone concentration (1.96 nmol/l vs. 2.52 nmol/l, $p = 0.269$) and free androgen index (FAI; 2.43 vs. 3.34) on the day of hCG administration (117). A negative correlation exists between day 12 postembryo transfer β-hCG levels and FAI. Through speculation, alleviation of hyperandrogenism and insulin resistance at the ovarian level may improve folliculogenesis and therefore the developmental potential of the embryo. Tang et al. showed no difference in average embryo score of the transferred embryos despite an improvement in CPR and live birth rate (LBR), hence the changes may be on a metabolomic level not yet classified (113). Serum VEGF and estradiol concentrations on the day of hCG administration are also greatly reduced in those on metformin. By ameliorating the expression of VEGF, the risk of OHSS can be reduced.

Thus, while there is variable data on the ability of metformin to not improve the "take home baby rate" after IVF, it does reduce the risk of moderate–severe OHSS in these high risk patients with PCOS.

IN VITRO MATURATION

In vitro maturation (IVM) has attracted a lot of attention as a new ART (125). Immature oocytes are retrieved transvaginally from antral follicles of either unstimulated or minimally stimulated ovaries (126). The oocyte matures in vitro in a specially formulated medium for 24–48 hours. The oocyte is then fertilized, usually with intra-cytoplasmic sperm injection (ICSI) and the selected embryo(s) transferred two to three days later. Although more labor-intensive, the potential clinical advantage is that patients generally require less monitoring and most importantly avoid the risk of OHSS. For those with PCOS, IVM offers a promising alternative to conventional IVF (127).

The maturation rate of oocytes retrieved from patients with PCOS has been lower than those with normal ovaries (128). However, priming with hCG before the retrieval has been shown to improve maturation rates from unstimulated polycystic ovaries (129). Child et al. (126) showed in a prospective observational study that significantly more immature oocytes are retrieved from the PCO than the normal ovary (10 ± 5.1 vs. 5.1 ± 3.7). The overall maturation and fertilization rate was comparable but the pregnancy and live birth rates were significantly higher in the PCO/PCOS groups. An explanation for this was the greater number of embryos available to select from but also the patients with PCOS were considerably younger within the study. Research continues into identifying prognostic indicators of the developmental potential of the embryos. Evaluating the cumulus layer is a potentially useful and simple procedure that may provide a scoring system in this evolving subject (130).

IVM as compared with conventional IVF yields significantly fewer mature oocytes (7.8 vs. 12, $p < 0.01$) with significantly lower implantation rates (131). The lower implantation rates may be due to a reduced oocyte potential, a higher frequency of abnormal meiotic spindle and chromosomal alignment, or reduced endometrial receptivity (132). It is important to ensure that infants born through such treatment remain healthy in the long term. A prospective observational study on 41 pregnancies showed no increase in preterm birth, birth weight, or major structural malformation as compared with those through conventional IVF (133). However, much larger studies are required to provide robust safety data on this new technology.

Siristatidis et al. concluded in a Cochrane Systematic Review, that no RCTs exist to base practice recommendations regarding IVM before IVF or ICSI in women with PCOS (134). There is an urgent need for randomized trials within this field. Continuous improvements in culture medium and synchrony between endometrial and embryonic development will hopefully result in improved success rates with IVM in the future.

CONCLUSION

Women with PCOS undergoing IVF cycles respond differently to women with normal ovaries. For the obese, weight loss and lifestyle modification should remain pivotal in the management of infertility, improving success rates and reducing potentially serious outcomes both in the short and long term. The GnRH antagonist protocol provides a safe alternative to the traditional GnRH agonist culminating in similar live birth rates but much reduced OHSS severity. Metformin remains a useful adjunct in the potential reduction of OHSS. IVM is a promising treatment that may ameliorate many of these issues for the notoriously difficult to manage polycystic ovary.

REFERENCES

1. Stein IF, Leventhal ML. Amenorrhoea associated with bilateral polycystic ovaries. Am J Obstet Gynecol 1935; 29: 181–91.
2. Polson DW, Wadsworth J, Adams J, Franks S. Polycystic ovaries – a common finding in normal women. Lancet 1988; 1: 870–2.
3. Balen A, Michelmore K. What is polycystic ovary syndrome? Are national views important? Hum Reprod 2002; 17: 2219–27.
4. Tsichorozidou T, Overton C, Conway GS. The pathophysiology of polycystic ovary syndrome. Clin Endocrinol (Oxf) 2004; 60: 1–17.
5. Diamanti-Kandarakis E, Papavassiliou AG. Molecular mechanism of insulin resistance in polycystic ovary syndrome. Trends Mol Med 2006; 12: 324–32.
6. Clark AM, Thornley B, Tomlinson L, Galletley C, Norman RJ. Weight loss in obese infertile women results in improvement in reproductive outcome for all forms of fertility treatment. Hum Reprod 1998; 13: 1502–5.
7. Amer SA, Li Tc, Metwally M, EMarh M, Ledger WL. Randomized controlled trial comparing laparoscopic ovarian diathermy with clomiphene citrate as a first-line method of ovulation induction in women with polycystic ovary syndrome. Hum Reprod 2009; 24: 219–25.
8. Laven JS, Fauser BC. What role of oestrogens in ovarian stimulation. Maturitas 2006; 54: 356–62.
9. Balen AH, Jacobs HS. A prospective study comparing unilateral and bilateral laparoscopic ovarian diathermy in women with polycystic ovary syndrome. Fertil Steril 1994; 62: 921–5.
10. Buyalos RP, Lee CT. Polycystic ovary syndrome: pathophysiology and outcome with in vitro fertilization. Fertil Steril 1996; 65: 1–10.
11. The Rotterdam ESHRE/ASRM-sponsored PCOS consensus workshop group. Revised 2003 consensus on diagnostic criteria and long-term health risks related to polycystic ovary syndrome (PCOS). Hum Reprod 2004; 19: 41–7.
12. Balen AH, Laven JSE, Tan SL, Dewailly D. Ultrasound assessment of the polycystic ovary: international consensus definitions. Hum Reprod update 2003; 9: 505–14.
13. Jonard S, Robert Y, Cortet-Rudelli C. Ultrasound examination of polycystic ovaries: is it worth counting the follicles? Hum Reprod 2003; 18: 598–603.
14. Michelmore KF, Balen AH, Dunger DB, Vessey MP. Polycystic ovaries and associated clinical and biochemical features in young women. Clin endocrinol (oxf) 1999; 51: 779–86.
15. Rodin DA, Bano G, Bland JM, Taylor K, Nussey SS. Polycystic ovaries and associated metabolic anormalities in Indian subcontinent Asian women. Clin Endocrinol (oxf) 1998; 49: 91–9.
16. Wijeyaratne CN, Balen AH, Barth J, Belchetz PE. Clinical manifestations and insulin resistance in PCOS among south Asians and Caucasians: is there a difference? Clin Endocrinol 2002; 57: 343–50.
17. Knochenhauer ES, Key TJ, Kahsar-Miller M, et al. Prevalence of the polycystic ovary syndrome in unselected black and white women of the Southeastern United States: a prospective study. J Clin Endocrin metab 1998; 83: 3078–82.
18. Dumesic DA, Padmanabhan V, Abbott DH. Polycystic ovary syndrome and oocyte developmental competence. Obstet Gynecol Surv 2008; 63: 39–48.
19. Weghofer A, Munne S, Chen S, Barad D, Gleicher N. Lack of association between polycystic ovary syndrome and embryonic aneuploidy. Fertil Steril 2007; 88: 900–5.
20. Rice S, Christoforidis N, Gadd C, et al. Impaired insulin-dependent glucose metabolism in granulosa-lutein cells from anovulatory women with polycystic ovaries. Hum Reprod 2005; 20: 373–81.
21. Skov V, Glintborg D, Knudsen S, et al. Reduced expression of nuclear-encoded genes involved in mitochondrial oxidative metabolism in skeletal muscle of insulin-resistant women with polycystic ovary syndrome. Diabetes 2007; 56: 2349–55.
22. Wood JR, Dumesic DA, Abbott DH, Strauss JF III. Molecular abnormalities in oocytes from women

with polycystic ovary syndrome revealed by micro-array analysis. J Clin Endocrinol Metab 2007; 92: 705–13.

23. Harris SE, Maruthini D, Tang T, Balen AH, Picton HM. Metabolism and karyotype analysis of oocytes from patients with polycystic ovary syndrome. Hum Reprod 2010; 25: 2305–15.

24. Hickey TE, Legro RS, Norman RJ. Epigenetic modification of the X chromosome influences susceptibility to polycystic ovary syndrome. J Clin Endocrinol Metab 2006; 91: 2789–91.

25. Li Z, Huang H. Epigenetic abnormality: a possible mechanism underlying the fetal origin of polycystic ovary syndrome. Med Hypotheses 2008; 70: 638–42.

26. Boomsma CM, Eijkemans MJ, Hughes EG, et al. A meta-analysis of pregnancy outcomes in women with polycystic ovary syndrome. Hum Reprod Update 2006; 12: 673–83.

27. Wax JR. Risks and management of obesity in pregnancy: current controversies. Curr Opin Obstet Gynecol 2009; 21: 117–23.

28. Teissier MP, Chable H, Paulhac S, Aubard Y. Comparison of follicle steroidogenesis from normal and polycystic ovaries in women undergoing IVF: relationship between steroid concentrations, follicle size, oocyte quality and fecundability. Hum Reprod 2000; 15: 2471–7.

29. Garcia-Velasco JA, et al. The aromatase inhibitor letrozole increases the concentration of intraovarian androgens and improves in vitro fertilization outcome in low responder patients: a pilot study. Fertil Steril 2005; 84: 82–7.

30. La Marca A, Morgante G, Palumbo M. Insulin-lowering treatment reduces aromatase activity in response to follicle-stimulating hormone in women with polycystic ovary syndrome. Fertil Steril 2002; 78: 1234–9.

31. Misajon A, Hutchinson P, Lolatgis N, Trounson AO, Almahbobi G. The mechanism of action of epidermal growth factor and transforming growth factor alpha on aromatase activity in granulosa cells from polycystic ovaries. Mol Human Reprod 1999; 5: 96–103.

32. Willis DS, Watson H, Mason HD. Premature response to luteinizing hormone of granulosa cells from anovulatory women with polycystic ovary syndrome: relevance to mechanism of anovulation. J clin endocrine Metab 1998; 83: 3984–91.

33. Weil S, Vendola K, Zhou J, Bondy C. Androgen and follicle-stimulating hormone interactions in primate ovarian follicle development. J Clin Endocrine Metab 1999; 84: 2951–6.

34. Vendola K, Zhou J, Wang J, Bondy CA. Androgens promote oocyte insulin-like growth factor 1 expression and initiation of follicle development in the primate ovary. Biol Reprod 1999; 61: 353–7.

35. Check JH, Nazari A, Dietterich C. Comparison of androgen levels in conception vs. non-conception cycles following controlled ovarian stimulation using the luteal phase gonadotrophin-releasing hormone agonist protocol. Gynae Endocrin 1995; 9: 209–14.

36. Kodaman P, Taylor H. Hormonal regulation of implantation. Obstet Gynaecol Clin North Am 2004; 31: 745–55.

37. Okon MA, Laird SM, Tuckerman EM, Li TC. Serum androgen levels in women who have recurrent miscarriages and their correlation with markers of endometrial function. Fertil Steril 1998; 69: 682–90.

38. Westergaard LG, Yding Andersen C, Erb K, et al. Placenta protein 14 concentrations in circulation related to hormonal parameters and reproductive outcome in women undergoing IVF/ICSI. Reprod Biomed Online 2004; 8: 91–8.

39. Tuckerman EM, Okon MA, Li T, Laird SM. Do androgens have a direct on endometrial function? AN in vitro study. Fertil Steril 2000; 74: 771–9.

40. Maliqueo M, Bacallao K, Quezada S. Sex hormone binging globulin expression in the endometria of women with polycystic ovary syndrome. Fertil Steril 2007; 87: 321–8.

41. Giudice LC. Endometrium in PCOS: implantation and predisposition to endocrine CA. Best Practice Res Clin ENdocrin Metab 2006; 20: 235–44.

42. Rose GL, Dowsett M, Mudge JE, White JO, Jeffcoate SL. The inhibitory effects of danazol, danazol metabolites, gestrinone and testosterone on the growth of human endometrial cells in vitro. Fertil Steril 1988; 49: 224–8.

43. Wass P, Waldenström U, Rössner S, Hellberg D. An android body fat distribution in females impairs the pregnancy rate of in vitro fertilization-embryo transfer. Hum Reprod 1997; 12: 2057–60.

44. Pasquali R, Pelusi C, Genghini S, Cacciari M, Gambineri A. Obesity and reproductive disorders in women. Hum Reprod Update 2003; 9: 359–72.

45. Fedorcsák P, Dale PO, Storeng R, Tanbo T, Abyholm T. The impact of obesity and insulin resistance on the outcome of IVF or ICSI in women with PCOS. Hum Reprod 2001; 16: 1086–91.

46. Jungheim ES, Lanzendorf SE, Odem RR. Morbid obesity is associated with lower clinical pregnancy rates after invitro fertilization in women with polycystic ovary syndrome. Fertil Steril 2009; 256–61.

47. Jungheim ES, Lanzendorf SE, Odem RR. Morbid obesity is associated with lower clinical pregnancy rates after invitro fertilization in women with polycystic ovary syndrome. Fertil Steril 2009; 256–61.

48. Brewer CJ, Balen AH. The impact of obesity on conception and implantation. Reproduction 2010; 140: 347–64.

49. Fedorcsák P, Dale PO, Storeng R, Tanbo T, Abyholm T. Impact of overweight and underweight on assisted reproduction treatment. Hum Reprod 2004; 19: 2523–8.

50. Dokras A, Bochner M, Hollinrake E. Screening women with polycystic ovary syndrome for metabolic syndrome. Obstet Gynecol 2005; 106: 131–7.

51. Dale PO, Tanbo T, Haug E, Abyholm T. The impact of insulin resistance on the outcome of ovulation induction with low dose follicle stimulating hormone in women with polycystic ovary syndrome. Hum Reprod 1998; 13: 567–70.

52. Loveland JB, McClamrock HD, Malinow AM, Sharara FI. Increased body mass index has a deleterious effect on in-vitro fertilisation outcome. J Assisted Reprod Genet 2001; 18: 382–6.

53. Centre for Maternal and Child Enquiries. Saving Mothers' Lives. Reviewing maternal deaths to make motherhood safer: 2006–2008. The Eighth report of the Confidential Enquiries into Maternal Deaths in the United Kingdom. BJOG 2011; 118 (Suppl 1): 1–203.

54. Balen A. The effects of ovulation induction with gonadotrophins on the ovary and uterus and implications for assisted reproduction. Hum Reprod 1995; 10: 2233–7.

55. Shoham Z, Conway GS, Patel A, Jacobs HS. Polycystic ovaries in patients with hypogonadotrophic hypogonadism: similarity of ovarian response to gonadotrophin stimulation in patients with polycystic ovary syndrome. Fertil Steril 1992; 58: 37–45.

56. Dor J, Shulman A, Levran D. The treatment of patients with polycystic ovarian syndrome by in vitro fertilization and embryo transfer: a comparison of results with those of patients with tubal infertility. Hum Reprod 1990; 5: 816–18.

57. MacDougall MJ, Tan SL, Balen A, Jacobs HS. A controlled study comparing patients with and without polycystic ovaries undergoing in-vitro fertilization. Hum Reprod 1993; 8: 233–7.

58. Kodama H, Fukuda J, Karube H. High incidence of embryo transfer cancellations in patients with polycystic ovarian syndrome. Hum Reprod 1995; 10: 1962–7.

59. Heijnen EM, Eijkemans MJ, Hughes EG, et al. A meta analysis of outcomes of conventional IVF in women with polycystic ovary syndrome. Hum Reprod Update 2006; 12: 13–21.

60. Ludwig M, Finas DF, al-Hasani S, Diedrich K, Ortmann O. Oocyte quality and treatment outcome in intracytoplasmic sperm injection cycles of polycystic ovarian syndrome patients. Hum Reprod 1999; 14: 354–8.

61. Balen AH, Tan SL, MacDougall J, Jacobs HS. Miscarriage rates following in-vitro fertilization are increased in women with polycystic ovaries and reduced by pituitary desensitization with buserelin. Hum Reprod 1993; 8: 959–64.

62. Fedorcsák P, Storeng R, Dale PO, Tanbo T, Abyholm T. Obesity is a risk factor for early pregnancy loss after IVF or OCSI. Acta Obstet Gynaecol Scand 2000; 79: 43–8.

63. Jonard S, Dewailly D. The follicular excess in polycystic ovaries, due to intra ovarian hyperandrogenism may be the culprit for the follicular arrest. Hum Reprod Update 2004; 10: 107–17.

64. Dewailly D, Catteau-Jonard S, Reyss AC. The excess in 2–5 mm follicles seen at ovarian ultrasonography is tightly associated to the follicular arrest of the polycystic ovary syndrome. Hum Reprod 2007; 22: 1562–6.

65. Pellatt L, Rice S, Mason HD. Anti-Mullerian hormone and polycystic ovary syndrome: a mountain too high? Reproduction 2010; 139: 825–33.

66. Webber LJ, Stubbs S, Stark J, et al. Formation and early development of follicles seen in the polycystic ovary. Lancet 2003; 362: 1017–21.

67. Webber LJ, Stubbs SA, Stark J, et al. Prolonged survival in culture of preantral follicles from polycystic ovaries. J Clin Endocrinol Metab 2007; 92: 1975–8.

68. Kezele PR, Nilsson EE, Skinner MK. Insulin but not insulin-like growth factor-1 promotes the primordial to primary follicle transition. Mol Cell Endocrinol 2002; 192: 37–43.

69. Vendola K, Zhou J, Wang J, Bondy CA. Androgens promote insulin-like growth factor1 and insulin-like growth factor1 receptor gene expression in the primate ovary. Hum Reprod 1999; 14: 2328–32.

70. Otala M, Mäkinen S, Tuuri T. Effects of testosterone, dihydrotestosterone and 17-beta-estradiol on human ovarian tissue survival in culture. Fertil steril 2004; 82(Suppl 3): 1077–85.

71. Brinsden PR, Wada I, Tan SL, Balen A, Jacobs HS. Diagnosis, prevention and management of Ovarian hyperstimulation syndrome. Br J Obstet Gynaecol 1995; 102: 767–72.

72. Delvigne A, Dubois M, Battheu B. The ovarian hyperstimulation syndrome in in-vitro fertilization: a Belgian multicentric study. Clinical and biological features. Hum Reprod 1993; 8: 1353–60.

73. Agrawal R, Conway G, Sladkevicius P. Serum vascular endothelial growth factor and Doppler blood flow velocities in in-vitro fertilization: relevance to ovarian hyperstimulation syndrome and polycystic ovaries. Fertil Steril 1998; 70: 651–8.

74. Whelan JG, Vlahos NF. The ovarian hyperstimulation syndrome. Fertil Steril 2000; 73: 883–96.

75. Pellicer A, Albert C, Mercader A, et al. The pathogenesis of ovarian hyperstimulation syndrome: in vivo studies investigating the role of interleukin-1 beta, interleukin-6, and vascular endothelial growth factor. Fertil Steril 1999; 71: 482–9.

76. Artini PG, Monti M, Matteucci C. Vascular endothelial growth factor and basic fibroblast growth factor in polycystic ovary syndrome during controlled ovarian hyperstiluation. Gynaec Endocrinol 2006; 22: 465–70.

77. Agrawal R, Tan SL, Wild S, et al. Serum vascular endothelial growth factor concentrations in in vitro fertilization cycles predict the risk of ovarian hyperstimulation syndrome. Fertil Steril 1999; 71: 287–93.

78. Herr F, Baal N, Reisinger K, et al. hCG in the regulation of placental angiogenesis. Results of an In Vitro Study. Placenta 2007; 28: 85–93.

79. Wang TH, Horng SG, Chang CL. Human chorionic gonadotrophin-induced ovarian hyperstimulation syndrome is associated with up-regulation of vascuular endothelial growth factor. J Clin Endocrinol Metab 2002; 87: 3300–8.

80. Miele C, Rochford JJ, Filippa N. Insulin and insulin-like growth factor-1 induce vascular endothelial growth factor mRNA expression via different signalling pathways. J Biol Chem 2000; 275: 21695–702.

81. Agrawal R, Jacobs H, Payne N, Conway G. Concentration of vascular endothelial growth factor released by cultured human leutinized granulosa cells is higher in women with polycystic ovaries than in women with normal ovaries. Fetil Steril 2002; 78: 1164–9.

82. Stanek MB, Borman SM, Molskness TA. Insulin and insulin-like growth factor stimulation of vascular endothelial growth factor production by luteinized granulosa cells: comparison between polycystic ovarian syndrome and non-PCOS women. J Clin Endocrin Metab 2007; 92: 2726–33.

83. Rutherford AJ, Subak-Sharpe RJ, Dawson KJ. Improvement of in vitro fertilisation after treatment with buserelin, an agonist of luteinising hormone releasing hormone. Br Med J (Clin Res Ed) 1988; 296: 1765–8.

84. Frydman R, Parneix I, Belaisch-Allart J. LHRH agonists in IVF: different methods of utilization and comparison with previous ovarian stimulation treatments. Hum Reprod 1988; 3: 559–61.

85. Fleming R, Coutts JR. LHRH analogues for ovulation induction, with particular reference to the polycystic ovary syndrome. Baillieres Clin Obstet Gynaecol 1988; 2: 677–87.

86. Salat-Baroux J, Alvarez S, Antoine JM. Comparison between long and short protocols of LHRH agonist in the treatment of polycystic ovary disease by in-vitro fertilization. Hum Reprod 1988; 3: 535–9.

87. Tan SL, Kingsland C, Campbell S. The long protocol of administration of gonadotropin-releasing hormone agonist is superior to the short protocol for ovarian stimulation for in vitro fertilization. Fertil Steril 1992; 57: 810–14.

88. Nugent D, Vandekerckhove P, Hughes E, Arnot M, Lilford R. Gonadotrophin therapy for ovulation induction in subfertility associated with polycystic ovary syndrome. Cochrane Database Syst Rev 2000: CD000410.

89. Marci R, Senn A, Dessole S. A low-dose stimulation protocol using highly purified follicle-stimulating hormone can lead to high pregnancy rates in in-vitro fertilisation patients with polycystic ovaries who are at risk of a high ovarin response to gonadotropins. Fertil Steril 2001; 75: 1131–5.

90. Teissier MP, Chable H, Paulhac S, Aubard Y. Recombinant human follicle stimulating hormone versus human menopausal gonadotropin induction: effects in mature follicle endocrinology. Hum Reprod 1999; 14: 2236–41.

91. van Wely M, Westergaard LG, Bossuyt PM, van der Veen F. Effectiveness of human menopausal gonadotropin versus recombinant follicle-stimulating hormone for controlled ovarian hyperstimulation in assisted reproductive cycles: a meta–analysis. Fertil Steril 2003; 80: 1086–93.

92. Anderson AN, Devroey P, Arce JC. Clinical outcome following stimulation wih highly purified hMG or recombinant FSH in patients undergoing IVF: a randomised assessor-blind controlled trial. Hum Reprod 2006; 21: 3217–27.

93. Al-Inany HG, Abou-Setta AM. Are all human-derived follicle-stimulating hormone products the same? A systematic review and meta-analysis using direct and asjusted indirect analyses to determine whether fostimon is more efficient than metrodin-HP. Gynaecol Endocrinol 2012; 28: 94–101.

94. The European Middle East Orgalutran® Study Group. Comparable clinical outcomes using the GnRh antagonist ganirelix or a long protocol of the GnRH agonist triptorelin for the prevention of premature LH surges in women undergoing ovarian stimulation. Hum Reprod 2001; 16: 644–51.

95. Al-Inany HG, Abou-Setta AM, Aboulghar M. Gonadotrophin-releasing hormone antagonists for assisted conception. Cochrane Database Syst Rev 2006; 3: CD001750.

96. Stadtmauer LA, Sarhan A, Duran EH. The impact of a gonadotropin-releasing hormone antagonist on gonadotropin ovulation induction cycle in women with polycystic ovary syndrome: a prospective randomized study. Fertil Steril 2011; 95: 216–20.

97. Lainas TG, Petsas GK, Zorzovilis IZ. Initiation of GnRH antagonist an Day 1 of stimulation as compared to compared with the long agonist protocol in PCOS patients. A randomised controlled trial: effect on hormonal levels and follicular development. Hum Reprod 2007; 22: 1540–6.

98. Bahçeci M, Ulug U, Ben-Shlomo I, Erden HF, Akman MA. Use of a GnRH antagonist in controlled ovarian hyperstimulation for assited conception in women with polycystic ovary disease: a randomised, prospective pilot study. J Reprod Med 2005; 50: 84–90.

99. Ragni G, Vegetti W, Riccaboni A, et al. Comparison of GnRH agonists and antagonists in assisted reproduction cycles f patients at high risk of ovarian hyperstimulation syndrome. Hum Reprod 2005; 20: 2421–5.

100. Griesinger G, Diedrich K, Tarlatzis BC, Kolibianakis EM. GnRH-antagonists in ovarian stimulation for IVF patients with poor response to gonadotropins, polycystic ovary syndrome and risk of ovarian hyperstimulation: a meta-analysis. Reprod Biomed Online 2006; 13: 628–38.

101. Lainas TG, Sfontouris IA, Zorzovilis IZ. Flexible GnRH antagonist protocol versus GnRH agonist long protocol in patients with polycystic ovary syndrome treated for IVF: a prospective randomised controlled trial (RCT). Hum Reprod 2010; 25: 683–9.

102. Papanikolaou EG, Pozzobon C, Kolibianakis EM. Incidence and prediction of ovarian hyperstimulation syndrome in women undergoing gonadotropin-releasing hormone antagonist in vitro fertilisation cycles. Fertil Steril 2006; 85: 112–20.

103. Engmann L, Siano L, Schmidt D. GnRH agonist to induce oocyte maturation during IVF in patients at high risk of OHSS. Reprod Biomed Online 2006; 13: 639–44.

104. Itskovitz-Eldor J, Kol S, Mannaaerts B. Use of a single bolus of GnRh agonist triptorelin to trigger ovulation after GnRh antagonist ganireliz treatment in women undergoing ovarian stimulation for assisted reproduction with special reference to the prevention of ovarian hyperstimulation syndrome: preliminary report. Hum Reprod 2000; 15: 1965–8.

105. Fauser BC, de Jong D, Olivennes F. Endocrine profiles after triggering of final oocyte maturation with GnRH agonist after cotreatment with the GnRH antagonist ganirelix duing ovarian hyperstimulation for in vitro fertilisation. J Clin Endocr Metab 2002; 87: 709–15.

106. Acevedo B, Gomez-Palomares JL, Ricciarelli E, Hernández ER. Trigerring ovulation with gonadotropin-releasing hormone agonists does not compromise embryo implantation rates. Fertil Steril 2006; 86: 1682–7.

107. Babayof R, Margalioth EJ, Huleihel M, et al. Serum inhibin A, VEGF and TNF-alpha levels after triggering oocyte maturation with GnRh agonist compared with HCG in women with polycystic ovaries undergoing IVF treatment: a prospective randomised trial. Hum Reprod 2006; 21: 1260–5.

108. Youssef MA, Van der Veen F, Al-Inany HG. Gonadotropin-releasing hormone agonist versus HCG for oocyte triggering in antagonist assisted reproductive technology cycles. Cochrane Database Syst Rev 2011: CD008046.

109. The European Recombinant LH Study Group. Human recombinant luteinizing hormone is as effective as, but safer than, urinary human chorionic gonadotrophin in inducing final follicular maturation and ovulation in in-vitro fertilization procedures: results of a multicenter double blind study. J Clin Endocrin Metab 2001; 86: 2607–18.

110. Tso Lo, Costello MF, Albuquerque LE, Andriolo RB, Freitas V. Metfomin treatment before and during IVF or ICSI in women with polycystic ovary syndrome. Cochrane Database Syst Rev 2009: CD006105.

111. Costello MF, Chapman M, Conway U. A systematic review and meta-analysis of randomized controlled trials on metformin co-administration during gonadotrophin ovulation induction or IVF in women with polycystic ovary syndrome. Hum Reprod 2006; 21: 1387–99.

112. Moll E, van der Veen F, van Wely M. The role of metformin in polycystic ovary syndrome: a systematic review. Hum Reprod Update 2007; 13: 527–37.

113. Tang T, Lord JM, Norman RJ, Yasmin E, Balen AH. Insulin-sensitizing drugs (metformin, rosiglitazone, pioglitazone, D-chiro-inositol) for women with polycystic ovary syndrome, oligoamenorrhoea and subfertility. Cochrane Database Syst Rev 2009: CD003053.

114. Rutter MK, Meigs JB, Sullivan LM, D'Agostino RB Sr, Wilson PW. Insulin resistance, the metabolic syndrome and incidence cardiovascular events in the Framingham offspring study. Diabetes 2005; 54: 3252–7.

115. Moran LJ, Misso ML, Wild RA, Norman RJ. Impaired glucose tolerance, type 2 diabetes and metabolic syndrome in polycystic ovary syndrome: a systematic review and meta-analysis. Hum Reprod Update 2010; 16: 347–63.

116. Hurd WW, Abdel-Rahman MY, Ismail SA, et al. Comparison of diabetes mellitus and insulin resicstance screening menthods for women with polycystic ovary syndrome. Fertil Steril 2011; 96: 1043–7.

117. Tang T, Glanville J, Orsi N, Barth JH, Balen AH. The use of metformin for women with PCOS undergoing IVF treatment. Hum Reprod 2006; 21: 1416–25.

118. Onalan G, Pabucca R, Goktolga U, et al. Metformin treatment in patients with polycystic ovary syndrome undergoing invitro fertilization: a prospective randomized trial. Fertil Steril 2005; 84: 798–801.

119. Kjotred SB, von During V, Carlsenve SM. Metformin treatment before IVF/ICSI in women with polycystic ovary syndrome: a prospective, randomized, double blind study. Hum Reprod 2004; 19: 1315–22.

120. Fedorcsak P, Dale PO, Storeng R, Abyholm T, Tanbo T. The effect of metformin on ovarian stimulation and in vitro fertilisation in insulin-resistant women with polycystic ovary syndrome: an open-label randomized cross-over trial. Gynaecol Endocrinol 2003; 17: 207–14.

121. Doldi N, Persico P, Di Sebastiano F, Marsiglio E, Ferrari A. Gonadotrophin-releasing hormone antagonist and metformin for treatment of polycystic ovary syndrome patients undergoing in vitro fertilization-embryo transfer. Gynaecol Endocrinol 2006; 22: 235–8.

122. Fleming R, et al. Metformin reduces serum mullerian-inhibiting substance levels in women with polycystic ovary syndrome after protracted treatment. Fertil Steril 2005; 83: 130–6.

123. Kjøtrød SB, Carlsen SM, Rasmussen PE, et al. Use of metformin before and during ART in non-obese young infertile women with PCOS: a prospective, randomised, double-blind, multi-centre study. Hum Reprod 2011; 26: 2045–53.

124. Swanton A, Lighten A, Granne I. Do women with ovaries of polycystic morphology without any other features of PCOS benefit from short term metformin co-treatment during IVF? A double-blind, placebo-controlled, randomised trial. Hum Reprod 2011; 26: 2178–84.

125. Trousen A, Wood C, Kausche A. In vitro maturation and the fertilization and developmental competence of oocytes recovered from untreated polycystic ovarian patients. Fertil steril 1994; 62: 353–62.

126. Child TJ, Abdul-Jalil AK, Gulekli B, Tan SL. In Vitro maturation and fertilization of oocytes from unstimulated normal ovaries, polycystc ovaries and women with polycystic ovary syndrome. Fertil Steril 2001; 76: 936–42.

127. Chian RC. In-vitro maturation of immature ooctes for infertile women with PCOS. Reprod Biomed Online 2004; 8: 547–52.

128. Child TJ, Phillips SJ, Abdul-Jalil AK, Gulekli B, Tan SL. A comparison of in vitro maturation and in vitro fertilization for women with polycystic ovaries. Obstet Gynaecol 2002; 100: 665–70.

129. Chian RC, Buckett WM, Tulandi T, Tan SL, et al. Prospective randomised study of human chorionic gonadotrophin priming before immature oocyte retrieval from unstimulated women with polycystic ovarian syndrome. Hum Reprod 2000; 15: 165–70.

130. Liu S, Jiang JJ, Feng HL. Evaluation of the immature human oocytes from unstimulated cycles in polycystic ovary syndrome patients using a novel scoring system. Fertil Steril 2010; 93: 2202–9.

131. Le Du A, Kadoch IJ, Bourcigaux N. In vitro oocyte maturation for the treatment of infertility associated with polycystic ovarian syndrome: the French experience. Hum Reprod 2005; 20: 420–4.

132. Li Y, Feng HL, Cao YJ. Confocal microscopic analysis of the spindle and chromosome configurations of human oocytes matured in vitro. Fertil Steril 2006; 85: 827–32.

133. Cha KY, Chung HM, Lee DR. Obstetric outcome of patients with polycystic ovary syndrome treated by in vitro maturation and in vitro fertilisation-embryo transfer. Fertil Steril 2005; 83: 1461–5.

134. Siristatidis CS, Maheshwari A, Bhattacharya S. In vitro maturation in sub fertile women with polycystic ovarian syndrome undergoing assisted reproduction. Cochrane Database Syst Rev 2009: CD006606.

57

Management of hydrosalpinx

Annika Strandell

INTRODUCTION

In the beginning of the in vitro fertilization (IVF) era, tubal factor infertility was the sole indication for the treatment. Today, other indications constitute the majority of treatments and tubal disease may account for as little as 20% in some centers. It is notable that tubal factor infertility is often reported to yield worse results than other causes of infertility. We reported tubal factor infertility to be an independently negative predictive factor of pregnancy and birth, as compared with all other indications, (1) in the debate on high multiple pregnancy rates in IVF.

Hydrosalpinx is the severe condition that has attained special interest in research and clinical practice. Tubal diseases like salpingitis isthmica nodosa and other types of proximal tubal occlusions have not been studied exclusively in connection with assisted reproductive techniques (ART) and will not be further explored here. This chapter will focus on the problems associated with hydrosalpinx and ART, including diagnosis, prognosis, possible mechanisms, and interventions.

DEFINITIONS AND METHODS OF DIAGNOSIS

Hydrosalpinx is a commonly used term to describe a heterogeneous spectrum of pathology of distal tubal occlusion. A strict definition is a collection of watery fluid in the uterine tube, occurring as the end stage of pyosalpinx. However, hydrosalpinx is used for any distal tubal occlusion regardless of the cause, implying that a non-tubal infection such as an adjacent appendicitis can also cause hydrosalpinx. Furthermore, the end stage of a tubal infection has different appearances: The *hydrosalpinx simplex* is characterized by excessive distension and thinning of the wall of the uterine tube, the plicae being few and widely separated, while the *hydrosalpinx follicularis* describes a tube without any central cystic cavity, the lumen being broken up into compartments as the result of fusion of the tubal plicae. Thus, the terminology is not consistent with the original translation since hydrosalpinx is also used in cases without any obvious fluid in the tubes. *Sactosalpinx* is also used as a synonym although the definition is slightly different: Dilation of the inflamed uterine tube by retained secretions (*saktos* = stuffed).

The diagnosis of hydrosalpinx can be suspected and, in many cases also confirmed by transvaginal ultrasound, if the tube is fluid-filled. Ultrasound has the obvious advantage to hysterosalpingography to detect the condition without the instillation of fluid that carries a high risk of subsequent infection (Figs. 57.1 and 57.2). Both methods, including instillation of contrast, can be used to diagnose a distally occluded tube without any fluid prior to instillation. Antibiotic prophylaxis is mandatory. Laparoscopy is obviously the ultimate method for diagnosis of hydrosalpinx and associated pathology of pelvic adhesions. However, the method is highly invasive, and advantage should be taken to perform all diagnostic and therapeutic procedures at the same time.

It has been proposed to establish cutoff values for the size of a hydrosalpinx, to decide when there is a need for intervention prior to IVF. However, the size of a hydrosalpinx, as measured by ultrasound, may vary during a cycle and it has not been possible to correlate IVF outcome to the precise size. Only two indices of size have been established – detection at ultrasound examination and bilateral affection – and these are discussed in the next section.

HYDROSALPINX – A SIGN OF POOR PROGNOSIS

Since 1994 there have been a large number of retrospective studies dedicated to the influence of hydrosalpinges on pregnancy results in IVF, most of them showing an impaired outcome (2). Patients with hydrosalpinges have been identified as having significantly lower implantation and pregnancy rates than patients suffering from other types of tubal damage. The retrospective data have been compiled and summarized in meta-analyses, of which one is shown in Figure 57.3 (3). There is a consistency in the results showing a reduction by half in clinical pregnancy and delivery rates and a doubled rate of spontaneous abortion in women with hydrosalpinx. In addition, thaw cycles demonstrated a significantly reduced pregnancy rate, which none of the separate studies has been able to show. The rate of ectopic pregnancy was nonsignificantly increased in hydrosalpinx patients [Odds ratio (OR) 1.3, 95% confidence interval (CI) 0.7–2.6]. Patients with tubal infertility have an increased risk of ectopic pregnancy after IVF compared

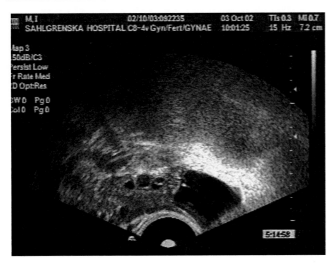

Figure 57.1 Typical appearance of a hydrosalpinx beside the ovary at transvaginal ultrasound investigation.

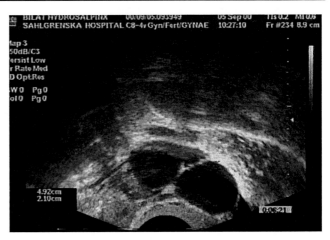

Figure 57.2 The folds of the tubal wall in a distended hydrosalpinx depicted as typical spikes into the lumen.

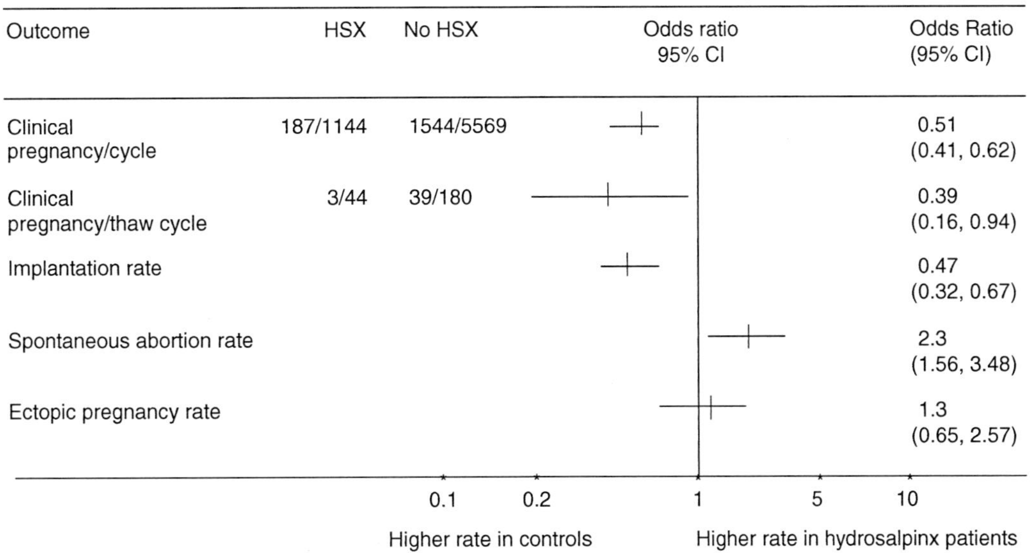

Outcome	HSX	No HSX	Odds ratio 95% CI	Odds Ratio (95% CI)
Clinical pregnancy/cycle	187/1144	1544/5569		0.51 (0.41, 0.62)
Clinical pregnancy/thaw cycle	3/44	39/180		0.39 (0.16, 0.94)
Implantation rate				0.47 (0.32, 0.67)
Spontaneous abortion rate				2.3 (1.56, 3.48)
Ectopic pregnancy rate				1.3 (0.65, 2.57)

```
        0.1    0.2          1       5    10
      Higher rate in controls   Higher rate in hydrosalpinx patients
```

Figure 57.3 Meta-analysis of retrospective studies on IVF outcome in hydrosalpinx patients compared with patients with other tubal infertility. *Abbreviation*: HSX, hydrosalpinx. Source: From Ref. 3.

with patients with other indications, but it has not been possible to establish that patients with hydrosalpinges have an increased risk of ectopic pregnancy compared with patients suffering from other types of tubal infertility. Although retrospective cohort studies are not the best quality of evidence, it is obvious from the overwhelming consistency in results that patients with hydrosalpinges have an impaired pregnancy outcome after IVF.

Some of the retrospective studies have attempted to characterize further and subdivide the different features of hydrosalpinx. The first publication showed that the size was important by demonstrating that only largely distended hydrosalpinges were associated with significantly reduced pregnancy and delivery rates (2). deWit et al. also demonstrated the importance of size by using ultrasound and allocated hydrosalpinges according to size depending on whether they were visible or not (4).

Pregnancy rates were significantly lower (15%) in patients with visible hydrosalpinges compared with patients in whom the hydrosalpinges were not visible (31%). Wainer et al. demonstrated that the presence of bilateral as opposed to unilateral hydrosalpinx was associated with significantly lower pregnancy (12% vs. 24%) and implantation rates (5% vs. 11%) (5). These findings suggest that the total amount of fluid in the hydrosalpinges is negatively correlated to the chance of achieving a pregnancy, and these aspects should be considered in the design of a prospective trial.

WHAT IS THE MECHANISM OF HYDROSALPINX IMPAIRING IMPLANTATION?

The hydrosalpinx fluid may act on two different target systems: Directly on the transferred embryos or on the endometrium and its receptivity for implantation, or both.

Embryotoxic Properties of Hydrosalpinx Fluid

Potential embryotoxic effects have been evaluated using either mouse or human embryos in human hydrosalpinx fluid. There is a discrepancy in the results of culture systems using human and murine models, but the results from different mouse studies are also diverging. In a review of hydrosalpinx studies, five out of eight studies using a murine model described embryotoxicity at low concentrations of human hydrosalpinx fluid, and three studies demonstrated impaired development, but in undiluted hydrosalpinx fluid only (6). There are only two studies on human embryos, neither of which have been able to demonstrate any obvious toxic effect on embryo development (7,8). The experimental models using mouse and human embryos do not seem to be comparable, and conclusions from studies based on mouse models are not obviously applicable to humans. From studies on embryo development, it may be concluded that hydrosalpinx fluid does not appear to host a common potent factor deleterious to embryo development, and the lack of essential substrates is more likely to be responsible for the impaired development of embryos in undiluted hydrosalpinx fluid.

Is Hydrosalpinx Fluid Toxic in Individual Cases?

Even though there may not be a common toxic factor in all fluids, the presence of factors inhibitory to embryo development in fluids from certain individuals cannot be excluded. Most experiments are based on small numbers of hydrosalpinx fluids, and individual variations in content may reflect the differences in embryo development. In a study on the effect of hydrosalpinx fluid on gametes and fertilization, one out of four fluids was directly cytotoxic to murine spermatozoa when incubated in 50% hydrosalpinx fluid during capacitation (9).

No pathogenic microorganisms have been detected in any of the published studies, but slightly elevated concentrations of endotoxin have been demonstrated in individual fluids as a sign of previous infection (7). If a toxic substance was responsible for the negative influence, assay of the aspirated hydrosalpingeal fluid before stimulation would be useful in selecting patients for salpingectomy.

An assay of mouse embryo culture in 50% hydrosalpinx fluid has been suggested to predict IVF outcome (10). In a population of 39 hydrosalpinx patients, the test had a sensitivity of 64%, a specificity of 86%, and a positive likelihood ratio of 4.5, suggesting the test to be fairly good in detecting toxicity. The diagnostic performance was not improved by including important factors like age and number of good quality embryos transferred. The use of this technique requires transvaginal puncture, preferably before the start of any stimulation, when the result may be helpful in the decision concerning prophylactic salpingectomy. The technique still awaits clinical evaluation.

The hydrosalpingeal fluid may also exhibit growth-promoting properties, as seen by a study in which the production of tropho-uteronectin by human cytotrophoblasts was significantly increased by the presence of hydrosalpinx fluid, suggesting promotion of early embryo-integrin interactions (11). Also, a significant increase in trophoblast cell viability, as well as in the production of β-human chorionic gonadotropin (HCG) in the presence of hydrosalpinx fluid, suggested growth-promoting properties of hydrosalpinx fluid.

Oxidative Stress

The presence of oxidative and antioxidant systems in various reproductive tissues has evoked interest in the role of oxidative stress in reproductive diseases. Oxidative stress has been defined as an elevation in the steady-state concentration of various reactive oxygen species on a cellular level and has been suggested to be of importance in hydrosalpinx cases. A first report on this issue described a positive effect of low levels of reactive oxygen in relation to blastocyst development, as compared with absence of reactive oxygen species in hydrosalpinx fluid (12). The low levels were suggested to be within a physiological range, and no high levels were detected to demonstrate a negative effect. This hypothesis will need further evaluation.

Endometrial Receptivity

The cross talk between the embryo and the endometrium, essential for allowing the embryo to implant, and mediated by the secretion and expression of certain cytokines and other substances during the implantation window, may be disturbed under the presence of hydrosalpinx fluid. Cytokines like interleukin-1 (IL-1), leukemia inhibitory factor (LIF), colony stimulating factor-1 (CSF-1), and the integrin $\alpha_v\beta_3$ are all factors that have been shown to be of importance to implantation; they and some of their receptors are secreted or expressed by either the embryo or the endometrium in an increased manner during the implantation window (13,14).

Chlamydia trachomatis is the most common pathogen, and antibodies to chlamydial heat-shock proteins were found to be more prevalent in patients with hydrosalpinx compared with women in couples of male infertility (15). Heat-shock proteins elicit intense immune and inflammatory reactions, and are thought to be responsible for a local immune response, leading to inflammatory reactions, impaired implantation, and immune rejection after embryo transfer (16).

One study has demonstrated impaired endometrial and sub-endometrial blood flow among hydrosalpinx patients, supporting the theory of simultaneous damage to the endometrium as the original infection (17).

Mechanical Explanations

Leakage of hydrosalpingeal fluid through the uterine cavity, resulting in embryo disposal, has been suggested as a mechanism by several authors (18–20). The clinical feature of hydrorrhea was shown to be a sign of poor prognosis among patients with hydrosalpinx undergoing IVF (19). The existence of a hydrosalpingeal fluid interface on the endometrial surface, sometimes seen during ART, has been suggested to be a hindrance to implantation (19,21). One study has demonstrated an association between endometrial cavity fluid and increased cancelation rates and lower clinical pregnancy rates in ART cycles, but without any association with hydrosalpinges visible on ultrasound (22). These findings suggest that leakage of hydrosalpingeal fluid through the uterine cavity is only one of several possible explanations of endometrial cavity fluid.

It has also been suggested that hydrosalpinx fluid may cause an increase in endometrial peristalsis. In one report, uterine dynamics of five patients with hydrosalpinx were analyzed by image-processing techniques and compared with healthy volunteers (23). The authors describe, from a mathematical simulation model, a reflux phenomenon (opposing the cervix-to-fundus intrauterine peristalsis) generated by a pressure gradient from tubal fluid accumulation. It was suggested that this reflux phenomenon could explain the reduced implantation rate associated with hydrosalpinx.

INTERVENTIONS AGAINST HYDROSALPINX IN CONJUNCTION WITH IVF

According to the theory that the hydrosalpingeal fluid plays a causative role in impairing implantation and/or embryo development, any surgical intervention interrupting the communication to the uterus would remove the leakage of the hydrosalpingeal fluid and restore pregnancy rates. Treatment with salpingectomy prior to IVF is the only surgical method that has been evaluated in a sufficiently large randomized controlled trial (RCT), supplying us with a high level of evidence to formulate our recommendation. Other suggested treatments for hydrosalpinges prior to IVF, such as tubal ligation and transvaginal aspiration may also be considered but they need further evaluation in large prospective trials.

Salpingectomy

Hitherto, salpingectomy is the only method of prophylactic surgery in patients with hydrosalpinx that has been properly evaluated in a large randomized trial (24). A multicenter study in Scandinavia compared laparoscopic salpingectomy to no intervention prior to the first IVF cycle; the study demonstrated a significant improvement in pregnancy and birth rates after salpingectomy in patients with hydrosalpinges that were large enough to be visible on ultrasound. Clinical pregnancy rates were 46% versus 22% ($p = 0.049$), and birth rates were 40% versus 17% ($p = 0.040$) in salpingectomized patients versus patients without any surgical intervention (Fig. 57.4B). The difference in outcome was not statistically significant in the total study population of 204 patients, which included patients with hydrosalpinges that were not visible on ultrasound (Fig. 57.4A), demonstrating that the benefit of salpingectomy is only evident if the tube is fluid-filled.

Within the group of hydrosalpinges visible on ultrasound, there can still be tubes that are suitable for reconstructive surgery, and the main rule must be that tubes with healthy-looking mucosa should not be removed (Figs. 57.5 and 57.6).

The psychological aspect of removing the tubes in an infertile patient is very important and has to be considered. Even if it is obvious that the patient would benefit from salpingectomy, it is crucial that she is psychologically prepared to undergo the procedure. In some cases, it takes one or several failed cycles before the patient is ready to give her consent.

There are four additional RCTs on salpingectomy prior to IVF (25–28), all of smaller sample sizes as compared to the Scandinavian study. A systematic review in the Cochrane Library (29) included meta-analyses demonstrating a significant improvement in ongoing pregnancy (OR 2.2, 95% CI 1.3–3.8) after IVF if salpingectomy was performed compared with no surgical intervention. If an additional study (26) (only published as an abstract) is also included in a meta-analysis, the common OR for ongoing pregnancy or live birth is 2.7 (95% CI 1.6–4.6) as shown in Fig. 57.7.

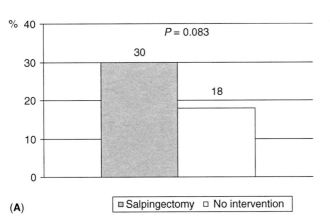

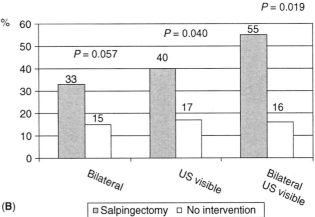

Figure 57.4 Live birth rates in the first transfer cycle of 204 patients in the Scandinavian multicenter trial on salpingectomy prior to IVF in hydrosalpinx patients. (**A**) The total study population. (**B**) The a priori decided subgroups of bilateral and/or ultrasound visible hydrosalpinges. *Abbreviation*: US, ultrasound.

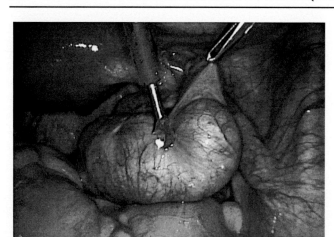

Figure 57.5 A hydrosalpinx without adjacent adhesions is easy to assess at laparoscopy.

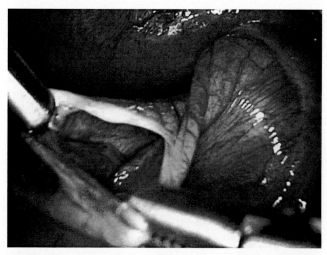

Figure 57.6 Assessment of mucosal status through a distal opening of the hydrosalpinx is recommended before the final decision of salpingectomy or distal tuboplasty is taken.

Author	Surgery Birth or ongoing pregnancy/ patients	No surgery Birth or ongoing pregnancy/ patients	Odds ratio 95% CI	Weight	Odds ratio (95% CI)
Déchaud 1998 (25)	13/30	6/30		20%	3.06 (0.97, 9.66)
Strandell 1999 (24)	31/116	15/88		49%	1.77 (0.89, 3.54)
Goldstein 1998 (26)	4/15	1/16		5%	5.45 (0.53, 55.80)
Kontoravdis 2006 (27)	23/47	1/14		26%	12.45 (1.51, 103.05)
Total	71/208	23/148		100%	2.66 (1.55, 4.56)

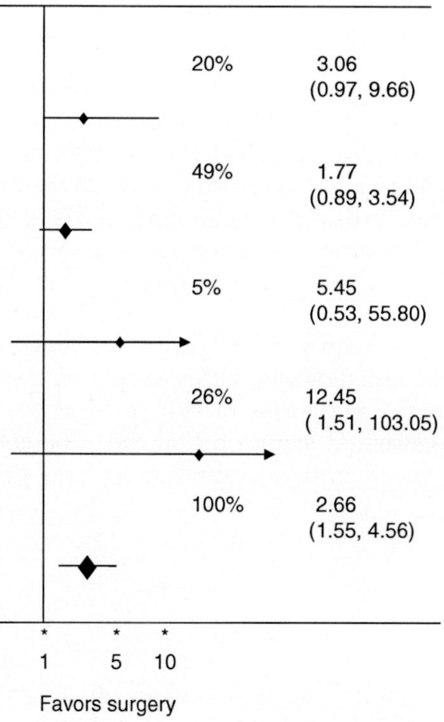

0.1 0.2   1   5   10

Favors control   Favors surgery

Figure 57.7 Meta-analysis of four randomized trials of laparoscopic salpingectomy versus no surgery in hydrosalpinx patients due to undergo IVF, with primary outcome live birth or ongoing pregnancy.

In the Scandinavian study, the cumulative result, including all subsequent cycles, was evaluated (30). Patients were offered up to three stimulated cycles, and those who were randomized to undergo salpingectomy achieved a cumulative birth rate of 55%. When all subsequent cycles were considered, including all patients regardless of the size of the hydrosalpinx, salpingectomy implied a doubled birth rate as compared to patients with persistent hydrosalpinges (hazard ratio 2.1, 95% CI 1.6–3.6, $p = 0.014$). This result, as well as the compiled data from the Cochrane Review, suggests that all patients with hydrosalpinx, regardless of size or fluid accumulation, should undergo salpingectomy. However, the cumulative data from the Scandinavian study revealed that the benefit of salpingectomy mainly affected patients with hydrosalpinges visible on ultrasound, and consequently,

Table 57.1 Summary of Studies Examining the Effect of Salpingectomy on Ovarian Function by Measuring the Number of Retrieved Oocytes after Controlled Ovarian Hyperstimulation. Controls are the Same Patients before Surgery, the Contralateral Ovary, or Patients Without Previous Tubal Surgery

| Author | No. of patients | Reason for surgery | No. of oocytes | | Study design |
			Ipsilateral vs. contralateral	Overall (two ovaries)	
Verhulst 1994 (32)	26 vs. 134	Ectopic pregnancy hydrosalpinx sterilization	Not studied	11.2 vs. 1.2 n.s.	Retrospective comparison with controls
Lass 1998 (33)	29 vs. 73	Ectopic pregnancy	3.8 vs. 6.0 p < 0.01	9.9 vs. 9.1 n.s.	Prospective comparison with controls
Strandell 1999 (24)	110 vs. 82	Hydrosalpinx	not studied	10.6 vs. 10.6 n.s.	Randomized trial
Dar 2000(34)	26	Ectopic pregnancy after IVF	6.1 vs. 5.3 n.s.	11.1 vs. 9.7 n.s.	Analysis before and after surgery
Tal 2002 (36)	26 vs. 52	Ectopic pregnancy	6.3 vs. 6.2 n.s.	8.6 vs. 8.4 n.s.	Comparison with matched controls
Gelbaya 2006 (37)	40 vs. 103	Hydrosalpinx	not studied	10.2 vs. 12.9	Retrospective cohort
Kontoravdis 2006 (27)		Hydrosalpinx	not studied	12.1 vs. 10.9 n.s.	Randomized trial
Orvieto 2011 (38)	15	Hydrosalpinx	not studied	11.6 vs. 10.2 n.s.	Analysis before and after surgery
Strandell 2001 (30)	26	Hydrosalpinx	not studied	9.4 vs. 8.7 n.s	Analysis before and after surgery

Abbreviation: n.s. = non significant.

those are the only patients to be recommended prophylactic salpingectomy prior to IVF.

A cost-effectiveness analysis, based on the Scandinavian RCT, showed that the strategy to perform salpingectomy prior to the first IVF cycle was more cost-effective than the strategy to suggest surgery after one or two cycles had failed (31).

Effect on Ovarian Function after Salpingectomy

The effect of salpingectomy on ovarian function has been debated, and the results of hitherto published studies are not entirely in consensus (24,27,32–38). A summary of studies is presented in Table 57.1. The close anatomical association of the vascular and nervous supply to the tube and ovary constitute the theoretical rationale for the risk of impaired ovarian function after surgery. Several studies have analyzed the ovarian performance in IVF cycles subsequent to salpingectomy due to ectopic pregnancy. None of them demonstrate an effect on the overall performance although one study has shown a decreased response in the ovary, ipsilateral to the salpingectomy (33). In the Scandinavian RCT on salpingectomy prior to IVF, there was no difference in the number of retrieved oocytes (Table 57.1) (24). In a subsequent analysis on a subset of patients, who underwent a stimulated cycle both before and after the salpingectomy, the effect of salpingectomy on the ovarian performance was examined by measuring the need for follicle-stimulating hormone (FSH) and the number of

retrieved oocytes (35). There were no significant differences in either the amount of FSH used or the number of retrieved oocytes. In the cycle after salpingectomy, in mean 0.7 fewer oocytes were retrieved compared with the cycle before surgery Table 57.1. In two studies, (27,37) different surgical methods for hydrosalpinx were compared. The finding from the retrospective study, (37) of significantly fewer retrieved oocytes after salpingectomy, in comparison with tubal ligation, was not confirmed in the randomized trial (27). One recent trial demonstrated fewer developed follicles on the ipsilateral side comparing the same ovary before and after surgery, but did not report on the number of retrieved oocytes from separate ovaries (38).

From the results, we cannot conclude that patients with a low ovarian reserve are at greater risk to suffer from poor response after salpingectomy. However, theoretically, it seems important to be very careful not to damage the vascular and nervous supply when performing a salpingectomy. A laparoscopic salpingectomy should be performed with cautious use of electrocautery, with no unnecessary excision of the mesosalpinx, but resection very close to the actual tube to avoid damage to the medial tubal artery; it is preferable to leave a portion of an adherent tube on the ovary rather than to perform an excessively radical salpingectomy. The risk of dehiscence in the uterine wall and subsequent protrusion of the fetus has been described; suggesting that resection not too close to the uterus is to be recommended (39).

Tubal Occlusion by Laparoscopy

Surgical treatment requiring laparoscopy also includes proximal ligation and salpingostomy. There is one randomized trial, in which 115 patients with hydrosalpinx were allocated to proximal tubal occlusion, salpingectomy, or no surgery prior to IVF (27). Salpingectomy but not tubal ligation demonstrated significantly higher ongoing pregnancy rates (49% and 38%, respectively) compared to women having no surgery (7%), analysed on an intention-to-treat basis. The Cochrane Review (29) included an additional small RCT (28) (published as an abstract) and a meta-analysis of these two studies demonstrated an OR for clinical pregnancy of 4.8 (95% CI 2.2–10.0). According to the theory of the hydrosalpingeal fluid affecting the endometrium negatively, the procedure of tubal ligation is likely to be effective in improving pregnancy results. The procedure is currently recommended when pelvic adhesions are too extensive to perform a salpingectomy.

Tubal Occlusion by Hysteroscopy

Tubal occlusion through hysteroscopy has been suggested when laparoscopy is contraindicated, like in cases with severe obesity or frozen pelvis. The first case report describing the use of microinsert sterilization device (Essure™) has been followed by a case series of 10 patients, reporting a live birth rate of 20% after one IVF cycle and/or frozen embryo transfer (40,41). The most recent report is a case series of 20 patients, in which successful occlusion was obtained in 19 (42). Results are reported as 12 births/20 patients. There are no controlled studies available. The obvious advantage is that the method can be performed in local anesthesia and thus avoiding complications related to laparoscopy and general anesthesia.

Salpingostomy

There are no separate studies on salpingostomy prior to IVF, although it has been performed in a few cases and reported to be part of a control group to hydrosalpinx patients in retrospective studies. Salpingostomy is naturally the method of choice if the tube is suitable for reconstructive surgery. The selection of patients suitable for surgical repair has to be based on the evaluation of the tubal mucosa through an endoscopic technique, and tubes with more than half of the mucosa in a good condition may have a fair chance of spontaneous conception (43). These patients should be given sufficient time to await spontaneous conception, although the woman's age may hasten the need for IVF.

Transvaginal Aspiration

Whatever the exact mechanism of the negative influence of hydrosalpinx fluid, the treatment options concern the disposal of the fluid. The simplest way, vaginal aspiration of fluid, has been evaluated in an RCT comparing transvaginal aspiration to no aspiration (44). Unfortunately, the study was stopped in advance due to recruitment difficulties. The study was thus underpowered including 66 patients and the difference in clinical pregnancy rate (31% vs. 18%) did not reach statistical significance.

There is a rapid reoccurrence of fluid already noticeable at the time of transfer in many cases, which most likely compromises any beneficial effect of drainage (45). Aboulghar et al. evaluated transvaginal aspiration before ovarian stimulation was initiated and demonstrated that there was no improvement in pregnancy rates (46). The occurrence of infections in association with puncture of hydrosalpinx seems to be rare when antibiotics have been given, according to the published reports. The method has the obvious advantage of being less invasive than the other available surgical methods.

It can be concluded that transvaginal aspiration of hydrosalpingeal fluid at the time of oocyte collection is a treatment option, particularly if there is a contraindication or nonacceptance for surgery, or if a hydrosalpinx develops during ovarian stimulation.

Antibiotic Treatment

The use of antibiotics has also been discussed, not only as prophylactics when a hydrosalpinx has been punctured, but also when given as a routine before oocyte retrieval to all patients. However, antibiotic treatment specifically in hydrosalpinx patients has never been prospectively evaluated. One retrospective study suggested that extended doxycycline treatment during an IVF cycle would minimize the detrimental effect of hydrosalpinx (47). When patients with hydrosalpinx who received extended doxycycline treatment during an IVF cycle were compared with patients with other indications (tubal occlusion/adhesions or endometriosis/unexplained infertility) who did not receive any antibiotics, implantation and pregnancy rates were similar in all groups. This design does not allow for any recommendation of antibiotic treatment as an effective treatment. The method is, however, advantageously cheap and simple, but its benefit still needs to be evaluated in a prospective trial.

Repeated Implantation Failure in Patients with Tubal Factor Infertility

The question whether salpingectomy is beneficial in patients without evident hydrosalpinx but with tubal factor infertility often arises if there is a repeated implantation failure after IVF. There is presently no data to support salpingectomy in this group. Indeed, the Scandinavian multicenter study (30) demonstrated that salpingectomy in comparison with no surgery did not increase pregnancy rates among patients with distally occluded tubes without fluid accumulation (OR 1.6, 95% CI 0.6, 4.8).

INTERVENTIONS AGAINST HYDROSALPINX WITHOUT IVF

As IVF developed and the results improved, the importance of using surgical methods for treating tubal infertility declined. It is well known that the success rate was closely related to the status of the tubal mucosa; the less damage to the tubes, the better chance of a subsequent intrauterine pregnancy. Today, IVF is often offered as a first-line treatment also to patients with mild tubal damage. Whether surgery is discussed or not, is mainly a question of surgical competence, availability of IVF, and the patient's financial situation, and is not primarily a medical issue.

The work-up of the subfertile couple has also changed over time, so that laparoscopy is no longer a compulsory investigation, due to limited resources and the fact that laparoscopy is a very invasive procedure. This new mode implies that fewer patients will be evaluated laparoscopically during the work-up, unless a hydrosalpinx is detected.

The result from the Scandinavian multicenter study to recommend salpingectomy prior to IVF has raised a number of concerns by Puttemans et al., (48) who fear that tubes that are suitable for functional surgery could be sacrificed. In the scenario where laparoscopy is not routinely used, this fear might be justified, if the tubes are not properly evaluated before a salpingectomy is performed. Even if a patient is scheduled for a laparoscopic salpingectomy, it is necessary to open the distally occluded tube for evaluation of the mucosa before a final decision of salpingectomy is taken. If it is appropriate to perform a salpingostomy, time for spontaneous conception should be given instead of immediate IVF.

Salpingectomy of a unilateral hydrosalpinx may imply an increased chance of spontaneous conception. Two women in the Scandinavian study (24) conceived spontaneously after long-lasting infertility followed by a unilateral salpingectomy and achieved a full term pregnancy; at least three additional case reports on the same theme have been published (49–51).

SUMMARY AND CONCLUSIONS

In patients with severe tubal disease presented as a hydrosalpinx on ultrasound and with a destroyed mucosa upon endoscopic inspection, IVF is the method of choice, but should be preceded by a discussion of laparoscopic salpingectomy, which will double the patient's chances of a subsequent birth after IVF. In cases of extensive adhesions, rendering the salpingectomy difficult and bearing a risk of complications, proximal ligation and distal fenestration is the preferred method. Psychological aspects of removing or interrupting the tubes are very important and always have to be considered. If no surgical intervention is performed prior to IVF, transvaginal aspiration of the fluid can be performed in conjunction with oocyte retrieval under antibiotic cover.

Patients with a preserved mucosa in the hydrosalpinx may have a good chance of spontaneous conception if salpingostomy is performed.

In the presence of a unilateral hydrosalpinx and a contralateral healthy tube, a unilateral salpingectomy can be recommended, followed by sufficient time to await spontaneous conception, before proceeding to IVF.

IMPLICATIONS FOR RESEARCH

The underlying mechanisms of impaired implantation and/or development of embryos in the presence of hydrosalpinx need further exploration. Basic research on endometrial receptivity and implantation are very intense research fields, and as more general knowledge is gained, more specific hypotheses may be directed to the negative role of hydrosalpinx. In addition, the formation of hydrosalpinx following pelvic infection needs to be elucidated. A better understanding of the mechanisms would provide prerequisites for a more rational therapy. As of today, we recommend very robust surgical methods, but it is possible that the treatment should be more individualized. Salpingectomy, tubal ligation, and transvaginal aspiration compared to no intervention have been evaluated in randomized trials, but only the former in a sufficiently large trial. Also comparisons between the methods have been underpowered. A trial designed to evaluate if hysteroscopic tubal occlusion or transvaginal aspiration is non-inferior to laparoscopic salpingectomy in terms of pregnancy and live birth rates after IVF would be of great clinical value.

REFERENCES

1. Strandell A, Bergh B, Lundin K. Selection of patients suitable for one-embryo transfer may reduce the rate of multiple births by half without impairment of overall birth rates. Hum Reprod 2000; 15: 2520–5.
2. Strandell A, Waldenström U, Nilsson L, Hamberger L. Hydrosalpinx reduces in-vitro fertilization/embryo transfer rates. Hum Reprod 1994; 9: 861–3.
3. Zeyneloglu HB, Arici A, Olive DL. Adverse effects of hydrosalpinx on pregnancy rates after in vitro fertilization-embryo transfer. Fertil Steril 1998; 70: 492–9.
4. deWit W, Gowrising CJ, Kuik DJ, et al. Only hydrosalpinges visible on ultrasound are associated with reduced implantation and pregnancy rates after in-vitro fertilization. Hum Reprod 1998; 13: 1696–701.
5. Wainer R, Camus E, Camier B, et al. Does hydrosalpinx reduce the pregnancy rate following in vitro fertilization. Fertil Steril 1997; 68: 1022–6.
6. Strandell A. The influence of hydrosalpinx on in-vitro fertilisation and embryo transfer – a review. Hum Reprod Update 2000; 6: 387–95.
7. Strandell A, Sjögren A, Bentin-Ley U, et al. Hydrosalpinx fluid does not adversely affect the normal development of human embryos and implantation in vitro. Hum Reprod 1998; 13: 2921–5.
8. Granot I, Dekel N, Segal I, et al. Is hydrosalpinx fluid cytotoxic? Hum Reprod 1998; 13: 1620–4.
9. de Vantéry Arrighi C, Lucas H, El-Mowafi D, et al. Effects of human hydrosalpinx fluid on in-vitro murine fertilization. Hum Reprod 2001; 16: 676–82.
10. Chen CD, Yang JH, Lin KC, et al. The significance of cytokines, chemical composition, and murine embryo development in hydrosalpinx fluid for predicting the in-vitro fertilization outcome in women with hydrosalpinx. Hum Reprod 2002; 17: 128–33.
11. Sawin SW, Loret de Mola JR, Monzon-Bordonaba F, et al. Hydrosalpinx fluid enhances human trophoblast viability and function in vitro: Implications for embryonic

implantation in assisted reproduction. Fertil Steril 1997; 68: 65–71.

12. Bedaiwy MA, Goldberg JM, Singh M, et al. Relationship between oxidative stress and embryotoxicity of hydrosalpingeal fluid. Hum Reprod 2002; 17: 601–4.

13. Lessey BA, Castelbaum AJ, Buck CA, et al. Further characterization of endometrial integrins during the menstrual cycle and in pregnancy. Fertil Steril 1994; 62: 497–506.

14. Sjöblom C, Wikland M, Robertson SA. Granulocyte-macrophage colony-stimulating factor promotes human blastocyst development in vitro. Hum Reprod 1999; 14: 3069–76.

15. Spandorfer SD, Neuer A, LaVerda D, et al. Previously undetected Chlamydia trachomatis infection, immunity to heat shock proteins and tubal occlusion in women undergoing in-vitro fertilization. Hum Reprod 1999; 14: 60–4.

16. Ajonuma LC, Ng EH, Chan HC. New insights into the mechanisms underlying hydrosalpinx fluid formation and its adverse effect on IVF outcome. Hum Reprod Update 2002; 8: 255–64.

17. Ng EH, Chan CC, Tang OS, Chung PC. Comparison of endometrial and subendometrial blood flows among patients with and without hydrosalpinx shown on scanning during in vitro fertilization treatment. Fertil Steril 2006; 85: 333–8.

18. Mansour RT, Aboulghar MA, Serrour GI, Riad R. Fluid accumulation of the uterine cavity before embryo transfer: A possible hindrance for implantation. J Vitro Fertil Embryo Transfer 1991; 8: 157–9.

19. Andersen AN, Lindhard A, Loft A, et al. The infertile patient with hydrosalpinges-IVF with or without salpingectomy. Hum Reprod 1996; 11: 2081–4.

20. Bloeche M, Schreiner T, Lisse K. Recurrence of hydrosalpinges after transvaginal aspiration of tubal fluid in an IVF cycle with development of serometra. Hum Reprod 1997; 12: 703–5.

21. Sharara FI. The role of hydrosalpinx in IVF: Simply mechanical? Hum Reprod 1999; 14: 577–8.

22. Levi AJ, Segars JH, Miller BT, Leondires MP. Endometrial cavity fluid is associated with poor ovarian response and increased cancellation rates in ART cycles. Hum Reprod 2001; 16: 2610–15.

23. Eytan O, Azem F, Gull I, et al. The mechanism of hydrosalpinx in embryo implantation. Hum Reprod 2001; 16: 2662–7.

24. Strandell A, Lindhard A, Waldenström U, et al. Hydrosalpinx and IVF outcome: A prospective, randomized multicentre trial in Scandinavia on salpingectomy prior to IVF. Hum Reprod 1999; 14: 2762–9.

25. Déchaud H, Daures JP, Arnal F, et al. Does previous salpingectomy improve implantation and pregnancy rates in patients with severe tubal factor infertility who are undergoing in vitro fertilization? A pilot prospective randomized study. Fertil Steril 1998; 69: 1020–5.

26. Goldstein DB, Sasaran LH, Stadtmauer L, Popa R. Selective salpingostomy-salpingectomy (SSS) and medical treatment prior to IVF in patients with hydrosalpinx. (Abstracts) Fertil Steril 1998; 70(3 Suppl 1): S320.

27. Kontoravdis A, Makrakis E, Pantos K, et al. Proximal tubal occlusion and salpingectomy results in similar improvement in in vitro fertilization outcome in patients with hydrosalpinx. Fertil Steril 2006; 86: 1642–9.

28. Moshin V, Hotineanu A. Reproductive outcome of the proximal tubal occlusion prior to IVF in patients with hydrosalpinx. (Abstracts) Hum Reprod 2006; 21: i193–4.

29. Johnson NP, Mak W, Sowter MC. Surgical treatment for tubal disease in women due to undergo in vitro fertilization. Cochrane Database of Systematic Reviews 2010: CD002125–DOI: 10.1002/14651858.CD002125.pub3.

30. Strandell A, Lindhard A, Waldenstrom U, Thorburn J. Hydrosalpinx and IVF outcome: Cumulative results after salpingectomy in a randomized controlled trial. Hum Reprod 2001; 16: 2403–10.

31. Strandell A, Lindhard A, Eckerlund I. Cost-effectiveness analysis of salpingectomy prior to IVF, based on a randomized controlled trial. Hum Reprod 2005; 20: 3284–92.

32. Verhulst G, Vandersteen N, van Steirteghem AC, Devroey P. Bilateral salpingectomy does not compromise ovarian stimulation in an in-vitro fertilization/embryo transfer programme. Hum Reprod 1994; 9: 624–8.

33. Lass A, Ellenbogen A, Croucher C, et al. Effect of salpingectomy on ovarian response to superovulation in an in vitro fertilization-embryo transfer program. Fertil Steril 1998; 70: 1035–8.

34. Dar P, Sachs GS, Strassburger D, Bukovsky I, Arieli S. Ovarian function before and after salpingectomy in artificial reproductive technology patients. Hum Reprod 2000; 15: 142–4.

35. Strandell A, Lindhard A, Waldenstrom U, Thorburn J. Salpingectomy prior to IVF does not impair the ovarian response. Hum Reprod 2001; 16: 1135–9.

36. Tal J, Paltieli Y, Korobotchka R, et al. Ovarian response to gonadotropin stimulation in repeated IVF cycles after unilateral salpingectomy. J Assist Reprod Genet 2002; 19: 451–5.

37. Gelbaya TA, Nardo LG, Fitzgerald CT, et al. Ovarian response to gonadotrophins after laparoscopic salpingectomy or the division of fallopian tubes for hydrosalpinges. Fertil Steril 2006; 85: 1464–8.

38. Orvieto R, Saar-Ryss B, Morgante G, et al. Does salpingectomy affect the ipsilateral ovarian response to gonadotropin during in vitro fertilization-embryo transfer cycles? Fertil Steril 2011; 95: 1842–4.

39. Inovay J, Marton T, Urbancsek J, et al. Spontaneous bilateral cornual uterine dehiscence early in the second trimester after bilateral laparoscopic salpingectomy and in-vitro fertilization. Hum Reprod 1999; 14: 2471–3.

40. Rosenfield RB, Stones RE, Coates A, et al. Proximal occlusion of hydrosalpinx bt hysteroscopic placement of microinsert before in vitro fertilization- embryo transfer. Fertil Steril 2005; 83: 1547–50.

41. Mijatovic V, Veersema S, Emanuel MH, Schats R. Essure hysteroscopic tubal occlusion device for the treatment of hydrosalpinx prior to in vitro fertilization-embryo transfer in patients with a contraindication for laparoscopy. Fertil Steril 2010; 93: 1338–42.

42. Galen DI, Khan NM, Richter KS. Essure multicenter off-label treatment for hydrosalpinx before in vitro fertilization. J Minim Invasive Gynecol 2011; 18: 338–42.

43. Vasquez G, Boeckx W, Brosens I. Prospective study of tubal mucosal lesions and fertility in hydrosalpinges. Hum Reprod 1995; 10: 1075–8.

44. Hammadieh N, Coomarasamy A, Ola B, et al. Ultrasound-guided hydrosalpinx aspiration during oocyte collection

improves pregnancy outcome in IVF: a randomized controlled trial. Hum Reprod 2008; 23: 1113–17.

45. Sharara FI, McClamrock HD. Endometrial fluid collection in women with hydrosalpinx after human chorionic gonadotrophin administration: a report of two cases and implications for management. Hum Reprod 1997; 12: 2816–19.

46. Aboulghar MA, Mansour RT, Serour GI, et al. Transvaginal ultrasonic needle guided aspiration of pelvic inflammatory cystic masses before ovulation induction for in vitro fertilization. Fertil Steril 1990; 53: 311–14.

47. Hurst BS, Tucker KE, Awoniyi CA, Schlaff WD. Hydrosalpinx treated with extended doxycyclin does not compromise the success of in vitro fertilization. Fertil Steril 2001; 75: 1017–19.

48. Puttemans P, Campo R, Gordts S, Brosens I. Hydrosalpinx and ART: hydrosalpinx-functional surgery or salpingectomy? Hum Reprod 2000; 15: 1427–30.

49. Choe J, Check JH. Salpingectomy for unilateral hydrosalpinx may improve in vivo fecundity. Gynecol Obstet Invest 1999; 48: 285–7.

50. Kiefer DG, Check JH. Salpingectomy improves outcome in the presence of a unilateral hydrosalpinx in a donor oocyte recipient: a case report. Clin Exp Obstet Gynecol 2001; 28: 71–2.

51. Aboulghar MA, Mansour RT, Serour GI. Spontaneous intrauterine pregnancy following salpingectomy for a unilateral hydrosalpinx. Hum Reprod 2002; 17: 1099–100.

58

Fertility preservation strategies

Stine Gry Kristensen, Tine Greve, and Claus Yding Andersen

OVERVIEW

Nowadays the chance of surviving a cancer disease is significantly increased as compared to the earlier times and the group of cancer survivors is constantly growing. This remarkable achievement is mainly due to the development of more aggressive treatment regimes, which unfortunately do carry the risk of unwanted side effects such as infertility, which can jeopardize the chance to have one's own biological children. For many girls and women, fertility preservation is of high priority and will improve their quality of life as cancer survivors.

Around 2% of women in their reproductive age suffer from invasive cancer and are in risk of ovarian failure after receiving sterilizing chemotherapy and radiotherapy (1). In contrast to the testis the ovary is equipped with a fixed number of oocytes without germ-stem cells leaving no possibility for replenishment of the pool of oocytes.

Until recently in vitro fertilization (IVF) and embryo transfer (ET) in combination with cryopreservation was considered the only possible option for women to conceive after recovery from a sterilizing cancer treatment. This method, however, cannot sustain long-time fertility, including support of functioning ovulatory cycles. In addition, it encompasses some disadvantages in the context of women with a current disease. Before IVF the women will normally undergo ovarian stimulation, which may be incompatible with an urgent cancer treatment. Moreover, more than 4000 children are exposed to potentially sterilizing treatment in the United States annually and they cannot currently be helped to maintain ovarian function and later fertility (2).

Cryopreservation and transplantation of ovarian tissue fulfill a number of these short-comings: Grafting of cryopreserved ovarian tissue can restore menstrual cyclicity to patients who entered menopause as a consequence of the treatment and the patient gets the possibility of a spontaneous conception (3,4). The technique does not require pretreatment and can be performed from one day to another independently of where the patient is in the menstrual cycle. Moreover, the method does not require male gametes, it is applicable even to prepubertal girls and ovarian tissue cryopreservation may be performed even in cases where chemotherapy has already been initiated in contrast to IVF and embryo freezing.

Fertility preservation in young women and men, who have experienced gonadotoxic treatment, is now a central topic to professionals and patients (5), and the different strategies will be discussed in this chapter. There is a special focus on cryopreservation of ovarian tissue, as this method is now gaining ground as a valid method of long-term fertility preservation in girls and women facing gonadotoxic therapy.

EFFECT OF CHEMO- AND RADIOTHERAPY ON THE OVARY

Chemotherapeutic agents differ in relation to their toxicity on ovarian function (6). The alkylating agents, such as cyclophosphamide and busulfan, are far more gonadotoxic than other chemotherapeutic agents. A study of young cancer patients found that the use of alkylating agents had an odds ratio (OR) of 4.0 for primary ovarian insufficiency (POI), which is significantly higher than when using platinum agents (OR = 1.8), plant alkaloids (OR = 1.2), or antimetabolites (OR < 1) (7). Cyclophosphamide is a cell cycle–nonspecific drug, and as such is more cytotoxic to the ovaries than cell cycle–specific drugs, as it may harm both resting and dividing cells. Studies on mice have shown that exposure to cyclophosphamide causes follicular destruction in exponential proportion to increasing dose (8).

The fact that ovaries of young girls contain a higher number of follicles than ovaries from older women makes them more resistant to chemotherapy. Thus, young girls tolerate higher doses of chemotherapy before entering POI (9).

Radiotherapy interrupts the normal cellular proliferation cycle and causes extensive cell damage. However, despite the fact that postnatal oocytes are mitotically inactive, they are still highly susceptible to the damage caused by radiotherapy. The high number of follicles in the prepubertal ovary makes it less vulnerable than in later reproductive life, but the risk of POI after abdominal radiotherapy is still high (10). It has been estimated that a total radiation exposure of 20 Gy fractionated over six weeks in younger women and children produces sterility with 95% confidence (11).

Finally, the high-dose chemo- and radiotherapy used prior to bone marrow transplantation (BMT) leave the vast majority of patients without ovarian function and fertility (7).

CANDIDATES FOR FERTILITY PRESERVING METHODS

In the Danish fertility preservation program, the criteria are a more than 50% risk of post-treatment infertility and an estimated higher than 50% chance of surviving five years after diagnosis. There is no strict upper age limit and in clinical practice women with a relative high number of antral follicles in her mid-thirties may be offered the procedure. However, new treatment regimes constantly develop and a precise prediction is impossible.

Risk Assessment

Most antineoplastic treatments in childhood are not hazardous to the immediate ovarian function of the affected girls, although they may reduce the future ovarian function and fertility potential. However, some treatments and cancer diagnoses are associated with a high risk of POI, and in these cases fertility preserving methods should be discussed with and offered to the woman or to the girl in cooperation with her parents if she is a minor (6). The different fertility preserving techniques (pros and cons) and their relevance to girls and young women according to the planned treatment are presented in Table 58.1. Patients with an almost 100% risk of POI are those in whom BMT is planned and those receiving abdominal radiation. In cases where high-dose chemotherapy is planned, the indication for fertility preservation should be evaluated individually in relation to the planned dose and type of drug used. In patients who have already received a relatively mild chemotherapy because of a malignancy, and who later experience a relapse, cryopreservation of ovarian tissue may be considered before the second round of chemotherapy, which usually includes more aggressive and gonadotoxic chemotherapeutics (6).

Fertility preservation was initially indicated only for cancer patients receiving sterilizing chemotherapy; however, today its indications are extended to cover patients receiving gonadotoxic chemotherapy for other systematic illnesses, such as autoimmune diseases, and those patients undergoing oophorectomy for benign ovarian conditions and for prophylactic purposes.

CURRENT OPTIONS FOR PRESERVATION OF FEMALE FERTILITY

When a patient faces a substantial risk of POI, the different methods for fertility preservation (Fig. 58.1), their advantages and disadvantages, their efficiency, and the possible experimental nature of the treatment needs to be taken into consideration.

Transposition of the Ovaries

The technique of moving the ovaries out of the field of radiation, also known as oophoropexy, is now used in most women that require pelvic irradiation. However, although the ovaries may be out of the field of direct radiation, the scatter dose may cause significant ovarian damage and in fact cause ovarian failure in 50–90% of the cases (12).

Hormonal Suppression

It has been suggested that co-treatment with gonadotropin-releasing hormone analogues (GnRHa) should protect the ovaries from the harmful effects of chemotherapy (13,14). Currently, there is no solid evidence to show a beneficial effect of GnRHa (15,16).

Cryopreservation of Mature Oocytes or Embryos

Mature oocytes, fertilized oocytes, as well as human embryos derived from couples undergoing IVF treatment

---

Table 58.1 Fertility Preserving Measures Applicable to Female Patients with a Malignant Diagnosis: Pros and Cons

Method	Planned treatment	Age group	Mode of obtaining future pregnancy	Advantages	Disadvantages
Oophoropexy	Abdominal radiation	P÷ girls P+ girls Adult women	Spontaneous or IVF	Standard procedure	Scatter radiation
Cryopreservation of oocytes and embryos	BMT, abdominal radiation, and high-dose AA	(P+ girls?) Adult women	Fertilization of oocytes and/or embryo transfer	Established technique	May incur delay Require sperm Fixed fertility potential Not appropriate for prepubertal girls
Cryopreservation of ovarian tissue	BMT, abdominal radiation, and high-dose AA	P– girls P+ girls Adult women	Spontaneous or IVF after transplantation of frozen–thawed tissue	Minimal delay Restores ovarian function → spontaneous and repeated conception No lower age limit	Requires surgery Risk of malignant cell contamination Efficacy unknown

Abbreviations: AA, alkylating agents; P÷, prepubertal; P+, postpubertal.
Source: Modified from Ref. 6.

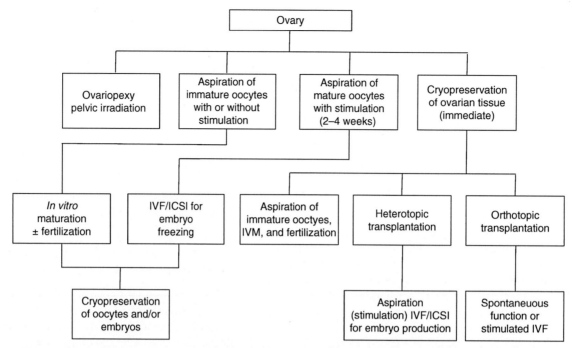

Figure 58.1 Options for fertility preservation in women. *Abbreviations*: IVM, in vitro maturation; IVF, in vitro fertilization; ICSI, intra-cytoplasmic sperm injection.

can be cryopreserved following standard procedures, and the results of thawing and replacing such oocytes and embryos are now good, with pregnancy rates of around 20% per thaw cycle (17–20). These techniques require two to four weeks for completion, and are therefore often not relevant in cancer patients, as a delay in the antineoplastic treatment is not desirable. Recently, however, a protocol has been described in which ovarian stimulation may start even during the luteal phase in cancer patients, thus requiring a maximum of two weeks before oocyte collection can be performed (21).

In vitro maturation (IVM) of immature oocytes with subsequent fertilization is still an experimental procedure with low success (22).

Cryopreservation of Ovarian Tissue

The success of ovarian cryopreservation is based on the high cryopreservation tolerance of small (resting) primordial follicles in contrast to the vulnerable, larger growing follicles. The vast majority of primordial follicles are located in the outermost 1 or 2 mm of the ovarian cortex, which is relatively easy to isolate from the rest of the ovarian tissue. When the ovarian cortex has been frozen it can be stored for years in liquid nitrogen allowing time for the patient to recover. After the patient is cured, some of the cryopreserved tissue can be re-transplanted to those who entered menopause and the ovarian grafts are able to reestablish a cyclic endocrine hormone milieu including appropriate conditions for conception, gestation, and parturition, possibly via IVF–ET (23–25). The efficacy by which this technique actually results in the birth of healthy children still needs to be established and a comparison to other techniques, which has also been

used in connection with cancer patients in a only limited number of cases, cannot presently be performed.

TECHNICAL ASPECTS OF OVARIAN TISSUE CRYOPRESERVATION

The Danish Fertility Preservation Program was initiated in 1999. Since then, more than 500 patients have had ovarian tissue cryopreserved for clinical purposes and currently 14 ovaries per year per million inhabitants are frozen. Since 2003, 25 autotransplantations have been performed in 18 women, resulting in nine pregnancies, of which three resulted in the birth of healthy babies (23,26), one ongoing pregnancy, and one legal abortion (27). Thus, the Danish protocol for ovarian tissue cryopreservation has proven quite robust, and is becoming a well-established method of fertility preservation in the Danish healthcare system.

The Danish Protocol

An entire ovary (Fig. 58.2A) or part of an ovary is removed surgically, often during laparoscopy. In a sterile bench, the ovary is placed in a 6-cm Petri dish containing 20 ml isotonic saline solution and the cortex is isolated using hooked forceps and scalpels (Fig. 58.3). When all medullar tissue is removed and the cortex has been trimmed to a thickness of 1–2 mm (Fig. 58.2B), it is cut into 5 × 5–15 mm pieces (Fig. 58.2C). During the trimming procedure, the tissue is rinsed several times in an isotonic saline solution. The pieces are transferred to a 50-ml plastic tube containing 30 ml of freezing solution [0.1 mol/l sucrose, 1.5 mol/l ethylene glycol, and 10 mg/ml human serum albumin (HSA, 200 mg/ml) in phosphate-buffered

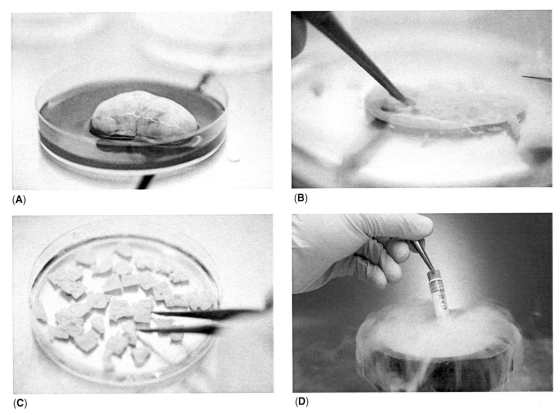

(A)   **(B)**

(C)   **(D)**

Figure 58.2 Cryopreservation of human ovarian tissue for fertility preservation. (**A**) One ovary or part of an ovary is surgically removed. (**B**) The medulla is removed and the cortex is trimmed to a thickness of 1–2 mm. (**C**) The cortex is then cut into pieces of 5 × 5 mm. The pieces of cortex equilibrate in cold freezing solution for 25 minutes on ice. (**D**) The cortex pieces are transferred to individual cryotubes and slow-frozen in liquid nitrogen.

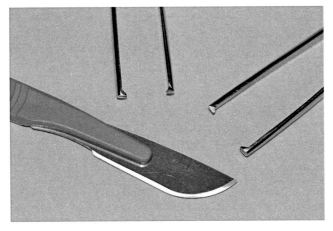

Figure 58.3 Instruments used for preparation of the ovarian cortex. Hooked forceps ensure a firm hold on the ovarian tissue during dissection, and a scalpel with a long cutting edge enables a smooth trimming of the cortex.

saline (PBS)], and equilibrated for approximately 25 min at 1–2°C on a tilting table. The fragments of cortex are transferred individually to 1.8-ml cryovials (Nunc A/S, Roskilde, Denmark) using sterile forceps, each containing 1 ml of fresh freezing solution and are cryopreserved using a programmable Planer freezer 360-1.7 (Planer Ltd, Middlesex, UK) (Fig. 58.2D). The following program is used: Starting temperature 1°C, then –2°C/min to –9°C, five minutes of soaking, followed by manual seeding for

ice crystal induction, –0.3°C/min to –40°C, –10°C/min to –140°C, and directly into liquid nitrogen. From the moment the tissue enters the freezing solution and until initiation of the cryoprogram exactly 30 minutes elapses and the temperature is constantly kept at around 1–2°C. Following freezing, the tubes are sealed in a second plastic holster (double sealing, Fig. 58.4A) and half of the tissue is long-term stored in each of two separate nitrogen tanks (Fig. 58.4B).

During the processing of the cortical tissue a small piece of cortex is taken for histology and used to estimate the follicular density.

Choice of Cryoprotectant

A number of different mixtures of cryoprotectant have successfully been used for cryopreservation of ovarian tissue. The use of permeating cryoprotectants such as dimethylsulfoxide (DMSO) or ethylene glycol with or without a non-permeating substance such as sucrose, have after replacement of frozen/thawed ovarian tissue to menopausal women resulted in regained ovarian function and the birth of healthy children (4,28–30). Thus, the ovarian tissue appears to be quite robust prior to cryopreservation (at least if kept at temperatures close to zero degrees) with a good fraction of the follicles surviving the freezing procedure. The combination of cryoprotectants that we use was based on a comparative study between different cryoprotection mixtures in which the

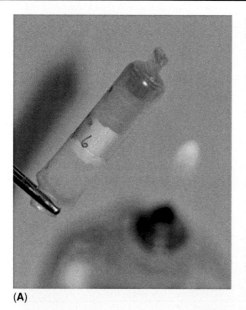
(A)

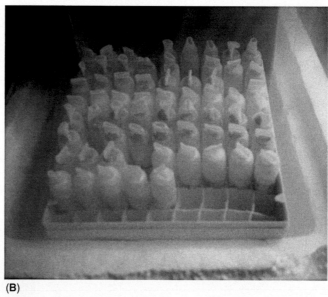
(B)

Figure 58.4 Dobbelt sealing and storage of cryotubes. (**A**) Once frozen, the cryotubes containing the ovarian tissue are double sealed in cryoflex. (**B**) Before long-term storage. Notice the different color codes for each patient.

survival of mouse follicles was evaluated histologically and by replacement of frozen/thawed ovarian tissue to immunodeficient mice (31).

Quality Control by Xenotransplantation of Human Ovarian Tissue

To qualitatively assess follicle survival following freezing, frozen–thawed ovarian cortical biopsies from 42 women were transplanted under the skin of oophorectomized immunodeficient mice, a total of 49 times in our program (31). From these women, 36 had a malignant diagnosis prior to cryopreservation: Breast cancer (n = 9); Hodgkin's and non-Hodgkin's lymphoma (n = 9); leukemia (acute lymphoblastic, chronic myeloid and acute myeloid; n = 7); sarcoma (n = 5); and miscellaneous (n = 6). The mice were killed after four weeks. (Fig. 58.5A). Histological evaluation showed healthy primordial follicles in all of the cortical biopsies and confirmed that follicular viability was maintained after thawing (Fig. 58.5B). Transplantation of frozen/thawed ovarian tissue to immunodeficient mice is still considered to be one of the best ways of evaluating the whole cryopreservation procedure.

Slow Freezing vs. Vitrification

The most widely used protocol for ovarian cryopreservation is the slow freezing method (32–36) and up until now all children born from replacement of frozen/thawed ovarian tissue is a result of the slow-freezing technique (30).

Two techniques are currently being tested as alternatives to the slow freezing method: (i) Vitrification, in which the tissue is exposed to high concentrations of cryoprotectants for a short time and immediately plunged in liquid nitrogen. Some reports favor the use of vitrification (37–39) while others find superior results

using slow freezing (40,41) and it is currently questionable whether vitrification offers any significant clinical benefit. (ii) Whole ovary freezing, in which the cryoprotectants are introduced through the vascular pedicles in vitro followed by cryopreservation, (42) may avoid the ischemia-induced follicle loss that occurs in connection with transplantation because anastomosis of ovarian vessels secure a fast blood supply (43). However, currently the ovarian vessels seem to become damaged during the freezing process.

Transportation of Ovarian Tissue Prior to Cryopreservation

Ovarian tissues remain viable after transportation for up to five hours on ice prior to freezing (23,34). This allows hospitals without cryopreservation expertise to treat women locally for the cancer disease and just send the ovarian tissue to the center that performs cryopreservation. This facilitates quality control, proper equipment, and personnel to fulfill clinical, legal, and scientific standards required for proper conduction of the procedure. The feasibility of centralized cryobanking has been proven by the Danish experience of transporting ovarian tissue prior to freezing and these principles have now been introduced in Germany and many other countries (4).

Actually, we have recently demonstrated good follicle survival after freezing and transplantation of human ovarian cortex to ovariectomized immunodeficient mice for a period of four weeks following a transport period of 20 hours on ice prior to cryopreservation (Fig. 58.5B) (31).

Cryopreservation of a Whole Ovary vs. Biopsy

In most Danish patients an entire ovary is removed for cryopreservation. The advantages of this approach are the

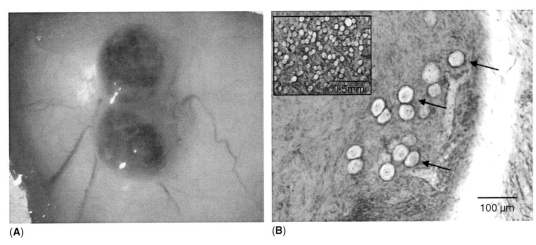

Figure 58.5   (**A**) Two pieces of frozen–thawed human ovarian cortex (5 × 5 mm) transplanted under the skin of an oophorectomized mouse. After two weeks, macroscopically visible revascularization was established. (**B**) Human ovarian cortex kept on ice for 20 hours prior to freezing. Thawed tissue was transplanted under the skin of an oophorectomized mouse for four weeks. Histology showed healthy primordial follicles (arrows) surrounded by small blood vessels. Insert shows histology of the fresh sample. Bars, 100 µm and 0.5 mm. (insert). *Source*: From Ref. 31.

minimized possibility of postoperational complications and the possibility of repeating the transplantation in case the tissue of the first transplantation becomes exhausted and prolonging the window of possible fertility from two to four years to possibly six to 10 years. Half an ovary or cortical biopsies may also be taken in case of prior unilateral oophorectomy or resection of one ovary. However, the decision of cryopreserving one whole ovary in contrast to parts of it remains a controversial issue (44).

There is little evidence to suggest that unilateral oophorectomy by itself has any major impact on the age of menopause. Women with a single ovary may have slightly elevated serum follicle-stimulating hormone (FSH) concentrations (45), but appear to have an unreduced fertility potential either through natural conception or via IVF (46).

AUTOTRANSPLANTATION OF CRYOPRESERVED OVARIAN TISSUE

Although ovarian tissue from thousands of girls and women has been cryopreserved, globally results from transplantation accumulate at a slow pace. Usually the patient needs at least two years for cure before receiving transplantation. Furthermore, fortunately merely around half of the women, who had one of her ovaries cryopreserved actually entered menopause immediately or shortly after termination of treatment (47). According to a recent review, around 29 women have had frozen/thawed tissue transplanted (4); however, in year 2012 this number is likely to exceed 60.

Thawing of Cryopreserved Ovarian Tissue

Thawing consists of a three-step procedure each of 10 minutes duration (Fig. 58.6). The vials containing the frozen tissue are placed in a 37°C water bath. Immediately when the solution becomes liquid, the cortical tissue is

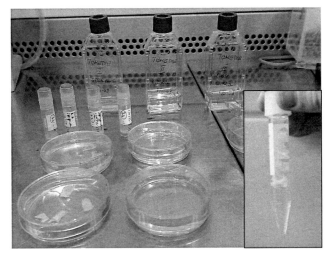

Figure 58.6   Three-step thawing procedure. Pieces of cortex is transferred to thawing solutions with decreasing concentrations of cryoprotectant. Insert shows the finale step of thawing and the tissue is subsequently brought to the operating theatre for transplantation.

removed and placed in the first thawing medium (0.75 mol/l ethylene glycol and 0.25 mol/l sucrose in PBS), and moved to the second medium with sterile forceps (0.25 mol/l sucrose in PBS) on a tilting table at room temperature. For the last 10 minutes of thawing, the tissue is transferred to PBS in a 10-ml plastic tube for 10 minutes (Fig. 58.6, insert), which is brought to the operating theatre for immediate reimplantation.

The period of time between transplantation and revascularization of the tissue appears to be critical to follicle survival, since 60–70% of follicles have been found to be lost in connection with transplantations in sheep, whereas only a small fraction is lost due to the actual cryopreservation procedure (48). To minimize the time period from thawing to reimplantation it is important to plan the transplantation in a way that allows immediate

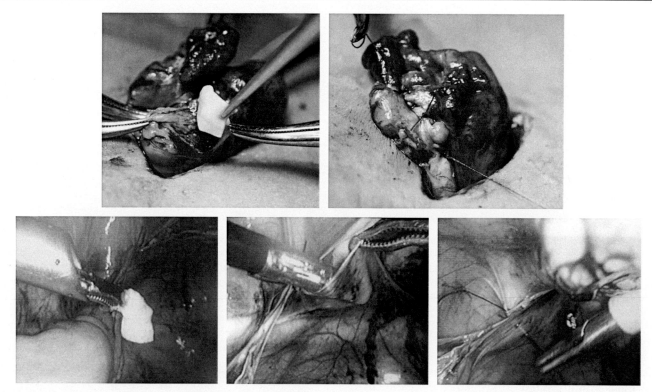

Figure 58.7 Transplantation of cryopreserved ovarian tissue. (*Top panel*) Orthotopic transplantation; pieces of thawed ovarian cortex being transplanted in a subcortical pocket in the in situ ovary. (*Bottom panel*) Heterotopic transplantation; pieces of thawed ovarian cortex being transplanted in a subperitoneal pocket corresponding to the pelvic wall. *Source*: Modified from Ref. 49.

grafting once the thawed pieces of ovarian cortex arrives in the operating theater.

Ortho- and Heterotopic Transplantation

In most Danish patients transplantation has been performed as a combined laparoscopy/mini-laparotomy to subcortical pockets of the remaining menopausal ovary (23,49). Under general anesthesia a 50 mm surgical incision to the lower abdomen is performed, and the remaining ovary is mobilized laparoscopically and made available on the surface. Longitudinal incisions in the ovarian cortex are made, thus creating small pockets just below the cortex on each side of the ovary (Fig. 58.7 Top panel). The fragments are aligned next to one another in the pockets with the cortex side outward (23,49). Normally six to 10 pieces of cortex can be positioned onto the remaining ovary depending on the size of the ovary.

Whenever possible the tissue is transplanted under the cortex of the remaining ovary left in situ (orthotopic transplantation, Fig. 58.7 Top panel); however, in some cases where the remaining ovary has been removed or the ovarian volume is significantly reduced, it is necessary to transplant the tissue to peritoneal pockets on the anterior abdominal wall or to the lateral pelvic wall (peritoneal orthotopic or heterotopic transplantation, Fig. 58.7 Bottom panel).

RESTORATION OF OVARIAN ACTIVITY

To date, 18 patients in the Danish program have received transplantation of the frozen/thawed tissue. In seven

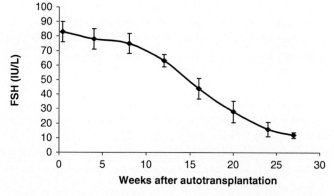

Figure 58.8 Restoration of ovarian function serum levels of FSH (IU/L) in 12 Danish patients after autotransplantation of frozen–thawed ovarian tissue (mean ± standard error of the mean). *Abbreviation*: FSH, follicle-stimulating hormone.

cases, the patients have received one additional transplant, either to increase the pool of available follicles or because the function of the tissue transplanted the first time was exhausted and the patient re-entered menopause. The ovarian tissue resumed endogenous hormone production and follicular development in all patients (31). However, in one patient with breast cancer who had ovarian tissue cryopreserved at the age of 36 years, the tissue only functioned for seven months after the first autotransplantation and never regained hormone production and follicular maturation after a second attempt. In Fig. 58.8, FSH concentrations after the first transplantations in 12 Danish patients shows that FSH concentrations remain high for a short period after transplantation until follicular growth reaches a stage in which estradiol and inhibin B is secreted and then starts to decline toward premenopausal concentrations. So far, the longest period of duration of the tissue is 66 months in a patient with Ewing's sarcoma who was 27 years at the time of cryopreservation of ovarian cortex. Another woman has had ovarian function for more than seven years in total after two concecutive transplantations.

Our studies have shown that a fairly constant period of around 20–25 weeks is required for the development of the first preovulatory follicle, irrespective of age, quantity of tissue replaced, or the number of follicles present in the transplant (31), thereby confirming and extending observations by Donnez and coworkers (24,30). This suggests that follicular growth and development is relatively unaffected by these factors. The transition time from the resting human primordial follicle to the preovulatory stage has been estimated to be almost half a year (50). If only the primordial and primary follicles survived cryopreservation, it would be expected that the period required for preovulatory follicular development would last somewhat longer than the four to five months as observed in the present study. This suggests that some growing follicles do survive the cryopreservation procedure and resume growth after transplantation. This notion is supported by our findings of morphologically normal growing follicles in histological sections of frozen/thawed ovarian tissue (data not shown) and corroborate results of previous studies (51,52). However, restoration of ovarian function following transplantation in patients receiving gonadotoxic chemotherapy immediately prior to cryopreservation may take up to eight months, which possibly reflect the presence of only nongrowing primordial follicles in the frozen/thawed tissue (53–55).

A recent review by Donnez et al. (30) showed that the duration of restored ovarian activity was shorter (one to two years) in the subgroup of women who had received chemotherapy immediately before cryopreservation, compared with those who had not (four years; Table 58.2). Indeed, in some patients, the duration of graft activity was less than two years, while in others, who had not received chemotherapy it was considerably longer (four years).

The age of patients at cryopreservation is also a predictive factor. The review by Donnez et al. (30) report that all the 13 women who have conceived following transplantation of cryopreserved ovarian tissue, except one, were under 30 years of age (19–28 years), and six of the 10 patients were under 25 years (mean 23 years; range 19–25 years).

Live Births

During the last 15 years, the technique has developed from the first successful report of live birth in sheep (56), to the resumption of follicular activity and menstrual cycle in humans (53,57,58), and finally in 2004, Donnez and coworkers reported the first live birth after autotransplantation of cryopreserved ovarian tissue in humans (35). Orthotopic reimplantation has so far led to the birth of 14 healthy babies in 11 women (23,26,30,35,36,59–64). Among the 14 live births, eight were girls and six boys (Table 58.2) and all were healthy. All singleton deliveries occurred after 37 weeks of gestation, and the one twin pregnancy ended in delivery of two boys at 33 weeks (62).

The majority of women conceived naturally following transplantation of cryopreserved ovarian tissue (Table 58.2), which constitutes a good argument in favor of orthotopic reimplantation. In connection with IVF it should be pointed out that in series published by Andersen et al. (23), Dolmans et al. (65), and Meirow et al. (36), an empty follicle rate as high as 29–35% was observed during the IVF procedure and the percentage of immature or degenerated oocytes is much higher (37%) in patients with frozen–thawed transplanted tissue than in the general population undergoing intracytoplasmic sperm injection (ICSI) (65).

Heterotopic transplantation has resulted in two biochemical pregnancies, but so far not in live births (66).

RISK OF MALIGNANT CELL CONTAMINATION

There may be a risk of reintroducing the original cancer in connection with transplantation of ovarian tissue, which is removed before the patients receive chemotherapy. Malignant cells in the ovarian cortex can thus occur in the frozen tissue and possibly, if transplanted, cause a relapse of the cancer.

Autopsy studies and case reports showed that indeed most tumors can metastasize to the ovaries (67). However, ovarian tissue cryopreservation is usually only offered to patients with a high chance of a long-term survival and these patients will typically have low stage and limited disease with a minimal risk of dissemination and ovarian involvement (31). One exception, however, is leukemia which is a disease of the blood and is hence believed to be present in all tissue.

Evaluation of Ovarian Tissue for Residual Disease

To minimize risk of grafting ovarian tissue to cancer survivors, a variety of different techniques may be used either separately or in combination: (i) The surgeon performing excision of the tissue should observe for possible gross pathology near and on the ovaries; (ii) Before reimplantation, a piece of the frozen/thawed tissue can be evaluated by histology and immunohistochemistry (IHC) using the markers that characterized the original tumor; (iii) If the cancer expresses a specific marker, reverse transcription and quantitative PCR (RT–PCR and qPCR) can detect very few copies of a disease-specific genetic marker; and (iv) Immunodeficient mice can be transplanted with ovarian tissue and kept for four to six months to detect whether the original human cancer develops. If the mice do not develop cancer it cannot be excluded that the tissue contains tumor cells as some human cancers do not grow well in mice.

Table 58.2   Fourteen Live Births After Orthotopic Transplantation of Frozen–Thawed Ovarian Tissue (July 2011)

Age at cryopreservation	Disease	Chemo before cryopreservation	Chemo± radio after cryopreservation	Time from reimplantation to restoration of ovarian function (mo)	Time from reimplantation to pregnancy (mo)	Natural/IVF	Gestation in weeks/ sex/weight in kg	Ref.
25	Hodgkin's	No	MOPP/ABV/38 Gy	4.5	11	N	39♀/3.720	(35)
19	Neurectodermic tumor	No	4 Anticancer agents, SCT	3.5	9	N	38♂/2.830	(30)
28	Non-Hodgkin's lymphoma	Yes	BEAM,SCT	6.5	11	IVF	38.5♀/3.000	(36)
24	Hodgkin's	Yes	ABVD (5c)	4.0	8	N	39♀/3.130	(59)
			EVA-CBV SCT		48	N	39♀/2.870	
27	Ewing sarcoma	No	VIDE	4.0	6	IVF	39♀/3.204	(23,26)
			VAI		25	N	39♀/3.828	
25	Hodgkin's	Yes	DHAP (3c), SCT	5.5	10	IVF	37♂/2.600	(23)
20	Hodgkin's	No	6 Anticancer agents, SCT	3.5	8	N	38♂/3.089	(60)
27	Microscopic polyangiitis	Yes	Cytoxan	4.5	11	IVF	37♀/2.030	(61)
36	Breast cancer	No	FEC (3c), docetaxel (3c)	3.5	10	IVF	33♂/1.650	(62)
							33♂/1.830	(63)
20	Sickle cell anemia	No	Busulfan, cytoxan, SCT	4.0	6	N	38♀/3.700	(63)
19	Thalassemia	No	3 Anticancer agents, PBSCT	3.5	10.5	IVF	39♂/3.026	(64)

Abbreviations: Chemo, chemotherapy; radio, radiotherapy; SCT, stem cell transplantation; cytoxan, cyclophosphamide; N, natural pregnant. MOPP/ABV: mechlorethamine, vincristine, procarbazine, prednisone, doxorubicin, bleomycin, vinblastine; BEAM: BCNU, etoposide, Ara-C, and melphalan; ABVD: doxorubicin 25 mg/m², bleomycin 10,000 IE/m², vinblastin 6 mg/m², dacarbazine 375 mg/m²; VIDE: vincristin 1.5 mg/m², ifosfamid 3 mg/m² (3 days), doxorubicin 20 mg/m² (3 days), ethoposide 150 mg/m² (3 days); VAI: vincristin 1.5 mg/m², actinomy-cin 0.75 mg/m² (2 days), ifosfamid 3 mg/m² (2 days); DHAP: dexametasone 40mg, cytarabine 4 g/m², cisplatin 100 mg/m²; FEC: fluorouracil, epirubicin, and cyclophosphamide; PBSCT: peripheral blood SCT. *Source:* Modified from Ref. 30.

As the piece of ovary used for any of the above methods cannot be used for transplantation, it is impossible to exclude completely that the pieces used for transplantation are not contaminated with malignant cells.

Risk of Malignant Cell Contamination

Risk evaluation for malignant cell infiltration of the ovaries in patients undergoing ovarian tissue cryopreservation for fertility preservation is presented in Table 58.3. The risk of reintroducing the cancer is considered high in leukemia patients (75–77), but is very unlikely in patients with lymphomas (3,72), except in the rare cases of Burkitt's lymphoma (78). Currently, there is no established method to regain fertility for patients who suffered from a leukemia, but in the future isolated follicle transplantation or IVM (79) may be become possible.

Most importantly, no relapses at the site of the transplant have so far been reported as a result of replacing frozen/thawed ovarian tissue to those around 30 women worldwide who had a previous malignant disease.

PRESERVATION OF MALE FERTILITY

The testis has been shown to be highly susceptible to the toxic effects of irradiation and chemotherapy at all stages of life (80). Young cancer survivors are approximately half as likely as their siblings to sire a pregnancy if they have been exposed to high-risk chemo- and/or radiotherapy (81).

Effect of Chemo- and Radiotherapy on the Testis

The impact of combination chemotherapy on the spermatogenic epithelium is dependent on the type and dosage of the drugs used (82–84). The threshold dose of cyclophosphamide, in relation to infertility, has been estimated to be between 7.5 and 9g/m² (85,86), or in postpubertal boys, 10g/m² (87). Recent observations suggest that slow recovery of spermatogenesis may occur even after these high doses and permanent sterility may appear from 19 to 20g/m² doses of cyclophosphamide and other alkylating agents (85,88).

The germinal epithelium is also very sensitive to irradiation damage and it depends on total dose and fractionation (89,90). In the prepubertal testis, germline stem cells are acutely and dose-dependently depleted following radiation exposure (91,92). Doses of more than six Gy are able to deplete the spermatogonial stem cell pool and lead to permanent infertility (93,94).

Recovery of spermatogenesis occurs from the remaining stem cells and relies on the type, dose, and fractionation of cytotoxic drugs and irradiation (95). In men, re-colonization of surviving spermatogonia can first be detected six months after a dose of 0.2 Gy, nine to 18 months after a dose of 1 Gy, and more than four years after a dose of 10 Gy (96,97).

Current Options for Preservation of Male Fertility

Cryopreservation of ejaculated sperm is the routinely used tool for fertility preservation in adult male patients (98). Success rates in achieving a pregnancy using cryopreserved sperm have greatly improved by ICSI (99). All pubertal boys with testis volumes above 10–12ml are encouraged to donate a semen sample prior to cancer therapy (98,99). Alternatively, electro-ejaculation, penile vibratory stimulation, search for spermatozoa in urine sample, or testicular sperm extraction from a biopsy can

Table 58.3   Risk Evaluation for Malignant Cell Infiltration of the Ovaries in Patients Undergoing Ovarian Tissue Cryopreservation for Fertility Preservation

Disease	Risk evaluation studies
Breast cancer	Histology/IHC showed no evidence of malignant cell involvement in ovarian tissue from 134 women with breast cancer (68–70).
Hodgkin's lymphoma	Xenotransplantation of histological negative tissue to SCID found no evidence of Hodgkin's lymphoma in 13 women (71). Light microscopy showed no evidence of malignant cells in ovarian tissue from 73 women with Hodgkin's lymphoma (3,53,71,72). However, a 19-year-old girl had to cortex pieces evaluated before cryopreservation and one showed ovarian involvement of Hodgkin's lymphoma (73). The remaining tissue from this girl was thawed and examined but showed no signs of tumor cells.
Non-Hodgkin's lymphoma	Cortical tissue from 21 women have been evaluated with light microscopy (3,71). PCR techniques have been used in 2 of the women (3) and xenotransplantation to SCID mice in 5 other women (71). None showed signs of malignant cells. However, ovarian metastasis of Burkitt's lymphoma has been identified (3)
Ewing's sarcoma	Histology/IHC did not identify malignant cells in 7 women (74). Five of these women had their tissue evaluated with PCR and 1 was positive for Ewing's sarcoma.
Leukemia	Ovarian cortex biopsies from 27 women were evaluated with histology and 26 with histology and IHC. None revealed leukemic infiltration (75,76). qPCR were also used in the 26 cases with specific genetic markers and 16 were positive (75,76). One study xenotransplanted frozen/thawed ovarian cortex to SCID mice and found viable malignant cells in 5 of 18 grafts (75).
Miscellaneous	A patient with rhabdomyosarcoma and enlarged cystic ovaries had tumor infiltration of the tissue. Biopsies from 5 women with cervical cancer have been evaluated histological and showed no signs of ovarian involvement (69). Light microscopy showed no signs of cancer in a biopsy from the ovary of 13 women with hematological malignancies (leukemia and lymphoma), 13 with sarcoma; one woman with colon cancer and one suffering from a medulloblastoma.

be used as a source to retrieve spermatozoa for boys unable to ejaculate (100).

Since prepubertal boys cannot benefit from sperm banking and cryopreserved samples are finite resources that do not offer the possibility of restoring natural fertility, a potential alternative strategy for preserving their fertility involves cryopreservation of immature and adult testicular tissue prior to cancer treatment. Since this tissue contains spermatogonial stem cells, the patients maintain their potential to use these cells at later time points to reestablish germ cell development in cases where no spontaneous initiation of spermatogenesis occurs after the patient has been cured of the disease (101). Several protocols have been developed for cryopreservation of cell suspensions and testicular fragments from adult and cryptorchid testes using propanediol, glycerol, ethylene glycol, or DMSO (91,102–104).

Testicular Grafting and Transplantation of Germ Cells

Prepubertal testicular tissue from different species (mice, hamster, and monkey) survives freezing surprisingly well and is after xenografting able to support sperm production that can be retrieved from the tissue for assisted reproductive technique procedures (105). However, no report of successful testicular autografting in men has been published as yet.

In mice, germ cell transplantation was for the first time successfully performed in 1994, where microinjection of spermatogonia into the seminiferous tubules prompted germ cell development up to complete spermatogenesis (106). The clinical potential of the technique was shown by the infusion of germ cell suspensions into the testes of nonhuman primates and man. Ultrasound guided infusion of germ cell suspensions via the intratesticular rete testis appears to offer a simple and rather noninvasive procedure for autologous infusion of germ cells back to the patient (107). However, concerns for the clinical use of germ cell transplantation are a potentially inefficient restoration of spermatogenesis as well as the risk to transfer tumor cells leading to relapse of the oncological disease. It has been shown that as few as 20 leukemic cells injected into a testis in a rat model can induce disease relapse (108).

CONCLUSIONS

Both established and experimental therapies can now be used to allow young women and men to overcome the infertility that may result from their gonadotoxic treatment.

It is now technically feasible to take out ovarian tissue prior to cancer treatment and cryopreserve the fertility potential. After having finished cancer treatment the tissue can be transplanted back to those who entered menopause and regain function. Secretion of hormones and reestablishment of menstrual cycles and fertility will follow and although this technique is in its infancy, the method may provide real hope to these patients.

In boys and men testicular tissue can be cryopreserved with good result but strategies for transplantation still needs to be established.

FUTURE ASPECTS

IVM of early follicles to stages from which mature fertilizable oocytes could be retrieved is an option to circumvent replacing the tissue in the woman. This has been achieved in mice (109) and recently a metaphase II oocyte was retrieved from a primate follicle cultured from an early stage of development (110). However, a lot of research is still required to establish this as a possible clinical application. Another approach that could be used in leukemia patients could be isolation of the primordial follicles, with a view to replacing these isolated follicles into the remaining ovary. Indeed, different isolation techniques have been developed for human follicles (111–113), and isolated primate secondary follicles developed to the antral stage in a 3D culture system (114).

REFERENCES

1. Jemal A, Siegel R, Ward E, et al. Cancer statistics. CA Cancer J Clin 2007; 57: 43–66.
2. Practice Committee of American Society for Reproductive Medicine. Practice Committee of Society for Assisted Reproductive Technology. Ovarian tissue and oocyte cryopreservation. Fertil Steril 2008; 90: S241–6.
3. Meirow D, Hardan I, Dor J, et al. Searching for evidence of disease and malignant cell contamination in ovarian tissue stored from hematologic cancer patients. Hum Reprod 2008; 23: 1007–13.
4. Von Wolff M, Donnez J, Hovatta O, et al. Cryopreservation and autotransplantation of human ovarian tissue prior to cytotoxic therapy – a technique in its infancy but already successful in fertility preservation. Eur J Cancer 2009; 45: 1547–53.
5. Lamar CA, Decherney AH. Fertility preservation: state of the science and future research directions. Fertil Steril 2008; 91: 316–19.
6. Schmidt KT, Larsen EC, Andersen CY, Andersen AN. Risk of ovarian failure and fertility preserving methods in girls and adolescents with a malignant disease. BJOG 2010; 117: 163–74.
7. Meirow D. Reproduction post-chemotherapy in young cancer patients. Mol Cell Endocrinol 2000; 169: 123–31.
8. Meirow D, Lewis H, Nugent D, Epstein M. Subclinical depletion of primordial follicular reserve in mice treated with cyclophosphamide: clinical importance and proposed accurate investigative tool. Hum Reprod 1999; 14: 1903–7.
9. Nicholson HS, Byrne J. Fertility and pregnancy after treatment for cancer during childhood or adolescence. Cancer 1993; 71: 3392–9.
10. Wallace WHB, Thomson AB, Saran F, Kelsey TW. Predicting age of ovarian failure after radiation to a field that includes the ovaries. Int J Radiat Oncol Biol Phys 2005; 62: 738–44.
11. Lushbaugh CC, Casarett GW. The effects of gonadal irradiation in clinical radiation therapy: a review. Cancer 1976; 37: 1111–20.

12. Wo JY, Viswanathan AN. Impact of radiotherapy on fertility, pregnancy, and neonatal outcomes in female cancer patients. Int J Radiat Oncol Biol Phys 2009; 73: 1304–12.

13. Badawy A, Elnashar A, El-Ashry M, Shahat M. Gonadotropin-releasing hormone agonists for prevention of chemotherapy-induced ovarian damage: prospective randomized study. Fertil Steril 2009; 91: 694–7.

14. Pereyra Pacheco B, Me´ndez Ribas JM, Milone G, et al. Use of GnRH analogs for functional protection of the ovary and preservation of fertility during cancer treatment in adolescents: a preliminary report. Gynecol Oncol 2001; 81: 391–7.

15. Blumenfeld Z, von Wolff M. GnRH-analogues and oral contraceptives for fertility preservation in women during chemotherapy. Hum Reprod Update 2008; 14: 543–52.

16. Meistrich ML, Shetty G. Hormonal suppression for fertility preservation in males and females. Reproduction 2008; 136: 691–701.

17. Desai N, Blackmon H, Szeptycki J, Goldfarb J. Cryoloop vitrification of human day 3 cleavage-stage embryos: post-vitrification development, pregnancy outcomes and live births. Reprod Biomed Online 2007; 14: 208–13.

18. Cobo A, Bellver J, Domingo J, et al. New options in assisted reproduction technology: the Cryotop method of oocyte vitrification. Reprod Biomed Online 2008; 17: 68–72.

19. Abdelhafez FF, Desai N, Abou-Setta AM, Falcone T, Goldfarb J. Slow freezing, vitrification and ultra-rapid freezing of human embryos: a systematic review and meta-analysis. Reprod Biomed Online 2010; 2: 209–22.

20. Cobo A, Diaz C. Clinical application of oocyte vitrification: a systematic review and meta-analysis of randomized controlled trials. Fertil Steril 2011; 96: 277–85.

21. von Wolff M, Thaler CJ, Frambach T, et al. Ovarian stimulation to cryopreserve fertilized oocytes in cancer patients can be started in the luteal phase. Fertil Steril 2008; 92: 1360–5.

22. Demirtas E, Elizur SE, Holzer H, et al. SL. Immature oocyte retrieval in the luteal phase to preserve fertility in cancer patients. Reprod Biomed Online 2008; 17: 520–3.

23. Andersen CY, Rosendahl M, Byskov AG, et al. Two successful pregnancies following autotransplantation of frozen/thawed ovarian tissue. Hum Reprod 2008; 23: 2266–72.

24. Donnez J, Squiffl et J, Van Eyck AS, et al. Restoration of ovarian function in orthopically transplanted cryopreserved ovarian tissue: a pilot experience. Reprod Biomed Online 2008; 16: 694–704.

25. Oktay K, Oktem O. Ovarian cryopreservation and transplantation for fertility preservation for medical indications: report of an ongoing experience. Fertil Steril 2008; 93: 762–8.

26. Ernst E, Bergholdt S, Jorgensen JS, Andersen CA. The first woman to give birth to two children following transplantation of frozen/thawed ovarian tissue. Hum Reprod 2010; 25: 1280–1.

27. Greve T, Ernst E, Markholt S, Schmidt KT, Andersen CY. Legal termination of a pregnancy resulting from transplanted cryopreserved ovarian tissue. Acta Obstet Gynecol Scand 2010; 89: 1589–91.

28. Hovatta O. Methods for cryopreservation of human ovarian tissue. Reprod Biomed Online 2005; 10: 729–34.

29. Newton H, Fisher J, Arnold JR, et al. Permeation of human ovarian tissue with cryoprotective agents in preparation for cryopreservation. Hum Reprod 1998; 13: 376–80.

30. Donnez J, Silber S, Andersen CY, et al. Children born after autotransplantation of cryopreserved ovarian tissue. A review of 13 live births. Ann Med 2011; 43: 437–50.

31. Rosendahl M, Schmidt KT, Ernst E, et al. Cryopreservation of ovarian tissue for a decade in Denmark: a view of the technique. Reprod Biomed Online 2011; 22: 162–71.

32. Hovatta O, Silye R, Krausz T, et al. RM. Cryopreservation of human ovarian tissue using dimethylsulphoxide and propanediol-sucrose as cryoprotectants. Hum Reprod 1996; 11: 1268–72.

33. Fuller B, Paynter S. Fundamentals of cryobiology in reproductive medicine. Reprod Biomed Online 2004; 9: 680–91.

34. Schmidt KL, Ernst E, Byskov AG, Nyboe Andersen A, Andersen CY. Survival of primordial follicles following prolonged transportation of ovarian tissue prior to cryopreservation. Hum Reprod 2003; 18: 2654–9.

35. Donnez J, Dolmans MM, Demylle D, et al. Livebirth after orthotopic transplantation of cryopreserved ovarian tissue. Lancet 2004; 364: 1405–10.

36. Meirow D, Levron J, Eldar-Geva T, et al. Pregnancy after transplantation of cryopreserved ovarian tissue in a patient with ovarian failure after chemotherapy. N Engl J Med 2005; 353: 318–21.

37. Keros V, Xella S, Hultenby K, et al. Vitrification versus controlled-rate freezing in cryopreservation of human ovarian tissue. Hum Reprod 2009; 24: 1670–83.

38. Amorim CA, Curaba M, Van Langendonckt A, Dolmans MM, Donnez J. Vitrification as an alternative means of cryopreserving ovarian tissue. Reprod Biomed Online 2011; 23: 160–86.

39. Ting AY, Yeoman RR, Lawson MS, Zelinski MB. In vitro development of secondary follicles from cryopreserved rhesus macaque ovarian tissue after slow-rate freeze or vitrification. Hum Reprod 2011; 26: 2461–72.

40. Isachenko V, Isachenko E, Weiss JM, Todorov P, Kreienberg R. Cryobanking of human ovarian tissue for anti-cancer treatment: comparison of vitrification and conventional freezing. Cryo Lett 2009; 30: 449–54.

41. Oktem O, Alper E, Balaban B, et al. Vitrified human ovaries have fewer primordial follicles and produce less antimüllerian hormone than slow-frozen ovaries. Fertil Steril 2011; 30; 95: 2661–4; e1.

42. Martinez-Madrid B, Camboni A, Dolmans MM, et al. Apoptosis and ultrastructural assessment after cryopreservation of whole human ovaries with their vascular pedicle. Fertil Steril 2007; 87: 1153–65.

43. Bromer JG, Patrizio P. Fertility preservation: the rationale for cryopreservation of the whole ovary. Semin Reprod Med 2009; 27: 465–71.

44. Anderson RA, Wallace WH. Fertility preservation in girls and young women. Clin Endocrinol (Oxf) 2011; 75: 409–19.

45. Cooper GS, Thorp JM Jr. FSH levels in relation to hysterectomy and to unilateral oophorectomy. Obstet Gynecol 1999; 94: 969–72.

46. Lass A. The fertility potential of women with a single ovary. Hum Reprod Update 1999; 5: 546–50.

47. Rosendahl M, Andersen CY, Ernst E, et al. Ovarian function after removal of an entire ovary for cryopreservation of pieces of cortex prior to gonadotoxic treatment: a follow-up study. Hum Reprod 2008; 23: 2475–83.

48. Baird DT, Webb R, Campbell BK, Harkness LM, Gosden RG. Long-term ovarian function in sheep after ovariectomy and transplantation of autografts stored at -196 C. Endocrinology 1999; 140: 462–71.

49. Schmidt KT, Rosendahl M, Ernst E, et al. Autotransplantation of cryopreserved ovarian tissue in 12 women with chemotherapy-induced premature ovarian failure: the Danish experience. Fertil Steril 2011; 95: 695–701.

50. Gougeon A. Regulation of ovarian follicular development in primates: facts and hypotheses. Endocr Rev 1996; 17: 121–55.

51. Newton H, Aubard Y, Rutherford A, Sharma V, Gosden R. Low temperature storage and grafting of human ovarian tissue. Hum Reprod 1996; 7: 1487–91.

52. Newton H, Illingworth P. In-vitro growth of murine pre-antral follicles after isolation from cryopreserved ovarian tissue. Hum Reprod 2001; 16: 423–9.

53. Radford JA, Lieberman BA, Brison DR, et al. Orthotopic reimplantation of cryopreserved ovarian cortical strips after high-dose chemotherapy for Hodgkin's lymphoma. Lancet 2001; 357: 1172–5.

54. Demeestere I, Simon P, Buxant F, et al. Ovarian function and spontaneous pregnancy after combined heterotopic and orthotopic cryopreserved ovarian tissue transplantation in a patient previously treated with bone marrow transplantation: case report. Hum Reprod 2006; 21: 2010–16.

55. Meirow D, Levron J, Eldar-Geva T, et al. Monitoring the ovaries after autotransplantation of cryopreserved ovarian tissue: endocrine studies, in vitro fertilization cycles, and live birth. Fertil Steril 2007; 87: 418–22.

56. Gosden RG, Baird DT, Wade JC, Webb R. Restoration of fertility to oophorectomized sheep by ovarian autografts stored at) 196C. Hum Reprod 1994; 9: 597–603.

57. Oktay K, Economos K, Kan M, et al. Endocrine function and oocyte retrieval after autologous transplantation of ovarian cortical strips to the forearm. JAMA 2001; 12: 1490–3.

58. Schmidt KL, Andersen CY, Starup J, et al. Orthotopic autotransplantation of cryopreserved ovarian tissue to a woman cured of cancer – follicular growth, steroid production and oocyte retrieval. Reprod Biomed Online 2004; 8: 448–53.

59. Demeestere I, Simon P, Emiliani S, Delbaere A, Englert Y. Fertility preservation: successful transplantation of cryopreserved ovarian tissue in a young patient previously treated for Hodgkin's disease. Oncologist 2007; 12: 1437–42.

60. Silber SJ, DeRosa M, Pineda J, et al. A series of monozygotic twins discordant for ovarian failure: ovary transplantation (cortical versus microvascular) and cryopreservation. Hum Reprod 2008; 23: 1531–7.

61. Piver P, Amiot C, Agnani G, et al. Two pregnancies obtained after a new technique of autotransplantation of cryopreserved ovarian tissue. In: 25th Annual Meeting of ESHRE, 28 June–1 July, 2009. Amsterdam, the Netherlands: Oxford University Press. Hum Reprod 2009: i15.

62. Sánchez-Serrano M, Crespo J, Mirabet V, et al. Twins born after transplantation of ovarian cortical tissue and oocyte vitrification. Fertil Steril 2010; 93: 268. e11–13.

63. Roux C, Amiot C, Agnani G, et al. Live birth after ovarian tissue autograft in a patient with sickle cell disease treated by allogeneic bone marrow transplantation. Fertil Steril 2010; 93: 2413.e15–19.

64. Revel A, Laufer N, Ben MA, Lebovich M, Mitrani E. Micro-organ ovarian transplantation enables pregnancy: a case report. Hum Reprod 2011; 26: 1097–103.

65. Dolmans MM, Donnez J, Camboni A, et al. IVF outcome in patients with orthotopically transplanted ovarian tissue. Hum Reprod 2009; 24: 2778–87.

66. Rosendahl M, Loft A, Byskov AG, et al. Biochemical pregnancy after fertilization of an oocyte aspirated from a heterotopic autotransplant of cryopreserved ovarian tissue: case report. Hum Reprod 2006; 21: 2006–9.

67. Kyono K, Doshida M, Toya M, et al. Potential indications for ovarian autotransplantation based on the analysis of 5,571 autopsy findings of females under the age of 40 in Japan. Fertil Steril 2010; 93: 2429–30.

68. Sanchez-Serrano M, Novella-Maestre E, Rosello-Sastre E, et al. Malignant cells are not found in ovarian cortex from breast cancer patients undergoing ovarian cortex cryopreservation. Hum Reprod 2009; 24: 2238–43.

69. Kim SS, Lee WS, Chung MK, et al. Long-term ovarian function and fertility after heterotopic autotransplantation of cryobanked human ovarian tissue: 8-year experience in cancer patients. Fertil Steril 2009; 91: 2349–54.

70. Rosendahl M, Timmermans WV, Nedergaard L, et al. Cryopreservation of ovarian tissue for fertility preservation: no evidence of malignant cell contamination in ovarian tissue from patients with breast cancer. Fertil Steril 2011; 95: 2158–61.

71. Kim SS, Radford J, Harris M, et al. Ovarian tissue harvested from lymphoma patients to preserve fertility may be safe for autotransplantation. Hum Reprod 2001; 16: 2056–60.

72. Seshadri T, Gook D, Lade S, et al. Lack of evidence of disease contamination in ovarian tissue harvested for cryopreservation from patients with Hodgkin's lymphoma and analysis of factors predictive of oocyte yield. Br J Cancer 2006; 94: 1007–10.

73. Bittinger SE, Nazaretian SP, Gook DA, et al. Detection of Hodgkin lymphoma within ovarian tissue. Fertil Steril 2011; 95: 803–6.

74. Abir R, Feinmesser M, Yaniv I, et al. Occasional involvement of the ovary in Ewing sarcoma. Hum Reprod 2010; 25: 1708–12.

75. Dolmans MM, Marinescu C, Saussoy P, et al. Reimplantation of cryopreserved ovarian tissue from patients with acute lymphoblastic leukemia is potentially unsafe. Blood 2010; 116: 2908–14.

76. Rosendahl M, Andersen MT, Ralfkiaer E, et al. Evidence of residual disease in cryopreserved ovarian

cortex from female patients with leukemia. Fertil Steril 2010; 94: 2186–90.

77. Sonmezer M, Oktay K. Fertility preservation in female patients. Hum Reprod Update 2004; 10: 251–66.

78. Osborne B, Robboy SJ. Lymphomas or leukaemia presenting as ovarian tumors an analysis of 42 cases. Cancer 1983; 52: 1933–43.

79. Dolmans MM, Yuan WY, Camboni A, et al. Development of antral follicles after xenografting of isolated small human preantral follicles. Reprod Biomed Online 2008; 16: 705–11.

80. Jahnukainen K, Ehmcke J, Hou M, Schlatt S. Testicular function and fertility preservation in male cancer patients. Best Pract Res Clin Endocrinol Metab 2011; 252: 287–302.

81. Green DM, Kawashima T, Stovall M, et al. Fertility of male survivors of childhood cancer: a report from the Childhood Cancer Survivor Study. J Clin Oncol 2010; 28: 332–9.

82. Wallace WH, Anderson. RA, Irvine DS. Fertility preservation for young patients with cancer: who is at risk and what can be offered? Lancet Oncol 2005; 6: 209–18.

83. Aubier F, Flamant F, Brauner R, et al. Male gonadal function after chemotherapy for solid tumors in childhood. J Clin Oncol 1989; 7: 304–9.

84. Siimes MA, Rautonen J. Small testicles with impaired production of sperm in adult male survivors of childhood malignancies. Cancer 1990; 65: 1303–6.

85. Ridola V, Fawaz O, Aubier F, et al. Testicular function of survivors of childhood cancer: a comparative study between ifosfamide- and cyclophosphamide-based regimens. Eur J Cancer 2009; 45: 814–18.

86. Meistrich ML, Wilson G, Brown BW, da Cunha MF, Lipshultz LI. Impact of cyclophosphamide on long-term reduction in sperm count in men treated with combination chemotherapy for Ewing and soft tissue sarcomas. Cancer 1992; 70: 2703–12.

87. Rivkees SA, Crawford JD. The relationship of gonadal activity and chemotherapy-induced gonadal damage. JAMA 1988; 259: 2123–5.

88. Gurgan T, Salman C, Demirol A. Pregnancy and assisted reproduction techniques in men and women after cancer treatment. Placenta 2008; 29(Suppl B): 152–9.

89. Brauner R, Czernichow P, Cramer P, et al. Leydig-cell function in children after direct testicular irradiation for acute lymphoblastic leukemia. N Engl J Med 1983; 309: 25–8.

90. Sklar CA, Robison LL, Nesbit ME, et al. Effects of radiation on testicular function in long-term survivors of childhood acute lymphoblastic leukemia: a report from the children cancer study group. J Clin Oncol 1990; 8: 1981–7.

91. Jahnukainen K, Ehmcke J, Schlatt S. Testicular xenografts: A novel approach to study cytotoxic damage in juvenile primate testis. Cancer Res 2006; 66: 3813–18.

92. Jahnukainen K, Ehmcke J, Nurmio M, et al. Irradiation causes acute and long-term spermatogonial depletion in cultured and xenotransplanted testicular tissue from juvenile nonhuman primates. Endocrinology 2007; 148: 5541–8.

93. Rowley MJ, Leach DR, Warner GA, Heller CG. Effect of graded doses of ionizing radiation on the human testis. Radiat Res 1974; 59: 665–78.

94. Centola GM, Keller JW, Henzler M, Rubin P. Effect of low-dose testicular irradiation on sperm count and fertility in patients with testicular seminoma. J Androl 1994; 15: 608–13.

95. van Alphen MMA, van den Kant HJG, de Rooij DG. Repopulation of the seminiferous epithelium of the rhesus monkey after Xirradiation. Radiat Res 1988; 113: 487–500.

96. Anserini P, Chiodi S, Spinelli S, et al. Semen analysis following allogeneic bone marrow transplantation. Additional data for evidence-based counselling. Bone Marrow Transplant 2002; 30: 447–51.

97. Hahn EW, Feingold SM, Simpson L, Batata M. Recovery from aspermia induced by low-dose radiation in seminoma patients. Cancer 1982; 50: 337–40.

98. Kamischke A, Jurgens H, Hertle L, et al. Cryopreservation of sperm from adolescents and adults with malignancies. J Androl 2004; 25: 586–92.

99. Baukloh V. German Society for Human Reproductive Biology retrospective multicentre study on mechanical and enzymatic preparation of fresh and cryopreserved testicular biopsies. Hum Reprod 2002; 17: 1788–94.

100. Meseguer M, Garrido N, Remohi J, et al. Testicular sperm extraction (TESE) and ICSI in patients with permanent azoospermia after chemotherapy. Hum Reprod 2003; 18: 1281–5.

101. Orwig KE, Schlatt S. Cryopreservation and transplantation of spermatogonia and testicular tissue for preservation of male fertility. J Natl Cancer Inst Monogr 2005; 34: 51–6.

102. Brook PF, Radford JA, Shalet SM, et al. Isolation of germ cells from human testicular tissue for low temperature storage and autotransplantation. Fertil Steril 2001; 75: 269–74.

103. Keros V, Rosenlund B, Hultenby K, et al. Optimizing cryopreservation of human testicular tissue: Comparison of protocols with glycerol, propanediol and dimethylsulphoxide as cryoprotectants. Hum Reprod 2005; 20: 1676–87.

104. Kvist K, Thorup J, Byskov AG, et al. Cryopreservation of intact testicular tissue from boys with cryptorchidism. Hum Reprod 2006; 21: 484–91.

105. Schlatt S, Kim SS, Gosden. R. Spermatogenesis and steroidogenesis in mouse, hamster and monkey testicular tissue after cryopreservation and heterotopic grafting to castrated hosts. Reproduction 2002; 124: 339–46.

106. Brinster RL, Zimmermann JW. Spermatogenesis following male germ-cell transplantation. Proc Natl Acad Sci USA 1994; 91: 11298–302.

107. Schlatt S, Rosiepen G, Weinbauer GF, et al. Germ cell transfer into rat, bovine, monkey and human testes. Hum Reprod 1999; 14: 144–50.

108. Jahnukainen K, Hou M, Petersen C, Setchell B, Söder O. Intratesticular transplantation of testicular cells from leukemic rats causes transmission of leukemia. Cancer Res 2001; 61: 706–10.

109. Xu M, Kreeger PK, Shea LD, Woodruff TK. Tissue-engineered follicles produce live, fertile offspring. Tissue Eng 2006; 12: 2739–46.

110. Xu J, Yeoman R, Lawson M, Zelinski M, Stouffer R. Survival, growth, and maturation of primary follicles from rhesus monkeys during encapsulated three-dimensional culture. ESHRE 2011; abstract O-081.

111. Kristensen SG, Rasmussen A, Byskov AG, Andersen CY. Isolation of pre-antral follicles from human ovarian medulla tissue. Hum Reprod 2011; 26: 157–66.
112. Telfer EE, McLaughlin M, Ding C, Thong KJ. A two-step serum-free culture system supports development of human oocytes from primordial follicles in the presence of activin. Hum Reprod 2008; 23: 1151–8.
113. Dolmans MM, Michaux N, Camboni A, et al. Evaluation of Liberase, a purified enzyme blend, for the isolation of human primordial and primary ovarian follicles. Hum Reprod 2006; 21: 413–20.
114. Xu J, Bernuci MP, Lawson MS, et al. Survival, growth, and maturation of secondary follicles from prepubertal, young, and older adult rhesus monkeys during encapsulated three-dimensional culture: effects of gonadotropins and insulin. Reproduction 2010; 140: 685–97.

59

Viral disease and Assisted Reproductive Techniques

Carole Gilling-Smith

INTRODUCTION

The last decade has seen a rapid rise in the number of Assisted Reproductive Technology (ART) centers electing to treat patients with blood borne viruses such as HIV, Hepatitis B and C. This chapter sets out the considerations to be given to planning and managing a cost-effective, safe and ethically sensitive service and reviews the evidence base for the proposed therapeutic regimes.

HIV: AN OVERVIEW

Worldwide, over 30 million men, women, and children are living with HIV or AIDS, with over a million in the United States alone. In the developed world, the introduction and development of highly active antiretroviral therapy (HAART) since the mid 90s (1) has led to the redefinition of HIV as a chronic disease (2). HIV, a retrovirus, leads to progressive CD4 (+) T-lymphocyte cell depletion. HAART consists of reverse transcriptase and protease inhibitors that interrupt viral replication and slow down and halt CD4 depletion. The triggers for initiating HAART are the presence or development of AIDS-related symptoms and/or a fall in CD4 count to below a critical level (<350 cells/µl), although guidelines for initiation of treatment vary widely across different geographical regions according to resources available (3). Subsequent monitoring of response to therapy is through regular serum CD4 and viral load (VL) measurements. Disease progression from initial seroconversion to development of symptoms can be slow, with lapses of up to 15 years allowing for timely intervention. With continued improvements in HAART, projected life expectancy is currently estimated to approach that of negative controls (4). In addition to improvements in life quality and expectancy, the use of selected antiretrovirals during pregnancy and at the time of delivery, elective caesarean section where appropriate and the avoidance of breastfeeding are all measures that have collectively led to a fall in the mother to child transmission (MTCT) risk from more than 30% to less than 2% (5). From a purely ethical perspective, the radical changes seen in the natural history of the disease over the last decade have led to numerous publications debating the arguments against denying HIV-infected men and women fertility treatment (6–12). Aside from the issues of not discriminating against those with a treatable viral illness, there are strong arguments to support the benefit of ART in such couples as a means of reducing horizontal viral transmission risk and improving the chances of bearing a healthy non-infected child. The net effect has been a rise in the demand for reproductive care in HIV-infected individuals (13) and the development of more structured services targeting this group of patients.

Service planning should broadly cover three objectives; to offer risk reduction strategies such as sperm washing to minimize viral transmission risk to the uninfected partner and future child; to offer the same spectrum of fertility treatments to HIV infected as non-infected individuals; to ensure all procedures undertaken are carried out in such a way as to avoid viral transmission risk to healthcare workers and other patients attending the center.

HIV: THE RISKS OF NATURAL CONCEPTION

The merits and risks of natural conception in HIV-positive men and women as compared to ART is currently a highly controversial topic in the literature (14,15) and one which cannot be ignored by reproductive specialists in the initial counseling of patients on their reproductive options. HIV is transmitted primarily through genital secretions during vaginal (or anal) intercourse. The risks of trying to conceive through unprotected intercourse carries a transmission risk for both HIV-serodiscordant couples, where one partner only is infected as well as in seroconcordant couples, where both are infected. In practice, horizontal transmission risk is extremely difficult to quantify precisely for a heterosexual couple in a stable relationship, limiting intercourse to the fertile time of the month.

In discordant couple, where the man is HIV positive, the risk of viral transmission is quoted as 0.1–0.5% per act of intercourse, provided the couples are in a stable monogamous relationship, not abusing intravenous drugs or participating in any other form of high-risk activity (16,17). Although mathematical models cite a risk of 1 in 100,000 per act of intercourse for those with an undetectable VL (18), in practice viral shedding in semen has been reported to occur even in men fully suppressed on HAART because of different compartmentalization of HIV in plasma and semen (19–21). A review of 19 studies analyzing the association between serum VL and semen VL found a large variation in estimated correlation (coefficients of 0.07–0.60) and confirmed a significant effect of the use of HAART with optimal penetration of the genital tract to strengthen the association and significant effect of co-existing sexually transmitted infections and viral resistance to weaken the association (22).

It has been proposed by a group from Switzerland that men with negative VLs, achieved through long-term use of HAART, are sexually non-infectious (23). The main weakness of this proposal is the paucity of prospective published data examining the risks of timed unprotected intercourse in serodiscordant couples trying to conceive where the male partner has been fully suppressed on HAART. Study sizes are small, no doubt due to ethical restrictions, and span a decade when HAART was not in widespread use. Mandelbrot in 1997 reported a seroconversion rate as high as 4% in couples who were in a stable monogamous relationship and not participating in any high-risk activity (24). In a retrospective study of discordant couples attempting to conceive where the HIV-positive partner had undetectable HIV through use of HAART for at least six months, no seroconversions were noted in the 77 couples who conceived (14). However, in addition to the fact the sample size was small, this study omitted to analyze seroconversions in couples who failed to conceive. There are no improvements in safety to be gained by inseminating ejaculated semen, which has been first tested for HIV, into the vagina or uterus as the detection of HIV-RNA and -DNA in ejaculated semen is unreliable (25). Since the Swiss proposal (23), there has been an increasing trend for couples to reconsider unprotected intercourse as a means of conceiving naturally, with some additional measures such as pre-exposure prophylaxis (PrEP) in the form of Tenofovir to be given at the time of the urine LH surge and 24 hours later. The only published evidence on safety and efficacy of such an approach comprises a small series of 53 serodiscordant couples in whom the HIV-positive man had been successfully treated with HAART for over six months and had undetectable levels of HIV-RNA in the plasma (<50 copies/ml) (26). Median female age was 33 years and 244 events of unprotected intercourse took place over the study period. Pregnancy rates were reported as 26% for the first attempt rising to 66% after five attempts and 75% after 12 attempts. It is interesting to note that these couples elected to restrict their acts of unprotected intercourse to the fertile time of the cycle, despite a growing trend in Swiss couples to have regular sex without condoms, which is a reflection of the high degree of anxiety that still exists over unprotected intercourse, even in couples electing to conceive naturally.

A single case report of HIV transmission to the female partner in a serodiscordant couple where the male had undetectable serum VL through long-term use of HAART (27) highlights the need for caution and, although it is well recognized that timed unprotected intercourse may be the only option for discordant couples unable to access, or finance, risk-reduction options such as sperm washing or donor insemination, the limited data on the safety of this approach must be emphasized and discordant couples planning parenthood must be fully counseled on the

alternative ART options such as sperm washing with intra-uterine insemination (IUI) or in vitro fertilization (IVF)/intracytoplasmic injection (ICSI) or donor sperm insemination to enable them to make an informed choice.

The risk of viral transmission through unprotected intercourse is significantly lower in serodiscordant couples where the woman is HIV positive. ART is not necessary in such couples, unless fertility issues exist, as conception can be achieved safely by collecting sperm in a condom (which is free of spermicidals) after intercourse and inseminating this into the woman's vagina using a syringe and, if preferred, a quill (18,28). This process of self-insemination should be discussed fully with the couple and advice given on how to identify the fertile period in a woman's cycle, using home urinary ovulation detection kits if necessary.

Couples who are both HIV positive can elect to conceive either through timed unprotected intercourse or through self-insemination but face the dilemma of superinfection. This is defined as reinfection with a second strain of HIV after the first infection has been established through seroconversion. The true risk is unquantifiable but documented to be very low in patients who are chronically infected with HIV (18). The risk of superinfection also depends on whether the man and woman are infected with the same HIV strain and whether or not either or both are on HAART. All seroconcordant couples should be counseled on the risk of superinfection by their HIV physician and sperm washing considered as a means of eliminating this risk wherever possible.

REPRODUCTIVE OPTIONS FOR SERODISCORDANT COUPLES WHERE THE MAN IS HIV POSITIVE

The therapeutic options if natural intercourse is to be avoided are:

1. Insemination using donor sperm: Donor sperm removes the risk of viral transmission, as sperm donors are screened for HIV and other blood–borne viruses, and the option of genetic parenting from the infected male.
2. Sperm washing: In this process, the female partner is treated with the infected partner's sperm, centrifuged first to separate spermatozoa from seminal fluid and associated non-sperm cells.
3. Adoption: This option is rarely chosen but available to couples who feel unable to use the above ART measures or consider natural conception.

SPERM WASHING

Sperm washing, pioneered and first proposed in 1992 by an Italian gynecologist in Milan (29), involves centrifugation of semen on a density gradient to separate live spermatozoa, which do not carry HIV, from seminal plasma and non-germinal cells which may carry virus followed by a swim-up. The processed sperm can then be used in ART. The technique rests on the observation that HIV is present in seminal fluid and as cell associated virus in

Table 59.1   Results of Assisted Reproduction Attempts in 1036 Couples Undergoing Sperm Washing in Europe According to Different Procedures Used

Procedures	IUI	IVF	ICSI	FET	Total	P[d]
Couples	853	76	262	40	1231[a]	–
Cycles	2840	107	394	49	3390	–
Pregnancy per cycle (%)[b]	15.1	29.0	30.6	20.4	17.5	<0.001
Multiple pregnancy rate (%)	4.9	17.2	20.8	20.0	9.12	<0.01
Delivery per cycle (%)[c]	11.5	20.8	15.8	14.3	12.3	<0.05
Pregnancy per couple (%)	42.7	38.2	43.1	25.0	41.9	>0.05
Delivery per couple (%)	35.1	26.3	21.0	17.5	30.9	<0.01

[a]The total was over 1036 couples as a couple could have different assisted reproduction procedures (e.g., four IUI + two IVF).
[b]Missing information in 66 IUI and seven IVF cycles.
[c]Missing information in 91 IUI, 11 IVF, and 40 ICSI cycles.
[d]*P*-value for comparison between procedure groups.
Abbreviations: FET, frozen embryo transfer; ICSI, intra cytoplasmic sperm injection; IUI, intrauterine insemination; IVF, in vitro fertilization.
Source: From Ref. 44.

leucocytes and non-spermatozoa cells (NSCs) but is not capable of attaching to, or infecting, spermatozoa. This is well supported by the literature on the subject, which is extensive (30–35).

As a laboratory process, sperm washing involves centrifugation of freshly ejaculated semen in a 40–80% colloidal, silica density gradient to separate progressively motile HIV-free sperm from NSC and seminal plasma which remain in the supernatant. The sperm pellet is resuspended in fresh medium. Subsequent processing varies between centers. Early published studies adopted the most cautious approach of washing the sample at least twice before final swim-up but this can lead to a substantial loss of viable sperm without necessarily conferring any added benefit in terms of safety (36). As a quality control for the procedure, and to protect the service from medicolegal action, it is recommended that an aliquot of washed sperm (~100 μl) should be tested for detectable HIV-RNA prior to the sample being used for treatment (37,38). A nucleic acid–based sequence amplification (NASBA, Biomerieux, Basingstoke, Hampshire, UK) or similar commercial assay can be used (39). The risk of the sample having detectable HIV has been reported to be as high as 3–6% (28,40,41). This risk exists even in the presence of an undetectable serum VL since in a small proportion of cases, centrifugation fails to remove all the seminal plasma and leucocytes. The number of washes should be limited as repeated centrifuging leads to loss of sperm quality and quantity. A modified approach of two washes with a swim-up only performed if the patient is not on HAART or if the sample prepares with significant debris such as white cells allows the post-wash sperm yield to be maximized with no increase in residual virus (36).

There have been no reported cases of infection of the female partner when sperm washing is carried out following published protocols in over 5000 published cycles of sperm washing combined with IUI, IVF, or ICSI (29,40,41, 42–46). ART outcome is reported to compare favorably to that in non-infected patients. The most relevant publication analyzing safety and efficacy of sperm washing as a

treatment was produced by the collaborative group "CREAThE" (Centres for REproductive Assisted Techniques for HIV in Europe). The study analysed 1036 serodiscordant couples from eight European Centers undergoing 3315 cycles of sperm washing with either IUI, IVF, or ICSI being performed according to fertility issues with a six-month post-treatment follow-up of the female partner with HIV testing (44). No seroconversions were reported and pregnancy rates in each category of treatment were comparable to those previously reported for HIV-negative patients (Table 59.1)

SPERM WASHING TREATMENT: CLINICAL PROTOCOLS

Patients should receive pre-conceptual counseling, both together and individually before embarking on treatment (37). Counseling should cover the nature and risks of sperm washing, the impact of possible treatment failure, the psychosocial issues of coping with a child when one parent is HIV positive, and the possibility of single parenting in the future if the infected partner were to die. The couples need to understand that sperm washing is a risk-reduction method and not a risk-free method as technically, the virus could still be present in the washed sample at a titer below the detection limit of the HIV assay. In order that couples make an informed decision about treatment, pre-conceptual counseling should include an open discussion about the risks of unprotected intercourse.

Clinical work-up prior to sperm washing should include a full medical and social history as well as a sexual health screen and fertility screen in both partners. The sexual health will ensure that the viral status of both partners is known at the time of treatment and that any genital lesions or infections are identified and treated before any fertility treatment is envisaged as these can increase the risk of viral transmission (28,47) and reduce pregnancy rates. The purpose of the fertility screen is to identify any co-existing fertility issues and thus define the optimum mode of treatment. It is recommended that the male partner has a semen analysis, and the female partner has an endocrine profile (follicle-stimulating hormone, luteinizing hormone, estradiol, and anti-Müllerian hormone) and baseline pelvic scan, to include an antral follicle count, in the early follicular phase of her cycle (day 2–4) together with a mid-luteal progesterone to confirm ovulation. A minimally invasive test of tubal patency is also advisable (e.g., hysterosalpingogram), unless there is a history of pelvic pain or infection in which case a laparoscopy is preferable to assess tubal patency (37).

Most couples electing to have sperm washing are voluntarily infertile and do not have significant fertility issues. In Europe, such couples would be initially offered IUI in a natural cycle using washed sperm. This is in contrast to Northern America where ICSI using washed sperm would be recommended as first line management (48). The major factor that has driven U.S. practice toward ICSI as a first line treatment modality, regardless of seminal or female factors, is the 1990 CDC recommendation against insemination of sperm from an HIV-positive man (49). This stems from a single reported case of HIV transmission to the female partner of an HIV-infected man after IUI of processed sperm. The sperm washing process in this case would not meet current standards of practice as it did not include a density gradient step or a post-wash viral test. A recent, 10-year review of sperm washing treatment by Sauer et al. from Colombia University, New York, reported that ICSI with sperm washing was exclusively utilized for fresh cycles without post-wash viral testing (45). The authors argued that ICSI in serodiscordant couples is best practice since it minimizes oocyte contact with seminal plasma and cells by exposing only a single sperm to each oocyte. The argument against post-wash testing is the inability to characterize the cells chosen for ICSI and a lack of evidence of HIV detection in previous swim-up samples used for ICSI (45). The counter-argument proposed by European centers is that ICSI is unnecessary based on scientific grounds of safety and has unnecessary cost implications, poses risks to the mother as a result of ovarian stimulation, and risks to the offspring in cases where multiple pregnancies are generated as well as having the potential for increased de-novo chromosomal abnormalities (50).

The inclusion of a swim-up or not is likely to continue to be debated but best practice in all scientific processes dictates a quality control step to ensure that the inseminated sample is free of detectable HIV. A recent analysis of 186 seminal samples from men with undetectable VL on long-term HAART identified that 18 (9.7%) had demonstrable virus (370–18,000 copies/ml) reinforcing the benefit of post-wash testing as well as the value of sperm washing in even the healthiest cohort of HIV-positive men (48). The various viral testing assays continue to undergo strict quality control monitoring (51) and efforts are being made to standardize assays and assay protocols between units.

In contrast to the policy in Northern America, the Dutch consensus of embryologists, virologists, and gynecologists has been not to perform ICSI in HIV-positive men because of the theoretical danger of producing a new endogenous retrovirus in the human genome and possible infection of the embryo as a consequence of injecting a single sperm potentially carrying an HIV-particle directly into the oocyte (52). There is little scientific support for such a policy which in practice excluded 33% of HIV-positive men in the Netherlands who had insufficient semen quality for an IUI procedure.

The recommended approach to treatment based on the evidence reviewed above is to offer IUI in a natural cycle as the first line treatment, unless the woman is anovulatory, where clomiphene or injectable gonadotropins should be used to induce ovulation. Ultrasound follicular tracking is advisable to time insemination accurately and, where possible, human chorionic gonadotropins administered to ensure the timing of ovulation is known precisely. Between three and six cycles of IUI should be undertaken before a couple is offered assisted conception with either superovulation and IUI or IVF. If there is evidence of tubal blockage, the couple should be advised to have IVF with washed sperm and if the semen analysis is poor then ICSI should be performed. There are reports of successful pregnancy outcome with sperm washing in HIV-positive azoospermic men where testicular sperm retrieval has been performed (53,54). However, the limitations to this approach are the quantity and quality of sperm available for washing and subsequent HIV-RNA testing.

Effect of HIV on Semen Parameters and Sperm Washing IUI Outcome

The majority of HIV-positive men have semen parameters within the defined WHO normal range. However, in the two largest studies to date of semen parameters in HIV-positive men, Nicopoullos et al. (55,56) consistently found all parameters to be significantly impaired compared to HIV-negative controls, with a significant negative correlation between CD4 count as a marker of HIV infection and immune status on sperm count, motility, and morphology. There was a significant decrease in volume, count, motility, morphology, and post-wash parameters when CD4 counts dropped below median levels (450 cells/mm^3) but had no effect of VL on any sperm parameter. This contrasts to earlier studies (57,58) that found VL to correlate with sperm motility and morphology.

Although early studies suggested that HIV parameters such as VL, CD4 count, and use of HAART were predictors of cycle outcome (55), re-analysis of a decade of treatment in the United Kingdom found seminal parameters to be the most important predictors of success in sperm washing with IUI (59). Currently there are insufficient data to recommend starting HAART purely to improve seminal parameters and IUI success rates with sperm washing and the decision to start medication should be primarily based on the health of the individual and established parameters such as CD4 counts.

Assisted Conception in the HIV-Positive Female

HIV-positive women need to address a number of issues when planning to conceive. The HIV physician is best placed to provide pre-conceptual advice on HAART, self-insemination methods, and measures that will need to be put in place during pregnancy to reduce MTCT risk, as well as advising on any long-term health issues related to viral illness, which might be a contraindication to pregnancy. Relatively few antiretroviral medications (e.g., Efavirenz) are contraindicated during pregnancy due to potential teratogenic effects on the fetus (5) but it should be borne in mind that the evidence on the safety of most antiretrovirals during pregnancy is still incomplete. Folic acid should be given antenatally to minimize the risk of neural tube defects as antiretrovirals are known to have a folate antagonist effect.

There is increasing evidence to suggest that HIV-positive women have reduced fertility (13,60). There are no data to suggest an increased incidence of cycle irregularity in positive women, but studies on positive women undergoing IVF suggest that HIV-positive women have lower IVF success rates than HIV-negative controls and require higher doses of gonadotropin stimulation (61–63). IVF outcome does not appear to be affected in HIV-positive women undergoing ovum donation, pointing toward an effect of HIV and/or immunosuppression on ovarian response and ovarian reserve rather than on implantation (64). Retrospective data from Sub-Saharan Africa (65,66) and prospective data from the United Kingdom indicate an increased incidence of tubal infertility in positive women (13,62) of at least twice that of HIV-negative controls. On the basis of increased risk of low ovarian reserve and increased tubal infertility, HIV-positive women trying to conceive should be referred sooner rather than later for fertility evaluation and certainly if they have not conceived within six to 12 months of self-insemination. Referral should be early if there is a history of pelvic inflammatory disease or in women over 35 years of age to assess tubal function and ovarian reserve.

Reducing Risk During ART in Positive Women

Minimizing risk in HIV-positive women lies primarily in reducing MTCT. There are no additional specific measures that can be taken during fertility treatment to further reduce this risk. There has been concern that invasive procedures such as IVF could increase the chances of the embryo becoming infected. The number of women treated so far is small and prospective data limited. A study of 10 women undergoing IVF or ICSI demonstrated that HIV was detectable in follicular fluid removed during vaginal egg collection in all patients with a detectable serum VL and in 60% of those with an undetectable serum VL (67). This raises the theoretical possibility of the embryo becoming infected at the laboratory stage of ART even before embryo transfer, although the likelihood is that viral infection would lead to embryo death. Longitudinal studies are needed to monitor outcome of ART cycles in positive women to identify if any such risk increases the chance of MTCT.

Management of HIV-positive women should involve a multidisciplinary team comprising HIV physician, fertility specialist, and obstetrician with a special interest in HIV. The couple should have a sexual health screen for the same reasons as couples undergoing sperm washing. Likewise they should have a fertility screen in a similar way to HIV-negative couples (early follicular phase endocrine profile and pelvic scan, mid-luteal progesterone, and test of tubal function) and the male partner should have a semen analysis (37). Couples concordant for HIV should be advised to conceive using sperm washing to prevent the risk of superinfection.

MANAGING PATIENTS WITH HEPATITIS

Hepatitis B (HBV) and Hepatitis C (HCV) viruses are major causes of chronic hepatitis, cirrhosis, and hepatocellular cancer. In cases where fertility treatment is required and one or both partners are HBV or HCV positive, samples should be treated as infectious and handled according to clinical and laboratory guidelines set out below.

In the case of hepatitis B, vertical transmission accounts for over 40% of cases of chronic infection and the sexual transmission risk is twofold higher than for HIV and sixfold higher than for HCV. Unlike HIV or HCV, an effective vaccine is available for HBV and all healthcare workers and partners of known infected individuals should be vaccinated. Uninfected women should only consider conception post-vaccination. Sperm washing should not be required as a means of reducing horizontal transmission risk unless a woman fails to develop adequate immunity through vaccination. If ART is required in HBV positive couples for fertility issues, similar clinical protocols to non-infected patients should be used. The Dutch view, as with HIV samples, is that if ART is required in a couple where the male is HBV positive, ICSI should be avoided due to the risk of introducing HBV into the oocyte (68). There are no substantive data to support this view.

Vertical transmission risk for an HBV positive woman during pregnancy is 2–15% if she is only HBsAg-positive, and 80–90% if she is also positive for HBeAg or is HBV DNA positive. Infection in the neonate can be minimized if immunoprophylaxis (HBV vaccination and one dose of Hepatitis B immunoglobulins) is given within 24 hours of birth with a further dose at one and six months. Breastfeeding does not appear to play a role in perinatal transmission (37).

HCV infection is primarily transmitted by parenteral spread (blood products, shared needles, needlestick injury). Sexual transmission risk is very low unless the patient is co-infected with HIV (69). There is no vaccine for HCV and sperm washing should be offered to HCV-discordant couples where the male is infected. The principles of treatment are the same as in HIV-infected discordant couples (70,71) and sperm washing is as effective in reducing transmission risk to the female partner as in discordant cases of HIV.

HCV-RNA positive men and women should be offered antiretroviral treatment prior to planning conception with the aim of clearing the virus. This is normally a decision taken in conjunction with their hepatologist and must take into consideration the risks of delaying conception (conception is contraindicated during treatment and for at least six months post-treatment) against the benefits of reducing viral transmission risks during conception and pregnancy and improving the health of the individual. Vertical transmission risk in HCV-RNA positive women can be as high as 11% and increases to 16% if there is coinfection with HIV but for HCV-RNA negative individuals, vertical transmission risk is <1% (72). In the absence of a vaccine, there are no specific measures available to protect the neonate and the administration of immunoglobulin offers little protection. There are no data to suggest HCV is transmitted during breastfeeding.

Data regarding ART outcome in patients infected with HBV or HCV are inconclusive as numbers studied are still small. Earlier studies suggested reduced ovarian response, implantation, and pregnancy rates (73,74) but a more recent study on HBV patients suggested improved outcome compared to non-infected controls (75).

REDUCING TRANSMISSION RISK IN THE ART CENTER

Handling and freezing gametes and embryos from patients who carry blood–borne viruses increases the potential risk of cross contamination to samples from viral-negative patients and health workers involved in assisted reproduction (76,77), although a recent study would suggest this risk to be very low (78). Universal precautions should be employed at all times and it is advisable that samples from patients with known or suspected blood–borne viruses are handled in a separate laboratory or laboratory area with equipment (e.g., incubators, flow hoods, and cryostorage tanks) dedicated to handling infected samples (76). It is also recommended that gametes and embryos from patients with known viral infections are cryopreserved in separate heat-sealed straws (79) and cryostorage tanks due to the possible risk of transmission in liquid nitrogen (80,81). It has been suggested that vapor phase storage would offer more security against the risk of cross-contamination as compared to liquid nitrogen, without affecting embryo and sperm survival (82), but there are no long-term data to assess safety and efficacy of this approach.

In the United Kingdom and most ART centers in Europe and North America, all patients planning to undergo assisted conception are required to be screened for HIV, hepatitis B, and hepatitis C. This has the benefit of identifying high-risk patients from the outset so that the risk reduction strategies discussed in this chapter can be implemented (76,83).

REFERENCES

1. Hogg RS, Heath KV, Yip B, et al. Improved survival among HIV-infected individuals following initiation of antiretroviral therapy. JAMA 1998; 279: 450–4.
2. Scandlyn J. When AIDS became a chronic disease. West J Med 2000; 172: 130–3.
3. Siegfried N, Uthman OA, Rutherford GW. Optimal time for initiation of antiretroviral therapy in asymptomatic, HIV-infected, treatment-naive adults. Cochrane Database Syst Rev 2010: CD008272.
4. Collaboration TATC. Life expectancy of individuals on combination antiretroviral therapy in high-income countries: a collaborative analysis of 14 cohort studies. Lancet 2008; 372: 293–9.
5. de Ruiter A, Mercey D, Anderson J, et al. British HIV Association and Children's HIV Association guidelines for the management of HIV infection in pregnant women 2008. HIV Med 2008; 9: 452–502.
6. Gilling-Smith C, Smith JR, Semprini AE, et al. HIV and infertility: time to treat. There's no justification for denying treatment to parents who are HIV positive ART in HIV-infected couples: has the time come for a change of attitude? BMJ 2001; 322: 566–7.
7. Ethics Committee of the American Society for Reproductive Medicine. Human immunodeficiency virus and infertility treatment. Fertil Steril 2002; 77: 218–22.
8. Minkoff H, Santoro N. Ethical considerations in the treatment of infertility in women with human immunodeficiency virus infection. N Engl J Med 2000; 342: 1748–50.
9. Lyerly AD, Anderson J. Human immunodeficiency virus and assisted reproduction: reconsidering evidence, reframing ethics. Fertil Steril 2001; 75: 843–58.
10. Ethics Committee of the American Society for Reproductive Medicine. Human immunodeficiency virus and infertility treatment. Fertil Steril 2010; 94: 11–15.
11. Sauer MV. Providing fertility care to those with HIV: time to re-examine healthcare policy. AJOB 2003; 3: 33–40.
12. Gilling-Smith C. Risking parenthood? Serious viral illness, parenting and welfare of the child. In: Shenfield F, Sureau C, eds. Ethical Dilemmas in Assisted Reproduction. Parthenon Publishing Group, Carnforth, 2006: 57–69.
13. Frodsham LCG BF, Barton S, Gilling-Smith C. Human immunodeficiency virus infection and fertility care in the United Kingdom – demand and supply. Fertil Steril 2006; 85: 285–9.
14. Barreiro P, Castilla JA, Labarga P, Soriano V. Is natural conception a valid option for HIV-serodiscordant couples? Hum Reprod 2007; 22: 2353–8.
15. Matthews LT, Baeten JM, Celum C, Bangsberg DR. Periconception pre-exposure prophylaxis to prevent HIV transmission: benefits, risks, and challenges to implementation. AIDS 2010; 24: 1975–82.
16. Gray RH, Wawer MJ, Brookmeyer R, et al. Probability of HIV-1 transmission per coital act in monogamous, heterosexual, HIV-1 serodiscordant couples in Rakai, Uganda. Lancet 2003; 357: 1149–53.
17. De Vincenzi I. A longitudinal study of human immunodeficiency virus transmission by heterosexual partners. N Engl J Med 1994; 331: 341–6.
18. Fakoya A, Lamba H, Mackie N, et al. British HIV Association, BASHH and FSRH guidelines for the management of the sexual and reproductive health of people living with HIV infection 2008. HIV Med 2008; 9: 681–720.
19. Luizzi G, Chirianni A, Clement M, et al. Analysis of HIV-1 load in blood, semen and saliva: evidence for different viral compartments in a cross-sectional and longitudinal study. AIDS 1996; 10: F51–6.

20. Coombs RW, Speck CE, Hughes JP, et al. Association between culturable human immunodeficiency virus type 1 (HIV-1) in semen and HIV-1 RNA levels in semen and blood: evidence for compartmentalisation of HIV-1 between semen and blood. J Infect Dis 1998; 177: 320–30.

21. Zhang H, Domadula G, Beumont M, et al. Human immunodeficiency virus type 1 in the semen of men receiving highly active antiretroviral therapy. N Engl J Med 1998; 339: 1803–9.

22. Kalichman SC, Di Berto G, Eaton L. Human immunodeficiency virus viral load in blood plasma and semen: review and implications of empirical findings. Sex Transm Dis 2008; 35: 55–60.

23. Vernazza P, Hirshel B, Bernasconi E, Flepp M. Les personnes séropositives ne souffrant d'aucune autre MST et suivant un traitement antirétroviral efficace ne transmettent pas le VIH par voie sexuelle. Bull Des Médecins Suisses 2008; 89: 165–9.

24. Mandelbrot L, Heard I, Henrion-Geant R, Henrion R. Natural conception in HIV-negative women with HIV-infected partners. Lancet 1997; 349: 850–1.

25. Dunne AL, Mitchell F, Allen KM, et al. Analysis of HIV-1 viral load in seminal plasma samples. J Clin Virol 2003; 26: 239–45.

26. Vernazza PL, Graf I, Sonnenberg-Schwan U, Geit M, Meurer A. Preexposure prophylaxis and timed intercourse for HIV-discordant couples willing to conceive a child. AIDS 2011; 25: 2005–8.

27. Sturmer M, Doerr H, Berger A, Gute P. Is transmission of HIV-1 in non-viraemic serodiscordant couples possible? Antivir Ther 2008; 13: 729–32.

28. Gilling-Smith C, Nicopoullos JDM, Semprini AE, Frodsham LC. HIV and reproductive care – a review of current practice. BJOG 2006; 113: 869–78.

29. Semprini AE, Levi-Setti P, Bozzo M, et al. Insemination of HIV-negative women with processed semen of HIV-positive partners. Lancet 1992; 340: 1317–19.

30. Bagasra O, Farzadegan H, Seshamma T, et al. Detection of HIV-1 proviral DNA in sperm from HIV-1 infected men. AIDS 1994; 8: 1669–74.

31. Vernazza PL, Gilliam BL, Dyer J, et al. Quantification of HIV in semen: correlation with antiviral treatment and immune status. AIDS 1997; 11: 987–93.

32. Quayle AJ, Xu C, Mayer KH, Anderson DJ. T lymphocytes and macrophages, but not motile spermatozoa, are a significant source of human immunodeficiency virus in semen. J Infect Dis 1997; 176: 960–8.

33. Quayle AJ, Xu C, Tucker L, Anderson DJ. The case against an association between HIV-1 and sperm: molecular evidence. J Reprod Immunol 1998; 41: 127–36.

34. Kim LU, Johnson MR, Barton S, et al. Evaluation of sperm washing as a potential method of reducing HIV transmission in HIV-discordant couples wishing to have children. AIDS 1999; 13: 645–51.

35. Baccetti B, Benedetto A, Burrini AG, et al. HIV particles detected in spermatozoa of patients with AIDS. J Submicrosc Cytol Pathol 1991; 23: 339–45.

36. Vourliotis M, Nicopoullos JDM, Gilling-Smith C, et al. A comparison of sperm yield following changes in HIV sperm washing laboratory practice. Hum Reprod 2009; 24(Suppl 1): i166.

37. Gilling-Smith C, Almeida P. HIV, hepatitis B and hepatitis C and infertility: reducing risk. Hum Fertil (Camb) 2003; 6: 106–12.

38. Semprini AE, Fiore S. HIV and reproduction. Curr Opin Obstet Gynecol 2004; 16: 257–62.

39. Burgisser P, Vernazza P, Flepp M, et al. Swiss Cohort Study: Performances of five different assays for the quantification of viral load in persons infected with various subtypes of HIV-1. J Aquir Immun Def Synd 2000; 23: 138–44.

40. Marina S, Marina F, Alcolea R, et al. Pregnancy following intracytoplasmic sperm injection from an HIV-1 seropositive man. Hum Reprod 1998; 13: 3247–9.

41. Marina S, Marina F, Alcolea A, et al. Human immunodeficiency virus type I-serodiscordant couples can bear healthy children after undergoing intrauterine insemination. Fertil Steril 1998; 70: 35–9.

42. Ohl JP, Partisani M, Wittemer C, et al. Assisted reproduction techniques for HIV serodiscordant couples: 18 months of experience. Hum Reprod 2003; 18: 1244–9.

43. Garrido N, Meseguer M, Simon C, Pellicer A, Remohi J. Assisted reproduction in HIV and HCV infected men of serodiscordant couples. Arch Androl 2004; 50: 105–11.

44. Bujan L, Hollander L, Coudert M, et al. Safety and efficacy of sperm washing in HIV-1-serodiscordant couples where the male is infected: results from the European CREAThE network. AIDS 2007; 21: 1909–14.

45. Sauer MV, Wang JG, Douglas NC, et al. Providing fertility care to men seropositive for human immunodeficiency virus: reviewing 10 years of experience and 420 consecutive cycles of in vitro fertilization and intracytoplasmic sperm injection. Fertil Steril 2009; 91: 2455–60.

46. Nicopoullos JD, Almeida P, Vourliotis M, Goulding R, Gilling-Smith C. A decade of sperm washing: clinical correlates of successful insemination outcome. Hum Reprod 2010; 25: 1869–76.

47. Fleming DT, Wasserheit JN. From epidemiological synergy to public health policy and practice: the contribution of other sexually transmitted diseases to sexual transmission of HIV infection. Sex Transm Infect 1999; 75: 3–17.

48. Nicopoullos JD, Almeida P, Vourliotis M, Gilling-Smith C. A decade of the United Kingdom sperm-washing program: untangling the transatlantic divide. Fertil Steril 2010; 94: 2458–61.

49. CDC. Center for Disease Control and Prevention: HIV-1 infection and artificial insemination with processed semen. MMWR 1990; 249: 55–6.

50. Bujan L, Gilling-Smith C, Hollander L, Semprini EA, Vernazza P. Lack of clinical and scientific evidence to justify the systematic use of ICSI in HIV-serodiscordant couples wishing to conceive where the male partner is infected. Fertil Steril 2009; 91: e1–2.

51. Pasquier C, Anderson D, Andreutti-Zaugg C, et al. Multicenter quality control of the detection of HIV-1 genome in semen before medically assisted procreation. J Med Virol 2006; 78: 877–82.

52. van Leeuwen E, Prins JM, Jurriaans S, et al. Reproduction and fertility in human immunodeficiency virus type-1 infection. Hum Reprod Update 2007; 13: 197–206.

53. Nicopoullos JD, Frodsham LC, Ramsay JW, et al. Synchronous sperm retrieval and sperm washing in an intracytoplasmic sperm injection cycle in an azoospermic man who was positive for human immunodeficiency virus. Fertil Steril 2004; 81: 670–4.

54. Bujan L, Daudin M, Moinard N, et al. Azoospermic HIV-1 infected patients wishing to have children: proposed strategy to reduce HIV-1 transmission risk during

sperm retrieval and intracytoplasmic sperm injection: Case Report. Hum Reprod 2007; 22: 2377–81.

55. Nicopoullos JD, Almeida PA, Ramsay JW, Gilling-Smith C. The effect of human immunodeficiency virus on sperm parameters and the outcome of intrauterine insemination following sperm washing. Hum Reprod 2004; 19: 2289–97.

56. Nicopoullos JD, Almeida P, Vourliotis M, Gilling-Smith C. A decade of the sperm-washing programme: correlation between markers of HIV and seminal parameters. HIV Med 2011; 12: 195–201.

57. Dulioust E, Du AL, Costagliola D, et al. Semen alterations in HIV-1 infected men. Hum Reprod 2002; 17: 2112–18.

58. Bujan L, Sergerie M, Moinard N, et al. Decreased semen volume and spermatozoa motility in HIV-1-infected patients under antiretroviral treatment. J Androl 2007; 28: 444–52.

59. Nicopoullos JDM, Vourliotis M, Wood R, Almeida P, Gilling-Smith C. A decade of the UK sperm-washing program: outcome, predictors of pregnancy and the way forward? Hum Reprod 2009; 24: 318.

60. Coll O, Lopez M, Vidal R, et al. Fertility assessment in non-infertile HIV-infected women and their partners. Reprod Biomed Online 2007; 14: 488–94.

61. Coll O, Fiore S, Floridia M, et al. Pregnancy and HIV infection: A European consensus on management. AIDS 2002; 16(Suppl 2): S1–S18.

62. Coll O, Lopez M, Hernandez S. Fertility choices and management for HIV-positive women. Currt Opin HIV AIDS 2008; 3: 186–92.

63. Martinet V, Manigart Y, Rozenberg S, et al. Ovarian response to stimulation of HIV-positive patients during IVF treatment: a matched, controlled study. Hum Reprod 2006; 21: 1212–17.

64. Coll O, Suy A, Figueras F, et al. Decreased pregnancy rate after in-vitro fertilization in HIV-infected women receiving HAART. AIDS 2006; 20: 121–3.

65. Brunham RC, Cheang M, McMaster J, Garnett G, Anderson R. Chlamydia trachomatis, infertility, and population growth in sub-Saharan Africa. Sex Transm Dis 1993; 20: 168–73.

66. Brunham RC, Garnett GP, Swinton J, Anderson RM. Gonococcal infection and human fertility in sub-Saharan Africa. Proc Biol Sci 1991; 246: 173–7.

67. Frodsham LCG, Cox AD, Almeida PA, Rozis G, Gilling-Smith C. In vitro fertilisation in HIV positive women: risk of mother to embryo viral transmission. Hum Reprod 2004; 9(Suppl 1): 138.

68. Lutgens SP, Nelissen EC, van Loo IH, et al. To do or not to do: IVF and ICSI in chronic hepatitis B virus carriers. Hum Reprod 2009; 24: 2676–8.

69. MacDonald M, Crofts N, Kaldor J. Transmission of hepatitis C virus: rates, routes, and cofactors. Epidemiol Rev 1996; 18: 137–48.

70. Pasquier C, Daudin M, Righi L, et al. Sperm washing and virus nucleic acid detection to reduce HIV and hepatitis C virus transmission in serodiscordant couples wishing to have children. AIDS 2000; 14: 2093–9.

71. Halfon P, Giorgetti C, Bourliere M, et al. Medically assisted procreation and transmission of hepatitis C virus: absence of HCV RNA in purified sperm fraction in HIV co-infected patients. AIDS 2006; 20: 241–6.

72. Steyaert SR, Leroux-Roels GG, Dhont M. Infections in IVF: review and guidelines. Hum Reprod Update 2000; 6: 432–41.

73. Pirwany IR, Phillips S, Kelly S, Buckett W, Tan SL. Reproductive performance of couples discordant for hepatitis B and C following IVF treatment. J Assist Reprod Genet 2004; 21: 157–61.

74. Englert Y, Moens E, Vannin AS, et al. Impaired ovarian stimulation during in vitro fertilization in women who are seropositive for hepatitis C virus and seronegative for human immunodeficiency virus. Fertil Steril 2007; 88: 607–11.

75. Lam PM, Suen SH, Lao TT, et al. Hepatitis B infection and outcomes of in vitro fertilization and embryo transfer treatment. Fertil Steril 2010; 93: 480–5.

76. Gilling-Smith C, Emiliani S, Almeida P, Liesnard C, Englert Y. Laboratory safety during assisted reproduction in patients with blood-borne viruses. Hum Reprod 2005; 20: 1433–8.

77. Lesourd F, Izopet J, Mervan C, et al. Transmissions of hepatitis C virus during the ancillary procedures for assisted conception. Hum Reprod 2000; 15: 1083–5.

78. Cobo A, Bellver J, de Los Santos MJ, Remohi J. Viral screening of spent culture media and liquid nitrogen samples of oocytes and embryos from hepatitis B, hepatitis C, and human immunodeficiency virus chronically infected women undergoing in vitro fertilization cycles. Fertil Steril 2011; 97: 74–8.

79. Benifla JL, Letur-Konirsch H, Collin G, et al. Safety of cryopreservation straws for human gametes or embryos: a preliminary study with human immunodeficiency virus-1. Human Reprod 2000; 15: 2186–9.

80. Tedder RS, Zuckerman MA, Goldstone AH, et al. Hepatitis B transmission from contaminated cryopreservation tank. Lancet 1995; 346: 137–40.

81. Clarke GN. Sperm cryopreservation: is there a significant risk of cross-contamination? Human Reprod 1999; 14: 2941–3.

82. Tomlinson M, Sakkas D. Is a review of standard procedures for cryopreservation needed? Safe and effective cryopreservation-should sperm banks and fertility centres move toward storage in nitrogen vapour? Hum Reprod 2000; 15: 2460–3.

83. Practice Committee of American Society for Reproductive Medicine. Guidelines for reducing the risk of viral transmission during fertility treatment. Fertil Steril 2008; 90(Suppl 5): S156–62.

60

Severe ovarian hyperstimulation syndrome

Zalman Levine, Inna Berin, and Daniel Navot

INTRODUCTION

Ovarian hyperstimulation syndrome (OHSS) is the gravest complication of so-called controlled (far too often uncontrolled) ovarian hyperstimulation (COH) (1). From a perspective of priorities in reproductive medicine in general and assisted reproductive techniques (ARTs) in particular, OHSS is second only to high-order multiple births on the list of adverse outcomes that need to be minimized or completely eliminated.

OHSS consists of ovarian enlargement accompanied by an overproduction of ovarian hormones and a host of other ovarian vasoactive substances, which alone or in concert may produce the hyperpermeability state responsible for the signs, symptoms, and complications of OHSS Fig. 60.1.

CLASSIFICATION

Like many other diseases, OHSS exists in a clinical spectrum. Some patients, at one end of the spectrum, exhibit only mild signs and symptoms of the disease; others, at the other extreme, require intensive management and may even be at risk for death from the disease (2–6). Diseases that can manifest in a range of severity need classification systems for two reasons. First, if clinicians are to evaluate and treat patients with the disease, parameters must exist which can be applied to each patient to assess the extent of disease and to plan an appropriate management strategy. Just as congestive heart failure is classified based on level of functional ability to help clinicians determine whether the patient can be managed medically or should be placed on a heart transplant list, so must OHSS be classified to help clinicians determine whether the patient should be managed supportively or intensively, medically or surgically, at home or in the hospital.

Second, if clinical researchers are to study disease epidemiology and investigate various strategies for treatment and prevention, a uniform classification scheme will ensure consistency by allowing researchers to speak in a common language about the disease and by enabling clinicians to apply the results of these studies to individual patients. Just as the revised American Fertility Society classification system for endometriosis enables standardized research into the disease and ensures the relevance of clinical trials for clinical practice, so must

OHSS be classified to ensure uniform definitions in clinical research and to maximize the application of the research into everyday clinical care.

CLASSIFICATION SCHEMES BY DISEASE SEVERITY

Over the past 25 years, several classification systems have been suggested to better categorize OHSS and disseminate uniform guidelines for prevention and treatment. Most of these classification systems are based on the severity of the disease – based on a combination of the severity of the patient's symptoms as well as the severity of the physical, laboratory, and radiologic signs of the disease. Five major severity-based schemes have been suggested to classify OHSS.

Rabau 1967

Although pregnant mare serum gonadotropin was used clinically as early as the 1930s to induce ovulation, the results of these early trials were disappointing. Gonadotropin treatments began to enter the clinical armamentarium in 1958, when a combination of follicle-stimulating hormone (FSH) derived from cadaveric human pituitary glands, and human chorionic gonadotropin (hCG), successfully induced ovulation and pregnancy (7). With the use of these agents, and with the later introduction of clomiphene citrate (8) and human menopausal gonadotropins (hMG) (9), experience with the spectrum of OHSS unfortunately grew.

The original classification, suggested by Rabau et al. in 1967 (10), categorizes the syndrome into six grades by levels of increasing severity. Grade 1 disease is defined by the presence of supraphysiologic levels of estradiol (E2) and pregnanediol, as measured by 24-hour urinary excretion greater than 150 µg and 10 mg, respectively. Grade 2 adds to these laboratory measurements the presence of enlarged ovaries and questionably palpable cysts. Interestingly, Rabau did not define grades 1 and 2 as OHSS at all, and felt that these grades were expected by-products of ovarian stimulation and required no attention or treatment.

In the Rabau classification system, grade 3 disease adds the presence of abdominal distention and definitively palpable ovarian cysts, and grade 4 includes vomiting and possibly diarrhea. To Rabau, patients with grades 3 and 4 OHSS are at possible risk for future worsening and complications, and require observation but no intervention. Grades 5 and 6, in this system, require hospitalization with aggressive observation and intervention. Grade 5 is defined by fluid shifts and third spacing leading to ascites and hydrothorax, and grade 6 is defined by hematologic changes in blood volume, blood viscosity, and coagulation time.

Schenker 1978

Schenker et al. (11) modified the Rabau classification system to group the grades into a less cumbersome mild/moderate/severe terminology, but maintained the grading system as well. In the Schenker scheme, grades 1 and 2 are termed mild OHSS, and include the same definitions – urinary excretion of E2 and pregnanediol for grade 1, and enlarged ovaries with small cysts for grade 2. Grades 3 and 4 are termed moderate OHSS, and include abdominal distention for grade 3, and nausea, vomiting, and/or diarrhea for grade 4. Grades 5 and 6 are defined as severe disease, including large ovarian cysts and ascites and/or hydrothorax for grade 5, and hemoconcentration, increased blood viscosity, and coagulation changes for grade 6.

Golan 1989

While the Rabau and Schenker classification systems seemed at the time to be comprehensive, they suffer from several drawbacks. First, they focus more on ovarian response, particularly in the lower grades of the disease, than on the clinical syndrome. Second, they are difficult to incorporate into the clinical setting, as 24-hour urinary hormones are not routinely measured. Third, they incorporate unnecessarily cumbersome subdivisions; simple classification as mild, moderate, and severe OHSS would be adequately descriptive and more clinically useful. Finally, these schemes were developed through observation of women undergoing ovulation induction. More recently, with the evolution of ART and routine use of COH in ART patients, the laboratory and clinical findings in the lower grades of the Rabau and Schenker classifications are routinely observed and may reflect not a syndrome but an acknowledgment that COH has indeed been achieved.

Therefore, there was a need for a simpler, more clinically useful, and more relevant system. Golan et al. (12) in 1989 attempted such a revision of these older systems by classifying OHSS into mild, moderate, and severe, eliminating hormone measurements from the system, and including in the mild category clinical symptoms previously classified as moderate disease prior to the days of routine COH for ART. Golan does maintain a grading scheme, defining grades 1 and 2 as mild OHSS, grade 3 as moderate OHSS, and grades 4 and 5 as severe OHSS. In the mild category, grade 1 includes abdominal discomfort and distention, and grade 2 adds enlarged ovaries to 5–12 cm and nausea, vomiting, and/or diarrhea.

For moderate OHSS, Golan introduces the use of ultrasound, defining ultrasound evidence of ascites as grade 3, even if the degree of ascites is not detectable clinically. Severe OHSS features respiratory symptoms such as dyspnea and tachypnea and clinical evidence of ascites and/or hydrothorax as grade 4, and hemoconcentration, oliguria, increased blood viscosity, coagulation abnormalities, hypotension, and renal hypoperfusion as grade 5. Perhaps one of the most important innovations of the Golan system is the introduction of ultrasound as a tool in classifying OHSS, encouraging the use of this technology, already in widespread use in the monitoring of ovarian response, for the evaluation and monitoring of OHSS as well. The moderate form of OHSS includes significant ovarian enlargement (5–12 cm), and accompanying symptoms such as abdominal pain, significant bloating, nausea, and diarrhea.

Navot 1992

The major deficiency of the Golan classification scheme is the absence of a distinction between forms of the disease that are severe but not life threatening, and forms that are critical and potentially fatal. If one of the major purposes of the classification scheme is to aid the clinician in appropriately managing the patient with OHSS, such a distinction would be of great clinical import. Additionally, clinicians routinely assess the severity and course of OHSS with laboratory measurements of hematologic parameters, electrolytes, and renal function, yet the classification system does not address these widely used measurements in a quantitative way.

To correct these deficiencies, Navot et al. (13) subdivided the "severe" category into "severe OHSS" and "critical OHSS." According to the Navot scheme, patients with severe OHSS have variably enlarged ovaries, massive ascites with or without hydrothorax, a hematocrit greater than 45%, a leukocyte count greater than 15,000, clinically measured oliguria, serum creatinine 1.0–1.5, creatinine clearance at least 50 mL/min, laboratory evidence of hepatic dysfunction, and anasarca. Patients with critical, life-threatening OHSS have a critically contracted blood volume and multiorgan failure. They exhibit more extreme forms of the same parameters, including a hematocrit greater than 55%, a leukocyte count greater than 25,000, serum creatinine at least 1.6, creatinine clearance 50 mL/min or less, prerenal azotemia, thromboembolic phenomena, and acute respiratory distress syndrome (ARDS) (Table 60.1).

Of note, unlike the earlier schema, the Navot system minimizes the significance of ovarian enlargement. In the past, ovulation induction was the primary cause of OHSS, and ovarian size may have been an important parameter in assessing the disease. However, now that much OHSS results from COH for ART, follicular aspiration and iatrogenic follicular trauma during oocyte retrieval may minimize ovarian size even in the face of severe OHSS. With COH, anasarca can frequently coexist with relatively minor ovarian enlargement. Therefore, the Navot scheme downplays ovarian enlargement,

Table 60.1 Classification of OHSS

Mild	Moderate	Severe	Critical
Bloating	Vomiting	Massive ascites	Tense ascites
Nausea	Abdominal pain	Hydrothorax	Hypoxemia
Abdominal distention	US evidence of ascites	Hct >45%	Pericardial effusion
Ovaries ≤5 cm	Hct >41%	WBC >15,000/mm^3	Hct >55%
	WBC >10,000/mm^3	Oliguria	WBC >25,000/mm^3
	Ovaries >5 cm	Creatinine 1–1.5 mg/dL	Oliguria or anuria
		Creatinine clearance ≥ 50 mL/min	Creatinine >1.5 mg/dL
		Hepatic dysfunction	Creatinine clearance <50 mL/min
		Anasarca	Renal failure
		Ovaries variably enlarged	Thromboembolic phenomena
			ARDS
			Ovaries variably enlarged

Abbreviations: Hct, hematocrit; WBC, white blood count; US, ultrasound; ARDS, acute respiratory distress syndrome; OHSS, ovarian hyperstimulation syndrome.

relying more on the general clinical picture and on common laboratory parameters.

Rizk 1999

In an attempt to further subdivide Golan's severe category, Rizk et al. (14) defined three grades of severe OHSS. Grade A severe OHSS features dyspnea, oliguria, nausea, vomiting, diarrhea, abdominal pain, clinical or ultrasound evidence of ascites, hydrothorax, and enlarged ovaries on ultrasound. Patients with grade A disease have a normal biochemical profile. Grade B severe OHSS adds massive ascites, markedly enlarged ovaries, severe dyspnea, severe oliguria, increased hematocrit, hepatic dysfunction, and elevated serum creatinine. Grade C OHSS, which features complications that Rizk feels can also occur in the setting of moderate disease, resembles Navot's "critical" category with end-organ complications such as renal failure, venous thrombosis, and ARDS.

CLASSIFICATION BY DISEASE ONSET: EARLY AND LATE OHSS

Since 1994, investigators (15–17) have recognized that what is commonly called OHSS actually includes two distinct disease entities: OHSS that occurs three to seven days after hCG triggering, and OHSS that occurs more than 10 days after hCG triggering. As a disease, OHSS seems to include these two distinct forms based on the timing of its onset, and can consequently be classified into early OHSS and late OHSS. Both forms of OHSS share a common pathophysiology; in both, hCG triggers granulosa cells to produce vasoactive substances which induce the capillary permeability that yields the clinical sequelae of OHSS. What distinguishes the early and late forms of the disease is the source of the hCG. In early OHSS, the exogenously-injected hCG drives the granulosa directly to secrete sufficient vasoactive substances to produce the syndrome within three to seven days, while in late OHSS, early pregnancy is responsible for the

granulosa cell activity, as the implanting trophoblast produces increasing levels of endogenous hCG.

Clinically, these two entities ought to be distinguished, because they are distinct. Early OHSS, but not late OHSS, is dependent on ovarian stimulation; higher peak E2 levels and greater gonadotropin doses are correlated with an increased incidence of early OHSS, but not of late OHSS. Therefore, criteria related to ovarian response can be used to predict early OHSS, but not late OHSS. Early OHSS can occur in any stimulated cycle, while late OHSS only occurs in the setting of a pregnancy. Late OHSS is more likely to be severe; in fact, late OHSS may account for almost 70% of all cases of severe OHSS. Late OHSS can occur with either a singleton or multiple pregnancy. While some authors have suggested that multiple pregnancy has a stronger association with late OHSS than singleton pregnancy by virtue of higher trophoblastic hCG production, a more recent report found an equal association of singleton and multiple pregnancies with late OHSS (18).

ETIOLOGY

While the exact etiological factor responsible for the pathogenesis of OHSS is unknown, the syndrome is known to be dependent on hCG. OHSS does not occur if hCG is withheld, and ongoing hCG stimulation by an early pregnancy is a significant risk factor for persistent and severe OHSS. This hCG dependence underlies some of the major preventive strategies for the syndrome. More recently, numerous vasoactive substances have been implicated in the pathophysiology of the disease, including prorenin, renin, prostaglandins, angiotensin II, vascular endothelial growth factor (VEGF), tumor necrosis factor α (TNFα), insulin-like growth factor 1 (IGF-1), epidermal growth factor (EGF), basic fibroblast growth factor (BFGF), platelet-derived growth factor (PDGF), transforming growth factors (TGF) α and β, and interleukins 1β, 2, and 6 (19–30). Many of these substances are proangiogenic, and are probably responsible for the physiologic neovascularization that occurs during folliculogenesis and leutinization within the ovary.

VEGF seems to play a particularly critical role in the patho-physiology of OHSS. Evidence for this critical role includes the facts that VEGF is secreted by granulosa cells, VEGF levels correlate with OHSS severity, recombinant VEGF has been shown to induce OHSS, and specific VEGF anti-serum has been shown to reverse the effects of VEGF-induced OHSS. Furthermore, hCG has been shown to increase VEGF secretion by granulosa cells, and to increase serum levels of VEGF (31–33). Indeed, many of the angio-genic factors implicated in the pathophysiology of OHSS probably act directly or indirectly through VEGF. Since angiogenic factors are so strongly associated with OHSS, ongoing research will likely identify anti-angiogenic strate-gies for prevention and treatment.

OHSS has been reported in several women with spon-taneous pregnancies, (34–36) and the cause of this OHSS seems to be a familial mutation in the FSH receptor, increasing its sensitivity to trophoblastic hCG. The muta-tion allows for constitutive stimulation of the FSH recep-tor by hCG, triggering the ovarian cascade responsible for OHSS. This form of OHSS clearly illustrates the distinc-tion noted above between early and late OHSS; these women did not have stimulated ovaries and did not have hCG triggering, yet developed OHSS due to endogenous production of hCG by the developing pregnancy. This spontaneous late OHSS in at least one report was severe, requiring hospitalization and intensive management. Whether FSH receptor mutations or polymorphisms will play a role in the onset or severity of iatrogenic OHSS will require further research.

Serum E2 also seems to play a role in the pathogenesis of OHSS, but the nature of this role is not clear because a high serum E2 level, while a known risk factor for OHSS, seems to be neither necessary nor sufficient for the devel-opment of the disease. On one hand, the fact that most patients with OHSS have high E2 levels (37) may suggest that high E2 is necessary in the development of OHSS; but on the other hand, OHSS can occur in hypoestro-genic patients such as those with hypogonadotropic hypogonadism (38). Similarly, the fact that a high serum E2 level is a definitive risk factor for OHSS may suggest that it is sufficient for the development of OHSS; but on the other hand, OHSS does not occur when hCG is with-held, despite high E2 levels (39). Estradiol itself does not have direct vasoactivity (40) and does not seem to cause the vascular dysfunction seen in OHSS (41). Recently, expression of the cystic fibrosis transmembrane conduc-tance regulator (CFTR) has been studied in OHS because of CFTR's known effects in increasing channel activity in the peritoneal cavity, which can cause fluid shifts and ascites. Estradiol is a known upregulator of CFTR expres-sion, which may provide a potential causative link between hyperestrogenemia and OHSS (42).

PREVENTION OF SEVERE OHSS

The Role of the Stimulatory Agent and Protocol

OHSS has intrigued clinicians for many years because of its devastating consequences in otherwise healthy young

Table 60.2 Risk Factors Associated with OHSS

High risk	Low risk
Young (<35 years)	Older (>35 years)
Polycystic-appearing ovaries	Hypogonadotropic
Asthenic habitus	Heavy build
High serum E2 (ART >4000 pg/ml, OI >1700 pg/ml)	Low serum E2
Multiple stimulated follicles (ART >20, OI >6)	Poor response to gonadotropins
Necklace sign	Few antral follicles
Pregnancy	Elevated baseline FSH
hCG luteal supplementation	Progesterone or no luteal supplementation
GnRH-agonist downregulatory protocol	Clomiphene citrate and/or hMG protocol
High serum anti-Müllerian hormone	

Abbreviations: E2, estradiol; FSH, follicle-stimulating hormone; hCG, human chorionic gonadotropin; hMG, human menopausal gonadotropin, ART, assisted reproductive techniques; OI, ovulation induction.

women. As an iatrogenic condition resulting from elective ovarian stimulation in the quest for pregnancy, the need to completely prevent the syndrome is evident. To promul-gate safe or controlled ovarian stimulation, it is essential to first define the "at-risk population." Table 60.2 delineates the risk factors for severe OHSS that should alert the clini-cian contemplating COH. Because oocyte retrieval for in vitro fertilization (IVF), presumably due to the follicular trauma inherent in the procedure, decreases the risk of OHSS, the criteria defining high versus low risk may differ depending on whether the COH is for the purpose of IVF or for conventional ovulation induction or superovulation. The single most important risk factor for OHSS is a polycys-tic appearance of the ovaries on transvaginal ultrasound, with a high antral follicle count and a "necklace sign" or "string of pearls" appearance (Fig. 60.2). In contrast, rela-tively quiescent ovaries with few antral follicles usually predict a slow COH response with little risk of OHSS.

Recently, serum concentrations of anti-Müllerian hor-mone (AMH) have been investigated as a risk factor for OHSS. AMH is secreted by ovarian granulosa cells in preantral and small antral follicles, and can be used to estimate ovarian reserve and predict ovarian response to gonadotropin stimulation (43). In one recent study, all cycle cancellations due to OHSS occurred in patients who were in the highest AMH quartile of greater than 7 ng/mL (44). Another recent cohort study found baseline serum AMH levels prior to stimulation to be highly cor-related with OHSS, with an AMH concentration of greater than or equal to 3.36 ng/mL yielding a sensitivity of 90.5% and specificity of 81.3% for the subsequent development of OHSS (45).

Early reports suggested a relationship between the type of gonadotropin preparation utilized and the risk of OHSS, but subsequent comparisons between recombinant FSH (rFSH) and hMG did not show significant differences among variable drug regimens. A large study by Bergh

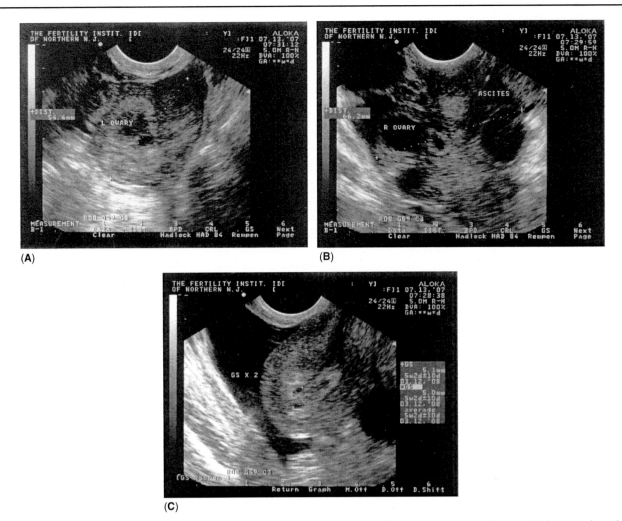

Figure 60.1 Transvaginal ultrasound depicting the ovaries and uterus of a 26-year-old woman who had undergone IVF for unexplained infertility. Peak E_2 was 2336 pg/ml on the ninth day of stimulation using a gonadotropin-releasing hormone (GnRH)-antagonist protocol. Human chorionic gonadotropin (hCG) 10,000 units were used for oocyte maturation. Twenty oocytes were retrieved, two blastocysts were transferred on the fifth day following oocyte retrieval, and six blastocysts were cryopreserved. Two days after embryo transfer, the patient presented with abdominal pain and nausea, and was found to have ovarian enlargement, moderate ascites, hemoconcentration, and leukocytosis. She was diagnosed with moderate ovarian hyperstimulation syndrome (OHSS) and treated as an outpatient with isotonic fluids. Serum hCG was positive 10 days after embryo transfer. A clinical twin intrauterine pregnancy was observed ultrasonographically on the 17th day after embryo transfer, as seen in (**C**). An enlarged left ovary can be seen in (**A**) and an enlarged right ovary with ascites in (**B**). The patient continued to be monitored as an outpatient until resolution of her OHSS, and was discharged to obstetric care with an ongoing twin pregnancy at 11 weeks gestational age.

et al. (46) compared 119 cycles of rFSH (Gonal-F) to 114 cycles of highly purified urinary FSH (uFSH-HP) (Metrodin HP). Both groups were downregulated by a long gonadotropin releasing hormone agonist (GnRH-a) protocol. All parameters studied, including E_2 serum concentrations, ampoules utilized, days of stimulation, number of oocytes retrieved, and number of embryos obtained, were significantly in favor of rFSH, and although clinical pregnancy rates and implantation rates were similar, significantly more embryos were frozen subsequent to rFSH stimulation. The respective rates of OHSS for rFSH and uFSH-HP were 5.2% and 1.7%, respectively. Another large study compared 585 patients receiving rFSH with 386 patients receiving urinary FSH (uFSH) (47). This report demonstrated similar advantages of rFSH regarding length of treatment and ampoules utilized, but also showed a significantly higher ongoing pregnancy rate for rFSH when frozen–thawed embryos were added to the equation. The rate of OHSS in this study was 3.2% versus 2.0% for rFSH and uFSH, respectively, and the difference was not statistically significant.

The capacity of rFSH to enhance both follicular recruitment and serum E_2 concentrations may indeed carry a slightly increased risk of OHSS. However, the seemingly increased risk in these studies may also be due to early inexperience with rFSH. With increased awareness and understanding of the unique features of rFSH, the actual rate of OHSS with rFSH use has since decreased, as has been borne out in subsequently published studies (48,49).

Indeed, numerous studies have shown that the method of stimulation (chronic low dose, step up, or step down) carries far more weight as a risk factor than the type of injectable gonadotropin used (50,51). Specifically, the so-called chronic low dose regimen is more likely to result

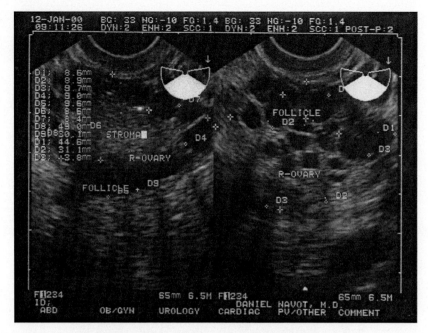

Figure 60.2 Transvaginal ultrasound depicting the right ovary of a 31-year-old woman with amenorrhea and polycystic ovarian syndrome. The picture features major high-risk factors for the development of severe ovarian hyperstimulation syndrome:

- "String of pearls" appearance of antral follicles on the *left panel*.
- Dense stroma occupying the center of the ovary.
- Enlarged ovary measuring 49 × 44.6 mm.
- Total of 60 antral follicles in one ovary.

in a mono- or bifollicular response and therefore a significantly lower rate of OHSS. Similarly, unlike a step-up protocol that continuously rescues follicles from atresia, a step-down protocol will allow more follicles to undergo atresia, thus reducing the overall number of follicles capable of secretory activity by the time hCG is administered. A reduction in the rate of OHSS will naturally follow.

An extension of the step-down concept is "coasting" or "controlled drift" championed by Sher et al. (52,53) and later widely practiced by several other researchers with variable results. Coasting may work to prevent or reduce the severity of OHSS by altering the capacity of the granulosa cells to produce VEGF (54), and seems to confer this benefit without compromising cycle outcomes. Benadiva et al. and Tortoriello et al., for example, reported a significant reduction in OHSS with coasting (55–58), and a 2003 review of 10 studies showed that <2% of women developed OHSS while maintaining acceptable pregnancy rates (36.5–63%) when coasting was continued until serum E_2 levels fell below 3000 pg/mL (59). A retrospective analysis by Kovács et al., in which gonadotropins were withheld for an average of 2.2 days, showed that pregnancy rates in the coasting group were comparable to those in non-coasted control cycles (60). Two other recent retrospective studies similarly demonstrate the absence of any adverse effect of coasting on cycle outcome, including implantation rate, pregnancy rate, and live birth rate (61,62). In contrast, however, other studies have found either no benefit in coasting (63,64), or have shown diminished oocyte collection rates (65) and implantation and pregnancy rates (66) when coasting is prolonged, particularly greater than three days (67). Most of these discrepancies in the benefit

and outcome of coasting likely stem from interstudy differences in coasting protocols. Additional research is required to evaluate the efficacy of coasting and to determine the optimal protocol for delaying hCG administration in high-risk patients (68).

The use of gonadotropin releasing hormone agonists (GnRH-a) in conjunction with COH, either as a "long" or "short" protocol, profoundly affects the risk of OHSS. GnRH-a play a paradoxical role in OHSS by virtue of the control they afford, despite their overall suppressive effect on ovarian stimulation. Both the long and the short GnRH-a protocols uniformly abolish the mid-cycle luteinizing hormone (LH) surge. This suppression of the LH surge allows continued stimulation by gonadotropins, which in turn will drive more follicles to either full or quasi maturation with a consequent rise in serum E2 values and a markedly increased risk of OHSS (13). In contrast, during cycles without GnRH-a suppression, either a significant LH surge or at least marked luteinization will limit continued gonadotropin stimulation and thus lead to a concomitantly lesser risk of OHSS. On the other hand, because of the suppressive effect of GnRH-a on ovarian function, some have advocated continuing GnRH-a administration for one week following HCG administration in GnRH-a downregulation cycles where all embryos are electively cryopreserved because of a high risk of OHSS (69). This strategy can be extended easily to oocyte donation cycles.

The Role of HCG and Its Substitutes

Once the prerequisite for severe hyperstimulation is established, namely a multifollicular, high-estrogenic milieu, the occurrence of OHSS is utterly hCG dependent; either exogenously-administered or pregnancy-derived hCG is absolutely essential for the development of OHSS. In contrast, avoidance of hCG or substitution by a low-affinity, shorter-acting compound are the mainstays for the prevention of OHSS. Indeed, the acknowledgment of the role of hCG in OHSS has led to all but complete discontinuation of the foul habit of hCG administration for luteal supplementation. Cessation of this practice eliminated a major risk factor for OHSS in assisted reproduction.

However, hCG as a surrogate for the mid-cycle LH surge is still universally used in COH for both ovulation induction and IVF. The standard dosage of hCG used to trigger ovulation is 5000–10,000 IU, or 250 µg of recombinant hCG (rhCG). hCG in these dosages takes six to nine days to clear from the circulation, thus exerting continuous ovarian stimulation up to the stage in which endogenous pregnancy-derived hCG is perceived. Since hCG has a very long half-life and high affinity for the ovarian LH receptor, it sustains the function of multiple corpora lutea to the point of rescue by endogenous hCG. This ovarian action of hCG exerts a stimulatory effect on the putative ovarian substances which directly promote, or may even be the causal factors in, ovarian hyperstimulation. Indeed, angiotensin II, VEGF, TNFα, and interleukins 1β, 2, or 6 are all either directly or indirectly enhanced by hCG (70,71). Because of these OHSS-promoting actions of hCG, one simple preventative strategy is to administer lower-dose hCG. As expected, triggering ovulation or oocyte maturation with lower-dose hCG on a sliding scale, with the administration of between 3300 and 5000 units depending on serum E2 concentration on the day of triggering, has been shown to decrease the risk of OHSS (72,73).

Recombinant LH and OHSS

The critical role of hCG in OHSS has prompted many researchers to look for an alternate substance to trigger ovulation while reducing the prolonged and often excessive stimulation of hCG. Although exogenous native LH would constitute a physiological replacement, it has several theoretical disadvantages, including its very short half-life of about 20 minutes. Because of this short half life, either huge doses or repeated administration would be needed to create a sustained surge of at least 24 hours. Recombinant LH (rLH) has been commercially available for several years now. A dose-finding study, in which rLH was utilized to trigger ovulation, showed the engineered product to be highly sialated, greatly extending its half-life in vivo. Because of this, the use of rLH as a mid-cycle substitute to the natural LH surge is now feasible in all kinds of COH, whether using gonadotropins alone, clomiphene citrate in conjunction with gonadotropins, downregulation with GnRH-a, or LH suppression with GnRH antagonists (GnRH-ant).

While this prolonged half-life, on one hand, allows rLH to be clinically useful, it might also theoretically render the rLH similar to hCG, and therefore may not substantially reduce the incidence of OHSS. One preliminary comparison of rLH and rhCG in IVF demonstrated a lower incidence of moderate to severe OHSS in women receiving a single dose of rLH (74). Loumaye et al. used doses of rLH between 5000 and 30,000 IU to compare with 5000 IU of hCG (75). All doses of rLH in the Loumaye et al. study successfully induced final follicular maturation and yielded similar numbers of oocytes and equal fertilization rates, but the incidence of ovarian enlargement and some ascites seemed to be directly dose dependent. Whereas no ovarian enlargement or ascites were seen with the administration of up to 10,000 IU of rLH, one of 26 women (3.8%) who took 30,000 IU rLH, and 13 of 121 women (10.7%) who took hCG, had ovarian enlargement, ascites, or accompanying symptomatology. One patient in the hCG group had severe OHSS. The group concluded that rLH may be safer than hCG as far as OHSS is concerned. This dose-finding study suggests that the rLH used probably has a relatively long half-life compared with native LH. Alternately, it is possible that a single peak of rLH is sufficient to induce final oocyte maturation as opposed to the 24-hour-long naturally occurring LH surge.

GnRH-Agonists and OHSS

Alternatively, final follicular maturation and ovulation may be triggered using a GnRH agonist to stimulate an endogenous LH surge in patients at risk for OHSS. Early attempts to elicit an LH surge with synthetic GnRH in an hMG-stimulated cycle yielded variable results (76,77). More recently, however, attempts to trigger ovulation with GnRH analogues have been more consistent in their results. Lanzone et al. (78) and Imoedemhe et al. (79) were the first to report the successful use of GnRH-a for induction of an endogenous LH/FSH surge for final follicular maturation following exogenous gonadotropin stimulation of the ovaries. Since then, there have been numerous reports of the successful use of GnRH-a to successfully induce follicular maturation in IVF cycles (80,81), as well as ovulation in non-IVF cycles (82,83).

Several authors have addressed the efficacy of GnRH-a in preventing OHSS. Most reports support the hypothesis that GnRH-a induces adequate ovulation while avoiding OHSS. Emperaire and Ruffie studied 37 of 126 cycles in 48 patients undergoing ovulation induction with a regimen of either hMG or hMG with clomiphene citrate (84). All cycles were considered to be at high risk for OHSS and/or multiple pregnancy (E2 level >1000–1200 pg/ml and >3 follicles of >17 mm mean diameter). In these at-risk cycles, an endogenous LH surge was provoked by intranasal buserelin 200 mg three times at eight-hourly intervals. Ovulation was documented in all cycles except one (97%). Eight pregnancies resulted (21.6%), and there were no cases of OHSS. Imoedemhe et al. (79) used two doses of GnRH-a (Suprefact 100 mg) by nasal spray eight hours apart to induce follicular maturation 34–36 hours prior to oocyte recovery in 38 women considered at risk of OHSS (E2 >4000 pg/ml) in an IVF program. Of the 707 oocytes recovered at egg retrieval, 93% were scored as mature, and 46% were successfully fertilized. Twenty-six women had embryos replaced; 11 pregnancies occurred (28.9%), and there were no cases of OHSS. Itskovitz et al. used buserelin acetate in dosages of either 250 mg or 500 mg injected subcutaneously in either a single or two divided doses, 12 hours apart (81). Approximately 78% of all eggs recovered were considered mature. Three of 13 patients conceived (21.4%), and none developed any signs or symptoms of OHSS. Shalev et al. (83) and Balasch et al. (85) used a single subcutaneous injection of triptorelin or leuprolide (0.5 mg), respectively, to trigger ovulation in gonadotropin-stimulated cycles which would otherwise have been cancelled due to a high risk for OHSS. Fifty percent and 17.4% Conception rates of 50% and 17.4% were achieved, respectively, while no patient developed OHSS. Kulikowski and colleagues used a single dose of 0.3 mg GnRH-a subcutaneously in 32 patients undergoing ovulation induction for IVF and in 16 patients undergoing ovulation induction for ovulatory disturbances, all of whom they felt were at risk of OHSS (E_2 > 2500 pg/ml) (86). All patients had ovulation induced with a clomiphene/hMG protocol. There were no cases of OHSS in the GnRH-a group, and four pregnancies occurred (12.5%). In the control IVF group, there were four cases of OHSS, and three pregnancies occurred (8.8%). In the 16 patients who had undergone ovulation induction with clomiphene/ hMG/GnRH-a, no OHSS was detected, while four patients became pregnant (25%). Engmann et al. randomized 66 IVF patients at risk for OHSS to a GnRH-antagonist (GnRH-ant) protocol with GnRH-a trigger, or a GNRH-a downregulatory protocol with hCG trigger (87). All patients received luteal support using intramuscular progesterone, and the GnRH-a trigger group received luteal estrogen supplementation as well. Thirty-one percent of patients in the hCG trigger group developed some form of OHSS, compared with none in the GnRH-a trigger group. Moreover, there were no significant differences in implantation, clinical pregnancy, and ongoing pregnancy rates. The study concluded that the use of a GnRH-a trigger reduces, if not eliminates, the risk of OHSS in high-risk patients, without compromising pregnancy outcomes. In summary, a number of investigators have used mid-cycle GnRH-a, in varying dosages and time intervals, for cycles considered to be at high risk for development of OHSS. Pregnancy rates of 12.5–50% were achieved, with a 0% incidence of OHSS. Because some studies have suggested a degradation in pregnancy outcomes with the use of GnRH-a triggers (88), Griesinger et al. proposed the use of a GnRH-a trigger to prevent OHSS, together with pronuclear cryopreservation and frozen–thawed embryo transfer at a later date. In their prospective observational study, cumulative ongoing pregnancy rates were high, and no cases of moderate or severe OHSS were observed (89).

In contrast to the above reports showing an absence of development of OHSS in high risk patients given GnRH-a for follicular maturation and ovulation, van der Meer et al. published a study in which three patients who used buserelin to induce a preovulatory endogenous LH surge in lieu of hCG nevertheless developed moderate OHSS (90). Severe ascites, hypovolemia, or electrolyte imbalance did not occur, and no patients were hospitalized.

These authors concluded that OHSS is due to a massive luteinization of the follicles after exaggerated follicular stimulation, and can occur independent of the ovulation triggering agent. Gerris et al. also reported the occurrence of moderate OHSS in one patient following GnRH-a administration (82), but in this case native GnRH was used, resulting in successful ovulation triggering but without the critical ovarian suppression which is thought to be at least equally important in the prevention of OHSS (91). Casper surveyed a total of 163 cycles in which GnRH-a was used to trigger ovulation in the context of preventing OHSS (92). He stipulated that 900 cycles should have been randomized to detect a significant difference between GnRH-a and hCG. However, his analysis relies on an assumed 2% risk for severe OHSS, and while a 2% risk may be applicable to the average woman undergoing COH, most women in his survey likely had far greater risk, possibly in the 10–20% range. The preponderance of evidence to date supports a decreased incidence of OHSS with GnRh-a compared with hCG as the triggering agent for ovulation, although a small possibility of moderate OHSS remains, particularly in conception cycles. Most importantly, there have been no reports of severe or critical OHSS after triggering ovulation with mid-cycle GnRH-a.

Clinicians using GnRH-a to trigger ovulation must realize that the ensuing luteal phase is dramatically deficient, with a premature luteolysis originally shown by Beckers et al. (93) Full luteal support must therefore be employed. Various regimens for luteal support have been suggested, such as supplementation with transdermal and/or oral E2 to maintain serum E2 levels above 200 pg/ml, together with intramuscular progesterone and/or vaginal progesterone to maintain serum progesterone levels above 20 ng/ml (87). In oocyte donation cycles, in cycles using a gestational carrier, and in cycles in which all embryos or oocytes are expected to be cryopreserved, luteal sufficiency is of no concern. In such cases, GnRH-a triggering is widely accepted, with all studies to date showing an absolute elimination of any risk of OHSS (94–96).

Clinicians must also be aware that because of pituitary desensitization, GnRH-a cannot be used as an ovulation trigger for cycles in which GnRH-a was previously used for downregulation. If a patient at high risk for OHSS is identified and GnRH-a triggering is contemplated, a GnRH-ant protocol, rather than a long-acting GnRH-a protocol, should be used for suppression of the endogenous mid-cycle LH surge.

GnRH-Antagonists and OHSS

GnRH antagonists seem to be associated with a decreased risk of OHSS compared with the GnRH-a long protocol in patients undergoing IVF. Although one meta-analysis found no differences in the incidence of OHSS with the use of GnRH-ant compared with long GnRH-a downregulatory protocols (97), another more recent meta-analysis of 27 randomized controlled trials revealed a significant reduction in the incidence of OHSS with the use of GnRH-ant compared with GnRH-a downregulation protocols, with a relative risk of 0.61 (98). Furthermore, fewer interventions to prevent OHSS were administered in GnRH-ant protocols versus GnRH-a protocols (odds ratio 0.44). Another meta-analysis confirmed a decreased risk of OHSS with the use of GnRH-ant, but particularly for cetrorelix and less so for ganirelix (99). A prospective multicenter study demonstrated a reduction in the incidence of OHSS, and a decreased cycle cancellation rate for OHSS risk, in high-risk IVF patients treated with a GnRH-ant protocol as compared with historical controls downregulated with GnRH-a (100). A recent meta-analysis of 45 randomized controlled trials also confirms a significant reduction in the incidence of OHSS with the use of GnRH-ant as compared with GnRH-a (101,102). Interestingly, since the degree of ovarian suppression with GnRH-ant may be more profound at high doses, the dose of GnRH-ant may thereby be adjusted to minimize the development of OHSS in high-risk patients. de Jong et al. employed this strategy when they used the GnRH-ant ganirelix to prevent OHSS by increasing the dose of the antagonist when target E_2 values were inadvertently exceeded (103). Indeed, E_2 values rapidly decreased with a concomitant decrease in ovarian size. Similarly, GnRH-ant may be administered in a downregulated GnRH-a cycle, as an alternative to coasting, to decrease E2 levels. Such a strategy, in comparison with coasting, has been shown to result in a lower incidence of OHSS with similar pregnancy rates (104,105).

Although these GnRH-ant strategies are novel, far more intriguing, as discussed in the previous section, is the potential use of GnRH-ant in conjunction with either rLH or GnRH-a to trigger ovulation. Because of the competitive nature of GnRH-ant suppression and lack of desensitization, it is possible to trigger ovulation with GnRH-a during co-treatment with gonadotropins and GnRH-ant. The respective dosages of each agent still awaits further studies, although 0.25 mg of ganirelix or cetrorelix daily seems to be sufficient to eliminate the LH surge, and seems to result in favorable clinical outcomes. Theoretically, a larger dose of GnRH-a would be needed to induce an LH surge in cycles suppressed by a GnRH-ant than in cycles using gonadotropins alone without a GnRH-ant. It cannot be reiterated enough that full progesterone support is mandatory throughout the luteal phase when GnRH-a is used to trigger ovulation.

Embryology Strategies

Liberal application of embryo cryopreservation for patients showing early signs of hyperstimulation can be an important safety net in guarding against severe OHSS (106), although the efficacy of cryopreservation as a preventive measure for OHSS has been questioned (107). With routine culture of embryos to the blastocyst stage, it is possible to accurately assess the degree of OHSS prior to embryo transfer; because blastocyst transfer takes place on the seventh day after hCG, absence of even a moderate degree of OHSS is reassuring, and one may safely proceed with embryo transfer (13). The higher implantation rates associated with blastocyst transfer have led some clinicians to

employ single blastocyst transfer in patients at risk of developing severe OHSS (108,109). Such a strategy results in a negligible multiple gestation rate, which purportedly is associated with more severe OHSS presumably secondary to higher hCG levels. Although theoretically plausible, the utility of such an approach remains to be confirmed.

Improvements in in vitro maturation of immature oocytes might also enable women, particularly those with polycystic ovarian syndrome (PCOS) who are at greatest risk of OHSS, to undergo assisted reproduction using minimal, if any, gonadotropin stimulation. This may dramatically reduce or eliminate the risk of OHSS (110,111).

Prophylactic Use of Colloid Agents to Prevent OHSS

Third spacing and intravascular volume depletion due to increased capillary leakage are hallmarks of OHSS. Several investigators have administered intravenous colloidal agents such as albumin and hydroxyethyl starch (HES) at the time of oocyte retrieval as prophylactic intravascular volume and oncotic pressure enhancers to minimize the risk of developing OHSS (112–114). In contrast to the significant value of albumin for treatment of the fully developed syndrome, colloids are of questionable benefit as preventive measures. A meta-analysis of five randomized clinical trials validated the use of intravenous albumin administration at the time of oocyte retrieval in high-risk patients (115). In this meta-analysis, albumin infusion to 18 at-risk women was necessary to prevent one case of severe OHSS. Another more recent meta-analysis of nine randomized clinical trials found limited evidence of benefit from intravenous albumin in reducing the incidence of OHSS in high-risk patients undergoing IVF, but did note a marked decrease in the incidence of OHSS with the preventive infusion of HES at the time of oocyte retrieval (116). Overall, because albumin treatment inheres risks such as allergic reactions and transmission of viruses and prions, the relative merits of albumin infusion compared with other preventive strategies remain unclear.

Miscellaneous Techniques to Prevent OHSS

Other modalities that have been suggested for the prevention of OHSS include unilateral or bilateral follicular aspiration as a rescue for cycles not otherwise intended to undergo oocyte retrieval (117). Egbase advocated ovarian diathermy prior to initiation of COH (118). Ovarian diathermy should, however, be reserved to young patients with severe PCOS who tend to hyperstimulate even on a prolonged low dose FSH regimen.

Metformin

Metformin, the second-generation biguanide insulin sensitizer, has been advocated for the treatment of women with severe PCOS and insulin resistance. Although a more favorable response to ovulation enhancement would be expected, it is unclear yet whether a reduction in the incidence of OHSS will follow. One small study comparing combined treatment using clomiphene and metformin with clomiphene alone showed a lower incidence of OHSS with the addition of metformin, although this difference did not achieve statistical significance (119). A randomized prospective trial showed that adding metformin to gonadotropin regimens for ovulation induction yields fewer large follicles, lower E_2 levels on the day of hCG administration, and a reduced rate of cycle cancellation for over-response (120). These effects would probably result in a reduced risk of OHSS as well. Indeed, a study of 287 women undergoing IVF demonstrated a significant reduction in the incidence of OHSS in those taking metformin (121). Clearly, though, more data are needed to fully elucidate the effects of metformin on OHSS in women with PCOS.

Ovarian suppression

Suppression of ovarian steroidal secretion, either through continued administration of GnRh-a following oocyte retrieval coupled with cryopreservation, or through administration of intramuscular hydroxy-progesterone caproate and estradiol valerate following embryo transfer, has been suggested to minimize the risk of developing OHSS. Both approaches currently remain experimental (69,122). Aromatase inhibitors administered in the luteal phase can be used to reduce luteal estradiol concentrations, and thus may be a promising approach in preventing OHSS or minimizing its attendant hyperestogenemia-related risks in patients such as oocyte donors whose luteal sufficiency is of no concern (123).

Corticosteroids

The anti-inflammatory action of corticosteroids has also been hypothesized to be beneficial in preventing OHSS. However, because of conflicting reports in the literature, there are currently insufficient data to recommend such an approach (124,125).

Calcium

Calcium infusion has also been hypothesized to prevent OHSS because of its inhibition of cyclic adenosine monophosphate (cAMP) synthesis and cAMP-dependent renin secretion from juxtaglomerular cells in the kidneys (126,127). Reduced renin secretion results in decreased angiotensin II production, with a consequent decrease in angiotensin II-mediated stimulation of VEGF synthesis. In two studies to date, IVF patients at risk for OHSS were infused intravenously with calcium gluconate 10%, 10 mL in 200 mL of normal saline, on the day of oocyte retrieval and for three days thereafter. Patients receiving the calcium infusion had a decreased incidence of both mild and severe OHSS (128,129). This prevention modality carries little risk and potential benefit, but because of insufficient data cannot yet be routinely recommended.

VEGF Antagonism

Recent novel research has focused on preventive strategies aimed particularly at VEGF as the critical ovarian mediator of the syndrome. Encouragingly, treatment with a VEGF receptor antagonist prevented the increase in capillary permeability seen in an OHSS rat model (130). Likewise, treatment with *fms*-like tyrosine kinase, a soluble agent which binds VEGF with high affinity and thus decreases its availability for its endothelial effects, demonstrated the same result in a similar OHSS rat model (131).

Dopamine Agonists

Dopamine agonists also decrease vascular permeability by preventing the phosphorylation of VEGF receptor 2 and thus reducing the release of vasoactive angiogenic agents (132,133). Cabergoline, a dopamine D2 receptor agonist, inactivates VEGF receptor 2 in animal models (134), and a recent prospective, randomized double blind study investigated the effects of daily cabergoline treatment (0.5 mg/day) in oocyte donors at risk for OHSS. The study showed more than a 50% reduction in the incidence of moderate OHSS with the use of cabergoline from the day of hCG administration through six days post oocyte retrieval (135). Several other studies and meta-analyses have demonstrated similar findings for cabergoline, as well as for the other dopamine agonists quinagolide and bromocriptine (136–142). Such novel options make pathophysiologic sense, and have the potential to play a future role in OHSS prevention.

Obviously, there are many strategic options for the prevention of OHSS in high-risk patients. The current increasing use of GnRH-ant in clinical practice holds great promise for preventing severe OHSS. As we master the complexity of GnRH-ant for LH surge suppression together with GnRH-a for triggering ovulation, ovarian stimulation will likely become better controlled, and severe OHSS will become a rare if not forgotten entity.

TREATMENT OF SEVERE OHSS

Medical Approach

There are two possible approaches to the treatment of OHSS, one pathogenesis oriented and one empiric. The former approach utilizes agents that specifically negate the putative causative factor(s) of OHSS. Indomethacin was hypothesized to be such an agent when prostaglandins were believed to play a role in OHSS. Angiotensin converting enzyme (ACE) inhibitors are another group of specific pharmacological agents which were thought to have potential use in the treatment of OHSS because they inhibit the production of angiotensin II, a probable pathogenic factor for the syndrome. Unfortunately, indomethacin did not benefit the syndrome, and ACE inhibitors are teratogenic and thus contraindicated whenever a pregnancy is contemplated. Just as VEGF antagonists may become useful for the prevention of

OHSS, similar cytokine inhibitors are being studied for treatment of the syndrome. To date, such therapies remain investigational, largely preclinical, and not yet compelling. One study found pentoxifylline, an inhibitor of the synthesis of TNFα, to be ineffective in limiting ascites formation in an OHSS rabbit model, although it did decrease ovarian weight compared with controls (143). In any case, until such interventions are validated in human trials, the treatment of OHSS remains largely empiric in nature.

The clinical manifestations of OHSS are a cascade of pathophysiologic events resulting from a global increase in vascular permeability. This increased vascular permeability causes a decrease in the colloid oncotic pressure (144), which results in a change in extracellular fluid equilibrium. Fluid consequently shifts into the extravascular or "third" space, depleting intravascular volume and causing hypotension. "Third spacing" causes abdominal ascites, pleural and pericardial effusions, and dependent edema. Cardiac preload falls due to a combination of hypovolemia caused by fluid shifts, and compression of the inferior vena cava from the increasing intraperitoneal pressure due to ascites accumulation. Falling cardiac preload reduces cardiac output, which, together with a decrease in peripheral vascular resistance due to an arterial vasodilatation (145), in turn leads to a decrease in renal perfusion. Decreasing renal perfusion increases proximal tubule reabsorption of salt and water, leading to decreased urinary sodium excretion and oliguria. The proximal sodium reabsorption, and consequently diminished exposure of the distal tubule to sodium, impairs the sodium–hydrogen/potassium exchange in the distal tubule, causing hyperkalemic acidosis. Decreasing renal perfusion also decreases glomerular filtration rate (GFR), which can result in oliguria or anuria and a full-blown prerenal azotemia. OHSS also produces a hypercoagulable state, possibly due to a combination of hemoconcentration, high levels of ovarian steroids, and changes in liver perfusion resulting in decreased hepatic protein synthesis with consequent depletion of circulating antithrombotic factors (146).

Individual treatment will depend on the severity of the syndrome. Mild forms of OHSS require little more than reassurance, since it is well established that mild symptoms usually resolve, in the absence of pregnancy, within two weeks after receiving hCG. If a pregnancy ensues, mild symptoms may progress but rarely more than one degree in severity. In patients with moderate ascites and mild hemoconcentration (hematocrit <45%), bed rest and abundant liquid intake should be prescribed. The tendency toward intravascular volume depletion and hyponatremia may be treated with oral isotonic electrolyte solutions; sports drinks, popular among athletes, are particularly suitable because they are engineered for optimal rehydration. The patient should be vigilant in noting any decreases in urine output, significant weight gain, or abdominal bloating as self-assessed by daily abdominal girth measurement. These findings, if present, may

be the first warning signals of accumulation of ascitic fluid and worsening hemoconcentration. A hematocrit >45%, or 30% increased over baseline, indicates that the condition has entered the category of severe OHSS and that hospitalization is required.

Dramatic clinical deterioration is most likely to manifest eight to nine days after hCG administration, when endogenous, pregnancy-derived hCG becomes perceptible. The single most important variable that indicates the severity of the OHSS is hemoconcentration, as reflected in the hematocrit. Because the hematocrit is actually the ratio between red cell volume and total blood volume, where total blood volume = red cell volume + plasma volume, the change in plasma volume must always be larger than the change reflected by the hematocrit (70). Thus, a change of two percentage points in the hematocrit from 42% to 44% is four times smaller than the actual 8% drop in plasma volume. This is extremely important to remember when one is treating patients with OHSS. Any increase in the hematocrit as it approaches 45% underestimates the magnitude of plasma volume depletion and thus the seriousness of the patient's condition. One should therefore not be lulled into a false sense of security when only a small incremental rise in hematocrit between 40% and 45% is observed. Similarly, in the face of hemoconcentration, small reductions in hematocrit may represent a significant improvement in plasma volume (13).

An additional measure of hemoconcentration is the magnitude of leukocytosis; white blood cell (WBC) counts higher than $25,000/mm^3$, largely reflecting a granulocytosis, may be seen. This massive neutrophilia may be attributed to hemoconcentration and generalized stress reaction. When oral isotonic fluid intake is insufficient to maintain plasma volume, intravenous fluid therapy becomes mandatory. Table 60.3 details the advantages and disadvantages of various therapies in the treatment of severe OHSS, and Figure 60.3 provides a clinical algorithm for the management of OHSS. Crystalloids alone, although seldom sufficient in restoring homeostasis because of massive protein loss through hyperpermeable capillaries, still remain the mainstay of treatment. Because of the tendency for hyponatremia, sodium chloride with or without glucose is the crystalloid of choice. The daily volume infused may vary from 1.5 L to greater than 3.0 L. Although some authors advocate fluid restriction to minimize the accumulation of ascites (147), one should rather deal with the discomfort of ascites than face the consequences of hemoconcentration with the attendant risks of thromboembolism and renal shutdown. To maintain fluid balance, the patient's urine output, oral and intravenous fluid intake, body weight, abdominal girth, hematocrit, and serum electrolytes must be monitored. In addition, coagulation parameters and liver enzymes should be periodically assessed. Intravenous volume replacement should aim to improve renal perfusion before fluid escapes into the peritoneal and/or pleural cavities; this transient hemodilution is achieved at the expense of increased third spacing and

Table 60.3 Pros and Cons of Various Therapies of OHSS

Therapy	Pros	Cons
IV crystalloids	Alleviates hemoconcentration Improves renal perfusion	Lost immediately from vascular tree Aggravates ascites
Fluid restriction	Controls ascites	Reduces renal perfusion Promotes hemoconcentration
Albumin	Improves colloid-oncotic pressure Improves renal perfusion	Risks of human blood product
Furosemide	Reduces total body water	Further reduces intravascular volume
Indomethacin	May block prostaglandin-induced hyperpermeability	Implicated in renal failure
ACE inhibitors	May block angiotensin II-induced hyperpermeability	Teratogenic
Paracentesis	Alleviates tense ascites Improves renal perfusion	Risks of hemorrhage, infection, and leakage
Heparin	Decreases risk of thromboembolic phenomena	Increases risk of hemorrhage
Peritoneovenous shunt	Replaces lost electrolytes and proteins	Risk of self-toxicity Elaborate setup and risk of infection
Dopamine drip	Improves renal perfusion	Need for Intensive Care Unit management

increased total body water. Whenever adequate fluid balance cannot be restored by crystalloid alone, plasma expanders should be utilized. Since albumin is the main protein lost in OHSS, human albumin is physiologic and thus the colloid of choice (Table 60.3). Albumin at doses of 50–100 g at 25% concentration should be administered intravenously and repeated every two to 12 hours until the hematocrit falls below 45% and urine output increases.

At a relatively advanced stage of OHSS, during treatment with crystalloids and colloids, gradual hemodilution is obtained at the expense of a tightening abdominal wall with the rapid accumulation of ascitic fluid. At this stage of restored intravascular volume and improved renal perfusion, there may occur a sudden, paradoxical onset of oliguria, with an increasing serum creatinine and a rapidly falling creatinine clearance (148). This sudden deterioration in fluid balance is probably the result of a significant rise in intra-abdominal pressure produced by tense ascites. Increased intra-abdominal pressure may in turn impede renal venous outflow, causing congestion, renal edema, and decrease in renal function. Such tense ascites is best treated surgically via therapeutic paracentesis, although diuretics may also be effective. When oliguria persists despite evidence of adequate hemodilution, intravenous furosemide at a 10–20 mg dose is often beneficial. In practice, an albumin-furosemide chase protocol seems to yield the best results. Two units of albumin, 50 g each, followed immediately by intravenous furosemide, will often result in diuresis. In states of volume contraction, hemoconcentration and hypotension, furosemide should be strictly avoided. In this precarious stage of OHSS, with impending renal failure, renal dose dopamine drip should be used for renal rescue.

Paracentesis

The single most important treatment modality in life-threatening OHSS that cannot be controlled by medical therapy is paracentesis. Because much of the clinical pathophysiology of OHSS stems from the increase in intra-abdominal pressure caused by ascitic fluid shifts, (149,150) OHSS can be considered to be an abdominal compartment syndrome (151). As such, reduction in intra-abdominal pressure alone can alleviate much of the clinical constellation of OHSS, and may even be considered the most important treatment modality for moderate or severe OHSS, and certainly for any OHSS with tense ascites. Rabau et al. first proposed the use of paracentesis in the treatment of severe OHSS (10). Paracentesis was temporarily discredited, but later regained popularity (Table 60.3 and Fig. 60.3) (11). Thaler (152), Borenstein (148), and Forman (153) have all promoted paracentesis as safe and exceptionally beneficial. Dramatic improvements in the clinical symptoms of severe OHSS, with almost instantaneous diuresis, were reported (148). In a series of seven patients in whom paracentesis was performed, urine output rose from 780 ± 407 ml to 1670 ± 208 ml (P < 0.05), creatinine clearance rose from 75.4 ± 16 ml/min to 101 ± 15 ml/min (P < 0.05), hematocrit decreased from $46.3\% \pm 2.2\%$ to $37.1\% \pm 2.5\%$ (P < 0.05), and a mean weight loss of 5.3 kg was observed (98). In the study by Forman et al. (153), 37 L of ascitic fluid with a protein content of 46 to 53 g/L (reflecting a total protein loss of 1.85 kg) was removed from a single patient, underscoring both the high protein content of ascitic fluid and the safety of the procedure.

The indications for paracentesis include the need for symptomatic relief, tense ascites, oliguria, rising serum creatinine concentration or falling creatinine clearance, and hemoconcentration unresponsive to medical

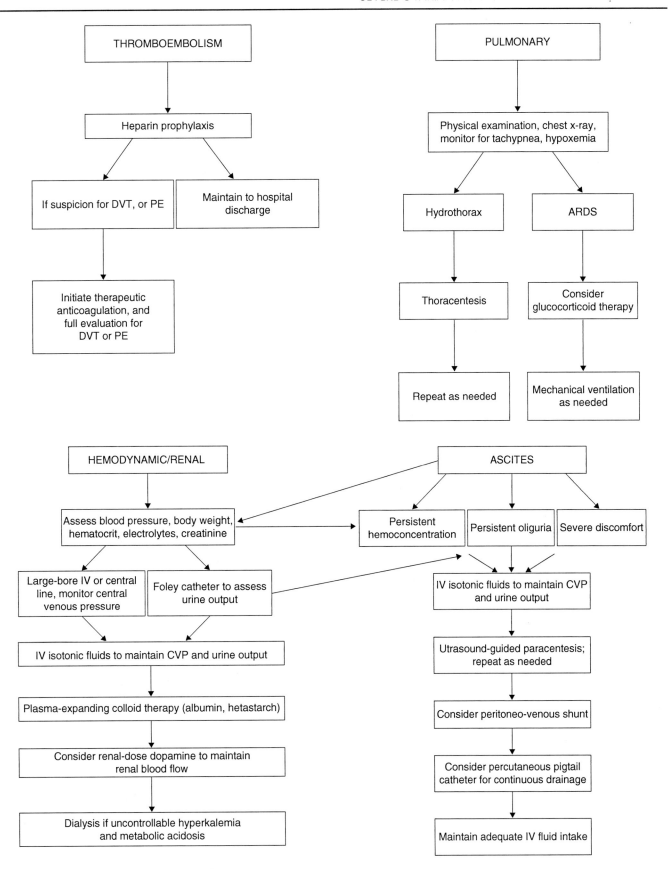

Figure 60.3 Algorithm for the intensive care of the patient with critical ovarian hyperstimulation syndrome. *Abbreviations*: IV, intravenous; CVP, central venous pressure; ARDS, acute respiratory distress syndrome; DVT, deep vein thrombosis; PE, pulmonary embolus.

treatment. Paracentesis should be performed aseptically under ultrasound guidance. Careful monitoring of hemodynamic stability is also mandatory. Rizk and Aboulghar advocated transvaginal ultrasonically guided aspiration of ascitic fluid as an effective and equally safe method (154), but a transabdominal approach can be used as well. Up to 4 L may be removed either by slow drainage to gravity, (152) or with negative pressure using large evacuated containers. Paracentesis is contraindicated in patients who are hemodynamically unstable, or in the presence of suspected hemoperitoneum.

With aggressive use of paracentesis, including repeated paracenteses when ascitic reaccumulation is noted, patients with even severe OHSS can be treated effectively and safely as outpatients, without the need for hospitalization (155). In fact, outpatient management of moderate or severe OHSS with early and frequent paracentesis has been recently shown to be more effective than traditional inpatient therapy (156) and should therefore be considered for all such patients.

A new and innovative treatment for severe OHSS was suggested by Koike et al. (147). These authors describe continuous peritoneovenous shunting in 18 patients with severe OHSS. This study group was compared with 36 control patients who had received intravenous albumin at a dose of 37.5 g/day. Recirculation of ascites fluid rich in proteins is not a novel idea (157); however, the reliance on a continuous shunt from the peritoneal cavity into the antecubital vein is a novel and logical way to replenish the vascular tree with the fluid, proteins, and electrolytes that were lost from the vasculature. The study reports faster hemodilution, shorter hospital stays, and prompt improvement in symptoms in the shunted patients due to diuresis and reduction in the amount of ascites. There are, however, some problems with the study besides for the complexity of the setup. First, the reinfused ascites may contain the very substances which might be responsible for the profound hyperpermeability of OHSS, and thus may exacerbate the syndrome. Second, the group advocates fluid restriction, which may aggravate hemoconcentration and thus contribute to renal failure and thromboembolic phenomena (147).

In addressing the hypercoagulable state of OHSS, most authors reserve anticoagulation for special circumstances in which thromboembolic events have already occurred, or in the setting of a hereditary coagulopathy. One study suggests that prophylactic screening for hereditary thrombophilias should perhaps be undertaken in all patients undergoing assisted reproduction, because of a higher prevalence of thrombophilia in women with severe OHSS (158). However, another conflicting study found no such increased prevalence, and recommends against screening the general IVF population for thrombophilias (159). In any case, although prophylactic treatment of women with OHSS with unfractionated or low-molecular-weight heparin is of some theoretical value, rapid alleviation of the patient's hemoconcentration is far more important.

Rarely, as a last resort, when the critical stage of OHSS is complicated by renal failure, thromboembolism, acute respiratory distress syndrome, and multiorgan failure, there is no choice but to perform a potentially life-saving termination of pregnancy.

REFERENCES

1. Abramov Y, Elchalal U, Schenker JG. An epidemic of severe OHSS; a price we have to pay? Hum Reprod 1999; 14: 2181–3.
2. Moses M, Bogowsky H, Anteby E, et al. Thromboembolic phenomena after ovarian stimulation with menopausal gonadotrophins. Lancet 1965; 2: 1213.
3. Esteban-Altirriba J. Le syndrome d'hyperstimulation massive des ovaries. Rev Fr Gynecol Obstet 1961; 56: 555.
4. Figueroa-Cases P. Reaccion ovarica monstruosa a las gonadotrofinas a proposito de un caso fatal. Ann Cirug 1958; 23: 116.
5. Cluroe AD, Synek BJ. A fatal case of ovarian hyperstimulation syndrome with cerebral infarction. Pathology 1995; 27: 344–6.
6. Semba S, Moriya T, Youssef EM, et al. An autopsy case of ovarian hyperstimulation syndrome with massive pulmonary edema and pleural effusion. Pathol Int 2000; 50: 549–52.
7. Gemzel CA, Diczfalusy E, Tillinger G. Clinical effect of human pituitary follicle-stimulating hormone. J Clin Endocrinol Metab 1958; 18: 1333.
8. Greenblatt RB, Barfield WE. Induction of ovulation with MRL/41. JAMA 1961; 178: 101.
9. Lunenfeld B. Treatment of anovulation by human gonadotropins. J Int Fed Gynecol Obstet 1963; 1: 153.
10. Rabau E, David A, Serr DM, et al. Human menopausal gonadotrophin for anovulation and sterility. Am J Obstet Gynecol 1967; 98: 92–8.
11. Schenker JG, Weinstein D. Ovarian hyperstimulation syndrome: a current survey. Fertil Steril 1978; 30: 255–68.
12. Golan A, Ron-El R, Herman A, et al. Ovarian hyperstimulation syndrome: an update review. Obstet Gynecol Surv 1989; 44: 430–40.
13. Navot D, Bergh PA, Laufer N. Ovarian hyperstimulation syndrome in novel reproductive technologies: prevention and treatment. Fertil Steril 1992; 58: 249–61.
14. Rizk B, Aboulghar MA. Classification, pathophysiology, and management of ovarian hyperstimulation syndrome. In: Brinsden P, ed. In-Vitro Fertilization and Assisted Reproduction. New York, London: The Parthenon Publishing Group, 1999; 131–55.
15. Dahl Lyons CA, Wheeler CA, Frishman GN, et al. Early and late presentation of the ovarian hyperstimulation syndrome: two distinct entities with different risk factors. Hum Reprod 1994; 9: 792–9.
16. Mathur RS, Akande VA, Keay SD, et al. Distinction between early and late ovarian hyperstimulation syndrome. Fertil Steril 2000; 73: 901–7.
17. Papanikolaou EG, Tournaye H, Verpoest W, et al. Early and late ovarian hyperstimulation syndrome: early pregnancy outcome and profile. Hum Reprod 2005; 20: 636–41.
18. De Neubourg D, Mangelschots K, Van Royen E, et al. Singleton pregnancies are as affected by ovarian

hyperstimulation syndrome as twin pregnancies. Fertil Steril 2004; 82: 1691–3.

19. Navot D, Margalioth EJ, Laufer N, et al. Direct correlation between plasma renin activity and severity of the ovarian hyperstimulation syndrome. Fertil Steril 1987; 48: 57–61.

20. McClure N, Healy DI, Rogers PA, et al. Vascular endothelial growth factor as a capillary permeability agent in ovarian hyperstimulation syndrome. Lancet 1994; 344: 235–6.

21. Friedlander MA, Loret de Mola JR, Goldfarb JM. Elevated levels of interleukin-6 in ascites and serum from women with ovarian hyperstimulation syndrome. Fertil Steril 1993; 60: 826–33.

22. Abramov Y, Schenker JG, Lewin A, et al. Plasma inflammatory cytokines correlate to the ovarian hyperstimulation syndrome. Hum Reprod 1996; 11: 1381–6.

23. Revel A, Barak V, Lavy Y, et al. Characterization of intraperitoneal cytokines and nitrates in women with severe ovarian hyperstimulation syndrome. Fertil Steril 1996; 66: 66–71.

24. Orvieto R, Ben-Rafael Z. The immune system in severe ovarian hyperstimulation syndrome. Isr J Med Sci 1996; 32: 1180–2.

25. Sealey JE, Atlas SA, Glorioso N, Manapat H, Laragh JH. Cyclical secretion of prorenin during the menstrual cycle: synchronization with luteinizing hormone and progesterone. Proc Natl Acad Sci USA 1985; 82: 8705–9.

26. Derkx FH, Alberda AT, Zeilmaker GH, Schalekamp MA. High concentrations of immunoreactive renin, prorenin and enzymatically-active renin in human ovarian follicular fluid. Br J Obstet Gynaecol 1987; 94: 4–9.

27. Geva E, Jaffe RB. Role of vascular endothelial growth factor in ovarian physiology and pathology. Fertil Steril 2000; 74: 429–38.

28. Whelan LG 3rd, Vlahos NF. The ovarian hyperstimulation syndrome. Fertil Steril 2000; 73: 883–96.

29. Warren RS, Yuan H, Matli MR, Ferrara N, Donner DB. Induction of vascular endothelial growth factor by insulin-like growth factor I in colorectal carcinoma. J Biol Chem 1996; 271: 483–8.

30. Ferrara N, Davis-Smyth T. The biology of vascular endothelial growth factor. Endocrinol Rev 1997; 18: 4–25.

31. Levin ER, Rosen GF, Cassidenti DL, et al. Role of vascular endothelial growth factor in ovarian hyperstimulation syndrome. J Clin Invest 1998; 102: 1978–85.

32. Neulen J, Yan Z, Raczek S, et al. Human chorionic gonadotropin-dependent expression of vascular endothelial growth factor/vascular permeability factor in human granulosa cells: importance in ovarian hyperstimulation syndrome. J Clin Endocrinol Metab 1995; 80: 1967–71.

33. Pellicer A, Albert C, Mercader A, et al. The pathogenesis of ovarian hyperstimulation syndrome: in vivo studies investigating the role of interleukin-1β, interleukin-6, and vascular endothelial growth factor. Fertil Steril 1999; 71: 482–9.

34. Smits G, Olatunbosun O, Delbaere A, et al. Ovarian hyperstimulation syndrome due to a mutation in the follicle-stimulating hormone receptor. New Engl J Med 2003; 349: 760–6.

35. Vasseur C, Rodien P, Beau I, et al. A chorionic gonadotropin-sensitive mutation in the follicle-stimulating hormone receptor as a cause of familial gestational spontaneous ovarian hyperstimulation syndrome. N Engl J Med 2003; 349: 753–9.

36. Montanelli L, Delbaere A, Di Carlo C, et al. A mutation in the follicle-stimulating hormone receptor as a cause of familial spontaneous ovarian hyperstimulation syndrome. J Clin Endocrinol Metab 2004; 89: 1255–8.

37. Haning RV Jr, Austin CW, Carlson IH, et al. Plasma estradiol is superior to ultrasound and urinary estriol glucuronide as a predictor of ovarian hyperstimulation syndrome during induction of ovulation with menotropins. Fertil Steril 1983; 40: 31–6.

38. Levy T, Orvieto R, Homburg R, et al. Severe ovarian hyperstimulation syndrome despite low plasma estrogen concentrations in a hypogonadotrophic, hypogonadal patient. Hum Reprod 1996; 11: 1177–9.

39. Schenker JG. Prevention and treatment of ovarian hyperstimulation syndrome. Hum Reprod 1993; 8: 653–9.

40. Delvigne A, Rozenberg S. Systematic review of data concerning etiopathology of ovarian hyperstimulation syndrome. Int J Fertil Womens Med 2002; 47: 211–26.

41. Manau D, Balasch J, Arroyo V, et al. Circulatory dysfunction in asymptomatic in vitro fertilization patients. Relationship with hyperestrogenemia and activity of endogenous vasodilators. J Clin Endocrinol Metab 1998; 83: 1489–93.

42. Ajonuma LC, Tsang LL, Zhang GH, et al. Estrogen-induced abnormally high cystic fibrosis transmembrane conductance regulator expression results in ovarian hyperstimulation syndrome. Mol Endocrinol 2005; 19: 3038–44.

43. Gnoth C, Schuring AN, Friol K, et al. Relevance of anti-Mullerian hormone measurement in a routine IVF program. Hum Reprod 2008; 23: 1359–65.

44. La Marca A, Giulini S, Tirelli A, et al. Anti-Mullerian hormone measurement on any day of the menstrual cycle strongly predicts ovarian response in assisted reproductive technology. Hum Reprod 2007; 22: 766–71.

45. Lee TH, Liu CH, Huang CC, et al. Serum anti-Mullerian hormone and estradiol levels as predictors of ovarian hyperstimulation syndrome in assisted reproductive technology cycles. Hum Reprod 2008; 23: 160–7.

46. Bergh C, Howles CM, Borg K, et al. Recombinant human follicle stimulating hormone (r-hFSH; Gonal-F) versus highly purified urinary FSH (Metrodin HP): results of a randomized comparative study in women undergoing assisted reproductive techniques. Hum Reprod 1997; 12: 2133–9.

47. Out HJ, Mannaerts BM, Driessen SG, Bennink HJ. A prospective, randomized, assessor-blind, multicentre study comparing recombinant and urinary follicle stimulating hormone (Puregon versus Metrodin) in in-vitro fertilization. Hum Reprod 1995; 10: 2534–40.

48. Frydman R, Howles C, Truong F. A double-blind, randomized study to compare recombinant follicle stimulating hormoun (FSH; Gonal-F) with highly purified urinary FSH (Medtrodin HP) in women undergoing assisted reproductive techniques including intracytoplasmic sperm injection: on behalf of The French Multicentre Trialists. Hum Reprod 2000; 15: 520–5.

49. Schats R, Sutter P, Bassil S, et al. Ovarian stimulation during assisted reproduction treatment: comparison of recombinant and highly purified urinary human FSH: on behalf of The Feronia and Apis study group. Hum Reprod 2000; 15: 1691–7.

50. Hedon B, Hugues JN, Emperaire JC, et al. A comparative prospective study of a chronic low dose versus a conventional ovulation stimulation regimen using recombinant human follicle stimulating hormone in anovulatory infertile women. Hum Reprod 1998; 13: 2688–92.

51. Homburg R, Levy T, Ben-Rafael Z. A comparative prospective study of conventional regimen with chronic low-dose administration of follicle-stimulating hormone for anovulation associated with polycystic ovary syndrome. Fertil Steril 1995; 63: 729–33.

52. Sher G, Salem R, Feinman M, et al. Eliminating the risk of life-endangering complications following overstimulation with menotropin fertility agents: a report on women undergoing in vitro fertilization and embryo transfer. Obstet Gynecol 1993; 81: 1009–11.

53. Sher G, Zouves C, Feinman M, Maassarani G. 'Prolonged coasting': an effective method for preventing severe ovarian hyperstimulation syndrome in patients undergoing in-vitro fertilization. Hum Reprod 1995; 10: 3107–9.

54. Tozer AJ, Iles RK, Iammarrone E, et al. The effects of 'coasting' on follicular fluid concentrations of vascular endothelial growth factor in women at risk for developing ovarian hyperstimulation syndrome. Hum Reprod 2004; 19: 522–8.

55. Benadiva CA, Davis O, Kligman I, et al. Withholding gonadotropin administration is an effective alternative for the prevention of ovarian hyperstimulation syndrome. Fertil Steril 1997; 67: 724–7.

56. Tortoriello DV, McGovern PG, Colon JM, Skurnick JH, Lipetz K, Santoro N. 'Coasting' does not adversely affect cycle outcome in a subset of highly responsive in vitro fertilization patients. Fertil Steril 1998; 69: 454–60.

57. Grochowski D, Wolczynski S, Kuczynski W, et al. Correctly timed coasting reduces the risk of ovarian hyperstimulation syndrome and gives good cycle outcome in an in vitro fertilization program. Gynecol Endocrinol 2001; 15: 234–8.

58. Al-Shawaf T, Zosmer A, Hussain S, et al. Prevention of severe ovarian hyperstimulation syndrome in IVF with or without ICSI and embryo transfer: a modified "coasting" strategy based on ultrasound for identification of high-risk patients. Hum Reprod 2001; 16: 24–30.

59. Levinson-Tavor O, Friedler S, Schachter M, et al. Coasting – what is the best formula? Hum Reprod 2003; 18: 937–40.

60. Kovács P, Mátyás S, Kaali SG. Effect of coasting on cycle outcome during in vitro fertilization/ intracytoplasmic sperm injection cycles in hyper-responders. Fertil Steril 2006; 85: 913–17.

61. Yilmaz N, Uygur D, Ozgu E, Batioglu S. Does coasting, a procedure to avoid ovarian hyperstimulation syndrome, affect assisted reproduction cycle outcome? Fertil Steril 2010; 94: 189–93.

62. Abdalla H, Nicopoullos JDM. The effect of duration of coasting and estradiol drop on the outcome of assisted reproduction: 13 years of experience in 1,068 coasted cycles to prevent ovarian hyperstimulation. Fertil Steril 2010; 94: 1757–63.

63. Shapiro D, Craven G, Mitchell-Leef J, et al. Allowing estradiol levels to fall in a controlled drift does not affect pregnancy rates and offers no protection against ovarian hyperstimulation syndrome. Fertil Steril 1997; 1997(Suppl): S169.

64. Lee C, Tummon I, Martin J, et al. Does withholding gonadotrophin administration prevent severe ovarian hyperstimulation syndrome? Hum Reprod 1998; 13: 1157–8.

65. Delvigne A, Kostyla K, Murillo D, Van Hoeck J, Rozenberg S. Oocyte quality and IVF outcome after coasting to prevent ovarian hyperstimulation syndrome. Int J Fertil Womens Med 2003; 48: 25–31.

66. Isaza V, Garcia-Velasco JA, Aragones M, et al. Oocyte and embryo quality after coasting: the experience from oocyte donation. Hum Reprod 2002; 17: 1777–82.

67. Ulug U, Bahceci M, Erden HF, Shalev E, Ben-Shlomo I. The significance of coasting duration during ovarian stimulation for conception in assisted fertilization cycles. Hum Reprod 2002; 17: 310–13.

68. D'Angelo A, Amso N. "Coasting" (withholding gonadotropins) for preventing ovarian hyperstimulation syndrome. Cochrane Database Syst Rev 2002; 3: CD002811.

69. Endo T, Honnma H, Hayashi T, et al. Continuation of GnRH agonist administration for 1 week, after HCG injection, prevents ovarian hyperstimulation syndrome following elective cryopreservation of all pronucleate embryos. Hum Reprod 2002; 17: 2548–51.

70. Bergh PA, Navot D. Ovarian hyperstimulation syndrome – a review of pathophysiology. J Assist Reprod Genet 1992; 9: 429–38.

71. Orvieto R, Ben-Rafael Z. Ovarian hyperstimulation syndrome: a new insight into an old enigma. J Soc Gynecol Investig 1998; 5: 110–13.

72. Chen D, Burmeister L, Goldschlag D, Rosenwaks Z. Ovarian hyperstimulation syndrome: strategies for prevention. Reprod Biomed Online 2003; 7: 43–9.

73. Kashyap S, Leveille M, Wells G. Low dose hCG reduces the incidence of early and severe ovarian hyperstimulation syndrome. Fertil Steril 2006; 86(Suppl 2): S182–3; (P-138).

74. European Recombinant LH Study Group. Human recombinant luteinizing hormone is as effective as, but safer than, urinary human chorionic gonadotropin in inducing final follicular maturation and ovulation in in vitro fertilization procedures: results of a multicenter double-blind study. J Clin Endocrinol Metab 2001; 86: 2607–18.

75. Loumaye E, Piazzi A, Engrand P. Results of a phase II, dose finding, clinical study comparing r-LH with hCG to induce final follicular maturation prior to IVF (Abst.O-236). Sixteenth World Congress on Fertility and Sterility, San Francisco, 1998.

76. Breckwoldt M, Czygan PJ, Lehmann F. Synthetic LH-RH as a therapeutic agent. Acta Endocrinol (Copenh) 1974; 75: 209–20.

77. Crosignani PG, Trojsi L, Attanasio A, Tonani E. Hormonal profiles in anovulatory patients treated with gonadotropins and synthetic luteinizing hormone releasing hormone. Obstet Gynecol 1975; 46: 15–22.

78. Lanzone A, Fulghesu AM, Apa R, Caruso A. LH surge induction by GnRH agonist at the time of ovulation. Gynecol Endocrinol 1989; 3: 213–20.

79. Imoedemhe D, Chan R, Sigue A, Pacpaco E. A new approach to the management of patients at risk of ovarian hyperstimulation in an in-vitro fertilization programme. Hum Reprod 1991; 6: 1088–91.

80. Gonen Y, Balakier H, Powell W. Use of gonadotropin-releasing hormone agonist to trigger follicular maturation for in vitro fertilization. J Clin Endocrinol Metab 1990; 71: 918–22.

81. Itskovitz J, Boldes R, Levron J, Erlik Y, Kahana L. Induction of preovulatory luteinizing hormone surge and prevention of ovarian hyperstimulation syndrome by gonadotropin-releasing hormone agonist. Fertil Steril 1991; 56: 213–20.

82. Gerris J, De Vits A, Joostens M. Triggering of ovulation in human menopausal gonadotrophin-stimulated cycles: comparison between intravenously administered gonadotrophin-releasing hormone (100 and 500 µg), GnRH agonist (buserelin, 500 µg) and human chorionic gonadotrophin (10000 IU). Hum Reprod 1995; 10: 56–62.

83. Shalev E, Geslevich Y. Induction of pre-ovulatory luteinizing hormone surge by gonadotrophin-releasing hormone agonist for women at risk for developing the ovarian hyperstimulation syndrome. Hum Reprod 1994; 9: 417–19.

84. Emperaire J. Triggering ovulation with endogenous luteinizing hormone may prevent the ovarian hyperstimulation syndrome. Hum Reprod 1991; 6: 506–10.

85. Balasch J, Tur R, Creus M, et al. Triggering of ovulation by a gonadotropin releasing hormone agonist in gonadotropin-stimulated cycles for prevention of ovarian hyperstimulation syndrome and multiple pregnancy. Gynecolog Endocrinol 1994; 8: 7–12.

86. Kulikowski M, Wolczynski S, Kuczynski W, Grochowski D. Use of GnRH analog for induction of the ovulatory surge of gonadotropins in patients at risk of the ovarian hyperstimulation syndrome. Gynecol Endocrinol 1995; 9: 97–102.

87. Engmann L, Diluigi A, Schmidt D, et al. The use of gonadotropin-releasing hormone (GnRH) agonist to induce oocyte maturation after cotreatment with GnRH antagonist in high-risk patients undergoing in vitro fertilization prevents the risk of ovarian hyperstimulation syndrome: a prospective randomized controlled study. Fertil Steril 2008; 89: 84–91.

88. Griesinger G, Dietrich K, Devroey P, Kolibianakis EM. GnRH agonist for triggering final oocyte maturation in the GnRH antagonist ovarian hyperstimulation protocol: a systematic review and meta-analysis. Hum Reprod Update 2006; 12: 159–68.

89. Griesinger G, von Otte S, Schroer A, et al. Elective cryopreservation of all pronuclear oocytes after GnRH agonist triggering of final oocyte maturation in patients at risk of developing OHSS: a prospective, observational proof-of-concept study. Hum Reprod 2007; 22: 1348–52.

90. Van der Meer S, Gerris J, Joostens M. Triggering of ovulation using a gonadotrophin-releasing hormone agonist does not prevent ovarian hyperstimulation syndrome. Hum Reprod 1993; 8: 1628–31.

91. Kol S, Lewit N, Itskovitz-Eldor J. Ovarian hyperstimulation: effects of GnRH analogues. Ovarian hyperstimulation syndrome after using gonadotrophin-releasing hormone analogue as a trigger of ovulation: causes and implications. Hum Reprod 1996; 11: 1143–4.

92. Casper RF. Ovarian hyperstimulation: effects of GnRH analogues. Does triggering ovulation with gonadotrophin-releasing hormone analogue prevent severe ovarian hyperstimulation syndrome? Hum Reprod 1998; 11: 1144–6.

93. Beckers NG, Macklon NS, Eijkemans MJ, et al. K, Bustion S, Loumaye E, Fauser BC. Nonsupplemented luteal phase characteristics after the administration of recombinant human chorionic gonadotropin, recombinant luteinizing hormone, or gonadotropin-releasing hormone (GnRH) agonist to induce final oocyte maturation in in vitro fertilization patients after ovarian stimulation with recombinant follicle-stimulating hormone and GnRH antagonist cotreatment. J Clin Endocrinol Metab 2003; 88: 4186–92.

94. Bodri D, Guillén JJ, Galindo A, et al. Triggering with human chorionic gonadotropin or a gonadotropin-releasing hormone agonist in gonadotropin-releasing hormone antagonist-treated oocyte donor cycles: findings of a large retrospective cohort study. Fertil Steril 2009; 91: 365–71.

95. Humaidan P, Kol S, Papanikolaou EG. GnRH agonist for triggering of final oocyte maturation: time for a change of practice? Hum Reprod Update 2011; 17: 510–24.

96. Youssef MA, Van der Veen F, Al-Inany HG, et al. Gonadotropin-releasing hormone agonist versus HCG for oocyte triggering in assisted reproductive technology cycles. Cochrane Database Syst Rev 2011: 1–55.

97. Griesinger G, Diedrich K, Tarlatzis BC, Kolibianakis EM. GnRH-antagonists in ovarian stimulation for IVF in patients with poor response to gonadotrophins, polycystic ovary syndrome, and risk of ovarian hyperstimulation: a meta-analysis. Reprod Biomed Online 2006; 13: 628–38.

98. Al-Inany H, Abou-Setta AM, Aboulghar MA. Gonadotropin-releasing hormone antagonists for assisted reproduction: a cochrane review. Reprod Biomed Online 2007; 14: 640–9.

99. Ludwig M, Katalinic A, Diedrich K. Use of GnRH antagonists in ovarian stimulation for assisted reproductive technologies compared to the long protocol. Arch Gynecol Obstet 2001; 265: 175–82.

100. Ragni G, Vegetti W, Riccaboni A, et al. Comparison of GnRH agonists and antagonists in assisted reproduction cycles of patients at high risk of ovarian hyperstimulation syndrome. Hum Reprod 2005; 20: 2421–5.

101. Al-Inany HG, Youssef MA, Aboulghar M, et al. Gonadotropin-releasing hormone antagonists for assisted reproductive technology. Cochrane Database Syst Rev 2011: 1–114.

102. Al-Inany HG, Youssef MA, Aboulghar M, et al. GnRH antagonists are safer than agonists: an update of a Cochrane review. Hum Reprod Update 2011; 17: 435.

103. de Jong D, Macklon NS, Mannaerts BM, Coelingh Bennink HJ, Fauser BC. High dose gonadotrophin-releasing hormone antagonist (ganirelix) may prevent ovarian hyperstimulation syndrome caused by ovarian stimulation for in-vitro fertilization. Hum Reprod 1998; 13: 573–5.

104. Gustofson RL, Segars JH, Larsen FW. Ganirelix acetate causes a rapid reduction in estradiol levels without adversely affecting oocyte maturation in women pretreated with leuprolide acetate who are at risk of

ovarian hyperstimulation syndrome. Hum Reprod 2006; 21: 2830–7.

105. Aboulghar M, Mansour RT, Amin YM, et al. A prospective randomized study comparing coasting with GnRH antagonist administration in patients at risk for severe OHSS. Reprod Biomed Online 2007; 15: 271–9.

106. Garrisi G, Navot D. Cryopreservation of semen, oocytes, and embryos. Curr Opin Obstet Gynecol 1992; 4: 726–31.

107. D'Angelo A, Amso NN. Embryo freezing for preventing ovarian hyperstimulation syndrome: a Cochrane review. Hum Reprod 2002; 17: 2787–94.

108. Kinget K, Nijs M, Cox AM, et al. A novel approach for patients at risk for ovarian hyperstimulation syndrome: elective transfer of a single zona-free blastocyst on day 5. Reprod Biomed Online 2002; 4: 51–5.

109. Trout SW, Bohrer MK, Deifer DB. Single blastocyst transfer in women at risk of ovarian hyperstimulation syndrome. Fertil Steril 2001; 76: 1066–7.

110. Child TJ, Phillips SJ, Abdul-Jalil AK, Gulekli B, Tan SL. A comparison of in vitro maturation and in vitro fertilization for women with polycystic ovaries. Obstet Gynecol 2002; 100: 665–70.

111. Tan SL, Child TJ. In vitro maturation of oocytes from unstimulated polycystic ovaries. Reprod Biomed Online 2002; 4(Suppl 1): 18–23.

112. Shalev E, Giladi Y, Matilsky M, Ben-Ami M. Decreased incidence of severe ovarian hyperstimulation syndrome in high risk in-vitro fertilization patients receiving intravenous albumin: a prospective study. Hum Reprod 1995; 10: 1373–6.

113. Isik AZ, Gokmen O, Zeyneloglu HB, Kara S, Gulekli B. Intravenous albumin prevents moderate-severe ovarian hyperstimulation in in-vitro fertilization patients: a prospective, randomized and controlled study. Eur J Obstet Gynecol Reprod Biol 1996; 70: 179–83.

114. Gokmen O, Ugur M, Ekin M, et al. Intravenous albumin versus hydroxyethyl starch for the prevention of ovarian hyperstimulation in an in-vitro fertilization programme: a prospective randomized placebo controlled study. Eur J Obstet Gynecol Reprod Biol 2001; 96: 187–92.

115. Aboulghar M, Evers JH, Al-Inany H. Intravenous albumin for preventing severe ovarian hyperstimulation syndrome: a Cochrane review. Hum Reprod 2002; 17: 3027–32.

116. Youssef MA, Al-Inany HG, Evers JL, Aboulghar M. Intra-venous fluids for the prevention of severe ovarian hyperstimulation syndrome. Cochrane Database Syst Rev 2011: 1–37.

117. Egbase PE, Al Sharhan M, Grudzinskas JG. Early unilateral follicular aspiration compared to coasting for the prevention of severe OHSS; a prospective randomized study. Hum Reprod 1999; 14: 1421–5.

118. Egbase PE. Severe OHSS; How many cases are preventable? Hum Reprod 2000; 15: 8–10.

119. Malkawi HY, Qublan HS. The effect of metformin plus clomiphene citrate on ovulation and pregnancy rates in clomiphene-resistant women with polycystic ovarian syndrome. Saudi Med J 2002; 23: 663–6.

120. DeLeo D. Effects of metformin on gonadotropin-induced ovulation in women with polycystic ovary syndrome. Fertil Steril 1999; 72: 282–5.

121. Khattab S, Fotouh IA, Mohesn IA, Metwally M, Moaz M. Use of metformin for prevention of ovarian

hyperstimulation syndrome: a novel approach. Reprod Biomed Online 2006; 13: 194–7.

122. Rjosk HK, Abendstein BJ, Kreuzer E, Schwartzler P. Preliminary experience with steroidal ovarian suppression for prevention of severe ovarian hyperstimulation syndrome in IVF patients. Hum Fertil 2001; 4: 246–8.

123. Garcia-Velasco JA, Quea G, Piró M, et al. Letrozole administration during the luteal phase after ovarian stimulation impacts corpus luteum function: a randomized, placebo-controlled trial. Fertil Steril 2009; 92: 222–5.

124. Lainas T, Petsas G, Stavropoulou G, et al. Administration of methylprednisolone to prevent severe ovarian hyperstimulation syndrome in patients undergoing in vitro fertilization. Fertil Steril 2002; 78: 529–33.

125. Tan SL, Balen A, el Hussein E, Campbell S, Jacobs HS. The administration of glucocorticoids for the prevention of ovarian hyperstimulation syndrome in in vitro fertilization: a prospective randomized study. Fertil Steril 1992; 58: 378–83.

126. Ortiz-Capisano MC, Ortiz PA, Harding P, Garvin JL, Beierwaltes WH. Decreased intracellular calcium stimulates renin release via calcium-inhibitable adenylyl cyclase. Hypertension 2007; 49: 162–9.

127. Beierwaltes WH. The role of calcium in the regulation of renin secretion. Am J Physiol Renal Physiol 2010; 298: F1–11.

128. Yakovenko SA, Sivozhelezov VS, Zorina IV, et al. Prevention of OHSS by intravenous calcium. Hum Reprod 2009; 24(Suppl 1): i61.

129. Gurgan T, Demirol A, Guven S, et al. Intravenous calcium infusion as a novel preventive therapy of ovarian hyperstimulation syndrome for patients with polycystic ovarian syndrome. Fertil Steril 2011; 96: 53–7.

130. Gomez R, Simon C, Remohi J, Pellicer A. Vascular endothelial growth factor receptor-2 activation induces vascular permeability in hyperstimulated rats, and this effect is prevented by receptor blockade. Endocrinology 2002; 143: 4339–48.

131. NcElhinney B, Ardill J, Caldwell C, McClure N. Preventing ovarian hyperstimulation syndrome by inhibiting the effects of vascular endothelial growth factor. J Reprod Med 2003; 48: 243–6.

132. Busso C. Symposium: update on prediction and management of OHSS. Prevention of OHSS – dopamine agonists. Reprod Biomed Online 2009; 19: 43–51.

133. Garcia-Velasco J. How to avoid ovarian hyperstimulation syndrome: a new indication for dopamine agonists. Reprod Biomed Online 2009; 19: 71–5.

134. Gomez R, Gonzalez-Izquierdo M, Zimmermann RC, et al. Low-dose dopamine agonist administration blocks vascular endothelial growth factor (VEGF)-mediated vascular hyperpermeability without altering VEGF receptor 2-dependent luteal angiogenesis in a rat ovarian hyperstimulation model. Endocrinology 2006; 147: 5400–11.

135. Alvarez C, Marti-Bonmati L, Novella-Maestre E, et al. Dopamine agonist cabergoline reduces hemoconcentration and ascites in hyperstimulated women undergoing assisted reproduction. J Clin Endocrinol Metab 2007; 92: 2931–7.

136. Spitzer D, Wogatzky J, Murtinger M, et al. Dopamine agonist bromocriptine for the prevention of ovarian

hyperstimulation syndrome. Fertil Steril 2011; 95: 2742–4.

137. Soares S, Gomez R, Simon C, Garcia-Velasco J, Pellicer A. Targeting the endothelial growth factor system to prevent ovarian hyperstimulation syndrome. Hum Reprod Update 2008; 14: 321–33.

138. Humaidan P, Quartarolo J, Papanikolaou G. Preventing ovarian hyperstimulation syndrome: guidance for the clinician. Fertil Steril 2010; 94: 389–400.

139. Carizza C, Abdelmassih V, Abdelmassih S, et al. Cabergoline reduces the early onset of ovarian hyperstimulation syndrome: a prospective randomized study. Reprod Biomed Online 2008; 17: 751–5.

140. Youssef M, van Wely M, Hassan MA, et al. Can dopamine agonists reduce the incidence and severity of OHSS in IVF/ICSI treatment cycles? A systematic review and meta-analysis. Hum Reprod Update 2010; 16: 459–66.

141. Busso C, Fernandez-Sanchez M, Garcia-Velasco J, et al. The non-ergot derived dopamine agonist quinagolide in prevention of early ovarian hyperstimulation syndrome in IVF patients: a randomized, double-blind, placebo-controlled trial. Hum Reprod 2010; 25: 995–1004.

142. Busso C, Fernandez-Sanchez M, Garcia-Velasco J, et al. Quinagolide is effective in preventing moderate/severe OHSS in IVF patients: a randomised, double-blind, placebo-controlled trial. Hum Reprod 2008; 23(Suppl): i60.

143. Serin IS, Ozcelik B, Bekyurek T, et al. Effects of pentoxifylline in the prevention of ovarian hyperstimulation syndrome in a rabbit model. Gynecol Endocrinol 2002; 16: 355–9.

144. Tollan A, Holst N, Forsdahl F, et al. Transcapillary fluid dynamics during ovarian stimulation for in vitro fertilization. Am J Obstet Gynecol 1990; 162: 554–8.

145. Balasch J, Arroyo V, Fábregues F, et al. Neurohormonal and hemodynamic changes in severe cases of ovarian hyperstimulation syndrome. Ann Intern Med 1994; 121: 27–33.

146. Fábregues F, Balasch J, Gìnès P, et al. Ascites and liver test abnormalities during severe ovarian hyperstimulation syndrome. Am J Gastroenterol 1999; 94: 994–9.

147. Koike T, Araki S, Minakami H, et al. Clinical efficacy of peritoneovenous shunting for the treatment of severe OHSS. Hum Reprod 2000; 15: 113–17.

148. Borenstein R, Elhalal U, Lunenfeld B, Shoham Z. Severe OHSS; a reevaluated therapeutic approach. Fertil Steril 1989; 51: 791–5.

149. Cil T, Tummon IS, House AA, et al. A tale of two syndromes: ovarian hyperstimulation and abdominal compartment. Hum Reprod 2000; 15: 1058–60.

150. Maslovitz S, Jaffa A, Eytan O, et al. Renal blood flow alteration after paracentesis in women with ovarian hyperstimulation. Obstet Gynecol 2004; 104: 321–6.

151. Grossman LC, Michalakis KG, Browne H, Payson MD, Segars JH. The pathophysiology of ovarian hyperstimulation syndrome: an unrecognized compartment syndrome. Fertil Steril 2010; 94: 1392–8.

152. Thaler I, Yoffe M, Kaftory JK, Brandes JM. Treatment of OHSS; the physiologic basis for a modified approach. Fertil Steril 1981; 36: 110–13.

153. Forman RG, Frydman R, Egan D, Ross C, Barlow DH. Severe OHSS using agonists of gonadotropin-releasing hormone for in vitro ferilization; a European series and a proposal for prevention. Fertil Steril 1990; 53: 502–9.

154. Rizk B, Aboulghar MA. Modern management of OHSS. Hum Reprod 1991; 6: 1082–7.

155. Smith LP, Hacker MR, Alper MM. Patients with severe ovarian hyperstimulation syndrome can be managed safely with aggressive outpatient transvaginal paracentesis. Fertil Steril 2009; 92: 1953–9.

156. Csokmay JM, Yauger BJ, Henne MB, et al. Cost analysis model of outpatient management of ovarian hyperstimulation syndrome with paracentesis: "Tap early and often" versus hospitalization. Fertil Steril 2010; 93: 167–73.

157. Fukaya T, Funamaya Y, Chiba S, et al. Treatment of severe OHSS by ultrafiltration and reinfusion of ascitic fluid. Fertil Steril 1994; 61: 561–4.

158. Dulitzky M, Cohen SB, Inbal A, et al. Increased prevalence of thrombophilia among women with severe ovarian hyperstimulation syndrome. Fertil Steril 2002; 77: 463–7.

159. Fabregues F, Tassies D, Reverter JC, et al. Prevalence of thrombophilia in women with severe ovarian hyperstimulation syndrome and cost-effectiveness of screening. Fertil Steril 2004; 81: 989–95.

61

The environment and reproduction

Machelle M. Seibel

I used to walk along the beach,
a favorite thing to do.
Until the plastic and the trash completely
spoiled my view.
The place I take my rod and reel to catch my
favorite dish.
Has elevated mercury, so I can't eat the fish.
From *Protect Environment* by Machelle M. Seibel

Al Gore may have been unsuccessful in running for U.S. president, but he has been a lightning rod in highlighting the impact of human industry on the environment, garnering an academy award for his documentary *An Inconvenient Truth*. Global warming, however, is not the only consequence of the 80,000 synthetic compounds used in the United States during the last half-century (1). One of our most basic human goals – reproduction – is also being affected.

It is estimated that over 1000 new chemicals are being introduced into the world every year, yet less than 5% have been investigated for their effect on reproduction. Fertility studies in Pennsylvania have shown decreased total fertility rates from 1901 to 1985 (2), and the overall U.S. pregnancy rate in 1996 was 9% lower than it was in 1990 (3). There is evidence that the quality and quantity of semen in normal men is also declining (4,5). What role do the thousands of compounds in our everyday environment play in these declining rates? What role does environmental exposure play in the spectrum of infertility patients that present to our clinics? What evidence is available for interpreting exposures, and what clinical considerations can we yield from such research?

To address these questions we will consider the environment not as the world at large, but rather as three *microenvironments*: the follicle, the seminal fluid, and the amniotic sac. From this vantage point, the inhabitants are the egg, the sperm, and the unborn child. In this way, the impact of the environment is not a story of what the world will be like decades from now but rather an increased awareness of the impact of the environment on our reproductive-aged patients and children today.

MECHANISMS OF ACTION

Direct damage to the cell membrane or intracellular components is the only one way compounds can cause tissue injury. Some compounds alter the communication between different cells by mimicking or blocking normal pathways. Endocrine-disrupting chemicals (EDCs) are thought to effect reproduction by directly or indirectly mimicking, stimulating, antagonizing, altering, or displacing natural hormones (6). Exposure to such agents at critical stages of development can have a significant impact upon cellular, and ultimately fetal, development. Incomplete development of DNA repair mechanisms, detoxification enzymes, and the blood–brain barrier can exacerbate a chemical's effect on the developing fetus. Moreover, there is an increasing body of research suggesting that epigenetic modulation may be an underlying mechanism of action. These effects, however, may not be seen for years.

The theory of EDCs can be traced back to the publication of *Silent Spring* (1962), by Rachel Carson (7). In a serialized printing in the *New Yorker* she proposed a connection between the population changes in wildlife ecology and the increasing rates of human cancer. She associated both changes with widespread use of agricultural and manufacturing chemicals. Her work eventually prompted a government investigation that culminated in the banning of the pesticide dichlorodiphenyltrichloroethane (DDT) in 1972. It was 20 years later that Theo Colborn and colleagues advanced the EDC theory that is now widely accepted (8–11): EDCs can exact more influence over the development of affected offspring than the genes they inherit. EDCs have been shown to have deleterious effects on animal and fish reproduction (12), but primary outcome data are still being gathered in establishing an association between human exposure and infertility. Nevertheless, compelling data exist on the role of EDCs in other hormone-driven diseases, such as the rising prevalence of endometriosis in industrialized countries (13).

BIOLOGICAL PLAUSIBILITY

Xenoestrogens, alkylphenolic chemicals [bisphenol A (BPA), polychlorinated biphenyls (PCBs)], phthalates, dioxins, lead, mercury, and pesticides are ubiquitous in the global environment. They are unavoidable for the majority of us and have been reported to have a myriad of effects (Table 61.1). Many of these toxicants came under increased scrutiny when animal experiments began to demonstrate biological plausibility for human harm. Sharpe et al. demonstrated that gestational and lactational

Table 61.1   Summary of Common Environmental Toxicants

	Phthalates	Pesticides	PCBs	Dioxins	PBDEs	Bisphenols	Heavy metals
Sources of exposure	Plastic toys, shampoos, soaps, nail polish, other personal care products, medical devices, timed-release drug coatings, flooring lacquers, and varnishes	DDE, DDT, organochlorides, and "nonpersistent pesticides." DDT is banned in most countries, save Mexico, China, India, and parts of Africa. It is found in fruits, vegetables, flowers, antimicrobial soap, and air exposure in agricultural areas	Banned in the United States and most countries. PCBs have dioxin-like properties. They were used for cutting oils, as lubricants, and as electrical insulators. Sources are contaminated fish and game consumption	Results from industrial activities and fires. Found in fatty meats, fish, and dairy products	Flame retardants in mattresses, furniture, pillows, carpets, electronic devices, TVs, DVDs, players, and computers	Polycarbonate plastics: Rigid water bottles, soda bottles, and plastic food containers	Lead: pre-1978 paint, old pipes. Mercury: Old thermometers and large fish such as tuna, shark, king mackerel, and swordfish, and as electrical tilefish. Pressure-treated wood can leach chromium and arsenic
Potential effects	↑ TTP ↑ AGD	↓ Fecundability ↓ Success with IVF ↑ Semen quality ↑ Spontaneous abortion ↑ Preterm birth ↑ SGA	↓ Response to ovulation induction ↓ Fecundability ↓ Lactation ↓ Sperm quality ↑ Endometriosis Altered menstrual cycle	↑ Cancer ↑ Birth defects Change in sex ratio ↑ Endometriosis	Reproductive development disruption	↑ Breast cancer Prostate changes	↓ IQ in offspring ↓ Semen quality/quantity ↑ Spontaneous abortion ↑ TTP ↑ Preterm labor
How to decrease exposure	Unavoidable	Wash produce well, buy organic vacuum frequently in agricultural areas	Avoid eating fish or game from areas known to be contaminated	Avoid fatty meats Avoid areas known to be contaminated	Unavoidable	Avoid hard plastic bottles and food containers, but likely unavoidable	Remove old paint and pressure-treated lumber. Be cautious/limit certain fish consumption

Abbreviations: PCBs, Polychlorinated biphenyls; PBDEs, polybrominated diphenyl ethers; DDE, dichlorodiphenyldichloroethylene; DDT, dichlorodiphenyltrichloroethane; IVF, in vitro fertilization; TTP, time to pregnancy; AGD, Anogenital distance; SGA, small for gestational age.

exposure of rats to xenoestrogens resulted in reduced testicular size and sperm production (14). Dicofol, an estrogenic organochloride pesticide, was observed to induce a significant decrease in ovarian follicles and the number of estrous cycles in rabbits (15), while follicle destruction has been reported in rhesus monkeys exposed to PCBs (16). The list of mammalian studies linking subfertility to environmental toxicants is extensive, including studies demonstrating embryotoxicity for DDT, methoxychlor, and hexachlorocyclohexane (17). Most human exposure is through food, air, or, in the case of trihalomethanes (THMs), absorption through skin. Exposure to the aforementioned compounds has been well documented, but is only now being monitored more closely. There were few data about nonoccupational exposure to potential toxicants until the Centers for Disease Control (CDC) began testing in 1999 (116 compounds) and 2003 (148 compounds) (18). *National Geographic* published an article in 2006 about a journalist who had his blood tested for levels of environmental toxicants to see what the average American accumulates in a lifetime. The tests, which cost around US$ 15,000, revealed 165 of 320 chemicals tested, including levels of a fire retardant used on airline seats 10 times higher than the average American, because of the many hours he spends in airplanes (19). The article highlights the fact that these chemicals are ubiquitous not only in the environment but also in our bodies.

The correlation between animal experiments and human experience was nicely demonstrated by Swan et al. when they examined the relationship between neonatal anogenital distance (AGD), a sexually dimorphic feature considered to be a sensitive indicator of masculinization and phthalate metabolites (20). Phthalates (diesters of 1,2-benzenedicarboxylic acid) are a ubiquitous group of chemicals found in hundreds of products ranging from soft plastic vinyl toys and flooring to shampoos, soaps, and nail polish. High-molecular-weight phthalates are used in the manufacturing of flexible vinyl for flooring, wall coverings, food contact applications, and medical devices. Low-molecular-weight phthalates are used in personal care products as solvents and plasticizers, for making lacquers, varnishes, and coatings used in pharmaceuticals for timed-release drugs. Humans rapidly metabolize phthalate diesters (their half-lives are generally less than 24 hours), and thus do not accumulate them. Urinary biomarkers (phthalate monoesters), therefore, represent exposure in the last one to two days only. Swan et al. evaluated mother–son pairs who had been recruited for an unrelated pregnancy cohort study ($n = 85$) and found a significant inverse relationship between the level of phthalate metabolites in the mother's third trimester urine and the son's AGD at birth. Higher prenatal phthalate metabolite levels correlated with a shorter AGD, which, in turn, was associated with incomplete testicular descent and smaller penile volume. These findings demonstrate the effect an environmental chemical can have on morphological development. Although implied, further investigation is needed to comment specifically on fertility or fecundity.

Making the jump from biological plausibility to biological truth can be a difficult task. The randomized controlled trial (RCT) is widely recognized as the gold standard in medical research, but the use of such trials poses distinct challenges when studying toxicity. RCTs would be unethical: Deliberately exposing individuals to potentially toxic chemicals is neither realistic nor to be condoned. Given these limitations, Stephen Genuis argues that clinical trials are not the only objective and credible way of establishing causality of a disease (21). He poses a simple analogy: It would be absurd to require an RCT to confirm the efficacy of parachutes to "prevent death and major trauma related to gravitational challenge" (22). In other words, not all research topics can be evaluated in identical manners.

There are other challenges for interpreting environmental toxicant studies. Time-lag bias is a limitation that is highlighted by our experience with in utero diethylstilbestrol (DES) exposure and vaginal cancer: Compounds can have devastating effects in the long term that are not immediately recognizable. Variations in genetic vulnerability and phenotypic response can also mask a compound's impact. For example, studies on BPA metabolism have shown induction of hepatic cytochrome p450s in humans (23,24). Individuals have p450 isoenzyme variation and thus will respond to bisphenols with different levels of metabolic activity. Furthermore, it can be difficult to interpret dose–response curves because hormonal toxicants do not always respond according to the classic dose–response curve. Estradiol, for instance, has a negative feedback mechanism upon gonadotropin-releasing hormone (GnRH) release from the hypothalamus until it reaches a critical concentration at which it begins to increase the release of GnRH. This culminates in the luteinizing hormone (LH) surge that initiates ovulation. If EDCs are hormone mimickers, they probably act in the same fashion: Effects may be seen at extremely low concentrations, but not at the higher concentrations used to test for chemical toxicity (25). This has been described as a nonmonotonic, hormetic, or "biphasic" dose–response curve (Fig. 61.1) and is described frequently in the endocrinology literature but not in the assessment of environmental agents.

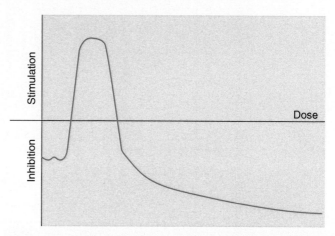

Figure 61.1 Hormetic/biphasic dose–response curve. The non-monotonic, hormetic, or "biphasic" dose–response curve describes the action of certain agents at different doses such that a very low dose of a chemical agent may trigger the opposite response to a very high dose.

Lastly, environmental health research is complicated by the phenomenon of bioaccumulation. Humans are exposed to thousands of compounds over a lifetime and it is therefore difficult to sort out the relationship between a specific compound and a specific outcome (26). The CDC's *National Report on Human Exposure to Environmental Chemicals* (14) is in its third edition and has only evaluated 148 compounds through blood and urine analysis of the known 80,000 synthetic compounds in our environment. With lag-time bias, phenotypic variation, the inability to perform RCTs, unpredictable dose– response mechanisms, and the bioaccumulation of multiple compounds at once, it is apparent how difficult "proof" of causality can be in environmental toxicology.

THE SEMINAL PLASMA MICROENVIRONMENT

At levels measured in parts per trillion (ppt) and parts per billion (ppb), hormones such as insulin and estradiol are bioactive in cells and tissue. EDCs appear to be bioactive at equally low levels found in our blood stream (25). Of great concern is the postulation that the seminal plasma acts as a chemical concentrator, increasing levels of various environmental toxicants in the fluid surrounding our next generation. Men living in agrarian areas where use of pesticides is high have higher pesticide levels in their blood and semen, and lower sperm counts and motility than men living further away (27).

As mentioned previously, humans rapidly metabolize phthalate diesters, and do not accumulate them. Despite fast metabolization, the omnipresence of phthalates in our environment raises concern. A study in 2003 from Columbia University Center for Children's Environmental Health found that among 60 pregnant women tested, 100% had measurable urinary phthalate levels despite being sampled from different areas of both New York City ($n = 30$) and Krakow, Poland ($n = 30$) (28). Concurrent research from the Harvard School of Public Health found a dose–response relationship between urine levels of phthalate metabolites and a decrease in sperm motility and concentration in a cohort of 168 infertile men (29). Additional studies demonstrated similar results (26,30). A conflicting study from Sweden, however, found no change in semen quality in 234 young men recruited at the time of their medical exam for entry into the military based on urine phthalate levels (31). Russ Hauser, a Harvard researcher, brings to light multiple methodological and analytical differences between these studies in a review article that calls into question the validity of the Swedish study and comparability of the study results (30). Most notable are the study population differences: The Swedish study recruited young men, and the American studies had older infertile patients. Although not conclusive, the data suggest phthalates play a role in decreased sperm quality and possibly fertility.

Conflicting data also exist for many other potential reproductive toxicants. The trihalomethanes are a group of chemical by-products of the chlorination processes used to disinfect drinking water. They have been a source of investigation for infertility and birth defects. One THM,

bromodichloromethane, has been associated with low sperm counts and increased abnormal semen morphology (32), but the majority of studies in both rats and humans have not found conclusive evidence that trihalomethanes decrease sperm quality or quantity (33). Additional investigations have questioned a relationship between THM exposure and spontaneous abortion (34,35). In 2000, an international workshop gathered to assess the impact of disinfectant by-products on reproduction and concluded that more research on methods of exposure assessment needed to be done to properly evaluate exposure risk (36). Since that time, a well-documented case–control study of over 2400 pregnancies in North Carolina did not find an association between THMs and spontaneous abortion (37). The study enrolled patients at seven weeks' gestation or less, sampled weekly drinking water from three distinct THM-profile regions, and specifically analyzed exposure during critical periods of fetal development.

Another chemical that causes concern is the pesticide dichlorodiphenyldichloroethylene (DDE), a persistent remnant of DDT, which, although no longer being produced in the United States, is sporadically used in Mexico (27), India, and China (38). Despite initially using pilot data, two studies were unable to demonstrate an association between sperm quality and DDE in both infertile U.S. patients ($n = 12$) and older Swedish fishermen ($n = 195$) (39,40). At this time, the evidence suggesting a risk of DDE to male fertility at casual exposure levels is still being evaluated.

PCBs, much like DDT, have been banned in the United States since the late 1970s. PCBs are synthetic, persistent, halogenated, lipophilic substances that are still ubiquitous in our environment today. They have varying hormonal functions: some act as weak estrogens and some are antiestrogenic. PCBs were used as early as 1881 in cutting or thinning oils, as lubricants, and as electrical insulators. In the 1930s they were reported to cause "chloracne" and even death from liver failure in occupational exposures (41). The Hudson River is perhaps the most famous site of PCB contamination from over 30 years of General Electric dumping PCBs until successfully sued to stop in 1975. We encounter PCBs primarily through the diet, but they can enter our systems by dermal contact (household dust) and inhalation. The half-life in some cases is >10 years; hence, their existence today (42).

Inhibition Stimulation

Dose

The connection between seminal plasma PCB levels and sperm quality was first shown in 1986 (43). It became clear in 2002 that PCBs were not the guilty molecules, but it was their active metabolites that were responsible for gamete abnormalities (44). Several environmental exposure studies show a consistent decrease in sperm quality in relation to seminal plasma PCB metabolite levels across different age groups: 18–21–year–olds (45), 30-year-old infertile couples, and 39- and 50-year-old fishermen (40). Russ Hauser at the Harvard School of Public Health has spent over six years studying PCBs and their effect on male factor infertility. He makes a strong case that the epidemiological data support an inverse association of PCBs with reduced semen quality, specifically reduced sperm motility. The associations found are generally consistent across studies, despite a range of PCB levels, methods of measuring PCB levels, and methods of measuring semen quality (30).

Nonpersistent pesticides or "contemporary-use" pesticides are those that are currently in use for killing insects, weeds, and other pests. While nonpersistent in the environment, heavy use of pest control in the developed world means that most people receive at least some exposure to low levels of these chemicals. Several epidemiological studies on occupational exposure to contemporary-use pesticides have been reported. In one cross-sectional study, greenhouse workers ($n = 122$) exposed to over a dozen pesticides were stratified into low, medium, or high exposure groups. The highest exposure group showed a higher proportion of abnormal sperm and lower median sperm counts in workers with more than 10 years of experience compared to those with less than five years (46). The study was appropriately adjusted for sexual abstinence and other potential cofounders. Juhler et al. investigated dietary exposure to pesticides and semen quality in a cross-sectional study of organic farmers compared to traditional farmers (47). Through food frequency questionnaires and pesticide monitoring programs they found that men with a lower intake of organic food had lower proportions of normally shaped sperm using strict criteria after controlling for various confounders (2.5 vs. 3.7%; $p = 0.003$). However, there were no differences between groups in 14 other semen parameters. Oliva et al. had similar results in Argentina (48), but Larsen et al. did not find significant differences in sperm quality between Danish farmers who sprayed pesticides and those who did not (49). Unfortunately for the sake of clarity, none of these studies looked at individual pesticide exposure, only exposure in general. This lack of specificity indicated the ever-present need for more controlled investigations that can link measurable quantities of these newer compounds to sperm quality and ultimately fertility.

Several studies have specifically investigated exposure to organophosphate pesticides (50,51) and found similar results to the broad cross-sectional studies mentioned previously. Whorton et al. (52) studied workers who packaged carbaryl (a common insecticide marketed under the name Sevin since 1958) and found an increased incidence of oligozoospermia (<20 million sperm/ml) compared with a reference group of chemical workers. Fifteen percent of exposed workers had sperm concentrations below the reference value of 20 million sperm/ml compared with 5.5% of nonexposed controls ($p = 0.07$). Wyrobek et al. (53) reported an association between carbaryl exposure and sperm morphology soon thereafter. The distribution of abnormal sperm morphology was significantly higher for exposed workers ($p < 0.005$), and the proportion of teratospermic men (>60% abnormal) was larger in the exposed group (29%; $n = 50$) compared with controls

(12%, $n = 34$; $p = 0.06$). Meeker et al. (54) found an inverse relationship between sperm concentration and motility in 272 men recruited from infertile couples and urinary levels of 1-naphthol, a metabolite of both carbaryl and naphthalene. They suggested that "an interquartile range increase in carbaryl metabolite levels in urine is associated with a 4% decrease in sperm motility," and may result in a significant increase in the number of subfertile men across the U.S. population. In summary, there are human data supporting the association between contemporary-use pesticides and decreased semen quality, but the public health implications are yet to be determined.

The estrogenic monomer BPA is used in the manufacture of polycarbonate plastic products, in resins lining metal cans, in dental sealants, and in blends with other types of plastic products. Typical products include polyvinyl chloride (PVC), medical tubing, water pipes, soda bottles, and baby bottles (Table 61.1). Over time, the ester bonds linking BPA molecules in polycarbonate and resins undergo hydrolysis, resulting in the release of free BPA into food, beverages, and the environment. This hydrolysis is accelerated by heat or contact with acidic and basic substances, such that repeated washing or contact with substances of different acidity leads to increased leaching of BPA from polycarbonate. BPA levels have been found in rivers and streams, drinking water, indoor air, and leaching out of landfills (55). Numerous monitoring studies now show almost ubiquitous human exposure to biologically active levels of this chemical (56).

The Food and Drug Administration (FDA) and Environmental Protection Agency (EPA) currently consider daily exposure of BPAs of <50 μg/kg to be safe based on megadose studies in which the lowest tested dose was 1000-fold higher. Now, over 40 studies have been published, reporting significant effects in rats and mice at doses <50 μg/kg (57). Previous "safe levels" of exposure are now under scrutiny as older studies are being recognized as limited because of assay sensitivity. Moreover, it is difficult, but not impossible, to conduct laboratory experiments and avoid contamination from polycarbonate lab plastics.

Mechanistically, BPAs exert estrogenic effects through the classic nuclear estrogen receptor, by acting as selective estrogen receptor modulators, and by initiating rapid responses via estrogen receptors presumably associated with the plasma membrane (55). BPAs bind very little to sex hormone-binding protein and thus have an unconjugated free fraction of 8% that can be delivered to cells more easily than estradiol, which has a free fraction of 3.5% (58). Additionally, pregnant women have a significantly higher affinity for BPAs than nonpregnant women (59). Indeed, BPAs have been detected in fetal cord serum, maternal serum during pregnancy, and amniotic fluid (60). For unclear reasons, the level of BPAs found in the amniotic fluid of 15–18-week gestations is five times higher than serum levels, but returns to a concentration similar to fetal and maternal serum in the third trimester (Fig. 61.2). Although the metabolism of BPAs is not completely understood, these findings can be explained by the development of fetal capacity to metabolize BPAs in the late second trimester, possibly by the liver. Metabolism

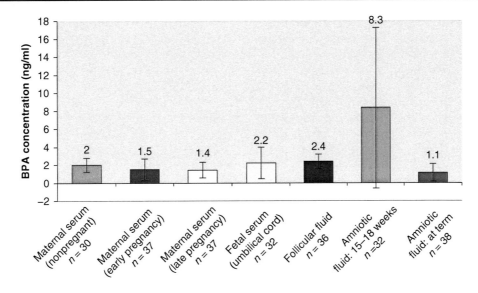

Figure 61.2 Bisphenol A concentrations in human biological fluids. Columns represent mean bisphenol A (BPA) values, and "whiskers" give the 95% confidence intervals of the values. The amniotic fluid at 15–18 weeks was significantly elevated ($p < 0.0001$) compared with other biological fluids. *Source*: From Ref. 61.

research, like epidemiological studies, is just beginning to be published to accompany a large body of animal research already accessible. Whereas BPAs are newer molecules, heavy metals have long been implicated in impairing fertility. The most frequently studied metals are lead and mercury. Physicians have recognized lead as a reproductive toxicant for well over a century. Lead salts, in fact, were once used as abortificants. The effects on reproduction were well summarized in 1944 (62):

It is generally agreed that if pregnancy does occur it is frequently characterized by miscarriage, intrauterine death of the fetus, premature birth and, if living children are born, they are usually smaller, weaker, slower in development, and have a higher infant mortality.

Beyond broad generalizations, however, there is little evidence supporting the claim that lead affects fertility per se. Animal studies have shown altered spermatogenesis at 35 μg/dl (the CDC-cited safe level is <10 μg/dl), and a few case reports have observed similar findings in humans with levels over 40 μg/dl (63). It has been demonstrated that lead crosses into the seminal fluid, but in general, studies focused on male fertility and lead exposure are lacking. In Denmark, a prospective cohort of workers in a battery manufacturing plant had average serum lead levels of 35.9 μg/dl, but no decrease in the birth rate [odds ratio (OR) = 0.98, 95% confidence interval (CI) 0.88–1.12] (64). A study of welders in Canada demonstrated a decrease in sperm quality, but did not correlate those findings with decreased fertility (65). Likewise, there is scant evidence of increased spontaneous abortion rates or increased time to pregnancy (TTP). No doubt, more information on the impact of lead on reproduction will be forthcoming as newer techniques of investigation are developed.

THE FOLLICLE MICROENVIRONMENT

One by-product of in vitro fertilization (IVF) has been access to follicular fluid for studies demonstrating the presence of toxicants (66–69). The pesticides DDE, mirex, hexachloroethane, and 1,2,4-trichlorobenzene, along with PCBs, BPA, and phthalates, have been implicated in infertility, but have not consistently demonstrated adverse IVF or pregnancy outcomes. Variables examined include number of oocytes retrieved, recovered, and fertilized, cleavage rates, and pregnancy rates. In a Canadian study of 21 IVF couples, higher DDE levels correlated with failed fertilization, but higher follicular PCB levels correlated with pregnancy success (66). A study of IVF patients in 1984 showed that oocyte recovery and embryo cleavage rates were inversely related to chlorinated hydrocarbon concentrations (69), although a subsequent study showed a positive relationship (68). Most remarkable, however, is the fact that in all of these studies, pesticides are present in follicular fluid at the time of resumption of meiosis when chromosome susceptibility is at its highest.

For the most part, follicular toxicant concentrations are lower than serum levels (59,66). Knowing the relationship between serum and follicle concentrations has allowed speculation on the fertility outcomes of non-IVF patients based on serum levels. Law et al. pulled frozen third trimester blood samples from 380 planned pregnancies recruited for the 1959–1965 Collaborate Perinatal Project and compared serum levels of PCBs and DDE with TTP and fecundability. Dose–response curves with proportional hazards suggested that as PCB and DDE levels increase, the probability of pregnancy decreases. Since DDE and PCBs are lipophilic, the serum levels obtained in this study were adjusted for maternal lipid volume (an appropriate adjustment not done in most published reports). Once adjusted, the increased TTP attributed to DDE disappeared and the PCB effect became considerably weaker, leaving no significant difference in TTP or fecundability based on either substance's concentration (70). These results echo the findings of a cohort of Swedish fishermen from which multiple papers have been published showing no relationship between fish consumption (including persistent organochlorine and PCB exposure) and TTP, miscarriage rate, stillbirths, or subfertility (71). In the end, there is little evidence to support the association between DDE, PCBs, and subfertility. Once again, however, the presence of such toxic substances bathing the preovulatory oocyte is worrisome given the protective barrier the reproductive organs have to passage of most substances. More studies will be required to understand if there is any adverse impact of these substances on oocyte DNA.

Just as paternal lead and mercury exposure is widely thought to impair fertility, so is maternal exposure. Lead has been shown to destroy oocytes and lead to follicular atresia in rodents and primates (72), but has only been measured in follicular fluid in two published human studies available on MEDLINE (73,74), while mercury measurement has not been reported at all. Various rodent and nonhuman primate studies have demonstrated suppression of menarche, decreased circulating progesterone levels, and less frequent menstrual cycles with lead exposure (63). Nevertheless, examination of human epidemiological data is less conclusive. First, the mechanism of lead's toxicity is not well understood: It is unclear if there is a direct toxic effect on the ovary, the effect is mediated through a central neuroendocrine dysfunction, or both. Second, older studies demonstrate an association between high-dose occupational exposure and spontaneous fetal loss (75), but a later study was unable to find an association between the two when 304 women living near a lead smelter in Yugoslavia were compared with 335 women from a nearby town with low serum lead levels (76).

As mentioned, mercury levels have not been reported in follicular fluid, but mercury's effect on the developing fetus in utero has been subject to a great deal of scrutiny.

Maternal tobacco use would seem to be one of the simplest areas to modify toxin accumulation in the ovarian follicular fluid. Objective measurements of tobacco compounds and their metabolites in follicular fluid correlate with subjective measures of lower quality of ovarian, gamete, and embryo quality in smokers and in those exposed to passive smoke (77). A range of chemical toxins, such as nicotine, carbon monoxide, and follicular fluid cadmium concentration is also reported to be higher in smokers than in nonsmokers (78).

THE AMNIOTIC SAC MICROENVIRONMENT

Over a decade ago, the endocrinologist Howard Bern of UC Berkeley in California coined the phrase the "fragile fetus" while explaining the vulnerability of the developing fetus in utero to insult and exposure. This phrase has proven true when it comes to lead and mercury exposure. For years it was assumed that the developing fetus was protected by the placenta. But a study in 2005 by the

Environmental Working Group tested the blood of 10 randomly selected infants and the results found 200 toxic elements in the cord blood of the babies. These included mercury, industrial chemicals, pollutants, and pesticides. http://www.ewg.org/reports/bodyburden2/execsumm. php Mercury is a common atmospheric element that is released from the earth's crust. Inorganic mercury gets converted to soluble forms that are deposited into soil and water by precipitation. Sources such as coal mining "rain down" mercury across the earth, depositing it on both land and sea. These soluble mercury forms are then methylated via microbes or nonenzymatic processes, and readily taken up by proteins. Methyl mercury then rapidly accumulates in the food chain through predatory fish. Humans, at the top of the food chain, acquire mercury through food consumption as well. The greatest concern with mercury is not fertility – there is little evidence correlating mercury poisoning and infertility – but the developmental effects of in utero exposure.

In theory, the fetus is particularly vulnerable to mercury (79). In adults, methyl mercury can be converted to inorganic mercury by intestinal flora and 90% eventually removed from our system through the feces. The fetus, with neither gut flora, nor a fully functional liver, nor the ability to defecate, is virtually guaranteed to rapidly accumulate this heavy metal. We must also consider the process of urination: In utero urine is cycled from the amniotic fluid into the developing fetus' nose and mouth, and back into the amniotic fluid, unlike in adults, where urination is an essential mechanism for clearing toxicants from the body. Couple higher toxicant levels with deficient excretion mechanisms and there is the potential for alarming toxicant accumulation. Moreover, because levels of circulating binding proteins are lower in the fetus, there is a higher concentration of circulating unbound toxicants. Lastly, the blood–brain barrier is more permeable during development and thus the developing brain proportionally receives greater exposure to toxicants than the adult brain. In theory, this can increase the vulnerability of the fetus to neurotoxins such as mercury.

We have known for decades that lead and mercury pass through the placenta, into the amniotic fluid, and directly to the baby in concentrations near maternal blood serum. Umbilical cord blood levels of lead are usually only 10–20% lower than maternal serum levels (80), but mercury (methyl mercury) levels are generally higher than maternal serum levels (63). Mercury has been the most publicized environmental toxicant in relation to reproductive health, and explains the FDA's recommended limitations on fish consumption in pregnancy. Current FDA recommendations are for women of childbearing age to avoid fish that are likely to contain high levels of methyl mercury (>1µg/g), including swordfish, shark, tilefish, and king mackerel. Fortunately, many U.S. sport fish have levels lower than this (Fig. 61.3). In Massachusetts, though, there are no bodies of water that have safe levels of mercury for fish consumption by women of childbearing age. A statement to this effect was issued by the Massachusetts Department of Public Health

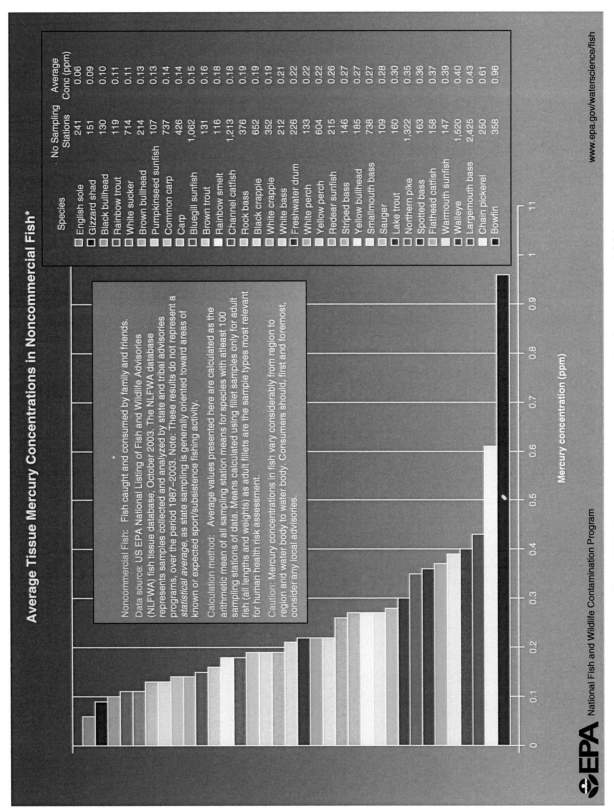

Figure 61.3   Average tissue mercury concentrations in noncommercial fish.

in 2004. This was an extension on an advisory from 1994 to 2001 (81):

> Previously issued statewide fish consumption advisory which cautioned pregnant women to avoid eating fish from all freshwater bodies due to concerns about mercury contamination ... now include women of childbearing age who may become pregnant, nursing mothers and children under 12 years of age.

Epidemiological studies show that an increase of only 1 ppm of mercury lowers the average cognitive score of a child (82), while high-dose exposure can lead to neonatal central nervous system (CNS) damage and even death. Minamata disease, mercury poisoning caused by dumping in Japan's Bay of Minamata, is an example of the potential effects of high-dose exposure (83).

However, fish are an important source of omega-3 fatty acids, which are essential for fetal neurodevelopment, and there is some evidence that higher fish consumption is correlative with greater cognitive development. A cohort study of 8947 women in England found that women who consumed over 340 g (12 oz) of fish per week during pregnancy had children with significantly greater outcomes on 14 of 23 neurodevelopmental measures, including various fine-motor, communication, social development milestones, and verbal IQ at eight years of age (84).

Unfortunately, recommendations about limiting fish consumption in pregnancy may overestimate the risk of chronic low-dose mercury intake and underestimate the benefit of omega-3 fatty acids. The challenge is to find the correct balance. Two important prospective observational studies, the Seychelles Child Development Study (85) ($n = 779$) and the Faroe Islands Cohort Study (86) ($n = 878$), followed fish consumption and cognitive function for nine and 14 years, respectively, and reported conflicting results. The Seychelles study has not shown an association between in utero methyl mercury levels and neurocognitive function, while the Faroe Islands Cohort has consistently shown a negative correlation after correcting for postnatal exposure. In response to these two studies, the World Health Organization (WHO) published a new maternal serum cutoff level of 5.6 µg/dl, and a tolerable weekly mercury intake of 1.6 µg/kg to "protect the developing fetus and embryo, the most sensitive subgroup of the population" (83).

A second way of evaluating fetal mercury exposure is by cord blood mercury levels. The U.S. National Research Council has issued concern for cord blood levels >58 ppm or (5.8 µg/l) (87). Large fish-consuming populations have been shown to have mercury levels average high above this. In Taiwan, 65 pregnant women filled out a questionnaire in the third trimester and gave blood samples, placenta tissue, and cord blood after delivery. Eighty-nine percent of the maternal blood mercury concentrations exceeded the U.S. National Research Council recommended value. Levels were highest in women who ate fish more than three times a week while pregnant (88). In Hawaii, a study of 308 newborns showed a mean cord blood concentration of 4.8 µg/l, with 28% above the recommended safety value (89). While it is clear that fish consumption is correlated with both maternal and fetal mercury levels, the developmental significance is still being evaluated.

Other amniotic sac microenvironment toxicants have been implicated in affecting fertility. Guo et al. studied one of the only prospective cohorts of high-dose PCB exposure when contaminated cooking oil was used in Taiwan in 1979 (90). In 1998 they contacted children exposed to PCBs in utero and performed sperm analysis. They found abnormal sperm motility, morphology, and decreased ability to penetrate hamster eggs. Fertility rates have yet to be reported.

The translation of subfertility across generations is one of the most interesting and concerning concepts to arise out of reproductive environmental health research. Belgian investigators failed to show a difference in serum concentration of the pesticide by-product DDE in fertile men ($n = 73$) and infertile men ($n = 82$), but a sub-analysis of the blood of mothers of the patients demonstrated higher serum pesticide levels in mothers of subfertile men ($n = 19$) than in those of fertile men ($n = 23$) (91). While these results can only offer hypotheses on the role of exposure to pesticides in utero and fertility, they do provide reason for caution toward potential toxicants and increase the need to verify their potential risks.

THE GLOBAL ENVIRONMENT

The global environment is the most difficult to deconstruct. In truth, the collection of studies presented here probably reflects alteration in the functionality of semen or ovarian follicles. There is, however, the potential for environmental agents to affect the systems that support pregnancy. For example, environmental estrogens may change the hormonal balance that allows sufficient endometrial growth, affect angiogenesis necessary to support a developing placenta, or cause/worsen endometriosis and tubal patency. These details are sure to be elucidated in the near future. Nevertheless, regional differences in fertility rates highlight the potential effect of the global environment on fertility (92).

A study that falls into this category of the "global environment" was published in 1999 by Khattak et al. Their prospective case-controlled trial on the effect of occupational maternal exposure to organic solvents involved pregnant women exposed to solvents and matched by age, gravity, smoking, and alcohol usage to comparable pregnant women exposed to a recognized nonteratogenic agent. In addition to an increased incidence of miscarriage [54/117 (46.2%) vs. 24/125 (19.2%); $p < 0.001$], the women in the exposure group were 13 times more likely to have children with major cardiovascular or CNS malformations (93). The authors concluded that occupational exposure to organic solvents in pregnancy is associated with increased risk of major fetal malformations. Where this effect takes place is not clear: it could be either the gametes or the amniotic microenvironment or both.

Animal research has demonstrated that fetal alterations may continue to impact future generations through persistent epigenetic changes. Genome methylation or histone

Table 61.2 The Fertility/Fecundity Impact of Chemical Exposure During Adulthood

Substance	Potential effect on females	Potential effect on males
Bisphenol A (BPA)	Oocyte chromosomal abnormalities, recurrent abortions	Poor semen quality
Chlorinated hydrocarbons	Menstrual abnormalities, reduced fertility, endometriosis, fetal loss	Poor semen quality and hormonal changes
Disinfection by-products	Fetal loss, irregular menses	
Ethylene oxide	Fetal loss	Poor semen quality and miscarriage in partner
Glycol ethers (paints, thinners, printing inks)	Fetal loss, reduced fertility	Decreased semen quality
Heavy Metals (Pb, Hg, Cd)	Fetal loss, reduced fertility, irregular menses	Abnormal sperm, reduced fertility
Pesticides	Irregular menses, reduced fertility, fetal loss	Poor semen quality, miscarriage in female partner
Phthalates (plastic additives)	Fetal loss, irregular menses, lower fertility	Decreased semen quality
Solvents (benzene, toluene xylene, and others)	Fetal loss, irregular menses, lower fertility	Reduced fertility, decreased semen quality
Cigarette smoke	Reduced fertility, miscarriage, early menopause	Reduced fertility, decreased semen quality

Source: Modified from "Challenged conceptions: Environmental chemicals and fertility"; http://www.rhtp.org/fertility/vallombrosa/documents/Challenged_Conceptions.pdf, pg 5.

acylation can alter gene expression without modifying the DNA sequence and can transmit from generation to generation with a higher penetrance than DNA mutations themselves (94). Anway et al. illustrated this concept when they observed that rats exposed to vinclozolin (an antiandrogenic compound that is used as a fungicide in wine vineyards) or methoxychlor (an estrogenic compound that has replaced DDT as a pesticide) resulted in increased male infertility in F1 generation rats and persisted in over 90% of all male rats through the next three generations (95). These kind of results in humans have only been hinted at by the association of elevated maternal serum levels of DDE with grown children's fertility rates, (88) and the transgenerational effect of DES and vaginal cancer (96).

Even more interesting (and complicating) are reports that environmental agents thought to be toxic may actually enhance reproduction. Higher follicular fluid levels of PCBs have been associated with better IVF outcomes (66), higher DDE levels associated with reduced TTP (97), and in vitro work has shown that DDE stimulates the aromatase enzyme system of granulosa cells in synergy with follicular-stimulating hormone (FSH) (98) and thus may speed follicle maturation. Additionally, in Denmark, 192 IVF couples with paternal exposure to pesticides, fungicides, and herbicides had a 21% spontaneous abortion rate compared with 28% in the reference population of 2925 (99). How these findings will ultimately be interpreted is not presently clear.

CLINICAL CONSIDERATIONS

It is relatively easy to accept research indicating the presence of environmental toxicants in the semen, the oocyte, and the amniotic fluid. Translation of the epidemiological and observational research to the bedside is challenging. Clinically, how do we counsel our patients? We agree that providers should be cautious, not alarming, given

that the literature is suggestive, not conclusive, of links between EDCs and decreased reproductive performance (Table 61.2) (100). One way to incorporate knowledge about environmental exposures is to include questions during history taking about exposure to solvents, pesticides, or heavy metals. Ask patients where they live and where they have lived, where they work, what they eat, how much fish they consume, and what exposures their parents may have had to plastics, heavy metals, pesticides, and industrial solvents. Several formal exposure evaluations have been published for this purpose (101,102). Encourage patients, particularly those thinking of starting a family, to eat organic. A summary of the 12 fruits and vegetables that contain the most pesticides, known as the "Dirty Dozen" is available from the Environmental Working Group (EWG) http://www.ewg.org/foodnews/summary/. If at all possible, these foods should be selected from an organic source. If organic options are either not available or are too expensive, the "Clean 15" list contains the fruits and vegetables that contain the least pesticides (Table 61.3) and make excellent substitutions. The knowledge gained from history-taking can be used to advise patients according to the precautionary principle: (103). Educate patients on potential toxic exposures, and let them make efforts to avoid them. The data gathered can also become the basis for observational research opportunities to understand better which substances are most deleterious, and at what levels.

The role of toxin decontamination is neither well studied nor reported, but certainly is not new. Hippocrates wrote of solariums; religious groups recommend fasting; Aborigines wrote of sweat lodges and hot baths; Egyptians applied body wraps; and some Scandinavian cultures utilized saunas and steam baths (21). None of these decontamination methods have been studied and reported upon in the scientific literature, despite the many services advertised in every community in the world.

Table 61.3 A Summary of the "Dirty Dozen" and "Clean 15" Lists of Fruits and Vegetables Containing the Most and Least Pesticides, Respectively

Dirty dozen	Buy these organic	Clean 15	Lowest in pesticide
1	Apples	1	Onions
2	Celery	2	Sweet corn
3	Strawberries	3	Pineapples
4	Peaches	4	Avocado
5	Spinach	5	Asparagus
6	Nectarines—imported	6	Sweet peas
7	Grapes—imported	7	Mangoes
8	Sweet bell peppers	8	Eggplant
9	Potatoes	9	Cantaloupe—domestic
10	Blueberries—domestic	10	Kiwi
11	Lettuce	11	Cabbage
12	Kale/collard greens	12	Watermelon
		13	Sweet potatoes
		14	Grapefruit
		15	Mushrooms

Source: From EWG's Shopper's Guide to Pesticides.

In the end, the scientific communities at large remain unimpressed with the impact of EDCs. The National Academy of Science report on "Hormonally Active Agents in the Environment" (104) was unable to come to a consensus opinion on the topic; the WHO state-of-the-science assessment in 2002 (105) concluded that organochlorines (PCBs, DDE) do affect pregnancy in wildlife, but was uncertain about the effect on humans. Congress mandated the EPA, through the advisory of the Endocrine Disruptor Screening and Testing Advisory Committee (EDSTAC), to expand its current mandate to test all food-use pesticides and drinking water contaminants for hormonal activity. This is to include evaluation of the 80,000+ registered chemicals under the toxic substances control act of 1998 – a daunting task that requires prioritization. Currently, the EPA is reporting on the first 200 of these chemicals.

There has been much progress and expansion in investigating the role that different compounds play in our reproductive health. There is much more work needed, however, to draw any definitive conclusions. We must ask ourselves: Why are we allowing an "innocent until proven guilty" approach for chemical agents dispersed into our environment, when we insist the opposite for all pharmaceuticals? (21).

REFERENCES

1. Trubo R. Endocrine-disrupting chemicals probed as potential pathways to illness. JAMA 2005; 294: 291–3.
2. Nonaka K, Miura T, Peter K. Recent fertility decline in Dariusleut Hutterites: an extension of Eaton and Mayer's Hutterite fertility study. Hum Biol 1994; 66: 411–20.
3. Ventura SJ, Mosher WD, Curtin SC, Abma JC, Henshaw S. Trends in pregnancies and pregnancy rates by outcome: estimates for the United States, 1976–96. Vital Health Stat 2000; 21: 1–47.
4. Auger J, Kunstmann JM, Czyglik F, Jouannet P. Decline in semen quality among fertile men in Paris during the past 20 years. N Engl J Med 1995; 332: 281–5.
5. Carlsen E, Giwercman A, Keiding N, Skakkebaek NE. Evidence for decreasing quality of semen during past 50 years. BMJ 1992; 305: 609–13.
6. Brevini TA, Zanetto SB, Cillo F. Effects of endocrine disruptors on developmental and reproductive functions. Curr Drug Targets Immune Endocr Metabol Disord 2005; 5: 1–10.
7. Carson R, Darling L, Darling L. Silent Spring. Cambridge, MA: Houghton Mifflin, Riverside Press, 1962.
8. Colborn T. Nontraditional evaluation of risk from fish contaminants. In: Ahmed F, ed. Proceedings of a Symposiumon Issues in Seafood Safety. Washington, DC: National Academy of Sciences, Institute of Medicine, Food, and Nutrition Board, 1991.
9. Colborn T, Vom Saal FS, Soto AM. Developmental effects of endocrine-disrupting chemicals in wildlife and humans. Environ Health Perspect 1993; 101: 378–84.
10. Colborn T. Pesticides – how research has succeeded and failed to translate science into policy: endocrinological effects on wildlife. Environ Health Perspect 1995; 103(Suppl 6): 81–5.
11. Colborn T, Dumanoski D, Myers JP. Our Stolen Future: Are We Threatening Our Fertility, Intelligence, and Survival? A Scientific Detective Story. New York: Dutton, 1996.
12. Damstra T. Potential effects of certain persistent organic pollutants and endocrine disrupting chemicals on the health of children. J Clin Toxicol 2002; 40: 457–65.
13. Heilier JF, Nackers F, Verougstraete V, et al. Increased dioxin-like compounds in the serum of women with peritoneal endometriosis and deep endometriotic (adenomyotic) nodules. Fertil Steril 2005; 84: 305–12.
14. Sharpe RM, Fisher JS, Millar MM, Jobling S, Sumpter JP. Gestational and lactational exposure of rats to xenoestrogens results in reduced testicular size and sperm production. Environ Health Perspect 1995; 103: 1136–43.
15. Jadarmkunti UC, Kaliwal BB. Effect of dicofol formulation on estrous cycle and follicular dynamics in albino rats. J Basic Clin Physiol Pharmacol 1999; 10: 305–14.
16. Muller WF, Hobson W, Fuller GB, et al. Endocrine effects of chlorinated hydrocarbons in rhesus monkeys. Ecotoxicol Environ Saf 1978; 2: 161–72.
17. Alm H, Tiemann U, Torner H. Influence of organochlorine pesticides on development of mouse embryos in vitro. Reprod Toxicol 1996; 10: 321–6.
18. CDC. Third National Report on Human Exposure to Environmental Chemicals. Atlanta, GA: CDC, 2005.
19. Duncan D. The pollution within. National Geographic 2006; 210: 116–43.
20. Swan SH, Main KM, Liu F, et al. Decrease in anogenital distance among male infants with prenatal phthalate exposure. Environ Health Perspect 2005; 113: 1056–61.
21. Genuis SJ. Health issues and the environment – an emerging paradigm for providers of obstetrical and gynaecological health care. Hum Reprod 2006; 21: 2201–8.

22. Smith GC, Pell JP. Parachute use to prevent death and major trauma related to gravitational challenge: systematic review of randomised controlled trials. BMJ 2003; 327: 1459–61.

23. Niwa T, Tsutsui M, Kishimoto K, et al. Inhibition of drug-metabolizing enzyme activity in human hepatic cytochrome P450s by Bisphenol A. Biol Pharm Bull 2000; 23: 498–501.

24. Niwa T, Fujimoto M, Kishimoto K, et al. Metabolism and interaction of Bisphenol A in human hepatic cytochrome P450 and steroidogenic CYP17. Biol Pharm Bull 2001; 24: 1064–7.

25. Welshons WV, Thayer KA, Judy BM, et al. Large effects from small exposures. I. Mechanisms for endocrine-disrupting chemicals with estrogenic activity. Environ Health Perspect 2003; 111: 994–1006.

26. Hauser R, Williams P, Altshul L, Calafat AM. Evidence of interaction between polychlorinated biphenyls and phthalates in relation to human sperm motility. Environ Health Perspect 2005; 113: 425–30.

27. Younglai EV, Holloway AC, Foster WG. Environmental and occupational factors affecting fertility and IVF success. Hum Reprod Update 2005; 11: 43–57.

28. Adibi JJ, Perera FP, Jedrychowski W, et al. Prenatal exposures to phthalates among women in New York City and Krakow, Poland. Environ Health Perspect 2003; 111: 1719–22.

29. Duty SM, Silva MJ, Barr DB, et al. Phthalate exposure and human semen parameters. Epidemiology 2003; 14: 269–77.

30. Hauser R. The environment and male fertility: recent research on emerging chemicals and semen quality. Semin Reprod Med 2006; 24: 156–67.

31. Jonsson BA, Richthoff J, Rylander L, Giwercman A, Hagmar L. Urinary phthalate metabolites and biomarkers of reproductive function in young men. Epidemiology 2005; 16: 487–93.

32. Fenster L, Waller K, Windham G, et al. Trihalomethane levels in home tapwater and semen quality. Epidemiology 2003; 14: 650–8.

33. Shaw GM, Ranatunga D, Quach T, et al. Trihalomethane exposures from municipal water supplies and selected congenital malformations. Epidemiology 2003; 14: 191–9.

34. Waller K, Swan SH, DeLorenze G, Hopkins B. Trihalomethanes in drinking water and spontaneous abortion. Epidemiology 1998; 9: 134–40.

35. Waller K, Swan SH, Windham GC, Fenster L. Influence of exposure assessment methods on risk estimates in an epidemiologic study of total trihalomethane exposure and spontaneous abortion. J Expo Anal Environ Epidemiol 2001; 11: 522–31.

36. Arbuckle TE, Hrudey SE, Krasner SW, et al. Assessing exposure in epidemiologic studies to disinfection by-products in drinking water: report from an international workshop. Environ Health Perspect 2002; 110(Suppl 1): 53–60.

37. Savitz DA, Singer PC, Herring AH, et al. Exposure to drinking water disinfection by-products and pregnancy loss. Am J Epidemiol 2006; 164: 1043–51.

38. Garcia AM. Pesticide exposure and women's health. Am J Ind Med 2003; 44: 584–94.

39. Hauser R, Chen Z, Pothier L, Ryan L, Altshul L. The relationship between human semen parameters and environmental exposure to polychlorinated biphenyls and p,p2-DDE. Environ Health Perspect 2003; 111: 1505–11.

40. Rignell-Hydbom A, Rylander L, Giwercman A, et al. Exposure to CB-153 and p,p2-DDE and male reproductive function. Hum Reprod 2004; 19: 2066–75.

41. Schroeder M. Did Westinghouse keep mum on PCBs? Business Week, 1991.

42. Phillips DL, Smith AB, Burse VW, et al. Half-life of polychlorinated biphenyls in occupationally exposed workers. Arch Environ Health 1989; 44: 351–4.

43. Bush B, Bennett AH, Snow JT. Polychlorobiphenyl congeners, p,p'-DDE, and sperm function in humans. Arch Environ Contam Toxicol 1986; 15: 333–41.

44. Dallinga JW, Moonen EJ, Dumoulin JC, et al. Decreased human semen quality and organochlorine compounds in blood. Hum Reprod 2002; 17: 1973–9.

45. Richthoff J, Rylander L, Jonsson BA, et al. Serum levels of 2,22,4,42,5,52-hexachlorobiphenyl (CB-153) in relation to markers of reproductive function in young males from the general Swedish population. Environ Health Perspect 2003; 111: 409–13.

46. Abell A, Ernst E, Bonde JP. Semen quality and sexual hormones in greenhouse workers. Scand J Work Environ Health 2000; 26: 492–500.

47. Juhler RK, Larsen SB, Meyer O, et al. Human semen quality in relation to dietary pesticide exposure and organic diet. Arch Environ Contam Toxicol 1999; 37: 415–23.

48. Oliva A, Spira A, Multigner L. Contribution of environmental factors to the risk of male infertility. Hum Reprod 2001; 16: 1768–76.

49. Larsen SB, Joffe M, Bonde JP. Time to pregnancy and exposure to pesticides in Danish farmers. ASCLEPIOS Study Group. Occup Environ Med 1998; 55: 278–83.

50. Padungtod C, Savitz DA, Overstreet JW, et al. Occupational pesticide exposure and semen quality among Chinese workers. J Occup Environ Med 2000; 42: 982–92.

51. Kamijima M, Hibi H, Gotoh M, et al. A survey of semen indices in insecticide sprayers. J Occup Health 2004; 46: 109–18.

52. Whorton MD, Milby TH, Stubbs HA, Avashia BH, Hull EQ. Testicular function among carbaryl exposed exployees. J Toxicol Environ Health 1979; 5: 929–41.

53. Wyrobek AJ, Watchmaker G, Gordon L, et al. Sperm shape abnormalities in carbaryl-exposed employees. Environ Health Perspect 1981; 40: 255–65.

54. Meeker JD, Ryan L, Barr DB, et al. The relationship of urinary metabolites of carbaryl/naphthalene and chlorpyrifos with human semen quality. Environ Health Perspect 2004; 112: 1665–70.

55. Welshons WV, Nagel SC, Vom Saal FS. Large effects from small exposures. III. endocrine mechanisms mediating effects of Bisphenol A at levels of human exposure. Endocrinology 2006; 147: S56–69.

56. Calafat AM, Kuklenyik Z, Reidy JA, et al. Urinary concentrations of bisphenol A and 4-nonylphenol in a human reference population. Environ Health Perspect 2005; 113: 391–5.

57. Vom Saal FS, Welshons WV. Large effects from small exposures. II. the importance of positive controls in low-dose research on Bisphenol A. Environ Res 2006; 100: 50–76.

58. Nagel SC, Vom Saal FS, Welshons WV. The effective free fraction of estradiol and xenoestrogens in human

serum measured by whole cell uptake assays: physiology of delivery modifies estrogenic activity. Proc Soc Exp Biol Med 1998; 217: 300–9.

59. Ikezuki Y, Tsutsumi O, Takai Y, Kamei Y, Taketani Y. Determination of bisphenol A concentrations in human biological fluids reveals significant early prenatal exposure. Hum Reprod 2002; 17: 2839–41.

60. Schonfelder G, Wittfoht W, Hopp H, et al. Parent bisphenol A accumulation in the human maternal–fetal–placental unit. Environ Health Perspect 2002; 110: A703–7.

61. Tsutsumi O. Assessment of human contamination of estrogenic endocrine-disrupting chemicals and their risk for human reproduction. J Steroid Biochem Mol Biol 2005; 93: 325–30.

62. Cantarow A, Trumper M. Lead Poisoning. Baltimore: Williams & Wilkins, 1944.

63. Miller R, Bellinger D. Metals. In: Paul M, ed. Occupational and Environmental Reproductive Hazards: A Guide for Clinicians. Baltimore: Williams & Wilkins, 1993.

64. Bonde JP, Kolstad H. Fertility of Danish battery workers exposed to lead. Int J Epidemiol 1997; 26: 1281–8.

65. Bigelow PL, Jarrell J, Young MR, Keefe TJ, Love EJ. Association of semen quality and occupational factors: comparison of case-control analysis and analysis of continuous variables. Fertil Steril 1998; 69: 11–18.

66. Younglai EV, Foster WG, Hughes EG, Trim K, Jarrell JF. Levels of environmental contaminants in human follicular fluid, serum, and seminal plasma of couples undergoing in vitro fertilization. Arch Environ Contam Toxicol 2002; 43: 121–6.

67. Foster WG, Jarrell JF, Younglai EV, et al. An overview of some reproductive toxicology studies conducted at health Canada. Toxicol Ind Health 1996; 12: 447–59.

68. Jarrell J, Villeneuve D, Franklin C, et al. Contamination of human ovarian follicular fluid and serum by chlorinated organic compounds in three Canadian cities. CMAJ 1993; 148: 1321–7.

69. Trapp M, Baukloh V, Bohnet HG, Heeschen W. Pollutants in human follicular fluid. Fertil Steril 1984; 42: 146–8.

70. Law DC, Klebanoff MA, Brock JW, Dunson DB, Longnecker MP. Maternal serum levels of polychlorinated biphenyls and 1,1-dichloro-2,2-bis (p-chlorophenyl) ethylene (DDE) and time to pregnancy. Am J Epidemiol 2005; 162: 523–32.

71. Axmon A, Rylander L, Stromberg U, et al. Polychlorinated biphenyls in serum and time to pregnancy. Environ Res 2004; 96: 186–95.

72. Vermande-Van Eck GJ, Meigs JW. Changes in the ovary of the rhesus monkey after chronic lead intoxication. Fertil Steril 1960; 11: 223–34.

73. Silberstein T, Saphier O, Paz-Tal O, et al. Lead concentrates in ovarian follicle compromises pregnancy. J Trace Elem Med Biol 2006; 20: 205–7.

74. Paksy K, Gati I, Naray M, Rajczy K. Lead accumulation in human ovarian follicular fluid, and in vitro effect of lead on progesterone production by cultured human ovarian granulosa cells. J Toxicol Environ Health 2001; 62: 359–66.

75. Rom WN. Effects of lead on the female and reproduction: a review. Mt Sinai J Med 1976; 43: 542–52.

76. Murphy MJ, Graziano JH, Popovac D, et al. Past pregnancy outcomes among women living in the vicinity of a lead smelter in Kosovo, Yugoslavia. Am J Public Health 1990; 80: 33–5.

77. Cooper AR, Moley KH. Maternal tobacco use and its preimplantation effects on fertility: More reasons to stop smoking. Semin Reprod Med 2008; 26: 204–12.

78. Hannoun A, Nassar AH, Usta M, Musa AA. Effect of female nargile smoking on in vitro fertilization outcome. Euro J Obstet gyneclol Repro Bio 2010; 150: 171–4.

79. Makri A, Goveia M, Balbus J, Parkin R. Children's susceptibility to chemicals: a review by developmental stage. J Toxicol Environ Health 2004; 7: 417–35.

80. Angell NF, Lavery JP. The relationship of blood lead levels to obstetric outcome. Am J Obstet Gynecol 1982; 142: 40–6.

81. Condon S. A public health response to mercury in fish. 2007. [Available from: http://www.mass.gov/]

82. Axelrad DA, Bellinger DC, Ryan LM, Woodruff TJ. Dose–response relationship of prenatal mercury exposure and IQ: an integrative analysis of epidemiologic data. Environ Health Perspect 2007; 115: 609–15.

83. FAO/WHO. Evaluation of certain food additives and contaminants: sixty-seventh report of the Joint FAO/WHO Expert Committee on Food Additives. Rome, Italy: WHO technical report series; no. 940, 2006.

84. Hibbeln JR, Davis JM, Steer C, et al. Maternal seafood consumption in pregnancy and neurodevelopmental outcomes in childhood (ALSPAC study): an observational cohort study. Lancet 2007; 369: 578–85.

85. Davidson PW, Myers GJ, Weiss B, Shamlaye CF, Cox C. Prenatal methyl mercury exposure from fish consumption and child development: a review of evidence and perspectives from the Seychelles child development study. Neurotoxicology 2006; 27: 1106–9.

86. Debes F, Budtz-Jorgensen E, Weihe P, White RF, Grandjean P. Impact of prenatal methylmercury exposure on neurobehavioral function at age 14 years. Neurotoxicol Teratol 2006; 28: 536–47.

87. NRC. National Research Council: Toxicological Effects of Methylmercury. Washington, DC: National Academy Press, 2000.

88. Hsu CS, Liu PL, Chien LC, Chou SY, Han BC. Mercury concentration and fish consumption in Taiwanese pregnant women. BJOG 2007; 114: 81–5.

89. Sato RL, Li GG, Shaha S. Antepartum seafood consumption and mercury levels in newborn cord blood. Am J Obstet Gynecol 2006; 194: 1683–8.

90. Guo YL, Hsu PC, Hsu CC, Lambert GH. Semen quality after prenatal exposure to polychlorinated biphenyls and dibenzofurans. Lancet 2000; 356: 1240–1.

91. Charlier CJ, Foidart JM. Comparative study of dichlorodiphenyldichloroethylene in blood and semen of two young male populations: lack of relationship to infertility, but evidence of high exposure of the mothers. Reprod Toxicol 2005; 20: 215–20.

92. Carpenter DO, Shen Y, Nguyen T, Le L, Lininger LL. Incidence of endocrine disease among residents of New York areas of concern. Environ Health Perspect 2001; 109(Suppl 6): 845–51.

93. Khattak S, K-Moghtader G, McMartin K, et al. Pregnancy outcome following gestational exposure to organic solvents: a prospective controlled study. JAMA 1999; 281: 1106–9.

94. Nakao M. Epigenetics: interaction of DNA methylation and chromatin. Gene 2001; 278: 25–31.

95. Anway MD, Cupp AS, Uzumcu M, Skinner MK. Epigenetic transgenerational actions of endocrine disruptors and male fertility. Science 2005; 308: 1466–9.

96. Crews D, McLachlan JA. Epigenetics, evolution, endocrine disruption, health, and disease. Endocrinology 2006; 147: S4–10.

97. Cohn BA, Cirillo PM, Wolff MS, et al. DDT and DDE exposure in mothers and time to pregnancy in daughters. Lancet 2003; 361: 2205–6.

98. Younglai EV, Holloway AC, Lim GE, Foster WG. Synergistic effects between FSH and 1,1-dichloro-2,2-bis(P-chlorophenyl)ethylene (P,P2-DDE) on human granulosa cell aromatase activity. Hum Reprod 2004; 19: 1089–93.

99. Hjollund NH, Bonde JP, Ernst E, et al. Pesticide exposure in male farmers and survival of in vitro fertilized pregnancies. Hum Reprod 2004; 19: 1331–7.

100. Giudice LC. Infertility and the environment: the medical context. Semin Reprod Med 2006; 24: 129–33.

101. Miller CS, Prihoda TJ. The Environmental exposure and sensitivity inventory (EESI): a standardized approach for measuring chemical intolerances for research and clinical applications. Toxicol Ind Health 1999; 15: 370–85.

102. Rea WJ. Chemical Sensitivity: Tools of Diagnosis and Methods of Treatment. Vol 4 Boca Raton, FL: Lewis Publishers, 1992.

103. Cranor CF. Toward understanding aspects of the precautionary principle. J Med Philos 2004; 29: 259–79.

104. NRC. National Research Council: Hormonally Active Agents in the Environment. Washington, DC: National Academy Press, 1999.

105. IPCS. International programme on chemical safety. In: Damstra T, Barlow S, Bergman A, Kavlock R, van der Kraak G, eds. Global Assessment of the State-of-the-Science of Endocrine Disruptors. Geneva, Switzerland: World Health Organization, 2002.

62

Bleeding, severe pelvic infection, and ectopic pregnancy

Raoul Orvieto and Zion Ben-Rafael

Transvaginal ultrasound-guided aspiration of oocytes is a well accepted and universally used method in assisted reproduction (1,2). Its major advantages include easy access to ovarian follicles with excellent oocyte yield and good visualization of the major pelvic vessels. It is done as a day care procedure, either under intravenous analgesia and sedation or under general anesthesia, and is usually traumatic. Nevertheless, there are some inherent risks, namely, puncture of blood vessels and hemoperitoneum, bleeding from the vaginal-vault puncture site, rupture of adnexal cystic masses, bowel perforation, trauma to pelvic organs, and pelvic infection. In addition, embryo transfer (ET) itself may be associated with complications such as pelvic infection, multiple pregnancy (which is directly related to the number of transferred embryos), spontaneous abortion, and extrauterine pregnancy (EUP). Maxwell et al. (3) have reported on the incidence of both serious and minor complications in young women undergoing 886 oocyte retrievals for oocyte donation. While the rate of serious complications, which included ovarian hyperstimulation syndrome, ovarian torsion, infection, and ruptured ovarian cyst, was 0.7%, the rate of minor complications severe enough to prompt the donor to seek medical attention after retrieval was 8.5%.

The aim of the present review is to discuss comprehensively three of these complications: bleeding, pelvic inflammatory disease (PID), and EUP.

BLEEDING

Vaginal Bleeding

During ultrasound-guided transvaginal oocyte aspiration, multiple punctures of the vaginal vault, or inappropriate handling and rotation of the ultrasound vaginal probe while inserting an aspiration needle through the vaginal vault can injure or tear the vaginal mucosa, ovaries, intra-abdominal organs, or blood vessels (1,4–8). Bleeding from the vaginal vault is a common consequence of ovum pick-up (OPU), with a reported incidence of 1.4–18.4% (5). In most cases, vaginal bleeding as a result of OPU stops spontaneously at the end of the procedure (6). In cases in which it does not, the bleeding site needs to be identified by vaginal exploration with a large speculum, followed by application of pressure with a sponge forceps or vaginal packing with a large gauze roll. If this is unsuccessful, or the tear is wide and deep, suturing is necessary.

Intraperitoneal or Retroperitoneal Bleeding

Transvaginal oocyte aspiration can also cause bleeding if intraperitoneal or retroperitoneal pelvic blood vessels are injured or if there is damage to the fine vascular network surrounding the punctured ovarian follicle. The reported incidence of severe intra- or retroperitoneal bleeding varies from 0% to 1.3% (1,6–9); a recent report described one case of intra-abdominal bleeding complicating aspiration of 1000 oocyte donors (10). Lean patients with polycystic ovary syndrome (PCOS) were specifically demonstrated to be at much higher risk for this complication (11). Intraperitoneal bleeding tends to be severe with acute hemodynamic deterioration, whereas retroperitoneal bleeding usually has a later and more indolent presentation. Yih et al. (12) studied serial complete blood counts before and after OPU in 93 in vitro fertilization (IVF) cycles and demonstrated a nonsignificant change in hematocrit levels, indicating that a clinically significant blood loss after OPU is actually uncommon.

Azem et al. (13) described a patient who presented to the emergency room 10 hours after OPU with severe lower abdominal pain, vomiting, and tenesmus. Examination revealed a distended abdomen with severe tenderness in the pouch of Douglas; on transvaginal sonography, a minimal, 3–4 cm collection of fluid was noted. Laparoscopy followed by laparotomy, which was performed on the basis of the clinical profile, revealed a retroperitoneal hematoma 7 cm in diameter. After evacuation and hemostasis, active bleeding from the mid-sacral vein occurred and was controlled by a metal clip. This case demonstrates the indolent course of retroperitoneal bleeding and physicians should be alerted to the possibility of retroperitoneal hematoma despite an absence of free fluid in the pouch of Douglas. Of notice, similar case with no significant intraperitoneal fluid collection was recently described as a result from ureteral injury with the consequent uro-retroperitoneum (14).

Intra-abdominal bleeding should be suspected immediately after OPU on the development of signs and symptoms of anemia – specifically, weakness, dizziness, dyspnea, or persistent tachycardia. Early management consists of intense hemodynamic monitoring, together with serial measurement of blood hemoglobin concentrations and ultrasonographic evaluation for the presence of intra-abdominal fluid. It should be emphasized, however, that intra-abdominal blood clots or retroperitoneal bleeding might be invisible even to an experienced ultrasound operator. A drop in hemoglobin concentration is an indication for prompt blood transfusion. If hemodynamic deterioration continues or acute abdominal pain develops, diagnostic laparoscopy or exploratory laparotomy with subsequent hemostatis of the bleeding site(s) are required. The clinician must make sure to handle the fragile overhyperstimulated ovaries very cautiously.

Our group described three cases of severe intra-abdominal bleeding from ovarian puncture sites during OPU, leading to acute abdominal complications (1). In two of the patients, symptoms developed three hours after OPU (hemoglobin 9.0 g/100 ml and 8.1 g/100 ml, respectively), and laparoscopic drainage and hemostatis were sufficient. The third patient became symptomatic after four hours (hemoglobin 7.3 g/100 ml) and required exploratory laparotomy and hemostatis in addition to the transfusion of four units of blood as a life-saving procedure. More recently, Battaglia et al. (15) reported severe intra-abdominal bleeding from the surface of both ovaries in a patient with coagulation factor XI deficiency. As expected, the patient became symptomatic three hours after OPU and required laparotomy, partial resection of stuffed ovaries, and hemostasis. Physicians should be aware of the presence of concomitant coagulopathy and might therefore consider intense coagulation-factor replacement before or during abdominal exploration.

Can we prevent severe intra-abdominal bleeding from ovarian puncture sites during OPU? In a recent cross-sectional retrospective study, Revel et al. (16) questioned the utility of coagulation screening before OPU. Among the 1032 patients evaluated, they found that 534 coagulation tests were needed to prevent one case of bleeding associated with an abnormal coagulation test result. Furthermore, despite the routine use of Doppler ultrasound during OPU, all cases with moderate peritoneal bleeding could not be predicted (17).

Description of the intraoperative measures needed to control intra-abdominal hemorrhage is beyond the scope of this text, and the reader is referred elsewhere for a detailed review (18).

PELVIC INFLAMMATORY DISEASE

Pelvic inflammatory disease is an infrequent complication of ultrasound-guided transvaginal aspiration of oocytes or ET, with a reported incidence of 0.2–0.5% per cycle (8,19–21). Signs or symptoms of pelvic infection, such as pyrexia, continuous low abdominal pain, dysuria, or offensive vaginal discharge, are infrequent (19). However, this does not exclude occult, subclinical bacterial colonization, which may influence the success of the IVF–ET treatment, or slowly progress throughout pregnancy (22). Our group evaluated the outcome of all IVF–ET procedures performed in our unit between 1986 and 1992 (21). Of the 4771 patients who underwent transvaginal OPU, 28 (0.58%) had symptoms of PID within one to seven days. The diagnosis was established by a rise in body temperature to 38°C for more than 48 hours, signs of pelvic peritonitis on physical examination, leukocyte count of >12,000 cells/m³, and elevated erythrocyte sedimentation rate. All patients were admitted to hospital for treatment with intravenous antibiotics. Of notice, ovarian abscess following oocyte retrieval may manifest late during pregnancy with low grade fever or vague abdominal pain (23).

OPU can also lead to severe abdominal complications. Our group reported on nine patients (0.24%) with tubo–ovarian or pelvic abscess after transvaginal-guided OPU (21). Three patients required laparotomy and adnexectomy, whereas in six patients, culdocentesis was performed for adequate pelvic abscess drainage. Kelada and Ghani (24) have recently described a case of bilateral ovarian abscesses following transvaginal oocyte retrieval, complicated by early signs of consumption coagulopathy. The latter is a serious and life-threatening complication of pelvic infection and sepsis, which should be diagnosed and corrected immediately.

Mechanisms Underlying Pelvic Infection

During transvaginal aspiration, accidental needle transport of cervicovaginal flora into ovarian tissue can cause unilateral or bilateral oophoritis, and accidental puncture of a contaminated or sterile hydrosalpinx can cause salpingitis. Some authors have attributed pelvic infection to infected endometriotic cysts or tubo–ovarian abscess after aspiration of endometriomas (25,26), or, rarely, to inadvertent puncture of the bowel. Pelvic infection can occur as a direct consequence of transcervical ET. This is evidenced by reported cases of PID following ET in an agonadal donor-egg recipient (27), or during cryopreserved ET (28); it may also occur as a result of the reaction of a silent or persistent subclinical infection, as seen occasionally after hysterosalpingography. Another possible cause during ET is catheterization of the uterus, which may force bacteria-laden air or fluid into one or both tubes by a piston-like effect.

Effect of Acute Pelvic Infection on IVF-ET Outcome

The first study of the impact of pelvic infection on IVF–ET outcome was reported by our group in 1994 (21). We found that the number of oocytes recovered, fertilized, and cleaved in 28 patients undergoing IVF in whom PID developed was similar to that of a comparison group with mechanical infertility. However, there were no

376 TEXTBOOK OF ASSISTED REPRODUCTIVE TECHNIQUES: CLINICAL PERSPECTIVES

pregnancies in the PID group, as compared with the 23–31% pregnancy rate per transfer in the whole group of patients treated by IVF, indicating that the appearance of PID at the critical time of implantation may cause a failure to conceive. This finding has several possible explanations, as outlined in detail below.

Endotoxemia

Endotoxin-releasing bacteria can be introduced into the peritoneal cavity during transvaginal oocyte recovery, and into the uterine cavity or tubes during ET. Ng et al. (29) described a case in which human oocytes were degenerated and fragmented, with no evidence of fertilization, in the presence of *Klebsiella*-derived endotoxin. In a study of the effects of endotoxin infusion on the circulating levels of eicosanoids, progesterone, and cortisol, and on abortions, Giri et al. (30) found that the first-trimester cows were more sensitive to the abortifacient effect of endotoxin than the second- and third-trimester cows. The mechanism of the endotoxin-induced abortion apparently involved the prolonged release of prostaglandin F2-α, which has a stimulant effect on uterine smooth muscle contractions and a luteolytic effect resulting in a gradual decline in the plasma level of progesterone (30). In addition, high endotoxin doses can induce the release of various autacoids, catecholamines, and cortisol, which directly or indirectly lead to metabolic and circulatory failures and, thereby, termination of pregnancy.

Local Inflammatory Reaction

Bacteria trigger a chain of events that lead to the activation, proliferation, and differentiation of lymphocytes, and the production of specific antibodies and various cytokines. This excessive production of cytokines may disrupt the delicate balance between the immune and reproductive systems and result in reproductive failure (31–33).

Temperature Elevation

Apart from their direct role on implantation and early embryonic development, cytokines may mediate temperature elevation and indirectly affect the outcome of IVF–ET. The febrile reaction is an integrated endocrine, autonomic, and behavioral response coordinated by the hypothalamus. The actions of circulating cytokines, such as interleukin (IL)-1 and tumor necrosis factor (TNF), on the central nervous system result in the secretion of prostaglandin E2, which initiates the elevation in body temperature together with corticosteroid secretion (34), also a component of the stress response. Some authors have suggested that fever is essential for amplifying the emergence of T-cell immunity in peripheral tissues (35). In vitro experiments have shown that temperature elevation leads to disintegration of the cytoskeleton (36) and may affect the transport of organelles. In pregnancy, maternal heat exposure can cause intracellular embryonic damage (37) and inhibit cell mitosis, proliferation, and migration,

resulting in cell death. In a study of guinea pig embryos, Edwards et al. (38) reported cell damage within minutes and cell death within hours after heating. Other mechanisms of heat-induced cell injury are microvascular lesions, placental necrosis, and placental infarction (39).

Treatment

The Role of Prophylactic Antibiotics in IVF–ET

The potential for intraperitoneal bacterial contamination during transvaginal oocyte recovery is well known and has led to the routine use of prophylactic antibiotics and vaginal disinfection (40). Meldrum (41) found no case of pelvic infection among 88 transvaginal retrievals with the use of intravenous cefazolin and vaginal preparation with povidone–iodine and saline irrigation; nor did Tsai et al. (42) in patients with ovarian endometrioma, using only vaginal douching with aqueous povidone–iodine followed by normal saline irrigation. Borlum and Maiggard (43) reported on two cases of serious pelvic infection in almost 400 transvaginal aspirations. They used only two vaginal douchings with sterile saline and noted that minimizing the number of repeated vaginal penetrations may have helped in lowering the risk of infection. However, the appropriate type of antibiotic administration, timing or duration of therapy, and the efficacy of therapy have not yet been established (41,44). Indeed, some authors claim that these measures may not only further reduce the incidence of PID after oocyte retrieval, but can even increase the risks of both an adverse reaction and of colonization with resistant organisms. Our experience with vaginal douchings with sterile saline in approximately 1100–1200 OPUs per year revealed a very low rate of PID after OPU. Peters et al. (45) suggested that only women with a tubal abnormality and a history of pelvic infection should receive prophylactic antibiotics before oocyte aspiration, and also possibly after ET. Others have suggested that such patients may benefit from transabdominal or transvesical rather than transvaginal procedures (46,47).

It is also noteworthy that Egbase et al. (48), in a study of the effect of prophylactic antibiotics in OPU on the endocervical microbial inoculation of the endometrium at ET, found that prophylactic antibiotics not only reduced the number of positive microbiology cultures of embryo catheter tips, but also significantly increased implantation and clinical pregnancy rates. On the other hand, in their prospective randomized study, Peikrishvili et al. (49) could not demonstrate any beneficial effects of antibiotic prescription (amoxicillin + clavulanic acid 1 g/125 mg) for six days following oocyte retrieval on implantation, pregnancy, or miscarriage rates.

Curative

Pelvic inflammatory disease or tubo–ovarian abscess after OPU require accurate diagnosis and prompt treatment with broad-spectrum antibiotics. In the presence of a pelvic abscess that is larger than 8 cm or unresponsive to medication, transvaginal or percutaneous drainage is the treatment of choice (50), with or without ultrasound-guided intracavitary instillation of a combination of antibiotics (51). Sometimes surgical laparoscopy or laparotomy is needed to evacuate the abscess or remove the infected tubes or adnexae.

Summary

The appearance of PID at the critical time of implantation results in failure to conceive. This effect may be mediated by bacterial endotoxins, a local inflammatory reaction against bacteria with the involvement of cytokines that affect implantation and early embryonic development, or temperature elevation that directly affects the conceptus. Although the role of prophylactic antibiotics is still controversial, they can be considered in the presence of risk factors for PID; aspiration of hydrosalpinx or endometriomas during OPU might be a risk factor for infection and should be avoided. Furthermore, to prevent total failure, if PID develops before ET, cryopreservation and ET in subsequent cycles should be considered. However, if PID develops after ET, the bacterial infection and fever should be treated rigorously to prevent reproductive failure.

EXTRAUTERINE PREGNANCY

EUP is the implantation of a blastocyst anywhere except in the endometrial lining of the uterine cavity. In recent years, EUPs have shown a marked increase in both absolute number and rate of occurrence (52). Already in 1992, almost 2% of all pregnancies in the United States were EUPs, and ectopic pregnancies accounted for 10% of all pregnancy-related deaths (52,53). The rates of abortions, multiple pregnancies, and EUPs are higher in pregnancies resulting from assisted reproductive techniques (ART) than in spontaneous pregnancies.

Other factors associated with the development of EUP include previous EUP, salpingitis, previous surgery to the fallopian tube, peritubal adhesions, pelvic lesions that distort the tube, developmental abnormalities of the tube, and altered tubal motility.

EUP after ART

The first IVF–ET pregnancy reported was an ectopic pregnancy (54). Today, the incidence of EUPs after IVF ranges from 2.1% to 9.4% of all clinical pregnancies (55,56). In 1996, the Society for Assisted Reproductive Technology (SART) (57) reported a decrease in the incidence of EUP to 0.8% of transfers and 1.6% of pregnancies, compared with 0.9% and 2.8%, respectively, in 1995. This finding was attributable to the decrease in the proportion of couples with tubal factor infertility undergoing IVF treatment and a concomitant increase in couples with male factor infertility. Recently, the SART reported the outcome of ART initiated in the United States in 2001 (58). The incidence of EUP for all ART procedures was 0.8% per transfer and 1.6% per clinical

pregnancy, which compares favorably with the estimated overall incidence of EUP in the United States of 2% per reported pregnancy (52).

Risk Factors

Data on risk factors for EUP after IVF are still unclear. Martinez and Trounson (59) failed to identify any risk factors, whereas Karande et al. (60) pointed to a prior ectopic pregnancy. Verhulst et al. (61) found a significantly higher rate of EUP after IVF in patients with tubal disease (3.6%) compared with those with normal tubes (1.2%); this finding was confirmed by several other studies (56,62–64). Cohen et al. (65) showed that the number of patent tubes at the time of transfer was a risk factor, with a higher EUP rate in patients with zero or two patent tubes than in patients with one. In an analysis of the Bourn Hall Clinic data, Marcus and Brinsden (66) noted that the main risk factor was a history of PID. Though they found EUP to be more prevalent in patients with tubal factor infertility, those who received a higher culture-medium volume and those with a higher progesterone/E2 ratio on the day of ET, had no associated history of EUP. Finally, Ankum et al. (67) in a meta-analysis of risk factors for EUP, concluded that the four most significant were previous EUP, documented tubal pathology, previous tubal surgery, and in utero exposure to diethylstilbestrol. These results were confirmed by Lesny et al. (68) who also added one more – a difficult ET on day 2 rather than day 3. Clayton et al. (69) have recently analyzed the EUP risk among 94,118 patients who conceived with ART procedures. Two thousand--nine (2.1%) were ectopic. In comparison with the ectopic rate (2.2%) among pregnancies conceived with IVF (fresh, non-donor cycles), the ectopic rate was significantly increased when zygote intrafallopian transfer (ZIFT) was used (3.6%) and significantly decreased when donor oocytes were used (1.4%) or when a gestational surrogate carried the pregnancy (0.9%). Among fresh non-donor IVF–ET procedures, the risk for ectopic pregnancy was significantly increased among women with tubal factor infertility, endometriosis, and other non-tubal female factors of infertility and significantly decreased among women with a previous live birth. Moreover, transfer of high quality embryos was associated with a decreased ectopic risk when two or fewer embryos were transferred, but not when three or more embryos were transferred.

There are many theories on the manner by which embryos implant in the fallopian tube following ET: By the hydrostatic force of the transfer medium containing the embryos in the fallopian tube ostia; by the gravitational pull of the embryos to the hanging tubes, which are located lower than the uterine fundus; and by reflux expulsion of the embryo due to embryonic migration to the fallopian tubes, either spontaneously or secondary to uterine contractions (70). The technique of ET itself may also be a culprit in EUP, although this is controversial (71). For example, while Yovich et al. (72) noted a significantly higher rate of EUP when the embryos were placed high near the uterine fundus or into the tube itself, rather than in the lower uterus, Friedman et al. (73) have demonstrated that blastocyst transfer closer to the fundus (<10 mm) is associated with higher pregnancy rate. However, although in the latter study no EUP occurred in the <10 mm group, this outcome should be monitored closely in larger studies.

The transfer volume of culture media containing embryos may play a role in embryonic migration into the fallopian tubes. While most clinicians contend that more than 80 μl of media are needed for the embryo to reach the fallopian tube (56), Knutzen et al. (74) using a mock intrauterine ET with 50 μl of radiopaque dye demonstrated easy passage of all or part of the material in 44% of patients. Lesny et al. (75) explained these findings by the propulsion of the embryo from the uterine fundus into the tubes by the junctional-zone contractions. Therefore, as the likelihood of tubal placement is very high, the development of tubal pregnancy is not due solely to embryos reaching the tubes, but rather to an additional pathological process that prevents their movement back into the uterine cavity. Potential mechanisms may be tubal disease affecting the luminal surface and thereby delaying or blocking embryonic passage into the uterine cavity, external factors that interfere with tubal motility, and abnormal embryos (62), such as those derived from chromosomally abnormal gametes (76).

To ameliorate the role of abnormal fallopian tubes in the pathogenesis of EUP after IVF, several authors have recommended that the tubes be occluded at the level of the uterotubal junction (77,78). However, this measure does not prevent the development of an interstitial pregnancy (64), although it certainly prevents the well-known phenomenon of spontaneous pregnancies after IVF treatment, which occurs in 30% of the patients with patent tubes (79).

Another potential interfering factor in tubal function and ET is the different hormonal milieus resulting from ovulation-induction protocols, particularly those including clomiphene citrate (61,80). This may result from the effect of the high E2 levels on tubal peristalsis through the control of tubal smooth muscle contractility and ciliary activity (72,80). Pygriotis et al. (64) however, did not demonstrate a difference in E2 levels on the day of human chorionic gonadotropin (hCG) administration between IVF patients with and without EUP. Furthermore, they found an increased proportion of EUPs in frozen ETs following natural cycles in which the E2 levels were comparatively low.

In summary, the reproductive health characteristics of infertile women, the different hormonal milieu, technical issues of IVF procedures, and the estimated embryo implantation potential were all suggested as possible risk factors (81), however, the mechanisms are still uncertain and need further investigation.

Heterotopic Pregnancy Following ART

The general incidence of combined intrauterine and extrauterine (heterotopic) pregnancy is 1:15,000–30,000, and it increases dramatically to 1:100 in pregnancies following ART or ovulation induction (82–84). Although a distorted pelvic anatomy is responsible for the predisposition to both extrauterine and heterotopic pregnancy (85–87), heterotopic pregnancies are associated with a greater number of embryos transferred, whereas EUP is not. Tummon et al. (88) reported that when four or more embryos were transferred, the odds ratio for the development of a heterotopic pregnancy versus EUP was 10. The difficult diagnosis of this potentially life-threatening complication is often made during emergency surgery following tubal rupture and hemoperitoneum. In about 70% of cases, the outcome of the intrauterine pregnancy is favorable (live birth) once the extrauterine pregnancy is terminated (89,90). A high index of suspicion and early intervention are mandatory to salvage the viable intrauterine pregnancy and prevent maternal mortality.

Diagnosis and Treatment

Noninvasive diagnostic measures using transvaginal ultrasonography combined with serum hCG monitoring have proved to be a reliable tool in the diagnosis of EUP. Since most pregnancies following ART are monitored at an early stage before the onset of symptoms, early diagnosis of the condition and improved management and care have resulted in a decline in the morbidity and mortality of EUP. Of note is the fact that treating EUP with methotrexate has no influence on patients' serum anti-Müllerian hormone levels (91), nor patients' performance in the following IVF cycle (92). The diagnosis and treatment of EUP are beyond the scope of this chapter, and readers are referred elsewhere for a detailed review (93,94).

BRIEF SUMMARY

Transvaginal ultrasound-guided aspiration of oocytes is a well accepted and universally used method in assisted reproduction. Its major advantages include easy access to ovarian follicles with excellent oocyte yield, and good visualization of the major pelvic vessels, and it is usually atraumatic. Nevertheless, there are some inherent risks, namely, puncture of blood vessels and intra-abdominal or retroperitoneal bleeding, bleeding from the vaginal-vault puncture site, rupture or perforation of pelvic organs, and pelvic infection. In addition, embryo transfer itself may be associated with complications such as pelvic infection, multiple pregnancy, or extrauterine pregnancy. This chapter has comprehensively presented and discussed three of these complications: bleeding, PID, and EUP.

REFERENCES

1. Dicker D, Ashkenazi J, Feldberg D, et al. Severe abdominal complications after transvaginal ultrasonographically-guided retrieval of oocytes for in vitro fertilization and embryo transfer. Fertil Steril 1993; 59: 1313–15.
2. Feldberg D, Goldman JA, Ashkenazi J, et al. Transvaginal oocyte retrieval controlled by vaginal probe for

in vitro fertilization: a comparative study. J Ultrasound Med 1988; 7: 726–8.

3. Maxwell KN, Cholst IN, Rosenwaks Z. The incidence of both serious and minor complications in young women undergoing oocyte donation. Fertil Steril 2008; 90: 2165–71.

4. Modder J, Kettel LM, Sakamoto K. Hematuria and clot retention after transvaginal oocyte aspiration: a case report. Fertil Steril 2006; 86: e1–2.

5. Tureck RW, Garcia C, Blasco L, Mastroianni L. Perioperative complications arising after transvaginal oocyte retrieval. Obstet Gynecol 1993; 81: 590–3.

6. Lenz S, Leeton J, Renou P. Transvaginal recovery of oocytes for in vitro fertilization using vaginal ultrasound. J In Vitro Fert Embryo Transf 1987; 4: 51–5.

7. Serour GI, Aboulghar M, Mansour R, et al. Complications of medically assisted conception in 3500 cycles. Fertil Steril 1998; 70: 638–42.

8. Govaert I, Devreker F, Delbaere A, et al. Short-term medical complications of 1500 oocyte retrievals for in vitro fertilization and embryo transfer. Eur J Obstet Gynecol Reprod Biol 1998; 77: 239–43.

9. Aragona C, Mohamed MA, Espinola MS, et al. Clinical complications after transvaginal oocyte retrieval in 7,098 IVF cycles. Fertil Steril 2011; 95: 293–4.

10. Sauer MV. Defining the incidence of serious complications experienced by oocyte donors: a review of 1000 cases. Am J Obstet Gynecol 2001; 184: 277–8.

11. Liberty G, Hyman JH, Eldar-Geva T, et al. Ovarian hemorrhage after transvaginal ultrasonographically guided oocyte aspiration: a potentially catastrophic and not so rare complication among lean patients with polycystic ovary syndrome. Fertil Steril 2010; 93: 874–9.

12. Yih MC, Goldschlag D, Davis OK, et al. Complete blood counts (CBC) after oocyte retrieval: what is normal? Fertil Steril 2001; 76: S115–16.

13. Azem F, Wolf Y, Botchan A, et al. Massive retroperitoneal bleeding: a complication of transvaginal ultrasonography-guided oocyte retrieval for in vitro fertilization-embryo transfer. Fertil Steril 2000; 74: 405–6.

14. Fiori O, Cornet D, Darai E, Antoine JM, Bazot M. Uro-retroperitoneum after ultrasound-guided transvaginal follicle puncture in an oocyte donor: a case report. Hum Reprod 2006; 21: 2969–71.

15. Battaglia C, Regnani G, Giulini S, et al. Severe intraabdominal bleeding after transvaginal oocyte retrieval for IVF-ET and coagulation factor XI deficiency: a case report. J Assist Reprod Genet 2001; 3: 178–81.

16. Revel A, Schejter-Dinur Y, Yahalomi SZ, et al. Is routine screening needed for coagulation abnormalities before oocyte retrieval? Fertil Steril 2011; 95: 1182–4.

17. Rísquez F, Confino E. Can doppler ultrasound-guided oocyte retrieval improve IVF safety? Reprod Biomed Online 2010; 21: 444–5.

18. Thompson JD, Rock WA. Control of pelvic hemorrhage. In: Rock JA, Thompson JD, eds. Te Linde's Operative Gynecology. 8th edn. Philadelphia: Lippincott-Raven, 1997: 197–232.

19. Howe RS, Wheeler C, Mastroianni L Jr, et al. Pelvic infection after transvaginal ultrasound-guided ovum retrieval. Fertil Steril 1988; 49: 726–8.

20. Curtis P, Amso N, Keith E, et al. Evaluation of the risk of pelvic infection following transvaginal oocyte recovery. Hum Reprod 1992; 7: 625–6.

21. Ashkenazi J, Farhi J, Dicker D, et al. Acute pelvic inflammatory disease after oocyte retrieval: adverse effects on the results of implantation. Fertil Steril 1994; 61: 526–8.

22. Al-Kuran O, Beitawi S, Al-Mehaisen L. Pelvic abscess complicating an in vitro fertilization pregnancy and review of the literature. J Assist Reprod Genet 2008; 25: 341–3.

23. Sharpe K, Karovitch AJ, Claman P, Suh KN. Transvaginal oocyte retrieval for in vitro fertilization complicated by ovarian abscess during pregnancy. Fertil Steril 2006; 86: 219.e11–13.

24. Kelada E, Ghani R. Bilateral ovarian abscesses following transvaginal oocyte retrieval for IVF: a case report and review of literature. J Assist Reprod Genet 2007; 24: 143–5.

25. Yaron Y, Peyser MR, Samuel D, et al. Infected endometriotic cysts secondary to oocyte aspiration for in vitro fertilization. Hum Reprod 1994; 9: 1759–60.

26. Nargund G, Parsons J. Infected endometriotic cysts secondary to oocyte aspiration for in vitro fertilization. Hum Reprod 1995; 10: 1555.

27. Sauer MV, Paulson RJ. Pelvic abscess complicating transcervical embryo transfer. Am J Obstet Gynecol 1992; 166: 148–9.

28. Friedler S, Ben-Shachar I, Abramov Y, et al. Ruptured tubo-ovarian abscess complicating transcervical cryopreserved embryo transfer. Fertil Steril 1996; 65: 1065–6.

29. Ng SC, Edirisinghe WR, Sathanathan AH, Ratnam SS. Bacterial infection of human oocytes during in vitro fertilization. Int J Fertil 1987; 32: 298–301.

30. Giri SN, Emau P, Cullor JS, et al. Effect of endotoxin on circulating levels of eicosanoids, progesterone, cortisol, glucose and lactic acid, and abortion in pregnant cows. Vet Microbiol 1990; 21: 211–31.

31. Ben-Rafael Z, Orvieto R. Cytokine involvement in reproduction. Fertil Steril 1992; 58: 1093–9.

32. Tartakovski B, Ben-Yair E. Cytokines modulate preimplantation development and pregnancy. Develop Biol 1991; 146: 345–52.

33. Romero R, Espinoza J, Mazor M. Can endometrial infection/inflammation explain implantation failure, spontaneous abortion, and preterm birth after in vitro fertilization? Fertil Steril 2004; 82: 799–804.

34. Saper CB, Breder CD. Endogenous pyrogens in the CNS: role in the febrile response. Prog Brain Res 1992; 93: 419–28.

35. Hanson DF. Fever and the immune response. the effects of physiological temperatures on primary murine splenic T-cell responses in vitro. J Immunol 1993; 151: 436–48.

36. Kitano Y, Okada N. Organization and disorganization of actin filament in human epidermal keratinocyte: heat, shock treatment and recovery process. Cell Tissue Res 1990; 261: 269–74.

37. Milunski A, Ulcickas M, Rothman KJ, et al. Maternal heat exposure and neural tube defects. JAMA 1992; 268: 882–5.

38. Edwards MJ, Mulley R, Ring S, Wanner RA. Mitotic cell death and delay of mitotic activity in guinea-pig embryos following brief maternal hyperthermia. J Embryol Exp Morphol 1974; 32: 593–602.

39. Hendricks AG, Stone GW, Hendrickson RV, Matayoshi K. Teratogenic effects of hyperthermia in the bonnet monkey (Macaca radiata). Teratology 1979; 19: 177–82.

40. Russell JB, DeCherney AH, Hobbins JC. A new trans-vaginal probe and biopsy guide for oocyte retrieval. Fertil Steril 1987; 47: 350–2.

41. Meldrum DR. Antibiotics for vaginal oocyte aspiration. J In Vitro Fert Embryo Transf 1989; 6: 1–2.

42. Tsai YC, Lin MY, Chen SH, et al. Vaginal disinfection with povidone iodine immediately before oocyte retrieval is effective in preventing pelvic abscess formation without compromising the outcome of IVF-ET. J Assist Reprod Genet 2005; 22: 173–5.

43. Borlum KG, Maiggard S. Transvaginal oocyte aspiration and pelvic infection. Lancet 1989; 2: 53(letter).

44. Van Os HC, Roozenburg BJ, Janssen-Caspers HAB, et al. Vaginal disinfection with povidone iodine and the outcome of in vitro fertilization. Hum Reprod 1992; 7: 349–50.

45. Peters AJ, Hecht B, Durinzi K, et al. Salpingitis or oophoritis: What causes fever following oocyte aspiration and embryo transfer? Obstet Gynecol 1993; 81: 876–7.

46. Wren M, Parson J. Ultrasound directed follicle aspiration in IVF. In: Chen C, Tan SL, Cheng WC, eds. Recent Advances in the Management of Infertility. New York: McGraw-Hill, 1989: 105–81.

47. Ashkenazi J, Ben-David M, Feldberg D, et al. Abdominal complications following ultrasonically-guided percutaneous transvesical collection of oocytes for in vitro fertilization. J In Vitro Fert Embryo Transf 1987; 4: 316–18.

48. Egbase PE, Udo EE, Al-Shharhan M, Grudzinskas JG. Prophylactic antibiotics and endocervical microbial inoculation of the endometrium at embryo transfer. Lancet 1999; 354: 651–2.

49. Peikrishvili R, Evrard B, Pouly JL, Janny L. Prophylactic antibiotic therapy (amoxicillin + clavulanic acid) before embryo transfer for IVF is useless. results of a randomized study. J Gynecol Obstet Biol Reprod 2004; 33: 713–19.

50. Russell JB, Decherney AH, Hobbins JC. A new trans-vaginal probe and biopsy guide for oocyte retrieval. Fertil Steril 1987; 47: 350–2.

51. Caspi B, Zalel Y, Or Y, et al. Sonographically-guided aspiration: an alternative therapy for tubo-ovarian abscess. Ultrasound Obstet Gynecol 1996; 7: 439–42.

52. Centers for Disease Control and Prevention. Ectopic pregnancy—United States, 1990–1992. MMWR Recomm Rep 1995; 1: 46.

53. Berg CJ, Atrash HR, Koonin LM, Tucker M. Pregnancy-related mortality in the United States, 1987–1990. Obstet Gynecol 1996; 88: 161.

54. Steptoe P, Edwards R. Reimplantation of a human embryo with subsequent tubal pregnancy. Lancet 1976; 1: 830–2.

55. Azem F, Yaron Y, Botchan A, et al. Ectopic pregnancy after in vitro fertilization-embryo transfer (IVF/ET): the possible role of the ET technique. J Assist Reprod Genet 1993; 10: 302–4.

56. Zouves C, Erenus M, Gomel V. Tubal ectopic pregnancy after in vitro fertilization and embryo transfer: a role for proximal occlusion or salpingectomy after failed distal tubal surgery. Fertil Steril 1991; 56: 691–5.

57. SART, ASRM. Assisted reproductive technology in the United States: 1996 results generated from the American society for reproductive medicine/society for assisted reproductive technology registry. Fertil Steril 1999; 71: 798–807.

58. SART, ASRM. Assisted reproductive technology in the United States: 201results generated from the American society for reproductive medicine/society for assisted reproductive technology registry. Fertil Steril 2007; 87: 1253–66.

59. Martinez F, Trounson A. An analysis of factors associated with ectopic pregnancy in a human in vitro fertilization program. Fertil Steril 1986; 45: 79–87.

60. Karande VC, Flood JT, Heard N, et al. Analysis of ectopic pregnancies resulting from in vitro fertilization and embryo transfer. Hum Reprod 1991; 6: 446–9.

61. Verhulst G, Camus M, Bollen N, et al. Analysis of the risk factors with regard to the occurrence of ectopic pregnancy after medically assisted procreation. Hum Reprod 1993; 8: 1284–7.

62. Herman A, Ron-El R, Golan A, et al. The role of tubal pathology and other parameters in ectopic pregnancies occurring in in vitro fertilization and embryo transfer. Fertil Steril 1990; 54: 864–8.

63. Correy JF, Watkins RA, Bradfield GF, et al. Spontaneous pregnancies and pregnancies as a result of treatment on an in vitro fertilization program terminating in ectopic pregnancies or spontaneous abortions. Fertil Steril 1988; 50: 85–8.

64. Pygriotis E, Sultan KM, Neal GS, et al. Ectopic pregnancies after in vitro fertilization and embryo transfer. J Assist Reprod Genet 1994; 11: 80–3.

65. Cohen J, Mayaux MJ, Guihard-Moscato ML. Pregnancy outcomes after in vitro fertilization. a collaborative study on 2342 pregnancies. Ann NY Acad Sci 1988; 54: 1–6.

66. Marcus SF, Brinsden PR. Analysis of the incidence and risk factors associated with ectopic pregnancy following in-vitro fertilization and embryo transfer. Hum Reprod 1995; 10: 199–203.

67. Ankum WM, Mol BW, Van der Veen, et al. Risk factors for ectopic pregnancy: a meta-analysis. Fertil Steril 1996; 66: 513–16.

68. Lesny P, Killick SR, Robinson J, Maguiness SD. Trans-cervical embryo transfer as a risk factor for ectopic pregnancy. Fertil Steril 1999; 72: 305–9.

69. Clayton HB, Schieve LA, Peterson HB, et al. Ectopic pregnancy risk with assisted reproductive technology procedures. Obstet Gynecol 2006; 107: 595–604.

70. Russell JB. The etiology of ectopic pregnancy. Clin Obstet Gynecol 1987; 30: 181–90.

71. Schoolcraft WB, Surrey ES, Gardner DK. Embryo transfer: techniques and variables affecting success. Fertil Steril 2001; 76: 863–70.

72. Yovich JL, Turner SR, Murphy AJ. Embryo transfer technique as a cause of ectopic pregnancies in in vitro fertilization. Fertil Steril 1985; 44: 318–21.

73. Friedman BE, Lathi RB, Henne MB, Fisher SL, Milki AA. The effect of air bubble position after blastocyst transfer on pregnancy rates in IVF cycles. Fertil Steril 2011; 95: 944–7.

74. Knutzen UK, Sotto-Albors CE, Fuller D, et al. Mock embryo transfer (MET) in early luteal phase, the cycle prior to in vitro fertilization and embryo transfer (IVF/ET). Proc 45th Annual Meeting of the American Fertility Society. San Francisco, CA, 13–16 Nov 1989. American Fertility Society, Program Supplement, pS152: 299.

75. Lesny P, Killick SR, Tetlow RL, et al. Embryo transfer—can we learn anything new from the observation of

junctional zone contraction? Hum Reprod 1998; 13: 1540–6.

76. Job-Spira N, Coste J, Boue J, et al. Chromosomal abnormalities and ectopic pregnancy? New directions for aetiological research. Hum Reprod 1996; 11: 239–43.

77. Svare J, Norup P, Grove Thomsen S, et al. Heterotopic pregnancies after in vitro fertilization and embryo transfer—A Danish survey. Hum Reprod 1993; 8: 116–18.

78. Tucker M, Smith D, Pike I, et al. Ectopic pregnancy following in vitro fertilization and embryo transfer. Lancet 1981; 2: 1278.

79. Ben-Rafael Z, Mashiach S, Dor J, et al. Treatment- independent pregnancy after in vitro fertilization and embryo transfer trial. Fertil Steril 1986; 45: 564–7.

80. Fernandez H, Coste J, Job-Spira N. Controlled ovarian hyperstimulation as a risk factor for ectopic pregnancy. Obstet Gynecol 1991; 78: 656–9.

81. Chang HJ, Suh CS. Ectopic pregnancy after assisted reproductive technology: what are the risk factors? Curr Opin Obstet Gynecol 2010; 22: 202–7.

82. Ben-Rafael Z, Carp HJ, Mashiach S, et al. The clinical features and incidence of concurrent intra and extra uterine pregnancies. Acta Eur Fertil 1985; 16: 199–202.

83. Dimitry ES, Subak-Sharpe R, Mills M, et al. Nine cases of heterotopic pregnancies in 4 years of in vitro fertilization. Fertil Steril 1990; 53: 107–10.

84. Tal J, Hadad S, Gordon M, et al. Heterotopic pregnancy after ovulation induction and assisted reproduction technologies: a literature review from 1971 to 1993. Fertil Steril 1996; 66: 1–12.

85. Goldman GA, Fisch B, Ovadia J, Tadpir Y. Heterotopic pregnancy after assisted reproductive technologies. Obstet Gynecol Surv 1992; 47: 217–21.

86. Molloy D, Deambrosis W, Keeping D, et al. Multiple-sited (heterotopic) pregnancy after in vitro fertilization and gamete intrafallopian transfer. Fertil Steril 1990; 53: 1068–71.

87. Li HP, Balmaceda JP, Zouves C, et al. Heterotopic pregnancy associated with gamete intra-fallopian transfer. Hum Reprod 1992; 7: 131–5.

88. Tummon IS, Whitmore NA, Daniel SAJ, et al. Transferring more embryos increases risk of heterotopic pregnancy. Fertil Steril 1964; 61: 1065–7.

89. Rizk B, Tan SL, Morcos S, et al. Heterotopic pregnancies after in vitro fertilization and embryo transfer. Am J Obstet Gynecol 1991; 164: 161–4.

90. Rojanski N, Schenker JG. Heterotopic pregnancy and assisted reproduction—an update. J Assist Reprod Genet 1996; 13: 594–601.

91. Oriol B, Barrio A, Pacheco A, et al. Systemic methotrexate to treat ectopic pregnancy does not affect ovarian reserve. Fertil Steril 2008; 90: 1579–82.

92. Orvieto R, Kruchkovich J, Zohav E, et al. Does methotrexate treatment for ectopic pregnancy influence the patient's performance during a subsequent in vitro fertilization/embryo transfer cycle? Fertil Steril 2007; 88: 1685–6.

93. Rock JA, Damario MA. Ectopic pregnancy. In: Rock JA, Thompson JD, eds. Te Linde's Operative Gynecology. 8th edn. Philadelphia: Lippincott-Raven, 1997: 501–27.

94. Yao M, Tulandi T. Current status of surgical and nonsurgical management of ectopic pregnancy. Fertil Steril 1997; 67: 421–33.

63

Iatrogenic multiple pregnancies: The risk of ART

Isaac Blickstein

INTRODUCTION

The common denominator of most assisted reproductive techniques (ART) is ovarian (hyper)stimulation. The scheme to expose excess female gametes to abundant sperm intended to increase fertilization may inadvertently produce multiple zygotes. In ovulation induction, the number of fertilized eggs is uncontrolled and unpredicted. By contrast, the number of zygotes transferred in ART has been always under control. Consequently, multiple pregnancies following ART are almost exclusively physician-made, i.e., iatrogenic multiple pregnancies (IMPs).

There are two exceptions to this statement. First, single embryo transfer (ET) may still be associated with an increased risk of monozygotic (MZ) twins since ART augments the rate of zygotic splitting (1,2). Second, observations from the East Flanders Prospective Twin Survey suggest that a genetic familial trait for spontaneous twins may also be involved in induced conceptions. Hence, women with "twins in the family" undergoing infertility treatment (3) may be at increased risk of having multiples as compared with women without that characteristic.

Regardless of the mechanism involved in IMP, ART undoubtedly increases the risk of multiple births. In 1998, the incidence of multiples in the UK was 25% twins and 5% triplets (4). Whilst globally there have been reductions over recent years in these rates following ART it is still an issue. Roughly, these reference figures represent a 20- and 50-times increased frequency for iatrogenic twins and triplets, respectively, as compared with naturally occurring multiples. Table 63.1 shows a simple model of an obstetrical service with 4000 live births/year, including 5% following iatrogenic pregnancies (5). In this model, the number of twins is doubled and that of triplets is 3.5-times increased. Importantly, 5% iatrogenic pregnancies will produce an excess of 31.5/1000 multiple pregnancy neonates over the expected rate in spontaneous pregnancies.

ART and ovulation induction, the major contributors to the epidemic of multiple pregnancies, did not arise ex vacuo. In a modern society, women rely on efficient modern fertility treatment when deciding on postponing childbirth. It follows that advanced maternal age, by itself an accepted risk factor for natural multiples, is also a significant risk factor for reduced fecundity and increased need for fertility treatment. Thus, social trends act in concert with available ART to increase the risk of multiple pregnancies. Figure 63.1 shows the ratio of spontaneous to induced twins in East Flanders over the last two decades. Except for the unexplained "hump" in 1980, there is a clear change in the rate of induced twins from 1:46 into 1 in every two to three twins (6). This population-based trend might be even more accentuated in hospital-based data.

The wide spectrum of issues encompassed in IMP deserves a separate volume (7,8). In this chapter, several risks of multiple pregnancies following ART will be specifically addressed.

Important information related to iatrogenic multiple pregnancies comes from the Israeli National registry of very low birth weight (VLBW, <1500 g) twins. Figure 63.2 shows that over the years, the frequency of VLBW twins as a result of ovulation induction did not increase. At the same time, however, the frequency of VLBW twins as a result of in vitro fertilization is steadily increasing, suggesting that the "disease burden" of small twins is clearly man-made and potentially avoidable.

THE PREGNANCY

It is beyond the scope of this chapter to describe in detail the risks associated with multiple pregnancies (9,10). It is generally accepted that the human female is programmed for mono-ovulation, monofetal development, and nursing only one neonate. Consequently, pregnancies with more than one fetus overwhelm the uterine capacity to adequately nurture the fetuses. Animal and human models have repeatedly demonstrated the reciprocal relationship between birth weight and gestational age at delivery and litter size. Using singleton standards, a significant proportion of twins and all high-order multiple pregnancies (HOMPs) will be delivered preterm and will be small for gestational age. In addition to absolute growth restriction, relative (discordant) growth is common (11).

As a result of the limited uterine capacity, natural reduction in fetal number is frequently seen. At the early stages, the embryo may disappear ("vanishing twin syndrome") in one of every six to seven twin pregnancies following ART (12,13). The vanishing twin syndrome,

Table 63.1   Estimating the Contribution of 5% Iatrogenic Conceptions in an Obstetrical Service with 4000 Deliveries/Year (Spontaneous, 1.2% twins and 0.1% triplets; iatrogenic, 25% twins, 5% triplets)

	Singles	Twins	Triplets	Births	Neonates
100% spontaneous	3948	48	4	4000	4056
5% iatrogenic	140	50	10	200	270
95% spontaneous	3750	46	4	3800	3854
Total	3890	96	14	4000	4124

Source: Adapted from Ref. 5.

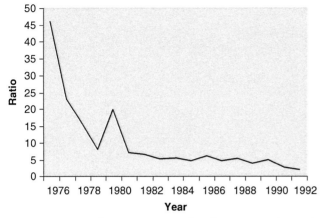

Figure 63.1   Ratio of spontaneous to induced twins. Since the implementation of effective infertility treatment the ratio changed from 1 induced for every 40–50 spontaneous twin pregnancies, to 1 induced for every two to three spontaneous twin pregnancies. *Source*: Adapted from the East Flanders Prospective Twin Survey Ref. 5.

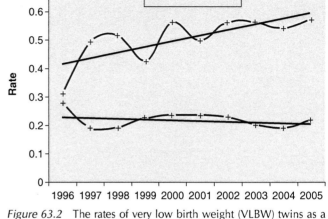

Figure 63.2   The rates of very low birth weight (VLBW) twins as a result of in vitro fertilization (IVF) and of ovulation induction (OI) (Isaac Blickstein, unpublished observation).

considered by many as natural multifetal pregnancy reduction (MFPR), gained special attention when Pharoah and Cooke hypothesized that single embryonic death may be implicated in cerebral palsy in the survivor (14,15). However, Matias et al. (16) summarized several case–control studies on plurality-dependent spontaneous embryonic loss rates after ART and found that twin pregnancies have a two to five times lower miscarriage rate of the entire pregnancy compared with singletons. At present, it is unclear if this advantage is a chance event or related to the presence of a higher placental (and hormonal) support of the early pregnancy.

Multiples are associated with higher frequencies of malformations of varied etiology. The yet unknown factor(s) that causes zygotic splitting has been implicated in causing structural malformations in MZs. In the subset with monochorionic (MC) placentas, also encountered in HOMPs, twin–twin transfusion syndrome (TTTS) may affect as many as 10–15% of the pairs and may result in major morbidity of one or both twins. Later in pregnancy, single fetal demise associated with MC placentas may result in severe end organ damage in the survivor.

Finally, it has been shown that the risk of cerebral palsy (CP) is five- to sixfold and 23-fold increased in twins and triplets, respectively, compared with singletons (17). A model based on British data related to transfer of two

and three embryos (4) and on British data related to CP in multiples (18) suggested a significantly lower estimated CP rate (2.7/1000 neonates) after spontaneous pregnancies compared with transfer of three embryos [odds ratio (OR) = 6.3], two embryos (OR = 3.3), and transfer of three embryos in which all triplets had been reduced to twins (OR = 3.8) (Fig. 63.3) (19).

Three additional aspects deserve further consideration. First, as mentioned above, there is an increased risk of zygotic splitting following ART. It is not known why MZs are more frequent in conceptions after ART. The most common cause and effect speculation suggests that the exposure of the zona pellucida to biochemical or mechanical trauma leads to herniation of the blastocyst and splitting of the zygote. Zygotic splitting is not only a biologic enigma but is also a major area of clinical importance, primarily because of the confirmed increased morbidity and mortality associated with MZ twinning.

Currently, zygotic splitting is inferred when the number of fetuses exceeds that of transferred embryos, or when monoamniotic twins are diagnosed. Evidently, the reported figures underestimate the true incidence, since bichorionic (BC) MZs cannot be clinically differentiated from same-sex BC dizygotic (DZ) twins. In addition, previous reports did not mention the number of transferred embryos and/or the method of ART. In an initial study (1), the data indicated that splitting is expected in 4.9% after in vitro fertilization (IVF) without intracytoplasmic sperm injection (ICSI) 12 times higher than the 0.4% rate of MZs in spontaneous conceptions. In a subsequent study (2), of a much larger data set from British IVF centers, Blickstein et al. found "only" a sixfold increased splitting rate. Blickstein and Keith (20) postulated that, given the remarkably constant frequency of MZ twins in different populations, there might be splitting-prone oocytes after fertilization. Thus, the higher the number of ovulation events (i.e., following ovarian stimulation), the greater the chance of recruiting a splitting-prone oocyte for ovulation, as is indeed the case with all methods of assisted conceptions. In addition, the more fecund patients with a better chance to conceive are significantly more likely to have MZ twins, as seen in those receiving a less "aggressive" regimen such as clomiphene citrate as the sole treatment, compared with other ovulation enhancing agents (21). It

follows that the chance of a follicle that contains an oocyte with a propensity to undergo splitting is quasi "dose–dependent," where the term "dose" refers to the combined effect of the patient's fecundity and the specific treatment administered. This finding is supported by the possibility that ovarian stimulation – the common denominator of all assisted procreation – may affect oocyte development which could predispose to splitting (Fig. 63.4).

Second, one must also reconsider mortality figures in HOMPs undergoing MFPR. There is little doubt that MFPR is among the ultimate paradoxes of medicine whereby infertile patients undergo intricate treatments and, when at last successful, may have to consider reduction (= termination) of their "surplus" fetuses (= success). At the same time, there is little doubt that MFPR may be the only solution for a potentially successful outcome of a high-order multiple gestation. MFPR, discussed elsewhere in this volume, is indeed associated with improved perinatal outcome, as expected from comparing HOMPs with twins or singletons. However, given that all fetuses have a similar survival potential, it is argued that the reduced fetus(es) should be included in the mortality figures of MFPR (22). Table 63.2 shows the minimal mortality rates associated with various MFPR procedures, which suggest, quite bluntly, that MFPR is, in fact, a lethal iatrogenic sequence of iatrogenic multiples.

The third point to consider is the frequently overlooked risk of chromosomal disorders in IMP. Although each of the fetuses in a polyzygotic multiple gestation has the same chance for an aberration, as does a singleton with similar risk variables, there is an increased risk for the mother that one of her multiples will be affected. Data have clearly substantiated older calculations that showed that a 31-year-old mother of DZs carries a similar risk of having one twin with Down's syndrome as a 35-year-old mother of a singleton (23). Given that IMPs are more common in older mothers and that biochemical markers are less useful for twins and unavailable for HOMPs, one must rely on nuchal translucency measurements (24,25) or on invasive cytogenetic procedures [amniocentesis or chorionic villus sampling (CVS)]. Regrettably, little information exists about the former in HOMPs and the latter carries increased risk for miscarriage in these premium pregnancies.

Considering all the risks associated with IMP, one undoubtedly should prefer a singleton to a multiple pregnancy. To minimize risks, no more than a single embryo should be transferred. This policy has been implemented in recent years in many countries and a full discussion of the results is beyond the scope of this chapter. In general, the balance between the risk of multiples, the success rate of single ET, and the potential need for reimbursement of

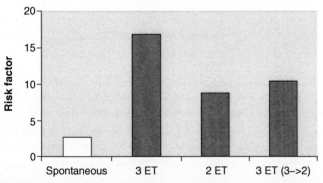

Figure 63.3 Estimated risk of cerebral palsy following transfer of three and two embryos, and following natural multifetal pregnancy reduction (MFPR) of all triplets to twins. A three- to sixfold increased risk of cerebral palsy is expected. *Abbreviation*: ET, embryo transfer. *Source*: Adapted from Ref. 19.

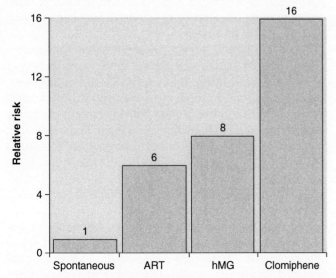

Figure 63.4 Zygotic splitting. Frequency of MZ twins following various methods of assisted reproduction. The accepted 0.4% of spontaneous zygotic splitting was used as reference. *Abbreviations*: ART, assisted reproductive technique; hMG, human menopausal gonadotropin. Data from the East Flanders Prospective Twin Survey. *Source*: Adapted from Ref. 1.

Table 63.2 Minimal Mortality Rates in Various Natural Multifetal Pregnancy Reduction (MFPR) Combinations

MFPR	$4 \rightarrow 2$	$5 \rightarrow 2$	$3 \rightarrow 2$	$4 \rightarrow 1$	$3 \rightarrow 1$	$2 \rightarrow 1$
Minimal mortality (%)	50	60	33	75	66	50

additional cycles has been considered and the net result seems to favor single ET. However, there are two additional partners to the triangle. IMP following ART is usually achieved after long-standing infertility and is usually the "end-stage" procedure. At this phase of reproductive life, most couples would consider a multiple pregnancy as compensation for their efforts (26). No wonder that most couples will support, or even persuade the physician, to increase the chances of pregnancy by increasing the number of transferred embryos.

THE PATIENT

The optimism at the beginning of ART changes quite often to severe psychological morbidity. From the outset, couples are faced with dilemmas that they have never faced before. For instance, couples initiating therapy were given questionnaires to determine attitudes regarding multiple pregnancy and MFPR (26,27). The results suggested declining ratings as the number of fetuses increased. Intrauterine insemination (IUI) patients felt more favorable than the IVF group toward all gestational outcomes and less favorable toward MFPR. Baor and Blickstein (26) suggested that young adults who postpone childbearing may presume that fertility is granted but, when all other measures fail, the use of ART is considered the ultimate salvation for these couples. However, ART is highly stressful and may lead to significant negative psychological consequences (loss of self-esteem, confidence, health, close relationships, security, and hope). The risks of multiple pregnancies is frequently overlooked or underappreciated by infertile couples. Despite the real risks associated with a multiple pregnancy and birth, infertile patients often express a desperate wish to have twins or triplets, thereby accomplishing an instant family. The authors highlighted the need to provide infertile couples with detailed information on the risks of multiple pregnancy and birth.

In the next step, couples may confront the dilemma to donate or destroy supernumerary embryos. This seeming impasse was investigated in 200 couples embarking on IVF–ET treatment (28). Couples' opinions on genetic lineage and education were determinant in their decision to destroy or to donate their supernumerary embryos than their opinions on the in vitro embryo status. The couples expressed various attitudes toward risks of twins and triplets, whereby twins were much more desired than triplets, which are often refused.

The psychological morbidity following MFPR and/or raising high-order multiples has been documented. When confronting the dilemma of potential loss of the entire pregnancy following MFPR, couples may experience considerable emotional distress. Nevertheless, many viewed this option as their "least bad" alternative (29). The French group that followed couples during pregnancy and for four years postpartum provided some important clues to understanding this complex situation (30,31). They first studied the effects of MFPR on the mothers' emotional well-being and the relationship with the children during the two years following intervention.

Then, at two years, they compared mothers who had a reduction with mothers who had not and had delivered triplets. At one year, a third of the women in the reduction group reported persistent depressive symptoms related to the reduction, mainly sadness and guilt. The others made medical and rational comments expressing no emotion. At two years all but two women seemed to have overcome the emotional pain associated with the reduction. The comparison with mothers of triplets indicated that the mothers' anxiety and depression, and difficult relationships with the children, were less acute in the reduction group. At four years after delivery, all mothers reported emotional distress, mainly fatigue and stress. One-third of the mothers had a high score of depression and used psychotropic medication. The relationships with the children and difficulties in coping with their behavior and conflicts were the main reason for psychological distress. Difficulties had not decreased over the years to the extent that one-third of the mothers spontaneously expressed regrets about having triplets.

A Swedish study found similar results (32). Couples ($n = 21$) with complete sets of triplets aged four to six years were interviewed about their experiences of being "triplet parents." The diagnosis of triplets had been a shock for most. All triplets were born prematurely. The first time at home was chaotic for most of the parents. Eventually, "triplet parents" spent more time organizing their lives and less time on emotional care than did parents of singletons.

The psychological effects are often superimposed on maternal complications, which are common in multiple pregnancies. The list of serious morbidity associated with twins and HOMPs has not been specified for IMP. However, risks of hypertensive disorders, eclampsia, complications of treatment for premature contractions, prolonged bed rest, prolonged hospitalization, and operative deliveries are significantly higher in multiples than in singletons. Thus, the possibility of serious maternal morbidity associated with IMP should be considered to the same extent that ovarian hyperstimulation syndrome (OHSS) is considered before ART.

Since maternal morbidity is undoubtedly increased in multiple gestations, it has been proposed that maternal mortality is also increased (33). However, since a multiple pregnancy is not registered as the direct cause of death, the risk is unknown. For example, eclampsia, tocolysis, and delivery related deaths were more common in twins (33). Data from the Perinatal Information System, including over 700 Latin America and Caribbean hospitals, have clearly shown that multiple pregnancy increases the risk of significant maternal morbidity in nulliparas and maternal mortality in multiparas (34). It is believed that IMPs are not spared these risks.

The epidemic of iatrogenic HOMPs enabled some insight into the increased maternal morbidity in these cases. The most significant morbidities found in triplets were pregnancy-induced hypertension (27–33%), HELLP [hemolysis, elevated liver enzymes, and low platelets syndrome; (9–10.5%)], anemia (27–58.1%), and postpartum hemorrhage (9–12.3%) (35,36).

Since maternal morbidity clearly increases with plurality, it is expected that maternal morbidity will decrease following MFPR. Skupski et al. (37) found that severe preeclampsia was more common among IVF triplet pregnancies (26.3%) than among IVF triplets reduced to twins (7.9%). The prevalence of all preeclampsia cases was also higher among the triplet group (44.7%) than among the twin group (15.8%). Since all pregnancies were successfully implanted triplets, this finding suggests that plurality and placental mass are probably more important to the development of preeclampsia than is successful implantation alone. Similar findings were reported on gestational diabetes (GDM) (38).

It was hypothesized that GDM, by its virtue to increase fetal size might have a beneficial effect in twins. A matched-control study found the pre-gravid obesity was associated with diabetes during a twin pregnancy. The twin neonates from the GDM group had more respiratory distress syndrome (OR 2.2; 95% CI 1.3, 3.7) and had a threefold, but not significantly increased perinatal mortality rate. Importantly, birth weight characteristics were similar in both groups (39).

Maternal morbidity should also be considered in the context of maternal age. ART has enabled pregnancies beyond the range of reproductive years, when underlying diseases are more common and pregnancy complications are expected to be intensified.

Data from the United States National Center for Health Statistics and the Center for Disease Control (NCHS/CDC Press release, September 14, 1999) suggest that (i) between 1980–82 and 1995–97 the twin birth rate rose 63% for women aged 40–44 years and nearly 1000% for women aged 45–49 years; (ii) the HOMP birth rate rose nearly 400% for women in their 30s and more than 1000% for women in their 40s. In 1997 there were more twins born to women aged 45–49 years than during the whole decade of the 1980s. Obviously, motherhood at or beyond the edge of reproductive age is a new aspect of what clinicians previously referred to as pregnancy in the "older gravida" (40). With ART, the boundary between "old" and "young" no longer exists. Generally, the majority of the published studies have been unanimous about the special and perhaps supercautious attitude required for the older mother, an approach that translates to higher rates of peripartum interventions. Despite the fact that some complications may occur more frequently in older mothers as a result of accumulated prior diseases, there is no direct evidence that older age, per se, complicates either gestation or parturition. Quite unexpectedly, Keith et al. found that older age has an advantage of better perinatal outcome (mainly in terms of birth weight) of twins and triplets (41). It is unclear if this is a result of a better socioeconomic status of older mothers or if it is related to some uterine "programming" effect.

In contrast to these skyrocketing rates, there are few series describing such "geriatric gravidas" and therefore, the true prevalence of various complications may be underestimated. In one study, 4.5 ± 1.1 cleaving embryos were transferred per cycle to 45–59-year-old patients, resulting in 74 delivered pregnancies (34.9%). There were 29 (39.2%) multiple gestations, including 20 twins, seven triplets, and two quadruplets. Two of the triplet and both of the quadruplet pregnancies underwent MFPR to twins. Antenatal complications occurred in 28 women (37.8%), including preterm labor, hypertension, diabetes, preeclampsia, HELLP syndrome, and fetal growth retardation. Cesarean section was done in 64.8% (42).

The age-related risk for trisomy, depending on the source of the female gametes, is of primary importance when ART is performed in the elderly. For those who conceive without donor eggs, this risk might be exceptionally high. However, in the case of a polyzygotic multiple gestation, the risk of pregnancy loss following cytogenetic studies might be unacceptably high. Thus, the timing of these studies becomes pertinent. In countries where feticide is permitted only before the 24th week of gestation, the only options are first-trimester chorionic villus sampling (CVS) or second-trimester amniocentesis. In some countries, feticide is not restricted to gestational age, and late feticide is a clear option. In such instances, amniocentesis is scheduled during the 30th–32nd week, with the possibility of feticide at 33–35 weeks. This logical scheme eliminates the risk of losing the entire pregnancy at an unsalvageable age. However, this scheme provokes two major problems: First, the patient might deliver during the time interval before the cytogenetic results; second, legitimization of third-trimester feticide is a formidable ethical dilemma and does not imply that physicians will agree to terminate a viable fetus. These intricacies may be settled if preimplantation diagnosis should become a useful option.

Surrogate motherhood is a good example how ART may change all we know about IMP: Consider the "Angela" case, in which two embryos of unrelated couples were transferred to a surrogate uterus. The newborn twins, whose parentage was confirmed postpartum, were non-siblings who shared no common genes and, of course, shared nothing with the surrogate mother (43).

It goes without saying that the most common and the most risky complication of multiple pregnancies is preterm birth, for which no remedy is available. However, irrespective of plurality, an association between preterm birth and ART has long been suspected and found to be related to causes such as iatrogenic preterm birth (in the so-called "premium" pregnancies), fertility history, and past obstetric performance, and to underlying medical conditions of the female partner (44). Data showed that singleton as well as multiple pregnancies resulting from IVF have increased rates of preterm birth compared with naturally conceived pregnancies (44). The most plausible explanation seems to be a more liberal use of elective preterm birth. In any case, the most appropriate endpoint after ART should also include preterm or term birth as a measure of success.

Finally, the patient with IMP should also be considered in evolutionary terms. Innumerable studies have shown that, over the millennia, evolutionary forces selected a female prototype for spontaneous twins. Black, fertile, older, taller, and heavily built women are more likely to have twins and the outcome is likely better than in women with other characteristics. Thus, the fact that ART involves no selection (except fertility), and certainly no selection for motherhood of multiples, makes the IMP in many ways an iatrogenic contraevolutionary phenomenon.

THE PHYSICIAN

Three types of physicians comprise the third part of the IMP triangle: those involved in ART, those caring for maternal–fetal issues, and the pediatricians. Each is in charge of a different phase.

The Reproduction Phase

Since there seems to be a direct relation between the number of transferred embryos and success rate of ART on the one hand and the IMP rate on the other hand, there seems to be an inherent conflict in the reproduction phase. An idea about the anticipated rates of IMP comes from centers in which all available embryos were transferred and MFPR is not used (Fig. 63.5) (45). Before the implementation of the 2004 Italian Reproduction Law (46), the Reggio Emilia (Italy) Center for Reproductive Medicine observed that 34.6% of the clinical pregnancies were multiples, comprising 20% twins and 14.6% HOMPs (45). Interestingly, implementation of the Italian Reproductive Law, which limited the number of fertilized oocytes to three but obliged transfer of all embryos, did not significantly change the incidence of multiples and somewhat improved the overall outcome (46). Some concern exists, however, regarding the group of patients >38 years.

Ethical, legal, religious, and technical (i.e., availability of cryopreservation) constraints that obviate selection and/or disposal of surplus embryos is the easy way for deciding on the number of embryos that should be transferred. The hard way is careful analysis of success (live birth) versus failure (IMP) rates using selected embryos. Genetic and biochemical markers would supplement morphological criteria as normal-appearing embryos may be genetically abnormal. Preimplantation genetic studies may also replace invasive procedures during pregnancy following ART. For the time being, the first step has already been done by implementing elective single ET in several countries without significantly reducing outcomes.

Many of the recommendations have been based on ET without specifying their quality and their implantation potential. In the meantime, it has become possible to culture embryos to the blastocyst stage, selecting the fittest embryos for transfer and synchronizing the embryonic with the endometrial stages. Blastocyst transfer has been associated with a much improved implantation rate than that of three-day embryos. It is expected that the high "take-home baby" rate following the excellent implantation rates would lead to transfer of one or two blastocysts only, with concomitant reduction of the IMP rate. However, not all embryos will become blastocysts and it is unknown which dividing embryo will become a blastocyst in vitro. Thus, physicians may not wait for the five-day stage and will first transfer three-day embryos and then, when blastocysts are successfully cultured, will transfer additional blastocysts, generating iatrogenic superfecundations.

To date, there are no data regarding the consequences of such protocols. Logically, mixed-stage ETs will necessarily increase the chance of IMPs by adding the successful implantation of the five-day to that of the three-day embryo(s). In addition, we do not know the influence of co-implantation at different embryonic ages on the risk of zygotic splitting. We, among others, have noticed some bizarre complex chorionicity arrangements that have never been seen with the usual IVF–ET protocols (unpublished data, Fig. 63.6).

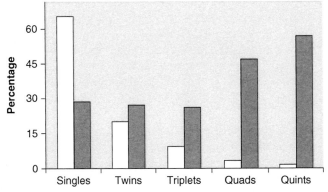

Figure 63.5 Spontaneous loss in iatrogenic multiple pregnancies (IMPs) when all available embryos are transferred and natural multifetal pregnancy reduction (MFPR) is not used. Light bars: Percentage of clinical pregnancies at 35 days post-transfer; dark bars: Percentage of disintegrated gestational sacs. Source: Adapted from Ref. 45.

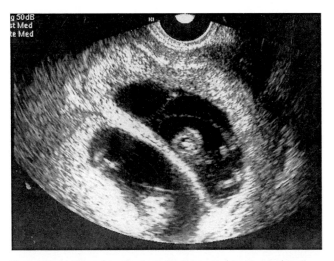

Figure 63.6 Complex chorionicity. Sonographic image showing a seven-week quadruplet pregnancy following sequential transfer of two embryos and one blastocyst. This bichorionic (BC) quadruplet pregnancy comprises monochorionic triamniotic triplets (upper sac) and a singleton (lower sac). Source: Image courtesy of B Caspi, MD.

It is therefore reasonable to conclude that demands from infertile couples and fertility clinics to maximize success rates conflict with the need to reduce the number of IMPs.

The Pregnancy Phase

Once pregnant, the woman is not infertile anymore and there should be no difference in the management of spontaneous as compared to iatrogenic pregnancies. However, the past reproductive history continues to follow the patient, albeit her pregnancy may be absolutely normal. When an IMP results, the designation of "premium gestation" seems appropriate, and most reproduction experts may refer the patient to a clinician involved in maternal–fetal medicine (MFM) conducting high-risk pregnancy clinics.

Couples frequently create a special attitude toward the "producer" and may feel abandoned when referred to another physician who takes over. Quite often the optimism involved in infertility treatment may change to pessimism or even to criticism (47). Then, the unprepared couples may consider MFPR or risky interventions as hostile suggestions. It follows that the dissociation between the reproductive and the MFM physician is by no means simple for any of the parties involved.

It is not yet accepted who should treat the IMP. Obviously, many subspecialties are involved: For example, the sonographer who makes the diagnosis may not be the one who will carry out the MFPR, and both may not take care of the preeclamptic patient. This complicated pregnancy follow-up is therefore never a one-man show, and a well-orchestrated teamwork is encouraged. Indeed, it has been shown that special multiple pregnancy clinics do have better results.

The extremely varied spectrum of IMPs is superimposed on the special patient–physician relationship. It is beyond the scope of this chapter to discuss in detail follow-up protocols tailored for the diverse presentations of IMP. A 32-year-old patient with premature ovarian failure and a 48-year-old perimenopausal woman may undergo similar egg or embryo donation, but are expected to run different age-related obstetric risks. Likewise, 20-year-old and 40-year-old women may need similar ICSI techniques for severe oligospermia, but differ in respect of anticipated age-related pregnancy complications.

The obligations for the fetus as a patient in a multiple pregnancy are quite complicated (48). In addition to the physician–mother–fetus relationship, there are feto–fetal relations that must be contemplated. The simplest example is a preterm multiple pregnancy in which fetal distress is suspected in one fetus. The obstetrician is faced with the dilemma to salvage one fetus by conferring risks of prematurity on the non-distressed fetus. A more complicated example is the consideration of MFPR in a BC triplet pregnancy (i.e., MC twins plus a singleton). Obviously, a three to two reduction will end with an MC twin gestation in which TTTS is a calculated risk. On the other hand, reducing the twins will increase the risk of losing the entire pregnancy. A third example is a single sac, remote from term, with rupture of the membranes in a triplet pregnancy. Should a delayed-interval delivery be performed (increasing the risk of amnionitis) or should the whole pregnancy be terminated?

It seems there is never a dull moment in caring for the mother with multiples, exemplified by conflicts between maternal condition and continuation of pregnancy. The lack of effective prophylactic measures against preterm labor and the risks associated with tocolysis is a good example of how the physiologic adaptation for a multiple gestation may complicate treatment with ®-mimetic drugs or with MgSO4. Thus, the risk in arresting preterm labor (to the mother) may be as significant as the risk (to the neonate) of delivering premature multiples.

It is beyond the scope of this chapter to describe the plethora of inefficient methods to reduce the preterm birth rate in multiple pregnancies. This pessimistic realization was reached by trying to carry multiple pregnancies to term (by singleton standards), whereas medicine is apparently unable to change the inherent inadequacy of the uteroplacental unit to accommodate and nurture multiples that long. In this respect, two points should be made. First, "term" in singletons is different than in twins or in HOMPs. Thus, it seems futile to aim for 38 weeks' gestation in multiples just to conclude that this target is unattainable. Second, it follows that a realistic gestational age based on related survival and morbidity rates should be set. For example, obstetricians should aim for 30 weeks' gestation if their neonatal service provides good outcome for neonates at this age. Thus, it seems reasonable to suggest that if prematurity in multiples is not preventable, efforts should be made to prevent extreme prematurity.

Finally, a time comes when the obstetrician and the patient consider the mode of delivery. There is little doubt that a planned (daytime), elective cesarean delivery offers a simple solution in terms of required personnel and safety to mother and neonates. This seems to be intuitively true for HOMPs and for small twins, although there are no prospective studies to support this assumption. For twins weighing at least 1500 g each, either route of delivery seems to be appropriate, irrespective of fetal presentation (49). However, as mentioned above, IMPs are frequently considered as "premium," high-risk pregnancies, and many will follow the dictum that "no high-risk pregnancy should end with a high-risk delivery" and opt for an elective abdominal birth.

The Neonatal Phase

There is no significant difference between treating three preterm singletons and a preterm triplet pregnancy, as each of these neonates deserves its own special care. However, the epidemic dimensions of IMP create consequential logistical problems that ideally should be separated from the purely medical problems. Regrettably, advances in ART have been much faster than the preparation of sufficient cribs in the neonatal intensive care unit (NICU). As a result, overproduction of preterm neonates overwhelms the capacity of many NICUs, leading to medical problems associated with over-crowded stations.

A Canadian study compared the preterm birth rates in two three-year periods, 1981–83 and 1992–94 (50). Preterm birth rate increased by 9% (from 6.3% to 6.8%). Importantly, the rate of preterm birth among live births resulting from multiples increased by 25% compared with 5% in singletons, confirming that the increase in preterm births is largely attributable to the increase in multiple birth rates.

HOMP births are at much greater risk than single births. An NCHS report on the final 1996 birth statistics for the United States found that infant mortality rates are 12 times higher for triplets than for singletons, triplets are 12 times more likely to die within the first year of life, the average birth weight of a triplet baby is half that of a singleton, and the gestational duration is, on average, seven weeks shorter. For 1995, 92% of triplets were preterm compared with about 10% of births in single deliveries.

Delivery of a multiple pregnancy should be a carefully planned event. A minimal neonatal team for a triplet delivery may include as many as 10 persons, including physicians, assistants, and a supervisor. Obviously, chaos prevails unless teamwork is harmonized. Neonatal transportation should be available if the expected number of neonates exceeds the number of available NICU cribs.

Logistic considerations do not end at delivery. Once at the nursery, all the multiples must be given equal opportunity to bond with their parents and, perhaps, according to psychological view, to continue their intrauterine contacts with their siblings. For instance, there is increasing evidence that co-bedding of twins in the NICU improves thermoregulation, feeding, and sleeping parameters (51). Indeed, the special and unique interaction between multiples during childhood and beyond seems to reflect the unique relationship that exists between fetuses that grow together in utero (Appendix).

Figure 63.7 shows mortality rates of twins, triplets, and higher-order multiples in England and Wales in 1993 relative to singletons, demonstrating the much increased incidence of stillbirth, perinatal, neonatal, and infant deaths in multiple pregnancy (52). Thus, parents of a multiple pregnancy are more likely to experience bereavement than those with singletons. The care that parents should receive when all fetuses/babies die is not different from that when a singleton dies. When one baby of a multiple birth dies, the loss is frequently underestimated; however, the loss of parents that are left "with something" is no less painful.

The time spent in the nursery may be the only opportunity for the parents to prepare for the future. At home, mothers may find the reality of coping with their multiples more demanding than they had expected. Needless to say, professional help is needed during infancy and childhood to the same extent that it had been needed before and during pregnancy.

Finally, it is well accepted that even perfectly normal multiples are a significant financial burden for every family.

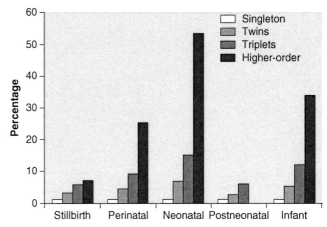

Figure 63.7 Mortality rates of twins, triplets, and higher-order multiples in England and Wales in 1993 relative to singletons. A much increased incidence of stillbirth, perinatal, neonatal, and infant deaths is shown in multiple pregnancy. *Source*: Adapted from Ref. 52.

Many studies have estimated the expenses involved in IMP. Given that costs involved in ART are similar to conceptions ending with a singleton, and given that costs of pregnancy surveillance of multiples are moderately increased as compared with singletons, the major financial impact of IMP evolves from raising premature infants in the expensive environment of the NICU. No mathematical skills are needed to establish the number of NICU days per IMP and to multiply the product by the daily cost of NICU hospitalization. Moreover, lifelong morbidity, which is significantly associated with preterm birth, has further implications on the expenses involved in caring for the handicapped children. Thus, from a financial perspective, IMP must be considered as a syndrome of an affluent society.

EPILOGUE: RE-DEFINING SUCCESS

Every day there are numerous healthy multiples delivered following ART conceptions. Almost every proud reproductive center documents this success in pictures of smiling parents, cute babies, and grinning physicians. The media love it as well and give prime time priority for items related to HOMP births. As a consequence, infertile couples exposed to these encouraging results are bound to push ART to its available limits, irrespective of the untoward outcome of a multiple pregnancy.

As stated previously and until proven otherwise, the human female is programmed by nature to have one child at a time. Consequently, success should have only one meaning – a "take-home baby" rate of one infant per pregnancy. Thus, there is an inherent absurdity in considering a HOMP in need of MFPR as a successful outcome, and it is likewise irrational to consider the delivery of triplets at 29 weeks' gestation as a successful event. Obviously, producing a three- to sixfold increased risk for a lifelong handicap such as cerebral palsy cannot be considered successful.

Two of the several solutions proposed to overcome the epidemic of IMP are relevant to ART. First, the dissociation between members of the "production line" should be minimal. Thus, both reproductive experts and their patients should have an accurate perspective of the potential obstetric, neonatal, and lifelong complications associated with IMPs. Second, the current changing trends from quantity to quality in ART, by transferring fewer but higher-quality embryos or blastocysts, may be the light at the end of the tunnel.

One should consider the international consensus statement on the perinatal care of multiples (Appendix), where many aspects related to ART are discussed. In any case, the apocalyptic views expressed in this chapter will remain pertinent as long as demands for better pregnancy rates by couples undergoing ART are accepted by overzealous reproduction centers without a clear definition of what should be considered successful.

APPENDIX

Recommendations and Guidelines for Perinatal Practice

The Istanbul international consensus statement on the perinatal care of multiple Pregnancy

Isaac Blickstein[1,**], Birgit Arabin[2], Frank A. Chervenak[3], Zehra N. Kavak[4], Louis G. Keith[5], Eric S. Shinwell[6], Alin Basgul[4], and Yves Ville[7]

[1] Department of Obstetrics and Gynecology, Kaplan Medical Center, Rehovot, Israel
[2] Department of Gynecology, Sophia Hospital Zwolle, Zwolle, The Netherlands
[3] Department of Obstetrics and Gynecology, New York Weill Cornell Medical Center, USA
[4] Department of Obstetrics and Gynecology, Marmara University Hospital, Istanbul, Turkey
[5] Department of Obstetrics and Gynecology, Northwestern University Medicine School, Chicago, USA
[6] Department of Neonatology, Kaplan Medical Center, Rehovot, Israel
[7] Department of Obstetrics and Gynecology, University Versailles St. Quentin, Poissy, France

Abstract

The purpose of this document is to expand the 1995 ISTS/COMBO Declaration of Rights that was initially produced to promote awareness of the special needs of multiple birth infants, children, and adults. It addresses the clinical and ethical dimensions of perinatal care of multiple pregnancies.

The ad hoc committee was chaired by Isaac Blickstein. The following individuals were present (in alphabetical order): Birgit Arabin (Zwolle, Netherlands/Berlin, Germany), Isaac Blickstein (Rehovot, Israel), Frank A. Chervenak (NY, USA), Zehra Nese Kavak (Istanbul, Turkey), Louis

G. Keith (Chicago, U.S.A), Eric S. Shinwell (Rehovot, Israel), and Yves Ville (Paris, France). Secretary of the meeting was Alin Basgul (Istanbul, Turkey).

This statement was endorsed by the International Society of Twin Studies (Ghent, Belgium, June, 2007) and by the World Association of Perinatal Medicine (Florence, Italy, September, 2007).

Consensus Statement

1. Multiples and their families, as any other individuals, have a right to full protection under the law and freedom from discrimination of any kind.
2. Pregnant women and their multiples have a right to be cared for by professionals who are knowledgeable regarding the management of multiple gestation and/or the lifelong special needs of multiples.
3. Individuals or couples seeking information and/or treatment for infertility have a right to full disclosure about clinically relevant information that might influence the conception of multiples, the associated risks, and the medically reasonable management alternatives for them. This disclosure should be specific to each potential intervention. Thus, if successive interventions are considered, multiple disclosures should be provided and consent obtained for each intervention.
4. When infertility treatment is contemplated, the a priori risks and consequences of having a multiple pregnancy secondary to each infertility treatment should be discussed. In settings where iatrogenic multiple gestations may result, the potential need for multifetal pregnancy reduction (MFPR) and its associated risks should be discussed.
5. Given the increased risk of any multiple pregnancy:

    (a) Infertility treatment should intend to prevent multiple pregnancies, in particular high-order multiples. This implies that a high-order multiple gestation after infertility treatment should be considered as a complication.
    (b) Infertility services should disclose their number of multiple pregnancies, both intentional and unintentional.
    (c) The economical justification of choosing a multiple pregnancy, especially high-order multiple pregnancy, should be discouraged.
    (d) The use of a multiple pregnancy as a potential cohort from which fetus of either sex can be selected is discouraged.
    (e) In the special case of inherited disease, pregestational diagnosis (PGD) to select embryos for transfer should be preferred to producing a multiple pregnancy in order to reduce the affected embryos.

---

*Constructed by an ad hoc committee, convened in Istanbul, January 26, 2007. Coordinator of WAPM Multiple Pregnancies Working Group: Isaac Blickstein.
** J. Perinat. Med. 35(2007) 465–467. Reproduced by permission.

6. MFPR should be considered as a destructive measure for reduced fetuses and a therapeutic measure for the remaining fetuses. It may also be traumatic for one or both parents. Its only role is to potentially promote a better outcome for the remaining embryo(s). It follows that:

    (a) The decision about MFPR is ultimately the pregnant woman's to make. The pregnant woman should be provided reliable information about institutional rather than national success rates of MFPR. The patient's beliefs and values are determinative in the decision making process regarding whether MFPR is to be performed and, if so, the number of embryos to be reduced.
    (b) Diagnostic evaluation of fetuses before MFPR is appropriate, as the resulting information is relevant to the pregnant woman's decision making.
    (c) MFPR should be considered as a relevant antenatal event and registries should be encouraged so that outcome can be appreciated.

7. Selective reduction of an anomalous fetus should be performed in a manner as to minimize the potential danger to the remaining fetus(es), taking chorionicity into consideration:

    (a) Screening, diagnosis, and selective reduction should be performed at a timing to optimize the outcome for the remaining fetus(es).
    (b) Selective reduction should be considered as a relevant antenatal event and registries should be encouraged so that outcomes can be appreciated.

8. A distinction must be made between a multiple pregnancy and a multiple birth. For epidemiological purposes, singleton births that started as a multiple pregnancy should be recorded in order to properly account for spontaneous and iatrogenic embryonic and fetal loss(es).

9. Ultrasound technology is critical for antenatal care in all multiple pregnancies. Chorionicity should be established by ultrasound as accurately and as early as possible in all multiple pregnancies. Information about chorionicity should be provided to the expectant mother along with its clinical significance. When this information is lacking, careful postpartum placental examination should be performed.

10. Zygosity determination should be a prerogative of the parents or of the multiples and not of the care providers (except for clearly defined research objectives in which informed consent has been given). Zygosity should be respected as any other human trait and deserves the same privacy rules. Involvement in registries of monozygotic twins should be absolutely voluntary on the part of the multiples.

11. Complex cases associated with monochorionic placentation, such as twin–twin transfusion syndrome (TTTS), twin reversed arterial perfusion (TRAP) sequence, and severe discordance, should be evaluated and treated in specialized centers based on scientific and ethical considerations. In the absence of the possibility of referral, consultation should be obtained requesting the best potential therapy in the local setting.

12. Following single perinatal demise within a set of multiples, parents may consider informing the survivor(s) that he/she/they were a sib of multiple pregnancy.

13. Whenever the clinical circumstance of one twin jeopardizes the other, care should be exercised to select a management plan that would optimize the outcome of both fetuses. The pregnant woman should be involved in such decision-making.

14. Fetal surveillance before and during labor should be carried out on all fetuses. It follows that each fetus should be adequately and appropriately monitored.

15. Delivery considerations should include the welfare of all fetuses. Mode of delivery should be based on medical considerations pertaining to each fetus, as well as on maternal health and preferences.

16. Delivery of multiples should ideally take place:

    (a) In a center that is equipped with neonatal intensive care facilities available simultaneously for each infant;
    (b) Where a medical care provider certified in neonatal resuscitation is present for each neonate; and with
    (c) Facilities for a high-risk delivery (such as availability of an experienced obstetrician, 24-h anesthesia coverage, blood availability, etc.). If this is not possible, in utero transfer may be preferable to postpartum transfer

17. Governments and private payers should be aware of the financial costs of multiple pregnancy and birth and the future upbringing of the multiples. Whenever possible, direct financial aid should be supplied to parents in proportion to plurality.

18. Any research involving multiples must be conducted using informed consent of the participants or their parents and must comply with accepted international codes of ethics and scientific standards for conducting human subject research.

19. In the instance when one or more of a set of multiples manifests a physical and/or mental handicap, management plans should respect the special needs of the handicapped member(s) in the setting of a multiple pregnancy while also giving attention to the special needs of the non-handicapped sib(s).

20. Public policy should support a set of multiples remaining together in foster care and adoptive families.

Acknowledgments

The committee acknowledges with thanks the assistance of Laurence B. McCullough, PhD (Huston, TX) in reviewing the preliminary draft of this document. The committee acknowledges with thanks the unrestricted educational grants provided by Philips Turk, EMA electronic devices, and Abdi Ibrahim Drug Company, Istanbul.

REFERENCES

1. Blickstein I, Verhoeven HC, Keith LG. Zygotic splitting after assisted reproduction. N Engl J Med 1999; 340: 738–9.

2. Blickstein I, Jones C, Keith LG. Zygotic-splitting rates after single-embryo transfers in in vitro fertilization. N Engl J Med 2003; 348: 2366–7.

3. Gielen M, Lindsey PJ, Derom C, et al. Modeling genetic and environmental factors to increase heritability and ease the identification of candidate genes for birth weight: a twin study. Behav Genet 2008; 38: 44–54.

4. Templeton A, Morris JK. Reducing the risk of multiple births by transfer of two embryos after in vitro fertilization. N Engl J Med 1998; 339: 573–7.

5. Blickstein I. Perinatal implications of iatrogenic multiple pregnancies. In: Voto LS, Margulies M, Cosmi EV, eds. 4th World Congress of Perinatal Medicine. Bologna: Monduzzi Editore, 1999: 167–72.

6. Leroy F. Les Jumeaux dans Tous Leurs Etats. Bruxelles: De Boeck-Wesmael, 1995: 87.

7. Blickstein I, Keith LG, eds. Iatrogenic Multiple Pregnancy: Clinical Implications. Lancaster, UK: Parthenon, 2000.

8. Blickstein I, Keith LG, eds. Multiple Pregnancy, 2nd edn. Oxford: Taylor & Francis, 2005.

9. Blickstein I, Smith-Levitin M. Twinning and twins. In: Chervenak FA, Kurjak A, eds. Current Perspectives on the Fetus as a Patient. Lancaster, UK: Parthenon, 1996: 507–25.

10. Blickstein I, Smith-Levitin M. Multifetal pregnancy. In: Petrikovsky BM, ed. Fetal Disorders: Diagnosis and Management. New York: John Wiley and Sons, 1998: 223–47.

11. Blickstein I, Goldman RD, Smith-Levitin M, et al. The relation between inter-twin birth weight discordance and total twin birth weight. Obstet Gynecol 1999; 93: 113–16.

12. Palermo GD, Cohen J, Alikani M, Adler A, Rosenwaks Z. Intracytoplasmic sperm injection: a novel treatment for all forms of male factor infertility. Fertil Steril 1995; 63: 1231–40.

13. Gavriil P, Jauniaux E, Leroy F. Pathologic examination of placentas from singleton and twin pregnancies obtained after in vitro fertilization and embryo transfer. Pediatr Pathol 1993; 13: 453–62.

14. Pharoah PO, Cooke RW. A hypothesis for the aetiology of spastic cerebral palsy – the vanishing twin. Dev Med Child Neurol 1997; 39: 292–6.

15. Blickstein I. Reflections on the hypothesis for the etiology of spastic cerebral palsy caused by the 'vanishing twin' syndrome. Dev Med Child Neurol 1998; 40: 358.

16. Matias A, La Sala GB, Blickstein I. Early loss rates of entire pregnancies after assisted reproduction are lower in twin than in singleton pregnancies. Fertil Steril 2007; 88: 1452–4.

17. Blickstein I. Do multiple gestations raise the risk of cerebral palsy? Clin Perinatol 2004; 31: 395–408.

18. Pharoah PO, Cooke T. Cerebral palsy and multiple births. Arch Dis Child Fetal Neonatal Ed 1996; 75: F174.

19. Blickstein I, Weissman A. Estimating the risk of cerebral palsy after assisted reproduction. N Engl J Med 1999; 341: 1313–14.

20. Blickstein I, Keith LG. On the possible cause of monozygotic twinning: lessons from the 9-banded armadillo and from assisted reproduction. Twin Res Hum Genet 2007; 10: 394–9.

21. Derom C, Leroy F, Vlietinck R, Fryns JP, Derom R. High frequency of iatrogenic monozygotic twins with administration of clomiphene citrate and a change in chorionicity. Fertil Steril 2006; 85: 755–7.

22. Blickstein I. Should the reduced embryos be considered in outcome calculations of multifetal pregnancy reduction? Am J Obstet Gynecol 1994; 171: 866–7.

23. Meyers C, Adam R, Dungan J, Prenger V. Aneuploidy in twin gestations: when is maternal age advanced? Obstet Gynecol 1997; 89: 248–51.

24. Sebire NJ, Snijders RJ, Hughes K, Sepulveda W, Nicolaides KH. Screening for trisomy 21 in twin pregnancies by maternal age and fetal nuchal translucency thickness at 10–14 weeks of gestation. Br J Obstet Gynaecol 1996; 103: 999–1003.

25. Maymon R, Jauniaux E, Holmes A, et al. Nuchal translucency measurement and pregnancy outcome after assisted conception versus spontaneously conceived twins. Hum Reprod 2001; 16: 1999–2004.

26. Baor L, Blickstein I. En route to an 'instant family': psychosocial considerations. Obstet Gynecol Clin North Am 2005; 32: 127–39.

27. Goldfarb J, Kinzer DJ, Boyle M, Kurit D. Attitudes of in vitro fertilization and intrauterine insemination couples toward multiple gestation pregnancy and multifetal pregnancy reduction. Fertil Steril 1996; 65: 815–20.

28. Laruelle C, Englert Y. Psychological study of in vitro fertilization–embryo transfer participants' attitudes toward the destiny of their supernumerary embryos. Fertil Steril 1995; 63: 1047–50.

29. Berkowitz RL, Lynch L, Stone J, Alvarez M. The current status of multifetal pregnancy reduction. Am J Obstet Gynecol 1996; 174: 1265–72.

30. Garel M, Stark C, Blondel B, et al. Psychological reactions after multifetal pregnancy reduction: a 2-year follow-up study. Hum Reprod 1997; 12: 617–22.

31. Garel M, Salobir C, Blondel B. Psychological consequences of having triplets: a 4-year follow-up study. Fertil Steril 1997; 67: 1162–5.

32. Akerman BA, Hovmolle M, Thomassen PA. The challenges of expecting, delivering and rearing triplets. Acta Genet Med Gemellol Roma 1997; 46: 81–6.

33. Blickstein I. Maternal mortality in twin gestations. J Reprod Med 1997; 42: 680–4.

34. Conde-Agudelo A, Belizan J. Maternal mortality and morbidity associated with multiple pregnancy. Twin Res 1999; 2: S3.

35. Malone FD, Kaufman GE, Chelmow D, et al. Maternal morbidity associated with triplet pregnancy. Am J Perinatol 1998; 15: 73–7.

36. Albrecht JL, Tomich PG. The maternal and neonatal outcome of triplet gestations. Am J Obstet Gynecol 1996; 174: 1551–6.

37. Skupski DW, Nelson S, Kowalik A, et al. Multiple gestations from in vitro fertilization: successful implantation alone is not associated with subsequent preeclampsia. Am J Obstet Gynecol 1996; 175: 1029–32.

38. Sivan E, Maman E, Homko CJ, et al. Impact of fetal reduction on the incidence of gestational diabetes. Obstet Gynecol 2002; 99: 91–4.

39. Simões T, Queirós A, Correia L, et al. Gestational diabetes mellitus complicating twin pregnancies. J Perinat Med 2011; 39: 437–40.

40. Blickstein I. Motherhood at or beyond the edge of reproductive age. Int J Fertil Womens Med 2003; 48: 17–24.

41. Keith LG, Goldman RD, Breborowicz G, Blickstein I. Triplet pregnancies in women aged 40 or older: a matched control study. J Reprod Med 2004; 49: 683–8.

42. Sauer MV, Paulson RJ, Lobo RA. Oocyte donation to women of advanced reproductive age: pregnancy results and obstetrical outcomes in patients 45 years and older. Hum Reprod 1996; 11: 2540–3.

43. Simini B. Italian surrogate twins. Lancet 1997; 350: 1307.

44. Blickstein I. Does assisted reproduction technology, per se, increase the risk of preterm birth? BJOG 2006; 113(Suppl 3): 68–71.

45. La Sala GB, Montanari R, Cantarelli M, et al. Iatrogenic multifetal pregnancies and SPIER. Twin Res 1999; 2: S6.

46. La Sala GB, Vilani MT, Nicoli A, et al. The effect of legislation on outcomes of assisted reproduction technology: lessons from the 2004 Italian law. Fertil Steril 2008; 89: 854–9.

47. Blickstein I. Litigation in multiple pregnancy and birth. Clin Perinatol 2007; 34: 319–27.

48. Chervenak FA, McCullough LB. Ethics in Obstetrics and Gynecology. New York: Oxford University Press, 1994.

49. Blickstein I. Cesarean section for all twins? J Perinat Med 2000; 28: 169–74.

50. Joseph KS, Kramer MS, Marcoux S, et al. Determinants of preterm birth rate in Canada from 1981 through 1983 and from 1992 through 1994. N Engl J Med 1998; 339: 1434–9.

51. Mazela JL, Gdzinowski J. Co-bedding twins and multiples – is there strong clinical evidence? Twin Res 1999; 2: S17.

52. Dunn A, MacFarlane A. Recent trends in the incidence of multiple births and associated mortality in England and Wales. Arch Dis Child 1996; 75: F10–19.

64

Egg and embryo donation

Mark V. Sauer and Matthew A. Cohen

INTRODUCTION

Human egg (oocyte) and embryo donation was first introduced in 1983 and has evolved over the past three decades into a relatively common procedure that addresses a variety of reproductive disorders. This method has provided key insights into the physiology and pathophysiology of reproduction and, like other assisted reproductive techniques (ART), has engendered its share of controversy. Furthermore, techniques introduced by egg donation, such as schemes for adequate hormonal preparation of the uterus for synchronizing embryos with a receptive endometrium, have been successfully applied to other fertility therapies, including the management of patients with cryopreserved embryos for transfer and those requiring in vitro maturation of immature oocytes.

The first report of a successful egg donation in a mammalian species involved rabbits. Heape in 1890 described the transfer of rabbit embryos from the uterus of a donor to the uterus of a synchronized recipient, followed by the delivery of healthy offspring (1). During the 1970s, mammalian embryo donation was applied to cattle to improve the reproductive efficiency of prize animals. By 1990 almost 19,000 calves were born annually in the United States as a result of embryo transfer procedures (2).

In 2007, approximately 40,000 calves, representing 11.5% of the total registered Angus cattle born that year, were a result of embryo transfer (3).

The vast majority of mammalian egg donations resulted from embryos fertilized in vivo, recovered from the donor by uterine lavage, and then transferred to the recipient uterus. Using a modification of this technique, in 1983 researchers at the University of California, Los Angeles fertilized an oocyte in vivo after the artificial insemination of a human donor and then transferred the recovered embryo into a synchronized recipient (4). A total of 14 insemination cycles resulted in two ongoing pregnancies (5). In 1984 the first delivery of a healthy male infant was reported (6).

During this same time period, researchers at Monash University in Melbourne began transferring embryos to infertile recipients as a result of eggs fertilized in vitro from donated oocytes obtained laparoscopically from infertile women (7). In 1984 they reported the first live birth following egg donation and in vitro fertilization (IVF) (8). Synchronization of the recipient and donor was achieved using oral estradiol valerate and intravaginal progesterone pessaries prescribed to the functionally agonadal recipient.

Donor uterine lavage was popular in the early 1980s since it was far less invasive than laparoscopy, but by 1987 uterine lavage was discontinued in humans because of the fear of human immunodeficiency virus (HIV) transmission and the inability to prevent occasional retained pregnancies in the embryo donors. Furthermore, around this time the introduction of transvaginal oocyte aspiration using ultrasound guidance enabled oocyte donation to be performed within an office setting, greatly reducing its inconvenience, improving its safety, and lessening its cost.

The popularity of egg and embryo donation is evidenced by the rapidly increasing demand for services. In the United States, 16,579 procedures involving fresh or frozen embryos procured through oocyte donation were reported to the Centers for Disease Control in 2008, nearly four times the number reported in 1996 (9). This increase is largely due to the rising percentage of women who remain childless past the age of 40 years old, a number that has sharply increased over the past 30 years (10). Many women are marrying later, or are pursuing education and vocation and deliberately delaying childbearing (11). Unfortunately, there is a natural decline in fertility associated with advancing age, and many healthy women later experience difficulties as a result of normal aging.

INDICATIONS FOR EGG AND EMBRYO DONATION

The indications for egg and embryo donation have expanded since its inception. Originally envisioned as a fertility treatment for women with premature ovarian failure (POF) (12), today women with many other reproductive disorders are considered prime candidates for therapy (Table 64.1).

Noniatrogenic POF, defined as women <40 years old with persistent amenorrhea and elevated gonadotropins, affects approximately 1% of the female population (13). The majority of cases are idiopathic, but about 20% are suspected of being autoimmune in nature or the result of concomitant glandular autoimmune disease (14). Thus, it is important to ensure that clinical or subclinical failure of the thyroid, parathyroid, and adrenal glands does not coexist, as well as diabetes mellitus and myasthenia gravis. Any

Table 64.1   Indications for Oocyte Donation

Premature ovarian failure
Gonadal dysgenesis
Repetitive IVF failure
Natural menopause
Inheritable disorders
Same sex couples

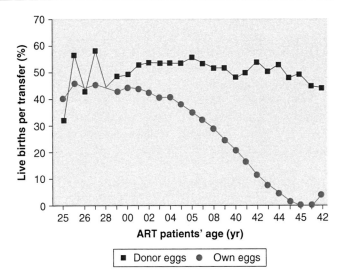

Figure 64.1   Live births per transfer for ART cycles using fresh embryos from own and donor eggs, by ART patient's age, 2008 (9). Abbreviation: ART, assisted reproductive technique.

of these conditions may adversely affect pregnancy outcome as well as impact upon the general health and well-being of the patient. If POF occurs <30 years old, a karyotype should also be requested to ascertain the presence of Y-chromosome mosaicism. Patients discovered to be mosaic are at risk of gonadal tumors and require extirpation of the abnormal gonad (15). In addition, a bone density evaluation is helpful to identify patients with osteopenia or osteoporosis, which may be present despite hormone replacement therapy (16). Turner Syndrome is the most common gonadal dysgenesis in women, with a prevalence of 1 in 2000 live born females. Both spontaneous puberty and spontaneous pregnancy are relatively rare in these patients occurring in less than 5% of affected individuals (17). Other rare conditions associated with POF include congenital thymic aplasia (e.g., DiGeorge syndrome) (18), galactosemia (19), and ataxia-telangiectasia (20), all of which require a more thorough and specific evaluation.

Chemotherapy and radiation treatments for cancer may also lead to POF. Gonadotoxicity is age and dose dependent, with younger patients being more resistant to damage (21,22). Removal of the ovaries is often required for treatment of malignancies, but surgical castration more commonly results from noncancerous conditions, including infection, torsion, or overly aggressive removal of intra-ovarian lesions (e.g., cystic teratomas, endometriomas).

Repetitive failure at IVF is common when a poor ovarian response to gonadotropins occurs. Occasionally patients are identified as poor candidates for IVF treatment prior to initiating care, thus sparing them the expense and psychological distress of multiple failed cycles. The first consideration is the age of the patient. It has long been known that natural fertility decreases with age, and this is also true with IVF (Fig. 64.1) (9). Many IVF centers have a maximum age limit beyond which they will not perform IVF without oocyte donation (47 years at Columbia University). Women of advanced reproductive age have far greater success with donated oocytes (23). Ovarian reserve is evaluated with serum follicle-stimulating hormone (FSH) levels on day 2 or 3 of the menstrual cycle (24). Values >15 mIU/ml are prognostic for a greatly reduced IVF success rate. Another useful serum marker is day 2 or 3 estradiol (25). Values >45 pg/ml are predictive of lower pregnancy rates and, if >75 pg/ml, the attempts usually end in failure. It is important that each laboratory determines the threshold values that are useful for their program.

Anti-Müllerian hormone (AMH) is produced in the granulosa cells from preantral and small antral follicles and serum levels are measurable and reflective of ovarian reserve. Higher levels of AMH are associated with greater number of retrieved oocytes in women undergoing IVF, while low levels appear to be reliable markers for diminished ovarian reserve (26). Thus, AMH testing may identify women at risk for either extreme (hypo- or hyper-) in ovarian responsiveness. Other tests are extant to assess ovarian reserve, but are more cumbersome than day 3 serum FSH and estradiol. The clomiphene challenge test measures serum FSH, luteinizing hormone (LH), and estradiol at baseline and again after five days (days 5–9) of 100 mg clomiphene citrate (27). Serum FSH values >15 mIU/ml post clomiphene are predictive of IVF failure. Day 2 or 3 serum inhibin B may also define ovarian reserve (28), but the commercially available assay is currently far more complex and time consuming than assays for FSH, estradiol, and AMH and not readily available.

In certain cases ovarian stimulation is adequate but fertilization rates are poor and often oocyte quality is marginal. Intracytoplasmic sperm injection (ICSI) may or may not be helpful, but if fertilization failure is persistent then oocyte donation is indicated. Similarly, successful fertilization may be present, but implantation does not occur. Assisted hatching may be helpful in these cases. Both ICSI and assisted hatching are discussed in detail in other chapters, but the belief is that recurrent implantation failure is often secondary to poor gametes and may be overcome by oocyte donation. Less clear is the patient with recurrent pregnancy loss, although at least one report suggests that oocyte donation is effective in these cases as well (29). Finally, in rare instances IVF failure may be due to ovaries that are inaccessible to either transvaginal or laparoscopic retrieval, and oocytes can be provided only through donation.

Although controversial, oocyte donation to treat infertility in women with physiological menopause is very effective (23). The Ethics Committee of the American Society for Reproductive Medicine (ASRM) stated that because of the physical and psychological risks involved (to both mother and child) oocyte donation in postmenopausal women should be discouraged (30). However, data on pregnancy outcome in these women, albeit after careful medical and psychological screening, do not reveal any unreasonable risks (31). Some have argued that postmenopausal pregnancy is "unnatural," but the same may be said of most ART. Furthermore, denying healthy older women donated oocytes while allowing older men complete access to reproductive care is considered by many to be both prejudicial and sexist (32).

Less controversial is the use of egg donation for inheritable conditions such as X-linked or autosomal traits and chromosomal translocations (33). However, with progress in preimplantation diagnosis, this reason for choosing egg donation may ultimately decrease (34).

Gay men and women are increasingly open in their relationships and seeking fertility care to have children. For gay males, and in cases of some lesbian couples, the use of oocyte donation and gestational carriers is required (35). The Ethics Committee of the ASRM has issued guidelines that call for a nondiscriminatory policy in treating homosexual patients requesting fertility assistance (36). As a result, a rising number of requests for oocyte donation services is coming from this population of patients.

RECIPIENT SCREENING

In addition to a complete history and physical examination, the suggested medical screening for recipients is shown in Table 64.2. Most of the tests are requisite standards for expectant mothers and IVF candidates. Patients of advanced maternal age are at higher risk for certain conditions such as diabetes mellitus, hypertension, and heart disease and therefore require additional testing focused on these disorders. Other recipients may warrant more comprehensive evaluations, such as a karyotype and autoimmune screen in patients with POF, or screening for anomalies of the aorta and urological system in patients with gonadal dysgenesis.

Psychological screening of recipient couples is also recommended. The stress that infertility places on relationships is well known (37). Furthermore, with respect to oocyte donation, the resulting child will not be genetically related to the mother. Most couples reconcile themselves to this, and research has shown that the desire to be parents is more important for positive parenting than a genetic link with the child (38). However, it remains important to address any grief, anxiety, and depression directly with the couple prior to proceeding. The role of the mental healthcare professional is usually one of support and guidance for the couple struggling with these issues. Occasionally, a couple is found to have greatly disparate ideas of what the pregnancy will accomplish. A pregnancy conceived merely to salvage a marriage or relationship is best deferred until the couple resolves their differences.

The presence of endometriosis does not affect the pregnancy rate of patients undergoing oocyte donation (39). However, a hydrosalpinx is probably deleterious, and surgical treatment to relieve the obstruction (tuboplasty) or remove the damaged tube (salpingectomy) is recommended (40). Recipients should have a normal uterine cavity free of adhesions, space-occupying lesions, and pathology. This is best assessed by a precycle sonohysterogram or diagnostic hysteroscopy.

A mock endometrial preparation cycle and timed endometrial biopsy is performed in many programs to ensure that an adequate response to endometrial priming is present. Glandular/stroma dyssynchrony is often found during endometrial stimulation (41), but apparently this does not adversely affect pregnancy rates (42). Other studies have evaluated endometrial thickness as a predictor of success with oocyte donation (42–45). An endometrium of <6 mm is associated with poor outcome. Another study showed that all endometrial biopsies were in phase if the thickness was >7 mm (46). A recent Cochrane Review failed to confirm any one particular protocol for optimizing endometrial preparation with regards to pregnancy rate in a retrospective analysis of 22 randomized controlled clinical trials (47). The great majority of women will have adequate responses to hormone replacement and, therefore, at Columbia University, we have chosen to forgo the mock cycle except in women in whom a poor response is anticipated, such as patients with prior pelvic radiation (48). Should a recipient have a thin endometrium on a previous attempt at egg donation or during a

Table 64.2 Suggested Medical Screening of Oocyte Recipient(s)

Oocyte recipient	Male partner
Complete blood count with platelets	Blood Rh and type
Blood Rh and type	Hepatitis screen
Serum electrolytes, liver, and kidney function	VDRL
Sensitive TSH (thyroid stimulating hormone)	HIV-1, HTLV-1
Rubella and hepatitis screen	Semen analysis and culture
VDRL	
HIV-1, HTLV-1	
Urinalysis and culture	
Cervical cultures for gonorrhea and chlamydia	
Pap smear	
Transvaginal ultrasound	
Uterine cavity evaluation (sonohysterogram, diagnostic hysteroscopy, or hysterosalpingogram)	
Electrocardiogram[a]	
Chest X-ray[a]	
Mammogram[a]	
Glucose tolerance test[a]	
Cholesterol and lipid profile[a]	

[a]If over 39 years of age.
Abbreviations: VDRL, Venereal Disease Research Laboratory; HTLV-1, Human T Lymphotropic Virus-1.

mock cycle, a trial of low-dose aspirin (81 mg daily) given at the time of the transfer cycle may increase pregnancy rates. Weckstein et al. found that in women with a previous endometrial thickness of <8 mm, the addition of low-dose aspirin increased the implantation rate from 9% in the untreated group to 24% in the treated group, despite a lack of increased endometrial thickness (49).

It has been argued that women of advanced reproductive age may demonstrate a higher percentage of out-of-phase biopsies (50), but both the biopsy and pregnancy outcome may be corrected with appropriate doses of progesterone (51). Of note, older women can expect pregnancy rates with oocyte donation comparable to younger recipients (52–54), whether or not mock cycles are performed.

OOCYTE DONOR RECRUITMENT

Perhaps the greatest obstacle to performing oocyte donation is the recruitment of suitable donors (55). Historically, donor eggs were obtained from women undergoing IVF with "excess oocytes." Many of these patients had ovarian abnormalities underlying their own infertility, making them imperfect donors. Furthermore, with the advent of increasingly successful embryo cryopreservation and the use of "softer" stimulation protocols, "extra oocytes" have became scarce. Obvious sources for oocytes are women undergoing tubal sterilization who might be willing to be hyperstimulated. However, very few of these women are eligible, since most are not willing to undergo fertility drug treatment, and many are >35 years old (56). Known designated donors are yet another option. Typically a family member (e.g., sister, niece) or very close friend is selected. The final sources of donors are women recruited from the general population at large, most often through advertisement.

There has been a long-standing debate as to whether it is ethical to pay oocyte donors for their eggs, and if so, how much. Areas of contention include the selling of body parts and exaggerated incentives that may represent an enticement for a procedure that carries risk and no direct medical benefit to the donor. For this reason, many countries do not permit oocyte donation (e.g., Germany, Norway, and Sweden) (57). Other countries allow only IVF patients with excess oocytes to donate. Israel, Great Britain, and Canada allow anonymous oocyte donation, but strongly discourage payment to the donor, except for verified expenses. The United States has no current regulation on payments to donors. The payments are construed as reimbursement for time and inconvenience (58), and indeed, without payment it is doubtful any country will recruit sufficient donors to meet demand (59). The amount of payment remains hotly debated (60).

Another area of controversy focuses on anonymity and identity disclosure. Most donors express a strong desire not to be identified by the children. In exchange for anonymity they willingly forfeit all legal obligations as parents. There is, however, an opposing view that, similar to adopted children, offspring of egg donation should have the same right to ultimately identify their genetic mother (61). As a result, the United Kingdom now mandates that donor identity be revealed to a child resulting from egg donation once he or she reaches the age of 18 years. In the United States there is little historic precedent for such a change in public policy, but should such legislation be enacted, a deleterious effect on donor recruitment can be expected (62).

OOCYTE DONOR SCREENING

Oocyte donors need to be provided full and comprehensive informed consent. The risks of participating in oocyte donation are few, and basically no different from those of standard IVF. Controlled ovarian hyperstimulation entails both known and theoretical risks. The risk of severe ovarian hyperstimulation syndrome (OHSS) is reported in approximately 1% of cases, although donors may be at less risk of severe OHSS compared with patients undergoing IVF, since pregnancy does not occur in the donor and moderate cases of OHSS are therefore not exacerbated (63). Using gonadotropin-releasing hormone (GnRH) agonist to trigger final oocyte maturation has shown to significantly reduce the occurrence of OHSS compared to using human chorionic gonadotropin (hCG) and represents a valid alternative for hyperstimulated egg donors to further reduce morbidity (64). In addition to a complete medical history and physical examination, the suggested medical screening of oocyte donors is shown in Table 64.3. Of utmost importance is the screening for infectious diseases. Unlike sperm, which are amenable to cryopreservation, oocytes have traditionally not been frozen for subsequent use. In sperm donation, cryopreservation allows a quarantine period and follow-up testing for infectious diseases. With respect to current practice, egg cryopreservation has not been universally adapted to oocyte donors. Transvaginal ultrasound examination is performed to detect pelvic pathology and determine ovarian morphology.

It is preferable that oocyte donors be under 30 years old, as younger donors appear to have higher pregnancy rates (52,65). Pregnancy rates of donors >30 years old are still acceptable, however, and other traits and characteristics (e.g., a close physical match to the recipient or advanced educational degree) may make a particular older donor desirable to a recipient. The prior fertility history of the donor does not appear to affect pregnancy outcomes (64,65). The concept of a "proven" donor is a popular myth, and lacks evidence-based support.

Table 64.3 Suggested Medical Screening of Oocyte Donors

Complete blood count with platelets
Blood type
Hepatitis screen
VDRL
HIV-1, HTLV-1
Cervical cultures for gonorrhea and chlamydia
Pap smear
Transvaginal ultrasound of pelvis
Appropriate genetic tests

Psychological evaluation by a licensed mental health practitioner is recommended for anonymous donors and is mandatory for known donors. Screening should focus on their motivation to donate, as well as their financial status to ensure that their participation is not overly influenced by monetary enticement. An assessment of coping skills and lifestyle are important to predict the donor's ability to participate in a lengthy and complicated process.

Occasionally, a history of psychiatric illness or drug and/or alcohol use in the donor or her family is elicited. These behaviors may have a genetic etiology and as such would exclude the potential donor from participation.

Genetic screening begins with a detailed history of the potential donor and her family. A sample history form is presented in Table 64.4 (66). The presence of any of the disorders should exclude her from participating. Donors

Table 64.4   Genetic Screening form Given to Oocyte Donors

Pregnancy history: Please list all the times you have been pregnant and the outcomes.

Family ethnic background:

Please indicate all relevant information in the following tables. When the requested information is unknown, please say so. If comments are needed, please make them. Remember that we are interested in your genetic background. If any relevant family member is adopted, please say so.

Relation	Age if living	Age at death	Cause of death
Grandfather (pat)			
Grandmother (pat)			
Grandfather (mat)			
Grandmother (mat)			
Father			
Mother			
Brothers			
Sisters			

Family Genetic History

Familial Conditions	Self	Mother	Father	Siblings	Comments
High blood pressure					
Heart disease					
Deafness					
Blindness					
Severe arthritis					
Juvenile diabetes					
Alcoholism					
Schizophrenia					
Depression or mania					
Epilepsy					
Alzheimer's disease					
Other (specify)					
Malformations					
Cleft lip or palate					
Heart defect					
Clubfoot					
Spina bifida					
Other (specify)					
Mendelian disorders					
Color blindness					
Cystic fibrosis					
Hemophilia					
Muscular dystrophy					
Sickle cell anemia					
Huntington's disease					
Polycystic kidneys					
Glaucoma					
Tay-Sachs disease					

Please take the time to explain any other problems or conditions in your family history that you feel could pertain to the health of future generations.

Source: From Ref. 66.

should be <35 years old to reduce the risk of aneuploidy in the offspring. Exceptions can be made in circumstances such as sister-to-sister donation where the benefits of shared genetic background may balance the known risks (which can be largely discovered by amniocentesis). Donors should also be tested for disorders common to their ethnic background. These include cystic fibrosis in whites, a sickle cell anemia test for blacks, and a complete blood count and mean corpuscular volume followed by hemoglobin electrophoresis in abnormal results for people of Mediterranean and Chinese ancestry to assess the risk of beta-thalassemia, and in people of Southeast Asian ancestry for alpha-thalassemia. Jews of eastern European ancestry should be screened for Tay–Sachs disease, Gaucher disease, mucolipidosis IV, Niemann–Pick disease, Bloom syndrome, familial dysautonomia, Fanconi anemia, fragile X syndrome, and Canavan disease. It is important to inform the recipient couples that even with appropriate screening 2–3% of babies are born with a major or minor malformation, and many genetic disorders cannot be detected or prevented with current testing methodology (67).

Guidelines for gamete and embryo donation have been periodically published and recently updated in an attempt to standardize screening policies and to incorporate recent regulations from the U.S. Food and Drug Administration (FDA) (68).

ENDOMETRIAL STIMULATION AND SYNCHRONIZATION

Endometrial preparation of the recipient is modeled on the natural menstrual cycle, using estrogen and progesterone (23). The initial estrogenic phase is most often maintained using either daily oral estradiol 4–8 mg or transdermal estrogen 0.2–0.4 mg. The initial results of oocyte donation cycles were significantly better than typically seen after standard IVF. The apparent detrimental effect of standard IVF on embryo implantation was felt to be secondary to the supraphysiologic concentrations of estrogen attained after controlled ovarian hyperstimulation (69,70). Transdermal estrogen adequately prepares the endometrium with overall lower serum concentrations of estrogens because of the lack of hepatic first-pass effect. However, the higher concentrations of serum estrogens noted following oral administration are of questionable clinical significance. Krasnow et al. found estradiol concentrations tenfold higher in the oral estrogen group and noted a higher rate of out-of-phase endometrial biopsies (71). Others, however, have shown no detriment with high levels of estrogen (72). Most programs continue to prescribe oral estradiol due to its ease of administration, lack of side effects, and long history of clinical success.

The length of estrogenic exposure may vary widely with little apparent clinical effect, again mimicking the variable follicular phase found in natural menstrual cycles. Anywhere from six to 38 days of prescribed estrogen prior to progesterone appears adequate (41,73,74). Most programs prescribe at least 12–14 days of estrogen

before initiating progesterone, but studies report that if it is necessary to prolong this period, perhaps because of a slow stimulation of the oocyte donor, no adverse effects are expected.

Synchronization of the recipient and donor is relatively easy to accomplish. The recipient begins estrogen several days prior to beginning ovarian stimulation in the donor to provide approximately 14 days of estradiol prior to progesterone administration. Ovulating recipients typically receive GnRH agonist for downregulation as in standard IVF cycles (e.g., 1 mg leuprolide acetate daily until suppressed, then 0.5 mg daily thereafter) to render them functionally agonadal. Alternatively, ovulating recipients are started on oral estrogen at the beginning of their menstrual cycle and maintained on estrogen, and a GnRH antagonist is used to block the LH surge, until the day of the donor's oocyte retrieval when progesterone is begun (Fig. 64.2) (73).

The timing of progesterone administration is more stringent. Navot et al. reported the optimal time for embryo transfer was two to four days after progesterone initiation for embryos at the two- to 12-cell stage (75). This corresponds to days 17–19 of the recipient's cycle, with day 15 defined as the day of progesterone initiation. No pregnancies were observed before two days or after four days of progesterone administration. These findings were confirmed by Prapas et al, who further delineated the optimal time for transfer of four- to eight-cell embryos to days 18 and 19 (76).

The dose of progesterone is typically 100 mg IM daily or 100–600 mg transvaginally daily. Many groups prefer the transvaginal approach because lower serum concentrations of progesterone are required to achieve target organ effect. Serum levels are low in these patients, but local tissue levels are high probably because of the absence of the hepatic first pass effect on clearance. As with estrogen, however, it is not resolved whether the mode of delivery of progesterone or its dose is of clinical significance. Most groups continue estrogen support through the progestational period, although at least one study has shown that continued estrogen use is not actually required (77).

Progesterone (and estrogen) administration can be discontinued once the placenta has established adequate steroidogenesis. Devroey et al. estimated this to occur at seven to nine weeks of gestation (78), while others have advanced this to the fifth week (79). Clinically, we begin weekly monitoring of serum progesterone concentrations 10 weeks after embryo transfer when a serum level of ≥30 ng/ml typically is attained. At that point, prescribing exogenous steroids is superfluous.

CLINICAL AND OBSTETRIC OUTCOMES

Recipients of donated eggs experience implantation and pregnancy rates similar to those normally seen in young women undergoing IVF. Thus, the ASRM recommends that no more than two high-quality embryos be transferred to patients to lessen the risk of multiple gestation. Oocyte donation has always been associated with the

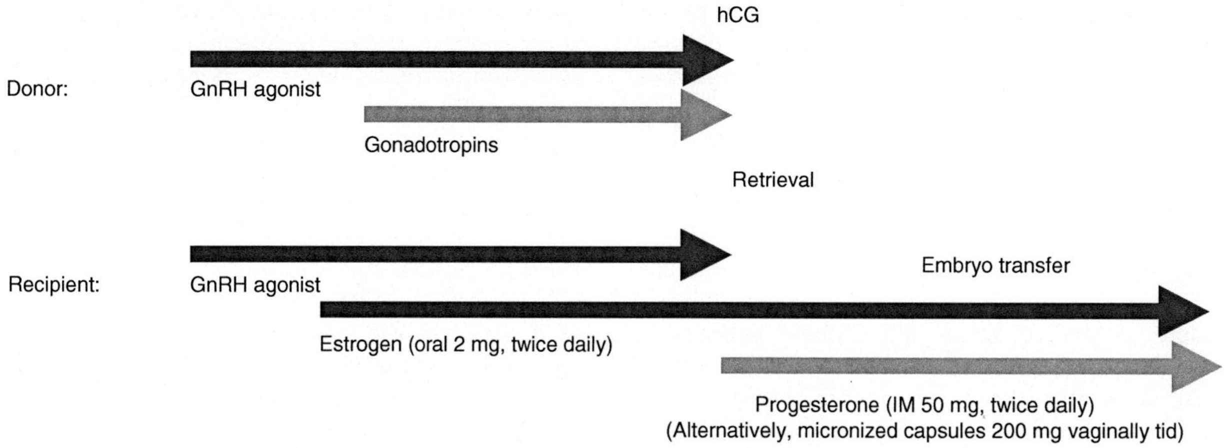

hCG

Donor: GnRH agonist

Gonadotropins

Retrieval

Recipient: GnRH agonist

Embryo transfer

Estrogen (oral 2 mg, twice daily)

Progesterone (IM 50 mg, twice daily)
(Alternatively, micronized capsules 200 mg vaginally tid)

Figure 64.2 Schematic representation of cycle synchronization using a GnRH agonist in both donor and recipient. GnRH agonists are used to downregulate the pituitary of recipients with evidence of ovarian activity prior to beginning oral estradiol. Oral estradiol is prescribed to the recipient four to five days in advance of the donor starting gonadotropin injections. Progesterone is administered starting the day after hCG injection in the donor, and one day prior to aspirating oocytes. Embryo transfer is performed three days following oocyte retrieval. Serum pregnancy testing occurs 12 days post transfer. Pregnant patients are maintained on estradiol and progesterone through 12 weeks of gestational age. *Abbreviations*: GnRH, gonadotropin-releasing hormone; hCG, human chorionic gonadotropin.

highest success rate among ARTs, and presently more than 50% of embryo transfers result in live births (9). Occasionally preimplantation genetic diagnosis (PGD) has also been used in an attempt to select better embryos for transfer since nearly half of biopsied normal appearing embryos selected from donors in their mid-twenties were aneuploid (80). In this study, transferring the PGD-selected embryos improved delivery rates and lowered the miscarriage rate of recipients, however, at an additional fiscal cost to the patient. Egg donation has been applied to treat infertility in women of advanced reproductive age (>45 years old) since 1990 and has soared in popularity as a result of its ability to reverse the inevitable loss of fertility in women approaching menopause (81). However, as demonstrated by a large retrospective review of 3089 cycles from Valencia, recipients >45 years old had lower pregnancy rates (49% vs. 44%), lower implantation rates (21% vs. 17%), and higher miscarriage rates (17% vs. 23%) than younger recipients (82). This trend is similarly apparent in reviewing the CDC/SART data from 2008 (Fig. 64.3). Therefore, the ability to totally restore uterine receptivity using estradiol and progesterone replacement remains uncertain in the presence of advancing reproductive age.

Several groups have evaluated the obstetric outcome of pregnancies following oocyte donation and concluded that results are favorable. (31,83–86) Common to all reports, however, were increases in the incidence of pregnancy-induced hypertension (PIH) and delivery by caesarean section. Soderstrom-Anttila et al. compared 51 oocyte donation deliveries to 97 IVF deliveries and noted a higher rate of PIH (31% vs. 14%) and cesarean section (57% vs. 37%) with oocyte donation (85). PIH was evaluated by the study of 72 pregnancies from donated gametes with age- and parity-matched controls (87). Preeclampsia was noted to be much higher in the donated gamete group (18.1% vs. 1.4%), suggesting an autoimmune component to the disorder. The increased risk of

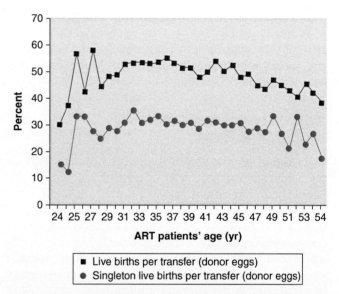

Figure 64.3 Live births per transfer and singleton live births per transfer for assisted reproductive technique (ART) cycles using fresh embryos from donor eggs, by ART patient's age, 2008 (9).

PIH appears to occur in younger recipients (<35 years old) as well (88). Two other studies evaluated older oocyte donation patients and found most complications, such as gestational diabetes and preterm labor, were associated with multiple pregnancies (31,83). Another clinical trial showed that 59 children of oocyte donation aged six months to four years had growth and development comparable to children from IVF and the general population (89). A review of pregnancy outcomes of 45 women >50 years old who delivered babies following egg donation at the University of Southern California demonstrated an increase in obstetric complications, with preeclampsia occurring in 35%, gestational diabetes in 20%, and multiple births in 35% (90). Antinori et al. described a 12-year experience with peri- and postmenopausal women aged between 45 years and 63 years in which

2729 women were screened (91). Only 42% of these women were suitable candidates, as the majorities were deemed too high risk for pregnancy due to underlying medical conditions. Overall, 1288 recipient cycles resulted in pregnancy in 38% of transfer events with 28% delivering per transfer. Antenatal complications were common (23.6%) in the ongoing pregnancies and included gestational hypertension, gestational diabetes, and preterm labor. A recent review of 101 consecutive pregnancies in women 50 years of age and older at Columbia University also noted an increased incidence of hypertensive disorders, gestational diabetes, premature rupture of the membranes, preterm labor and abnormal placentation similar to rates also seen in younger women (<42 years) undergoing egg donation (92). In summary, oocyte donation pregnancies should be considered high risk. However, in well-screened patients, the complications are manageable and parents can reasonably expect healthy children.

EMBRYO DONATION

Embryo donation has become more common as social attitudes toward single women and assisted reproduction have relaxed and the enhanced efficiency of cryopreservation has led to the banking of a large number of human embryos. The deliberate use of donor gametes, utilizing both sperm and egg, was described in 1995 as a means of "preimplantation adoption" (93). A programmed approach for creating embryos using donor gametes in single women of advanced reproductive age was suggested again in 1999 as a highly efficient and cost effective means for establishing pregnancy (94). More often, donated embryos are obtained from couples who have successfully conceived through IVF and now wish to give their cryopreserved supernumerary embryos to clinical programs for use in infertile women (95). Interestingly, couples and women who did not use frozen embryos after pregnancy with donor gametes were more likely to donate them for use in other women than women who had embryos banked following standard IVF with their own eggs. Original guidelines for embryo donation were published by the ASRM in 1998 (96). Recommendations include that the embryos undergo a minimum of six months' quarantine and that all donors are retested for infectious diseases prior to their use. Proper documentation of chain-of-custody of donated embryos and witnessed written relinquishment of embryos is also suggested. Although the program may charge professional fees for the service, embryos cannot be "sold," and donors cannot receive compensation.

FUTURE DIRECTIONS

The next frontier in oocyte donation may include the use of enucleated donor oocytes, which would allow recipients to use their own genetic material. This has been successful in cattle and other mammals, but has not been successful as yet in humans (97). Improvements in oocyte freezing may soon permit "egg banks" to be set up, reducing the need to synchronize patients while allowing for quarantine (98–100). Meanwhile, traditional oocyte donation continues to benefit many infertile women who would not otherwise become biological mothers.

REFERENCES

1. Heape W. Preliminary note on the transplantation and growth of mammalian ova in a foster mother. Proc R Soc London 1890; 48: 457.
2. Hasler JF. Current status and potential of embryo transfer and reproductive technology in dairy cattle. J Dairy Sci 1992; 75: 2857–79.
3. Grimes JF. Utilization of embryo transfer in beef cattle. Fact sheet Agriculture and Natural Resources ANR-17–08, The Ohio State University Extension, 2008. [Available from: http://ohioline.osu.edu]
4. Buster JE, Bustillo M, Thorneycroft I, et al. Nonsurgical transfer of an in-vivo fertilised donated ovum to an infertility patient. Lancet 1983; 1: 816–17.
5. Buster JE, Bustillo M, Thorneycroft IH, et al. Nonsurgical transfer of in vivo fertilised donated ova to five infertile women: report of two pregnancies. Lancet 1983; 2: 223–4.
6. Bustillo M, Buster JE, Cohen SW, et al. Delivery of a healthy infant following nonsurgical ovum transfer. JAMA 1984; 251: 889.
7. Trounson A, Leeton J, Besanko M, et al. Pregnancy established in an infertile patient after transfer of a donated embryo fertilised in vitro. Br Med J (Clin Res Ed) 1983; 286: 835–8.
8. Lutjen P, Trounson A, Leeton J, et al. The establishment and maintenance of pregnancy using in vitro fertilization and embryo donation in a patient with primary ovarian failure. Nature 1984; 307: 174–5.
9. Centers for Disease Control and Prevention. 2008 Assisted Reproductive Technology Success Rates. National Summary and Clinic Reports Department of Health and Human Services, December 2010.
10. Ventura SJ. First births to older mothers, 1970–86. Am J Public Health 1989; 79: 1675–7.
11. Hollander D, Breen JL. Pregnancy in the older gravida: how old is old? Obstet Gynecol Surv 1990; 45: 106–12.
12. Bustillo M, Buster JE, Cohen SW, et al. Nonsurgical ovum transfer as a treatment in infertile women. preliminary experience. JAMA 1984; 251: 1171–3.
13. Coulam CB, Adamson SC, Annegers JF. Incidence of premature ovarian failure. Obstet Gynecol 1986; 67: 604–6.
14. Coulam CB. Premature gonadal failure. Fertil Steril 1982; 38: 645–55.
15. Manuel M, Katayama PK, Jones HW Jr. The age of occurrence of gonadal tumors in intersex patients with a Y chromosome. Am J Obstet Gynecol 1976; 124: 293–300.
16. Cohen MA, Chang PL, Lindheim SR, Sauer MV. Diminished bone density in menopausal women undergoing ovum donation. Annual Meeting of the American Society for Reproductive Medicine, San Francisco, California, 1998 (abstract).
17. Chevalier N, Letur H, Lelannou D, et al. Maternal-Fetal cardiovascular complication in turner syndrome after oocyte donation: insufficient prepregnancy

screening and pregnancy follow-up are associated with poor outcome. J Clin Endocrinol Metab 2011; 96: E260–7.

18. Moncayo R, Moncayo HE. Autoimmunity and the ovary. Immunol Today 1992; 13: 255–8.

19. Kaufman FR, Donnell GN, Roe TF, Kogut MD. Gonadal function in patients with galactosaemia. J Inherit Metab Dis 1986; 9: 140–6.

20. Christin-Maitre S, Vasseur C, Portnoi MF, Bouchard P. Genes and premature ovarian failure. Mol Cell Endocrinol 1998; 145: 75–80.

21. Byrne J, Mulvihill JJ, Myers MH, et al. Effects of treatment on fertility in long-termsurvivors of childhood or adolescent cancer. N Engl J Med 1987; 317: 1315–21.

22. Gradishar WJ, Schilsky RL. Ovarian function following radiation and chemotherapy for cancer. Semin Oncol 1989; 16: 425–36.

23. Sauer MV, Paulson RJ, Lobo RA. A preliminary report on oocyte donation extending reproductive potential to women over 40. N Engl J Med 1990; 323: 1157–60.

24. Scott RT, Toner JP, Muasher SJ, et al. Follicle-stimulating hormone levels on cycle day 3 are predictive of in vitro fertilization outcome. Fertil Steril 1989; 51: 651–4.

25. Licciardi FL, Liu HC, Rosenwaks Z. Day 3 estradiol serum concentrations as prognosticators of ovarian stimulation response and pregnancy outcome in patients undergoing in vitro fertilization. Fertil Steril 1995; 64: 991–4.

26. LaMarca A, Sighinolfi G, Radi D, et al. Anti-Mullerian hormone as a predictive marker in assisted reproductive technology. Hum Reprod Update 2010; 16: 113–30.

27. Navot D, Rosenwaks Z, Margalioth EJ. Prognostic assessment of female fecundity. Lancet 1987; 2: 645–7.

28. Seifer DB, Lambert-Messerlian G, Hogan JW, et al. Day 3 serum inhibin-B is predictive of assisted reproductive technologies outcome. Fertil Steril 1997; 67: 110–14.

29. Remohi J, Gallardo E, Levy M, et al. Oocyte donation in women with recurrent pregnancy loss. Hum Reprod 1996; 11: 2048–51.

30. Ethics Committee of the American Society for Reproductive Medicine. Ethical considerations of assisted reproductive technologies. Fertil Steril 1997; 67(Suppl 1): 1S–9S.

31. Sauer MV, Paulson RJ, Lobo RA. Oocyte donation to women of advanced reproductive age: pregnancy results and obstetrical outcomes in patients 45 years and older. Hum Reprod 1996; 11: 2540–3.

32. Paulson RJ, Sauer MV. Pregnancies in postmenopausal women. Oocyte donation to women of advanced reproductive age: 'how old is too old?' Hum Reprod 1994; 9: 571–2.

33. Van Voorhis BJ, Williamson RA, Gerard JL, et al. Use of oocytes from anonymous, matched, fertile donors for prevention of heritable genetic diseases. J Med Genet 1992; 29: 398–9.

34. Munné S, Chen S, Colls P, et al. Maternal age, morphology, development and chromosome abnormalities in over 6000 cleavage-stage embryos. Reprod Biomed Online 2007; 14: 628–34.

35. Greenfield DA, Seli E. Gay men choosing parenthood through assisted reproduction: medical and psychosocial considerations. Fertil Steril 2011; 95: 225–9.

36. Ethics Committee of the American Society for Reproductive Medicine. Access to fertility treatment by gays, lesbians, and unmarried persons. Fertil Steril 2006; 86: 1333–5.

37. Burns L. An overview of the psychology of infertility. Infertil Reprod Med Clin N Am 1993; 3: 433–54.

38. Golombok S, Cook R, Bish A, Murray C. Families created by the new reproductive technologies: quality of parenting and social and emotional development of the children. Child Dev 1995; 66: 285–98.

39. Bustillo M, Krysa LW, Coulam CB. Uterine receptivity in an oocyte donation programme. Hum Reprod 1995; 10: 442–5.

40. Cohen MA, Lindheim SR, Sauer MV. Hydrosalpinges adversely affect implantation in donor oocyte cycles. Hum Reprod 1999; 14: 1087–9.

41. Navot D, Anderson TL, Droesch K, et al. Hormonal manipulation of endometrial maturation. J Clin Endocrinol Metab 1989; 68: 801–7.

42. Navot D, Bergh PA, Williams M, et al. An insight into early reproductive processes through the in vivo model of ovum donation. J Clin Endocrinol Metab 1991; 72: 408–14.

43. Abdalla HI, Brooks AA, Johnson MR, et al. Endometrial thickness: a predictor of implantation in ovum recipients? Hum Reprod 1994; 9: 363–5.

44. Antinori S, Versaci C, Gholami GH, et al. Oocyte donation in menopausal women. Hum Reprod 1993; 8: 1487–90.

45. Shapiro H, Cowell C, Casper RF. The use of vaginal ultrasound for monitoring endometrial preparation in a donor oocyte program. Fertil Steril 1993; 59: 1055–8.

46. Hofmann GE, Thie J, Scott RT Jr, Navot D. Endometrial thickness is predictive of histologic endometrial maturation in women undergoing hormone replacement for ovum donation. Fertil Steril 1996; 66: 380–3.

47. Glujovsky D, Pesce R, Fiszbajn G, et al. Endometrial preparation for women undergoing embryo transfer with frozen embryos or embryos derived from donor oocytes (Review). Cochrane Database Syst Rev 2010: CD006359.

48. Li TC, Dockery P, Ramsewak SS, et al. The variation of endometrial response to a standard hormone replacement therapy in women with premature ovarian failure. An ultrasonographic and histological study. Br J Obstet Gynaecol 1991; 98: 656–61.

49. Weckstein LN, Jacobson A, Galen D, et al. Low-dose aspirin for oocyte donation recipients with a thin endometrium: prospective, randomized study. Fertil Steril 1997; 68: 927–30.

50. Potter DA, Witz CA, Burns WN, et al. Endometrial biopsy during hormone replacement cycle in donor oocyte recipients before in vitro fertilization–embryo transfer. Fertil Steril 1998; 70: 219–21.

51. Meldrum D. Female reproductive aging – ovarian and uterine factors. Fertil Steril 1993; 59: 1–5.

52. Balmaceda JP, Bernardini L, Ciuffardi I, et al. Oocyte donation in humans: a model to study the effect of age on embryo implantation rate. Hum Reprod 1994; 9: 2160–3.

53. Abdalla HI, Wren ME, Thomas A, Korea L. Age of the uterus does not affect pregnancy or implantation rates; a study of egg donation in women of different ages sharing oocytes from the same donor. Hum Reprod 1997; 12: 827–9.

54. Stolwijk AM, Zielhuis GA, Sauer MV, Hamilton CJ, Paulson RJ. The impact of the woman's age on the success of standard and donor in vitro fertilization. Fertil Steril 1997; 67: 702–10.

55. Marina S, Exposito R, Marina F, et al. Oocyte donor selection from 554 candidates. Hum Reprod 1999; 14: 2770–6.

56. Feinman M, Barad D, Szigetvari I, Kaali SG. Availability of donated oocytes from an ambulatory sterilization program. J Reprod Med 1989; 34: 441–3.

57. Gunning JH. Oocyte donation: the legislative framework in Western Europe. Hum Reprod 1998; 13(Suppl 2): 98–104.

58. Sauer MV. Reproductive prohibition: restricting donor payment will lead to medical tourism. Hum Reprod 1997; 12: 1844–5.

59. McLaughlin EA, Day J, Harrison S, et al. Recruitment of gamete donors and payment of expenses. Hum Reprod 1998; 13: 1130–2.

60. Sauer MV. Indecent proposal: $5,000 is not "reasonable compensation" for oocyte donors. Fertil Steril 1999; 71: 7–10.

61. Annas GJ. The shadowlands – secrets, lies, and assisted reproduction. N Engl JMed 1998; 339: 935–9.

62. Sauer MV. Further HFEA restrictions on egg donation in the UK: two strikes and you're out! Reprod Biomed Online 2005; 10: 431–3.

63. Maxwell K, Cholst IN, Rosenwaks Z. The incidence of both serious and minor complications in young women undergoing oocyte donation. Fertil Steril 2008; 90: 2165–71.

64. Humaidan P, Kol S, Papanikolaou EG. GnRH agonist for triggering of final oocyte maturation: time for a change of practice? Hum Reprod Update 2011; 17: 510–24.

65. Cohen MA, Lindheim SR, Sauer MV. Donor age is paramount to success in oocyte donation. Hum Reprod 1999; 14: 2755–8.

66. Brown S. Genetic aspects of donor selection. In: Sauer MV, ed. Principles of Oocyte and Embryo Donation. New York: Springer-Verlag, 1998: 53–63.

67. Baird PA, Anderson TW, Newcombe HB, Lowry RB. Genetic disorders in children and young adults: a population study. Am J Hum Genet 1988; 42: 677–93.

68. The Practice Committee of the American Society for Reproductive Medicine and the Practice Committee of the Society for Assisted Reproductive Technology. 2006 Guidelines for gamete and embryo donation. Fertil Steril 2006; 86(Suppl 4): S38–50.

69. Edwards RG. Why are agonadal and post-amenorrhoeic women so fertile after oocyte donation? Hum Reprod 1992; 7: 733–4.

70. Check JH, Nowroozi K, Chase J, Nazari A, Braithwaite C. Comparison of pregnancy rates following in vitro fertilization–embryo transfer between the donors and the recipients in a donor oocyte program. J Assist Reprod Genet 1992; 9: 248–50.

71. Krasnow JS, Lessey BA, Naus G, et al. Comparison of transdermal versus oral estradiol on endometrial receptivity. Fertil Steril 1996; 65: 332–6.

72. de Ziegler D. Hormonal control of endometrial receptivity. Hum Reprod 1995; 10: 4–7.

73. Serhal PF, Craft IL. Ovum donation – a simplified approach. Fertil Steril 1987; 48: 265–9.

74. Younis JS, Mordel N, Ligovetzky G, et al. The effect of a prolonged artificial follicular phase on endometrial development in an oocyte donation program. J In Vitro Fert Embryo Transf 1991; 8: 84–8.

75. Navot D, Scott RT, Droesch K, et al. The window of embryo transfer and the efficiency of human conception in vitro. Fertil Steril 1991; 55: 114–18.

76. Prapas Y, Prapas N, Jones EE, et al. The window for embryo transfer in oocyte donation cycles depends on the duration of progesterone therapy. Hum Reprod 1998; 13: 720–3.

77. Lewin A, Benshushan A, Mezker E, et al. The role of estrogen support during the luteal phase of in vitro fertilization–embryo transplant cycles: a comparative study between progesterone alone and estrogen and progesterone support. Fertil Steril 1994; 62: 121–5.

78. Devroey P, Camus M, Palermo G, et al. Placental production of estradiol and progesterone after oocyte donation in patients with primary ovarian failure. Am J Obstet Gynecol 1990; 162: 66–70.

79. Scott R, Navot D, Liu HC, Rosenwaks Z. A human in vivo model for the luteoplacental shift. Fertil Steril 1991; 56: 481–4.

80. Reis Soares S, Rubio C, Rodrigo L, et al. Does preimplantation genetic diagnosis improve the outcome of egg donation cycles? Presented at the 19th Annual Meeting of ESHRE, 2003; P-568, xviii, 189.

81. Sauer MV, Kavic SM. Oocyte and embryo donation 2006: reviewing two decades of innovation and controversy. Reprod Biomed Online 2006; 12: 153–62.

82. Reis Soares S, Troncoso C, Bosch E, et al. Age and uterine receptiveness: predicting the outcome of oocyte donation cycles. J Clin Endocrinol Metab 2005; 90: 4399–404.

83. Pados G, Camus M, Van Steirteghem A, et al. The evolution and outcome of pregnancies from oocyte donation. Hum Reprod 1994; 9: 538–42.

84. Wolff KM, McMahon MJ, Kuller JA, et al. Advanced maternal age and perinatal outcome: oocyte recipiency versus natural conception. Obstet Gynecol 1997; 89: 519–23.

85. Soderstrom-Anttila V, Tiitinen A, Foudila T, Hovatta O. Obstetric and perinatal outcome after oocyte donation: comparison with in-vitro fertilization pregnancies. Hum Reprod 1998; 13: 483–90.

86. Abdalla HI, Billett A, Kan AK, et al. Obstetric outcome in 232 ovum donation pregnancies. Br J Obstet Gynaecol 1998; 105: 332–7.

87. Salha O, Sharma V, Dada T, et al. The influence of donated gametes on the incidence of hypertensive disorders of pregnancy. Hum Reprod 1999; 14: 2268–73.

88. Keegan DA, Krey LC, Chang HC, Noyes N. Increased risk of pregnancy-induced hypertension in young recipients of donated oocytes. Fertil Steril 2007; 87: 776–81.

89. Soderstrom-Anttila V, Sajaniemi N, Tiitinen A, Hovatta O. Health and development of children born after oocyte donation compared with that of those born after in-vitro fertilization, and parents' attitudes regarding secrecy. Hum Reprod 1998; 13: 2009–15.

90. Paulson RJ, Boostanfar R, Saadat P, et al. Pregnancy in the sixth decade of life. obstetric outcomes in women of advanced reproductive age. JAMA 2002; 288: 2320–3.

91. Antinori S, Gholami GH, Versaci C, et al. Obstetric and prenatal outcome in menopausal women: a 12-year clinical study. Reprod Biomed Online 2002; 6: 257–61.

92. Kort DH, Gosselin J, Choi JM, et al. Pregnancy after age 50: defining risks for mother and child. Am J Perinatol 2012; 29: 245–50.

93. Sauer MV, Paulson RJ, Francis MM, et al. Preimplantation adoption: Establishing pregnancy using donated oocytes and spermatozoa. Hum Reprod 1995; 10: 1419–22.

94. Lindheim SR, Sauer MV. Embryo donation: a programmed approach. Fertil Steril 1999; 72: 940–1.

95. Sehnert B, Chetkowski RJ. Secondary donation of frozen embryos is more common after pregnancy initiation with donated eggs than after in vitro fertilization–embryo transfer and gamete intrafallopian transfer. Fertil Steril 1998; 69: 350–2.

96. The American Society for Reproductive Medicine. Guidelines for gamete and embryo donation. guidelines for embryo donation. Fertil Steril 1998; 70(Suppl 3): 7S–8S.

97. Dominko T, Mitalipova M, Haley B, et al. Bovine oocyte cytoplasm supports development of embryos produced by nuclear transfer of somatic cell nuceli from various mammallian species. Biol Reprod 1999; 60: 1496–502.

98. Tucker MJ, Morton PC, Wright G, et al. Clinical application of human egg cryopreservation. Hum Reprod 1998; 13: 3156–9.

99. Nagy ZP, Chang CC, Shapiro DB, et al. Clinical evaluation of the efficiency of an oocyte donation program using egg cryo-banking. Fertil Steril 2009; 92: 520–6.

100. Cobo A, Meseguer M, Remohi J, Pellicer A. Use of cryo-banked oocytes in an ovum donation programme: a prospective, randomized, controlled, clinical trial. Hum Reprod 2010: 2239–46.

65

Gestational Surrogacy

Peter R. Brinsden

OVERVIEW

Surrogacy has been practiced as a means of helping women who are unable to bear children for centuries. The earliest mention is in the Old Testament of the Bible (1). Before the advent of modern assisted conception techniques, "natural surrogacy" was the only means of helping certain barren women to have babies. Before the introduction of artificial insemination, babies were conceived the "natural way," as practiced by Abraham (1). Later, with the introduction of artificial insemination techniques, it became more socially acceptable to use these than "natural means." Later still, when assisted conception techniques, such as in vitro fertilization (IVF) were introduced, embryos created entirely from the gametes of the "genetic" or "commissioning couple" could be transferred to the "surrogate host," who therefore provided no genetic contribution to any child that resulted from the arrangement. She bore the child and handed it over to the full "genetic parents."

"Gestational surrogacy," otherwise known as "IVF surrogacy" or "full surrogacy" is now generally accepted in many countries as a treatment option for infertile women with certain clearly defined medical problems. The first report of a baby being born by gestational surrogacy was from the United States in 1985 (2).

Gestational surrogacy is now accepted in the United Kingdom as a treatment option for infertile women, provided there are clearly defined medical indications. A report commissioned by the British Medical Association (BMA) in 1990 (3), provided the first evidence that surrogacy was formally accepted as a legitimate treatment option. However, in1984 the Warnock Committee (4) had recommended to the U.K. government that surrogacy should be prohibited. Opinions then started to change in 1985, when the annual representative meeting of the BMA passed a resolution – "This meeting agrees with the principle of surrogate births in selected cases with careful controls" (5). However, the BMA then published a further report in 1987 (6) which stated that surrogacy was not an acceptable form of treatment and at the Annual General Meeting later that year, the concept of surrogacy was further rejected, in spite of the 1985 resolution. The 1987 report made it clear that doctors "should not participate in any surrogacy arrangements" (6). However, a working party which subsequently reported to the BMA

in 1990 (3), stated that – "It would not be possible or desirable to seek to prevent all involvement of doctors in surrogacy arrangements, especially as the Government does not intend to make the practice illegal." This report proposed guidelines for doctors making it clear that only after intensive investigation and counseling, and very much as a last resort option, should IVF surrogacy be used as a treatment to overcome a couple's infertility problem. In the same year, the Human Fertilisation and Embryology Act (1990) (7) was passed through the U.K. Parliament and did not ban surrogacy. The most recent report of the BMA (8) states that "surrogacy is an acceptable option of last resort in cases where it is impossible or highly undesirable for medical reasons for the intended mother to carry a child herself."

During the years of this protracted debate in the United Kingdom, most other European countries had decided to ban the practice of surrogacy of any kind. The largest experience of both natural and gestational surrogacy is in the United States, where commercial surrogacy arrangements are allowed. Relatively few publications of experience with gestational surrogacy appeared in the literature in the early years, and there were few long-term follow-up studies of the babies or of the couples involved in surrogacy arrangements (9–12) in spite of strong recommendations to do so (13,14). However, more recently, a number of studies have been published on couples' long-term experiences and their children, which are reassuring, and which are further discussed in the Results section of this chapter.

In 1986 at Bourn Hall Clinic, despite opposition from the BMA and the recommendation of the Warnock report, Mr. Patrick Steptoe and Professor Robert Edwards, the pioneers of IVF, first proposed treating a patient by IVF surrogacy. After extensive discussions with the independent Ethics Committee to the Clinic, they undertook treatment of the first couple in the United Kingdom (15). Following an IVF treatment cycle, embryos from the "genetic couple" were transferred to the sister of the woman and a child was born to them in 1989. In the same year, the Ethics Committee to Bourn Hall drew up guidelines for the treatment of women by IVF surrogacy and the full program was formalized in 1990. The outcomes of the treatment of 49 genetic couples treated at Bourn Hall since then are detailed later in this chapter, together with a review of the results of clinics in the United States, where there is the largest experience of gestational surrogacy.

METHODS

Definitions of Terms

There has always been confusion among patients, practitioners, and between different countries on the definition of the different forms of surrogacy. It is common practice to use the term "surrogate mother" or "surrogate" for the woman who carries and delivers a baby. Others would argue, however, that it is the woman who rears the child, rather than the one who gives birth who is the surrogate mother, and the women who gives birth is the mother not the surrogate. Since the woman who gives birth is initially the legal mother of that child, further confusion is added.

"Gestational surrogacy," "full surrogacy," or "IVF surrogacy" is defined as treatment by which the gametes of the "genetic couple," "commissioning couple," or "intended parents" in a surrogacy arrangement are used to produce embryos and these embryos are subsequently transferred to a woman who agrees to act as a host for these embryos. The "surrogate host" is therefore genetically unrelated to any offspring that may be born as a result of this arrangement.

With "natural surrogacy" or "partial surrogacy" the intended host is inseminated with the semen of the husband of the "genetic couple." Any resulting child is therefore genetically related to the host.

In this chapter, only treatment by "gestational surrogacy" is considered and the couple who initiates the surrogacy arrangement and whose gametes are used will be known as the "genetic couple" and the woman who subsequently carries the child will be known as the "surrogate host."

Indications for "Gestational Surrogacy"

The principal indications for treatment by "gestational surrogacy" in our practice at Bourn Hall are shown in Table 65.1. Absence of a uterus following hysterectomy for uterine or cervical carcinoma, or following hemorrhage or congenital absence are the main indications. Other women who have suffered repeated miscarriages and are deemed to have little or no chance of carrying a child to term are considered for treatment. Repeated failure of treatment by IVF is also an indication for treatment, but it has only been used for women who have

Table 65.1 Indications for Treatment by Gestational Surrogacy

- Congenital absence of the uterus
- Following hysterectomy for cancer, postpartum hemorrhage, or menorrhagia
- Repeated failure of IVF treatment
- Recurrent abortion
- Severe medical conditions incompatible with pregnancy

never shown any signs of implanting normal embryos in an apparently normal uterus after at least six to eight IVF–embryo transfer (ET) cycles. There are certain medical conditions that would threaten the life of a woman were she to become pregnant, such as severe heart disease or renal disease, which are also indications. Discussion is always held with the specialist looking after the medical problems of these women, and the Ethics Committee require evidence that the female partner of the "genetic couple" will be able to look after the child adequately and that her life expectancy is reasonable. Women who request it purely for career or social reasons are not considered for treatment.

Because the indications for treatment are relatively limited, the actual need for treatment by gestational surrogacy is also limited. In our own practice, treatment by surrogacy accounts for <1% of the total annual throughput of cases, out of a total of about 1400 IVF and frozen embryo replacement cycles. It is practiced in only a limited number of IVF centers both in the United Kingdom (16) and in the United States. In a worldwide survey on behalf of the International Federation of Fertility Societies (IFFS), Jones et al. (17) reported that of the 57 countries surveyed, 20 allowed and/or practiced surrogacy.

Selection of Patients for Treatment

In our own practice, all "genetic couples" are referred by their General Practitioners or Gynecologists and are therefore already selected as probably being suitable for treatment. The "genetic couple" are seen alone in the first instance and in-depth consultation and counseling on all medical aspects of the treatment are carried out. If they are considered to be medically suitable for treatment and fall within the guidelines laid down by the independent Ethics Committee to Bourn Hall Clinic and they comply with the Code of Practice of the Human Fertilisation and Embryology Authority (HFEA) (18), particularly with regard to the welfare of any child born as a result of treatment, the couple are informed that they are required by Law in the United Kingdom (19) to find a host for themselves. They are told that the host may be a member of the "genetic couples" family, a close friend, or that they could find a suitable host through one of the patient infertility support groups in the United Kingdom set up to help couples seeking hosts, and for potential hosts seeking couples to help. Other groups have also reported using sisters (20), mothers, (21) and support groups or other agencies (10,22). All groups practicing gestational surrogacy are adamant about the need for in-depth medical and psychological screening of all "genetic couples," the surrogate hosts, and other members of the family, especially any existing children of the surrogate host, and possibly also the parents of the hosts and genetic couples (22,23).

In our own practice, when a suitable host has been found, she and her partner are interviewed at length and a full explanation of the implications of acting as a surrogate host explained to them. If the host is thought to be suitable, then both the genetic and host couples are counseled in depth. If this process is satisfactory and there are no obvious reasons why the arrangement should not be allowed to proceed from a medical and counseling standpoint, a report is prepared and submitted to the independent Ethics Committee to this clinic. The Committee then either approves the arrangement, holds it over for further information and discussion, or rejects it. In every case, the clinic acts in accordance with the recommendations of the Ethics Committee.

It must be stressed that, in all surrogacy arrangements, the welfare of any child born as a result of treatment and of any existing children of a family is given the utmost importance. This is in accordance with the Code of Practice of the Human Fertilisation and Embryology Authority (18) drawn up by the HFEA as a result of the Act of Parliament passed by the U.K. government in 1990 (8).

Counseling

In-depth counseling of all parties engaged in surrogacy arrangements is of paramount importance and aims to prepare all parties contemplating this treatment of last resort to consider all the facts which will have an influence on the future lives of each of them. They must be confident and comfortable with their decisions and have trust in each other, so that no one party is felt to be taking advantage of the other. The BMA in its 1990 report (3) produced a most useful statement: "The aggregate of foreseeable hazards should not be so great as to place unacceptable burdens on any of the parties – including the future child." Many issues must be discussed with both the genetic couple and the proposed host surrogate. These include:

For the Genetic Couples (8):

- A review of all alternative treatment options
- The need for in-depth counseling
- The need to find their own host (United Kingdom)
- The practical difficulty and cost of treatment by gestational surrogacy
- The medical and psychological risks of surrogacy
- Potential psychological risk to the child
- The chances of having a multiple pregnancy
- The degree of involvement that the host may wish to have with the child
- The possibility that a child may be born with a handicap
- The risks to the baby of the host smoking and drinking during a pregnancy
- The possibility that the host may wish to retain the child after birth and the fact that surrogacy contracts in the United Kingdom are not enforceable
- The importance of obtaining legal advice
- The genetic couples are advised to take out insurance cover for the surrogate host

For the Host (8):

- The full implications of undergoing treatment by IVF surrogacy
- The possibility of multiple pregnancy

- The possibility of family and friends being against such treatment
- The need to abstain from unprotected sexual intercourse during and just before the treatment
- The normal medical risks associated with pregnancy and the possibility of caesarian section
- Implications and feelings of guilt on both sides if the host should spontaneously abort a pregnancy
- The possibility that the host will feel a sense of bereavement when she gives the baby to the genetic couple
- The possibility that the child may be born with a handicap
- The fact that hosts in the United Kingdom are expected to only claim "reasonable expenses"

Other issues that must be discussed with both parties to a surrogacy arrangement include in-depth discussions on whether and what both parties will tell the children born as a result of treatment in the future about their origins and also what the host mother will tell any children she has. There is an increasing willingness of all couples involved with treatment by assisted reproductive techniques (ARTs) to be more open about their treatment, whether by IVF, the use of donor gametes, or surrogacy. It is felt by most workers in the area that it is better for couples to be open with their children about their origins rather than to try and cover them up.

Another issue that is often raised in counseling is whether the genetic mother may be able to breast-feed her baby when it is given to her by the host surrogate. There is a belief that the genetic mother may be able to provide some breast milk, which will almost certainly require bottle supplementation, if she puts the child to the breast regularly. It has been proposed that the genetic mother who receives the baby should prepare for the possibility of breast-feeding by stimulating secretion of milk manually, or with a breast pump, in the few weeks leading up to delivery of her child. If there is an enthusiasm to breast-feed then it is worth an attempt, but there is a strong possibility of disappointment.

Patient Management

Management of the Genetic Mother

The majority of "genetic mothers" treated in this clinic are fully assessed by their gynecologist before referral. The work-up usually includes a laparoscopy, if there are congenital anomalies, but it is not necessary after hysterectomy. Evidence of ovarian function can often be obtained from a history of cyclical premenstrual symptoms or symptoms of ovulation. This can be confirmed by one or more estimations of serum follicle-stimulating hormone (FSH) and luteinizing hormone (LH), and possibly timed progesterone levels in the estimated luteal phase. The blood groups of the genetic parents are requested in case the host is rhesus negative and both the genetic parents are tested for hepatitis B (HBV), hepatitis C (HCV), and human immunodeficiency virus (HIV) status. Ultrasound scanning of the ovaries is carried out on some patients to confirm the presence of one or both ovaries, their position, and possible evidence of their activity. Other investigations are carried out as necessary on an individual basis.

On completion of the full medical assessment, the counseling process and when the approval of the Ethics Committee has been obtained, treatment of the genetic couple is started, provided the host has already been identified, fully counseled, and approved. Since most women requesting treatment by gestational surrogacy are perfectly normal with regard to their ovarian function, the management of their IVF treatment cycles is straightforward. Ovarian follicular stimulation, monitoring, and oocyte recovery methods as practiced in this clinic have previously been described (24–26). Oocytes are collected by the standard transvaginal ultrasound-guided technique originally described by Wikland et al. in 1985 (27), and by our own group (28). In all treatment cycles in the United Kingdom, the embryos obtained from the genetic couple must be frozen for a six-month "quarantine" period for HIV status prior to their transfer to the uterus of the surrogate host. However, where a delay in treatment is expected, the semen of the husband of the genetic couple may be frozen for six or more months and, after a further test of HIV status, the embryos are then transferred "fresh" to the host. This policy is in line with the regulation of the HFEA that the sperm used in surrogacy cases should be treated in the same way as donor sperm, which by law must be frozen and quarantined for six months before it can be used (26).

Management of the Surrogate Host

In the United Kingdom, the recruitment of a surrogate host must be carried out by the genetic couple themselves. In our own Unit, only normal fit women who are 38 years of age or less and who have had at least one child are considered. Other groups will consider any woman less than 45 years of age who are willing to act as hosts (29). The relationships between the surrogate hosts and the genetic mothers in our own series are shown in Table 65.2. The Ethics Committee have recommended that hosts should be married or in a stable heterosexual relationship and that the husband or partner should be made fully aware during the counseling process of the implications of his partner acting as a surrogate host.

Fertility investigations of the proposed host have not been necessary. All hosts and their partners are tested for

Table 65.2   Relationship of Genetic Mothers to Surrogate Hosts in the Bourn Hall Gestational Surrogacy Program, with Proportions in Each Group

• Relations	
– Sister to sister	35%
– Sister to sister-in-law	20%
– Step-daughter to step-mother	5%
• Friend to friend	15%
• Through an organization (COTS)	25%

Abbreviation: COTS, Childlessness Overcome Through Surrogacy

HBV, HCV, and HIV status before the embryo transfer is carried out, and the HIV status of the "genetic couple" is re-tested. If the surrogate host is taking the oral contraceptive pill, it is discontinued one cycle before the replacement cycle and barrier methods of contraception or abstinence from intercourse are strongly recommended.

Embryo transfer to the surrogate host may either be carried out in a natural menstrual cycle or in a cycle controlled with exogenous hormone treatment. The latter is recommended if the menstrual cycles of the host are irregular, if they are found not to be ovulating normally, or if luteal phase insufficiency is suspected. In the early days of our own program, all fertile hosts who relied on barrier methods of contraception were placed on a LH-releasing hormone (LH-RH) analogue regimen, combined with hormone replacement therapy (HRT) to prevent any chance of natural conception. More recently, however, with proper advice on barrier contraception and an awareness of the strong motivation of hosts, this method has largely been discontinued. The management of the hormone controlled cycles for the transfer of frozen/thawed embryos has been described previously (30,31).

RESULTS

Treatment by gestational surrogacy generally achieves satisfactory pregnancy and delivered baby rates per genetic couple and per surrogate host; however, there are few published series reported in the literature. In our own series, live birth rates of between 37% and 43% per genetic or commissioning couple and 34% and 39% per host surrogate have been achieved, with a mean of two embryos transferred (26,32). Another U.K. series in which all the female partners in the "genetic couple" had had a hysterectomy achieved a pregnancy rate of 37.5% per surrogate host and 27.3% (6/22) per cycle of treatment begun (33).

In the original series reported by Utian and colleagues (9), a clinical pregnancy rate of 18% (7/59) per cycle initiated and 23% clinical pregnancy rate per embryo transfer was achieved. A later series of 180 cycles of IVF gestational surrogacy, reported by the same group, gave an overall pregnancy rate per cycle of 24% (38/138) and a live birth rate of 15.8% (25/158) (34). Another larger series from the United States showed ongoing or delivered pregnancy rates of 36% (172 of 484 surrogate hosts) (35), with a mean of 5±1.3 embryos transferred. Corson and colleagues reported a clinical pregnancy rate of 58% per commissioning couple and 33.2% per embryo transfer in women where the genetic women were less than 40 years of age (36).

What has recently become apparent is that very little investigation of the immediate and long-term outcome of the babies born as a result of gestational surrogacy has been carried out. However, Parkinson et al. (37) have reviewed the perinatal outcome of pregnancies from IVF surrogacy and compared them to the outcome of pregnancies resulting from standard IVF. As would be expected, the surrogate hosts who carried twin and triplet gestations delivered substantially earlier than those who gestated singleton pregnancies and the twin newborns were significantly lighter than singleton infants born through IVF surrogacy. Interestingly, the occurrence of pregnancy-induced hypertension and bleeding in the third trimester of pregnancy was up to five times lower in the surrogate hosts than in the standard IVF patient controls. Apart from birth weights and prematurity, little other information is given about the outcome of the babies.

There have been very few long-term follow-up studies of women who have acted as surrogate hosts, but there is little to suggest any long-term harm or regret among them (12,13,38). The most recent studies of hosts and commissioning couples show reassuring data and positive outcomes, particularly for the hosts (39–42).

COMPLICATIONS

Problems Encountered with Gestational Surrogacy

The major problems that have been reported with surrogacy arrangements have almost entirely arisen from "natural surrogacy" arrangements. The major problems have been legal and mostly revolve around the "ownership" and rights of both the "genetic couple" and the birth mothers. These are not further considered in this chapter but they are well documented in a number of papers published on the subject (3,13,14,43–46). The main reason these problems have arisen is that the majority of the arrangements were largely unsupervised and did not involve careful clinical and psychological assessment, counseling, and discussion with lawyers. With gestational surrogacy, professionals in all of these areas are invariably involved and, as a consequence, the number of complications arising out of these treatments is very few. In the past 22 years of our own experience, no serious clinical, ethical, or legal problems have been encountered. The major ethical and practical problems that might be encountered with IVF surrogacy include:

- The host may wish to keep the child. This is the complication that all practitioners in this area worry about most but, with proper counseling and legal advice, it has not occurred in our own series. The cases that have come to light have invariably involved "natural surrogacy."
- An abnormal child may be rejected by both the genetic and host parents. This is of course a major concern, but has not yet occurred in our own experience nor has any other group published on the occurrence of this complication.
- The question of whether it is ethical to pay hosts and if so how much has always caused concern. In the United States, payment is "up front" and revealed, whereas in the United Kingdom and most of Europe, altruistic surrogacy is what everyone aspires to, but it is in effect impractical and payment is often hidden as "reasonable expenses." Many also consider it

unethical not to pay hosts for the sacrifices that they make to help other couples. The European Society of Human Reproduction and Embryology (ESHRE) Task Force on Ethics and the Law (2005) (29) states that payment for (surrogacy) services is unacceptable," while the "IFFS Surveillance Report 2010" (17) states only that "The payment to the surrogate raises special concerns."
- The long-term effects on the children born as a result of gestational surrogacy are not known. The American Society of Assisted Reproduction (ASRM) (13) and BMA (8) strongly recommend long-term follow-up studies. However, these issues have been addressed more recently and, to date, the outcomes are reassuring (38–42).
- The long-term psychological effect on both the "genetic couple" and "host surrogates" is not known, nor is the effect on the hosts' existing children. Again long-term studies do need to be carried out and are also strongly advocated by the ASRM (14) and BMA (9).

In our own series, a number of relatively minor complications have occurred:

- A few of our "genetic women" have responded poorly to follicular stimulation and achieved relatively small numbers of oocytes. The mean number of oocytes recovered following the stimulation cycle has been 10 but the range has been two to 24. In the series of Meniru and Craft (33), three of their 11 patients failed to respond to ovulation induction and two other patients produced only very few oocytes, which failed to fertilize. In the posthysterectomy cases, this reduced follicular response may be due to reduced vascular supply to the ovaries (47).
- The follicular responses of women with the Rokitansky-Kuster-Hauser (RKH) syndrome were remarkably good. Four women with RKH syndrome underwent 10 stimulation cycles in the program of Ben Raphael and colleagues (48) with human menopausal gonadotropin (hMG), two to three ampoules per day. A mean of 14.6 oocytes (range 8–24) was collected and the fertilization rate was 71%. Of considerable interest and reassurance for this particular group of young women, has been a study to follow up the children born to women with congenital absence of the uterus and vagina (RKH syndrome). Petrozza and colleagues (49) sent questionnaires to all treatment centers performing surrogacy procedures and asked them to follow-up the frequency of congenital abnormalities among the progeny born to RKH syndrome women. Results of 162 IVF cycles produced 34 live born children, half of whom were female. No congenital anomalies were found amongst these females. These results appear to suggest that congenital absence of the uterus and vagina, if it is genetically transmitted, is not inherited commonly in a dominant fashion.

In a survey of all licensed clinics performing surrogacy in the United Kingdom (16), 29 of 113 licensed clinics perform or have performed surrogacy. In general, very few problems were reported, the most significant of which were:

- There was one report of a surrogate who failed to surrender the baby after the birth, but did so subsequently.
- One surrogate asked for more money from the "genetic couple" once she had achieved a pregnancy.
- One couple separated just before treatment started.
- There was unwelcome newspaper publicity in one case.
- A number of couples pulled out of treatment during the counseling phase.
- Poor response rates to follicular stimulation were noted in several clinics, particularly after Wertheim's hysterectomy.
- One patient changed her mind during the treatment and actively attempted not to get pregnant. She did not conceive and this led to friction within the family, despite many hours of counseling.

When questioned for this survey, most clinics felt that there should be greater control of surrogacy, particularly of natural surrogacy and that it should be performed within licensed clinics where appropriate health screening and counseling may be provided.

FUTURE DIRECTIONS AND CONTROVERSIES

In the United Kingdom and the United States, the public generally accepts that treatment by surrogacy, particularly gestational surrogacy, is a reasonable treatment option if there are good clinical indications. Because there are a number of countries, particularly in Europe, where surrogacy is not permitted, and as the ease of travel around the world increases, there are concerns that couples will travel around the world for treatment that is unavailable in their own countries. The concern is that these practices may lead to disputes and exploitation of desperate couples seeking this particular treatment (8). As an example of these concerns, there have been press reports of women from Eastern Europe taken and exploited as surrogate hosts in wealthier countries where gestational surrogacy is allowed. As a result of this, a number of countries have completely banned surrogacy. Existing controls by the HFEA and proposed changes which may be instituted, which are discussed later in this chapter, should prevent such exploitation in the United Kingdom.

There is evidence, certainly in the United Kingdom, that there is an increasing level of sympathy and support for the proper use of treatment by "gestational surrogacy" from the media and general public (50). With increasing education and awareness, the public has been able to better judge the benefits of this treatment when there are proper indications. Similarly, in the United States there is much greater acceptance of "gestational surrogacy," especially now that it is superseding "natural surrogacy" as the treatment option of choice for most couples.

In the surrogacy program at Bourn Hall, the main principle by which we have been guided is consideration of the welfare of any child that may be born as the result of treatment and of the existing children. This is enshrined in the Code of Practice (18) of the Human Fertilisation and Embryology Act 1990 (7) and also followed by the independent Ethics Committee to Bourn Hall.

If the best interests of the child are considered at all times as the priority, then the other issues will invariably fall into place. For instance, the fitness and welfare of the proposed host to go through with the treatment; the age, physical and psychological "fitness" of the female partner in the commissioning couple, and the seeking of proper legal advice, will nearly always become apparent if due consideration is given to the welfare of the child.

Legal Issues

The majority of the legal problems that have arisen as a result of surrogacy have been associated with cases of "natural surrogacy." There have been two cases that have received particular publicity – the "baby M case" (51,52) and also the case of Smith versus Jones (53,54). In the "baby M case," the final decision was that the genetic couple would have precedence for custody of the child over the birth mother. In the case of Smith versus Jones, which involved "gestational surrogacy" the District Court recognized the genetic parents to be the legal parents and gave them the right to put their names on the birth certificate of the baby (53,54). In the United States, a number of states have specific regulations regarding surrogate motherhood, but some are more specific than others about the rights of the "genetic mother" over those of the "birth mother." The complex differences between states have been well summarized by Schuster (45,46). Similarly, in the case of Johnson versus Calvert in the California Superior Court, where Johnson was the "gestational surrogate," the Calverts, the "genetic parents" of the child, were ruled to be the natural parents of the child (55).

Following a widely reported case in 1997 of a natural surrogacy arrangement that experienced severe difficulties, U.K. Health Ministers decided to seek views on certain aspects of the existing legislation relating to surrogacy and to "take stock and reassess the adequacy of existing law in this difficult area" (56). A review body was appointed and was asked specifically to address the following issues:

- to consider whether payments, including expenses, to surrogate mothers should continue to be allowed, and if so on what basis;
- to examine whether there is a case for the regulation of surrogacy arrangements through a recognized body or bodies; and if so to advise on the scope and operation of such arrangements; and
- in light of the above, to advise whether changes are needed to the Surrogacy Arrangements Act 1985 (19) and/or Section 30 of the Human Fertilisation and Embryology Act 1990 (7).

The Minister for Public Health at that time stated: "My aim is to ensure that the government provides a sensible and sensitive way forward, within a framework that inspires public confidence, in an area of personal life where feelings are inevitably raw and highly charged for those involved" (56). The review panel comprised three Professors – of Law, Psychology, and Ethics.

In response to the Health Minister's request, the report of the Surrogacy Review Team (57) was presented to the U.K. Parliament and published in October 1998. The following is a summary of their recommendations:

1. Payments to surrogate mothers should cover only genuine expenses, which should be supported with documentary evidence. Additional payments should be prohibited to prevent surrogacy arrangements being entered into for financial benefit.

2. Agencies involved in surrogacy arrangements should be registered by the U.K. Health Department and operate in accordance with a Code of Practice to be prepared for record keeping and the reporting of specified statistics on surrogacy and guidelines on research should be established by the Health Departments.

3. The existing Surrogacy Arrangements Act 1985 and Section 30 of the Human Fertilisation and Embryology Act 1990 should be replaced with a new Surrogacy Act which would address in one statute the main legal principles governing surrogacy arrangements in the United Kingdom:

    (a) to continue the current provision relating to nonenforceability of surrogacy contracts;

    (b) the continuation of current provisions prohibiting commercial agencies from assisting in the creation of surrogacy arrangements and prohibiting advertisements in relation to surrogacy;

    (c) new statutory provisions defining and limiting lawful payments to surrogate mothers;

    (d) provision for promulgation of a Code of Practice governing surrogacy arrangements generally;

    (e) provision for the registration of nonprofit making surrogacy agencies would be required to comply with the departments' Code of Practice on surrogacy arrangements to prohibit the operation of unregistered agencies; and

    (f) to make new provisions for the granting of parental orders to commissioning couples.

4. Parental orders should only be obtained in the High Court and judges should be able to order DNA tests and guardians' ad litem should be able to check criminal records.

5. For a parental order to be granted, the commissioning couple should be habitually resident in the United Kingdom, the Channel Islands, or the Isle of Man for a period of twelve months immediately preceding the application for a parental order.

Still, at the time of writing in 2011, these recommendations by the Surrogacy Review Team have not been implemented.

Treatment by "gestational surrogacy" is already fully regulated in the United Kingdom, since it can only be practiced in centers licensed by the HFEA. This should be sufficient to ensure that proper clinical and scientific services, counseling, and legal advice are provided to both commissioning couples and host surrogates. If "gestational surrogacy" is to be allowed to continue, which there is a general consensus that it should be (50), then the existing regulations are probably sufficient. However, "natural surrogacy" is completely unregulated in the United Kingdom and we believe should be brought under the control of a regulatory body, probably the HFEA.

As in the United States, Australian States have different regulations. Surrogacy is freely available in New South Wales, Western Australia, and the Australia Capital Territory. In Tasmania, South Australia, and Victoria, it is not illegal, but very strict controls on payment and the lack of binding legal arrangements make it almost impossible to carry out (58). There is a tendency, therefore, for couples seeking surrogacy arrangements to move from state to state (59).

The most recent issue concerning the provision of treatment by surrogacy is the ethical question of whether or not it is acceptable to provide this treatment, hitherto only recommended for heterosexual couples, to gay and lesbian couples. The Ethics Committee Report of the ASRM in 2006 carefully considered "the changing nature of reproduction and the family." They concluded that "... there is no sound basis for denying to single persons and gays and lesbians the same rights to reproduce that other individuals have," and they finally state: "As a matter of ethics, we believe that the ethical duty to treat persons with equal respect requires that fertility programs treat single persons and gay and lesbian couples equally with married couples in determining which services to provide" (60).

Religious Issues

Religious attitudes toward surrogacy differ widely:

The Catholic Church is strongly against all forms of assisted conception, particularly those that involve gamete donation and surrogacy (61). The Anglican Church is less rigid in its view on surrogacy and has not condemned it.

The Jewish religion, which is very much family orientated and puts a duty on Jewish couples to have children, does not forbid the practice of gestational surrogacy (62). From the religious point of view, a child born through gestational surrogacy to a Jewish couple will belong to the father who gave the sperm and to the woman who gave birth (63–65).

The Islamic view appears absolute and, in the same way that the use of donor gametes is strictly forbidden, so surrogacy is not allowed. It is suggested that it may be permissible between wives in the same marriage, but the debate continues (66).

CONCLUSION

It is now 26 years since the birth of the first child following a gestational surrogacy arrangement in the United States (2). In the 22 years of our own experience at Bourn

Hall, we have shown that the treatment of young women with very specific indications is successful and relatively free of complications. The practice of gestational surrogacy is almost entirely confined to the United Kingdom, where it can only be carried out in clinics licensed by the HFEA, a very few countries in Europe and in the United States.

The indications for treatment by gestational surrogacy are limited to a small group of women who have no uterus, suffer recurrent abortions, or suffer from certain medical conditions which would threaten the life of a woman were she to become pregnant. Times are changing, however, and recently gestational surrogacy has been used to help gay couples who wish to have families.

The treatment process in itself is straightforward. The woman from the "genetic couple" undergoes a normal stimulated IVF cycle and, unless the sperm of her partner has previously been frozen for six months, any embryos that are retrieved are frozen and later transferred to a selected surrogate host. The difficult aspects of the treatment concern the extreme care with which the surrogate host must be selected by the genetic couple to ensure complete compatibility and also the in-depth counseling that is required, both in the short and the long term, on all aspects of the treatment. The support and advice of an independent counselor and lawyer are absolutely essential and we believe the advice of an independent Ethics Committee is also essential in assessing the suitability of individual cases. As clinicians and counselors, we are inclined to become so deeply involved in the problems of individual couples that some of the more obvious pitfalls in the social, religious, or ethical aspects of treating a particular couple may easily be overlooked.

During the past 22 years of our experience, no serious clinical, ethical, or legal problems have been encountered. In one sister-to-sister arrangement, failure of the treatment caused some disagreement and unhappiness between the sisters and support counseling was necessary for more than three years. Another more minor problem that we have encountered has been that both parties very often have unreasonably high expectations of the success of treatment, in spite of very frank explanations and counseling being provided to them. Because the host is fit, young, and known to be fertile, she and the genetic parents invariably expect success and they feel badly let down if this is not achieved. An interesting problem that has arisen is that the miscarriage rate has been higher than expected, ~40% of the pregnancies have aborted spontaneously (26,32) in our own series, an outcome which obviously causes severe stress to both parties. The host feels guilt that she has lost the genetic couple's hard won pregnancy and the genetic couple feels guilt that the host has been through the stress of a miscarriage and possible curettage. Full support counseling for both couples is essential when this occurs.

At Bourn Hall we believe that a gestational surrogacy service should be part of a comprehensive infertility treatment program that most larger centers should offer now that it is an ethically accepted form of treatment in the United Kingdom and certain countries worldwide

(17). In our own practice surrogacy accounts for less than 1% of all the assisted conception cycles that we carry out. With a policy of careful selection and screening of both genetic and host couples, together with independent counseling, good success rates can be achieved. Long-term follow-up of the babies born as a result of this treatment is being carried out at present, as is the long term follow-up of the genetic parents and hosts of these arrangements.

ACKNOWLEDGMENTS

I would like to thank Reverend Dr. Tim Appleton (now deceased) for his help and support in the past as an independent counselor with the surrogacy program at Bourn Hall, and more recently to Mrs. Linda Koncewicz. Sincere thanks also go to my medical and nursing colleagues who, through their dedication in caring for couples going through the surrogacy program, have ensured its success and the happiness of many deserving couples.

REFERENCES

1. Holy Bible The Book of Genesis; 16: 1–15; 17: 15–19; 21: 1–4.
2. Utian WH, Sheean LA, Goldfarb JM, Kiwi R. Successful pregnancy after in vitro fertilisation and embryo transfer from an infertile woman to a surrogate. N Engl J Med 1985; 313: 1351–2.
3. British Medical Association. Surrogacy: Ethical Considerations. Report of the Working Party on Human Infertility Services. London: BMA Publications, 1990.
4. Committee of Enquiry. Report of the Committee of Inquiry into Human Fertilisation and Embryology. London: Her Majesty's Stationery Office, 1984.
5. British Medical Association. Annual Representative Meeting Report. 1985.
6. British Medical Association. Surrogate Motherhood. Report of the Board of Science and Education. London: BMA Publications, 1987.
7. Human Fertilisation and Embryology Act. London: Her Majesty's Stationery Office, 1990.
8. British Medical Association Report. Changing Conceptions of Motherhood. The Practice of Surrogacy in Britain. London: BMA Publications, 1996.
9. Utian WF, Goldfarb JM, Kiwi R, et al. Preliminary experience with in vitro fertilization-surrogate gestational pregnancy. Fertil Steril 1989; 52: 633–8.
10. Marrs RP, Ringler GE, Stein AL, Vargyas JM, Stone BA. The use of surrogate gestational carriers for assisted reproductive technologies. Am J Obstet Gynecol 1993; 168: 1858–63.
11. Fisher S, Gillman I. Surrogate motherhood: attachment, attitudes and social support. Psychiatry 1991; 54: 13–20.
12. Blyth E. Interviews with surrogate mothers in Britain. J Reprod Infert Psychol 1994; 12: 189–98.
13. Ethics Committee of the American Fertility Society. Ethical considerations in the new reproductive technologies. Fertil Steril 1986; 46(Suppl 1): 62–8.
14. American College of Obstetricians and Gynecologists. Committee on Ethics: Ethical Issues in Surrogate Motherhood. Washington, DC: American College of Obstetricians and Gynecologists, 1990.

15. Steptoe P. Surrogacy. Br Med J (Clin Res Ed) 1987; 294: 1688–9.

16. Balen AH, Hadyn CA. British fertility society survey of all licensed clinics that perform surrogacy in the UK. Hum Fert 1998; 1: 6–9.

17. Jones HJ, Cooke I, Kempers R, Brinsden PR, Saunders D. IFFS Surveillance 2010. Fertil Steril 2011; 95: 491. [Available from: http://www.iffs-reproduction.org]

18. Human Fertilisation and Embryology Authority. Code of Practice for Clinics Licensed by the Human Fertilisation and Embryology Authority. 7th edn. London: Human Fertilisation and Embryology Authority, 2007.

19. Surrogacy Arrangements Act. London: Her Majesty's Stationery Office, 1985.

20. Leeton J, King C, Harman J. Sister – sister in vitro fertilisation surrogate pregnancy with donor sperm: the case for surrogate gestational pregnancy. J In Vitro Fert Embryo Trans 1988; 5: 245–98.

21. Michello MC, Bernstein K, Jacobsen MJ, et al. Mother – daughter in vitro fertilisation triplet surrogate pregnancy. J In Vitro Fert Embryo Trans 1988; 5: 31–4.

22. Sheean LA, Goldfarb JM, Kiwi R, Utian WH. In vitro fertilisation (IVF) – surrogacy: application of IVF to women without functional uteri. J Invitro Fert Embryo Trans 1989; 6: 134–7.

23. Ethics Committee of the American Fertility Society. Surrogate gestational mothers: women who gestate a genetically unrelated embryo. Fertil Steril 1990; 53: 64S–7S.

24. Marcus SF, Brinsden PR, Macnamee MC, et al. Comparative trial between an ultrashort and long protocol of luteinising hormone-releasing hormone agonist for ovarian stimulation in in-vitro fertilization. Hum Reprod 1993; 8: 238–43.

25. Brinsden PR. Superovulation strategies in assisted conception. In: Brinsden PR, ed. A Textbook of In Vitro Fertilization and Assisted Reproduction. London, New York: Taylor and Francis, 2005: 177–88.

26. Brinsden PR. IVF Surrogacy. In: Brinsden PR, ed. A Textbook of in vitro Fertilization and Assisted Reproduction. London, New York: Taylor and Francis, 2005: 393–404.

27. Wikland M, Enk L, Hamberger L. Transvesical and transvaginal approaches for the aspiration of follicles by the use of ultrasound. Ann NY Acad Sci 1985; 442: 683–9.

28. Brinsden PR. Oocyte recovery and embryo transfer techniques for in vitro fertilization. In: Brinsden PR, ed. A Textbook of In Vitro Fertilization and Assisted Reproduction. London, New York: Taylor and Francis, 2005: 177–88.

29. Shenfield F, Pennings G, Cohen J, et al. ESHRE Task Force on Ethics and Law Chap 10. Surrogacy. Hum Reprod 2005; 20: 2705–7.

30. Sathanandan M, Macnamee M, Rainsbury P, et al. Frozen-thawed embryo replacement in artificial and natural cycles; a prospective study. Hum Reprod 1991; 5: 1025–8.

31. Marcus SF, Brinsden PR. Oocyte donation. In: Brinsden PR, ed. A Textbook of In Vitro Fertilization and Assisted Reproduction. Carnforth, New York: Parthenon, 1999: 343–54.

32. Brinsden PR, Appleton TC, Murray E, et al. Treatment by In Vitro fertilisation with Surrogacy – The experience of a single centre in the United Kingdom. Br Med J 2000; 320: 924–8.

33. Meniru GI, Craft IL. Experience with gestational surrogacy as a treatment for sterility resulting from hysterectomy. Hum Reprod 1997; 12: 51–4.

34. Goldfarb JM, Austin C, Peskin B, et al. Fifteen years of experience with an in-vitro fertilization surrogate gestational pregnancy programme. Hum Reprod 2000; 15: 1075–8.

35. Batzofin J, Nelson J, Wilcox J, et al. Gestational surrogacy: it is time to include it as part of ART? (abstract). ASRM 1999(Programme Suppl): P-017.

36. Corson SL, Kelly M, Braverman A, English ME. Gestational carrier pregnancy. Fertil Steril 1998; 69: 670–4.

37. Parkinson J, Tran C, Tan T, et al. Peri-natal outcome after in vitro fertilization – surrogacy,. Hum Reprod 1999; 14: 671–6.

38. Van den Akker OBA. Organisational selection and assessment of women entering a surrogacy agreement in the UK. Hum Reprod 1999; 14: 262–6.

39. Jadva V, Murray C, Lycett EJ, et al. Surrogacy: the experience of surrogate mothers. Hum Reprod 2003; 18: 2196–024.

40. Kleinpeter CB. Surrogacy: the parent's story. Psychol Rep 2002; 91: 201–19.

41. Golombok S, Murray C, Jadva V, et al. Families created through a surrogacy arrangement: parent-child relationships in the first year of life. Dev Psychol 2004; 40: 400–11.

42. MacCallum F, Lycett E, Murray C, et al. Surrogacy: the experience of commissioning couples. Hum Reprod 2003; 18: 1334–42.

43. Cohen B, Friend TL. Legal and ethical implications of surrogacy mother contracts. Clin Perinatal 1987; 14: 281–92.

44. Brazier M, Golombok S, Campbell A. Surrogacy: Review for the UK Health Minister of Current Arrangements for Payments and Regulation. Report of the Review Team. London: Department of Health, 1998.

45. Shuster E. Non-genetic surrogacy: no cure but problems for infertility? Hum Reprod 1991; 6: 1176–80.

46. Shuster E. When genes determine motherhood: Problems in gestational surrogacy. Hum Reprod 1992; 7: 1029–33.

47. Siddle N, Sarrel P, Whitehead M. The effect of hysterectomy on the age at ovarian failure: identification of a subgroup of women with premature loss of ovarian function and literature review. Fertil Steril 1987; 47: 94–100.

48. Ben-Raphael Z, Barr-Hava I, Levy T, Orvieto R. Simplifying ovulation induction for surrogacy in women with Mayer-Rokitansky-Kuster-Hauser syndrome. Hum Reprod 1998; 13: 1470–1.

49. Petrozza JC, Gray MR, Davies AJ, Reindollar RH. Congenital absence of the uterus and vagina is not commonly transmitted as a dominant genetic trait: outcomes of surrogate pregnancies. Fertil Steril 1997; 67: 387–9.

50. Bromham DR. Surrogacy: the evolution of opinion. Br J Hosp Med 1992; 47: 767–72.

51. Rothenberg KH, Baby M. The surrogacy contract, and the healthcare professional: unanswered questions. Law Med Health care 1988; 16: 113–20.

52. Andrews LB. The stork market: the Law of the new reproductive technologies. Am Bar Assoc J 1984; 78: 50–6.

53. Annas G. Using genes to define motherhood: the California solution. N Engl J Med 1992; 326: 417–20.

54. Smith VJ. Los Angeles Superior Court, Los Angeles County. 1987: No CF 025653.

55. Oxman RB. California's experiment in surrogacy. Lancet 1993; 341: 1468–9.

56. Warden J. Surrogacy to be reviewed in United Kingdom. Br Med J 1997; 314: 1782.

57. Surrogacy. Review for the UK Health Ministers of current arrangements for payments and regulation. Consultation Document. London: Department of Health, 1997.

58. Leeton J. The current status of IVF surrogacy in Australia. Aust NZJ Obstet Gynaecol 1991; 31: 260–2.

59. Johnson I. Regulation of assisted reproductive technology: the Australian experience. In: Brinsden PR. A Textbook of In Vitro Fertilization and Assisted Reproduction. Carnforth, New York: Parthenon, 1999: 424–7.

60. The Ethics Committee of the American Society for Reproductive Medicine. Access to treatment by gays, lesbians, and unmarried persons. Fertil Steril 2006; 86: 1333–5.

61. McCormick RA. Surrogacy: a catholic perspective. Creighton Law Rev 1992; 25: 1617–25.

62. Schenker JG. Assisted reproduction practice in Europe: legal and ethical aspects. Hum Reprod Update 1997; 3: 173–84.

63. Hirsh AV. Infertility in Jewish couples, biblical and rabbinic law. Hum Fertil (Camb) 1998; 1: 14–19.

64. Schenker JG. Infertility evaluation and treatment according to Jewish Law. Em J Obstet Gynaecol Reprod Biol 1997; 71: 113–21.

65. Benshushan A, Schenker JG. Legitimizing surrogacy in Israel. Hum Reprod 1997; 12: 1832–4.

66. Hussain FA. Reproductive issues from the Islamic perspective. Hum Fertil 2000; 3: 124–8.

The evolving role of the ART nurse: A contemporary review

Joanne L. Libraro

INTRODUCTION

Advances in reproductive technologies continue to offer millions of infertile patients, couples, and families around the world the opportunity to become parents despite significant limitation of infertility. As the "ART" of assisted reproductive techniques advance, multifaceted changes are noted in the roles, responsibilities, and commitments of each member of the infertility team. Clinical programs continue to modify their policies and procedures to meet the needs of the changing culture of medicine, science, and research that surrounds the field of reproductive medicine. The term "IVF" or in vitro fertilization has become synonymous with hope for those patients and couples that seek the advances in care options with the hope of fulfilling the dream of parenthood. In early days, treatment was considered something available only for the privileged or wealthy. Today, even more patients seek and successfully pursue treatment at one of many available IVF programs. The "ART" was seen as a "laboratory science," research oriented and experimental. As time passed, physicians, nurses, lab personal, and researchers have developed the prerequisite skills necessary to remain current in the field of reproductive endocrinology and infertility (REI). Additionally, the available technologies have become accepted as standard treatment modalities.

Dating back nearly 50 years ago at Bourne Hall under the guidance of Drs Robert Edwards and Patrick Steptoe, the future role of ART nurses was conceived and established (1). Jean Purdy (Fig. 66.1), the first recognized "nurse" of distinction in the field of REI, created and established the foundation for clinical growth, scientific development, holistic supportive therapies, and nursing research. The birth of Louise Brown – the first "test-tube" baby – on July 25, 1978 not only thrilled her parents, but also introduced the world to the future of ARTs. This triangle of success included Drs Edwards, Steptoe, and Jean Purdy. On the basis of their early commitment to the advancement of research and science surrounding infertility options, many groundbreaking discoveries have evolved further supporting today's scientists and professionals to continue.

The current trends in reproductive health support the need for nursing professionals to assume an ongoing, visionary, scientific, and academic approach to advancement. Nurses remain a primary influence in the industry, and define the future of nursing standards in reproductive health. As Jean Purdy demonstrated her determination to partner with many scientific professionals and focus on the goals of success, many of today's eager professionals seed the same alignment with clinical and research teams.

Many nursing roles in REI have evolved in recent years to assume a significantly more comprehensive responsibility that is in alignment with the rapidly changing trends in research, science, and treatment options. Since the early days, nursing roles have transformed, further defining the need for specialized education, training, and competencies. Now, more than ever, those professionals seeking success as an REI professional must support their clinical and theoretical knowledge base and remain current with regulatory and ethical trends. The critical role of the REI–ART nurse is reviewed in this chapter and reflects the ongoing change in trends.

ART: A RAPIDLY PROGRESSING FIELD

Many in the field of ARTs phrase the comprehensive clinical, emotional, and scientific process of infertility treatment as a journey. The arduous "journey" to success challenges many patients and couples as they strive for the goal of parenting. Couples face the challenge of accepting the need for assisted technology and the associated failures it stems from. Many layers of decision making – emotional, cultural, ethical, financial, and religious – are involved before initiating treatment. In many cases these challenges lead to the development of unique relationships established with the couple seeking treatment; the ART nurse plays a critical role in their care. Since the 1980s, significant changes in the process of REI have stimulated the need for reflection as professionals adapt to the changing trends. Technology advances, research initiatives, and the influences linked to regulatory influences drive the role of today's nursing professional.

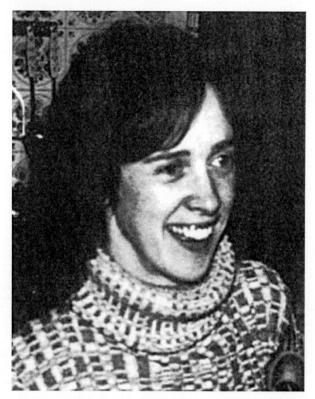

Figure 66.1 Jean Marion Purdy, 1945–1985. *Source*: From Ref. 1.

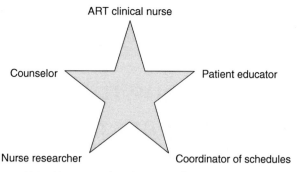

Figure 66.2 Nurses working in assisted reproductive techniques (ARTs) today have many roles.

The comprehensive staff contribution that includes REI physicians, nurses, psychologists, embryologists, andrologists, reproductive urologists, genetic counselors, financial counselors, reproductive endocrine laboratory staff, and administrative staff support the rapidly changing culture of REI and positively impact the role of nurses. Additional support in many IVF centers with academic affiliations includes the three-year fellowship for OB/GYNs interested in pursuing reproductive endocrinology and infertility. Educational and scientific advances expand for all involved in patient care as the team grows to meet the national trends. As the team melds their efforts on coordination, tremendous improvements are noted in the process of patient care. The collaborative nature of REI professional team-driven focuses further support the goal to provide supportive, clinically necessary care to patients and increases successes.

REI NURSING ROLE

The number of REI centers across the country continues to increase. This growth is in alignment with the number of nurses that support the clinical needs of the centers. The active roles of nurses in REI centers have continued to witness the same growth in their professional involvement in patient care. Many advanced professionals are now expanding roles in leadership, clinical, research, and administrative roles than in years past. This growth in partnership with physician teams has allowed nurses to extend their clinical role far beyond that of the traditional nursing model. In many ART centers, significant increases in autonomy are noted as supported by the framework of a highly specialized team of professionals. The resulting multidisciplinary responsibilities of today's REI nurse expand to include a variety of roles including (Fig. 66.2):

1. ART clinical nurse;
2. patient educator;
3. IVF coordinator;
4. regulatory compliance officer;
5. counselor;
6. nurse researcher;
7. egg donor coordinator;
8. preimplantation genetic diagnosis (PGD) coordinator;
9. fertility preservation coordinator;
10. male factor infertility coordinator.

REI nurses nationally support both large and small ART centers with similar goals for success. The diverse roles of today's REI nurses describes the vast need for education and competency in the medical aspects of care, the vast psychological support needs, quality assurance factors, and patient education. Experienced REI practitioners bring many of these core skills from other areas of nursing. Specific training at the center-specific level in the field of infertility embellishes these transferable skills. Furthermore, the treatment of infertility, through the use of IVF and other related techniques, has an ethical and religious dimension that may provoke considerable challenge for nurses and patients, for example, the use of donor sperm, directed donor sperm, donor oocytes or embryos, PGD, fertility preservation, or issues related to multiple pregnancies. It is this diversity in the role of the ART nurse, combined with the fact that patients or couples rely primarily on the nurse for education and, importantly, support, that ART nursing should not be the goal of a recent nursing school graduate. Those most likely to succeed as ART nurses are mature, experienced, flexible, and professional individuals who consistently seek to redefine their own role within a rapidly evolving field.

To remain successful in this highly demanding and constantly changing environment, REI nurses must support their professional commitment to education, certifications, and the development of coworkers. Training others enhances the team's ability to grow, supports the vision of the center to offer current technology with the guidelines of care, and supports the clinical needs for the team and patient population. Included in this training is a specific emphasis on resilience for the emotional and physical pressure of the role. At a minimum, nurses working in this specialty must require the confidence to provide accurate information, support emotional and clinical needs of the patients, while ensuring the governance of regulatory aspects of care. Each of these diverse, dynamic pieces develops the groundwork for success in REI. Personality traits that may be described as "shy," "apprehensive and reactive" are more likely to suffer burnout and be less successful professionally as well as to the patient. Indeed, there is evidence suggesting that ART nurses are at high risk of burnout. This is positively correlated to the length of time spent working in reproductive endocrinology and to a low perceived sense of emotional support [2]. As the nursing shortage in the United States continues, ART nursing positions remain difficult to fill. Thus, the workload carried by many ART nurses can be compounded by this resource challenge. In addition, the complexity of contemporary ART adds to the challenges that many programs face when hiring and retaining nursing staff.

ART CLINICAL NURSE

The traditional role of the nursing professional remains in contrast to the role of today's REI nurse. The academic structure that creates the ART center and the long-term needs of the patient populations determines the specific roles, education, and training necessary for success. Nurses have traditionally performed – or at least participated in – many of the technical steps involved in initiating a patient's ART cycle. Following initial consultation with the physician, the ART nurse becomes intimately involved in each patient's treatment cycle. In addition to their role in patient education, counseling, and treatment planning and coordination, nurses have commonly performed certain technical aspects of IVF treatment cycles, including:

1. REI and significant medical history with record review;
2. pretreatment evaluation of required diagnostic testing and screening;
3. evaluation of daily laboratory results;
4. medication administration and instruction;
5. preoperative, intraoperative, and postoperative care;
6. pregnancy evaluation and follow-up;
7. ovulation induction monitoring and intrauterine insemination (IUI) partner and donor programs [3].

PATIENT EDUCATOR

Reproductive endocrinology nurses are foundational resources for patients and couples seeking ART treatments. The comprehensive, individualized care needs declare the specific educational approaches used to direct treatment, evaluation, and follow-up care. As a key source of information to infertile couples, continuing education is a primary requirement for the professional

REI nurse, with the understanding that advances in technology have continued to positively impact clinical and research successes. However, with the advancing technology comes the need for extensive, global education across the REI centers. Each center differs in the available techniques, successes, and outcomes, yet the need for nurses to remain current on clinical, research, and regulatory trends is extensive. Through such education, nurses are best set to provide information related to current techniques and practices specific to their program.

Comprehensive patient education and support should be considered mandatory at every ART clinic. The goal of IVF patient orientation and education is to ensure that patients understand the "big picture" of their treatment. Ultimately, successful patient education fosters confidence in couples undergoing treatment. As a result, patients are more likely to be confident about providing informed consent, to be satisfied with their treatment and to be more inclined to accept its final outcome [4].

Key aspects of patient education include discussions that focus on:

1. the couple's specific infertility challenge;
2. overview of program practices (i.e., who's who, how the clinic runs, etc.);
3. available ART technologies including intracytoplasmic sperm injection (ICSI), genetic screening and testing (preimplantation genetic diagnosis – PGD), assisted hatching, testicular sperm extraction (TESE), third party reproduction, fertility preservation, etc.;
4. timing of the patient's cycle, including drug injections, overview of hospital experience from oocyte recovery to embryo transfer, etc.
5. preparation of the cycle, including prestimulation protocols, stimulation protocols, and possible adverse events;
6. post-transfer management, such as pregnancy testing, follow-up appointments, etc.
7. medication education for injection and reconstitution;
8. available support services that are center-specific, center-supported, or outside advocacy groups;
9. possible IVF concerns, such as premature ovulation, poor ovarian response, ovarian hyperstimulation syndrome (OHSS), etc.;
10. regulatory considerations specific to the individual cycles.

ART remains a complex specialty with ever changing medical terminology, a wide number of acronyms and abbreviations, and intricate drug regimens and protocols. For this reason, it is important for the ART nurse to prepare patients fully for what is to come during the ART process. These professionals focus on alleviating anticipated stress and fear associated with ART treatment, and fosters a sense of confidence to succeed.

In many ART centers, training occurs in a one-on-one approach, and includes both the patient and partner and is in addition to, or as a substitute for, group classes. The importance of involving the partner or spouse in the educational process cannot be overemphasized. Fortunately, the unique relationship that develops between the patient and the nursing team in conjunction with the support team enhances the communication needs and educational successes are noted. During the educational sessions, the nurse evaluates the patients' understanding of clinical needs and gains insight into each patient's specific treatment requirements. Nurses support educational needs specific to their treatment cycle including specific clinical applications for relating to the patient's religious, cultural, psychological, and medical needs.

Increases in clinical successes and outcomes are linked to increased patient compliance with drug regimens and clinical needs. Educational programs and patient comprehension increases understanding of protocols and procedures. The literature continues to support that success or failure of treatment depends on a clear understanding of the current treatment regimen, regardless of the patient's prior experience with the process. For example, human chorionic gonadotropin (hCG) is the single most important injection of the patient's treatment cycle. Nonetheless, errors in hCG administration have been attributed to poor cycle outcome. Patients have made reconstitution errors, such as injection of one-tenth of the dose or administration of diluent only, or timed the injection incorrectly (5). A recent report found that 10 patients (15.2%) undergoing IVF or ovulation induction treatment received hCG incorrectly, and in these cycles only one pregnancy occurred (6).

Historically, an REI nurse could expect to conservatively spend near two hours for a patient education session. Today, with the recent improvements to the instruments used for medication administration, nurses have noted a significant time saving associated with education and follow-up questions during stimulation. By example, urinary products required intramuscular administration and therefore necessitated comprehensive educational sessions. These products were exclusive to REI medication protocols and included preparations of human menopausal gonadotropins (hMG) and hCG. In the mid-1990s, with improvements in laboratory procedures, the movement from sub-zonal injection to ICSI, the evolution from urinary to recombinant medications, improvements in PGD procedures, and the expansion of other available technologies, the time and complexity of patient education increased dramatically. In particular, the late 1990s saw the introduction of recombinant follicle-stimulating hormone (FSH), followed by other recombinant gonadotropins. These medications were suitable for subcutaneous self-injection by the patient or her partner. In recent years, the advancement of endometrial coculture techniques, the broadening application of PGD testing, the addition of gonadotropin-releasing hormone antagonists as an alternative to the agonists for the prevention of a premature luteinizing hormone (LH) surge, and the development of new and more complicated protocols involving techniques such as testicular sperm extraction/aspiration have brought additional patient education challenges to the ART nurse. All these advances are associated with the need for nurses to provide appropriate and accurate education to patients, which of course requires the ART nurse to update her knowledge continually.

Despite a continued willingness to extend therapeutic options for patients, there are ongoing efforts to simplify treatment regimens and, thus, minimize confusion. ART nurses frequently consult with colleagues on ways to streamline the educational process for patients, which ultimately improves quality of patient care.

EDUCATIONAL RESOURCES

The provision of center-specific ART materials outlines the procedures, policies, and requirements of each center. Nurses respond to the changing trends in REI clinical, research, and treatment aspects as necessary to each center. The revision to educational materials is critical to supporting the needs of the patient, couples, and clinical team. Written materials support the in-person educational sessions and enhance the at home reference for patients. Demonstration remains an educational format that serves the population well. The steps involved in reconstitution support the benefits of demonstration with return demonstration. In more recent years, the introduction of liquid formulations and medication injection devices significantly improved and changed the process of education. The diversity of preparations available support the need for comprehensive, individualized education that values both demonstration and written material resources. The most obvious example of this is the education provided to patients and partners to self-inject medications. Nurses use hands-on, tactile-type teaching with instructional materials, such as injection buttocks, videos, etc., to encourage patients' understanding of the process. Utilizing this method also allows the nurse to assess the patient's comprehension and ability to perform medication administration and/or reconstitution. Today, nurses value the additional support of industry-driven resources to add to the educational setting. The use of CDs and DVDs has accented the at-home references for patients with great success.

Additionally, web-based accesses and industry supported written instructions are available for distribution to patients. Several of the national patient organizations also provide written materials (books, newsletters, fact sheets), CD/DVD, and reliable websites that are constantly being updated with current treatment options, support sessions, education related to insurance and provider information.

IVF NURSE COORDINATOR

The ART nursing coordinator remains an integral component of the care team in REI. The role of the ART Nurses Coordinator is extensive, and includes the evaluation of each research, clinical, and regulatory component of care. The nurse as a coordinator is part of the traditional nursing role that continues to this day. In ART programs, the overall goal of the nurse coordinator is to serve as a clinical liaison to provide close contact between scientists, clinicians, nurses, and patients to assist couples to move

Table 66.1   Coordinating the Assisted Reproductive Techniques Team: Some Aspects to Consider

Alerting the pharmacy regarding drug requirements
Scheduling interventional procedures (e.g., ultrasound examinations, oocyte retrievals)
Documenting treatment results and outcomes
Updating patient records
Communicating results to patients
Amending existing protocols or developing new ones
Updating the staff counselor on specific patient needs
Obtaining legal consents for new or updated procedures

smoothly through a treatment cycle. This requires a great deal of flexibility, as well as extreme attention to detail and good delegation skills. As clinical advances continue, ART programs need well informed coordinators and support staff to meet the needs of the patients. Timing, scheduling, and pre-testing requirements are complex and require specific detail-oriented staff to meet the needs. On-going education and staff reinforcement is essential to this success. Rather humorously, the role of nurse coordinator has been described as "organizing the world based on another woman's menstrual cycle ... or organized chaos" (4).

Coordinating the Unit

The success of an ART program is dependent upon the coordination of the collective team of professional, scientists, support staff, and nurses. The inclusive evaluation of clinical and academic responsibilities, prior commitments, such as lectures, vacations, and conferences are essential for timing and supporting the team. Table 66.1 highlights some of the aspects of treatment that must be incorporated into the overall treatment plan for all patients.

Nationally, ART centers continue to grow and expand the available services to include additional services and satellite-based centers. Such accesses enable couples greater access to care when they live significant distances from the main center and support their desire to remain at home and/or working for as long as possible during treatment. Additionally, the success of specific technologies achieved by some ART centers has attracted potential patients from both near, and as far as international countries. Coordinating care for patients who live abroad is much more complex than for those who live in closer proximity to the ART center. The requirements for long-distance coordination vary according to the couple's situation and selected treatment options. All in all, well-organized management of care contributes to the smooth running of an efficient unit, ensuring patient satisfaction and overall success.

PATIENT COORDINATION: FOCUS ON COMMUNICATION

As ART programs continue to grow, both in numbers and in expertise, there are ongoing initiatives to ensure quality of care and patient satisfaction initiatives. Patients are increasingly focused on communication, privacy, and

accuracy of information. Maintaining communication is essential to the process for both the center and the patient. Supporting the need for communication among the team is essential. The development of "nursing teams" in many ART centers has supported the goals for communication throughout the centers and highlights the benefits resulting from such commitments. Limiting the number of staff that interface with patients increases confidence, limits errors, and increases satisfaction for both the team and the patient. Continuity of care and team collaboration remains effective tools in the goal of communication in an REI program. Building confidence through communication influences patient satisfaction and successes within the REI programs.

In ART centers that have expanded to include satellite offices, the establishment of primary care nursing teams (an IVF coordinator and assistant coordinator assigned to each physician) structure supports goals for improved communication and team building. Patients seek access to members of the care team to support their personal goals. With advances in communication practices by way of IT systems, written and verbal communication trails, and team collaboration, ART centers support their practice mission to expand with the confidence that patient care is accented, that patients are treated safely, and within both regulatory guidelines and the recommendations of the American Society for Reproductive Medicine (ASRM).

REI nurses in ART centers engage other members of the care team in the process of treatment and support the goal of access to the primary physician. The nursing team handles the medical aspects of the treatment cycle, while other coordinators such as third-party liaisons, finance teams, and research nurses manage other issues related to the nonmedical, more administrative aspects of care (e.g., consents and contracts). Following comprehensive evaluations of such revisions to practice, it is noted that accountability and communication improved, both within the teams and with the center, and there were fewer complaints from patients regarding communication and callback issues (7).

Other centers have adapted a more modified approach with much success, designing nurse and doctor teams that coordinate phases of the treatment cycles. Once the patient is fully engaged in treatment, a more coordinated approach is utilized among the members of the team. Nurses tend to benefit from this practice as well through the development of a closer rapport with patients and increased job satisfaction. More subtly, they tend to be able to empathize better with patients and to develop a greater insight into patients' physical and emotional needs (8).

PATIENT COUNSELOR

REI professionals eagerly recognize the impact that infertility treatment has on the emotional state of patients and partners. Considerable emotional demands are noted in those seeking treatment. While infertility itself is recognized as a "life-crisis," provoking a variety of emotional responses, the range of ART treatment options now available to couples also raises complex emotional issues. These options may present significant medical, legal, religious, and/or ethical implications. As patients proceed along the treatment journey, the psychological impact may become increasingly more important. Several studies have suggested that emotional and psychological factors may be a leading cause of patient dropout (9). In fact, there are several reports suggesting that up to 60–65% of patients who begin treatment with an REI may drop out before treatment completion (10–12). In addition, the percentage of patients dropping out of treatment appears to increase with each subsequent failed cycle (13). Although emotional/psychological factors are important, other factors may also contribute to patient dropout (13). In recognition of the importance of psychological factors in treatment success, many clinics offer supportive counseling on a routine basis. Since the ART nurse is often the first to recognize the couples' need for counseling, she serves as an important advocate on their behalf.

NURSE VS. COUNSELOR

Although there is significant overlap noted in the emotional support provided by the ART nurse and a professional counselor, in general, counseling involves the use of psychological interventions based on theoretical frameworks for which specialized training is required. The nurse's perspective includes a thorough understanding of the patient's clinical scenario. The ART nurse is in a unique position to provide emotional support to the patient and her partner because of the close relationship that develops, based on a high level of trust, sensitivity, and discretion. This is very different from other clinical settings, because infertile patients rarely discuss the "private" side of their infertility outside of the nurse/counselor relationship.

Specific areas that the nurse can focus on to help promote psychological well-being include:

1. talking through individuals' emotional responses to their infertility;
2. identifying couples' sources of stress, such as the success of procedures like ICSI for severe male factor, PGD for the diagnosis of chromosomal and genetic abnormalities or donor gametes, and the associated issues of disclosure, ethical, and religious ramifications;
3. providing support to infertility patients' concerns and emotions;
4. discussion of therapeutic options, including:
   (a) guidance on realistic expectations;
   (b) anticipatory emotional responses;
   (c) ethical and religious concerns;
5. helping patients to maintain self-esteem and interpersonal relationships;
6. encouraging patients to continue with "life" outside of infertility.

In many instances, there will be an overlap between the nurse as "educator" and the nurse as "counselor." For example, as nurses discuss treatment options and verify patient understanding through appropriate questions and monitoring feedback, patients are able to provide informed consent, and ultimately feel more in control, therefore reducing potential anxiety. In addition, nurses collaborate with the psychological support team to offer patients additional services. ART nurses can take on a supportive role, drawing on clinical experiences to guide the couple in the decision-making process related to other treatment options or for those couples seeking closure after treatment failure.

SPECIALIST COUNSELING

Some ART centers require patients to undergo psychological counseling prior to pursuing treatment. Certainly in cases where third-party parenting options are being considered, all ART programs mandate patient counseling. This trend toward emotional wellness is on the rise and is seen to offer tremendous advantages to the patient and the couple. With the increase in third party reproduction, donor sperm, and gestational carrier settings, the risks are greater and suggest that more counseling opportunities benefit outcomes. Additionally, some patients will require support that extends beyond the type required by most couples undergoing "routine" ART procedures, and it is imperative that this should be recognized.

Research indicates that three particular groups of patients are likely to benefit from specialist counseling. They are patients:

1. experiencing high levels of stress (e.g., after a failed treatment, during a multiple pregnancy, undergoing PGD, TESE, failed ICSI, etc.);
2. requiring donated gametes, directed-donor settings, surrogacy, or adoption (third party reproduction);
3. seeking fertility services because of their special social or ethical circumstances (14).

NURSING RESEARCH

The driving force behind the acceptance of ART nursing as a separate specialty is nursing-directed research, ideally inspired, motivated, and supported through collaborations with physician colleagues. While the outcomes of nursing interventions are already used as sources for nursing-based research, generally the type of research undertaken by nurses has a more subjective approach, including investigation of the psychological, nurturing, and educational aspects of ART. This contrasts with the more objective research likely to be conducted by physicians. For example, a nurse-based study considering administration of progesterone for luteal phase support would focus more on the tolerability of the drugs administered than would a physician-driven study that would be more likely to concentrate on aspects such as in-phase endometrial development. Regardless of topic, nurses are already participating in clinical care research in partnership with other healthcare professionals, and are benefiting from the support given to them by the National Institute of Nursing Research and Nursing Research Mentors.

Increased acceptance of nursing driven research will come through translation of their research into practice. Thus, it is clear that forums are needed to allow nurses to disseminate the knowledge they are acquiring. Every opportunity should be afforded to nurses to present their studies, both at a local and at an international level, including the annual meetings of major societies such as the ASRM. In addition, there is a need for a specialized journal devoted to ART nursing. Such a journal could play an important role in stimulating ART nursing research, and in setting high standards for the publication of research studies.

THE ROLE OF AN EFFECTIVE REI NURSE LEADER

The nurse leader role in REI is an interesting meld of mentoring, leadership, clinical expertise, nurturing, and vision. As part of the daily practice, REI leaders focus on coordinating and directing teams on the clinical and administrative tasks to assure that the center functions effectively and efficiently on all levels. Frequently, the nurse leader manages administrative roles and interacts on a personal level with each member of staff as well as individual patients. Nurse leaders are an integral member of the center's quality assurance program, quality control, research, patient satisfaction team, clinical, and financial focus. As such, the responsibility of the ART nurse manager is not only to assure that their staff receives the training needed, but also to monitor and assess their activities continually so that the training standards are maintained. This ensures that the ongoing concerns of the patients and the ART center are addressed.

ART nurse leaders have the opportunity to contribute to all aspects of patient care, from the moment the patient enters the clinic to the time they leave, whereas in other areas of medicine the patients often receive "segmented" and often disjointed and confusing information. The quality of care, for which the nurse leader provides, offers overall responsibility, and contributes directly to the success of the ART program both in clinical terms and in terms of patient satisfaction. Many times the role is mentoring, nurturing, and reassuring on clinical, research, and personal levels. Burnout is a significant concern to the ART nurse leaders, as the differences between ART nursing and the traditional nursing role. Contrary to most areas of medicine, where nurses can adopt a more detached attitude, ART nurses are more likely to become personally involved with the infertile couple, regardless of inconvenience to themselves. Teaching ART staff nurses how to allocate time to particular tasks, to organize their day, and to seek personal education and supportive care from physicians and staff psychologists is an ongoing role of the ART nurse manager. With the right support, nurses will not only remain healthy but also remain in a position to do their job effectively. Nurse Managers' interactions in center-specific quality-assurance concerns assist with the evaluation of the ongoing needs of the department and its staff, and

therefore assure that a healthy clinical balance is maintained. The ability to recognize staff educational needs and offer the appropriate materials and opportunities to address these is another way to assure quality of care provided, as well as addressing issues of burnout. Since ART is such a specialized field, the ART nurse manager not only becomes the nurse educator within the ART center (e.g., to other new nurses), but is also called upon to educate other specialties, such as the neonatal intensive care unit (ICU) or high-risk ante partum staff, on issues pertinent to ART.

ART: NURSE TRAINING

As technology advances, the need for ongoing educational support within ART centers has increased. As previously mentioned, ART nurses benefit tremendously from supportive physicians and colleagues within their center. Furthermore, many ART nurses are fortunate to gain educational support or insight for their research interests through participation in or attendance at educational symposia or being supported in their research endeavors through sponsored ART clinics. ART nurses are also supported in their evolving role by a number of organizations that offer professional development advice, research mentors, conferences, lecturing opportunities, information on policies, procedures, and position statements, state-of-the-art medical information, and networking opportunities (Table 66.2). For example, the Nurses Professional Group (NPG) of the ASRM provides a forum for networking and information exchange among nurses. It also offers continuing medical education (CME) opportunities (through roundtables, seminars, etc.) at its annual meeting. The NPG has developed Protocols and Procedures for Nurses, a publication that encompasses a variety of topics such as:

1. nursing management of patients undergoing ART;
2. patient preparation for infertility-related treatments;
3. protocols on procedures performed in reproductive medicine practice.

While such resources are a valuable aid to the ART nurse, they are not a substitute for the one-on-one instruction that remains key to the successful training of a new ART nurse. Introductory training must include a review

Table 66.2 Professional Organizations Supporting the Assisted Reproductive Techniques Nurse

American Infertility Association (AIA; patient support group)
Nurses Professional Group (NPG) of the American Society for Reproductive Medicine (ASRM)
Regional nursing associations
RESOLVE (patient support group)
Biosymposia
Society for Assisted Reproductive Technology (SART)
Fertile Hope (patient support group)

of basic gynecology, including the integration of the reproductive/endocrine cycle, the characteristics of normal and abnormal cycles, and physical anomalies which interfere with fertility, together with a less academic but equally important overview of the responsibilities of key ART team functions. It is crucial that each member of the team knows not only their own responsibilities, but also those of their fellow team members and importantly how these roles interact. Ultimately, it is the practical experience of patient management and the experience gained through repeatedly performing assigned tasks that form the basic core of the ART nurse's education and training.

While expanding the skills of nurses will obviously increase the number of tasks they can perform competently within a treatment program, less obvious are the benefits such as increased job satisfaction and greater continuity of patient care. Well-defined responsibilities, standards, and protocols for clinical practice are required and should be continually refined. As an example, the recent inception of FDA regulations established National guidelines for ART centers, which required ongoing education for the experienced ART nurse and the development of new nurse training.

THE FUTURE OF ART

The role of the REI continues to see significant expansion. Clinical responsibilities are expanding in part due to the continued introduction and revision of techniques and treatment modalities, clinical goals, and patient focuses. Much of the significant changes involve nursing allocations of time and education, further supporting the need for visionary learning and goals. Despite the rapid advances made in ART and the constantly evolving role of nurses working in this field, there is currently no specific certification that officially recognizes IVF/ART nursing as a specialty. The NPG continues to support the development of education modules, and is currently supporting a certificate program for REI nurses. Unlike neonatal and high-risk ante partum nurses, who receive specialty training in an academic setting and who can qualify for certification, ART nurses have more limited educational resources. There is inadequate exposure to the field of infertility at any level of academic training, and when it is offered, often as a one-day course, the level of its content is highly variable. As outlined earlier, ART nursing is emotionally demanding, and is not recommended as an entry-level position due to the level of autonomy that is required in this field. A certain level of professional maturity is mandatory; infertility treatment is elective and couples are usually well educated in terms of options in infertility treatment, and are often able to make informed decisions on their treatment regimen. The nurse needs to be confident enough to face the challenges presented by often very determined but very well informed couples. As research and treatment options evolve for patients, so does the role of the nurse in reproductive medicine. In turn, the prospects for a variety of professional opportunities will develop, providing broader career options and greater job satisfaction.

CONCLUSIONS

REI nurses remain in a unique position professionally. The autonomous, interdisciplinary role that many nurses support, allows for an extended, participative role with both the patient and the clinical team. Nurses provide a deep empathy for a patient's infertility struggle, and play a critical role in the patients' treatment success. With the indicated education, mentoring from others on the team including physicians, and scientists, nurses continue to frame the profession with an eager sense of pride and determination. Appropriate continuing education and opportunities for clinical certification are essential to support this determined group of nursing professionals. Professional growth and clinical expertise comes to those that seek excellence, show a willingness to improve, and further expand the future of REI nursing practice. Continued participation in nursing research initiatives offers professionals a collaborative role with others in the field interested in the development of state-of-the-art standards. These goals are in alignment with the deep desire of professionals focused on desire to ensure patients benefit from the ongoing emotional, educational, and practical support offered by the contemporary ART nurse. Although ART nursing may be perceived as "stressful," it remains a profoundly rewarding career that offers tremendous value, satisfaction, and a future of unknown dimension.

REFERENCES

1. Edwards R, Purdy JM, Steptoe P. Implantation of the Human Embryo. London: Academic Press, 1985.
2. Rausch DT, Braverman AM. Burnout rates among reproductive endocrinology nurses: the role of personality and infertility attitudes. Presented at the 56th Annual Meeting of the American Society for Reproductive Medicine. San Diego, California, 21–26 October 2000; abstract.
3. D'Andrea KG. The role of the nurse practitioner in artificial insemination. J Obstet Gynecol Nurs 1984; 13: 75–8.
4. James CA. The nursing role in assisted reproductive technologies. NAACOGS Clin Issu Perinat Women's Health Nurs 1992; 3: 328–34.
5. Ludwig M, Doody KJ, Doody KM. Use of recombinant human chorionic gonadotropin in ovulation induction. Fertil Steril 2003; 79: 1051–9.
6. Markle RL, King PI, Martin DB, et al. Characteristics of successful human chorionic gonadotropin (hCG) administration in assisted reproduction. Presented at the 58th Annual Meeting of the American Society for Reproductive Medicine. Seattle, Washington, 13–16 October 2002; abstract.
7. Norbryhn G, Fontanilla T, Rogoff R, et al. Establishment of a primary care nursing team in a rapidly expanding multi-site reproductive endocrine center. Presented at the 56th Annual Meeting of the American Society for Reproductive Medicine. San Diego, California, 21–26 October 2000; abstract.
8. Muirhead M, Lawton J. A team approach to assisted conception treatment. Hum Fertil 1998; 1: 40–3.

9. Domar AD. Impact of psychological factors on drop-out rates in insured patients. Fertil Steril 2004; 81: 271–3.

10. Land JA, Courtar DA, Evers JLH. Patient drop out in an assisted reproductive technology program: implication for pregnancy rates. Fertili Steril 1997; 68: 278–81.

11. Olivius C, Friden B, Borg G, et al. Why do couples discontinue in vitro fertilization treatment? A cohort study. Fertil Seril 2004; 81: 258–61.

12. Malcom CE, Cumming DC. Follow-up of infertile couples who dropped out of a fertility specialist clinic. Fertil Steril 2004; 81: 269–70.

13. Rajkhowa M, Mcconnell A, Thomas GE. Reasons for discontinuation of IVF treatment: a questionnaire study. Hum Reprod 2006; 21: 358–63.

14. Boivin J, Appleton TC, Baetens P, et al. Guidelines for counseling in infertility: outline version. Hum Reprod 2001; 16: 1301–4.

67

Patient support in the ART program

Sharon N. Covington

OVERVIEW

Reproduction is considered the most basic of human needs, propelled by powerful biological and psychological drives. When the ability to reproduce is thwarted, a crisis ensues – the life crisis of infertility. The psychological crisis of infertility has been well documented in the literature. It is considered an emotionally difficult experience that impacts on all aspects of a couple's or an individual's life: relationships with others, life goals, social roles, self-image, self-confidence, and sexuality, to name a few (1). The losses associated with infertility are multifaceted, including the loss of hopes, dreams, future plans, marital satisfaction, self-esteem, sense of control, belief in the fairness of life, health, and well-being, and, most important, the "dream child" (2). Further, these losses evoke feelings of grief – shock, disbelief, sadness, anger, guilt, blame, and depression – which occur in a repetitive and predictable process as patients move through medical diagnosis and treatment. It is through the experience and expression of emotions involved in the grieving process that the infertile couple moves toward an acceptance of their infertile state, engages in the exploration of alternative plans, and begins to move forward with their lives (3).

During the past 50 years, we have seen a shift from the psychogenic infertility model, in which demonstrable psychopathology was thought to play an etiologic role in infertility, to a psychological sequelae model, in which numerous psychological factors were considered the result of infertility (4). In this concept, infertility is viewed as an emotionally difficult experience affecting all aspects of an individual's and a couple's life. Thus, emotional distress is a consequence and not a cause of infertility, as conceptualized previously. The application of a broader spectrum of theoretical approaches has led to a less individualistic perspective and a more holistic approach to infertility. In this sense, the interactions among individuals/couples and social/medical components are considered and must be factored into medical treatment. These perspectives have also increased understanding of individual and couple differences and resilience, the impact of reproductive medical treatments, and the efficacy of therapeutic psychological interventions.

Research examining the psychosocial context of infertility has burgeoned during this period. In a recent comprehensive review of the literature, Greil and associates (5) expanded on earlier work (6) by assessing research published in the last 10 years to determine how it has changed, where methodological progress has been made, and what generalizations can be drawn about the experience of infertility. They note the change from viewing infertility as a medical condition with psychological consequences to placing infertility within a larger sociocultural construct that shapes the experience. Methodologically, progress has been made with increased research attention on the male and couple experience from earlier work focusing primarily on the female. The authors identify two research traditions: One characterized by the quantitative analysis of clinic patients to improve service delivery and assess the psychological need for counseling, while the other tradition is based on qualitative research looking to capture the experience of infertile people outside the clinic context, both in developed and developing societies. They call for continued integration of the two research traditions in the development of a distinctly sociological approach to infertility.

Stress and Assisted Reproductive Techniques

Assisted reproductive techniques (ARTs), while opening up expanded opportunities for the treatment of infertility, have generated their own psychological challenges for patients. For most couples, ARTs are the last, best option for having a child, and occur after long months, and sometimes years, of treatment failure, often at tremendous emotional, physical, and financial cost. Patients entering ART programs usually do so with the burden of grief and disappointment from infertility, acting depressed, angry, tired, dependent, and anxious. Although emotionally depleted, couples are attracted to a technology that offers hope where, a few years ago, none existed. They find themselves drawn into a new emotional turbulence of contrasting feelings of hope and despair, which seem to be generated in part by the experience of the technology itself. The intensity and high-tech nature of ART create a stressful atmosphere, where the stakes are high and the chance of success may be relatively low. ART is a gamble, and, like gamblers, patients may have unrealistically high expectations of success (7,8) or feel compelled to try "just one more time," finding it difficult to end treatment without success. Of all infertility treatments, in vitro fertilization (IVF) is considered the most stressful, (9,10) with 80% of IVF patients ranking it as "extremely" to "moderately" stressful (11). Furthermore, after a failed cycle, almost all couples report acute depression, (12) with elevated anxiety and anger levels persisting weeks later (13). Despite the stressful consequences of infertility and ART, numerous studies report that the vast majority of patients are generally well-adjusted (14–17). In one of the most extensive reviews of scientifically rigorous research on the psychological effects of infertility, Stanton and Danoff-Burg concluded that the majority of infertile men and women are psychologically resilient and maintain adequate psychosocial functioning (18). Boivin found little evidence that infertile patients, as a group, experience significant, long-term maladjustment on measures of anxiety, psychiatric disturbance, marital conflict, and sexual dysfunction, when compared with population norms (19). Overall, this group reports marital adjustment in the normal range, and that the crisis of infertility may actually improve marital communication and emotional intimacy (20–23).

Gender Differences and ART Stress

The majority of studies of stress during ART are in women, and, overall, women react more intensely to infertility and ART than do men (24). Prior to IVF, women report more anxiety and depression, less life satisfaction, lower self-esteem, and more anticipatory stress than their male partners (21). During IVF, the intensity of a demanding treatment protocol – daily ultrasound monitoring, blood draws for hormone levels, injections, invasive procedures for oocyte retrieval, and embryo transfer – is frequently given by women as a cause of psychological distress (10). If treatment fails, depression persists longer for women than for their partners, lasting up to six months (13). Years later, women will recall the stress of IVF as more stressful for them than for their partner, regardless of the success or failure of treatment.

In one of the few studies examining men's distress during IVF, Boivin et al. found that men who were undergoing intracytoplasmic sperm injection (ICSI) reported more distress on the days prior to retrieval than did other IVF men (25). However, in all other areas, ICSI and IVF men were similar in their adjustment to infertility and in their distress during the treatment cycle. These findings were in contrast to those of early studies of distress among men with male factor diagnosis, as these infertile men reported more negative feelings and psychiatric distress (12,26). The discrepancy between these studies may have been due to the fact that ICSI could circumvent the infertility, whereas at the time of the earlier studies the only medical option available was donor insemination. While the intensity of emotional reactions to particular aspects of ART may differ between men and women, the types of reactions are the same, with both experiencing a significant increase in anxiety and depressive symptoms from pre- to posttreatment (21). In addition, both men and women rank the relative stresses of each stage of IVF equally, and tend to overestimate the chances of success of IVF in general, showing a high level of hopefulness in their own cases (13).

Men and women tend to cope differently with the stress of ART and infertility (20). As frequently noted, women are more expressive of feelings, and are more likely to seek emotional and social support during ART by informal activities such as talking to spouse, family, and friends. In terms of the effects of coping post-IVF treatment, Hynes et al. found that women who used problem-focused coping had a higher level of well-being than those who used avoidance-coping or social support (27). Men, on the other hand, who are often action-oriented and solution-focused, frequently cope with infertility through greater involvement in work or sports-related activities. While men and women may have different coping strategies, the use and effectiveness of these techniques may be influenced by the point in the infertility process and the existence of a gender-specific infertility diagnosis (28).

Gender differences may, also, be impacted by the perception of psychosocial support during ART (29). Since the nature of ART treatment is focused on women, men can feel more isolated and less emotionally supported then their partner, especially from family and friends. Increased distress may arise when infertile people do not get the emotional support they need during infertility (30). Psychosocial support and intervention are equally beneficial for both men and women (31) and, thus, recommended as part of treatment.

Levels of Stress during ART

While general assumptions may be made about stress levels during ART, the experience for infertility patients will be personal and unique: Each patient will experience the stress differently, based upon his or her own personality and life experiences. Newton et al. noted that stress has been conceptualized both as a stimulus or event (distressing circumstances outside the person) and as a response (internal disturbance) (24). A contrasting approach describes stress as neither an event nor a response, but rather a combination of factors: The perceived meaning of the event and self-appraisal of the adequacy of coping resources (32). Thus, it is not the stress itself but the perception of the stress that determines how ART patients experience and handle it.

The aspects of ART perceived to be stressful to patients are multifaceted and affect all parts of their life: marital, social, physical, emotional, financial, cultural, and religious. Time is stressful, both in the time commitment to an intense treatment which leads to disruption in family, work, and social activities, and, for some, in long waiting periods for IVF or third-party reproduction. ART stress impacts on the marital relationship with an emotionally laden experience, and, by removing the conjugal act for procreation, sexual intimacy is lost. Also, couples are stretched financially, paying for the high cost of ART treatment with a relatively low probability of success. Dealing with the medical staff and with the side effects or potential complications of medical treatment has its own stress: Hot flushes, headaches, mood fluctuations, shots, sonograms, future health concerns, and decision-making about embryos and multiple pregnancies. Religious, social, cultural, and moral issues may also make ART stressful, especially for those dealing with third-party reproduction, when these values are in conflict with the choice of treatment.

The first treatment cycle has been found to be the most stressful for patients, with high levels of confusion, bewilderment, and anxiety (7,10,13). This may be due to inexperience with the process, or possibly inadequate preparation of the patient by staff in terms of information and discussion of care. Slade et al. found that for couples attempting three cycles of IVF, distress diminished during the middle cycle but rose after they discovered that the intervention had not been successful, with the last cycle being as stressful as the first (13).

Within a treatment cycle, patients view IVF/ART as a series of stages which must be successfully completed before moving on to the next phase of treatment: monitoring, oocyte retrieval, fertilization, embryo transfer, waiting period, and pregnancy test stages. The level of stress, anxiety, and anticipation rises with each stage, peaking during the waiting period. A number of studies have confirmed what clinicians have known anecdotally: In order of perceived stress for patients, waiting to hear the outcome of the embryo transfer is the most stressful, followed by waiting to hear whether fertilization has occurred, and then the egg retrieval stage (11,33). Patients are aware of the importance of these key phases in the IVF process, and the uncertainty of the outcome is highly distressing.

Understandably, patients who are experiencing emotional distress from infertility will have their quality of life impacted. To identify these patients, several years ago an international effort was undertaken by the ASRM, ESHRE, and Merck-Serono to develop a psychometric tool that would be reliable, cross-cultural, and easy to access and interpret. Recently published, the Fertility Quality of Life (FertiQoL) is able to measure treatment quality (interactions with staff, quality of information) and treatment tolerability (effects on mood, disruptions to daily life), and could prove to be an invaluable tool for clinicians (34). It will be offered in a number of languages and is now available without cost online (www.fertiqol.org).

METHODS

Who Provides Patient Support Services in ART?

Given the host of research on the emotional consequences of infertility and on the distressing nature of ART, it is clear that patients need psychological support as an integrated part of the medical treatment process. Technology has become more complex and so have the psychological, social, and ethical issues related to treatment, which challenges the resources of staff and patients. As a result

of technologic advances in ART and recognition of the psychosocial issues and demands facing infertile patients, mental health professionals have become increasingly important members of the reproductive medical team (33,35). The specialization of "infertility counseling" has emerged, combining the fields of reproductive health psychology and reproductive medicine, for mental health professionals including social workers, psychologists, psychiatrists, marriage and family therapists, counselors, and psychiatric nurses.

Infertility counselors serve as a resource to patients and staff by providing specialized psychological services that support and enhance quality care. For example, the complex medical and psychological issues in third-party reproduction have social and legal implications that must be assessed carefully, and warrant involvement of a qualified mental health professional experienced in infertility counseling. In addition, the psychosocial impact on the offspring created by ART needs to be considered, and assistance given to families dealing with these issues pre- and post-treatment (35).

Nonetheless, the responsibility for patient support in the ART program is the duty of all staff members, not just the domain of nurses or infertility counselors (36). Interactions with each staff member, from administrative staff to physician, influence a patient's perception of care and, in turn, his or her stress level. Sensitivity, warmth, patience, and responsiveness create an environment of support. Also, general clinic routine and ambience reflect support and respect of patients when it is provided in an efficient, organized, clean, uncrowded, and esthetically pleasing atmosphere. All staff need to be sensitive to and knowledgeable about the psychological needs and stress of ART patients. While the primary focus of physicians, nurses, laboratory scientists, and other healthcare staff is the medical diagnosis and treatment of infertility, it must also entail "treating the patient, not the disease."

Types of ART Support Services

ART patient support services can be generalized from overall clinic administration and environment to specialized services which need to be provided by a mental health professional experienced in infertility counseling. For the purpose of this chapter, while specialized services provided by an infertility counselor are described, a detailed explanation of methodology is not addressed (4). Moving from specific to general, the method of providing patient support services can be categorized as:

1. Psychological assessment and evaluation
2. Therapeutic counseling
3. Supportive counseling
4. Information and education
5. Clinic administration.

Psychological Assessment and Evaluation

Psychological screening of participants using ART often varies from program to program, as currently only two countries (Australia and Canada) mandate counseling prior to ART treatment. While the Human Fertilisation and Embryology Authority (HFEA), which regulates assisted reproduction in the United Kingdom, has stipulated that psychosocial counseling must be offered to patients seeking IVF or donor gametes, (37) one study found that less than 25% of patients took up the suggestion (38). In the United States, recommendations and guidelines for the provision of psychological services to ART participants are voluntary, (39) and the decision concerning which patients should be screened or counseled, and for what procedures, is left to each individual fertility practice. Thus, available guidelines for assessment and evaluation are usually tailored to the specific requirement or preference of a particular program. Whether a clinic adopts formal or recommended guidelines or chooses to develop its own, the program's policy regarding infertility counseling, screening, exclusion criteria, and so on should be clearly defined for the protection of the medical team, the infertility counselor, and patients (40).

Notwithstanding the voluntary nature of screening ART participants, it has become the standard of care to require psychological evaluation and psychoeducational preparation of oocyte donors, surrogates, and gestational carriers by experienced mental health professionals. The evaluation usually involves both psychological testing of the donor/carrier, with the Minnesota Multiphasic Personality Inventory-2 (MMPI-2) being used most often, (41) and clinical interviews with donor/carrier and, when available, her partner. Assessment and counseling of recipients of donor gametes is also strongly recommended or required by many programs, especially when the donor/carrier is known or related. Other situations where programs may require screening and assessment involve patients undergoing IVF who are considered psychologically or physically vulnerable, previous IVF patients donating frozen embryos, single recipients of gamete donation, and older infertility patients (42).

The established protocol for psychological evaluation and assessment within the author's program includes:

1. All recipients of anonymous donor eggs, sperm, and embryos, and genetic parents using a gestational carrier, are required to see a staff infertility counselor. The psychoeducational counseling and assessment usually takes place in one or two counseling sessions, reading materials and support resources are provided, and issues related to raising children conceived through third-party reproduction are discussed.

2. Psychological evaluation of all anonymous oocyte donors is mandatory. Psychological testing (MMPI-2) is administered, and then scored and interpreted. A minimum of two clinical interviews, one with the donor and one with her and her partner, are conducted with a staff infertility counselor to assess psychological functioning and the process, motivations, and implications of gamete donation are discussed.

3. All known donors or gestational carriers and recipients are required to undergo evaluation and counseling, which includes administering the MMPI-2 to the donor and gestational carrier. Clinical interviews are held with the donor or carrier and patient separately, including their partners, and a joint "group" session is conducted to discuss how they will deal with issues in known donation. Legal consultation and contracts are also strongly recommended with gestational carriers.

4. Assessment and counseling of any infertility patient is required when the physician is concerned about psychological vulnerability or marital instability, or if a situation is presented to our internal ethics committee where additional psychosocial information is needed before a decision about treatment can be made.

Our mental health professional staff follow the criteria established for acceptance or rejection of participants in the recommended guidelines for "Psychological assessment of oocyte donors and recipients" and the "Psychological guidelines for embryo donation" developed by the Mental Health Professional Group of the American Society for Reproductive Medicine (ASRM) (39). When a recommendation to withhold or postpone treatment is made by the infertility counselor, a team meeting takes place so that a decision is made by team consensus, rather than one member (usually the physician or the infertility counselor) being seen by the patient as the "gatekeeper." It is useful to view and interpret these recommendations to the patient as protection of the parties involved rather than rejection, since it is the first responsibility of all healthcare providers "to do no harm."

Therapeutic Counseling

Another aspect of patient support services involves intervention and treatment for the consequences of infertility, or for underlying mental disturbances that could affect medical treatment. Treatment modalities of individual, couple, and group counseling provide an opportunity to assist patients in understanding and handling the emotional sequelae of infertility, identifying and developing a coping mechanism to deal with treatment, managing the effects of infertility or psychosocial history on interpersonal functioning (anxiety, depression, etc.) and on marital, sexual, and social relationships, considering the implications of ART treatment, decision making on treatment options and alternative family building, pregnancy and parenting following treatment, and ending treatment and building a life after infertility. Group counseling has been shown to be a highly effective, cost-efficient intervention for producing positive change when education and skills training (e.g., relaxation techniques) are emphasized (31).

ART programs may provide psychological assessment and therapeutic counseling services through an infertility counselor on the staff (an employee) or on site (an independent contractor), or may choose to refer to a qualified mental health professional who works independent of the clinic (43). Guidelines for when to refer patients for psychological assessment and intervention are displayed in Table 67.1.

Supportive Counseling

Supportive counseling involves reproductive healthcare providers giving both advice (counsel) and comfort (console) to their patients. Although nurses often assume primary responsibility for patient support, a team approach to advising and consoling is optimal. Services combine supportive and psychoeducational counseling, and may include:

1. Pre-IVF preparation session with an infertility counselor, which is offered as part of the treatment package.
2. Monthly support groups for IVF participants, patients considering or using donor gametes, and those with general infertility (non-ART), secondary infertility, miscarriage, and pregnancy after infertility. These groups are open-ended, of no cost to patients, and are run by a staff infertility counselor and, if needed, a nurse.

Table 67.1   When to Refer to an Infertility Counselor

Situations
The following situations serve as guidelines for referral for psychological assessment, counseling, and/or intervention (44):
- the use or consideration of third-party reproduction
- psychiatric illness (past or present)
- history of pregnancy complications or loss
- significant physical illness (past or present)
- sexual or physical abuse (past or present)
- conflicted gender identity, homosexuality, or bisexuality
- chemical abuse or dependency
- marital instability or chaotic social functioning
- single patients
- older patients

Symptoms
Referral to a mental health professional should also be considered when there is a change in current mental status and/or exacerbation of symptoms that are affecting normal functioning and relationships, including:
- depression or persistent sadness and tearfulness
- high levels of anxiety or agitation
- increased mood swings
- obsessive–compulsive behaviors
- strained interpersonal relationships
- social isolation
- loss of interest in usual activities
- diminished ability to accomplish tasks
- difficulty concentrating or remembering
- difficulty making decisions
- change in appetite, weight, or sleep patterns
- increased use of drugs or alcohol
- persistent feelings of pessimism, guilt, worthlessness
- persistent feelings of bitterness or anger
- thoughts of or reference to death or suicide

---

3. A monthly discussion series on infertility topics identified through a patient survey, such as adoption, donor issues, staff–patient communication, drug side effects, dealing with family and friends, decision making, marriage enhancement, and when to end treatment. These informal groups are facilitated by an infertility counselor, physician, nurse, and/or an invited guest from the community who is knowledgeable on the subject.
4. Stress management and relaxation classes taught by an infertility counselor and/or a nurse. Relaxation tapes and guided imagery tapes are also available to lend to patients for use before, during, and after retrieval and transfer.
5. Referral resources within the community for patients who request alternative approaches to help with quality of life during infertility, such as mind–body programs, yoga classes, acupuncture, and homeopathy.
6. Providing a network for patient-to-patient contact about aspects of treatment. Well-adjusted patients who have been through a procedure or have a specific diagnosis volunteer, or are asked by a staff member if they would be willing to speak one-on-one with other patients who request this contact. Common requests for contact are situations where patients have had a child via donor gametes, or who have undergone selective reduction or carried multiple pregnancies.
7. Giving each patient current information about local and national infertility support groups (e.g., RESOLVE, Inc.), such as monthly updates on meetings, support groups, living room sessions, telephone counseling, newsletters, and articles.

Information and Education

Probably the most far-reaching opportunity for ART support is through patients' easy access to written information and education about the medical and psychological aspects of infertility. Patients rely heavily on the educational materials that document the process and procedure of ART, and search out information at the clinic, through the media (TV, magazines, books, etc.), and on the internet. One study found that patients identified informational materials as their primary source of support, after talking with spouse, family, or friends (45).

Computer-based technology has become a powerful source of information, education, and support for patients. There is increasing evidence that the Internet can provide an effective intervention in helping patients manage the distress of infertility (46) and receiving direction from the medical staff on reliable Internet sites for information is needed (47). Social media, such as Facebook and Twitter, may become resources for support, interaction, and information for infertile patients when managed by the clinic, as well as providing a marketing tool for the practice. Multimedia methods, such as a CD-ROM that uses audio, video, interactive tasks, and personalized feedback, can serve as an effective psychosocial intervention (48) and should be considered by clinics as resource for patients. Finally, providing Internet access to personal health records and medical data is increasingly being considered within reproductive clinics to improve patient empowerment and satisfaction with care (49,50).

Any information and treatment packets sent out to new patients should include material on the emotional aspects of infertility and on support resources available through the clinic, in the community, and via the Internet. A clinic's website is also an important source of support information, and could connect to other internet resources, such as RESOLVE, for easy patient access. Examples of information and education support services from the author's program include:

1. Online, interactive webcasts (webinars) on medical and psychosocial topics of infertility (i.e., preparing for IVF, deciding on ovum donation, miscarriage, etc.). These webinars are live and allow patients to ask questions, which are then archived on the clinic website for patients to access and review at a later time.
2. Monthly IVF and donor egg recipient preparation classes for new patients beginning a cycle. Presentations are made by a member of each treatment team – physician, embryology/laboratory, nurse, infertility counselor – and the administrative/finance office, who discuss protocol and process, describe treatment services, and answer questions. These classes are held in the evening, a light dinner is provided, written materials on the medical and emotional aspects of IVF or donor egg are distributed, and the informal atmosphere allows for easy exchange with patients.
3. Ready access to pamphlets, articles, and written materials on the medical and emotional aspects of infertility, which are displayed in patient waiting areas. Ample supplies of these materials are available in the nursing, physician, and infertility counseling offices, as well as with administrative staff. For example, billing staff found that as patients were checking out from office visits they often talked about their stresses, and being able to give patients flyers on clinic support services or educational pamphlets was greatly appreciated.
4. A "fact sheet" of resources for patients with names, telephone numbers, and Internet websites about clinic and community support services relating to infertility, endometriosis, premature ovarian failure, polycystic ovary syndrome, adoption, pregnancy, pregnancy loss or termination, multiple gestation and parenting, and single parenting.
5. One-page "tip sheets" on topics that offer suggestions about coping with the emotional aspects of infertility (IVF, marital relationships, etc.) and "summary sheets" on medical treatments/procedures. Patient information "fact sheets" are also available through the ASRM's website (http://www.reproductivefacts. org/FactSheetsandBooklets), and can easily be downloaded and given to patients. These summary sheets are especially helpful, as the volume of information given to patients may be overwhelming, and research has shown that patients retain only a small portion of information verbally given to them.
6. A patient lending library of infertility-related books, videos, and audiotapes of instruction and information ranging from topics on sexual dysfunction and adoption to medical diagnosis and treatment of infertility.
7. Resources that can be accessed or downloaded from the clinic's website. These may include articles written by staff members on psychological and medical aspects of treatment, an "ask the expert" column for patients to write in questions, and online webcasts to present information on treatment programs and psychosocial issues of infertility.

Clinic Administration

The manner in which an ART program is administered, along with the physical environment of the clinic, affects both patients' stress levels and their perception of support. An esthetically pleasing, clean, well-maintained office staffed by friendly, professionally dressed, well-trained people goes a long way in communicating an impression of professional competence, caring, and confidence. A recent study found that patient satisfaction can be improved with organizational shifts, when the patient was assigned a primary physician as well as being seen by a fertility-trained nurse (50). Ways in which the author's program provides support through clinic administration includes:

1. Patient waiting areas, with access to reading materials, water, telephones, and restrooms. During weekend monitoring, a continental breakfast is available for patients in this area while patients wait to see the physician. (If a clinic shares space with an obstetrics and gynecology department, sensitivity needs to be considered, and reasonable efforts made to separate pregnant patients and small children from infertility patients by adjusting appointments/schedules and/or seating arrangements).
2. Private rooms where nurses or other clinical staff can instruct or consult with patients.
3. Private sections where billing and scheduling issues can be discussed by administrative staff with patients in a confidential manner.
4. A quiet, secure "donor room" for men to give semen samples, with erotic magazines/materials, video player, and a comfortable chair or bed.
5. Private recovery areas after egg retrieval and embryo transfer with safe places to store belongings, television/video player or music, and a comfortable chair for husbands.
6. Soothing, calming background music piped throughout the office.
7. An annual or biannual "baby party" for patients to come back with their children and celebrate with staff.
8. Miscarriage/pregnancy loss cards sent by the clinical staff when it is learned that, after a patient has been discharged from care, a pregnancy has been lost.

9. Primary care nursing, where a patient is assigned to one nurse, facilitating better continuity and coordination of treatment.
10. A staff member "patient advocate/ombudsman," who patients may talk to when they perceive a problem with their care, or other conflicts with the clinic that cannot be resolved.
11. Patient surveys, suggestion boxes, and written feedback, which encourage open communication regarding satisfaction, thoughts on improving care or services, and constructive criticism.
12. In-service training of all staff on the emotional needs of infertility patients, communication skills, stress management techniques, and on strategies to deal with difficult, demanding patients.
13. Staff support offering confidential assistance, direction, and referral for personal problems and professional burnout, by the staff mental health professional, or through an employee assistance program (EAP). Ultimately, happy staff members are productive workers, who give the best support and service to patients.

RESULTS

Although most patients undergoing ART are well adjusted and will cope adequately with the process, all will benefit from, and indeed need, emotional support during treatment. Numerous studies show that most patients believe psychosocial counseling is beneficial and that they would avail themselves of it, were it offered during treatment (19,51,52). While a minority of patients experience significant emotional distress and use formal counseling services, the vast majority of those who use formal counseling report having found it helpful (19).

The efficiency of psychosocial interventions impacting mental health issues (i.e., depression, anxiety, and distress) and pregnancy rate during infertility is still being debated. Boivin's comprehensive review of 380 studies found that psychosocial interventions were effective in reducing negative affective but did not affect pregnancy rates (31). However, Hammerli and associates (53) conducted a meta-analysis of 384 studies from 1978 to 2007 and found the opposite: Psychological interventions had little effect on negative affect yet improved some patients' chances of achieving pregnancy, but only if they were not receiving ART.

Several studies of patient satisfaction suggest that many patients are dissatisfied with support services (or the lack thereof) offered by their IVF centers (54–57). This information, coupled with the high dropout rates in ART programs, most likely due to psychological reasons, (58–60) suggests that IVF programs need to provide better and more comprehensive psychosocial support services. Studies have indicated that even when cost is not a factor in pursuing treatment, over half of patients drop out of treatment before depleting entitled insurance benefits (61–63). Cross-culturally, the most common reason given for treatment termination is psychological burden and distress (61–65). Providing integrated psychological support services may be an important step in diminishing a patient's depression and anxiety, lowering dropout rates, and possibly even increasing pregnancy rates – the goal of all fertility programs (59,66,67). It may also increase patients' overall sense of satisfaction with care, even when pregnancy is not achieved (68).

Simple strategies for managing patients can help a great deal (69). Olivius and colleagues (61) found that ease in contacting the clinic or clinician by telephone, seeing the same doctor during treatment, and receiving sufficient oral and written information about treatment and complications helped with patient distress. At the very least, written materials and educational resources on the medical and psychosocial aspects of infertility need to be readily available and given to patients by their programs. Further, the more holistically a patient is handled – supported medically and emotionally – the more likely she/he is to be treatment-compliant and satisfied with care, despite the outcome of treatment. In fact, the true mark of success of a program may be in the ability of the team to help patients feel that they, the patients, have done their best when treatment has failed (see Table 67.2 for a summary of strategies for ART patient support).

FUTURE DIRECTION

Reproductive medicine will continue to change as advancing technology presents increasingly complex options and choices for patients. As reproductive technology continues to advance and push the boundaries of social, psychological, religious, and ethical acceptance, the need for comprehensive support services for ART patients will continue to grow. Patients will request a more holistic approach to medical treatment, where their bodies and their emotions are treated with equal importance. As "educated consumers," ART patients will search for the most effective and comprehensive care program, often choosing a practice on the basis of whether psychological support services are integrated into treatment. There will continue to be a growing need for specialized clinical skills and services of mental health professionals trained in infertility counseling to provide this assistance to patients and staff. ART programs that have the foresight to integrate comprehensive support services with specialized mental health professionals as part of the treatment team will succeed.

CONCLUSION

Infertility is an emotionally exhausting, psychologically demanding experience for patients and, at times, their caregivers. Since ART is considered the most stressful of all infertility treatments, patients who undergo it need as much support psychologically as they do medically from their clinical team. Specialized support services are needed for psychosocial preparation, assessment, and treatment of patients who are faced with the unique issues associated with and/or the consequences of assisted reproduction. Experienced mental health professionals trained in infertility counseling must provide these specialized psychological services as part of, or in

Table 67.2 Strategies for Assisted Reproductive Techniques (ARTs) Patient Support

Before
- Educational classes presented by each member of the treatment team on IVF
- Pretreatment counseling session with a mental health professional/infertility counselor
- Psychosocial preparation and assessment of gamete donors, recipients, and surrogates with a mental health professional/infertility counselor
- Extensive written materials available and distributed on the medical, emotional, and financial aspects of ART
- Educational videos on the medical and emotional aspects of infertility and ART
- Support groups
- Stress management, relaxation, and guided imagery classes and CD/DVDs
- Resource lists of community support services including RESOLVE, Inc.

During
- Access to the mental health professional/infertility counselor and other team members
- Telephone support with a primary care nurse
- If a patient has met with an infertility counselor before starting the cycle, a brief visit in the OR on retrieval and/or transfer day
- Stress management, relaxation, and guided imagery classes and audio tapes
- Computer-based technology, including clinic website with resource materials and interactive social media (e.g., Facebook and Twitter); online educational webinars; written materials identifying reliable Internet sites for information and support; and educational CD-ROMs
- Support groups

After
- Psychosocial follow-up after a failed cycle or pregnancy loss
- Decision-making counseling regarding alternative therapies or ending treatment
- Counseling on alternative family building through adoption or third-party reproduction
- Counseling and support for the decision to remain child-free after infertility
- Counseling and preparation for multiple pregnancy, including selective reduction
- Counseling and follow-up for pregnancy after infertility, including support groups
- Counseling and follow-up for issues in parenting after infertility, including families created through donor gametes
- Support groups
- Patient feedback survey

Abbreviations: OR, operating room

close collaboration with, the treatment team (43). Finally, patient support is the responsibility of all employees of an ART program, and staff must be knowledgeable about and sensitive to the emotional needs of their patients.

REFERENCES

1. Menning BE. The emotional needs of infertile couples. Fertil Steril 1980; 34: 313–19.
2. Mahlstedt PP. The psychological component of infertility. Fertil Steril 1985; 43: 335–46.
3. Stanton AL, Dunkel-Schetter C. Psychological adjustment to infertility. In: Stanton AL, Dunkel Schetter C, eds. Infertility: Perspectives from Stress and Coping Research. New York: Plenum Press, 1991: 3–16.
4. Burns LH, Covington SN. Psychology of infertility. In: Covington SN, Burns LH, eds. Infertility Counseling: A Comprehensive Handbook for Clinicians, 2nd edn. New York: Cambridge University Press, 2006: 1–19.
5. Greil AL, Slauson-Blevins K, McQuillan J. The experience of infertility: a review of recent literature. Soc Health Ill 2010; 32: 140–62.
6. Greil A. Infertility and psychological distress: a critical review of the literature. Soc Sci Med 1997; 45: 1679–704.
7. Reading AE. Decision making and in vitro fertilization: the influence of emotional state. J Psychosom Obstet Gynecol 1989; 10: 107–12.
8. Visser A, Haan G, Zalmstra H, et al. Psychosocial aspects of in vitro fertilisation. J Psychosom Obstet Gynecol 1994; 15: 35–45.
9. Kopitzke EJ, Berg BJ, Wilson JF, Owen D. Physical and emotional stress associated with components of the infertility investigation: professional and patient perspectives. Fertil Steril 1991; 55: 1137–43.
10. Boivin J, Takefman J. The impact of the in vitro fertilization – embryo transfer (IVF–ET) process on emotional, physical, and relational variables. Hum Reprod 1996; 11: 903–7.
11. Connolly KJ, Edelmann RJ, Bartlett H, et al. An evaluation of counselling for couples undergoing treatment for in vitro fertilization. Hum Reprod 1993; 8: 1332–8.
12. Litt MD, Tennen H, Affleck G, Klock S. Coping and cognitive factors in adaptation in in vitro fertilization failure. J Behav Med 1992; 15: 171–87.
13. Slade P, Emery J, Lieberman BA. A prospective, longitudinal study of emotions and relationships in in vitro fertilization treatment. Hum Reprod 1997; 12: 183–90.
14. Connolly KJ, Edelmann RJ, Cooke ID, Robson J. The impact of infertility on psychological functioning. J Psychosom Res 1992; 36: 459–68.
15. Paulson JD, Haarmann BS, Salerno RL, Asmar P. An investigation of the relationship between emotional maladjustment and infertility. Fertil Steril 1988; 49: 258–62.
16. Downey J, Husami N, Yingling S, et al. Mood disorders, psychiatric symptoms and distress in women presenting for infertility evaluation. Fertil Steril 1989; 52: 425–32.
17. Edelmann RJ, Connolly KJ, Cooke ID, Robson J. Psychogenetic infertility: some findings. J Psychosom Obstet Gynecol 1991; 12: 163–8.
18. Stanton AL, Danoff Burg S. Selected issues in women's reproductive health: psychological perspectives. In: Stanton AL, Gallant SJ, eds. The Psychology of Women's Health: Progress and Challenges in Research and Application. Washington, DC: American Psychological Association, 1996: 261–305.
19. Boivin J. Is there too much emphasis on psycholosocial counselling for infertile patients? J Assist Reprod Genet 1997; 14: 184–6.
20. Freeman EW, Rickels K, Tausig J, et al. Emotional and psychosocial factors in follow-up of women after IVF–ET treatment. Acta Obstet Gynecol Scand 1987; 66: 517–21.
21. Newton CR, Hearn MT, Yuzpe AA. Psychological assessment and follow-up after in vitro fertilization: assessing the impact of failure. Fertil Steril 1990; 54: 879–86.

22. Berg BJ, Wilson JF. Psychological functioning across stages of treatment for infertility. J Behav Med 1991; 14: 11–26.

23. Lalos A, Lalos O, von Schoultz B. The psychosocial impact of infertility two years after completed surgical treatment. Acta Obstet Gynecol Scand 1985; 65: 599–604.

24. Newton CR, Sherrard W, Glavac I. The Fertility Problem Inventory: measuring perceived infertility- related stress. Fertil Steril 1999; 72: 54–62.

25. Boivin J, Shoog-Svanberg A, Andersson L, et al. Distress level in men undergoing intracytoplasmic sperm injection versus in vitro fertilization. Hum Reprod 1998; 13: 1403–6.

26. Nachtigall RD, Becker G, Wozny M. The effects of gender-specific diagnosis on men's and women's response to infertility. Fertil Steril 1992; 57: 113–21.

27. Hynes GJ, Callan VJ, Terry DJ, et al. The psychological well-being of infertile women after a failed IVF attempt: the effects of coping. Br J Med Psychol 1992; 65: 269–78.

28. Stanton AL, Burns LH. Behavioral medicine approaches to infertility counseling. In: Burns LH, Covington SN, eds. Infertility Counseling: A Comprehensive Handbook for Clinicians. New York: Parthenon Publishing, 1999: 129–47.

29. Agostini F, Monti F, De Pascalis L, et al. Psychosocial support for infertile couples during assisted reproductive technology treatment. Fertil Steril 2011; 95: 707–10.

30. Mindes EJ, Ingram KM, Kliewer W, et al. Longitudinal analysis of the relationship between unsupportive social interactions and psychological adjustment among women with fertility problems. Soc Sci Med 2003; 56: 165–80.

31. Boivin J. A review of psychosocial interventions in infertility. Soc Sci Med 2003; 57: 2325–41.

32. Cohen SJ, Kessler RC, Underwood GL. Strategies for measuring stress in studies of psychiatric and physical disorders. In: Cohen SJ, Kessler RC, Underwood GL, eds. Measuring Stress: A Guide for Health and Social Scientist. New York: Oxford University Press, 1995; 3–25.

33. Boivin J, Takefman J. Stress level across stages of in vitro fertilization in subsequently pregnant and non-pregnant women. Fertil Steril 1995; 64: 802–10.

34. Boivin J, Takefman J, Braverman A. The Fertility Quality of Life (FertiQoL) tool: Development and general psychometric properties. Fertil Steril 2011; 96: 409–15.

35. Covington SN. The role of the mental health professional in reproductive medicine. Fertil Steril 1995; 64: 895–7.

36. Covington SN. Reproductive medicine and mental health professionals: the need for collaboration in a brave new world. Orgyn 1997; 3: 19–21.

37. Human Fertilisation and Embryology Authority. Code of Practice, 2nd edn. London: HFEA, 1995.

38. Hernon M, Harris CP, Elstein M, et al. Review of organized support network for infertility patients in licensed units in the UK. Hum Reprod 1995; 10: 960–4.

39. American Society for Reproductive Medicine. Guidelines for gamete and embryo donation. Fertil Steril 2006; 86(Suppl 4): S38–50.

40. Klock SC, Maier D. Guidelines for the provision of psychological evaluations for infertile patients at the University of Connecticut Health Center. Fertil Steril 1991; 56: 680–5.

41. Klock SC, Covington SN. Minnesota Multiphasic Personality Inventory (MMPI-2) profiles in the assessment of ovum donors. Fertil Steril 2010; 94: 1684–8.

42. Covington SN. Preparing the patient for in vitro fertilization: psychological considerations. Clin Consider Obstet Gynecol 1994; 6: 131–7.

43. Covington SN. Infertility counseling in practice: a collaborative reproductive healthcare model. In: Covington SN, Burns LH, eds. Infertility Counseling: A Comprehensive Handbook for Clinicians, 2nd edn. New York: Cambridge University Press, 2006: 493–507.

44. Burns LH. An overview of the psychology of infertility. Infertil Reprod Med Clin North Am 1993; 4: 433–54.

45. Boivin J, Scanlan LC, Walker SM. Why are infertile patients not using psychosocial counselling? Hum Reprod 1999; 14: 1384–91.

46. Cousineau TM, Green TC, Corsini E, et al. Online psychoeducational support for infertile women: a randomized controlled trail. Hum Reprod 2008; 23: 554–66.

47. Kahlor L, Mackert M. Perceptions of infertility information and support sources among female patients who access the Internet. Fertil Steril 2009; 91: 83–90.

48. Cousineau TM, Lord SE, Seibring AR, et al. A multimedia psychosocial support program for couples receiving infertility treatment: a feasibility study. Fertil Steril 2004; 81: 532–8.

49. Tuil WS, Verhaak CM, Braat D, de Vries Robbe P, Kremer J. Empowering patients undergoing in vitro fertilization by providing Internet access to medical data. Fertil Steril 2007; 88: 361–8.

50. Van Emple I, Hermens R, Akkermans R, et al. Organization determinants of patient-centered fertility care: a multilevel analysis. Fertil Stert 2011; 95: 513–19.

51. Baram D, Tourtelot E, Muechler E, et al. Psychosocial adjustment following unsuccessful in vitro fertilization. J Psychosom Obstet Gynecol 1988; 9: 181–90.

52. Mazure CM, Greenfeld DA. Psychological studies of in vitro fertilization/embryo transfer participants. J In Vitro Fert Embryo Transf 1989; 6: 242–56.

53. Hammerli K, Hansjorg Z, Barth J. The efficacy of psychological interventions for infertile patients: a meta-analysis examining mental health and pregnancy rate. Hum Reprod Update 2009; 15: 279–95.

54. Sabourin S, Wright J, Duchesne C, Belisle S. Are consumers of modern fertility treatments satisfied? Fertil Steril 1991; 56: 1084–90.

55. Laffont I, Edelmann RJ. Perceived support and counselling needs in relation to in vitro fertilization. J Psychosom Obstet Gynecol 1994; 15: 183–8.

56. Sundby J, Olsen A, Schei B. Quality of care for infertility patients. An evaluation of a plan for a hospital investigation. Scand J Soc Med 1994; 22: 139–44.

57. Souter VL, Penney G, Hopton JL, Templeton AA. Patient satisfaction with the management of infertility. Hum Reprod 1988; 13: 1831–6.

58. Land JA, Courtar DA, Evers JL. Patient dropout in an assisted reproductive technology program: implications for pregnancy. Fertil Steril 1997; 68: 278–81.

59. Domar AD. Impact of psychological factors on dropout rates in insured infertility patients. Fertil Steril 2004; 81: 271–3.

60. Penzias AS. When and why does the dream die? Or does it? Fertil Steril 2004; 81: 274–5.

61. Olivius C, Friden B, Borg G, Bergh C. Why do couples discontinue in vitro fertilization treatment? A cohort study. Fertil Steril 2004; 81: 258–61.

62. Smeenk JMJ, Verhaak CM, Stolwijk AM, Kremer JA, Braat DD. Reasons for dropout in an in vitro fertilization/intracytoplasmic sperm injection program. Fertil Steril 2004; 81: 262–8.

63. Malcolm CE, Cumming DC. Follow–up of infertile couples who dropped out of a specialist fertility clinic. Fertil Steril 2004; 81: 269–70.

64. Brandes M, van der Steen J, Bokdam S, et al. When and why do subfertile couples discontinue their fertility care? Hum Reprod 2009; 24: 3127–35.

65. Domar AD, Smith Conboy L, Iannone M, Alper M. A prospective investigation into the reasons why insured United States patients drop out of in vitro fertilization treatment. Fertil Steril 2010; 94: 1457–9.

66. Terzioglu F. Investigation into the effectiveness of counseling on assisted reproductive techniques in Turkey. J Psychosom Obstet Gynaecol 2001; 22: 133–41.

67. Smeenk JMJ, Verhaak CM, Stolwijk AM, Kremer JAM, Braat DDM. Psychological interference in in vitro fertilization treatment. Fertil Steril 2004; 81: 277.

68. Mourad SM, Nelen W, Akkermans R, et al. Determinants of patients' experiences and satisfaction with fertility care. Fertil Steril 2010; 94: 1254–60.

69. Olivius C, Friden B, Borg G, Bergh C. Psychological aspects of discontinuation of in vitro fertilization treatment. Fertil Steril 2004; 81: 276.

68

The relationship between stress and in vitro fertilization outcome

Andrea Mechanick Braverman

OVERVIEW

The impact of patient stress on the process of in vitro fertilization (IVF) is a complex and multifaceted interplay between the mind and the body. The old model of psychogenic causation, for example, the Freudian approach that speaks of the woman's fear of impregnation or motherhood, has long been supplanted by the careful exploration of the interplay of stress on the endocrine system. Considerations of dispositional characterological factors such as optimism (1) or happiness (2) have also led to the hypothesis that such factors may play a role in treatment outcome.

Many studies have considered the relationship between stress (or other psychosocial variables) and its effect on pregnancy outcome per treatment cycle (1–5). The results have been mixed, and have often been confounding factors when the concepts of stress reduction and support as agents of cause or intervention in infertility and pregnancy outcomes are considered. In a comprehensive review of psychosocial interventions in infertility, Boivin noted that "analysis of these studies showed that psychosocial interventions were more effective in reducing negative affect than in changing interpersonal functioning," and that pregnancy rates were not likely to be affected by these interventions (6). Boivin also noted that counseling interventions that focused on affective expression regarding the emotional aspects of infertility were significantly less effective in producing a positive change than were education and skills training. Psychosocial intervention has looked at pregnancy and implantation rates (7,8), but not at treatment persistence and retention.

Some of the major confounds that occur while considering psychological distress and pregnancy outcome include: The relationship between distress and anxiety/depression; influences of diagnosis or influence of information or attitudes of the medical team; habituation effects of chronic stress; other life stressors; coping styles; and baseline psychological issues. In Domar's (8) review of the association of psychological distress and pregnancy outcome, the author concludes: "Women undergoing ART procedures report significant levels of negative psychological symptoms, both prior to beginning and especially after experiencing an unsuccessful cycle. Most of the research conducted with women undergoing ART treatment supports the theory that emotional distress is associated with treatment success." However, the author notes the limitations of many of these studies, including lack of control groups or small sample sizes.

More recently, studies have turned their attention away from the tremendously complex relationship between stress or depression and pregnancy outcome, focusing instead on the causes behind the discontinuation of treatment and treatment perseverance. These studies clearly demonstrate that treatment dropout is associated with psychological factors (1–5). Given the high pregnancy rates using IVF over cycles, even involving patients with poorer prognoses, the ability for patients to remain in treatment, that is, treatment persistence, gives a patient her best opportunity for achieving a pregnancy. Treatment persistence will allow a patient to optimize her biological potential.

RECENT RESEARCH

In their 2010 review, Boivin, Griffiths, and Venetis (9) performed a meta-analysis on prospective psychosocial studies that examined the association between pretreatment emotional distress, defined as anxiety or depression, and pregnancy. The subjects received one cycle of assisted reproductive technique (ART); effect size was determined by comparing those who achieved a pregnancy and those who did not. The authors found that there was no association between pretreatment emotional distress and pregnancy outcome. Limitations of the meta-analysis were due to the heterogeneity of the study designs.

Other research identifies infertility as a stressful event and has looked at its impact on the dyadic relationship. Some studies (10–12) have found that the infertility experience can strengthen a couple's relationship, and a 2011 study (13) explored whether there can be relational benefit from the infertility journey. In this prospective study, couples were followed for a five-year period of unsuccessful treatments. Women experienced a greater percentage of high levels of marital benefit. Different coping strategies were employed but the cause of infertility did not significantly contribute. Overall, a third of the couples experienced a longitudinal positive effect on the marital relationship over a five-year period.

Researchers have also begun to look at stress from the biomarkers and how such stress affects fertility (14). In a longitudinal prospective study, researches assess salivary cortisol and α-amylase levels and their relationship to female fecundity. The study found a statistically significant relationship for lowered probability of conception during the fertile follicular window as the woman's salivary α-amylase concentrations rise but offers no explanation of what the mechanism of impact is. This new research direction for understanding how stress impacts the body and fecundity may offer new directions for interventions for stress affecting infertile individuals.

SOURCES OF STRESS

The experience of infertility transcends borders and socioeconomic status. Nearly every society throughout history has produced art and literature that has spoken of the desire for offspring and the pain (or shame) that ensues when pregnancy does not occur. For many individuals, infertility is among the first life crises that they may face, having previously dealt with pregnancy's counterpoint (the prevention of pregnancy) through vigilant contraception. Messages from friends, family, and society reinforce the notion that fertility is within an individual's control. Public figures or movie stars who pursue infertility treatment with success at ages well into their 40s and 50s only contribute to some individual's incredulity that there may be a fertility issue with either or both partners. The inevitable fact that age may play a substantive role in fertility may be lost within these competing social messages.

The stress of infertility is felt in many ways by men and women and may change over time and as individuals experience failure in the cycles. In a groundbreaking 1985 study, Freeman and colleagues (15) evaluated 200 couples experiencing infertility. Half the women and 15% of the men endorsed the notion that infertility was the worst event of their lives. In a more recent study, Verhaak and colleagues (16) surveyed 148 IVF patients along with their 71 partners and measured numerous psychological factors (anxiety, depression, personality characteristics, the meaning of fertility problems, coping, marital relationship, and social support) at pre-treatment, post-treatment, and final treatment stages. Six months later, participants were assessed for anxiety and depression. Among women, anxiety and depression increased after unsuccessful treatment and decreased after successful treatment. There was no change in anxiety and depression levels for men after either successful or unsuccessful treatment.

Some of the major categories of stress that have been traditionally recognized are addressed below, but none of these factors unequivocally demonstrate a clear role in pregnancy outcome. Without question, entering into medical treatment for fertility places the individual and couple into a "patient" mode. The stress of being in medical care alone can be a psychological burden for some patients. Contributing to this stress may be the language of infertility to which patients are regularly exposed, such as the use of pejorative terms like "failed cycle," "incompetent cervix," "shooting blanks," and "advanced maternal age" that may impact patients' self-esteem and body image, and which may serve to reinforce the potentially stress-inducing notion that the individual is a patient with medical problems.

Self-Esteem and Body Image

For many individuals, being in "patient" mode means that their bodies are not working correctly; this circumstance can take a toll on their self-esteem as well as on their body image. The disappointment in their own bodies felt by the patient may be exacerbated by their unconscious belief that fertility should "come naturally," that it should be in their exclusive control. The stated message by friends, family, and others to "just relax and you'll get pregnant" serves to reinforce the notion that individuals are failing if they cannot make their bodies work correctly. Doubts may arise in a patient's mind regarding his or her sense of masculinity or femininity. For example, a man who has low motility may confuse emotionally the diagnosis with personal feelings of the loss of virility. The evaluation and scrutiny of the intimate and private areas of a relationship contributes to the pressure of being evaluated for adequacy (17).

Sexuality and Intimacy

Sexuality can also be affected by infertility. Sexual enjoyment has been found to be lessened during certain required tests, such as a postcoital (18). Sexuality may be linked with procreation during fertility treatment and is often divorced from recreation or intimacy. Timed intercourse can add to the burden of feeling measured, pressured, and stressed. Some women report feeling distanced from their bodies because of procedures or timed intercourse; men report feeling performance pressure with timed intercourse. Adding to these stressors are the feelings associated with unhappiness, anger, or disappointment in one's own body. None of these feelings or stressors enhances the sense of being a sexual person with sexual desires. This further adds to the burden on the relationship.

Relationship with Partner

Research has demonstrated that men and women experience, and are affected by, infertility in different ways, and that their coping strategies may differ as well (19). Repeated treatment failure may take its toll on the relationship. Partners may disagree about the timing of when to seek evaluation or pursuit of treatment; couples may also need to navigate differing levels of optimism about treatment outcome. Congruence can depend upon the degree to which the partners perceive the severity of the stress of the infertility; lack of congruence may in itself add to stress within the relationship.

Partners may adopt different coping strategies which may be intra-personally effective but may add to the relationship burden. In a study of German men, researchers found that men tended to suppress their emotions and had more difficulty communicating and identifying their emotions (20). Take, for example, the situation in which one partner feels great relief by being able to process the thoughts and feelings which arise and where another finds discussion stressful and anxiety producing. The very coping strategies that bring personal relief only adds to the relationship stress where one partner may feel "shut down" and the other partner feels unfairly burdened depending on which coping strategy is utilized. Couples may also experience lack of congruence with regard to disclosure or non-disclosure of their fertility issues. If one partner has been diagnosed, s/he may feel stigmatized by the disclosure; the other partner may feel burdened by the demands of not sharing the information with important support persons.

Overall, men with infertility tend to somaticize their reactions; this has been observed across cultures. Some cultures are protective of the stress infertility places on men because only female factor infertility is recognized in those cultures. In Western cultures, men may repress their feelings related to the infertility; this repression may correlate with sexual dysfunction during treatment (21).

The Burden of Infertility and Its Treatment

Many different emotions have been identified as arising from infertility: anger, denial, grief, guilt, anxiety, and depression. The literature remains equivocal about the impact that the length of diagnosis has on psychological burden and adaptation. Issues from the past may weigh emotionally on the individual, for example, previous pregnancy termination(s) or sexually transmitted diseases that may have contributed to the fertility problem. The constant cycle of hope and disappointment has led to the description of infertility as an "emotional roller coaster."

Treatment for infertility places very concrete demands on the individual and couple, which adds to the stress and burden. For some, the time demands of physician consultation, monitoring, inseminations, or IVF may present real problems on a patient's demanding job or upon an individual who is juggling childcare. Women must choose between being open or private about their treatment, not just with those in their personal lives but also within their careers; too many unexplained absences from work may result in a poor performance review. Many individuals and couples may also feel that they are in limbo, foregoing new jobs or promotions due to concerns about access to treatment or even financial coverage (depending on the country).

For all, the decision about being open or private about their fertility situation can frequently arise from simple questions such as "do you have children," often asked innocently in social situations. Social situations are sometimes avoided to escape painful stimuli such as encountering pregnant women or having contact with babies. This social isolation can also add to feelings of being different or of being cut-off from the usual support structures that the individual or couple typically depends upon. Families may fail to understand why the individual does not participate in expected family events such as visits to the maternity ward after a delivery, attending baby showers, or even attending holiday events.

OVERVIEW OF STRESS AND PREGNANCY OUTCOME DATA

A primary consideration of the stress and pregnancy outcome inquiry must focus on whether stress is causative of factors that would prohibit pregnancy or whether it is the diagnosis and/or treatment of infertility that causes stress. This consideration is further complicated by the issue of how stress is defined by researchers and mediated by patients. Studies that have addressed stress as it is activated by the hypothalamic–pituitary–adrenal (HPA) axis have been unable to clearly delineate the exact pathways or mechanisms (22–25).

Patients are bombarded with the adage to "just relax and you'll get pregnant," which leads to the integration of the assumption that stress has an immediate and direct impact upon their fertility. Despite the conflicting literature, it is generally concluded that stress does have an impact on the body (6,7). Stress also has an impact on energy level, optimism, patience, and perseverance. Stress is also mediated by personal coping styles. For example, one person's reaction to a very stressful event, e.g., public speaking, may elicit a large stress response. Yet, the intrapersonal experience of that stress may be energizing and allow the individual to feel that he is performing better. In a different study (26), the authors concluded that infertile women have a different personality profile and their stress levels (as measured by their prolactin and cortisol levels) were elevated compared to the controls.

Coping with stress may ultimately provide assistance to conception through stress reduction. Developing more effective coping strategies helps people reduce treatment termination, thereby allowing patients to truly maximize their biological potential. Improved coping strategies may also reduce relationship stress and improve communication, leading to more congruence between partners in pursuing treatment. Stress reduction should also lead to an improved sense of well-being (6). The relationship between stress and outcome is multifactorial – both complicated and curvilinear.

Take, for example, the individual who experiences anxiety during the waiting period between insemination and the pregnancy test. If the anxiety increases over time, the patient's desire to avoid the distress may grow greater than her desire to achieve pregnancy. Or the negative experience of anxiety may lead to avoidance behaviors with treatment tasks and reduce the efficacy of treatment, for example, missed monitoring appointments, or poor timing with coitus or medication.

Another conflict that may prevent good coping strategies is when an individual's belief conflicts with his or her needs. Dysfunctional beliefs lead to poor choices in coping strategies. For example, consider the patient who believes that medical intervention is "unnatural." This belief may lead that person to pursue treatment slowly and, for many medical reasons, this slowness may be costly. A 39-year-old woman who operates on the belief that medical intervention is unnatural may delay more aggressive treatment for a critical year or longer, thereby missing more optimal fertility opportunities. In another example, if a male partner believes that conception can take place without a doctor's intervention and his partner is ready to pursue treatment, conflict can quickly arise and tax the couple's communication skills.

Cognitive Therapy

Cognitive therapy is an effective tool for understanding how stress can arise when a person's beliefs are dysfunctional. The formulation of the patient's dysfunction is based on his or her internal experiences and how those experiences are distorted through negative beliefs, assumptions, inferences, and conclusions. Change is mediated by the task of examining the accuracy of these beliefs (27). In cognitive therapy, the therapeutic relationship takes a "back seat" as compared to a psychodynamic approach. It is the empirical investigation of these internal experiences and the opportunity to test the automatic thoughts, assumptions, and negative beliefs that yield the opportunity to correct the faulty dysfunctional constructs (28). It is the ability to change the person's underlying cognitive structures that will in turn change his or her affective state and pattern of behavior. Behavioral techniques and homework help to elicit cognitions that contribute to or cause problematic behavior and also help the patients test their maladaptive cognitions and assumptions, thus mobilizing the patients into constructive activities and enabling them to develop better coping strategies (9).

In contrast to the psychoanalytic approach (which works by making the patient conscious of his or her unconscious past), cognitive therapy identifies current thinking and behavior (29). For example, the combination of helping the patient understand the narcissistic injury of his or her infertility, as well as its impact on his or her interpersonal relationships and life planning, is critical. An individual may feel stress or inadequacy when her belief that "I cannot be a real woman unless I get pregnant" leads her to avoid interpersonal relationships to escape the painful feelings that arise from feeling isolated from the fertile world.

In addition, the recognition, as well as differentiation, of infertility as a crisis leads to stress. For some clients, infertility awakens or aggravates long-term issues in their lives, for example, anxiety about intimacy, poor communication skills, etc. The cyclic nature of infertility treatment creates the feeling in the patient of an immediate infertility crisis, rather than the patient identifying it as a chronic condition. In many situations, a woman may present as if she has persistent depressive symptoms, but in reality these symptoms remit during the two weeks of the follicular stage of her cycle. The stress may be chronic in that it exists all the time, but the woman experiences it intensely during the waiting period post ovulation.

Understanding that feelings of worthlessness, purposelessness, poor self-esteem, poor body image, isolation, and withdrawal (because of painful stimuli relating to fertility), among others, are inherent in the infertility experience is important for a thorough understanding of how change in the individual's reactions can be made by identifying these dysfunctional cognitions and exchanging them for functional ones. For example, a woman who has always struggled with body image issues may find that infertility exacerbates these feelings; educating and disentangling the issues with the patient by identifying the dysfunctional thoughts gives her the opportunity to diminish the emotional impact and substitute other thoughts and behaviors.

The stresses of infertility arise from many sources. Below are some examples of how dysfunctional thoughts are identified and responded to within a cognitive therapy model.

- *All-or-nothing thinking*:
  I can never feel like a real woman if I can't be pregnant; or
  My ability to gestate a pregnancy is a small part of my femininity.
- *Overgeneralization*:
  Everyone will think differently of my child because of the gestational carrier; or
  Some people may be curious about the gestational carrier pregnancy; or
  My child will still have the same genetics as it would, had I carried the pregnancy.
- *Selective negative focus*:
  I cannot care for my own child in utero; or
  I can care for my child by selecting the best gestational carrier and building a positive working relationship.
- *Disqualifying the positive:*
  I will never carry my own baby; or
  I will miss the pregnancy experience but I have the rest of my child's life to experience; or
  I will not carry a pregnancy but I can still have my own genetic child.
- *Arbitrary inference*:
  People think I'm selfish because I don't have any children; or
  People simply think we have not chosen to start our family yet.
- *Emotional reasoning*:
  Because I feel sad about not being pregnant, my child will feel sad that I couldn't carry him or her.
- *"Should" statements*:
  I should not feel sad, therefore I am not handling this well; or
  It is alright to feel sad and handling this event means working through the sadness.

Behavioral Medicine

Behavioral medicine offers many strategies for coping with and managing stress. Employing a variety of strategies, the intervention will focus on introducing techniques such as cognitive behavioral strategies, relaxation techniques, and guided imagery. Patients also consider how nutrition, acupuncture, massage therapy, and yoga may effectively manage their stress. Another potential aspect of infertility stress management involves communication training in that patients communicate more effectively with the medical professionals involved in their care. Better communication increases the ability to receive and understand information as well as allows the patients to feel that they can effectively negotiate meeting their needs.

COMPLEMENTARY ALTERNATIVE MEDICINE: ACUPUNCTURE, AND OTHER ALTERNATIVES

Infertility treatment has come a long way since the days when psychogenic reasoning placed the blame for their infertility on the infertile women themselves. Modern medicine has begun to consider the mind–body connection in the treatment of infertility. Hotly and passionately debated within the mental health and medical professional communities, the mind–body connection is sometimes considered an entity or process with a commonly understood definition when in fact, the mind–body connection is still more conjecture than fact. Yet, in a recent study, when asked to what extent religion and spirituality influenced patients' health, (56%) responded "much or very much;" yet only 6% believed that it changed "hard" medical outcomes. With regard to ways of coping with health issues, 75% felt that religion and spirituality helped patients cope and 75% felt it gave patients a positive state of mind (30).

It is estimated that, in the United States alone, complementary and alternative medicine (CAM) is utilized by at least one-third of all adults (31). That number increases to 62% of adults when prayer, used specifically for health reasons, is included. Other research clearly shows that globally, CAM is either a standard part of patient care or an emerging option (32). Treatment for infertility has evolved to include an understanding that the most effective treatment involves treating both the mind and the body.

Although evidence-based studies are still emerging for treatments such as acupuncture and relaxation approaches, more programs are opening their doors and their referrals to CAM. Accompanying the concept of treating the whole person is the paradigm of collaborative care in the treatment of the patient. A team approach comprised of a physician, nurse, mental health professional, acupuncturist, yoga instructor, or other professional represents the new model for providing patient care. Patient associations are emerging as leaders in providing these models for collaborative care. For example, in the United States, the American Fertility Association and Resolve regularly bring these diverse providers together for the benefit of patients, through the use of forums, in-person seminars, or internet seminars.

CAM has different meanings in different cultures and different countries. What is complementary in one country may be an accepted staple of regular treatment in another. Research internationally is expected to begin to integrate all these approaches and lead us to a more global understanding of how harmony between the mind and body can facilitate good health, and conversely, how disharmony or dysfunction between the mind and body can contribute to poorer results for the patient.

Acupuncture

The literature about the efficacy of acupuncture has been equivocal. The basic tenets of acupuncture posit that its efficacy is achieved by balancing the flow of Qi (energy) through the patient's body (33). Fertility mechanisms for women undergoing acupuncture involve the stimulation of the B-endorphin secretion that has its impact on the GnRH pulse generator and then upon gonadotropin and steroid secretion. This process creates a favorable environment within the uterus for implantation of the embryos by virtue of the increased blood flow (34). Although some studies have demonstrated a higher clinical pregnancy rate for acupuncture (34–36), others studies have shown no positive effects (33,37). Acupuncture's efficacy has been explored by comparing traditional acupuncture (needle insertions along the meridians and points), to electroacupuncture, to laser acupuncture, and to sham acupuncture. Criticism of the comparability of all these approaches has been made in the Western medical community and in traditional Chinese medical communities alike (38).

The first published study of a prospective, randomized trial of acupuncture was published in 2002 (36) which demonstrated a significantly higher pregnancy rate in the acupuncture group (n = 80) versus the controls (n = 80) with pregnancy rates being 42.5% and 26.3%, respectively. In a later study that was not published but presented at the European Society for Human Reproduction and Embryology (39), Paulus used sham acupuncture in a group, and compared the results to a group where traditional acupuncture was used, and no significant difference was observed. The authors noted that the pressure from the sham needles could indeed have created an effect. As Domar (38) observed, concerns were raised because the study was not ultimately published; Domar also goes on to suggest that studies should account for the effect that the belief by the patient that acupuncture is effective must be controlled for; he argues that it may be the belief which is the agent of change leading to increased pregnancy rates rather than the acupuncture itself.

In a recent study (34), patients were randomized into three groups: A control group, patients who received acupuncture on the day of embryo transfer, and patients who received acupuncture on the transfer day and then two days later. Clinical ongoing pregnancy rates were higher in both treatment groups than in the control group, but did not reach statistical significance. The authors concluded that acupuncture significantly improves the outcome for IVF but that adding treatment two days after offered no other improvement. In a different study, 225 patients were randomized to receive either luteal-phase acupuncture or placebo acupuncture (40). Both clinical and ongoing pregnancy rates were higher in the acupuncture group. The authors concluded that acupuncture was safe and effective for women undergoing IVF.

In another recent study of 228 patients, patients were randomized to receive acupuncture treatment or noninvasive sham acupuncture (33). The acupuncture group received three treatments. Traditional Chinese medicine was used to diagnose the infertility and treatment was rendered accordingly. In the sham acupuncture group, points near but not on the actual acupuncture points were used. No significant differences were found between the groups, but the authors suggested that a small treatment effect could not be excluded because the odds were 1.5 higher for the treatment group. The authors concluded that acupuncture was safe for women undergoing embryo transfer.

Finally, in a review article by Stener-Victorin and Hamaidan (41), the authors reviewed four studies and noted that three of these found a higher efficacy rate for the acupuncture groups. They cautioned that the different study protocols created challenges in drawing conclusions, but could state that acupuncture has a positive effect and no adverse effects on pregnancy outcome.

CONCLUSION

Many factors contribute to the stresses placed on, and experienced by, women and men who have fertility problems. Research has yet to disentangle and adequately address the relationship between stress and infertility. Counseling with cognitive or behavioral approaches offers tools for individuals and couples in coping with their infertility. There is emerging literature suggesting that patients are utilizing complementary alternative medical approaches and that acupuncture may be a safe and effective tool for assisting with infertility treatment.

REFERENCES

1. Smeenk JMJ, Verhaak CM, Stolwijk AM, Kremer JAM, Brat DDM. Reasons for dropout in an in vitro fertilization/intracytoplasmic sperm injection program. Fertil Steril 2004; 81: 262–8.
2. Olivius C, Friden B, Borg G, Bergh C. Why do couples discontinue in vitro fertilization treatment? A cohort study. Fertil Steril 2004; 81: 258–61.
3. VanderLaan B, Karande V, Krohm C, et al. N Cost considerations with infertility therapy: outcome and cost comparison and preferred provider organization care based on physician and facility cost. Hum Reprod 1998; 13: 1200–5.
4. Sharma V, Allgar V, Rajikhowa M. Factors influencing the cumulative conception rate and discontinuation of an in vitro fertilization treatment for infertility. Fertil Steril 2002; 78: 40–6.
5. Roest J, van Heusden AM, Zeilmaker GH, Verhoef A. Cumulative pregnancy rates and selective drop-out patients in in-vitro fertilization treatment. Hum Reprod 1998; 13: 339–41.
6. Boivin. J. A review of psychosocial interventions in infertility. Soc Sci Med 2003; 57: 2325–41.
7. Domar AD, Clapp D, Slawsby EA, et al. The impact of group psychological interventions on distress in infertile women. Health Psychol 2000; 19: 568–75.
8. Domar AD, Clapp D, Slawsby EA, et al. Impact of group psychological interventions on pregnancy rates in infertile women. Fert Steril 2000; 73: 805–11.
9. Freeman EW, Boxer AS, Rickels K, Tureck R, Mastrionni L Jr. Psychological evaluation and support in a program of in vitro fertilization and embryo transfer. Fertil Steril 1985; 43: 48–53.
10. Boivin J, Griffiths E, Venetis CA. Emotional distress in infertile women and failure of assisted reproductive technologies: meta-analysis of prospective psychosocial studies. BMJ 2011; 342: d223.
11. Greil AL. Infertilty and psychological distress: a critical review of the literature. Soc Sci Med 1997; 45: 1679–704.
12. Drosdzol A, Skrzypulec V. Evaluation of marital and sexual interactions of Polish infertile couples. J Sex Med 2009; 6: 3335–46.
13. Greil AL, Slauson-Blevins K, McQuiollan J. The experience of infertilitiy: a review of recent literature. Sociol Health Illn 2009; 32: 140–62.
14. Buck GM, Lum KJ, Sundaram R, et al. Stress reduces conception probabilities across the fertile window: evidence in support of relaxation. Fert Steril 2011; 95: 2184–9.
15. Peterson BD, Pirritano M, Block JM, Schmidt L. Marital benefit and coping strategies in men and women undergoing unsuccessful fertility treatments over a 5-year period. Fertil Steril 2011; 95: 1759; 1763.
16. Verhaak CM, Smeenk JM, van Minnen A, Kremer JA, Kraaimaat FW. A longitudinal, prospective study on emotional adjustment before, during and after consecutive fertility treatment cycles. Hum Reprod 2005; 20: 2253–60.
17. Keye WR. The impact of infertility on psychosexual function. Fertil Steril 1980; 34: 308–9.
18. Boivin J, Takefman JE, Brender W, et al. The effects of female sexual response in coitus on early reproductive process. J Behav Med 1992; 15: 509–18.
19. Newton CR. Counseling the infertile couple. In: Covington SN, Burns LH, eds. Infertility Counseling a Comprehensive Handbook for Clinicians. 2nd edn. New York: Cambridge University Press, 2006.
20. Conrad R, Schilling G, Langenbuch M, et al. Alexithymia in male infertility. Hum Reprod 2001; 16: 587–92.
21. Petok WD. The psychology of gender-specific infertility diagnoses. In: Covington SN, Burns LH, eds. Infertility Counseling A Comprehensive Handbook for Clinicians, 2nd edn. New York: Cambridge University Press, 2006.
22. Berga SL. Functional hypothalamic chronic anovulation. In: Adashi EY, Rock JA, Rosenwaks Z, eds. Reproductive Endocrinology, Surgery, and Technology. Vol 1, Philadelphia: Lippincott-Raven, 1996.

23. Chrousos GP, Torpy DJ, Gold PW. Interactions between the hypothalamic pituitary-axis and the female reproductive system: clinical implications. Ann Intern Med 1998; 129: 229–40.

24. Ferrin M. Clinical review 105: Stress and the reproductive cycle. Clin Endocrinolog Metab 1999; 2: 309–14.

25. Haimovice F, Hill JA. The role of psycho-neuro-endocrine-immunology in reproduction. In: Hill JA, ed. Cytokines in Reproduction. Austin: Landes Bioscience, 1998.

26. Cxemickzy G, Landgren BM, Collins A. The influence of stress and state anxiety on the outcome of IVF-treatment: psychological and endocrinological assessment of Swedish women entering IVF-treatment. Acta Obstet Gynecol Scand 2000; 79: 113–18.

27. Beck AT, Rush AJ, Shaw BF, Emery G. Cognitive Therapy of Depression. New York: Guildford, 1979.

28. Clark DM, Fairburn CG, eds. Science and Practice of Cognitive Behavior Therapy. New York: Oxford University Press, 1997.

29. Bergin AE, Garfield SL, eds. Handbook of Psychotherapy and Behavior Change, 4th edn. New York: Wiley & Sons, 1994.

30. Farr AC, Sellergren SA, Lantos JD, Chin MH. Physician's observations and interpretations of the influence of religion and spirituality on health. Arch Intern Med 2007; 167: 649–54.

31. Barnes PM, PowellGriner E, McFann K, Nahin RL. Complementary and alternative medicine use among adults: United States. Adv Data 2004; 27: 1–19.

32. Astin JA. Why patients use alternative medicine: results of a national study. JAMA 1998; 279: 1548–53.

33. Smith C, Meaghan C, Norman RJ. Influence of acupuncture stimulation on pregnancy rates for women undergoing embryo transfer. Fertil Steril 2006; 85: 1352–8.

34. Westergaard LG, Maol QM, Krogslund M, et al. Acupuncture on the day of embryo transfer significantly improves the reproductive outcome in infertile women: a prospective, randomized trial. Fertil Steril 2006; 85: 1341–5.

35. Margarelli PC, Cridenda DK. Acupuncture and IVF poor responders: a cure? Fertil Steril 2004; 81: S20.

36. Paulus WE, Zhang M, Strehler E, El-Danasouri I, Sterzik K. Influence of acupuncture on the pregnancly rate in patients who undergo assisted reproduction therapy. Fertil Steril 2002; 77: 721–4.

37. Quintero R. A randomized, controlled, double-blind cross-over study evaluating acupuncture as an adjunct to IVF. Fertil Steril 2002; 81: S11–12.

38. Domar AD. Acupuncture and infertility: we need to stick to good science. Fertil Steril 2006; 85: 1359–61.

39. Paulus WE, Zhang M, Strehler E, Seybold B, Sterzik K. Placebo controlled trial of acupuncture effects in assisted reproductive therapy. Hum Reprod 2003; 18(Suppl 1): xviii18.

40. Dieterle S, Ying G, Hartzmann W, Neuer A. Effect of acunpuncture on the outcome of in vitro fertilization and intracytoplasmic sperm injection: a randomized, prospective, controlled clinical study. Fertil Steril 2006; 85: 1347–51.

41. Stener-Victorin E, Hamaidan P. Use of acupuncture in female infertility and a summary of recent acupuncture studies related to embryo transfer. Acupunct Med 2006; 24: 157–63.

69

The impact of legislation and socioeconomic factors in the access to and global practice of assisted reproduction

Fernando Zegers-Hochschild, Karl G. Nygren, and Osamu Ishihara

INTRODUCTION

Throughout the world, the availability of infertility services is the result of public health policies associated with a variety of socioeconomic, political, and in many occasions, religious influences. Wide disparities exist in the access, quality, and delivery of infertility services within developed countries, but most of all between developed and developing countries. Relatively few of the world's infertile population have complete equitable access to the full range of infertility treatment at affordable levels. Even in wealthy countries, such as Japan and the United States, access to assisted reproductive techniques (ARTs) is, or has been marked by high disparity and inequality in the access to treatment, partly due to high costs and legislative decisions.

Access of men and women to health care and specifically to the treatment of infertility requires not only awareness of being infertile and the knowledge that there are treatment alternatives; large amounts of funds are also required, irrespective of whether they are provided by national health authorities, by individuals themselves, or by a combination of both.

In countries where access to infertility treatment is granted by law, fertility is understood as a right to which all women and men have equal access. Centralized policies are then established to have access to these goods. An example of policies regulating whom and under what conditions is access granted is reflected in the establishment of an age limit of women where treatment will be provided. Another example is a restriction in the number of embryos to be transferred in ART.

When access to infertility treatment is not part of a governmental policy, individuals must rely on their personal wealth and or private insurances covering medical care. Under this scenario, what regulates access to diagnosis and treatment is left to a free market policy, leaving out of reach, all those who cannot afford the costs involved. Furthermore, in most countries, companies providing private health insurances do not cover the costs involved in the treatment of infertility.

Coverage of infertility treatments offers some additional difficulties. While nobody would discuss the use of all available tools to save the lives of people with cancer, the use of modern reproductive technology is controversial and many legislators wonder whether specific treatments should be available or funded to generate a new life. Interestingly, there is much more social acceptance and legislative agreement in saving lives than in generating new ones.

Irrespective as to whether a country is over or under populated, there seems to be less public concern in prolonging the lives of the elder than in generating new young lives.

It is a rule of life that those promoting laws and regulations have already passed by the burden of existing; all they need to worry is the quality of their aging and death. On the other hand, for those who have not yet come to existence there are no chances of influencing policy makers unless the latter themselves have experienced infertility or have been moved by someone with this condition.

Countries around the world either have no regulations or regulate the practice of ART in a variety of different ways. It is the purpose of this chapter, to review how different legislation as well as socioeconomic, demographic, and religious factors influence access to and the way ART is practiced.

Most of the information concerning ART procedures will be related to treatment cycles initiated in 2006.

FACTORS INFLUENCING WORLDWIDE CONTRIBUTION TO ART CYCLES

Information on the number of ART procedures performed is now available thanks to worldwide data collected by the International Committee Monitoring Assisted Reproductive Technology (ICMART) (1,2). While in 2002, 48 countries reported 584,072 cycles, in the year 2006 51 countries reported 848,585 cycles, representing an increment of 33.3% in five years. The major contributor to ART cycles continue to be Europe with

53%, followed by Asia with 20%, and North America with 16% of initiated cycles reported in 2006. In the decade between 1996 and 2006 the number of initiated cycles increased by 70%, however, neither the relative contribution nor the percentage increment in cycles follows a homogeneous pattern, since by 2006, Latin America and the Middle East altogether represented only 4.9% of cycles performed worldwide (Fig. 69.1). In many ways, the proportion of ART cycles is a reflection of a balance between availability and access to this expensive form of infertility treatment.

INEQUALITY IN THE ACCESS TO ART

When access is expressed as the number of ART cycles per million women in reproductive age (25 to 40 years), the proportion of treatment cycles fluctuates between 17,000 and 23,000 cycles per million women in reproductive age in Nordic countries, such as Sweden and Denmark, and between 5000 and 7000 cycles in the United Kingdom and Germany. The disproportion is even greater between European countries and other regions of the world. Using the same calculations, access in United States is 3000 cycles per million, 8000 in Japan. With much low access to ART

treatments, countries in Latin America such as Argentina, Brazil, and Chile, perform between 400 and 1000 cycles per million. Similar numbers are found in other developing countries in the world such as Egypt with 800 cycles per million women in reproductive age.

Another way to look at the disparity in access to treatment in different populations is obtained by looking at the relative proportion of treatments performed in a certain population and its theoretical need. This proportion (Fig. 69.2) is calculated by dividing the number of initiated cycles per country, by the number of women aged 25 to 40 years assuming 10% infertility and 30% of those requiring ART (3% of all women aged 25 to 40 years). Using this calculation, differences between Sweden and Denmark on the one hand and Latin American countries and Egypt are vast. Interestingly, the major source of difference in access to modern reproductive technology does not only lay on the wealth of the country. It is also a reflection of the distribution of wealth. An example is United States, one of the wealthiest countries, with a disproportionate poor access to ART treatments in its population. Another reality is that of Israel where for a mixture of social and geopolitical reasons, access to ART is facilitated to an extent which provides free access to all those in need.

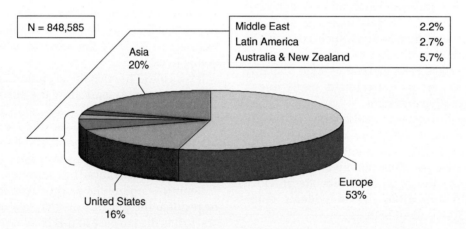

Figure 69.1   Regional contribution of ART cycles to the World Report (2006).

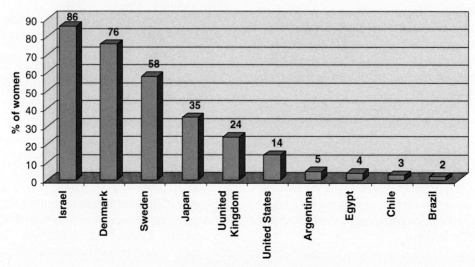

Figure 69.2   Access to ART.

FACTORS AFFECTING ACCESS TO ART

Access to ART can be the result of multiple variables. Table 69.1 describes the relationship between availability of ART and the ways funds allocated to health are distributed among the population. Countries from Northern Europe allocate 13% to 15% of their gross domestic product (GDP) to health expenditure, and more than 80% of it is allocated into public as opposed to private health expenditure. On the other hand, United States, with one of the highest GDP per capita of USD 44,000 also allocates the highest percentage of funds to health (19.1%) but due to a different economic policy, only 46.4% goes to public health expenditure. Countries in Latin America and Egypt are not only much poorer; they also follow trends similar to United States, allocating the majority of their restricted funds into private rather than public health. The consequence of this is that coverage of infertility treatments is reduced in these countries. While in the past, Japan and other Asian countries allocated a high proportion of their GDP to health and most of it as public health expenditure, its low coverage for ART treatments was the result of a political decision to refrain from funding infertility treatments altogether. However, in 2005 and 2006, Japan and Korea respectively introduced a policy consistent in governmental reimbursement for ART treatments, and although ART remains to be privately funded in Japan, approximately 50% to 60% of costs are reimbursed in women under a certain level of income. This resulted in reimbursement of 65,468 out of 190,690 (34.3%) cycles performed in 2008. This policy is in great part responsible for a rise in ART procedures from 125,277 in 2005 to 187,715 in 2008.

An opposite direction has driven Germany, where severe restrictions in public coverage of ART treatments have been imposed, resulting in a drop in the number of initiated cycles from 80,434 in 2003 to 54,695 in 2006. These two realities are a crude reflection that above cultural and ethnic differences, it is economy that has the largest impact in a couple's decision or capacity to use modern reproductive technology to procreate.

The first conclusion would be that access to ART treatment is strongly influenced by socioeconomic policies. Countries where infertility treatment is considered a right, to which all individuals are entitled as equals, distribute their wealth through public facilities and have a much higher coverage of treatments. On the contrary, countries where access to infertility treatments is partly regulated by the market, requiring out of pocket funding, have a much lower coverage of fertility treatments, which in turn, decreases the number of treatment cycles.

ACCESS TO ART TREATMENT AND INSURANCE COVERAGE

Indeed, access to health care and insurance coverage is intimately related. Very few countries in the world have national health plans covering full range of treatment. These are Australia, Belgium, France, Israel, Slovenia, and Sweden. Differences between them reside in the number of ART cycles that are covered by the national health plan and in the regulation imposed to have access to this facility (age limit of the female partner, maximum number of embryos to be transferred, etc.). An interesting observation results from the fact that countries with full coverage also deal with the costs involved in pregnancy, delivery, and neonatal care. Today, single embryo transfer (SET) is the rule in Sweden and in young women in Belgium. Therefore, the costs they have absorbed by covering ART have been compensated by decreasing the number of multiple births and high costs involved in the care of preterm babies. Some other countries in Europe and Middle East have only partial coverage from public sources like the United Kingdom, Denmark, Finland, and Tunisia, and today, Japan and Korea. What is more striking is that in Latin America, a region strongly influenced by Catholic tradition which opposes ART, access to infertility treatments is left out of coverage both by public and private insurances. A minor exception is Chile where 11% of treatment cycles are covered by public insurance. In 2011, the province of Buenos Aires, Argentina mandated free

Table 69.1   Number of ART Cycles (2006) According to Public/Private Health Expenditure (2006)

GDP per capita (dollars)	Country (% general government exp)		Public (%)	Private (%)	ART cycles/million women in reproductive age (25–40 yr)
34–50,000	Sweden	(13.2%)	82.6	17.4	17.527
	Denmark	(14.9%)	84.1	15.9	22.842
	United Kingdom	(15.7%)	81.9	18.1	7.218
	Australia	(17.1%)	66.6	33.4	19.948
	Japan	(17.5%)	81.3	18.7	10.424
44,000	United States	(19.1%)	46.4	53.6	4.130
5–8000	Brazil	(5.1%)	41.7	58.3	557
	Argentina	(14.4%)	55.8	44.2	1.482
	Chile	(14.0%)	42.1	57.9	819
1400	Egypt	(6.4%)	44.2	55.8	1.051

Abbreviations: GDP, gross domestic product; ART, assisted reproductive technique.

coverage of ART treatments to persons having social security, which is a public health system.

When ART treatment is covered by out of pocket funding, it results in a source of inequality and disparity in the availability of health resources. The absence of insurance coverage determines that only wealthy couples can get access to treatment and as will be seen later in this chapter, this factor is strongly associated with high rates of multiple births.

ACCESS TO ART AND DEMOGRAPHIC FACTORS

It is interesting to observe that coverage of infertility treatments in many countries or regions is strongly associated with the mean age of women, the fertility rate (ratio between the number of births and the number of women exposed to the risk of pregnancy), and the population growth rate (the rate at which the number of individuals in a population, increases). Table 69.2 describes in different countries, the association between access to ART, and the median age of the female population, fertility rate, and population growth rate.

Countries having the highest access to ART treatments are those with the lowest population growth rate and highest age of women. In contrast, younger populations with higher fertility rate as in most countries in Latin America and Middle East have less coverage or no coverage at all. Again, as discussed before, Japan has in recent years reacted to the high median age of their female population (almost 45 years) and low population growth rate. As referred before, Japan established a partial reimbursement policy, which immediately increased the use of ART, contributing to the renewal of its population through women who otherwise would have stayed childless or with fewer children than desired.

Perhaps the underlying factor responsible for these disparities is that in countries with an older female population and a negative growth rate, the nation as a whole needs to deal with population renewal. On the contrary, in countries with young female population and high growth rate, it is not the country but the individual who has to deal with his/her reproductive needs. This might perhaps explain why no Latin American countries consider infertility as a disease and therefore, infertility treatments do not fall into the public health agenda.

The desire to have more children is not a national priority in regions with young female population and high fertility rate. Furthermore, in the absence of a legislation regulating the practice of ART, access to fertility treatments is not on the agenda of national health policies and companies responsible for health insurance do not cover expenses related to fertility treatments. Furthermore, for many legislators in Latin America, procedures such as in vitro fertilization (IVF) and ET are considered morally unacceptable and a luxury that should not be sustained with state funds. An extreme example of this moral dictatorship is Costa Rica where the High Courts decided that IVF was morally unacceptable and illegal, forbidding the practice of ART in the country. The result of this policy is that a small proportion of wealthy citizens could afford travelling abroad while the vast majority of couples requiring ART remained childless. It was not until mid-2010 that a group of infertile couples won a pledge against the state of Costa Rica at the Inter American Court of Human Rights. As a result, the court obliged Costa Rica to provide ART treatment in that country. Today, the fight is for a reasonably liberal law regulating the practice of ART in that country.

INFLUENCE OF TRADITION AND RELIGION IN THE PRACTICE OF ART

It is often difficult to ponder the influence of religion, tradition, and other cultural factors in the application of laws regulating reproductive health. The difficulty is not necessarily the result of an imposition of certain religious morality, many times, economic and political forces are strongly bound to religious organizations, which at the end, influence legislative processes.

Christian Tradition

Although religion and public laws have been separated for centuries in countries in Western Europe and the Americas, Christianity, and most of all, the Roman Catholic Church is by far the most outspoken religious body when it comes to moral behavior concerning sex and reproduction. Catholic tradition has a strong influence in Latin America, less in United States, and even though most European countries have more rational,

Table 69.2 Access to ART (2006) According to Age of Female Population and Fertility Rate

Country	Female median age (years)	Total fertility rate	Population growth rate	Access % (25 to 40 yr) ref (Fig. 69.2)
Sweden	42.0	1.66	0.16	58
Denmark	40.7	1.74	0.33	76
United Kingdom	40.4	1.66	0.28	24
Japan	44.7	1.4	0.02	35
United States	37.8	2.09	0.91	14
Brazil	29.0	1.91	1.04	2
Argentina	30.7	2.16	0.96	5
Chile	31.4	2.00	0.94	3
Egypt	24.3	2.83	1.75	4

evidence-based approach to ethics in reproductive health issues, the Catholic tradition can still exert strong influence. A recent example was Italy's law regulating the practice of ART.

The fundamental basis for the Catholic opposition to any form of ART starts in the late 60s, when Pope Paul VI established in his Encyclical Humane Vitae that the uniting and procreative meanings of the conjugal act should not be voluntarily dissociated. Consequently, both contraception and assisted reproduction are considered immoral as they voluntarily dissociate these two meanings; one by allowing sexual intercourse devoid of its procreative meaning, and the other, by allowing procreation not mediated by sexual intercourse. Later, in 1987, the Vatican published a document "Donum Vitae," which contained an "Instruction on respect for human life," issued by the Congregation for the doctrine of faith and signed by Cardinal Joseph Ratzinger, today, Pope Benedict XVI. This document stated that a person, as we understand it, exists from conception onward and therefore, condemned all forms of assisted reproduction, irrespective of its intention, the source of gametes and marital status. This principle carried such power that later, the vast majority of countries in the Americas, signed the "American convention on human rights, pact of Costa Rica" which states that "laws should protect the lives of those to be born – in general – from conception onwards." Based on this principle, the Supreme Court of Costa Rica stopped ART in that country. In the rest of Latin America ART is performed but no laws are available, in spite of the fact that most countries have law projects sitting in their parliaments. In the majority of cases, this is mainly because no agreements are reached between legislators as to whether preimplantation embryos are entitled to rights of their own. Needless to say that any form of embryo manipulation, genetic diagnosis, or research, is performed in few countries without the possibility of discarding abnormal embryos.

The influence of Catholicism concerning ART is less evident in United States, where more value is placed in the right to autonomy, both from the perspective of couples and providers. It must be said, however, that the opposition of U.S. government to therapeutic cloning, and embryonic stem cell research, which lasted until the new president was elected, was mainly the result of lobbying by the Catholic Church under the argument that a preimplantation embryo is entitled with the same rights of an existing person.

For various reasons, the council of bishops in Europe has been more liberal in the application of directives arising from the Vatican. An example is the Catholic University of Leuven, Belgium, where ART, including embryo cryopreservation, is offered openly. A reverse example, however, is the recent law passed in Italy, which forbids fertilization of more than three oocytes, embryo cryopreservation, use of donor gametes, genetic diagnosis, etc. The reason behind this restrictive law is the result of pressure from the Catholic Church on the bases of human rights attributable to embryos from conception onward.

In a different attitude toward reproduction, all protestant denominations (Baptist, Methodist, Lutheran, Mormon, Presbyterian, Episcopalian, and others) are very liberal concerning infertility treatments and the promotion of reproductive science. ART is accepted as long as gametes belong to spouses and embryos are not intended to be destroyed.

Islamic Tradition

Different to religious laws regulating the Western world, Sharia law, which constitutes the bases for Islamic religion also, regulates political, public, and private lives. Its teachings and directions are open for interpretation as science and technology discovers new routes and they serve humankind and society (3).

Concerning reproduction, almost all scholars agree that it is legitimate for infertile couples to pursue any form of therapy as long as both male and female gametes belong to the couple and pregnancy takes place in the woman's uterus (4). Consistent with this concept of genetic heritage, Islam does not approve adoption. Thus, it is the duty of physicians to help infertile couples achieve conception with the freedom to use technology as long as this takes place inside the married couple (5). The embryo is entitled to due respect and genetic diagnosis can be practiced as long as it does not harm the embryo (4). Although law allows for preimplantation genetic diagnosis (PGD) in Islamic countries, couples cannot practice their autonomy to decide upon the fate of their embryos. In Islam, embryos cannot be discarded.

Jewish Tradition

The application of the Jewish tradition is circumscribed to the teachings found in the Torah, subsequently followed by a compilation of traditions and interpretations, such as the Talmud and other ancient religious documents. Israeli laws are secular and rule public affairs while private matters are the domain of Judaic law, enforced by special rabbinical courts. When it comes to procreation, both secular and religious laws are pragmatic and favor the stability and strength of the family and in agreement with the first commandment "Be fruitful and multiply," laws allow almost any form of assisted reproduction. Although marriage and/or a stable relationship are required to have access to ART, single mothers can also receive fertility treatments. Different religious branches of Judaism have marked differences in the interpretation of the law; nonetheless, at the end, the decision to use modern reproductive technology is dealt with freedom by infertile couples and provided by the government. Israeli law allows gamete donation (with strict regulations on the source of male gamete), any form of ART, PGD, even for sex selection, oocyte donation, etc.

Israel holds the highest number of IVF clinics per capita and the National Health Insurance Fund provides IVF treatment for up to two live births for childless couples and for single mothers.

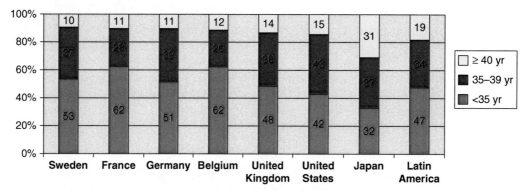

Figure 69.3   Age distribution of patients undergoing ART.

The coexistence of Jewish religion and law represents a remarkable example of equilibrium and tolerance between the strength found in tradition and the need to use science and technology to bear children and strengthen the family.

The purpose of reviewing religious morality is that specially in the developing world, religion can have a strong influence in political decisions. In countries dominated by Catholic tradition, which today are concentrated mainly in Latin America, much of the discussion is not centered in the rights of infertile women and men. On the contrary, most of the discussion is centered on the moral rights of an embryo. As a consequence of the above, ART is accepted because it is there, but no country has been able to reach a consensus on minimal standards to regulate the practice of ART. This lack of pragmatism in confronting biomedical and social realities is at least in part responsible for the low access to treatment generating inequality, lack of autonomy, and therefore absence of diagnostic and therapeutic procedures, such as PGD and other forms of preventing the inheritance of genetic diseases. In countries where the influence of religion in public policies has been restricted, it is the right of persons that prevails in as much as it does not affect the society as a whole.

In general, the more separation there is as to how and who is entitled to impose religious and public laws, the more respect there is for the needs of women, men, and for the children to be born.

HOW LEGISLATION AND CULTURE INFLUENCE THE PRACTICE OF ART

Age of Female Population Receiving ART Treatments

The age of the female partner has a great impact in the outcome of any fertility treatment and therefore in the mean number of embryos transferred. Therefore, when comparing ART policies and outcomes between countries or between different years, it is important to adjust the results by age. In 2006, the proportion of women ≥ 40 yeas ranged from 31% in Japan to 19% in Latin America and only 11% in Sweden (Fig. 69.3). While in Latin America the high proportion of older women probably results from economic variables, in Japan there is a mix of economic, cultural, and demographic reasons. Contrarily, in Nordic

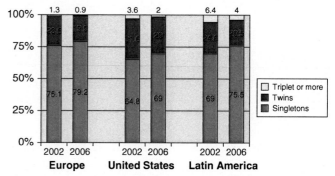

Figure 69.4   Regional variability in multiple birth IVF & ICSI (2002–2006).

countries in Europe, women request infertility treatment much earlier in their life because access is easier. This impacts success rates as well as the way ART is practiced. It is indeed easier to implement programs such as mild controlled ovarian stimulation (COS) protocols and elective single embryo transfers (eSET) in younger and therefore more fertile populations.

But the easiness for access to treatment is not all. Both Sweden and Japan share similar policies toward ETs; in fact, both countries have reached 70% of SET, in spite of major differences in population structure, reimbursement policies, and law.

Number of Embryos Transferred and Multiple Births

The issue of multiple births is one of the most serious complications generated by ART. The risks related to multiple birth do not only involve maternal and perinatal complications, they also generate financial and social problems, the majority of which have to be dealt with by the family alone. The rate of multiple births varies in different countries and regions. For 2006 the proportion of twins and triplets and more in Europe was 20.8%, compared with 24.5% in Latin America, and 31% in the United States. In the past five years, every region has moved in a similar direction, toward reducing the number of embryos transferred (Fig. 69. 4).

Perhaps, the most remarkable difference is in the number of triplets and more, which increased from 0.9% in Europe to 2% in United States and 4% in Latin America. The differences in high order multiple births in Latin

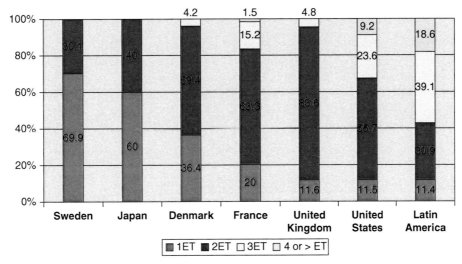

Figure 69.5 Percentage Transfer cycles according to the number of embryos transferred (2006). *Abbreviation:* ET, embryo transfer.

Table 69.3 Source of Funding Influences the Number of Transferred Embryos and High Order Multiple Births (2006)

Source of funding	Country	Mean N° embryos transf.	High order multiple births (%)
Public or private with partial/total reimbursement	Denmark	1.7	0.1
	Sweden	1.3	0[a]
	United Kingdom	1.9	0.3
	France	2.1	0.5
Out of pocket	Brazil	3	4
Out of pocket	Chile	2.5	1.8
Out of pocket + private insurance	United States	2.6	1.8
Out of pocket	Japan	1.4[a]	0
Out of pocket	Australia	1.6	0.4[a]
Out of pocket	Egypt	2.8	2[a]

[a]Data corresponds to cycles performed in 2005 and 2006.

America and United States is in part the result of embryo reduction in the latter.

Reports by the Latin American Registry of ART show that between 1990 and 2009, a total of 92,791 babies were born, 42,290 had cohabitated with at least one other fetus with a direct impact in perinatal mortality, which increased 2.8 times with twin births and 6.4 times with the birth of triplets and 18.7 times with the birth of quadruplets (6).

There is no doubt that the number of embryos transferred has a direct effect on the chances of becoming pregnant, and is the one single factor which by itself increases the risk of multiple gestation and birth. Indeed, this risk also increases as the age of woman decreases. In 2006, 57.7% of transfer cycles in Latin America included three or four embryos; compared with 32.8% in United States, 16.7% in France, 4.8% in the United Kingdom, and none in Sweden and none in Japan in the year 2007 (Fig. 69.5).

Many factors can be responsible for these regional differences, but the pressure for success placed by the couple and their family plays an important role. This pressure increases due to economic constraints. Thus, if for economic reasons, the couple can afford only one treatment cycle, the risk/benefit evaluation of multiple births as opposed to no birth is pondered differently than if couples have six cycles for free. Table 69.3 compares the number of embryos transferred and the proportion of high order multiple births in different countries during 2006. Data is presented according to whether the source of funding was public or out of pocket.

There is no doubt that the most efficient way to decrease the number of multiple births is by reducing the number of embryos transferred and this is easier to do when the high costs are totally or partially covered by public or private sources other than her/his own pocket.

The Experience with eSET in the Nordic Countries and Japan

These two different cultural and ethnic realities have dealt with the burden of multiple births using a similar strategy, which is prioritizing SET. In the case of countries like Sweden, infertile couples receive a substantial reimbursement (approximately 60% of costs) and 70% of transfers are SET while the rest are dual embryo transfers (DET). The results of this policy, implemented in

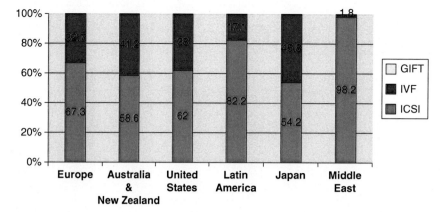

Figure 69.6   Type of assisted fertilization according to region (2006). *Abbreviations*: GIFT, gamete intrafallopian transfer; IVF, in vitro fertilization; ICSI, intracytoplasmic sperm injection.

Sweden and Finland in the early 2000, is that 94.2% of births are singletons, only 5.7% twins, and only 0.1% high order multiple births. It took approximately five years for Japan to start ART treatments in similar directions but in the absence of or with little reimbursement. The main motives to implement the SET policy were its benefit in the prevention of multiple births without severely affecting success rates. Thus, in 2008, 60% to 70% of ART treatments performed in Japan were SET. Differently to the Nordic experience, in Japan, where there are no laws regulating this treatment, it was the Japanese professional society which decided to implement this therapeutic strategy, and it has been followed by the majority of today's 500 institutions providing ART treatments.

Mode of Fertilization – ICSI vs. IVF

Since its introduction, the use of intracytoplasmic sperm injection (ICSI) has increased yearly. Today, in certain regions of the world, ICSI is used in more than 70% of ART cycles. Worldwide, the proportion of ICSI over IVF increased from 24% in 1995 to 56.2% in 2003. However, this proportion has regional variations, which similarly to what happens with the number of embryos transferred, is influenced by different legislations, specially by socioeconomic variables such as who is responsible for the costs of treatment. In countries where ART is subsidized by public funds, the proportion of ICSI is relatively low: 58.6% in Australia and 67.3% in Europe. In regions where ART is paid directly by consumers, the proportion of ICSI rises to over 80% in Latin America and 98.2% in the Middle East (Fig. 69.6) (7,8). Irrespective as to whether it is right or wrong, there is a tendency to avoid unexpected failed fertilization or low fertilization rate with regular IVF; and centers tend to use more ICSI to "ensure" fertilization.

EXAMPLES OF THE EFFECT OF LAWS ON THE OUTCOME OF ART TREATMENTS

Perhaps the best examples of the impact of legislation in the outcomes of ART can be found with the implementation of the new laws in Belgium and twice now in Italy.

The Belgium Example

In July 2003, the Belgium health authorities introduced legislation to improve financial access to ART treatments and to reduce multiple births. The main decision included that laboratory costs would be refunded for six cycles in a lifetime for women under the age of 43 years. This benefit is conditioned by the number of embryos that can be transferred, which varies from one to three depending on the age of women and the cycle number. Furthermore, it obliges each center to report all its data to a centralized registry who can evaluate trends. This policy not only eliminates inequality in access, it also decreases the risks of multiple births. In this way, the reduced neonatal costs should be enough to cover the costs of treatment.

This is perhaps one of the best examples on how a legislative body examines the available data and implements a solution that brings equality and benefit to all members of society. Belgium is a multireligious community cohabiting with a proportion of nonreligious community. The important fact is that this policy does not enter in the philosophical discussion of when does personhood begin. On the contrary, it looks at the economic, social, and biologic evidence with pragmatism and implements a legislation that can deal with them in the best possible way, allowing individuals to decide by themselves. The consequences of this legislation are still in evaluation, but so far, at least two conclusions can be extracted. First, the policy does not jeopardize the chances of a couple to have a baby. It can take more cycles to achieve the goal, but the cumulative birth rate is not affected. Second, there is a marked reduction in the rate of multiple births. A good review of this data can be found in a publication by L. van Landuyt (9).

The Italian Example

In March 2004 a new Italian law imposed a number of limitations to the medical profession and to infertile couples. In fact, no more than three oocytes could be inseminated because no more than three embryos could be generated. Furthermore, all embryos needed to be transferred since embryo cryopreservation, PGD, or any form of embryo manipulation was not allowed. In a different dimension, only married couples or heterosexual couples living a stable relationship, had access to ART treatment. No treatment is available for gay couples or single women.

This law establishes the right of an embryo over the rights of her and/or his progenitor. This is especially confusing in a country where the termination of a clinical pregnancy is legal. Furthermore, by restricting ART to only married and cohabiting, heterosexual couples, it specifically discriminates against infertile women since if they were fertile, they could become pregnant without requiring a stable heterosexual relationship. This discrimination is only restricted to those infertile women requiring ART; since infertile women are not required to have a heterosexual stable partner to have access to ovarian stimulation or pelvic surgery or any other form of infertility treatment. The ethical and clinical implications of this law have been discussed by Benagiano and Gianaroli (10).

Fortunately, after extensive lobbying and the use of scientific evidences, the right of women and men prevailed and in May 2009 the Italian Constitutional Court declared that the statement "the prevision of the creation of a number of embryos in any case not exceeding three and the mandatory transfer of all the embryos created for a maximum of three" was "unconstitutional." Today, the law says "ART techniques must not create a number of embryos exceeding the one strictly necessary," entrusting the decision of the right number of embryos to be created to the doctor, according to different patients' conditions.

With the Italian national registry created in 2005, it will now be possible to evaluate the effect on multiple births and success rates of the restrictive law passed in 2004 and at the same time, evaluate its reversal in 2009 (Giulia Scaravelli MD, personal communication).

These examples represent two different ways of legislating in areas related with sex and reproduction.

In the Italian experience in 2004, the main intention of legislators was to defend a moral principle "The respect of a person from conception (fertilization) onwards"; irrespective of the effects this might cause in actual persons (men and women) in the family and in society.

In the Belgian experience the main intention of legislators was to defend the right of actual persons to receive medical treatments. It was also an objective to protect the quality of life of those to be born by facilitating the birth of singletons.

There is a world tendency to procure safety over efficacy by lowering the number of embryos transferred, even if this decreases the overall pregnancy rates, particularly in countries where access to ART is guaranteed or at least facilitated by public resources. In the search for safety, a SET policy has been established in Sweden, Finland, and Belgium. There is more than one strategy to reach this goal, and these three countries have arrived to a SET policy by different roads.

In Sweden, currently in the lead of the SET transition, 70% of all ETs are now SET, with the eradication of triplets, and a reduction of twinning from over 25% before, to now only 5%. This transition is a result of a combination of several factors – a professional decision, soon supported by the national patient organization, and later followed by governmental regulation. The process took four years, from 2002 to 2005.

The main factor behind this move was a cooperative effort between the professional societies of gynecologists and pediatricians and governmental authorities, where the medical risks for IVF children were thoroughly investigated. A national IVF register of all women giving birth after IVF was formed and, using the personal identification number given to each Swedish citizen, crosslinks were made to five different population-based health registers already in operation. Very convincing evidence emerged, showing that the much higher risk profile of IVF children was caused not by the IVF technique per se, but to an elevated multiple delivery rates. A large randomized clinical study followed by national data demonstrated that pregnancy rates did not drop after a substantial increase in the proportion of SET. This finally made the case for SET as the norm. A very important driver for the transitions was the backup by the lay press.

In the midst of this process the law was changed to say that SET must be the norm. The change of law merely confirmed what was already happening, and was therefore welcomed in the country. Discussion on economy was never involved.

In Finland, the transition to SET as the norm was the result of professional decision only, with no governmental interference, and again economy was not an issue.

In Belgium, on the other hand, economical arguments on high national costs for postnatal health care of prematurely born multiple birth IVF children convinced the government to change reimbursement policies to strongly favor SET.

There is thus not one single road to procure an equilibrium between safety and efficacy; in this case through the SET policy: in Sweden, national data on safety and efficacy, followed by governmental regulation of the practice of IVF did it, in Finland the same process but with no governmental intervention, and in Belgium a change of governmental reimbursement policies. But the effect is the same: a much-reduced risk for the children.

The most recent example of a national change toward a balance between safety and efficacy has been established in Japan. In contrast with the Nordic countries, reimbursement in Japan covers less than 40% of ART cycles, 30% of women are ≥40 years compared to 11% in Sweden and Finland, and a large proportion of women receive mild forms of COS which include clomiphene citrate and alternative injections of human menopausal gonadotropin (hMG) or rFSH. Similarly to what took place in Sweden, in Japan there are no laws regulating the practice of ART. The Japanese Society of Obstetrics Gynecology took the decision and the vast majority of institutions followed its recommendation.

It is interesting to note that countries where the influence of religious morality is well balanced by strong and independent lay organizations, laws tend to follow realistic and sensible evaluation of reality and public decisions are adopted after incorporating the lay public and society as equals in the discussion of public policies. On the contrary, countries with strong religious influence, tend to moralize in such a way that the value of embryos become the dominating issue overlooking the rights of actual persons, in this case, infertile couples in the pursue of effective and safe treatment of infertility.

The examples of the Nordic countries in contrast with countries in Latin America and now Italy are true reflection of this reality.

REFERENCES

1. Adamson GD, de Mouzon J, Lancaster P, et al. World collaborative report on in vitro fertilization, 2000. International Committee for Monitoring Assisted Reproductive Technology (ICMART). Fertil Steril 2006; 85: 1586–622.
2. De Mouzon J, Lancaster P, Nygren KG, et al. International Committee for Monitoring Assisted Reproductive Technology (ICMART). World Collaborative Report on Assisted Reproductive Technology 2002. Hum Reprod 2009; 1: 1–11.
3. Serour GI. Traditional sexual practices in Islamic world. Global Bioethics 1995; 1: 35–47.
4. Yepren S. Current assisted reproduction treatment practices from an Islamic perspective. Reprod BioMed Online 2007; 14(Suppl 1): 44–7.
5. Serour GI. Medically assisted conception dilemma of practice and research. Islamic views. In: Serour GI, ed. Proceedings of the First International Conference on Bioethics in Human Reproduction Research in the Muslin World. Cairo. Egypt, 11CPSR 2, 1992; 235–42.
6. Zegers-Hochschild F, Schwarze JE, Crosby J, do Carmo Borges de Souza M. Twenty years of assisted reproductive technology (ART) in Latin America. JBRA Assist Reprod 2011; 15: 19–30.
7. Nygren KG, De Mouzon J, Adamson D, et al. World preliminary report on ART 2006. In: 26th Annual Meeting of ESHRE. Rome: Italy, 2010.
8. De Mouzon J, Goossens V, Bhattacharya S, et al. The European IVF-monitoring (EIM) Consortium, for the European Society of Human Reproduction and Embryology (ESHRE). Assisted Reproductive Technology in Europe, 2006: results generated from European Registers by ESHRE. Hum Reprod 2010; 25: 1851–62.
9. Van Landuyt L, Verheyen G, Tournaye H, et al. New Belgian embryo transfer policy leads to sharp decrease in multiple pregnancy rate. Reprod BioMed Online 2006; 13: 765–71.
10. Benagiano G, Gianaroli L. The new Italian IVF legislation. Reprod BioMed Online 2004; 9: 117–25.

70

Religious perspectives in human reproduction

Raphael Ron-El and Botros Rizk

Religion is an outcome of beliefs and heritage, which are strongly related to history and folklore that are influenced by environment, education, and interaction between people. Based on this definition, there is no wonder that views are different from one to another religion which is part of human culture. This is true, also, when it comes to procreation, especially in what is connected to human reproduction in nonnatural ways.

Since the extraordinary achievement of a baby by extracorporeal fertilization by Edwards and Steptoe in 1978, (1) the argument between the different views on the matter of human reproduction in the nonnatural ways has tremendously increased.

The core of the differences among the religions lies in the definition of what is a "human being." Is it an oocyte or sperm, or is a zygote (fertilized oocyte) a human being? Is a cleaved fertilized oocyte, i.e., two- or four-cell stage embryo, a human being? Or can a blastocyst or a fetus without or with heartbeats be defined as a human being?

Christianity claims that an embryo and fetus are considered as persons. Research on embryos, cryopreservation, and abortion is strongly disapproved (2,3). According to the Judaism, the Jewish religion, the embryo is considered to be mere water until the fortieth day when the soul enters the body (Yevamot 69 b, the Babylonian Talmud). This means that here the human being is defined as such on the eighth week of pregnancy (4). In Islam, the fetus is first a "Nutfa" for 40 days, then an "Alaqa" for 40 days, and last a "Mudgha " for another 40 days. At the end of this period of 120 days the soul enters the body (5). The old threshold of 40 days and upward from conception has been brought back to 14 days, because the new embryology has established this embryonic period of cellular activity before which individuation cannot begin.

In Hinduism, the soul is eternal. It has to live many earthly lives to purify itself to reach perfection and higher state of existence called "Mokasa." In Buddhism, the long string of reincarnation and final purification of the soul which enters in a superior state into the body is called "Nirvana."

Is the zygote or embryo a human being? This question is a real basis for discussion among ethicists. Dr Iglesias, a Roman Catholic philosopher (6), claims that an embryo is a biological entity with the potentiality of morality and personality. Thus, given that the embryo has this potentiality, it should be considered as a human being from the very beginning of its creation. Dr Mill (7) completely opposes this concept by stressing that an embryo, being a biological entity, has a long process of developing to the stage of morality. Morality means the attitude of a person to another person and or toward its environment process. As long the embryo has no morality, it is a biological material, a result of fusion of two biological gametes, not a human being.

Since this definition of "human being" is also not the same in every religion (8), there is a clear diversity of permissions up to when manipulation can be performed on gametes, embryo, or fetus. Moreover, the permissions vary from section to section in the same religion. All religions, anyhow, accept the principle that manipulation is prohibited on human beings.

CHRISTIANITY

The Christians in the world today are divided into more than 700 million Catholic, 325 million Protestants of different denominations, and 200 million Orthodox Christians.

The Roman (Catholic) Church

The main laws of the Catholic Church emerge from: The holy book, the Bible, and the "Tradition," which are the Church's decisional boards, priests, and dogmatic teachings.

According to the latter, the three leading principles related to the family, the child, and reproduction are:

1. The protection of the human being from the moment of its conception;
2. God commands husband and wife to have children. The child is the fruit of marriage;
3. Integrity and dignity norms must be taken into consideration in all these matters.

In 1956, the Pope Pius XII reemphasized these principles by stating that artificial fecundation is immoral and illegal, because it separates procreation and sexual normal functions of the married couple.

Therefore, it was clear that the procedures of infertility treatment as intrauterine insemination (IUI), in vitro fertilization (IVF), intracytoplasmic sperm injection (ICSI), embryo transfer (ET), and surrogate motherhood are not accepted. Moreover, the Catholic Church offers its respect and protection to the human being, starting with its first seconds of existence; it considers the embryo and fetus as persons and strongly disapproves research on embryos, cryopreservation, and abortion. Some of the mentors of the Catholic Church consider even the zygote as human being, as was mentioned by Dr. Iglesias (6).

The Eastern Orthodox Church

In a critical moment in Church history, the Church began to be pulled in two directions along the lines of East and West. At that time "East" meant Greece, Asia, Alexandria, and the Middle East and "West" referred to Europe. The causes of this rift were many, among which were language and culture, Latin versus Greek (9).

In 1054, Patriarch Michael Cerularius refused to recognize the Church of Rome's claim to be the head and mother of the churches. As Pope Leo IX had died, Cardinal Humbert excommunicated Cerularius, while Cerularius in return excommunicated Cardinal Humbert.

Thus, the "East–West Schism," or "The Great Schism," divided Christianity into the Eastern (Greek) Orthodox Church and the Roman (Latin) Catholic Church.

The primary locations of Orthodoxy in the world today are: Greece, Russia, Eastern Europe, Egypt, and the Middle East as in Syria, Lebanon, Palestine, and Israel. The Orthodox Church is larger in number than any of the Protestant denominations individually.

The Eastern (Greek) Orthodox Church is not as strict as the Roman (Latin) Catholic Church.

It allows the medical and surgical treatment of infertility, including IUI, but is against IVF and other assisted reproductive techniques (ARTs), surrogate motherhood, and sperm and embryo donation.

The Protestant Church

Protestants vary in their beliefs on IVF. Unlike the Catholic Church, there is not one set of ethical guidelines for Protestant couples to follow regarding the use of ART.

Those who support IVF, limit its use to married couples. All the embryos must be replaced into the uterus, meaning that no embryo wastage is permitted. Selective reduction is not allowed (10).

The Anglican Church

The Anglican Church, allows ARTs, IVF, and ET and allows the use of sperm obtained after masturbation. However, it forbids gamete donation.

The Anglican Church does not see the embryo with a moral status. A moral status can only be given to an individual with a well established personality. This attitude toward the status of the zygote and embryo is,

of course, a major difference from the other churches, which permits the manipulation of the zygote, embryo, and blastocyst.

The Coptic Church

The word "copt" derives from the Greek Aigyptios "Egyptian" via Coptic kyptaios and Arabic Qibti. Aigyptios derives from hikaptah, house of the Ka (spirit) of Ptah, one of the names for Memphis, the first capital of Ancient Egypt (11). The Arabs, upon arriving to Egypt in 640 A.D., called Egypt dar al Qibt (home of the Egyptians) and since Christianity was the official religion of Egypt, the word Qibt came to refer to the practitioners of Christianity as well as to the inhabitants of the Nile Valley.

The first book on the opinion of the Coptic Orthodox Church on IVF and transfer of embryos was published by His Grace, the late Bishop Gregorios, the Bishop of theological studies, Coptic culture, and scientific research (12). The introduction of his book starts by ascertaining that the success of IVF represents a great success for science by alleviating a great obstacle for married couples wishing to conceive a child. Although having children is not the only reason for marriage, it represents nature's first goal of marriage in all beings including humans. He fully acknowledges that motherhood is the strongest instinct that a woman could have and that having children is the first wish for any mother and certainly infertile women are among the unhappiest people even if they were married to the richest, wealthiest, and most famous. He also acknowledges that the success of IVF has brought happiness to thousands of married couples and settled lives among many families.

The second chapter focuses on the pitfalls of IVF and assisted conception. He emphasizes that a key issue is the fertilization of a woman's oocyte by her husband's sperm, and extreme accuracy should be exercised in this important issue. He stresses the role of the treating physician in honesty so that there is no question that fertilization has occurred between the husband and wife and not any third party. He acknowledges that in certain situations fertilization might not occur but does not accept that fertilization should be attempted between the wife's oocyte and any other man's spermatozoa, whether it is from a known or unknown donor. He does not accept the establishment of embryo banks and the buying and selling of gametes with money. This is fully unacceptable because it brings down the relation of the value of marriage and conception and having children to a low level.

ISLAM

The teaching of Islam covers all the fields of human activity; spiritual and material, individual and social, educational and cultural, economic and political, and national and international. Instruction which regulates everyday activity of life to be adhered to by good Muslims is called Sharia. There are two sources of Sharia in Islam: primary and secondary. The primary sources of Sharia in chronological order are: The Holy Quran, the very word of God, the Sunna and Hadith, which are the authentic traditions and sayings of the Prophet Mohamed. The secondary sources of Sharia are Istihsan, the choice of one of several lawful options, views of Prophet's companions, current local customs, if lawful; public welfare and rulings of previous divine religions if they do not contradict the primary sources of Sharia. A good Muslim resorts to secondary sources of Sharia in matters not dealt with in the primary sources. Even if the action is forbidden, it may be undertaken if the alternative would cause harm. The Sharia is not rigid. It is flexible enough to adapt to emerging situations in different items and places. It can accommodate different honest opinions as long as they do not conflict with the spirit of its primary sources and are directed to the benefit of humanity (11,13–15). Islam is a religion of Yusr (ease) not Usr (hardship) as indicated in the Holy Quran (16). The Broad Principles of Islamic Jurisprudence are permissibility unless prohibited by a text, (Ibaha), no harm and no harassment; necessity permits the prohibited and the choice of the lesser harm. ART was not mentioned in the primary sources of Sharia. However, these same sources have affirmed the importance of marriage, family formation, and procreation (11). Adoption is not acceptable as a solution to the problem of infertility. Islam gives legal precedence to purity of lineage and known parenthood of all children. The Quran explicitly prohibits legal adoption but encourages kind upbringing of orphans (17).

In Islam, infertility and its remedy with the unforbidden is allowed and encouraged. The prevention and treatment of infertility are of particular significance in the Muslim World. The social status of the Muslim women, her dignity, and self-esteem are closely related to her procreation potential in the family and in the society as a whole. Childbirth and rearing are regarded as family commitments and not just biological and social functions. As ART was not mentioned in the primary sources of Sharia, patients and Muslim doctors alike thought that by seeking ART for infertility treatment, they are challenging God's will trying to make the barren woman fertile, and handling human gametes and embryos. ART was only widely accepted after prestigious scientific and religious bodies and organizations issued guidelines that were adopted by Medical Councils or concerned authorities in different Muslim countries and controlled the practices in ART centers.

These Guidelines which played a role in the change of attitude of society and individuals in the Muslim World included Fatwa from Al-Azhar, Cairo (1980) (7), and Fatwa from Islamic Fikh Council, Mecca (1984), the Organization of Islamic Medicine in Kuwait (1991), Qatar University (1993), the Islamic Education, science and culture organization in Rabaat (2002), the United Arab Emirate (2002), and the International Islamic Center for population studies and research, Al Azhar University (14–19). These bodies stressed the fact that Islam encouraged marriage, family formation, and procreation in its primary sources. Treatment of infertility, including ART when indicated, is encouraged to preserve humankind within the frame of marriage, in otherwise incurable infertility.

In family affairs, particularly reproduction, the decisions are usually taken by the couple. However, not uncommonly the husband's decision is the dominating one. Today the basic guidelines for ART in the Muslim World are: If ART is indicated in a married couple as a necessary line of treatment, it is permitted during validity of marriage contract with no mixing of genes. If the marriage contract has come to an end because of divorce or death of the husband, artificial reproduction cannot be performed on the female partner even using sperm cells her former husband. The Shi'aa Guidelines has "opened' the way to a third party donation, via Fatwa from Ayatollah Ali Hussein Khomeini in 1999. This Fatwa allowed third party participation including egg donation, sperm donation, and surrogacy. The Fatwa is gaining acceptance in parts of the Shi'ite world. Recently, there has been some concern about sperm donation among Shi'aa. All these practices of third party participation in reproduction are based on the importance of maintaining the family structure and integrity among the Shi'aa family. They are allowed within various temporary marriage contract arrangements with the concerned donors.

Surrogacy is not Permitted

Cryopreservation is permitted and the embryos may be transferred to the same wife in a successive cycle but only during the validity of the marriage contract (7,8,16–18). The strict view is that marriage ends at death, and procuring pregnancy in an unmarried woman is forbidden.

Multifetal pregnancy, particularly high order multifetal pregnancy (HOMP) should be prevented in the first place. Should HOMP occur, in spite of all preventive measures, then multifetal pregnancy reduction may be performed applying the jurisprudence principles of necessity that permits the prohibited and the choice of the lesser harm. Multifetal pregnancy reduction is only allowed if the prospect of carrying the pregnancy to viability is small. Also it is allowed if the life or the health of the mother is in jeopardy (16,20–22). It is performed with the intention not to induce abortion but to preserve the life of remaining fetuses and minimize complications to the mother.

Embryo research, for advancement of scientific knowledge and benefit of humanity, is therefore allowed before 14 days after fertilization on embryos donated for research with the free informed consent of the couple. However, these embryos should not be replaced in the uterus.

Sex Selection

The use of sperm sorting techniques or preimplantation genetic diagnosis (PGD) for nonmedical reasons such as sex selection or balancing sex ratio in the family is forbidden. However, universal prohibition would itself risk prejudice to women in many present societies, especially while births of sons remain central to women's well-being. Sex ratio balancing in the family is considered acceptable, for instance, where a wife had borne three or four daughters or sons and it was in her and her family's best interests that another pregnancy should be her last. Employing sex selection techniques to ensure the birth of a son or a daughter might then be approved, to satisfy a sense of religious or family obligation and to save the woman from increasingly risk-laden pregnancies (18,19). Application of PGD or sperm sorting techniques for sex selection should be disfavored in principle, but resolved on its particular merits with guidelines to avoid discrimination against either sex, particularly the female child.

The possibility of postmenopausal pregnancy is now possible using one's own cryopreserved embryos or even oocytes and possible in future cryopreserved ovaries.

JUDAISM

At Mount Sinai, 3500 years ago, The "Torah" was given to Moses who had to deliver it to the people of Israel. The Torah is viewed as a single divine text that includes moral values and practical laws. The first commandment out of the 10 in the Torah instructs the people to "Be Fruitful and Multiply, fill the earth and subdue it" (20).

The Torah brings the story of infertility and its impact of the life of family. The first known story was of Sara who asked Abraham to marry her maid servant to enable him fatherhood.

The second story was of Rachel who used desperate measures. She declared to Jacob: "Give me children, otherwise I am dead." Rachel's next act was even more desperate. Reuven, the firstborn son of Leah, brought to his mother some plants known to enhance conception "dudaim" (21). Rachel begged her sister for the plants and made a deal: she would allow Leah to spend one night with Jacob in return for the plants. Lea's fifth-born son was the result of this deal. Rachel was finally "remembered" by God and she conceived and bore Joseph. She then stated: "God has taken away my disgrace."

The commandment and the knowledge that the soul enters the body at 40 days of gestation cause, in the Jewish tradition, to use and promote the fertility treatments when needed. Thus, ovulation induction and all ART are permitted. The orthodox Jewish legal system supports the constant questioning process which takes place when a new situation arises.

Therefore, the Orthodox Jews, who are about 15% of the inhabitants in Israel, consult themselves with the Rabbi to get his advice on what treatment should they take for their specific problem, also if a treatment was already suggested and discussed by their physician (4). The Rabbi's views on the suggested treatment, may not always coincide with those of the physician. A Jewish couple will definitely ask for the Rabbi's advice when it comes to decide to accept gamete donation or surrogacy.

Selective reduction is acceptable as the goal is to enhance the possibility of life as determined by doctors. Embryo research to promote life is acceptable. Therapeutic cloning is acceptable and even obligatory to do

research which can promote life-saving treatment (e.g., stem cell and cellular replacement therapy).

However, there are some controversial issues. Among them, spilling of seed in vain is forbidden. Some Rabbis insist that the husband should not ejaculate to provide semen specimen. Therefore, the knowledge about sperm quality will come only via sperm sampling extracted from the vagina following an intercourse. Collection of sperm for therapeutic procedure will be permitted by collection of sperm following an intercourse performed with a condom without antisperm agents (medical condom). The Talmud (the written instructions collected over the years from verbal tradition) specifically forbids "cutting the sperm ducts." Therefore, most of the Rabbis will not permit in cases of azoospermia the biopsy from the testes but would prefer the trial of aspiration from the testes. Only when aspiration results in no sperm, they would allow performing a biopsy (22).

Gamete donation is another debatable issue. There is no clear announcement from Rabbinic authorities. Most Rabbis will not allow sperm or egg donation. It is not adultery but strongly discouraged. However, if the Rabbi is convinced that this will be the only way to enable the couple parenthood, some Rabbis will agree on it. In this way, the couple has to search for the "right Rabbi," namely, the more open minded one.

If donor sperm is allowed and since Jewishness is conferred through the mother's side, most conservative Rabbis will prefer a non-Jewish donor sperm to prevent adultery between a Jewish man and a Jewish woman and to prevent future genetic incest among the offspring of anonymous donors.

It is well known that the ancient Israelis were divided into three sections according to the function of their antecedents fulfilled in the Temple: Kohen, Levi, and Israel. The Kohanim were the more prestigious people who were eligible to enter the holy holiest in the temple and bless the present prayers. Since the destruction of the Temple, the blessing of the Kohanim entered as part of the pray in the Synagogue. When an orthodox Jew who is a Kohen who needs to use donor sperm, he has the right to perform gendering on the resulting embryos to have a girl. In this way, he will not have consciously disgrace by risking the prayers with a blessing given by his virtual son from the donor sperm who is not a Kohen. This issue of gendering for this religious indication was decided by the Israeli Ministry of Justice in 2006. The Israeli Ministry of Health also permits gendering in couples who have at least four children of the same sex, once a national committee for sex selection for nonmedical reason has approved it in light of decided guidelines.

Recently, some Rabbis decided to permit egg donation with oocytes of non-Jewish donors. Again, the reason is to prevent incest among the offspring. They overcame the problem of conferring the Jewishness through the mother's side by deciding that the Jewish religion will be conferred by the religion of the parturient.

Surrogacy is still debatable. For the Rabbis who allow it, single Jewish women are preferred as surrogates, both

Table 70.1   The Permitted Procedures of Assisted Reproductive Techniques (ARTs) in the Different Religions

	IUI	IVF\ICSI	PGD	Surrogacy	Gamete donation	Fetal reduction
Christianity						
Catholic	No	No	No	No	No	No
Greek Orthodox	Yes	No	No	No	No	No
Protestant	Yes	Yes	No	No	No	No
Anglicans	Yes	Yes	No	No	No	No
Coptic	Yes	Yes	Yes	No	No	No
Judaism	Yes	Yes	Yes	Yes	Yes[a]	Yes[b]
Islam	Yes	Yes	No	No	No	Yes[b]

[a]Some of the Rabbis will agree on – sperm donation from a non-Jewish donor; - egg donation from a divorced woman.
[b]In cases with risk to mother's health.
Abbreviations: IUI, intrauterine insemination; IVF, in vitro fertilization; ICSI, intracytoplasmic sperm injection; PGD, preimplantation genetic diagnosis.

to avoid the implications of adultery for married surrogate women and to confer Jewishness through a Jewish woman's gestation of the fetus.

In summary, the procedures that are currently used in ART are not universally permitted in the three religions: Christianity, Islam, and Judaism. Table 70.1 shows the procedures and their availability according to different religions.

CURRENT PERMISSIONS FOR ART IN DIFFERENT COUNTRIES

The availability of different procedures of ARTs varies from country to country according to the relationships between the religion, laws, and traditions in each place as appears in Table 70.2.

This diversity of permissions for reproductive treatments causes patients to search for their desired treatment outside the boundaries of their home country. Thus, a huge movement of "Cross Border Reproductive Care," which is called also Medical Tourism started to be established (23).

With globalization doctors and patients alike are moving around to different parts of the world; it becomes not uncommon that physicians may have to provide medical services to patients with ethical precepts, which are different from that of their own. However, conscientious objection to offer certain required treatment to patients by their physicians should not deprive them from the right of being referred to other physicians who would provide such treatment. It becomes, therefore, mandatory to be aware of various religious perspectives on various practices.

The main desired treatments in this Cross Border Reproductive Care are mainly gamete donations, gendering, surrogacy, and treatments in postmenopausal and homosexual patients. In the last years this phenomenon has tremendously increased. For this reason more and more professional meetings, bylaws, and instructions are coming out by professional societies, governments, parliaments, and courts in different parts in the world.

Table 70.2   Procedures that Are Not Permitted in Some of the European Countries

Forbidden procedures	Countries	Limitations
Access to ART	France	Singles, Lesbians
	NL	Age >41 yr
Sperm donation	France	Singles, Lesbians
Oocyte donation	Germany	
	Italy	
	Norway	
TESE\PESA	NL	Limited to only 2 clinics
		Since 2007 – part of research program
PGD	Germany	Permitted only in PB
	NL	Except for: - one center (Maastricht)
		- BRCA
Surrogacy	Germany	
	Norway	
	Spain	
Embryo freezing	Italy[a]	
	Germany	

[a]Recently, the court instructed to enable the freezing procedure.
Abbreviations: TESE, testicular sperm extraction; PESA, percutaneous epididymal sperm aspiration; PGD, preimplantation genetic diagnosis.

Epilogue

On 14 October 2010 the Nobel Assembly in Sweden announced that the 2010 Nobel Prize in Physiology or Medicine was awarded to Dr Robert G Edwards for his achievements in IVF. The Roman Catholic Church reacted to the announcements by couple of declarations. Monsignor Carrasco de Paula said that the decision of the Nobel Prize Committee was completely wrong. Without the achievements of Dr Edwards there would not have been huge trade of millions of oocytes, full freezers of embryos, and surrogates waiting for them (24).

Also other prominent persons from Catholic Universities and catholic members of the European Parliament have criticized the choice of Dr Edwards for the same arguments (25).

Benagiano et al. (26) tries to combat these arguments with the following facts. First, by analyzing the treatment given to achieve the pregnancy of Louise Brown, only one oocyte was collected to achieve one embryo, which was transferred to the uterus. This was the original target of Dr Edwards. Not only this, Dr Edwards always preached in his presentations in professional meetings, to reduce the intense ovarian stimulations, which indeed were the ideological and professional basis for the "soft" ovarian stimulation of today. The fact that many embryos are created with the IVF treatments was a later phenomenon, when centers had the emerging interest to improve the rates of pregnancies achieved. The second argument, which is also discussed in the forward of this chapter, is that theology cannot resolve the issue when ensoulment takes place in the human being. Certainly, when a "human life-form" becomes a "potential human person," he must be protected (27).

In conclusion, the diversity in the approaches of the different religions to the definition of a "human being" is still a valid argument for endless debates. However, the strength of the technology of extracorporeal procreation, with all the problematic questions that have been raised and the strong natural desire of having offspring demand all involved parts to continue enabling the couples who need our help to give them our support and aid.

ACKNOWLEDGMENT

The authors wish to thank Hassan N. Sallam, MD, FRCOG, PhD (London), Professor and Chair, Department of Obstetrics and Gynecology, The University of Alexandria, for his excellent contribution toward the writing of this chapter.

REFERENCES

1. Steptoe PC, Edwards RG. Birth after reimplantation of human embryo. Lancet 1978; 12: 366.
2. Singer P, Wells D. In vitro fertilization: the major issues. J med Ethics 1983; 9: 192.
3. Abou Abdalla M. The Vatican view on human procreation: Religious perspectives of ethical issues in infertility and ART Chapter 73. In: Rizk B, Garcia-Velasco J, Sallam HN, Makrigiannakis A, eds. Infertility and Assisted Reproduction. Cambridge, UK: Cambridge University Press, 2008: 741–5.
4. Silber SJ. Infertility, IVF and Judaism: Religious perspectives of ethical issues in infertility and ART Chapter 73. In: Rizk B, Garcia-Velasco J, Sallam HN, Makrigiannakis A, eds. Infertility and Assisted Reproduction. Cambridge, UK: Cambridge University Press, 2008: 728–31.
5. Serour GI. Ismamic perspectives of ethical issues in ART: religious perspectives of ethical issues in infertility and ART Chapter 73. In: Rizk B, Garcia-Velasco J, Sallam HN, Makrigiannakis A, eds. Infertility and Assisted Reproduction. Cambridge, UK: Cambridge University Press, 2008: 737–40.
6. Iglesias T. In vitro fertilization: the major issues. J med ethics 1984; 10: 32–7.
7. Mills JE. Some comments to Iglesias's paper, 'in vitro fertilisation: the major issues'. J Med Ethics 1986; 12: 32–5.
8. Dunstan GR. The moral status of the human embryo: a tradition recalled. J Med Ethics 1984; 10: 38.
9. Dunaway M. What is the Orthodox Church? A Brief Overview of Orthodoxy. Ben Lomond, CA: Conciliar Press, 1995.
10. Mohler A. Christian Morality and Test Tube Babies, Part II. [Available from: www.albertmohler.com].
11. Serour GI. Ethical considerations of assisted reproductive technologies: A Middle Eastern Perspective. Opin Middle East Fertile Soc J 2000; 5: 1–13.
12. Bishop Gregorios HG. The Christian Opinion in In vitro Fertilization and Embryo Transfer. Bisphoric of Higher Studies. Cairo, Egypt: Coptic Culture and Scientific Research Publications, 1988.
13. Gad El-Hak AGH. In vitro fertilization and test tube baby. Dar El Iftaa Cairo Egypt 1980; 1225: 1:115: 3213–3228.
14. Gad El Hak AGE, Serour GI, ed. Some gynecological problems in the context of Islam. The International Islamic Center for Population Studies and Research. Cairo: Al Azhar University, 2000.
15. Serour GI. Attitudes and cultural perspective on infertility and its alleviation in the middle east area. In: Vaycnna E, ed. Current Practices and Controversies in Assisted Reproduction. Report of WHO Meeting. Geneva: WHO, 2002: 41–9.
16. Sura Al Bakara 2: 185, Holy Quaraan.
17. Sura Al Ahzab 32: 4–5, Holy Quraan.
18. Scrour GI. Transcultural issues in gender selection. In: Daya S, Harrison R, Kampers R, eds. Recent Advances in Infertility and Reproductive Technology. International Federation of Fertility Societies (IFFS) 18th World Congress on Fertility and Sterility, Montreal: Elsevier, 2004.
19. Serour GI. Family and sex selection. In: Healy DL, ed. Reproductive Medicine in the Twenty-First Century. Proceedings of the 17th World Congress on Fertility and Sterility. Melbourne, Australia: The Parthenon Publishing Group, 2002: 97–106.
20. Genesis 1: 28.
21. Genesis 30: 14.
22. Schenker JG. Assisted reproductive practice: religious perspectives. RBM online 2005; 3: 310.
23. Pennings G. International evolution of legislation and guidelines in medically assisted reproduction. RBM Online 2009; 21: 159.
24. ANSA News Agency, Nobel al padre della fecondazione in vitro, 2010.
25. Casini C. Nobel medicina Ci offende come membri della famiglia Umana. 2010.[Available from: www.toscanaoggi.it].
26. Benagiano G, Carrara S, Filippi V. Robert G Edwards and the Roman Catholic Church. RBM Online 2011; 22: 665.
27. Ford NM. The Prenatal Person: Ethics from Conception to Birth. Oxford: Blackwell Publishing, 2002.

Index

Page numbers in bold indicate Figures, page number in italic indicate Tables